CLINICAL CRITICAL CARE MEDICINE

CLINICAL CRITICAL CARE MEDICINE

Richard K. Albert, MD
Professor of Medicine
University of Colorado Health Sciences Center
Chief, Medical Service
Denver Health Medical Center
Denver, Colorado

Arthur S. Slutsky, MD
Professor of Medicine, Surgery, and Biomedical
   Engineering
Director, Interdepartmental Division of Critical Care
University of Toronto Faculty of Medicine
Vice President (Research), St. Michael's Hospital
Toronto, Ontario, Canada

V. Marco Ranieri, MD
Professor of Anesthesiology and Intensive Care
   Medicine
Università di Torino
Chairman, Sezione di Anestesiologia e Rianimazione
S. Giovanni Battista–Molinette Hospital
Turin, Italy

Jukka Takala, MD
Chief Physician
Professor of Intensive Care Medicine
Department of Intensive Care Medicine
University Hospital
Bern, Switzerland

Antoni Torres, MD
Cap de Servei de Pneumologia i Al-lèrgia Respiratòria
Institut Clínic del Tórax
Hospital Clínic de Barcelona
Facultat de Medicina
Universitat de Barcelona
Barcelona, Spain

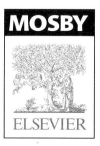
MOSBY
ELSEVIER

1600 John F. Kennedy Boulevard
Suite 1800
Philadelphia, PA 19103-2899

CLINICAL CRITICAL CARE MEDICINE   ISBN-13: 978-0-323-02844-8
Copyright © 2006 by Mosby, Inc., an affiliate of Elsevier Inc.   ISBN-10: 0-323-02844-6

Library of Congress Cataloging-in-Publication Data

Clinical critical care medicine / [edited by] Richard K. Albert . . . [et al.].
     p. ; cm.
     Includes bibliographical references and index.
     ISBN-13: 978-0-323-02844-8
     ISBN-10: 0-323-02844-6
     1. Critical care medicine. I. Albert, Richard K.
     [DNLM: 1. Critical Care—methods. 2. Intensive Care Units. WX 218 C641 2006]
  RC 86.7.C52 2006
  616.02′5—dc22
                                        2006044894

Acquisitions Editor: Dolores Meloni
Developmental Editor: Mary Beth Murphy
Project Manager: Cecelia Bayruns
Design Direction: Karen O'Keefe Owens

Printed in China

Last digit is the print number: 9 8 7 6 5 4 3 2 1

An education isn't how much you have committed to memory, or even how much you know. It's being able to differentiate between what you know and what you don't know.

—Anatole France

Contributors

Sheila Adam, MScN, BN, RGN
Nurse Consultant, Critical Care, Intensive Care Unit, University College London Hospitals Trust, London, United Kingdom

Neill Adhikari, MD, CM
Department of Critical Care Medicine, Sunnybrook and Women's College Health Sciences Centre; Interdepartmental Division of Critical Care, University of Toronto, Ontario, Canada

William C. Aird, MD
Department of Medicine, Harvard Medical School; Beth Israel Deaconess Medical Center, Boston, Massachusetts

Amalia Alcón, MD, PhD
Staff Especialista Sènior, Anesthesiology Department, Surgical Intensive Care Unit, Hospital Clínic, Barcelona, Spain

Peter Andrews, MD, FRCA
Director, Intensive Care Unit, Western General Hospital; Reader in Anaesthesia, Intensive Care and Pain Management, University of Edinburgh, Scotland

Massimo Antonelli, MD
Istituto di Anestesiologia e Rianimazione, Università Cattolica del Sacro Cuore, Policlinico A. Gemelli, Rome, Italy

Soja Anubkumar, MD
Research Fellow, Division of Nephrology, Columbia University College of Physicians and Surgeons, New York, New York

Andrea Arcangeli, MD
Istituto di Anestesiologia e Rianimazione, Università Cattolica del Sacro Cuore, Policlinico A. Gemelli, Rome, Italy

Vicente Arroyo, MD
Department of Medicine, University of Barcelona Medical School; Institute of Digestive Diseases, Hospital Clínic, Barcelona, Spain

Andrew J. Baker, MD, FRCPC
Medical Director, Trauma and Neurosurgery Intensive Care Unit, St. Michael's Hospital; Associate Professor, Departments of Anesthesia and Surgery, University of Toronto, Toronto, Ontario, Canada

Robert P. Baughman, MD
Professor of Internal Medicine, University of Cincinnati, Cincinnati, Ohio

Judith Bellapart, MD
Clinical Fellow, Trauma and Neurosurgery Intensive Care Unit, St. Michael's Hospital, University of Toronto, Toronto, Ontario, Canada

Rinaldo Bellomo, MBBS, MD, FACCP, FRACP, FJFICM
Department of Intensive Care and Department of Medicine (Melbourne University), Austin Hospital, Melbourne, Victoria, Australia

Mette M. Berger, MD, PhD
Department of Intensive Care, University Hospital, Lausanne, Switzerland

Maria Grazia Bocci, MD
Istituto di Anestesiologia e Rianimazione, Università Cattolica del Sacro Cuore, Policlinico A. Gemelli, Rome, Italy

Malte Book, MD
Department of Anaesthesiology and Intensive Care Medicine, University of Bonn, Bonn, Germany

Josep M. Bordas, MD
Institut de Malalties Digestives i Metabòliques, Hospital Clínic, IDIBAPS, Barcelona, Spain

Luca Brazzi, MD
Assistant Professor in Anesthesia and Intensive Care, Istituto di Anestesia e Rianimazione, Ospedale Maggiore di Milano IRCCS, Milan, Italy

Timothy G. Buchman, MD, PhD
Edison Professor of Surgery, Professor of Anesthesiology and of Medicine, Washington University School of Medicine, St. Louis, Missouri

Christian Byhahn, MD
Department of Anesthesiology, Intensive Care Medicine and Pain Therapy, J.W. Goethe-University Medical School, Frankfurt, Germany

B. Cabello, MD
Servei de Medicina Intensiva, Hospital Sant Pau, Barcelona, Spain

Pietro Caironi, MD
Istituto di Anestesia e Rianimazione, Università degli Studi di Milano; Servizio di Anesthesia e Rianimazaione, Ospedale Maggiore Policlinico-IRCC, Milan, Italy

Anselmo Caricato, MD
Istituto di Anestesiologia e Rianimazione, Università Cattolica del Sacro Cuore, Policlinico A. Gemelli, Roma, Italy

Andre F. Charest, MD
Renal Division, York Central Hospital, Richmond Hill, Ontario, Canada

René L. Chioléro, MD
Head, Department of Adult Critical Care Medicine, University Hospital (CHUV), Lausanne, Switzerland

Davide Chiumello, MD
Istituto di Anestesia e Rianimazione, Università degli Studi di Milano; Servizio di Anesthesia e Rianimazaione, Ospedale Maggiore Policlinico-IRCC, Milan, Italy

Chung-Wai Chow, MD, PhD
The Division of Respirology, Multi-Organ Transplant Unit, Department of Medicine, University of Toronto, Toronto General Hospital Division of the Research Institute of the University Health Network, Toronto, Ontario, Canada

Contributors

Vanessa Cobb, BSc, MRCP
Intensive Care Unit, St. James Wing, St. George's Hospital, London, United Kingdom

Stephen M. Cohn, MD, FACS
Professor and Chairman, The Dr. Witten B. Russ Professor, Department of Surgery, University of Texas Health Science Center, San Antonio, Texas

Timothy Cross, MD
Institute of Liver Studies, Kings College Hospital, Denmark Hill, London, United Kingdom

Marc de Moya, MD
Fellow, Divisions of Trauma and Critical Care, Jackson Memorial Medical Center, University of Miami School of Medicine, Miami, Florida

Yves Debaveye, MD
Department of Intensive Care Medicine, University Hospital Gasthuisberg, Leuven, Belgium

Paul Dorian, MD, FRCPC
Professor, University of Toronto, Faculty of Medicine; Staff Cardiologist, Department of Medicine, Division of Cardiology, Section of Cardiac Electrophysiology, St. Michael's Hospital, Toronto, Ontario, Canada

Gregory P. Downey, MD
Director, Division of Respirology, Professor and Vice Chair, Department of Medicine, University of Toronto, Toronto General Hospital Division of the Research Institute of the University Health Network, Toronto, Ontario, Canada

Philippe Eggimann, MD
Staff Physician and Junior Faculty, Department for Intensive Care Medicine and Burn Center, Centre Hospitalier Universitaire Vaudois, Lausanne, Switzerland

Björn Ellger, MD
Department of Intensive Care Medicine, University Hospital Gasthuisberg, Leuven, Belgium

E. Wesley Ely, MD, MPH
Division on Allergy, Pulmonary, and Critical Care Medicine, Center for Health Services Research, Vanderbilt University Medical Center and the VA Tennessee Valley Geriatric Research Education Clinical Center, Nashville, Tennessee

Àngels Escorsell, MD
Institut de Malalties Digestives i Metabòliques, Hospital Clínic, IDIBAPS, Barcelona, Spain

Neus Fábregas, MD, PhD
Staff Consultor, Anesthesiology Department, Surgical Intensive Care Unit, Hospital Clínic; Associate Professor, Universitat de Barcelona, Barcelona, Spain

Vito Fanelli, MD
Azienda Ospedaliera San Giovanni Battista, Servizio di Anestesia e Rianimazione, Turin, Italy

Faust Feu, MD
Institut de Malalties Digestives i Metabòliques, Hospital Clínic, IDIBAPS, Barcelona, Spain

Bernard G. Fikkers, MD
Department of Intensive Care, University Medical Centre Nijmegen, Nijmegen, The Netherlands

Joseph A. Fisher, MD, FRCPC
Professor, Faculty of Medicine University of Toronto; Staff, Department of Anesthesiology, Toronto General Hospital, Chief Scientist, Thornhill Research, Toronto, Ontario, Canada

Marco Fontanella, MD
Università di Torino, Dipartimento di Neuroscienze, Sezione di Neurochirurgia, Ospedale S. Giovanni Battista, Turin, Italy

Ognjen Gajic, MD
Division of Pulmonary and Critical Care Medicine, Mayo Clinic, Rochester, Minnesota

Luciano Gattinoni, MD
Consultant Physician, Istituto di Anestesia e Rianimazione, Milan, Italy

Gordon Giesbrecht, PhD
Professor, Laboratory for Exercise and Environmental Medicine and Department of Anesthesia, University of Manitoba, Winnipeg, Manitoba, Canada

Pere Ginès, MD
Senior Research, University of Barcelona Medical School, Hospital Clínic, Barcelona, Spain

Salvatore Grasso, MD
Dipartimento di Emergenza e Trapianti d'Organo, Sezione di Anestesiologia e Rianimazione, Ospedale Policlinico, Universitá di Bari, Bari, Italy

Thorsteinn Gunnarsson, MD, MSc
Clinical Fellow in Cerebrovascular Surgery and Interventional Neuroradiology, Division of Neurosurgery, University of Toronto, Toronto, Ontario, Canada

Richard Haddon, FRCA
Specialist Registrar in Anaesthetics, South East Scotland School of Anaesthesia, Edinburgh, Scotland

Mitchell L. Halperin, MD, FRCPC, FRS
Renal Divisions, St. Michael's Hospital, University of Toronto, Toronto, Ontario, Canada

C. William Hargett, MD
Fellow in Pulmonary, Allergy, and Critical Care Medicine, Division of Pulmonary, Allergy, and Critical Care Medicine, Duke University Medical Center, Durham, North Carolina

Michael Hiesmayr, MD
Cardiothoracic and Vascular Anaesthesia and Intensive Care, Medical University, Vienna, Austria

Ken Hillman, MBBS, FRCA, FANZCA, FJICM
Professor of Intensive Care, University of New South Wales; Area Medical Director, Sydney South West Area Health Service, Liverpool Hospital; Director, The Simpson Centre for Health Services Research, Sydney, New South Wales, Australia

Frank Hubbell, DO
Attending Physician, Director of Ambulatory Care, Saco River Medical Group and SOLO; Clinical Professor for the University of New England College of Osteopathic Medicine, Conway, New Hampshire

Rolf D. Hubmayr, MD
Division of Pulmonary and Critical Care Medicine, Mayo Clinic, Rochester, Minnesota

Leonard D. Hudson, MD
Professor of Medicine, Pulmonary and Critical Care Medicine, Harborview Medical Center, Seattle, Washington

Richard L. Hughes, MD
Division of Neurology, Department of Internal Medicine, Denver Health and Hospitals, Denver, Colorado

Robert M. Kacmarek, MD
Director, Respiratory Care, Massachusetts General Hospital; Professor of Anesthesiology, Harvard Medical School, Boston, Massachusetts

Kamel S. Kamel, MD
Renal Divisions, St. Michael's Hospital, University of Toronto, Toronto, Ontario, Canada

Catherine L. Kelleher, MD
Assistant Professor of Medicine, University of Colorado; Division of Nephrology, Denver Health Medical Center, Denver, Colorado

Sungmin Kiem, PhD
School of Pharmacy, University at Buffalo, Buffalo, New York; CPL Associates, Amherst, New York

Sven Klaschik, MD
Department of Anaesthesiology and Intensive Care Medicine, University of Bonn, Bonn, Germany

Anil Kumar, MBBS, MS, FRCS (Glasgow)
Clinical Fellow, Trauma and Neurosurgery Intensive Care Unit, St. Michael's Hospital, University of Toronto, Toronto, Ontario, Canada

Donald W. Landry, MD, PhD
Professor of Medicine, Director, Division of Nephrology, Columbia University, College of Physicians and Surgeons, New York, New York

Stephen E. Lapinsky, MD
Site Director, Intensive Care Unit, Mount Sinai Hospital and Interdepartmental Division of Critical Care, University of Toronto, Toronto, Ontario, Canada

Lutz Eric Lehmann, MD
Department of Anaesthesiology and Intensive Care Medicine, University of Bonn, Bonn, Germany

Mitchell M. Levy, MD
Brown University and Rhode Island Hospital, Providence, Rhode Island

Patricia C. Y. Liaw, PhD
Department of Medicine, McMaster University, and The Henderson Research Centre, Hamilton, Ontario, Canada

Shih-Hua Lin, MD
Renal Division, National Defense Medical Center, Taipei, Republic of China

Stuart L. Linas, MD
Professor of Medicine, Rocky Mountain Professor of Renal Research, University of Colorado Health Sciences Center; Chief, Renal Division, Denver Health Medical Center, Denver, Colorado

José A. Lorente, MD
Hospital Universitario de Getafe, Madrid, Spain

John M. Luce, MD
Professor of Medicine and Anesthesia, University of California, San Francisco; Chief Medical Officer, San Francisco General Hospital, San Francisco, California

Thomas Luecke, MD
Department of Anesthesiology and Critical Care Medicine, University Hospital of Mannheim; Faculty of Clinical Medicine, University of Heidelberg, Mannheim, Germany

Edward H. Maa, MD
Division of Neurology, Department of Internal Medicine, Denver Health and Hospitals, Denver, Colorado

Sheldon Magder, MD
McGill University Health Centre, Royal Victoria Hospital, Montreal, Canada

Atul Malhotra, MD
Assistant Professor of Medicine, Harvard Medical School; Attending Pulmonologist, Beth Israel Deaconess Medical Center, Boston, Massachusetts

Jordi Mancebo, MD
Unit Director and Associate Professor of Medicine, Servei de Medicina Intensiva, Hospital Sant Pau, Barcelona, Spain

Iqwal Mangat, MD, FRCPC
Assistant Professor, University of Toronto Faculty of Medicine; Staff Cardiologist, Department of Medicine, Division of Cardiology, Section of Cardiac Electrophysiology, St. Michael's Hospital, Toronto, Ontario, Canada

John C. Marshall, MD
St. Michael's Hospital, University of Toronto, Toronto, Ontario, Canada

Antoni Mas, MD
Senior Consultant, Liver Unit, Institut de Malalties Digestives i Metabòliques, Hospital Clínic, IDIBAPS, Barcelona, Spain

Luciana Mascia, MD, PhD
Università di Torino, Dipartimento di Discipline Medico-Chirurgiche, Sezione di Anestesiologia e Rianimazione, Ospedale S. Giovanni Battista, Turin, Italy

Eric M. Massicotte, MD, MSc, FRCSC
Associate Professor, Division of Neurosurgery, University of Toronto, Ontario, Canada

Greg McAnulty, BA, BSc, FRCA
Intensive Care Unit, St. James Wing, St. George's Hospital, London, United Kingdom

Maureen Meade, MD
Associate Professor, Clinical Epidemiology and Biostatistics, and Medicine, McMaster University, Faculty of Health Sciences, Hamilton, Ontario, Canada

Thomas John Morgan, MBBS, FJFICM
Senior Specialist, Intensive Care Unit, Mater Adult Hospital, South Brisbane, Queensland, Australia

Matthew T. Naughton, MD, FRACP
Associate Professor, Head, General Respiratory and Sleep Medicine, Department of Allergy, Immunology, and Respiratory Medicine, Alfred Hospital and Monash University, Melbourne, Victoria, Australia

Santiago Nogué-Xarau, MD
Intensive Care Unit, Hospital Clínic, Barcelona, Spain

Contributors

James O'Beirne, MD
Institute of Liver Studies, Kings College Hospital, Denmark Hill, London, United Kingdom

Juan A. Oliver, MD
Associate Professor of Clinical Medicine, Division of Nephrology, Columbia University, College of Physicians and Surgeons, New York, New York

Ilkka Parviainen, MD, PhD
Department of Anesthesiology and Intensive Care, Kuopio University Hospital, Kuopio, Finland

Paolo Pelosi, MD
Dipartimento Ambiente, Salute e Sicurezza, Università degli Studi dell'Insubria, Varese; Servizio di Anestesia e Rianimazione B, Ospedale di Circolo, Fondazione Macchi, Varese, Italy

Michael R. Pinsky, MD
Professor of Critical Care Medicine, Bioengineering and Anesthesiology, Department of Critical Care Medicine, University of Pittsburgh Medical Center, Pittsburgh, Pennsylvania

Margaret A. Pisani, MD, MPH
Department of Internal Medicine, Yale University School of Medicine, New Haven, Connecticut

Didier Pittet, MD, MS
Infection Control Program, University of Geneva Hospitals, Geneva, Switzerland

Christian Putensen, MD
Professor, Anesthesiology and Intensive Care Medicine, University of Bonn, Bonn, Germany

Graham Ramsay, MD
Atrium Medical Centre, Heerlen, The Netherlands

Andrew Rhodes, MRCP, FRCA
Consultant Anaesthetist, Intensive Care Unit, St. James Wing, St. George's Hospital, London, United Kingdom

Claudio Ronco, MD
Department of Intensive Care and Department of Medicine (Melbourne University), Austin Hospital, Melbourne, Victoria, Australia; Divisione di Nefrologia, Ospedale San Bortolo, Vicenza, Italy

Charis Roussos, MD, PhD
Professor and Chairman, Critical Care and Pulmonary Department, University of Athens Medical School, Evangelismos Hospital, Athens, Greece

Gordon D. Rubenfeld, MD, MSc
Associate Professor of Medicine, Pulmonary and Critical Care Medicine, University of Washington, Harborview Medical Center, Seattle, Washington

Lewis Rubinson, MD, PhD
Health Officer, Deschutes County Health Department; Division of Pulmonary and Critical Care Medicine, Bend Memorial Clinic, Bend, Oregon

Joshua Rucker, MD, BSc, FRCPC
Department of Anesthesia, Mount Sinai Hospital, Toronto, Ontario, Canada

Miguel Sánchez, MD, PhD
Unidad de Cuidados Intensivos, Hospital Universitario Principe de Asturias, Alcala de Henares (Madrid), Spain

Eduardo Sanjurjo-Golpe, MD
Intensive Care Unit, Hospital Clínic, Barcelona, Spain

Hugo Sax, MD
Infection Control Program, University of Geneva Hospitals, Geneva, Switzerland

Jerome J. Schentag, PharmD
School of Pharmacy, University at Buffalo, Buffalo, New York; CPL Associates, Amherst, New York

Jens-Christian Schewe, MD
Department of Anaesthesiology and Intensive Care Medicine, University of Bonn, Bonn, Germany

Daniel Schmidlin, MD
Hirslanden Klinik im Park, Zürich, Switzerland

Paul T. Schumacker, PhD
Department of Pediatrics, Northwestern University, Chicago, Illinois

Dror Soffer, MD
Director, The Yitzhak Rabin Trauma Division; Assistant Professor of Surgery, Tel-Aviv Sourasky Medical Center; University of Tel-Aviv, Sackler School of Medicine, Tel-Aviv, Israel

Ludivine Soguel, RN
Department of Intensive Care, University Hospital, Lausanne, Switzerland

Ulrike Stamer, MD
Department of Anaesthesiology and Intensive Care Medicine, University of Bonn, Bonn, Germany

R. Scott Stephens, MD
Department of Medicine, Johns Hopkins School of Medicine, Baltimore, Maryland

Frank Stüber, MD
Department of Anaesthesiology and Intensive Care Medicine, University of Bonn, Bonn, Germany

Peter M. Suter, MD
Professsor and Chief, Surgical Intensive Care, University Hospitals, Geneva, Switzerland

Jukka Takala, MD, PhD
Chief Physician, Professor of Intensive Care Medicine, University Hospital, Bern, Switzerland

Victor F. Tapson, MD
Professor of Medicine; Director, Center for Pulmonary Vascular Disease, Division of Pulmonary, Allergy, and Critical Care Medicine, Duke University Medical Center, Durham, North Carolina

Charles H. Tator, MD, MA, PhD, FRCSC, FACS
Professor of Neurosurgery and Robert Campeau Family Foundation Chair; President, Think First Canada; Chair, Canadian Brain and Nerve Health Coalition, Division of Neurosurgery, University of Toronto, Toronto, Ontario, Canada

Carlos Terra, MD
Research Fellow, University of Barcelona Medical School, Hospital Clínic, Barcelona, Spain

Aldo Torre, MD
Fellow Research, University of Barcelona Medical School, Hospital Clínic, Barcelona, Spain

Antoni Torres, MD
Cap de Servei de Pneumologia i Al·lèrgia Respiratòria, Institut Clínic del Tórax, Hospital Clínic de Barcelona, Facultat de Medicina, Universitat de Barcelona, Barcelona, Spain

David V. Tuxen, MB BS, FRACP, Dip DHM, MD, FJFICM
Associate Professor, Senior Intensivist, Department of Intensive Care and Hyperbaric Medicine, Alfred Hospital and Monash University, Melbourne, Victoria, Australia

Ilker Uçkay, MD
Infection Control Program, University of Geneva Hospitals, Geneva, Switzerland

Franco Valenza, MD
Assistant Professor in Anesthesia and Intensive Care, Istituto di Anestesia e Rianimazione, Ospedale Maggiore di Milano IRCCS, Milan, Italy

Greet Van den Berghe, MD, PhD
Professor of Medicine, University of Leuven; Director, Department of Intensive Care Medicine, University Hospital Gasthuisberg, Leuven, Belgium

Theodoros Vassilakopoulos, MD
Assistant Professor, Department of Critical Care and Pulmonary Services, University of Athens Medical School, Evangelismos Hospital, Athens, Greece

Jesús Villar, MD, PhD, FCCM
Director, Research Institute, Hospital N.S. de Candelaria, Tenerife, Canary Islands, Spain; Adjunct Scientist, Research Centre, St. Michael's Hospital, Toronto, Ontario, Canada

Christopher Wallace, MD, MSc, FRCSC, FACS
Head, Division of Neurosurgery, Krembil Neuroscience Centre, University Health Network, Toronto, Ontario, Canada

Stefan Weber, MD
Department of Anaesthesiology and Intensive Care Medicine, University of Bonn, Bonn, Germany

Jeffrey I. Weitz, MD
Departments of Medicine and Biochemistry, McMaster University, and the Henderson Research Centre, Hamilton, Ontario, Canada

Julia Wendon, MD
Senior Lecturer, Clinical Lead Liver Intensive Care, Institute of Liver Studies, Kings College Hospital, Denmark Hill, London, United Kingdom

Charles M. Wiener, MD
Professor of Medicine and Physiology, Vice Chairman, Department of Medicine; Director, Osler Medical Training Program, Johns Hopkins School of Medicine, Baltimore, Maryland

Stephan Windecker, MD
Invasive Cardiology, Department of Cardiovascular Diseases, University Hospital, Bern, Switzerland

Hermann Wrigge, MD
Assistant Professor, Anesthesiology and Intensive Care Medicine, University of Bonn, Bonn, Germany

Richard G. Wunderink, MD
Feinberg School of Medicine, Northwestern University, Chicago, Illinois

Preface

The purposes of this book are to present clinically relevant information that is encompassed in the discipline of critical care medicine, to do so from the perspective of the international community of critical care, and to emphasize a visual, as opposed to a textual, presentation of material as allowed by newer computer graphics and publishing capabilities.

Perhaps as a result of a number of recurring meetings that have drawn international attendance for many years, the global community of critical care is stronger than most other disciplines in medicine. We sought to draw this community together even more strongly by drawing on the combined expertise of 112 authors from 14 different countries (64 from Europe, 52 from North America, and 6 from Australia).

Mortimer J. Adler, a 20th-century American philosopher and educator, suggested that the point of good books was not how many of them you could get through, but rather how many could get through to you. We have structured this book such that each chapter contains numerous graphs, figures, and tables in the hope that more of the information will get through to you.

The book is directed to house officers, critical care trainees, and critical care practitioners, as well as to hospitalists, pulmonologists, anesthesiologists, general internists, and family physicians whose practice encompasses critically ill patients. The opening section considers generic issues that pertain to inflammation, genetics, control of vascular tone, the biologic response to stress, and cellular metabolism and tissue hypoxia. In addition to chapters that review commonly encountered organ-based conditions, we have included discussions on severity of illness scoring systems, end-of-life care, nursing issues, heart–lung interactions, and bioterrorism. Because of the ease of Web-based searching, we have reduced the number of references provided to "Suggested Reading."

RICHARD K. ALBERT, MD

ARTHUR S. SLUTSKY, MD

V. MARCO RANIERI, MD

JUKKA TAKALA, MD

ANTONI TORRES, MD

Introduction: What Is Critical Care Medicine?

Critical (or intensive) care medicine has become an integral part of the modern health care system. In a broad sense, intensive care has two main functions: first, to take care of emergency patients who have or are at risk for acute, potentially reversible life-threatening organ dysfunction, and second, to provide organ function support or intensive monitoring of vital organ functions for elective patients who are undergoing complex surgical or other interventional procedures and who have or are at high risk for organ function instability.

The roots of intensive care can be traced at least as far back as the beginning of the 19th century, when a room was reserved in Newcastle, UK, for severely ill patients and those who had recently had major surgery. In the United States, a postoperative recovery room was introduced at the Massachusetts General Hospital in 1873, and the concept of high-dependency care units for special groups of patients evolved in the United States during the first half of the 20th century.

The polio epidemic in the 1950s triggered a major development in intensive care in both Europe and the United States. Until 1952, negative-pressure ventilation with the "iron lung" or negative-pressure cuirass or tank ventilators was the only established way to provide prolonged mechanical ventilatory support. Due to the large number of polio victims in Denmark, manual positive-pressure ventilation through tracheostomy was applied on a large scale in patients concentrated in a facility that was the predecessor of the modern intensive care unit (ICU). It soon became apparent that positive-pressure ventilation substantially reduced mortality. This accelerated the development of intensive care units and facilitated the introduction of positive-pressure ventilators and other organ support technologies for intensive care.

Over the next 2 decades, intensive care units gradually were established for the care of seriously ill patients, patients with multiple injuries, and patients undergoing major surgery. ICUs became commonplace in the 1970s. Thus, even though the roots of intensive care medicine go back to the 1800s, intensive care in its current form and as a distinct medical specialty is young.

In theory, the diagnosis and management of critically ill patients is similar to that of less critically ill patients cared for in an acute care hospital ward. In practice, however, there are important differences. The greater severity of the ICU patient's illness or injuries poses a higher and more immediate risk of death. The diseases and treatments common to the ICU also place patients there at considerably higher risk for developing complications, many of which are also potentially life threatening. All of these factors have practical implications for patient management. Perhaps the greatest factor in the management of ICU patients is the condensed time course of the disease processes, which in turn requires more frequent assessments and changes in therapy.

Initial assessment of the critically ill patient often must be rapid, with initiation of treatment for life-threatening conditions taking place before a complete evaluation and database can be generated and before a full understanding of the patient's conditions can be developed. Also, the disease process may be rapidly evolving. This requires frequent reassessments, which may include returning to the patient's family or friends for a more detailed history, continuous monitoring of some organ functions such as hemodynamic function, and intermittent but frequent monitoring of other organ systems, including biochemical measurements that reflect organ function. More frequent physical examinations, by both physicians and nurses, may also be needed.

The treatment plan in critical care often consists of a therapeutic trial with predetermined treatment goals and predetermined responses to possible complications. Limits are set; when crossed, they result in a reassessment of the therapy and a possible therapeutic change. Critically ill patients are at higher risk for iatrogenic complications than are the less critically ill, in part because the life-threatening disease processes may require treatments with more possible side effects and in part because critically ill patients' organ dysfunctions predispose them to complications. Assessment of potential and developing iatrogenic complications is an important part of the management plan.

A specialized body of knowledge about critical illness, in which critical care physicians must be experts, has developed. This body of knowledge includes pathophysiology, understanding of mechanisms, special management modalities and techniques, and optimal organization for the delivery of critical care. Knowledge of the interactions among organ systems is accruing. For example, evidence is accumulating that ventilator-induced lung injury may lead to dysfunction of other organs through the systemic release of proinflammatory cytokines and other mediators of inflammation produced by respiratory cells, a process that has been called *biotrauma*. Such organ interactions are an important part of the special body of knowledge in critical care medicine.

Critical care medicine is, by nature, multidisciplinary. Physicians from several specialties with special critical care training and expertise—including surgery, internal medicine, anesthesiology, neurology, and neurosurgery, as well as some of their subspecialties—are involved in providing intensive care. There are also multiple categories of caregivers with special knowledge and skills required for the optimal delivery of critical care. The role of critical care nurses is especially key. Early ICUs were developed around the concept of providing a higher intensity of nursing care, with special training for these nurses. The specialty of critical care nursing subsequently developed. In North America, the profession of respiratory therapy, delivered by respiratory care practitioners, developed in large part as a result of the evolution of critical care. These professionals have special skills in ventilatory management and the setup and maintenance of mechanical ventilators, delivery of inhaled medications, and removal of respiratory secretions. Other specialists in critical care include pharmacists, nutritionists, social workers, and physical therapists. Recently, a new group of experts—those specializing in palliative care—has begun to play a role in critical care, providing expertise in comfort measures and end-of-life care.

As seriously ill patients began to survive longer with the advent of intensive care units, a spectrum of new problems evolved. Patients who would previously have died of single organ failure began to survive the acute phase of their critical illness and to progress to dysfunction of multiple organs. This pattern was first described by Arthur Baue in 1975. Today, dysfunction and failure of multiple organs is the most common final pathway to death for patients in intensive care.

The patient population treated in intensive care units has also changed. Due to the aging population, improvements in the treatment of malignancies, advances in surgical and other interventional techniques, and the expectations of the public and the medical profession, among other factors, intensive care patients today are likely to be older than before and to have complex comorbidities. Sepsis and other severe infections have become a major challenge, and despite major efforts from the intensive care community and the pharmaceutical industry, improvements in outcome from sepsis must be considered moderate at best. Although aspects of the complex pathophysiology of sepsis and multiple organ failure are much better understood today than they were 20 years ago, therapeutic breakthroughs have yet to be found. In contrast, and somewhat paradoxically, major advances have been made in reducing the harmful iatrogenic effects of intensive care life support; the best example of this is probably the introduction of lung-protective mechanical ventilation.

The vast spectrum of vital organ support and monitoring technologies and pharmacological interventions has made the modern intensive care unit a very complex facility. At the same time, the intensive care community is confronted with several apparently conflicting expectations: limited availability of resources and the demand for high quality of care, best care for individual patients and ethically acceptable allocation of available resources, treatment relying on complex and impersonal new technologies countered by a need to preserve human interaction with the critically ill patient and family, and efforts to provide acceptable quality of life without prolonging death. These are among the major challenges for today's intensive care specialist.

Today, intensive care is a complex multidisciplinary system at the intersection of diverse patient care processes. A better understanding of these patient care processes has clearly revealed that process and organizational improvements within as well as outside of the intensive care unit have at least as great potential for improving patient-centered outcomes as do many novel therapeutic interventions.

Some of the following improvements may sound self-evident but are still not systematically applied: the presence of a medical director with specialist training in intensive care medicine in the ICU; the 24-hour-a-day, 7-day-a-week availability of physicians trained in intensive care; and the availability of sufficient numbers of trained nursing personnel. Outcomes improve when a written summary of the treatment plan for each day is developed during morning rounds and posted at the bedside for all members of the critical care team to see. Other improvements are related to optimization of some components of the intensive care "package": protocolized delivery of mechanical ventilation, sedation protocols, and daily stops of sedation. Early involvement of intensive care personnel in the evaluation and treatment of patients outside the intensive care unit by "medical emergency" or "outreach" teams aims at avoiding delays in the care of patients with vital organ dysfunction ("intensive care without walls"). The combination of organizational optimization for early interventions outside the intensive care unit and treatment protocols has successfully been applied to improving the outcome of septic patients.

Cost constraints and the demand for efficiency in health care have shortened the length of stay throughout the hospital, and the number of traditional hospital beds has decreased. This tendency is likely to continue in the future as well: Patients who do not need therapeutic intervention, monitoring, or complex nursing care will not be hospitalized. Accordingly, the proportion of intensive care and high-dependency care beds is bound to increase, and this puts even more pressure on process integration and optimization. Flexible adjustment of the intensity of treatment will be necessary throughout the hospitalization, from intensive care to other high-dependency care areas and discharge.

Ultimately, success in process optimization and the provision of "intensive care without walls" requires great leadership, administrative, communication, and organizational skills. Quality control and continuous process improvement must be integrated in the daily practice of intensive care. These are just some of the challenges facing practitioners of the specialty of intensive care medicine today.

JUKKA TAKALA
LEONARD D. HUDSON

Contents

Introduction   What is Critical Care Medicine?   **xv**
Jukka Takala and Leonard D. Hudson

SECTION 1: BASIC BIOLOGY AND CRITICAL CARE MEDICINE

CHAPTER 1 Inflammation   1
Chung-Wai Chow and Gregory P. Downey

CHAPTER 2 Genetics   13
Frank Stüber, Lutz Eric Lehmann,
Jens-Christian Schewe, Ulrike Stamer, Stefan Weber,
Sven Klaschik, and Malte Book

CHAPTER 3 Stress and the Biology of the Responses   21
Timothy G. Buchman

CHAPTER 4 Vascular Tone   31
Donald W. Landry, Soja Anubkumar, and Juan A. Oliver

CHAPTER 5 Cell Metabolism and Tissue Hypoxia   41
Paul T. Schumacker

SECTION 2: PRACTICE OF CRITICAL CARE

CHAPTER 6 Monitoring and Treatment of Pain,
Anxiety, and Delirium in the ICU   51
Margaret A. Pisani and E. Wesley Ely

CHAPTER 7 Antibiotics in the ICU   61
Sungmin Kiem and Jerome J. Schentag

CHAPTER 8 Nonantimicrobial Measures to Prevent
Infections in Critical Care   71
Didier Pittet, Ilker Uçkay, Philippe Eggimann, and
Hugo Sax

CHAPTER 9 Antibiotic Prophylactic Strategies in the
ICU   87
Miguel Sánchez

CHAPTER 10 Severity of Illness Measures   95
Gordon D. Rubenfeld

CHAPTER 11 Hemodynamic Monitoring   101
Ognjen Gajic and Rolf D. Hubmayr

CHAPTER 12 Modes of Mechanical Ventilation   109
Robert M. Kacmarek, Jesús Villar, and Atul Malhotra

CHAPTER 13 Noninvasive Ventilation   121
B. Cabello and Jordi Mancebo

CHAPTER 14 Tracheostomy   131
Bernard G. Fikkers, Graham Ramsay, and
Christian Byhahn

CHAPTER 15 Monitoring Mechanical Ventilation   137
Salvatore Grasso and Vito Fanelli

CHAPTER 16 Patient–Ventilator Interaction
and Weaning   149
Christian Putensen and Hermann Wrigge

CHAPTER 17 Ventilator-Associated Lung Injury   161
Jesús Villar and Robert M. Kacmarek

CHAPTER 18 Weaning   169
Maureen Meade and Neill Adhikari

CHAPTER 19 Ventilator-Associated Pneumonia   175
Antoni Torres, Amalia Alcón, and Neus Fábregas

CHAPTER 20 Clinical Assessment of the Acutely
Unstable Patient   187
Jukka Takala

CHAPTER 21 Nursing Issues in the Critically Ill   199
Sheila Adam

CHAPTER 22 Nutritional Support   205
René L. Chioléro, Ludivine Soguel, and Mette M. Berger

CHAPTER 23 End-of-Life Care in the Intensive
Care Unit   217
John M. Luce and Mitchell M. Levy

SECTION 3: PULMONARY PROBLEMS

CHAPTER 24 Acute Exacerbations of Chronic
Obstructive Pulmonary Disease and Asthma   223
Matthew T. Naughton and David V. Tuxen

CHAPTER 25 Acute Respiratory Distress Syndrome   237
Luciano Gattinoni, Paolo Pelosi, Luca Brazzi, and
Franco Valenza

CHAPTER 26 Pulmonary Embolism   253
C. William Hargett and Victor F. Tapson

CHAPTER 27 A Physiologically Based Approach to
Perioperative Management of Obese Patients   263
Paolo Pelosi, Thomas Luecke, Pietro Caironi, and
Davide Chiumello

Contents

CHAPTER 28 Neuromuscular Respiratory Failure 275
Theodoros Vassilakopoulos and Charis Roussos

SECTION 4: CARDIOVASCULAR PROBLEMS

CHAPTER 29 Pathophysiology of Cardiovascular
Failure 283
Sheldon Magder

CHAPTER 30 Acute Coronary Syndromes 301
Stephan Windecker

CHAPTER 31 Arrhythmias in the Critical Care
Setting 319
Iqwal Mangat and Paul Dorian

CHAPTER 32 Hypertensive Emergencies 343
Catherine L. Kelleher and Stuart L. Linas

CHAPTER 33 Acute Cardiovascular Emergencies 355
Vanessa Cobb, Greg McAnulty, and Andrew Rhodes

CHAPTER 34 Heart–Lung Interactions 369
Michael R. Pinsky

SECTION 5: NEUROLOGIC PROBLEMS

CHAPTER 35 Intracranial Pressure and Cerebral
Blood Flow Autoregulation 383
Marco Fontanella and Luciana Mascia

CHAPTER 36 Management of Traumatic Brain Injury 395
Andrew J. Baker, Judith Bellapart, and Anil Kumar

CHAPTER 37 Management of Subarachnoid
Hemorrhage 405
Thorsteinn Gunnarsson and Christopher Wallace

CHAPTER 38 Seizures 415
Edward H. Maa and Richard L. Hughes

CHAPTER 39 Management of Spinal Injury 431
Charles H. Tator and Eric M. Massicotte

CHAPTER 40 Brain Death and Management of
the Organ Donor 439
Richard Haddon and Peter Andrews

SECTION 6: RENAL AND METABOLIC PROBLEMS

CHAPTER 41 Acid–Base Disorders 445
Thomas John Morgan

CHAPTER 42 Disorders of Water, Sodium, and
Potassium Homeostasis 459
Kamel S. Kamel, Andre F. Charest, Shih-Hua Lin, and
Mitchell L. Halperin

CHAPTER 43 Acute Renal Failure 475
Rinaldo Bellomo and Claudio Ronco

CHAPTER 44 Hepatorenal Syndrome 489
Vicente Arroyo, Pere Ginès, Carlos Terra, and Aldo Torre

CHAPTER 45 Acute Endocrine Disorders 497
Yves Debaveye, Björn Ellger, and Greet Van den Berghe

CHAPTER 46 Diabetic Ketoacidosis and Hyperosmolar
Nonketotic Coma 507
Ken Hillman

SECTION 7: GASTROINTESTINAL PROBLEMS

CHAPTER 47 Gastrointestinal Bleeding 517
Josep M. Bordas, Àngels Escorsell, Faust Feu, and Antoni Mas

CHAPTER 48 Pancreatitis 525
John C. Marshall

CHAPTER 49 Acute Liver Failure 531
Timothy Cross, James O'Beirne, and Julia Wendon

SECTION 8: HEMATOLOGIC PROBLEMS

CHAPTER 50 Coagulation Overview 543
Patricia C. Y. Liaw and Jeffrey I. Weitz

CHAPTER 51 Interaction of Coagulation and
Inflammation 555
William C. Aird

CHAPTER 52 Blood Product Replacement 561
Dror Soffer, Marc de Moya, and Stephen Cohn

SECTION 9: INFECTIOUS DISEASE PROBLEMS

CHAPTER 53 Community-Acquired Pneumonia 569
Richard G. Wunderink

CHAPTER 54 Pneumonia in the Immunocompromised
Patient 581
Robert P. Baughman

CHAPTER 55 Sepsis 589
José A. Lorente and John C. Marshall

SECTION 10: OTHER CRITICAL CARE PROBLEMS

CHAPTER 56 Multitrauma, Including Peripheral
Compartment Syndrome 603
Massimo Antonelli, Andrea Arcangeli, Maria Grazia Bocci,
and Anselmo Caricato

CHAPTER 57 Burns, Inhalation, and Electrical Injuries 613
Ilkka Parviainen

CHAPTER 58 Hypothermia and Hyperthermia   621
Gordon Giesbrecht and Frank Hubbell

CHAPTER 59 Pregnancy-Related Critical Care   625
Stephen E. Lapinsky

CHAPTER 60 Intensive Care after Cardiac Surgery   639
Michael Hiesmayr and Daniel Schmidlin

CHAPTER 61 Intensive Care after Major Surgery   657
Peter M. Suter

CHAPTER 62 Alcohol and Drug Ingestions   665
Santiago Nogué-Xarau and Eduardo Sanjurjo-Golpe

CHAPTER 63 Carbon Monoxide Poisoning   679
Joshua Rucker and Joseph A. Fisher

CHAPTER 64 Bioterrorism and the Intensive Care Unit   685
R. Scott Stephens, Charles M. Wiener, and Lewis Rubinson

Index   **697**

Section 1 Basic Biology and Critical Care Medicine

Chapter 1

Inflammation

Chung-Wai Chow and Gregory P. Downey

KEY POINTS

- Inflammation is a normal physiologic response to infection and injury and is integral to homeostasis and function of the innate immune system.
- Dysregulation of the inflammatory response resulting in perpetuation of inflammation is a common cause of organ dysfunction and failure in critically ill patients.
- Acute lung injury (ALI) and acute respiratory distress syndrome (ARDS) are pulmonary manifestations of inflammatory organ dysfunction and multiorgan failure that reflect widespread endothelial injury.
- Epithelial injury with failure of epithelial barrier and ion transport functions contributes to respiratory, renal, and gastrointestinal dysfunction.
- Although intensive research efforts have yielded molecularly targeted therapies for the treatment of inflammation that have been effective in animal models of sepsis and ALI, these strategies, with the exception of activated protein C for the treatment of sepsis, have not shown a clear benefit in clinical trials in patients with sepsis, ALI, and ARDS. Treatment of the underlying cause, supportive care, and mechanical ventilation using a lung protective strategy are the most effective therapeutic interventions in minimizing inflammatory lung injury.

Inflammation is a normal physiologic response to infection or tissue injury. It is characterized by vasodilatation, increased vascular permeability, and recruitment of inflammatory cells such as neutrophils, monocytes, macrophages, and, in some cases, lymphocytes. These physiological events, in conjunction with the release of soluble cytotoxic, inflammatory, and chemotactic mediators, function to contain, destroy, and remove the invading pathogen or agent. In the later stages of the inflammatory response, in which the focus is repair of the injured tissue, recruitment and activation of mesenchymal cells and fibroblasts are observed. In general, localized inflammatory responses are self-limited and result in resolution of injury. The outcome of a more widespread (systemic) inflammatory response, however, depends on the balance of the pro- and anti-inflammatory signals.

The inflammatory response is normally a tightly regulated process that coordinates microvascular responses with the sequential activation and recruitment of different leukocyte and other cell populations. Paradoxically, in certain circumstances, such as overwhelming infection in genetically predisposed hosts, these same responses can be detrimental and lead to damage to the host when dysregulation of the inflammatory response results in accentuation and perpetuation of inflammation. Clinically, this is manifest as multiorgan dysfunction, which if allowed to progress can result in multiorgan failure, a common disorder seen in more than 50% of patients admitted to medical–surgical intensive care units.

PATHOPHYSIOLOGY

The early reaction following an infection or injury is a carefully orchestrated inflammatory response involving endothelial cells, epithelial cells, neutrophils, monocytes, and macrophages. Activation of endothelial cells results in the production and release of vasoactive substrates, cytokines, chemokines, and cytotoxic mediators. Furthermore, activated endothelial cells display increased numbers of adhesion molecules, such as intercellular adhesion molecule-1 (ICAM-1) and E-selectin, on their plasma membranes. The adhesion molecules interact with specific ligands on circulating leukocytes and, in conjunction with local juxtacrine mediators such as platelet-activating factor (PAF) and interleukin (IL)-8, stimulate both adhesion and activation of the leukocytes, facilitating their transmigration across the endothelium to sites of injury and infection.

Contemporaneously, there is production of acute phase proteins, such as C-reactive protein (CRP) and activated protein C (APC). There is also activation of the complement system, resulting in production of additional inflammatory mediators, such as complement fragments (e.g., C3a and C5a) and kinins, and in release of leukocyte-derived proteases (e.g., elastase and cathepsins) and proteases of the coagulation cascade, such as thrombin (see also Chapters 50 and 51). In concert, these systems and mediators contribute to the magnitude and duration of the inflammatory response.

Although the initial inflammatory response tends to remain localized to the site of infection and/or injury and be self-limited, the production and release of soluble inflammatory mediators can spill over into the circulation, leading to a systemic inflammatory response syndrome (SIRS; Table 1.1). SIRS is characterized by hyper- or hypothermia, tachycardia, tachypnea, hypotension, and leukocytosis but is a relatively nonspecific response and can be seen in response to a variety of infectious or noninfectious insults. When an infectious agent is responsible for initiating SIRS, the syndrome is called sepsis. SIRS and

Basic Biology and Critical Care Medicine

Table 1.1 Definitions	
SIRS (system inflammatory response syndrome)	Two or more of 1. Temperature > 38°C or < 36°C 2. Tachycardia > 90 beats/min 3. Respiratory rate > 20 breaths/min or $Paco_2$ < 4.3 kPa 4. White blood count > 12×10^9/liter or < 4×10^9/liter or > 10% immature (band) forms No end organ damage
Sepsis	SIRS with a defined infectious etiology
MODS (multiorgan disorder syndrome)	SIRS or sepsis in association with dysfunction of multiple organs (renal, hepatic, cardiac, neurologic)
ALI	1. Acute onset 2. Bilateral infiltrates on chest x-ray 3. Pulmonary arterial pressure ≤ 18 mm Hg 4. Pao_2/Fio_2 ≤ 300 but > 200
ARDS	1. Acute onset 2. Bilateral infiltrates on chest x-ray 3. Pulmonary arterial pressure ≤ 18 mm Hg 4. Pao_2/Fio_2 ≤ 200

sepsis are normal physiological inflammatory responses to injury and infection. However, when unregulated, the disorder may progress to the multiorgan dysfunction syndrome (MODS; Fig. 1.1). Regardless of the cause of the original inciting event, the pathophysiology of MODS is a reflection of an ongoing and uncontained inflammatory response and is frequently accompanied by acute lung injury and ARDS.

Specific Cell Responses

Many different cell populations are activated during the inflammatory response (Table 1.2 and Figs. 1.2 and 1.3). The contributions of some of the major cells types are discussed next.

Immune Cells (Table 1.3)

Neutrophils (PMNs)

The primary function of PMNs in the innate immune response—to contain and kill invading microbial pathogens—is achieved through a series of rapid and coordinated responses culminating in phogocytosis and killing of the pathogens (Fig. 1.4). PMNs have a potent antimicrobial arsenal that includes oxidants, powerful proteinases, and cationic peptides.

Oxidants such as O_2^- and H_2O_2 are produced by a multicomponent enzyme termed the *phagocyte nicotinamide adenine dinucleotide phosphate (NADPH) oxidase*. Granules within the cytoplasm of PMNs contain potent proteolytic enzymes and cationic proteins that can digest a variety of microbial substrates. These compounds are released directly into the phagosome, compartmentalizing both the pathogen and the cytotoxic products. However, in pathological circumstances, these compounds are released into the extracellular space and can damage host tissues.

Monocytes/macrophages

Macrophages, an essential component of the innate immune system, are present within the interstitial tissues and on mucosal

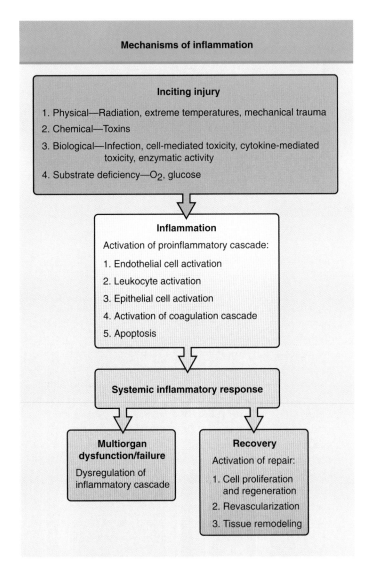

Figure 1.1. Mechanisms of inflammation. Development of local inflammation and subsequent systemic inflammatory response is a normal physiological response to injury and infection. Progression of the systemic inflammatory response to multiorgan dysfunction or resolution of inflammation with tissue repair and remodeling is determined by a complex interplay of host factors, the type and intensity of the inciting cause, and other mitigating factors.

Table 1.2 Cells Mediating the Inflammatory Response		
	Immune Cells	**Nonimmune Cells**
Early phase	Monocyte/macrophages Eosinophils Mast cells Neutrophils Natural killer cells	Endothelial cells Epithelial cells
Late phase	Lymphocytes Dendritic cells	Endothelial cells Epithelial cells Fibroblasts Mesenchymal cells

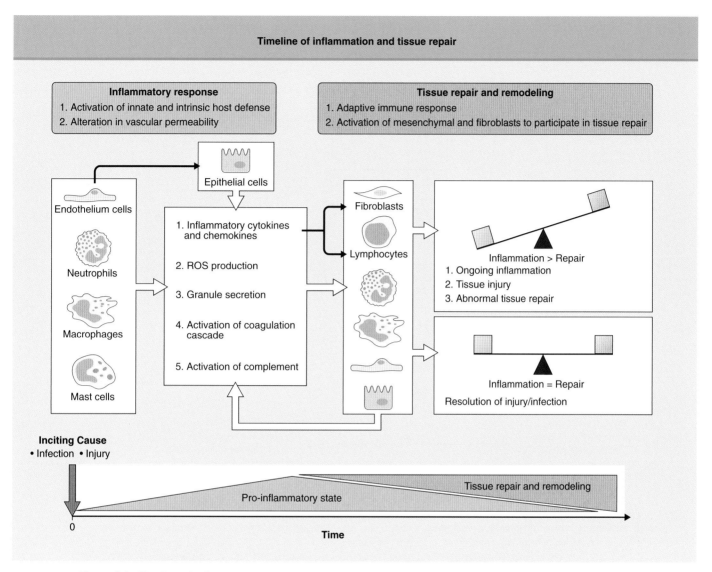

Figure 1.2. Timeline of inflammation and tissue repair. The initial response following infection or injury is a proinflammatory phase that is characterized by activation of leukocytes and endothelial and epithelial cells to promote destruction and removal of the inciting pathogen, particulate matter, or pollutant. In the later stages, resolution of inflammation and tissue repair predominate. This phase is characterized by the development of adaptive immunity and tissue repair and remodeling. Activation and proliferation of fibroblasts and mesenchymal cells are seen at this stage.

surfaces throughout the body. They function to provide (1) constant immune surveillance, (2) orchestration of the immune response, and (3) a bridge between the innate and adaptive arms of the immune system.

Macrophages are derived from myeloid precursors in bone marrow, spleen, and fetal liver. Precursor cells, termed monocytes, leave the vascular space in response to chemokines or other tissue-specific homing factors.

The environment into which the monocytes/macrophages migrate extensively influences the function of macrophages such that macrophages resident in different tissues display different patterns of function. Upon inflammatory insult to the tissue, these resident tissue macrophages can contribute to the innate immune response by synthesis and release of a variety of inflammatory and effector activities, the pattern of which is

differentially regulated by the microenvironment of the different tissues.

In early phases of a simple inflammatory response, macrophages display inflammatory and tissue-destructive activities, including release of metalloproteinase and oxidative radicals. Moreover, subsets of macrophages (dendritic cells) function in antigen recognition, processing, and display to cells of the adaptive immune system (lymphocytes).

As the inflammatory response progresses, later stages are dominated by macrophages displaying tissue-restructuring activities. Whether these phenotypes represent two distinct, sequential cellular infiltrates or a single infiltrate that progressively changes its function has important implications for the design of rational approaches to therapy for diseases involving chronic inflammation.

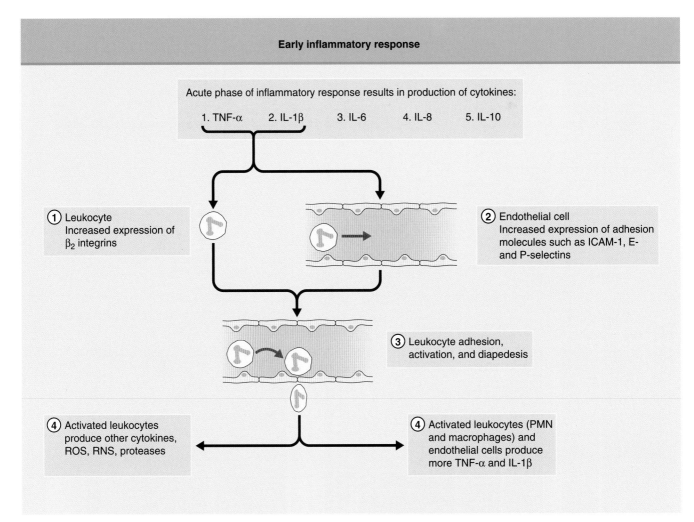

Figure 1.3. Early inflammatory response. Propagation of the inflammatory cascade is rapidly achieved by signaling events mediated by the early inflammatory cytokines, particularly TNF-α, IL-1β, and IL-6. They activate different cell populations to promote leukocyte adhesion and recruitment. This includes induction of β₂ integrins expression and activation in leukocytes (1) and upregulated expression of adhesion molecules on endothelial cells (2). The subsequent diapedesis of leukocytes across the endothelium (3) results in further activation of the leukocytes and endothelial cells and the perpetuation of inflammatory cytokine production (4).

Table 1.3 Role of Immune Cells in Inflammation		
Immune Cell	**Primary Role(s)**	**Primary or Unique Inflammatory Mediators**
Neutrophils	Kill and eliminate invading organisms	Reactive oxygen and nitrogen species
		Proteolytic enzymes and cationic proteins
		TNF-α, IL-1β, IL-6
Macrophages	Immune surveillance	TNF-α, IL-1β, IL-6
	Kill and contain invading microorganisms	TGF-β
	Removal of particulate matter	ICAM-1
	Antigen presentation	Reactive oxygen and nitrogen species
Mast cells	"Antennae" of immune response	Granule release (mediated via Fcε receptors)
		TLRs
		PAF, leukotrienes, and prostaglandins
		IL-1, IL-3, IL-4, IL-5, IL-6, IL-8, IL-10, IL-13, IL-16, TNF-α, VEGF, TGF-β, MIP-1α and MCP-1
Dendritic cells	Antigen presentation	TNF-α, IL-1β
Eosinophils	Allergic response	Eosinophil-specific granules
	Removal of parasites	Cationic proteins
		Major basic protein
		Eosinophil peroxidase
		Eosinophil-derived neurotoxin
		Lipid mediators—leukotriene C4 and PAF

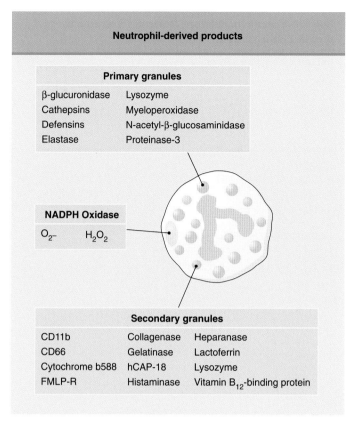

Neutrophil-derived products

Primary granules

β-glucuronidase	Lysozyme
Cathepsins	Myeloperoxidase
Defensins	N-acetyl-β-glucosaminidase
Elastase	Proteinase-3

NADPH Oxidase

O_2- H_2O_2

Secondary granules

CD11b	Collagenase	Heparanase
CD66	Gelatinase	Lactoferrin
Cytochrome b588	hCAP-18	Lysozyme
FMLP-R	Histaminase	Vitamin B$_{12}$-binding protein

Figure 1.4. Neutrophil-derived products. O_2- and H_2O_2 are produced by a multicomponent enzyme termed the phagocyte NADPH oxidase, which is unique to neutrophils (PMNs). Furthermore, they also contain unique secretory granules, called the primary and secondary granules, that contain potent proteolytic enzymes and cationic proteins that can digest a variety of microbial substrates.

Mast cells

Mast cells are key elements in the innate immune system and have been termed the "antennae" of the immune response. Mast cells are located throughout the body in close proximity to epithelial surfaces, near blood vessels, nerves, and glands, placing them at strategic locations for detecting invading pathogens. In addition, mast cells express a number of receptors that allow them to recognize diverse stimuli.

In sensitized individuals, IgE is bound to Fcε receptors (FcεRI) on the mast cell surface and binding of antigen to surface-bound IgE results in mast cell activation. Thus, multiple stimuli (foreign antigens) may trigger the same class of receptor. However, there is specificity in this system as a result of multiple signal transduction pathways that are differentially activated based on antigen size and receptor location, number, and subtype.

In addition, human mast cells also express toll-like receptors TLR-1, TLR-2, TLR-6, and TLR-4. TLRs are pattern recognition receptors that recognize specific molecular patterns of microorganisms. Expression of TLRs, in combination with other receptors, allows the mast cell to recognize many potential pathogens and generate a specific response. Importantly, mast cells are capable of releasing many immune-modulating molecules that stimulate inflammation and the adaptive immune response and can polarize T-cell subpopulations toward Th1 or Th2 subtypes. Mast cell products include the following:

1. Preformed mediators that are granule associated (e.g., histamine)
2. Mediators synthesized de novo (e.g., leukotriene C$_4$, PAF, and prostaglandin D$_2$)
3. Vast array of cytokines and chemokines, including IL-1, IL-3, IL-4, IL-5, IL-6, IL-8, IL-10, IL-13, IL-16, tumor necrosis factor-α (TNF-α), vascular endothelial growth factor (VEGF), transforming growth factor-β (TGF-β), macrophage inflammatory protein-1α (MIP-1α), and monocyte chemoattractant protein-1 (MCP-1).

In summary, the strategic location of mast cells in the body and their diversity of receptors and cytokines indicate an important role in regulating innate and adaptive immunity.

Dendritic cells

Dendritic cells can be viewed as conductors of the immune response. These cells, resident within tissues, develop in vivo from hematopoietic precursor cells. Dendritic cells bind, internalize, and process antigens and then display them on their surface in conjunction with human leukocyte antigen (HLA) molecules. These antigens are then "presented" to cells of the innate immune system (lymphocytes), along with other requisite activation signals, resulting in activation of lymphocytes, a pivotal process in the adaptive immune response.

Eosinophils

Eosinophils are primarily viewed as effector cells of allergic responses and of parasite elimination. These bone marrow–derived cells contain four distinct granule cationic proteins:

1. Major basic protein
2. Eosinophil peroxidase
3. Eosinophil cationic protein
4. Eosinophil-derived neurotoxin

During allergic inflammation, eosinophils release granule contents as well as inflammatory mediators, including lipid mediators such as leukotriene C4 and PAF, which may cause dysfunction and destruction of other cells.

Epithelial Cells

Epithelial cells line organs that are in continuous contact with the external environment, including the lung, the kidneys, and the gastrointestinal tract. These cells have multiple roles in maintaining homeostasis; they are crucial for the uptake of vital metabolites (O$_2$ and nutrients), for excretion of waste products, and for maintaining appropriate fluid and salt homeostasis. Because epithelial cells of the lung and gastrointestinal tract are in constant contact with the external environment, they are also subject to insult, injury, and infection with a plethora of inhaled or ingested materials and organisms.

Epithelial cells actively participate in the modulation of inflammation and are capable of mounting an immune response by internalization of organisms and secretion of cytotoxic and antimicrobial peptides. Epithelial cells are induced by bacterial components, such as lipopolysaccharide, and by cytokines, such as TNF-α and IL-1β, to express various gene products (via the NF-κB and IκB signaling pathways) that modulate the inflammatory response (Fig. 1.5). These include

Basic Biology and Critical Care Medicine

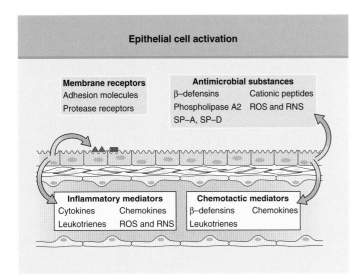

Figure 1.5. Epithelial cell activation. When activated, epithelial cells produce and secrete inflammatory and chemotactic mediators, and they induce surface expression of adhesion molecules and protease receptors that leads to activation and recruitment of leukocytes to the site of injury/infection. In addition, pulmonary epithelial cells secrete a number of soluble antimicrobial substances.

1. Cytokines such as IL-8, TNF-α, and IL-1β
2. Chemokines such as MIP-2, CXC chemokines, MCP-1, IL-7, and IL-15
3. Nitric oxide and reactive nitrogen molecules
4. Adhesion molecules such as β integrins and ICAM-1
5. TLRs such as TLR-2 and TLR-4
6. TNF-α receptors, TNFR1 and TNFR2
7. Growth factor receptors such as epidermal growth factor receptor and platelet-derived growth factor receptor
8. Plasminogen activator receptors

In addition to these molecules, pulmonary epithelial cells express a number of antimicrobial mediators that are unique to the lung, including the surfactant proteins SP-A and SP-D (members of the collectin family) and the β-defensins (Box 1.1).

Dysregulation of the pulmonary epithelium as a result of systemic inflammation results in depletion of surfactant and impaired fluid and salt transport, leading to interstitial edema and alveolar dysfunction (Fig. 1.6). Often, therapeutic strategies such as mechanical ventilation, which are meant to improve patient outcome, can also perpetuate the inflammatory response due to mechanical injury and shear forces (Fig. 1.7).

Endothelial Cells

Endothelial cells play a pivotal role in the regulation and propagation of the inflammatory response. Activated endothelial cells enhance the expression of numerous proteins involved in different pathways that contribute to inflammation, including the following:

1. Reactive nitrogen and oxygen species, including nitric oxide, peroxynitrite, superoxide (O_2^-), and hydrogen peroxide (H_2O_2), that are cytotoxic to microorganisms and cells
2. Inflammatory cytokines such as TNF-α, IL-1β, and IL-6, as well as chemokines such as IL-8, RANTES (regulated

---

Box 1.1 Immunomodulatory Molecules Secreted by Airway Epithelial Cells

Inflammatory Mediators

Cytokines
Chemokines
Leukotrienes
Calprotectin

Chemotactic Mediators

LL-37/CAP-18
b-Defensins
Chemokines
Leukotrienes

Antimicrobial Substances

β-Defensins
LL-37/CAP-18
Lysozyme
Lactoferrin
SLPI (secretory leukocyte proteinase inhibitor)
Elafin
Calprotectin
Phospholipase A2
SP-A, SP-D
Anionic peptides

upon *a*ctivation, *n*ormal *T* cell *e*xpressed and *s*ecreted), and MIP-1, to activate and recruit leukocytes
3. Cytokine and chemokine receptors such as TFNR1 and IL-1R
4. Adhesion molecules, including ICAM-1, ICAM-2, PECAM, VCAM-1, E-selectin, and P-selectin, that have differential specificities for different leukocyte populations
5. TLRs
6. Procoagulants and protease-activated receptors

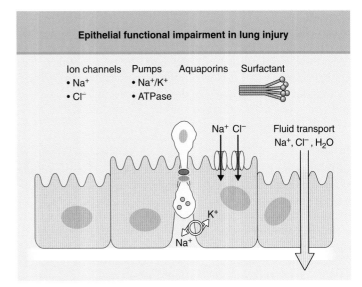

Figure 1.6. Epithelial functional impairment in lung injury. In lung injury, there is dysregulation of the ions channels, aquaporins, and the Na$^+$/K$^+$ pump such that the normal vectoral transport of salt and water across the pulmonary epithelium is impaired. There is also depletion of surfactant resulting in atelectasis and interstitial edema.

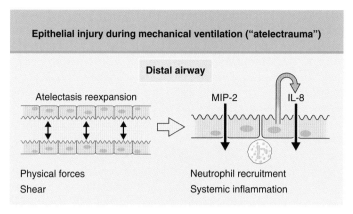

Epithelial injury during mechanical ventilation ("atelectrauma")

Distal airway

Atelectasis reexpansion

MIP-2   IL-8

Physical forces
Shear

Neutrophil recruitment
Systemic inflammation

Figure 1.7. Epithelial injury during mechanical ventilation (atelectrauma). During mechanical ventilation, atelectasis and subsequent reexpansion of the distal airways induce physical and sheer stress on the epithelial cells and activate them to produce MIP-2 and IL-8, leading to leukocyte recruitment and development of system inflammation.

7. Proteases
8. Leukotrienes and prostaglandins
9. Growth factors such as VEGF and TGF-β
10. Alterations in the cytoskeleton and in intercellular (junctional) proteins to allow for leukocyte transmigration and changes in vascular permeability

Far from being a homogeneous population, there are marked differences in the endothelial cell structure, surface phenotype, and profile of protein expression and secretion depending on the location of the vascular bed. For example, the vascular endothelium of organs such as the lung recruits primarily neutrophils in disorders such as ALI and ARDS, whereas inflammation of the central nervous system results in recruitment of mostly lymphocytes. Furthermore, in the central nervous system, in which maintenance of the blood–brain barrier requires tight control of transport of fluid and proteins across the endothelial bed, endothelial cells do not possess fenestrae.

Fibroblasts

Fibroblasts are classically viewed as structural cells and passive responders to exogenous influences. On the contrary, fibroblasts are integrally involved in regulation and perpetuation of inflammatory disorders. Matrix-degrading proteases, such as matrix metalloproteinases and cytokines such as IL-1 and TNF, are strongly expressed by fibroblasts. Conversely, fibroblasts synthesize extracellular matrix proteins such as collagen, which is required for tissue repair but, if laid down in an abnormal manner or excessive amount, contributes to organ dysfunction.

Inflammatory Mediators
Cytokines

Cytokines are soluble, low-molecular-weight proteins that play important roles in the regulation and propagation of the inflammatory response (Table 1.4). Originally described as products of

Table 1.4 Cytokines, Chemokines, and Their Functions		
Cytokine	**Function**	**Other Clinical Roles**
TNF-α	Proinflammatory Neutrophil activation in ARDS	Proximate cytokine released in response to inflammatory stimulus
IL-1β	Proinflammatory Neutrophil activation in ARDS Upregulation of adhesion molecules on leukocytes, endothelium, and airway epithelium	One of first cytokines to be released in response to inflammatory stimulus
IL-6	Proinflammatory Leukocyte activation Promotes proliferation of myeloid progenitor cells Induces pyrexia Acute phase reactant	Circulating levels are a marker of severity of ARDS of different etiologies
IL-10	Anti-inflammatory Inhibits release of TNF-α, IL-1β, and IL-6 from monocyte/macrophages Stimulates the production of IL-1ra and soluble p75 TNF receptor	
GM-CSF	Alveolar macrophage function Lung host defense Surfactant homeostasis	Low circulating levels associated with poor prognosis in sepsis
PAF	Acts via receptors on platelets, leukocytes, and endothelial cells Increases vascular permeability Leukocyte recruitment Primes and triggers leukocyte secretion	
ICAM-1	Leukocyte recruitment and retention	Increased in inflammation
C5a	Product of classical and alternate complement cascade Potent anaphylatoxin and chemoattractant Acts via C5aR Can be both pro- and anti-inflammatory	
Substance P	Neuropeptide that acts via its receptor NK1R Proinflammatory and associated with development of lung injury	
CC chemokines	Chemotactic and activator of monocytes	
CXC chemokines	Chemotactic and activator of neutrophils	

lymphocytes, cytokines are now known to be produced and secreted not only by leukocytes but also by a variety of cell populations, including endothelial cells, epithelial cells, and fibroblasts. Expression and secretion of cytokines are transcriptionally regulated and can be quickly enhanced following cell stimulation.

Signaling through cognate receptors, cytokines exert distinct responses in specific cell populations, stimulating some populations to activate, proliferate, and differentiate while having an inhibitory effect on other cells types. In this way, cytokines play a major role in regulating the intensity and duration of the inflammatory response. The cytokines that play important roles in inflammation, particularly in the early proinflammatory phase, include TNF-α, IL-1β, IL-6, and IL-8. Significant elevations of these cytokines are observed in generalized inflammatory states and particularly in gram-negative sepsis.

Activated macrophages are the major source of TNF-α and IL-1β in the proinflammatory state. Indeed, IL-1β and TNF-α work synergistically during the proinflammatory phase to induce transcriptional activation of a variety of genes, including those encoding cytokines, chemokines, adhesion molecules, proteases, and enzymes of the prostaglandin synthesis pathway. They exert their biological function via specific receptors: TNF-α via its two receptors, TNFR1 and TNFR2, whereas IL-1β transmits its signals primarily through IL-1R1. These receptors are expressed in various cell populations that include leukocytes, endothelial cells, epithelial cells, and fibroblasts and are subject to regulation by a variety of cytokines. Furthermore, there is differential expression of the receptors in different cell populations as well as in different tissue beds. In this way, specific cytokines exert divergent effects on different cell populations.

TNF-α elicits an early and a late response in inflammation. In the initial stages of inflammation, TNF-α induces a plethora of downstream signals that amplify the inflammatory response. Acting on macrophages, lymphocytes, and endothelial and epithelial cells, TNF-α induces expression of cytokines, chemokines, growth factors, and cell surface receptors that recruit hematopoietic cells, neutrophils, T lymphocytes, monocytes, and macrophages to sites of infection and injury. TNF-α also regulates changes in the vascular permeability and vascular endothelial cell proliferation by inducing the expression of angiogenic cytokines such as VEGF and TGF-β and by inducing plasminogen activator and its receptor.

In later stages of the inflammatory response, in which tissue remodeling and repair predominate, TNF-α also has a regulatory role by significantly upregulating the expression of matrix metalloproteinase (MMP)-9, a collagenase that plays a major role in tissue degradation and wound healing. Concomitantly, TNF-α suppresses the expression of the MMP-9 antagonist, tissue inhibitor of metalloproteinase-3.

IL-6 is another proinflammatory cytokine that plays an important role in the early phase of inflammation. Its production is stimulated by endotoxin, TNF-α, and IL-1β and is enhanced by stimulation of the plasminogen activator receptors (uPAR). IL-6 stimulates the synthesis of C-reactive protein and induces pyrexia. Regardless of the underlying etiology of inflammation, high circulating levels of IL-6 correlate with the severity of ARDS.

IL-10 is primarily an anti-inflammatory cytokine that acts to downregulate proinflammatory signals by inhibiting lymphocytic

and phagocytic function. In animal models of generalized sepsis, mice in which IL-10 expression has been knocked out experienced more pulmonary injury with higher levels of TNF-α, IL-1α, and IL-6 expression and increased leukocyte extravasation into the alveolar spaces. In patients with ARDS, low concentrations of IL-10 in the bronchoalveolar lavage fluid correlate highly with mortality.

Chemokines

Chemokines are 8- to 10-kDa glycoproteins that, although structurally related to cytokines, are distinct from them as a result of their ability to bind and signal G protein-coupled receptors (see Table 1.5). Chemokines are both chemotatic and cellular activating factors for leukocytes and can be classified into two groups:

1. CC chemokines
   These include MCP-1, MIP-1α, and RANTES.
   They act primarily on monocytes, lymphocytes, basophils, and eosinophils.
2. CXC chemokines
   These differ from CC chemokines by the presence of a single amino acid, X, between two amino-terminal cysteine (C) residues.
   Examples of CXC chemokines include IL-8, GRO-α (growth-related oncogene α), and NEA-78 (epithelial-derived neutrophil-activating peptide).
   CXC chemokines act primarily on neutrophils.

The chemokine receptors are structurally related heptaspannning transmembrane proteins that transmit their signals through heterotrimeric G proteins. Like cytokines, the effect of chemokine activation results in diverse physiological responses that are cell and stimulus specific. The binding specificity of individual chemokine receptors is determined by a region in the amino terminus of the protein. Some receptors are highly specific, whereas others bind multiple chemokines of both CC and CXC families. Differential regulation and expression of the chemokines receptor in different cell types play an important role in determining the biological result of chemokine activation.

Growth Factors

Various growth factors are also produced during the inflammatory response (Table 1.5). In general, these are produced in the

Table 1.5 Growth Factors and Functions	
Growth Factor	**Function**
VEGF	Regulates vascular permeability
	Induces vascular endothelial cell proliferation
	Upregulates tissue and urokinase plasminogen activator expression
IGF-1	Profibrotic
	Produced by macrophages
TGF-β	Mediator of tissue repair and fibrosis
	Regulates cell growth, death, and apoptosis; cell differentiation; and extracellular matrix synthesis
	Induces vasculogenesis
	Enhances mesenchymal cell proliferation
KGF	Epithelial cell specific
	Proinflammatory and fibrotic
HGF	Proinflammatory and fibrotic

later stages of inflammation and regulate cell growth, tissue repair, and angiogenesis.

ETIOLOGY

Inflammation is a normal physiologic response to tissue injury, infection, and exposure to exogenous materials. Whether inflammation remains localized and self-limited or whether sepsis develops into MODS with accompanying ALI and ARDS is the result of a complex interplay between the specific inciting cause, its intensity and duration, the genetic background of the host, the presence of other comorbid illnesses, and mitigating conditions that all interact to determine the magnitude of the inflammatory response (see Fig. 1.1). In many instances, in patients admitted to the intensive care unit, the primary cause leading to admission to the intensive care unit is obvious. Nonetheless, a systemic approach in identify the underlying etiology or etiologies that are contributing to the inflammatory state will guide treatment and offer prognostic value.

A number of classification systems are used to outline differential diagnosis of specific diseases. An approach to the etiology of inflammation, SIRS, and MODS is outlined in Table 1.6.

PRESENTATION

Clinical

When inflammation is localized, the classical signs of redness (*rubor*), swelling (*tumor*), warmth (*calor*), pain (*dolor*), and loss of function (*functio laesa*) are usually present. As inflammation proceeds to SIRS, the patient will develop systemic symptoms and signs, including fever, chills, sweats, tachypnea, hyperpnea, and tachycardia. Hypotension may ensue and may become more pronounced as multiorgan dysfunction worsens. Depending on the underlying cause of the inflammatory response, other signs and symptoms will be present.

Laboratory Tests

There are no specific laboratory tests that are diagnostic for inflammation per se, although some inflammatory disorders, such as autoimmune disorders, are associated with the presence of specific circulating markers (e.g., antinuclear antibodies). The systemic inflammatory response is associated with leukocytosis and the presence of immature (or band) neutrophils due to the recruitment of both mature and immature precursor cells from the bone marrow into the circulation. These cells are sequestered in systemic and pulmonary microvascular beds and may contribute to the pathogenesis of ALI/ARDS and multiorgan failure. Metabolic acidosis is often observed and is a reflection of inadequate tissue perfusion at a microvascular level. Although elevations of various cytokines and chemokines are observed in inflammation and can be indicative of disease severity, these tests remain primarily in the research realm and do not offer specific guidance in patient management.

A systemic search for the underlying cause, such as a thorough search for infection and other potential causes on the list of differential diagnoses, is the most helpful strategy in developing a treatment plan for patients with evidence of inflammation.

Radiographic

There is no specific radiographic presentation for inflammation. The presentation will differ depending on the etiology. However, when MODS has developed and is associated with ALI and ARDS, characteristic radiographic alterations of the chest x-ray with diffuse, bilateral infiltrates are observed.

DIAGNOSIS

A diagnosis of inflammation is made in the appropriate clinical setting of infection or injury. Specific definitions of clinical syndromes are defined in Table 1.1.

TREATMENT

Management of the patient with inflammation will depend on the source and the extent and severity of the inflammatory response. A general approach is outlined as follows:

1. Treat the underlying cause. If the source or etiology such as infection can be identified, treat it with appropriate antibiotics, surgical drainage, or repair.
2. Reverse any metabolic abnormalities. Replace fluids and electrolytes, and supply nutrients such as glucose.
3. Maintain adequate blood pressure using fluids, colloids, and, if necessary, vasopressors.
4. Maintain good tissue oxygenation with ventilatory support as needed.
5. Maintain adequate nutrition using enteral or parental feeding.
6. Prevent iatrogenic complications by preventing deep venous thrombosis and instituting infection control measures to prevent nosocomial infections.

In many instances in which the patient has developed multiorgan dysfunction, treatment of the underlying cause and good supportive care as outlined previously are not sufficient to halt the overexuberant inflammatory response and the associated

Table 1.6 Causes of Inflammation	
Exogenous causes	
Infections	Viruses, bacteria, atypical bacteria, fungi, parasites, prions, others
Allergens	Inhaled, ingested, topical
Chemicals	Inhaled, ingested, topical, drugs
Gaseous agents	Environmental exposure, work-related injuries
Burns	
Trauma	Accidental and iatrogenic
	Blunt and penetrating injuries
Radiation	
Hypo-/hyperthermia	
Endogenous causes	
Autoimmune diseases	Primary presentation or acute exacerbations of indolent disease
Coagulopathies	Intrinsic: sickle cell anemia, hypercoagulable states, thromboembolic disease
	Iatrogenic: multiple transfusions, cardiopulmonary bypass, hemodialysis, etc.
Metabolic dysequilibrium states	Hypoxia, hypo- and hyperglycemia, alcohol (ethanol, methanol) poisoning, rhabdomyolysis, drug overdose, drug interactions

Table 1.7 Treatment	
Specific treatment	Antibiotics
	Fluid and colloid replacement
	Diuretics
Anti-inflammatory treatment	Nonsteroidals
	Steroids
	Replacement Rx
	Surfactant
	N-acetyl cysteine/antioxidants
	Nitric oxide
	Biologicals
	Anticytokines
	Anti-IL2
	IL-1 receptor antagonists
	TNF receptor fusion protein
	Anti-TNF
	Anti-IgE
	Antithrombin
	Activated protein kinase C
	Leukotriene antagonists
	GM-CSF
	Anti-PAF
Supportive treatment	Ventilation
	Nutrition
	DVT prophylaxis

inflammatory-mediated tissue damage. During the past decade, a number of treatment options directed at modulation of the inflammatory response have become available. In general, these agents target specific inflammatory pathways or mediators in an attempt to downregulate the inflammatory cascade. Although many of these agents have been shown to be effective in vitro and in animal models of sepsis, few have shown beneficial results in clinical trials. A list of currently available specific anti-inflammatory agents is shown in Table 1.7. Those that have shown beneficial results in clinical trials are discussed here.

Steroids
Rationale and Outcome
Glucocorticoids (corticosteroids) have potent anti-inflammatory effects and have an important therapeutic role in the treatment of diverse inflammatory diseases. Their role in the management of sepsis and septic shock has been extensively evaluated and, indeed, reevaluated during the past several decades. Glucocorticoids were initially thought to be beneficial in the treatment of septic shock, but subsequent clinical trials conducted from the 1950s to the present day have shown that high-dose steroids have no impact (and, in some trials, have a detrimental effect) on survival of patients with sepsis. However, physiological doses (equivalent to 200–300 mg of hydrocortisone daily) given over 5 to 7 days with a tapering dose conferred significant survival benefit in patients with vasopressor-dependent shock (Minneci and colleagues, 2004) and should be administered in this clinical setting.

Nitric Oxide
Rationale and Outcome
Exogenous administration of inhaled nitric oxide (NO) is a clinically effective treatment in the management of respiratory failure in the newborn and has shown promise in the ameliora-

tion of pulmonary hypertension in different clinical settings that include idiopathic pulmonary hypertension, postcardiac transplant, and cor pulmonale. It was postulated that NO, acting as a selective pulmonary vasodilator, would be an effective treatment modality in the setting of ALI and ARDS by improving ventilation–perfusion mismatch, hypoxemia, and pulmonary hypertension. However, in three large clinical trials of patients with ALI and ARDS, inhaled NO failed to demonstrate any clinical benefit. In these trials, a transient improvement in oxygenation was observed, and this leaves open the possibility that NO may have a role as a rescue treatment modality in ARDS patients with severe and refractory hypoxemia. However, there are no definitive clinical data to support the use of NO in this setting.

Anti-TNF Therapies
Rationale
TNF-α is an important cytokine that is rapidly synthesized and released in the early phases of inflammation. This pivotal cytokine plays a significant role in propagation of the inflammatory cascade through its role in activating macrophages, neutrophils, and lymphocytes, as well as endothelial and epithelial cells. Markedly elevated levels of TNF-α are observed in a variety of inflammatory diseases, and serum levels of TNF-α correlate with patient outcomes. Initial studies in animal models of generalized sepsis revealed that anti-TNF therapies significantly improved mortality.

Outcome
Clinical trials of therapy targeting excessive levels of TNF have been conducted in patients with sepsis. Two anti-TNF products are available. One is a soluble fusion protein of p55–TNF receptor (also called p55–IgG or lenercept) that binds to TNF-α before it can activate TNF receptors on target cells. The second is a F(ab)2 fragment of a mouse monoclonal antibody (afelimomab) that binds to human TNF-α with high specificity and affinity. Both products have been shown to neutralize the biological effects of TNF-α in vivo and in vitro and are given as an intravenous infusion. A randomized, placebo-controlled clinical trial of patients with severe sepsis compared the outcomes of 87 patients who received a single dose of lenercept at the therapeutic dose of 0.083 mg/kg with the outcome of 78 patients who were treated with placebo alone (Pittet and coworkers, 1999). Patient outcomes on day 28 revealed that the treatment group had a lower overall mortality (36% reduction) with a trend toward shorter length of stay in the intensive care and more days free of ARDS and other organ failure. None of these outcomes, however, reached statistical significance.

Clinical trials with the afelimomab monoclonal antibody in patients with sepsis yielded similar results. Initial phase 2 open-label clinical trials (Reinhart and associates, 1996) suggested that patients with elevated serum IL-6 levels (i.e., those with a hyperinflammatory response) may benefit from afelimomab in a dose-dependent manner. A subsequent double-blind, randomized, placebo-controlled multicenter trial enrolled only patients with sepsis and high IL-6 levels (1000 pg/mL) (Reinhart and associates, 2001). A total of 222 patients received placebo and 224 were treated with afelimomab at 1 mg/kg TID for 3 days. Analysis at 28 days revealed no significant differences in patient outcome, although there was a trend to lower mortality (54%

vs. 57.7%) and an earlier resolution of organ dysfunction in the treatment group. Taken together, these results suggest that anti-TNF therapies are not beneficial in the management of patients with sepsis and MODS.

Activated Protein Kinase C [Drotrecogin-α (Activated)]

Rationale

During the early proinflammatory phase when significant elevations of TNF-α, IL-1β, and IL-6 are observed, there is concomitant activation of the coagulation cascade with production of activated protein C (APC). APC is an endogenous anticoagulant protein produced by the action of thrombin–thrombomodulin on its precursor, protein C. Importantly, APC has a number of anti-inflammatory activities that appear to be crucial for limiting the extent of inflammation and inflammatory-mediated tissue injury (Fig. 1.8), including the following:

1. Inhibition of monocyte/macrophage production of TNF-α, IL-1, and IL-6
2. Binding to endothelial selectins and therefore inhibiting leukocyte adhesion and recruitment
3. Limiting production of thrombin by inactivating factors Va and VIIIa
4. Acts via the coreceptor, endothelial cell protein C, to activate PAR-1 receptor, leading to production of the cell-protective chemokine, MCP-1.

In sepsis, the production of APC is impaired, in part due to downregulation of thrombomodulin by inflammatory cytokines. In the majority of patients with sepsis, decreased APC levels are observed and appear to correlate with increased mortality (see also Chapters 50, 51, and 55).

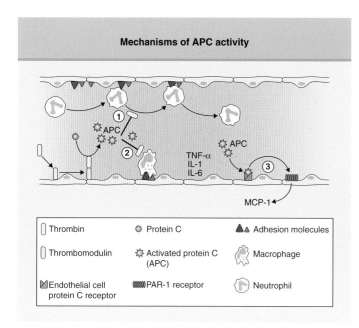

Figure 1.8. Mechanisms of APC activity. APC downregulates the inflammatory response by a number of mechanisms: It (1) impairs leukocyte adhesion, (2) abrogates cytokine expression in activated macrophages, and (3) activates PAR-1 receptor via the endothelial cell protein C receptor and induces monocyte chemotactic protein (MCP)-1.

Outcome

Clinical trials with APC indicate that this therapeutic modality may be of benefit in patients with sepsis. One of the largest placebo-controlled, randomized, double-blind trials (the PROWESS study; Bernard and colleagues, 2001) compared 1690 patients with severe sepsis. A total of 840 patients were in the placebo arm, and 850 in the treatment arm received 24 µg/kg/hr of APC as a continuously intravenous infusion for 96 hours. Outcome at 28 days revealed a reduction of 6.1% in overall mortality and 19.4% in relative risk of death in the treatment group. However, there was a significant risk of bleeding in the treatment group (3.5% vs. 2.0% in the placebo group). Although primarily seen in patients who had comorbidities such as gastroduodenal ulcers, increased PT/PT, and thrombocytopenia, this adverse reaction is potentially life threatening.

A follow-up study (the ENHANCE US trial; Bernard and coworkers, 2004) was a multicenter prospective single-arm clinical study of 273 patients with severe sepsis to assess all-cause mortality and drug safety at 28 days. The comparison groups were the controls of two previous placebo-controlled, double-blind studies, including the PROWESS trial totaling 449 patients. This trial revealed that there was a 6% higher survival rate in the treatment group compared with the control group, and younger patients (age < 75 years; mortality, 23.8%) derived more benefit from treatment than older patients (age ≥ 75 years; mortality, 35.6%).

Again, the major serious adverse reaction noted was bleeding, with an overall incidence of 4% in the treatment group. Most of these represented bleeding into the gastrointestinal tract, skin, soft tissue, and joints. Up to 69% of the bleeding was attributable to invasive procedures performed on the patient. Although not statistically significant, there was a trend of fewer thrombotic events, such as myocardial infarctions and stroke, in patients receiving APC.

Overall assessment of these clinical trials suggests that APC is beneficial in patients with sepsis. Due to the high incidence of bleeding, particularly in association with invasive procedures, it is recommended that the agent be discontinued 2 hours prior to a procedure, and that the infusion be resumed 12 hours postprocedure and only when good hemostasis has been achieved.

SUMMARY

Inflammation is an important physiological response to infection and injury, and it is crucial for maintaining homeostasis and innate immunity. However, inflammation can also result in detrimental effects since severe infections and insults can lead to an overexuberant response, leading to system inflammation, multiorgan failure, and ALI/ARDS. During the past several decades, we have learned much about the molecular mechanisms that are involved in the inflammatory cascade and have come to appreciate the complexity of the system. Of the specific (targeted) anti-inflammatory therapies that have undergone clinical trials in patients with sepsis or ALI/ARDS, only APC has been proven to be of benefit. Administration of physiological doses of glucocorticoids has also been shown to be beneficial in patients with sepsis. Future investigations in this area will need to consider this complexity and ensure that the beneficial effects of the inflammatory response are not compromised.

SUGGESTED READING

Bernard GR, Vincent JL, Laterre PF, et al: Recombinant Human Protein C Worldwide Evaluation in Severe Sepsis (PROWESS) study group. Efficacy and safety of recombinant human activated protein C for severe sepsis. N Engl J Med 2001;344:699–709.

Bernard GR, Margolis BD, Shanies HM, et al: Extended Evaluation of Recombinant Human Activated Protein C United States Investigators. Extended evaluation of recombinant human activated protein C United States Trial (ENHANCE US): A single-arm, phase 3B, multicenter study of drotrecogin alfa (activated) in severe sepsis. Chest 2004;125: 2206–2216.

Donnelly SC, Strieter RM, Reid PT, et al: The association between mortality rates and decreased concentration of IL-10 and IL-1 receptor antagonist in the lung fluids of patients with ARDS. Ann Intern Med 1996; 125:191–196.

Minneci PC, Deans KJ, Banks SM, Eichacker PQ, Natanson C: Meta-analysis: The effect of steroids on survival and shock during sepsis depends on the dose. Ann Intern Med 2004;141:47–56.

Pittet D, Harbarth S, Suter PM, et al: Impact of immunomodulating therapy on morbidity in patients with severe sepsis. Am J Respir Crit Care Med 1999;160:852–857.

Reinhart K, Menges T, Gardlund B, et al: Randomized, placebo-controlled trial of the anti-tumor necrosis factor antibody fragment afelimomab in hyperinflammatory response during severe sepsis: The RAMSES Study. Crit Care Med 2001;29:765–769.

Reinhart K, Wiegand-Lohnert C, Grimminger F, et al: Assessment of the safety and efficacy of the monoclonal anti-tumor necrosis factor antibody-fragment, MAK 195F, in patients with sepsis and septic shock: A multi-center, randomized, placebo-controlled, dose-ranging study. Crit Care Med 1996;24:733–742.

Riedemann NC, Guo R-F, Ward PA: Novel strategies for the treatment of sepsis. Nat Med 2003;9:517–524.

Chapter 2

Genetics

Frank Stüber, Lutz Eric Lehmann, Jens-Christian Schewe,
Ulrike Stamer, Stefan Weber, Sven Klaschik, and Malte Book

KEY POINTS

- The need for risk profiling as well as individualized drug therapy in the pharmacogenetic context motivates genetic studies in critically ill patients.
- New approaches for studying genetic predisposition to complex diseases involve associations between carriage of certain alleles and phenotype (disease) independent of the relationships of the subjects studied.
- Choice of candidate genes is critical because sound knowledge of the pathophysiology of a given disease is needed as well as data on genomic variations and their frequency and possible impact on gene function.
- An individual's predisposition to the effects of inflammatory insults is determined, at least in part, by genetic variants of endogenous mediators that constitute the pathways of inflammation.
- Understanding the genetic determination of the inflammatory process will allow the development of valuable diagnostic tools and new therapeutic approaches in severe sepsis.
- Genetic variants can modify pharmacokinetics and pharmacodynamics of drugs and, therefore, predispose to adverse drug reactions or reduced efficacy.

Genetics and intensive care medicine are medical disciplines that appear quite distant from each other in terms of common mutual understanding of geneticists and intensivists. As such, a natural question is, "Why should genetics be integrated into intensive care medicine?" The answer is rather simple: incidence and outcome. We need to understand endogenous as well as exogenous causes leading to conditions requiring intensive care and contributing to poor outcome in critically ill patients. Endogenous causes are to be found in the patient—in his or her genes. Genes contribute to the determination of the phenotype of any individual. Interindividual variation of the primary DNA sequence of genes can modulate gene function. Genes involved in disease processes relevant for intensive care are therefore candidate genes to explain the endogenous (i.e., genetic) predisposition to adverse outcomes in intensive care medicine.

The need for risk profiling as well as individualized drug therapy in the pharmacogenetic context motivates genetic studies in critically ill patients. Therefore, genetic studies currently represent an expanding field of interest for basic and clinical research. Integration of this topic into functional genomics is mandatory. Gene function is well considered even in genome analyses. Genomic promoter variants may predict the interindividual variability in response to inflammatory stimuli such as infection and trauma due to altered promoter activity and transcription. Genomic variations may affect gene expression profiles as well as protein structure and quantities. The genes involved in inflammation are numerous and so are genomic variations within many of those genes. The challenge of current genetic studies in intensive care is to define patterns of genomic variations that identify patients at risk for adverse outcomes in the intensive care unit (ICU) or, on the other hand, patients who benefit from specific therapies.

BASIC CONCEPTS OF GENETICS

Mendel published his "laws of heredity" in 1866 and demonstrated with experiments on peas that parents pass discrete elements of heredity to their offspring. Specific characteristics, visible as the so-called phenotype, like the color of flowers or color of mammal skin, are determined by genes called alleles that exist in a variety of forms. Black- or white-colored mice have different alleles of the same gene depending on the dominance relationship of the inherited parent alleles. A variety of genetic variations, the alleles, exist in genes, contributing to or modulating complex diseases, such as diabetes, hypertension, coronary artery disease, or susceptibility to infection. However, distinct genetic characteristics, such as individual variations in the base sequence of genes, most often occur as low informative markers. Only a few of those markers are considered to be highly informative markers because they represent major causes for inherited diseases (e.g., Huntington's disease and cystic fibrosis).

Genomic variations occur as single base variations or single nucleotide polymorphism (SNP), as insertion/deletion variants, or as more complex variants involving longer stretches of DNA sequence and higher allele numbers (Fig. 2.1). These complex variants comprise micro- and minisatellites and variable numbers of tandem repeats (see Fig. 2.1). Even alleles defined by different copy numbers of a whole functioning gene are targets for genotyping because the number of gene copies may closely relate to protein expression levels.

Genomic variations

Single Base Changes: i.e. SNP
(single nucleotide polymorphism)

CGATGCAACT
CGATCCAACT

Deletion/Insertion of Single Bases

ACGTCGCTGAG
ACGTCG TGAG

Variable Number of Tandem Repeats
(VNTR) mini/Microsatellites

TAACGCGCGCGATGC

Repeats of longer motifs

TGACAAC...GTCATTAC...GTCATTAC...GTCATTTAC...

Figure 2.1. Genomic variations.

STUDYING GENETICS IN COMPLEX DISEASES: STUDY DESIGN

Traditional genetic epidemiologic analyses have focused on segregation analysis of genetic variations (alleles) using well-characterized families in order to estimate the contribution of inherited alleles to disease. Family trees were analyzed and phenotypes (disease states) of carriers and noncarriers of certain alleles were compared. In many acute complex diseases present in the intensive care setting, family studies are extremely difficult to perform, especially when exogenous factors (trauma and infection) are major triggers of the disease. New approaches for studying genetic predisposition to complex diseases involve associations between carriage of certain alleles and phenotype (disease) independent of the relationships of the subjects studied. There are concerns about association studies because of possible low statistical power and the detection of spurious (false-positive) associations. These traditional concepts demand study designs similar to the transmission disequilibrium test (TDT) used in today's state-of-the-art genetic epidemiologic studies. All members of a given family do not face the same environmental risks in life to form a comparable study group within the TDT design. Many experts in genetic epidemiology now favor association study designs in complex diseases with a phenotype depending on an environmental impact such as injury or infection. This design does not require sampling of DNA from family members. There is a problem, however, in so-called "negative" association studies, in which genomic markers show very low and insignificant odds ratios (relative risks) when associated with disease phenotypes. Achievement of adequate statistical power $(1 - \beta = 0.8)$ in these studies is often impossible because required case numbers increase exponentially with decreasing relative risk (Fig. 2.2). The combination of genetic epidemiologic results with functional studies concerning a specific genomic marker may help to differentiate between valuable markers and those not needed in future studies and diagnostics.

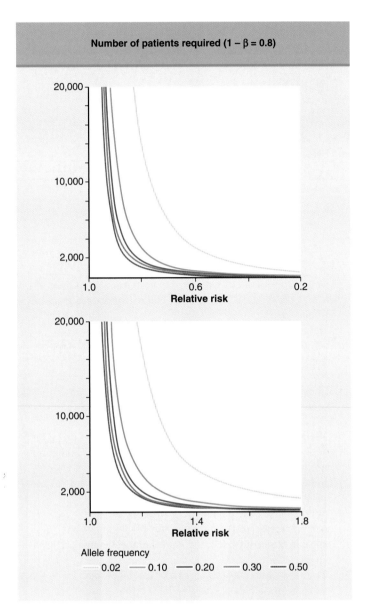

Figure 2.2. Case numbers required in genetic epidemiologic association studies. Statistical power of 80% requires enormous numbers of cases when the impact of a genomic variation (relative risk) and/or allele frequency is rather low.

Genetic epidemiologic tools designed to overcome the phenomenon of spurious association comprise structured analysis as well as the use of genomic controls (i.e., SNPs from "genomic deserts" indicating population substructure within groups).

Genes to Be Studied
Genetic association studies of complex diseases currently focus on candidate genes because genomewide scanning for genomic variants is too costly to perform in large numbers of individuals. The choice of candidate genes is critical because sound knowledge of pathophysiology of a given disease is needed as well as data on genomic variations and their frequency and possible impact on gene function (Table 2.1). The locations of genomic variations within a candidate gene determine the possible impact on gene function (Fig. 2.3): Variations within the coding sequence may alter the primary amino acid sequence, whereas

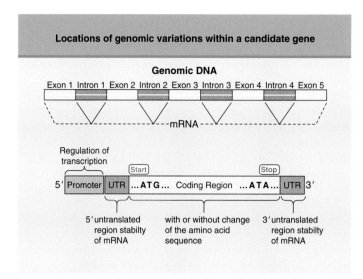

Figure 2.3. Genomic regions where introduction of base sequence variation may implicate altered gene expression levels (promoter), altered mRNA stability (UTR), or amino acid sequence changes (coding region).

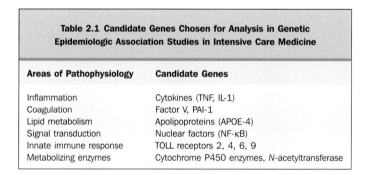

Table 2.1 Candidate Genes Chosen for Analysis in Genetic Epidemiologic Association Studies in Intensive Care Medicine	
Areas of Pathophysiology	Candidate Genes
Inflammation	Cytokines (TNF, IL-1)
Coagulation	Factor V, PAI-1
Lipid metabolism	Apolipoproteins (APOE-4)
Signal transduction	Nuclear factors (NF-κB)
Innate immune response	TOLL receptors 2, 4, 6, 9
Metabolizing enzymes	Cytochrome P450 enzymes, *N*-acetyltransferase

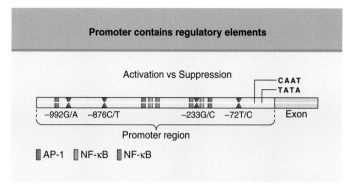

Figure 2.4. Promoter region with known genomic variants at four base positions (−72, −233, −876, and −992). *cis*-Acting elements (binding sites in the promoter for DNA binding proteins) are close to some variations but remain unchanged by polymorphisms.

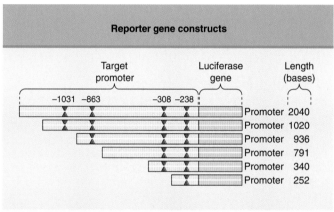

Figure 2.5. Promoter constructs of different fragment length. Sequence variations are introduced by site-directed mutagenesis at positions −238, −308, −863, and −1031.

variants in the untranslated regions of the mRNA may alter mRNA stability in the cytosol, possibly leading to low translation rates of mRNA into protein. Variations in the promoter region are of particular interest because this is where regulation of gene transcription occurs (Fig. 2.4). Promoters contain so-called *cis*-acting elements representing short sequence motifs that represent binding sites for DNA binding proteins (nuclear factors), also called *trans*-acting elements. Variation of these sequences may cause altered binding of nuclear factors, leading to decreased or increased gene transcription, depending on the activating or suppressing effects of a particular nuclear factor. Methods to test the impact of promoter variants on promoter activity comprise reporter gene constructs of different lengths containing base variants at defined positions that have been introduced by site-directed mutagenesis (Fig. 2.5). Indicator genes are usually luciferase or chloramphenicol transferase (Fig. 2.6).

Alternatives to the Candidate Gene Approach?

To some genetic epidemiologists, the candidate gene and association study approaches to the genetic predisposition in complex diseases have major weaknesses. In their view, the choice of candidate genes is determined by preexisting assump-

tions that bias the findings. Furthermore, by definition, these approaches will not identify any novel genes. Therefore, a genomewide approach is a frequent recommendation by genetic epidemiologists. Analysis of all currently detectable genomic variations (i.e., >300,000 SNPs) in an individual is possible by different approaches to genome scanning. The cost is the major factor excluding genomewide scanning as a feasible method in cohorts of hundreds or even thousands of patients.

Devlin and colleagues, as well as Koening and coworkers, are genetic epidemiologists who have suggested possible study designs to be used in implementing the candidate gene approach in complex diseases. Group sequential designs in combination with measures to detect spurious, false-positive association and correction for multiple testing help reduce genotyping costs and produce reliable results at adequate statistical power. Within this context, the candidate gene approach is practical but may be not be necessary when the use of genomewide approaches becomes widespread at reasonable cost.

Candidate Examples: Cytokine Genes with Promoter Variations

Systemic inflammatory reactions are common in intensive care patients and contribute substantially to morbidity and

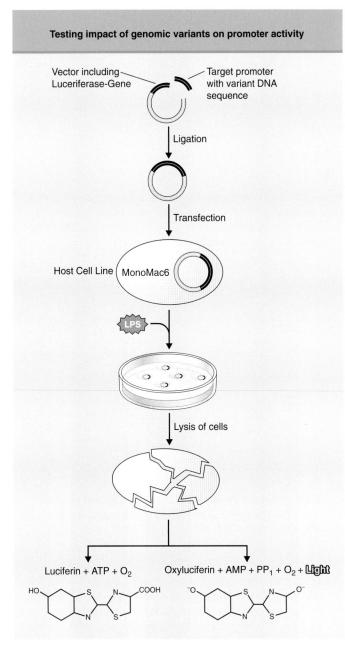

Testing impact of genomic variants on promoter activity

Figure 2.6. Testing promoter activity in vitro by reporter gene assay. The emitted light signal is quantified and relates directly to the promoter activity.

injury. The capacity of mediator production and release shows remarkable interindividual variation and may contribute to a wide range of clinical manifestations of inflammatory disease.

Which are important candidate genes and what genomic variations are to be used as diagnostic markers? Will certain subgroups of patients benefit more than others from antimediator strategies because they are genetically "programmed" to produce high mediator release in response to a given inflammatory response? Because resources for research are restricted, choice of candidate markers is critical. The knowledge of pathophysiologic processes leading to sepsis and organ failure has directed the search for candidate genes. Briefly, pro- and anti-inflammatory responses contribute to the outcome of patients with systemic inflammation and sepsis. Therefore, many genes encoding proteins involved in the transduction of inflammatory processes are candidate genes to determine the human genetic background that is responsible for interindividual differences in systemic inflammatory responses to injury.

Cytokines play a major role in mediating immune responses. Many cytokine genes involved in inflammatory cascades, and not just genes encoding proteins such as tumor necrosis factor-α (TNF-α) that directly cause the syndrome of extensive hyper-inflammation (i.e., septic shock), are important candidate genes that may determine the extent of an individual's response to injury.

Understanding the genetic determination of the inflammatory process will allow the development of valuable diagnostic tools and new therapeutic approaches in severe sepsis. Cytokine promoter variants may contribute substantially to studies on genetic predisposition to sepsis because they impact a gene region of high regulatory activity (see Fig. 2.4). In this view, researchers may be able to advance diagnostics and therapy of sepsis in the near future.

The group of candidate genes comprises but is not restricted to cytokines and includes numerous other effector molecules involved in inflammatory processes. Genes of the coagulation system, heat shock proteins or signal transduction molecules, and others are candidate genes for sepsis that show genomic variation. Cytokines released from immunocompetent cells are major mediators of the inflammatory response to infection. Primary proinflammatory cytokines, such as TNF-α and interleukin-1 (IL-1), induce secondary pro- and anti-inflammatory mediators, such as IL-6 and IL-10. They have been shown to contribute substantially to the host's primary response to infection.

An Important Candidate: Tumor Necrosis Factor

Many cytokines and related genes display variations in their promoter sequence (Box 2.1). Major interest has focused on the genomic variations of the TNF locus: Biallelic polymorphisms defined by restriction enzymes (NcoI and AspHI) or other single base changes within the promoter (−308 and −238) as well as multiallelic microsatellites (TNFa–e) have been investigated. Functional importance for regulation of the TNF gene has been described for polymorphisms within the TNF promoter region. The rare allele TNF2 (A at position −308) was suggested to be linked to high TNF promoter activity tested by reporter gene assays (see Fig. 2.6).

In contrast to genomic variations located in the promoter region, intronic polymorphisms are more difficult to associate

mortality. An individual's predisposition to the effects of inflammatory insults is determined, at least in part, by genetic variants of endogenous mediators that constitute the pathways of inflammation. This is particularly important in the intensive care setting, where many of the diseases that intensivists treat have a major inflammatory component (e.g., sepsis and acute respiratory distress syndrome). Genetic heterogeneity is clearly important as clinicians consider why apparently similar insults cause such marked differences in responses among patients. Genes encoding proteins involved in the transduction of inflammatory processes are among candidate genes to determine the human genetic background responsible for interindividual differences in systemic inflammatory responses to infection and

Box 2.1 Cytokines and Related Molecules with Reported Genomic Variations within the Promoter Region

TNF
IL-1α; -β; IL-2, -4, -6, -8, -9, -10, -11, -12, -13, -15, -16, -18
TGF-β
INF-γ
Fcγ-RIIIA
MIF
MCP-1, -4
MMP-1
RANTES, CCR5, TACR
CRP
NRAMP-1
TBX21
CTLA-4
TRAIL

Genetic predisposition for outcome of severe sepsis

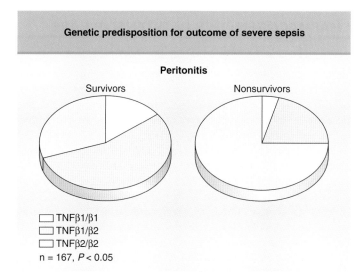

Peritonitis

Survivors   Nonsurvivors

☐ TNFβ1/β1
☐ TNFβ1/β2
☐ TNFβ2/β2
n = 167, $P < 0.05$

Figure 2.7. Genetic predisposition for outcome of severe sepsis. Genotype frequencies of the NcoI TNF-β polymorphism in surviving and nonsurviving peritonitis patients with severe sepsis differ significantly.

with a possible functional relevance. Initial studies reported an impact of well-known single nucleotide polymorphisms on the incidence and/or outcome of sepsis (Fig. 2.7). Also, various studies have related TNF polymorphisms to phenotypes of sepsis. Genomic TNF variants have been associated with mediastinitis or the development of organ dysfunction induced by systemic inflammation following major surgery. Genetic epidemiologic studies have examined the incidence and outcome of severe sepsis and septic shock; that is, researchers reported positive associations with a composite outcome they described as severe complications in a study of patients undergoing major surgery.

PROMOTER VARIANTS AND GENE FUNCTION

The question of which genotype is clearly associated with a high proinflammatory response in the clinical situation of severe gram-negative infection and severe sepsis has been analyzed in

ex vivo studies. Different cell culture conditions and cytokine induction contributed to differing results. Bayley and colleagues published a review on the functional impact of genomic variations within the TNF locus and asked whether there is a future for TNF promoter polymorphisms. Most of the genomic TNF variants demonstrated no impact on TNF expression or presented conflicting results. As more genetic information on different markers from different candidate genes becomes available, combined gene effects or gene–gene interaction studies will become an additional tool to study genetic predisposition. A combination of high TNF responders and low IL-10 responders (i.e., intermediate responders) had the highest death rate in a study of patients with acute renal failure. Clearly, genetic predisposition will ultimately be described by a set of genomic markers that may even differ between various causes of severe sepsis (e.g., pancreatitis and nosocomial pneumonia).

IL-1 is a very potent proinflammatory cytokine released by macrophages involved in the systemic inflammatory response. IL-1 is capable of inducing the symptoms of septic shock and organ failure in animal models and is regarded as a primary mediator of the systemic inflammatory response. Despite the finding that a homozygous genotype correlates with high IL-1β secretion, genotyping of patients with severe sepsis did not reveal any association with incidence or outcome of the disease.

IL-6 has a promoter variation at position −174 that has also been the subject of association studies. Although some studies have demonstrated positive association with sepsis in adults or even sepsis in low-birth-weight neonates, large confirmatory studies are needed. This promoter variant apparently predicts inducibility of IL-6 in peripheral blood cells. CG heterozygotes demonstrated the highest levels. Carriers of the G allele have elevated cytokine responses upon stimulation. This site displays strong binding of nuclear protein in electromobility shift assays. In addition, GC heterozygotes are prone to hay fever and sensitization to inhalant agents. IL-6 genotypes are also able to predict IL-6 plasma levels following extracorporeal circulation in coronary artery bypass graft patients.

ANTI-INFLAMMATORY CYTOKINES

IL-10 is a major anti-inflammatory cytokine and carries several promoter variants. Three haplotypes consisting of three single nucleotide polymorphisms at positions −592, −819, and −1082 are defined by ATA, ACC, and GCC, respectively. Haplotype ATA is associated with elevated IL-10 mRNA expression in peripheral blood cells following stimulation by *Streptococcus pneumoniae* and is also associated with death in children. In contrast, carriage of the −592 AA genotype in children is associated with the risk of hospitalization due to bronchiolitis caused by respiratory syncytial virus. This study also defines a gene–gene interaction of IL-10 with variants of the IL-4 gene, which also has strong anti-inflammatory effects. On the other hand, combination with TNF has led to a definition of a "TNF high producer:IL-10 low producer" risk genotype in inflammatory diseases. Even longevity has been associated with an "anti-inflammatory genotype" by characterizing the −1082 variant in the IL-10 promoter.

A great deal of research examining cytokine responses has been performed to identify the detrimental mechanisms of

Basic Biology and Critical Care Medicine

endotoxin. It is important to note, however, that there are a number of noncytokine mediators that contribute significantly to the toxicity of endotoxin (e.g., nitric oxide).

Potential benefit and protection against cellular stress induced by endotoxin and its mediators are provided by intracellular heat shock proteins. These proteins are capable of playing a role as molecular chaperones, facilitating protein synthesis and folding as well as restructuring partially denatured proteins. The diagnostic relevance of heat shock protein polymorphisms for determining predisposition to sepsis still has to be proved.

LESSONS LEARNED IN GENETICS

How do we find the "needle in the haystack"? We will probably not be able to depend on a single needle (i.e., genomic marker), but we will have to find and define a combination of these. Genotyping technology has advanced significantly so that there are now reliable microarray systems. The development of a "genomic ICU chip" for risk assessment as well as pharmacogenomics is near, but important information on genomic markers is still lacking. Fortunately, major funding agencies at the national (e.g., United States, France, and Germany) and international level (European Commission) have started to recognize genetic epidemiologic studies in sepsis and intensive care medicine as an important part of science with great potential to ultimately improve health care. The first large-scale genotyping studies have been completed, and results are eagerly awaited. It is hoped that they will help to resolve the initial confusion caused by statistically underpowered small-scale studies. Results of these studies should be used to design prospective studies to validate various classification models of predisposition. In addition, inclusion criteria may comprise genotype information in future therapeutic studies on sepsis.

GENETICS IN INTENSIVE CARE MEDICINE: CLASSIFICATION OF PREDISPOSITION

Major causes of critical illness-related morbidity and mortality are sepsis and its sequelae. Evidence-based efforts to improve standard care of sepsis patients are included in major campaigns, such as the surviving sepsis campaign of the Societies of Inten-

sive Care Medicine of Europe and North America as well as the International Sepsis Forum. In addition, new definitions and diagnostic concepts are being evaluated in order to facilitate early diagnosis and evidence-based therapies. These advances include the PIRO concept, which is designed to classify states of sepsis. The PIRO concept's "P" stands for predisposition. Genetic predisposition to the development of and outcome from sepsis has been recognized and suggested as a possible powerful tool for future risk stratification and even as inclusion criteria for therapeutic trials. Genomic research and genotyping in critically ill patients will be integrated into the field of functional genomics. Genomic variants in gene promoters are important genomic markers because they may influence the individual phenotype by altering gene expression levels and patterns as well as protein levels. Therefore, they should be included preferentially in lists of genomic markers to be evaluated in association studies as long as genomewide scans are not feasible in larger numbers of patients.

PHARMACOGENETICS IN INTENSIVE CARE

Occasionally, drugs unexpectedly have no effect or produce serious adverse effects, which can be life-threatening for some patients. A meta-analysis of 39 prospective studies estimated an overall incidence of serious adverse drug reactions of 6.7%. The occurrence of adverse drug reactions is associated with morbidity and mortality and substantial costs. Genetic variants can modify pharmacokinetics and pharmacodynamics of drugs and, therefore, predispose to adverse drug reactions or reduced efficacy. Variations in DNA sequences of relevant genes can have an impact on metabolic pathways or binding to receptors. Polymorphisms of genes encoding cytochrome P450 enzymes, drug receptors, ion channels, drug transporters, and other targets of pharmacotherapy are well recognized and account for some of the varying responses to sedatives such as benzodiazepines, opioids, antiarrhythmics, antibiotics, and others (Tables 2.2 and 2.3). The recent availability of genomic microarray testing for cytochrome P450 variants may help to predict efficacy of metabolism of drugs used for sedation, antimicrobial treatment, and others. There is a potential to reduce adverse drug reactions and better predict future pharmacotherapy in intensive care patients by genomic testing.

Table 2.2 Examples of Cytochrome P450 Polymorphisms and Their Impact on Pharmacotherapy

Cytochrome P450 Isoenzymes	Drugs Metabolized	Side Effects in Case of Altered Enzyme Activity
CYP2C9	Warfarin	Bleeding
	Phenytoin	Ataxia
	NSAIDs	Gastrointestinal bleeding
	Tolbutamide	Hypoglycemia
CYP2C19	Proton pump inhibitors (omeprazole)	
	Diazepam	Sedation
CYP2D6	Tricyclic antidepressants	Sedation, cardiotoxicity
	β-Blocker	Overdose
	Antiarrhythmic drugs	Arrhythmia
	Haloperidol	Parkinsonism
	5-HT₃-antagonists, ondansetron, tropisetron	Nausea, emesis
	Analgesics: codeine, tramadol	No analgesia/reduced analgesia

		Frequency (%)			
CYP2D6 Allele Variants	**Enzyme Function**	**Caucasian**	**Asian**	**African American**	**Ethiopian, Saudi Arabian**
*2xN	Genduplication: increased enzyme activity	3–5	0–2	2	10–16
*4	Splicing defect: inactive enzyme	12–21	1	2	1–4
*5	Deletion: no enzyme	2–7	6	4	1–3
*10	Unstable enzyme	1–2	51	6	3–9
*17	Reduced affinity to substrate	0	No data	34	3–9

Table 2.3 Allele Frequencies of Selected CYP2D6 Polymorphisms in Different Ethnic Populations

OUTLOOK

The application of genetics in the intensive care setting is very promising. Diagnostics based on genetics for risk assessment, as well as for patient-specific pharmacotherapy including more specific treatment options (e.g., immunomodulatory therapies), will likely impact daily decisions in routine intensive care procedures in the future. Improvement of patient outcome remains the ultimate goal. Genetic testing has the clear potential to help achieve this goal.

SUGGESTED READING

Angus DC, Burgner D, Wunderink R, et al: The PIRO concept: P is for predisposition. Crit Care 2003;7(3):248–251.

Bayley JP, Ottenhoff TH, Verweij CL: Is there a future for TNF promoter polymorphisms? Genes Immun 2004;19:315–329.

Cariou A, Chiche JD, Charpentier J, Dhainaut JF, Mira JP: The era of genomics: Impact on sepsis clinical trial design. Crit Care Med 2002;30(5 Suppl):S341–S348.

Cohen J: The immunopathogenesis of sepsis. Nature 2002;420(6917): 885–891.

Devlin B, Roeder K, Wasserman L: Genomic control, a new approach to genetic-based association studies. Theor Popul Biol 2001;60(3):155–166.

Freeman BD, Buchman TG: Gene in a haystack: Tumor necrosis factor polymorphisms and outcome in sepsis. Crit Care Med 2000;28(8): 3090–3091.

Koenig IR, Schafer H, Ziegler A, Muller HH: Reducing sample sizes in genome scans: Group sequential study designs with futility stops. Genet Epidemiol 2003;25(4):339–349.

Mira JP, Cariou A, Grall F, et al: Association of TNF2, a TNF-alpha promoter polymorphism, with septic shock susceptibility and mortality: A multicenter study. JAMA 1999;282(6):561–568.

Stuber F, Petersen M, Bokelmann F, Schade U: A genomic polymorphism within the tumor necrosis factor locus influences plasma tumor necrosis factor-alpha concentrations and outcome of patients with severe sepsis. Crit Care Med 1996;24(3):381–384.

Wunderink RG, Waterer GW: Genetics of sepsis and pneumonia. Curr Opin Crit Care 2003;9(5):384–389.

Chapter 3

Stress and the Biology of the Responses

Timothy G. Buchman

KEY POINTS

- The primary role of the clinician in managing the patient with a stress response is to limit the stress through prompt and definitive control of the cause/source. Without source control—relieving critical stenoses, draining pus, control of bleeding—recovery cannot and will not occur.
- The secondary role of the clinician in managing the patient with a stress response is to create an environment conducive to recovery, including optimal nutritional supplementation and control of pain.
- The "wasting syndrome" of chronic critical illness is associated with substantial changes not only in hormone levels but also in their dynamics, and conventional restitution schedules that do not restore those dynamics may be ineffective or perhaps even harmful.
- Stress and response cause sequential and characteristic changes that form a predictable trajectory away from and returning to physiologic normalcy; it is more important to recognize patients who are off-trajectory, to search for and correct the cause of the deviation, and thereby allow patients to return to a recovery course with a more predictably favorable outcome.
- There is a pressing clinical need for new mathematical and biological theory that could allow clinicians to discriminate between adaptive and maladaptive physiologic responses.

From birth to death, all living things continuously interact with their environment. The responses to environmental stress are collectively termed the stress response. Some human stress and response are ordinary, such as skin reddening after spending time outdoors on a sunny day. Some stress and response are temporally and physiologically trivial, such as the transient skin vasoconstriction that occurs when leaving a ski lodge en route to the slopes on a cold day. The focus of this chapter is nontrivial stresses (e.g., loss of 25% of circulating blood volume) and their responses.

Stress and response are dyadic, meaning that their biologic consequences to the organism as a whole are not readily separable. Our focus is not on separation but rather on failure of the dyad that, uncorrected, leads to the death of the organism. The dyad can fail in one of two generic ways: (1) The response can fail to compensate for the stress, and (2) the stress response can cause harm independent of and superimposed on the stress itself.

WHAT IS STRESS? MECHANISMS, INTENSITY, AND REVERSIBILITY

It is intuitive to classify stressors by mechanism into three broad exposures: physical (e.g., temperature shift or the application of force), chemical (e.g., exposure to oxidants or metabolic substrate starvation), and biological (e.g., virus or bacterial infection). It is more difficult to define the intensity at which exposure constitutes a "stress" worthy of the label. Skipping lunch risks only slight hunger pangs (and even has the potential benefit of shrinking a too generous waistline). However, a fortnight's starvation (which is still common among hospitalized patients despite expert exhortations for early nutritional support) not only modifies the pattern of fuel burn but also cannibalizes essential proteins, suppresses the immune system, and enervates responses to subsequent stressors. At what intensity does an event become a stress?

Embedded in the comparison between transient and prolonged starvation are two principles that provide a framework for thinking about stress in critically ill patients. The first idea is that the depth and duration of a stress affect not only the physiologic disturbance but also the physiologic response. Quantitating the disturbance and isolating the response and the effects of therapy remain elusive in the clinical setting; this is perhaps the strongest argument for continuing to focus on stress–response dyads. The second idea is that of ready reversibility. Mild dyspnea after climbing several flights of stairs, perhaps a little lightheadedness from the skipped lunch, and similar day-to-day stresses are readily (and usually spontaneously) corrected, appearing to induce no sustained changes in the human subject. This is not to say that repetition of such ordinary stresses has no cumulative effect. Exercise tolerance can improve, and weight can be lost. However, the individual events are not only readily reversible but also show no hysteresis in the reversal; that is, the physiologic path back from the stressed state mirrors the path from basal to that stressed state. For example, using a cardiovascular exercise machine like the kind that are ubiquitous in fitness centers will acutely elevate heart rate and oxygen consumption; stepping off typically allows those parameters to fall to preexercise values on about the same time course as their rise.

For this chapter, we choose an operational definition of stress restricted to those events that are not readily reversible but, rather, trigger a two-phase canonical response.[1] The first, shorter phase of the response redirects physiology toward immediate preservation of vital functions. Assuming the individual survives (either through intrinsic compensation or through the provision of critical care), the second phase further directs physiology toward repair of the damage caused by the stressor. This operational definition has a couple of corollaries. First, stresses can be sorted not only by the depth and duration of the exposure but also by the depth and duration of the systemic responses. The second corollary is perhaps even more important, namely that additional stresses during the period of systemic responses can have unexpected consequences.[2] For example, a wound and a soft tissue infection that might be independently survivable can prove lethal if one is temporally layered on the other.

A SCHEMA OF STRESS RESPONSES SCALED TO TIME AND DISTANCE

Humans (and other mammals that serve as experimental models for humans) display nested organization. Cells can replicate and differentiate but cannot be separated into component parts without losing their capacities for metabolism and repair. As such, they constitute root components in the nested organization. At the next level are tissues, which are collections of cells organized to perform a specific function, such as a muscle fiber. Tissues have characteristic metabolisms and also possess the capacity for functional repair: Workouts at the fitness center generally aim to tear down muscle in order to induce functional repair responses that also induce hypertrophy. Tissues are grouped into organs that have the capacity not only for functional compensation and restoration but also often for structural repair. A unique example of this structural repair is the liver, which is capable not only of scarring but also of regenerating functional mass. Finally, the organism as a whole must have the capacity for structural and functional repair, as is commonly observed during recovery from major trauma.

Pertinent to the issue of stress and biological response is the notion that responses are necessarily scaled (temporally and spatially) to the granularity of the organizational component. Reactions within or at the surface of a mammalian cell (a lymphocyte is approximately 10 μm in diameter) occur over a distance of nanometers and over diffusion-limited time scales (as short as a few microseconds in a synaptic cleft). In contrast, coordinate organismal responses must occur over distances of several meters and time scales sufficient to make large-scale repairs (Fig. 3.1).

The consequences of irreversible injury are also scaled. An injured cell typically has a small repertoire of responses. Some cells can locally signal the occurrence of an injury (e.g., by release of cytokines). All cells can execute an internal stress response (formerly known as the heat shock response) that repairs or replaces damaged components. However, since no particular cell is essential to the survival of a complex organism, a common response to severe cell injury is execution of a death program (apoptosis) that ordinarily suppresses local injury signals. When collections of cells in tissues are incapacitated, the common response is isolation and compensation by adjacent functional units. The fractal architecture of tissue functional units (pulmonary alveoli, renal nephrons, pancreatic acini, muscle fascicles, etc.) and of their nutritional support systems (blood and lymphatic channels) facilitates such isolation. Even permanent incapacitation of large numbers of functional units can sometimes escape clinical significance provided there is sufficient reserve. By definition, such problems are handled locally.

This chapter and this book focus on critical illness and critical care. Intrinsic mechanisms that facilitate recovery from moderate stress have been evolutionarily refined. Those endogenous responses are called into play irrespective of the application of organ supports commonly employed in critical care units. Exogenous organ supports were unanticipated in evolutionary time. Thus, the interventions of critical care are superimposed on and do not directly limit the endogenous responses.[3] This superimposition, however well intentioned, may therefore have unintended consequences.

The interventions of critical care are of two general types: care aimed directly at the cause of the critical illness (e.g., source control in management of bacterial sepsis) and care that is "supportive." The necessity of source control (neutralization of whatever triggered the critical illness) is not debated. Application of a "support" creates an unanticipated triad of stress–endogenous response–intervention. Whether the effect of the triad is salutary or injurious may depend on timing.

ACUTE STRESS AND THE CANONICAL RESPONSE

In the face of stress that overwhelms immediate compensation, humans have three sequential physiologic imperatives: escape to limit further injury, survive the threat to life, and repair the damage. Care neither replaces nor amplifies any particular response but, rather, interacts to supplement all these responses.

---

[1] Physiology functions in conditions far from equilibrium and uses energy to impose order and reduce entropy in comparison with the environment. Nonlinear and nonequilibrium systems, such as physiologic systems at any level of resolution (cells, tissues, and organs), by definition display time irreversibility. The fact that small, moment-to-moment perturbations are not only reversible but also appear to retrace the path toward the original condition (e.g., changes in heart rate and blood pressure with mild exercise and cessation of that exercise) is not evidence of temporal symmetry. Rather, it is evidence that given a sufficiently small perturbation, nonlinear and nonequilibrium systems often appear to be linear and in equilibrium. Appearance of a stress response is evidence that the linear–equilibrium approximation is no longer useful to describe the stress or model the stress–response dyad.

[2] This is a direct consequence of the nonlinearity of physiology. It is worthwhile to remember that physiology does not distinguish between an inadvertent additional event (e.g., a pulmonary embolism) and an intentional event (e.g., atelectasis of posterior pulmonary segments consequent to enforced supine position and monotonously regular mechanical breaths). Both have unexpected consequences for the patient recovering from, for example, community-acquired pneumonia.

[3] The stress responses are robust yet fragile. They are robust in the sense that they have evolved to respond to common and frequent perturbations encountered before modern times, yet they are otherwise fragile. Large-scale consequences of this fragility are commonly manifested as pandemics (plague, influenza, etc.); individual-scale consequences manifest as admissions to critical care units. Another way of expressing this idea is that stress responses have rendered us tolerant of common stresses but left us intolerant of rare events. Such tolerance is thus highly optimized; Doyle and Carlson (1999) suggested that highly optimized tolerance is a design principle of biological systems.

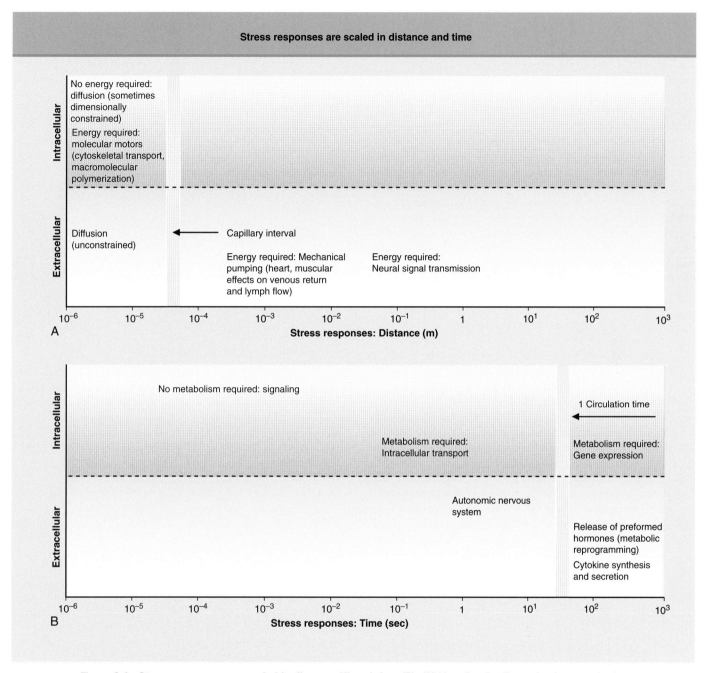

Figure 3.1. Stress responses are scaled in distance (*A*) and time (*B*). Within cells, signaling molecules are poised to respond to environmental changes and can reprioritize cellular programs by posttranslational modification of existing proteins, alterations in transcriptional programs, or selective posttranscriptional events. The diffusion-limited events may or may not require energy transfer; events that require transport (even within cells) require energy. All events that require cell–cell interactions, even those that involve release of preformed hormones, consume metabolic resources. Thus, redirection of energy stores is an essential feature of stress responses over multiple scales of distance and time.

Escape is facilitated by at least three mechanisms. Activation of the sympathetic nervous system to release preformed epinephrine and norepinephrine redirects blood flow toward vital organs and provides vasoconstriction to limit bleeding if present. Release of cortisol begins metabolic reprogramming to make sufficient carbohydrate fuel available to tissues. Pain sensations are temporarily attenuated so that even injured parts can be employed to escape the stress.

After escape, survival becomes the priority. Two of the physiologic mechanisms activated in the escape phase—secretion of catecholamines and cortisol—persist to produce a decrease in global metabolic activity even while redirecting protective blood and nutrient flow to the brain and heart. Temperature and total nutrient consumption fall. Pain and discomfort become prominent so that the metabolic costs invoked by movement are minimized. Thirst is prominent. The clinical correlate is shock.

Basic Biology and Critical Care Medicine

Although modern critical care confers survival on some patients who would otherwise die in this phase, many more survive with or without life supports. The original studies of this phase performed by Cuthbertson (who called this the "ebb" or hypometabolic phase of the stress response) included patients with femur fractures without attempts to control bleeding or to replenish blood products (blood banking had yet to be invented) or life support of any kind.

Once immediate survival is assured, repair of the injury becomes the priority for the patient and the focus of critical care. "Injury" here is used in a very broad sense to denote a tissue disturbance with little distinction made between an external wound, a fracture with local internal hemorrhage, a sterile internal injury such as pancreatitis, or tissue infection such as pneumonia. All require (in some measure) lysis of the injured tissue followed by rebuilding. The normal, successful rebuilding process that culminates in full functional recovery can be divided into four phases, all of which are hypermetabolic:

1. The first phase is deeply catabolic. In order to mobilize the building blocks necessary for repair, quantities of nitrogen (for protein synthesis) and potassium (for new cell synthesis) appear in the plasma. Utilization is inefficient, and both are wasted in the urine. With moderate injury and without critical care, this phase usually lasts approximately 4 days.

2. The second phase is also catabolic. Nitrogen is still mobilized and still wasted, but potassium is used more efficiently. Importantly, cortisol levels in plasma begin to diminish. With moderate injury and without critical care, this phase lasts approximately 3 days.

3. In the third phase, nitrogen wastage ceases. Hypermetabolism continues but with a spontaneous conversion to anabolism. It is during this third phase that the majority of tissue repair is performed. Ordinary functions such as intestinal transit become normal. It typically lasts 3 weeks with moderate injury and, again, without critical care.

4. The fourth and final phase includes restoration of lean muscle mass and especially fat stores. It can require 1 month or more of mild hypermetabolic, anabolic activity (Fig. 3.2).

The problem most commonly faced in the intensive care unit is apparent failure to progress from the first stage to the second. In order to understand the failure of progression, it is necessary to further characterize the normal progression and to describe the endocrine events that accompany it (Fig. 3.3).

1. Beginning as early as the escape phase, the stress response is coordinated by the central nervous system (CNS). The paraventricular neurons of the hypothalamus secrete corticotrophin-releasing hormone (CRH) and thereby activate the hypothalamic–pituitary–adrenal (HPA) axis. The CRH is delivered to the anterior pituitary and stimulates the secretion of ACTH from resident corticotrophs. ACTH secretion can be synergistically stimulated by arginine vasopressin (AVP), but AVP has little independent ACTH-releasing activity. ACTH and other neuroactive peptides (e.g., β-endorphin) are not stored but, rather, released by proteolytic cleavage of pro-opiomelanocortin. Once released into the general circulation, ACTH directly stimulates the adrenal cortex to produce glucocorticoids, miner-

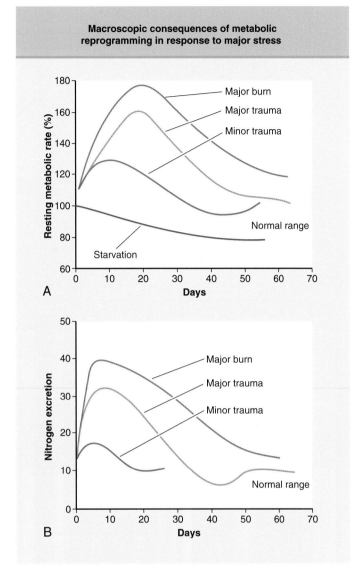

Macroscopic consequences of metabolic reprogramming in response to major stress

Figure 3.2. Macroscopic consequences of metabolic reprogramming in response to major stress. Metabolic rate *(top)* and nitrogen excretion *(bottom)* show a dose–response relationship with respect to the severity of the stress. Critical care can ameliorate but cannot obviate these changes. This figure, adapted from data obtained nearly half a century ago, emphasizes the long-lasting consequences of major physiologic stress. (Data from Kinney JM: Energy deficits in acute illness and injury. In Morgan AP (ed): Proceedings of a Conference on Energy Metabolism and Body Fuel Utilization. Cambridge, MA, Harvard University Press, 1966, p. 174).

alocorticoids, and adrenal androgens. Thus, ACTH levels are preserved and augmented during the early phase of acute stress. Glucocorticoids, primarily cortisol, ordinarily regulate their secretion by negative feedback on both the hypothalamus and the pituitary.

2. Glucocorticoids are pleiotropic molecules. Skeletal muscle breaks down under the influence of excess glucocorticoids. Glucocorticoids modulate the stress response at the molecular level, primarily by inhibiting expression of proinflammatory cytokines such as interleukin (IL)-1, IL-6, and tumor necrosis factor. Glucocorticoids also affect growth,

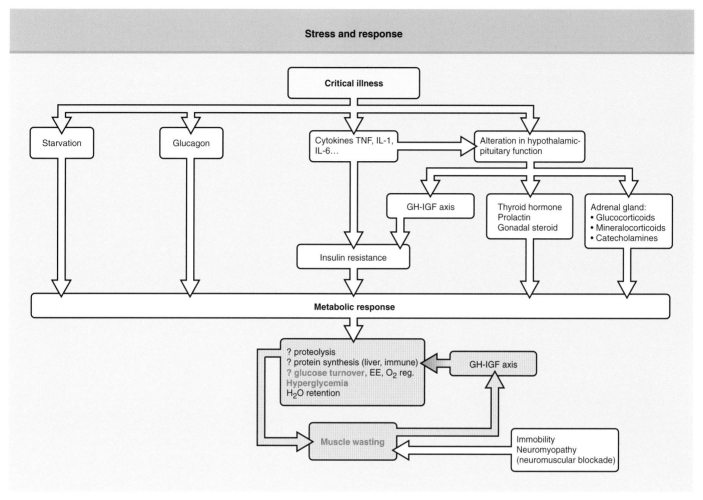

Figure 3.3. Stress and response. The alterations in the hormonal milieu following major stress shown in the upper half of the figure conspire to create a metabolic response that has significant consequences. The focus of this diagram is on the muscle wasting that is the most long-lasting effect of critical illness and has the greatest adverse effect on quality of life among survivors. (Adapted from Hadley JS, Hinds CJ: Anabolic strategies in critical illness. Current Opin Pharmacol 20022(6):700–707.)

reproductive functions, and the thyroid axis in acute stress. Glucocorticoids initially promote growth hormone (GH) secretion, suppress gonadotrophin-releasing hormone (GnRH) secretion from the hypothalamus, and inhibit gonadal tissues.

3. The second major axis, activated in the brain stem as early as the escape phase, is the peripheral autonomic nervous system (ANS). Since the primary activation in stress is the sympathetic (as opposed to parasympathetic) limb of the ANS, this is sometimes referred to as sympathetic nervous system (SNS) activation. Stress causes the rapid release of epinephrine and norepinephrine (which together are termed catecholamines) from the SNS–adrenal medullary system into blood. Although such release is the major SNS contribution to the stress response, there are other components. First, there is direct innervation from efferent cholinergic preganglionic fibers projecting from the intermediolateral column of the spinal cord. After synapsing in the sympathetic ganglia that lie outside the spinal cord, the postganglionic sympathetic fibers—mostly noradrenergic—project out to smooth muscle of the vasculature, heart, gut, kidney,

skeletal muscles, and even fat. Second, the ANS—here specifically including both sympathetic and parasympathetic limbs—has additional selective (and neurochemically coded) projections whose neurons express neuropeptides (e.g., neuropeptide Y) and may also selectively use ATP, nitric oxide, or lipid mediators of inflammation.

4. A third axis, the somatotropic axis, is stimulated by stress. The secretion of somatotropin (more commonly known as GH) from the somatotrophs of the pituitary gland is regulated by two hypothalamic hormones: GH-releasing hormone, which stimulates release, and somatostatin, which inhibits release of GH. In response to acute stress, average plasma GH levels rise. It is important to look beyond the average, however. In unstressed humans, GH levels are undetectable except for a couple of large-amplitude pulses daily. In acute stress, GH baseline levels rise, and additional pulses appear. The principal effector downstream of GH is insulin-like growth factor-1 (IGF-1), which instructs cells to grow and divide, generally helping the functional integrity of muscle and bone (Fig. 3.4A). IGF-1 levels fluctuate much less than GH levels over the course of a day, and for this

25

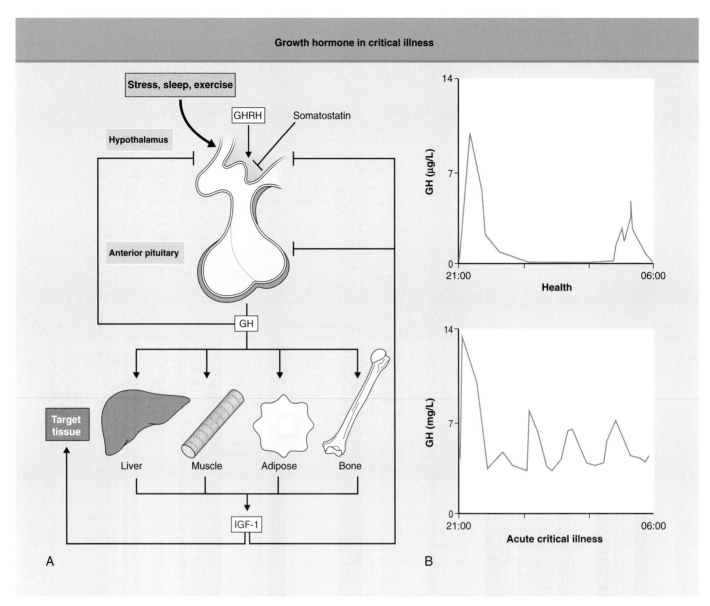

Figure 3.4. Growth hormone in critical illness. Structure *(A)* and dynamics *(B)*. Stress promotes secretion of growth hormone-releasing hormone (GHRH) from the hypothalamus, which stimulates release of growth hormone from the anterior pituitary gland into the general circulation. The targets include, at a minimum, liver, muscle, fat, and bone. Compared with normal health, dynamic secretion of growth hormone in acute critical illness is associated with elevations in both average level and pulsatility. *(B,* Adapted from data in van den Berghe G, de Zegher F, Bouillon R: Acute and prolonged critical illness as different neuroendocrine paradigms. J Clin Endocrinol Metab 1998;83(6):1827–1834.)

reason, students of GH often report IGF-1 levels as a surrogate for GH production (Fig. 3.4*B*).

5. When activated in concert, the HPA, the SNS, and the somatotropic axes elicit an acute and coordinate response that is colloquially termed the "stress response." This affects nearly all bodily functions, including direct effects on arousal, cardiac performance, vascular tone, ventilation, respiration, and intermediary metabolism.

6. In order to manage stress-induced metabolic disequilibrium, fuels are mobilized from stores for immediate use. Mobilization of this ready reserve activation of lipolysis, glycogenolysis, and gluconeogenesis is a consequence of glucagon release from pancreatic A cells. Glucagon release is mediated in part by the ANS. (Catecholamines and

cortisol assist with lipolysis, cortisol assists with gluconeogenesis, and epinephrine assists with glycogenolysis, but only glucagon uses all three paths to mobilize sugar and free fatty acids that constitute the immediately oxidizable fuels that are required in the initial phases of the stress response.)

7. These fuels are not just mobilized, they are oxidized in great quantities. This oxidation is the underlying cause of the hypermetabolic state. The oxidation necessarily causes an increased production of both carbon dioxide and heat.

8. Muscle proteolysis is a prominent feature of the stress response to injury and distinguishes the stress response from that muscle atrophy that accompanies starvation. In starvation, synthesis is depressed and catabolism does not occur.

In injury, synthesis is prominent but catabolism is over-whelming. Energy is "wasted" in the process of protein turnover. Left unchecked, muscle wasting becomes a prominent feature of the stress response. Ordinarily, excess proteolysis abates as cortisol levels fall. Whether the asso-ciation is causal or casual is uncertain.

9. If the perception of stress of blocked, the stress response is attenuated. Thus, for example, lower limb or lower abdom-inal surgery performed under neuraxial (epidural or spinal) anesthesia features a stress response markedly less than that of similar operations performed under general anesthesia. The role of the CNS in coordinating and perpetuating the stress response is evident.

10. Simulation of stress in normal animals or human subject vol-unteers by, for example, simultaneous infusion of cortisol, epinephrine, and glucagons induces metabolic changes similar to those caused by injury or other acute stress. Metabolic rates increase, glucose levels rise, amino acids are mobilized from skeletal muscle, and so on.

11. Cortisol, the catecholamines, and glucagon are collectively known as counterregulatory hormones because all act to mobilize fuels. The hormone that they "counterregulate" is insulin, whose primary purpose is to remove building blocks (sugar, fat, and amino acids) from the circulation into cells for storage. As long as counterregulatory hormones over-whelm the actions of insulin, the patient appears to be insulin resistant. Abatement of insulin resistance is neces-sary to shift from catabolism to anabolism.

12. The earliest descriptions of the counterregulatory response excluded the somatotropic axis. This was probably in error. As mentioned previously, the profile of GH secretion changes in response to acute stress and elevates both the baseline and the frequency of superimposed pulses. This augmentation of GH secretion may be in response to a decrease in GH receptors in peripheral tissues. Levels of IGF-1 (again, IGF-1 is a key effector hormone in the soma-totropic axis), along with levels of the GH-dependent binding protein IGF-BP3 and its acid labile subunit, fall in parallel with the GH receptors. Collectively, the picture is one of peripheral GH resistance. GH drives direct lipoly-tic, insulin-antagonizing, and immune stimulatory actions—actions that appear to prioritize essential fuels (glucose, free fatty acids, and glutamine) for hypermetabolic, if catabolic, survival.

13. Within a few hours of acute stress, and persisting through the first and second hypermetabolic phases, serum levels of the active form of thyroid hormone, triiodothyronine, are depressed. Thyroid-stimulating hormone (TSH) sustains release of T_4 from the thyroid gland, but peripheral con-version to T_3 is suppressed in favor of conversion to the inac-tive reverse T_3 form. This appears to favor conservation of metabolic effort in the hypometabolic phase of the stress response and to focus energetics on local repair of tissue during the early hypermetabolic phases. Pertinent to subse-quent discussions of chronic critical illness, the pattern of TSH secretion in health is markedly pulsatile—a pattern that is sustained (albeit at lower amplitude) during the acute (but not chronicc) response to stress.

14. Within minutes of acute stress, an immediate decrease in testosterone production by Leydig cells is thought to pre-serve energy stores and focus attention on survival. During the acute phase of critical illness, the pulsatile release of luteinizing hormone that is essential to bioactivity is preserved even though release of testosterone is suppressed.

15. Prolactin, which is secreted by lactotrophs in the anterior pituitary gland, is thought to enhance immune function during acute stress. Prolactin levels are elevated in acute stress, and the normal pulsatility of prolactin release is preserved.

In summary, the early hypermetabolic, catabolic phases of acute stress are characterized by preserved and enhanced anterior pituitary secretion that continues to feature normal pulsatile variation. Resolution of hypercortisolism marks the transition from catabolism to anabolism, both predicting and heralding spontaneous recovery. These patients typically respond to observation and adequate nutrition and tolerate rapid weaning from life supports.

Unfortunately, a significant minority of patients remain hypermetabolic and catabolic, stuck somewhere between the first and second phases of the canonical response to stress. These patients have chronic critical illness, which can be pragmatically (if arbitrarily) defined as more than 10 days of multisystem support. Their metabolic picture deterio-rates in characteristic ways. The most obvious is cannibal-ism of skeletal and visceral protein that results in a generalized wasting syndrome. A typical critically ill adult loses approximately 100 g of protein daily. Fatty acids are no longer used efficiently as metabolic substrates, and feeding of fat can cause deposition into the pancreas, liver, and other organs. Bedside assessment shows a familiar constellation of intracellular depletion (of water and potassium), insulin resistance, hypertriglyceridemia, hypercalcemia, hyperlactatemia, and widespread hypo-proteinemia.

What has become clear in recent years is that the endocrine profile also undergoes characteristic changes as the patient lapses into sustained multiple organ dysfunction (Fig. 3.5).

16. The first and perhaps most familiar endocrine change in chronic critical illness is that secretion of glucocorticoids becomes independent of ACTH. Whether the secretion is autonomous or whether there are undiscovered physiologic secretagogues is not known. Neither is it understood why ACTH levels fall, although roles for atrial naturietic peptide and substance P have been postulated. What is clearer, however, is that sustained hypercortisolism is accompanied by a reciprocal decline in adrenal androgens and mineralo-corticoids. Inspection of a biochemical pathway diagram suggests that the general fate of pregnenolone in the adrenal steroid biosynthetic pathway has been altered.

17. Secretion of other anterior pituitary hormones also falls, with reduced pulsatility. For example, whereas GH remains detectable, the amplitude of pulses is markedly reduced. In the face of reduced levels of GH, circulating IGF-1 and the acid labile subunit of the ternary complex continue to decline.

18. TSH levels fall to subnormal levels. Pulsatility gives way to monotony. Both peripheral T_4 and T_3 levels fall. Increases in TSH levels may herald recovery.

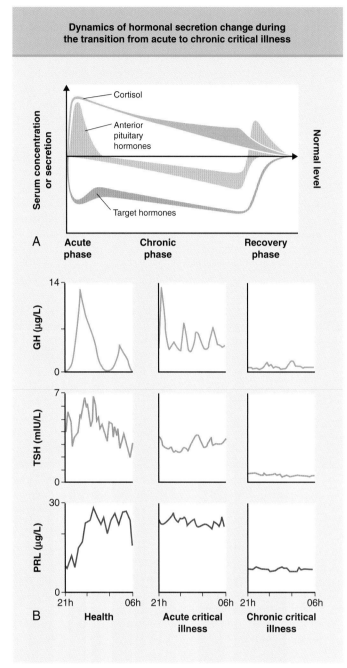

Figure 3.5. The dynamics of hormonal secretion change during the transition from acute to chronic critical illness. *A,* Coarse-grained view of changes in hormonal secretion during acute, chronic, and recovery phases. Despite persistent elevations of cortisol, anterior pituitary and target organ hormones decline in concentration and secretion. *B,* The changes are both qualitative and quantitative. There is a striking change in pulsatile secretion, suggesting collapse of the regulatory network that governs expression and secretion of these pituitary hormones. (*A,* Adapted from van den Berghe G, de Zegher F, Bouillon R: Acute and prolonged critical illness as different neuroendocrine paradigms. J Clin Endocrinol Metab 1998;83(6):1827–1834. *B,* Data from van den Berghe G: The neuroendocrine stress response and modern intensive care: The concept revisited. Burns 1999;25(1):7–16.)

19. Release of luteinizing hormone is also compromised in acute critical illness. Levels fall sharply. The frequency of pulsatility increases but amplitude falls close to undetectable levels. This appears to be an inadequate response to very low peripheral testosterone levels.
20. Baseline prolactin levels, which are markedly elevated in acute critical illness, fall markedly and well below those encountered in normal health. Pulsatility is nearly absent. This may be due to endogenous release of dopamine, and it may be exacerbated by the administration of dopamine as a drug.

Collectively, the hormonal phenotype of chronic critical illness is suppressed and hormones monotonously secreted by the anterior pituitary.

An intervention that appeared promising in animal trials, replacement of a suppressed pituitary hormone, was tried. Restoration of natural "stress levels" of GH by injection into critically ill patients resulted in excess death, suggesting that the change in GH profile is a marker for the transition from acute to chronic critical illness and not the cause.

Several approaches have been proposed to guide the patient toward anabolism and recovery.

Stop the stress. Such measures include control of hemorrhage, drainage of pus, and removal of necrotic tissues.

Do not make the patient's stress any worse than it already is. Such preventative measures include assurance of adequate oxygen delivery, management of pain and anxiety, and use of appropriate aseptic techniques when performing invasive procedures.

Specific metabolic interventions: These specifics are commonly tested on examinations:

A. Nutritional support: In order to attenuate the catabolic, nitrogen-wasting processes, many nutritional principles have been proposed. Few have withstood careful evaluation. The following can be safely recommended:
  1. Early nutritional support is desirable, starvation is not.
  2. The gut should be used whenever possible.
  3. If the gut cannot tolerate feeding for a week or so, parenteral nutrition is preferable to no nutrition. (A gut that cannot tolerate feeding for a week probably is outside of the realm of an acute stress response.)
  4. To minimize the catabolism of acute stress, give 25 to 30 kcal/kg/day of carbohydrate and fat. Fat should never exceed 30% of the total. Carbohydrate should not exceed 5 mg/kg/min, or approximately 25 kcal/kg/day. There is evidence that low-fat feedings in the acute stress period may reduce infection risks. For this reason, the earliest feedings are sometimes fat-free and slightly hypocaloric, delivering 3 or 4 mg/kg/min carbohydrate.
  5. To minimize the nitrogen wasting of acute stress, give at least 1.25 g protein/kg/day. If there is extensive tissue destruction associated with the acute stress (e.g., an extensive burn), give up to 2 g protein/kg/day. There is no evidence that protein supplementation beyond this level can be utilized in ordinary patients, and there is some concern that further nitrogen loading is harmful.

B. Immunonutritional modulation
　1. The benefits of immunonutritional modulation are much less certain than the benefits of ordinary nutritional support.
　2. Glutamine becomes conditionally essential during acute stress. Glutamine supplementation appears to reduce the risk of infection during acute stress, whether or not the acute stress is septic.[4]
　3. Arginine supplementation may improve outcome in general acute stress, but there is evidence-based concern (but not definitive proof) that it is harmful when given enterally to patients who are frankly septic.

C. Control of body temperature
　1. Fever commonly accompanies the response to stress.
　2. Correction of modest fever (<38.5°C) has never been shown to improve outcome.
　3. Attenuation of high fever (>39°C) may be beneficial in brain-injured patients.

D. Control of glycemia
　1. Hyperglycemia is a clinical sequela of insulin resistance brought on by acute stress. In the past, clinicians tolerated significant stress-induced hyperglycemia using the teleologic argument that stressed tissues required a ready supply of energy.
　2. There are no data demonstrating that tight control of glycemia to a normal range affects patient outcome following limited stress, such as that induced by minor or moderate elective surgery.
　3. There are data showing that correction of hyperglycemia following serious and sustained stresses of diverse types, including myocardial infarction, ischemic brain injury, and major cardiac surgery,

improves outcome. The association between improved outcome and tight glycemic control is strongest in surgical (as opposed to medical) patients. There is a debate as to whether the hyperglycemia should be fully corrected to a normal range (80–110 mg/dL) versus a less stringent correction (to 110–145 mg/dL). Irrespective of the debate, evidence suggests that insulin therapy to correct glucose to near-normal values improves outcome following some serious stresses.

GENETIC AND MOLECULAR DETERMINANTS OF MUSCLE TISSUE DYNAMICS

Perhaps the major unsolved problem in management of the biological response to stress in critically ill patients is the wasting syndrome. Irrespective of the energy balance and the intensity of nutritional support, patients with prolonged critical illness lose lean muscle mass and develop generalized weakness affecting both voluntary and involuntary muscle function. The descriptive term is critical illness myopathy (CIM). There are three morphologically distinct types: myopathy with unspecific morphologic alterations, myopathy with selective loss of myosin filaments (thick filament myopathy), and acute necrotizing myopathy of critical care. It is not clear whether the morphologies share a common pathogenesis.

Regardless of the mechanism, CIM perpetuates immobility and its complications, including (but not limited to) bedsores, venous thromboembolism, pneumonia, cardiac deconditioning, and further muscle wasting that conspire to prolong critical illness. Whether there is a meaningful association—casual or causal—between CIM and mortality is unclear because up to 80% of patients who survive prolonged critical illness have CIM, and presumably an even greater fraction who die have CIM. Amelioration or prevention of CIM in critical illness appears to be a significant goal. In pursuit of this goal, and in addition to optimizing nutrition and other parameters, several pharmacologic approaches have been proposed (Table 3.1).

---

[4]Whether glutamine should be classified primarily as an immunomodulator is debated. It lies at the nexus of several key metabolic, immunologic, and antioxidant pathways. In addition, it appears to function as a signaling molecule. Regardless, in trauma and burn patients, enteral administration of glutamine consistently reduces infectious complications and appears to reduce mortality.

Table 3.1 Metabolic Support Strategies in Critical Illness[a]

Support Class	Support	Effect
First-generation, nutritional	Increasing caloric intake	Does not prevent/reverse muscle wasting
	Increasing protein supply	Fat accretion
	>2 g nitrogen	Increased nitrogen loss
	Glutamine	Reduces infections
		May improve survival
	Arginine	Reduces infections
		Once sepsis established, may increase mortality
First-generation, hormonal	β-Blockade (propranolol)	Preserves lean body mass in burned children
	Insulin	Reduces protein degradation, improves synthesis; anabolic effects independent of IGF-1
	Thyroid hormones	Mixed effects; may aggravate muscle wasting
	Androgens	Reduces protein catabolism in young men with severe burns; effects on immune system uncertain
	Growth hormone	Despite predicted benefits of increasing IGF-1 levels and improved nitrogen balance, increased mortality in nonseptic critically ill patients
Second-generation, hormonal	Hypothalamic-releasing hormones (GHRH-2, TRH, GNRH)	Reactivates somatotropic and thyrotropic axes, restores pulatility; nitrogen balance improved; mortality effect uncertain

[a]Decades of research suggest that nutritional excess is counterproductive and that nutritional modulation (e.g., a specific amino acid supplement) may provoke helpful or harmful responses depending on the specific patient contest. Direct hormonal replacement/blockade also appears to have mixed effects. Manipulations aimed at the network of hypothalamic molecules that regulate release of pituitary hormones have shown some promise in reversing adverse metabolic effects of stress.

Basic Biology and Critical Care Medicine

First-generation approaches included administration of GH, testosterone, and the testosterone analog oxandrolone to critically ill patients. In general, studies showed that these agents either had negligible effect or caused adversity. (There are some exceptions, such as apparent salutary effects of oxandrolone on pediatric burn patients.)

Second-generation approaches focused on upstream regulators and downstream effectors of GH. An example of upstream regulatory strategy might include the infusion of hypothalamic-releasing molecules such as GH-releasing peptide, TRH, and GnRH. A downstream effect strategy might include the coadministration of IGF-1 and its binding protein IGF-BP3. Again, although there are promising results in unique populations (e.g., pediatric burn patients), there is neither promising animal data nor any human data to support such a second-generation approach in the general critically ill adult population.

Breakthroughs in understanding of the genetics and regulation of muscle development suggest a third-generation approach. There are three key observations. The first is that muscle atrophy is not merely a passive response to lack of electro-mechanical stimulus or an inflammatory milieu but, rather, involves activation of specific programs of gene expression involving the FOXO transcription factors as well as the ubiquitin protein ligases MuRF1 and MAFbx. The transcriptional activity of FOXO proteins is regulated by Sir2, an NAD^+-dependent deacetylase, and several FOXO targets are expressed at lower levels following Sir2 activation/overexpression. Sir2 can be activated by a spectrum of small molecules, such as resveratrol (a polyphenol found in red wine), that could be tested for their efficacy in shutting down the "atrophy pathway." The second is that the muscle atrophy/hypertrophy response of IGF-1 depends on the binding protein so that whereas binding to IGF-BP3 may cause hypertrophy, binding to IGF-BP4 may cause atrophy. IGF-BP5 has dual effects when bound to IGF-1. This suggests that IGF-1 therapy may have unpredictable and context-dependent effects. The third is that muscle atrophy is also regulated by a member of the transforming growth factor-β family, myostatin. Whereas direct myostatin inhibition (to prevent atrophy) is not possible, myostatin's natural inhibitor (follistatin) can be activated by blocking the activity of class I and II histone deacetylases (e.g., with valproic acid). A humanized monoclonal antibody to myostatin is in clinical trials to prevent and reverse the effects of heritable myopathies. Although none of these compounds or their molecular strategies has reached clinical evaluation in critical illness, they represent the third-generation approaches to prevention of the wasting syndrome.

SUGGESTED READING

Carlson JM, Doyle J: A mechanism for power laws in designed systems. Phys Rev E 1999;60:1412–1427.

Hadley JS, Hinds CJ: Anabolic strategies in critical illness. Curr Opin Pharmacol 2002;2(6):700–707.

Kinney JM: Energy deficits in acute illness and injury. In Morgan AP (ed): Proceedings of a Conference on Energy Metabolism and Body Fuel Utilization. Cambridge, MA, Harvard University Press, 1966, p 174.

van den Berghe G: The neuroendocrine stress response and modern intensive care: The concept revisited. Burns 1999;25(1):7–16.

van den Berghe G, de Zegher F, Bouillon R: Acute and prolonged critical illness as different neuroendocrine paradigms. J Clin Endocrinol Metab 1998;83(6):1827–1834.

Chapter 4

Vascular Tone

Donald W. Landry, Soja Anubkumar, and Juan A. Oliver

KEY POINTS

- Cellular mechanisms controlling vascular tone: The basic understanding of the intracellular mechanisms that mediate and modulate vascular tone are outlined with particular emphasis on recent findings with potential clinical relevance.
- Neurohormonal factors regulating vascular tone: The neuronal and hormonal agents that are clinically important for the regulation and modulation of vascular tone are reviewed.
- Autoregulation of vascular tone: The mechanisms intrinsic to vascular smooth muscle that mediate autoregulation of blood flow are outlined.

The degree of constriction/relaxation of the vascular smooth muscle (VSM) determines the diameter of blood vessels. In resistance arteries, smooth muscle tone in great part determines not only the level of arterial pressure but also the amount of blood that arrives at each capillary and the pressure at which it arrives. Clearly, in multiorgan organisms, effective function of VSM is a requisite for life, and given the variable metabolic needs of different organs, this function must be finely and individually tuned. Hence, it is not surprising that even our limited understanding of VSM function already shows an astonishing level of complexity. VSM function can be regulated by multiple signaling pathways, and VSMs from different organs use different pathways, thereby allowing organ-specific regulation of the circulation. Work with the patch clamp technique and molecular biology methods such as gene deletion have provided a large amount of new information. These studies are beginning to provide a variety of pharmacologic probes to explore the mechanisms of VSM function in health and disease, as well as to define targets for medication development.

CELLULAR MECHANISMS THAT CONTROL VASCULAR TONE

Mechanochemical Cycle of VSM

Constriction of VSM, like that of striated muscle, is produced by the cyclical interaction of the myosin molecule with actin filaments, and this interaction can be visualized as the heads of the myosin molecule "rowing" along the actin filaments. The myosin of smooth muscle, smooth muscle myosin II, has ATPase activity and translocating activity. As shown in Figure 4.1, at the end of the last constriction cycle, the heads of myosin are at their most forward positions and in contact with the actin filament. Binding of ATP by myosin separates it from actin, and the subsequent hydrolysis of ATP by the catalytic subunit of myosin induces a conformational change of the myosin head, which assumes a cocked conformation ("charged"). The subsequent binding of myosin to actin, followed by the release of inorganic phosphate (Pi) and ADP, generates the power stroke that, relative to myosin, moves the actin filament. Thus, contraction is produced by the intermittent power strokes of the myosin molecule rowing along the actin filaments. Binding of a new molecule of ATP by myosin will again release its head from actin and initiate another cycle.

Basic Mechanisms of Constriction and Relaxation of VSM

Constriction

In the circulation, a large number of signals of neuronal, humoral, mechanical, and ionic origin are capable of inducing VSM constriction. In addition to these vasoconstrictor factors, many other signals can actively dilate blood vessels so that vascular constriction can also be achieved by removal of vasodilator influences. However, for purposes of clarity, we review these two processes independently.

Like all muscle cells, VSM uses calcium (Ca^{2+}) as the signal for contraction. A 10^4-fold Ca^{2+} gradient exists across the VSM plasma membrane and across the membrane between the cytosol and the sarcoplasmic reticulum (SR). Cytosolic Ca^{2+} is kept at very low levels (~100 nM) by a variety of mechanisms, including a Ca^{2+}-Na^+ exchanger in the plasma membrane and a Ca^{2+}-ATPase in the SR that pumps calcium into this organelle. As shown in Figure 4.2, in most conditions, VSM constriction is initiated by the binding of a vasoconstrictor ligand (e.g., angiotensin II or norepinephrine) to its receptor and the subsequent interaction of the receptor with members of the G_q family of G proteins (i.e., it is a G protein-coupled receptor). This leads to activation of an isoform of the enzyme phospholipase C (PLC) and generation of inositol 1,4,5-triphosphate (IP_3), which binds to its receptor in the SR and causes Ca^{2+} release. As shown in Figure 4.2, calcium also enters the cell by voltage-gated L-type Ca^{2+} channels that open because the initial rise in cytoplasmic Ca^{2+} activates Cl^- channels and the exit of Cl^- depolarizes the cell membrane. At high concentrations, Ca^{2+} in the cytosol binds to calmodulin (CaM), which in turn binds to the key enzyme for muscle contraction, myosin light chain kinase (MLCK). A complex of Ca^{2+}, CaM, and MLCK allows this enzyme to phosphorylate two of the light chains of myosin. This critical step of phosphorylation of the MLCs triggers the cycling

Basic Biology and Critical Care Medicine

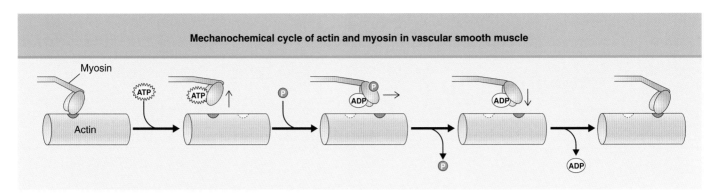

Figure 4.1. Mechanochemical cycle of actin and myosin in vascular smooth muscle. Binding of ATP to the myosin head separates it from the actin filament, and the subsequent hydrolysis of ATP displaces the myosin head along the filament. A new interaction of the myosin head with actin releases the inorganic phosphate and generates the power stroke.

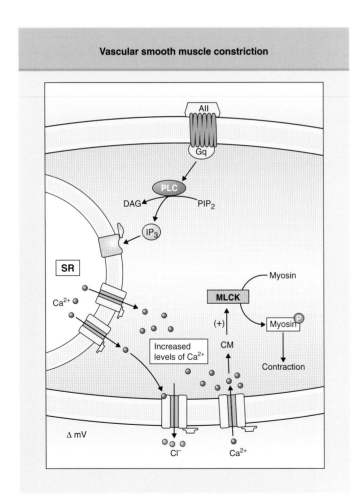

Figure 4.2. Vascular smooth muscle constriction. Schematic overview of signal transduction during vascular constriction upon activation by a vasoconstrictor ligand (e.g., angiotensin II or norepinephrine). Increased cytoplasmic calcium activates myosin light chain kinase (MLCK), which phosphorylates myosin and causes constriction. Intracellular calcium increases because it is released from the sarcoplasmic reticulum (SR) upon its activation by inositol triphosphate (IP$_3$). More critically, calcium also increases because membrane depolarization activates voltage-gated calcium channels and allows entry of extracellular calcium.

of myosin along the actin filaments (see Fig. 4.1) with the development of force and muscle contraction.

Relaxation
Because phosphorylated MLC can be dephosphorylated by the enzyme myosin light chain phosphatase (MLCP) (Fig. 4.3), decreasing cytoplasmic Ca^{2+} concentration allows MLC dephosphorylation to dominate, resulting in relaxation. This will occur when the vasoconstrictor agent causing the constriction is removed from the circulation. The Ca^{2+}-Na$^+$ exchanger in the plasma membrane translocates cytoplasmic Ca^{2+} to the outside and a Ca^{2+}-ATPase in the SR pumps the ion into this organelle.

As shown in Figure 4.3, active relaxation (i.e., relaxation initiated by a circulating ligand) is initiated, much as in the case of vasoconstrictors, by binding of a ligand (e.g., ANP) to its G protein-coupled receptor and subsequent activation of a cyclic nucleotide-dependent pathway. Two such pathways have been described. In the case of epinephrine and the β$_2$ receptor, the pathway is mediated by adenylate cyclase, which generates cyclic adenosine monophosphate (cAMP). In the case of ANP, it is a guanylate cyclase (not shown) that generates the cyclic nucleotide, cyclic guanyl monophosphate (cGMP). Interestingly, nitric oxide (NO) also induces generation of cGMP, but its method of action does not require a G protein-coupled receptor because it directly activates a soluble form of guanylate cyclase. In turn, both cAMP and cGMP activate their respective kinases, protein kinase A (PKA) for the former and protein kinase G (PKG) for the latter, which initiate a cascade of events leading to relaxation. Although the PKA-mediated pathway was discovered more that 30 years ago, much more is known about the more recently discovered PKG-mediated pathway, likely because the magnitude of its effect is substantially greater than that of PKA. Thus, we restrict our comments to it. As shown in Figure 4.3, PKG (or more specifically, its isoform cGK$_1$) has a multitude of actions, but its most prominent is its interaction with MLCP; it is capable of phosphorylating one of the subunits of this phosphatase, which results in its activation. As detailed previously, this will result in dephosphorylation of the MLC and relaxation. In addition, PKG/cGK$_1$ phosphorylates a protein

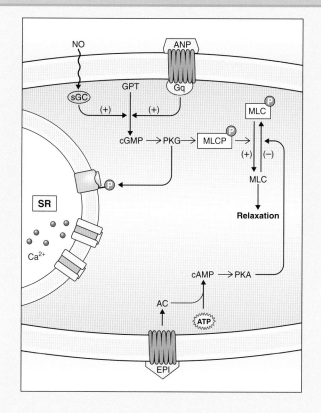

Figure 4.3. Vascular smooth muscle relaxation. Schematic overview of signal transduction during vascular relaxation upon activation by dilator ligands. Some ligands (e.g., atrial natriuretic peptide and nitric oxide) generate cGMP, and others (e.g., epinephrine and adenosine) generate cAMP. These nucleotides activate respective kinases, which in turn phosphorylate myosin light chain phosphatase (MLCP). Activation of MLCP dephosphorylates myosin light chains and thus causes relaxation. Note that activation of the cGMP-dependent kinase also prevents release of calcium from the sarcoplasmic reticulum (SR).

associated with the IP$_3$ receptor, thereby preventing the release of Ca^{2+} by the SR.

Calcium Sensitization

Although the concentration of cytoplasmic Ca^{2+} plays a central role in determining vascular tone, it has long been known that contraction force in VSM can vary independently of the level of this ion in the cytoplasm. Agonist-induced contractile force by angiotensin II, for example, is often greater than force induced by depolarization of the VSM cell membrane (by increasing extracellular K$^+$ and opening the voltage-gated Ca^{2+} channels) at identical or even lower concentrations of Ca^{2+} in the cytosol. The reason for this is that vasoconstrictor agonists can induce a signal transduction cascade that increases the "sensitivity" of the calcium sensor and effector molecules that control the machinery of contraction. The most important mechanism whereby Ca^{2+} sensitization modulates vascular smooth muscle tone is by regulating the activity of the enzyme that dephosphorylates the

light chains of myosin, MLCP. This Ca^{2+}-independent regulation of VSM tone involves a GTP-binding protein, RhoA, which is related to the Ras family of proteins and can function as a GTPase. RhoA works as a molecular switch in several cell processes, shuttling from an inactive GDP-bound state to an active form bound to GTP. As shown in Figure 4.4, a vasoconstrictor ligand such as thromboxane interacts with its G protein-coupled receptor and, by activation of guanine nucleotide exchange factors, leads to activation of RhoA and its associated kinase (ROK). In turn, ROK phosphorylates the regulatory subunit of MLCP, inhibiting its phosphatase activity and ability to induce relaxation. This pathway is of potential clinical interest as a target of drug development, and it has already been shown that administration of the ROK inhibitor Y27632 reduces blood pressure in several forms of experimental hypertension in the rat.

Two other, less well-defined mechanisms of inhibition of MLCP include the G protein-coupled release of arachidonic acid, which dissociates MLCP into its three subunits, thereby preventing its action. The other mechanism is mediated by diacyl glycerol, generated during activation of PLC, which activates protein kinase C (PKC). This kinase phosphorylates a 17-kDa protein called PKC-potentiated inhibitor protein (CPI-17),

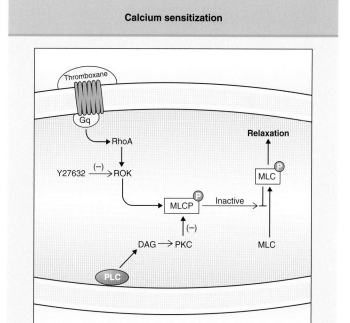

Figure 4.4. Calcium sensitization. Schematic overview of signal transduction during vascular smooth muscle constriction due to calcium sensitization. In this example, thromboxane binds to its receptor and activates RhoA and its associated kinase (ROK). This kinase phosphorylates myosin light chain phosphatase (MLCP), thereby preventing dephosphorylation of myosin and relaxation. Y27632 directly inhibits ROK and thus causes vasodilation and lowers arterial pressure. Activation of phospholipase C (PLC) (see also Fig. 4.2) and generation of diacylglycerol (DAG) also lead to an inhibition of MLCPP and constriction.

33

Basic Biology and Critical Care Medicine

which is specific to vascular smooth muscle and inhibits the catalytic subunit of MLCP. Contraction induced by phorbol esters is due to PKC phosphorylation of CPI-17 and subsequent inhibition of MLCP.

VSM Membrane Potential

The membrane potential of VSM ranges from −30 to −70 mV, depending on the cell type. As noted previously, an important part of the rise in cytoplasmic Ca^{2+} during ligand-mediated vasoconstriction is due to entry of extracellular Ca^{2+} via voltage-gated Ca^{2+} channels, which are inhibited by dihydropyridines and are also known as type L Ca^{2+} channels. The entry of Ca^{2+} is due to channel activation in response to a small depolarization of the plasma membrane resulting from opening of Cl^- channels by the Ca^{2+} released by the SR (Fig. 4.5). When the SR is depleted of Ca^{2+} there is also entry of Ca^{2+} by store-operated Ca^{2+} channels, which are activated by undefined mechanisms. In fact, sustained constriction of VSM is not possible unless Ca^{2+} entry into the cell from the extracellular space is facilitated.

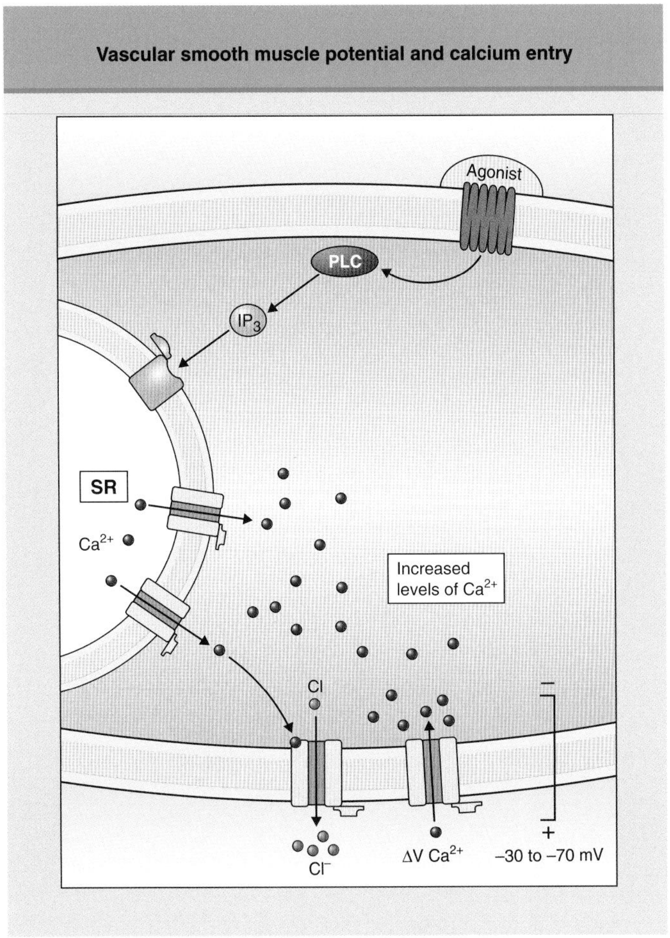

Figure 4.5. Vascular smooth muscle potential and calcium entry. Entry of extracellular calcium into the vascular smooth muscle (VSM) cytosol is critical for sustained contraction. Upon activation by a vasoconstrictor ligand, the initial increase in intracellular calcium is due to release of this ion from the sarcoplasmic reticulum (SR). This leads to activation of a chloride channel in the plasma membrane and subsequent depolarization. This slight change in membrane potential allows calcium entry via voltage-gated calcium channels.

Work with the patch clamp technique and molecular biology methods has revolutionized our understanding of the role of membrane potential in the control of VSM tone.

As shown in Figure 4.6, a more positive potential (depolarization) opens voltage-gated Ca^{2+} channels and, by increasing cytoplasmic Ca^{2+}, causes vasoconstriction. Conversely, hyperpolarization of the membrane causes vasodilation. Indeed, as detailed later, in some pathophysiological states, hyperpolarization of the VSM membrane vasodilates and causes hypotension even in the presence of vasoconstrictor ligands, providing a stark example of the important role of the membrane potential in the control of vascular tone. Several channels permeable to potassium that are critically involved in determining the membrane potential have been characterized.

Ca^{2+}-Regulated Large Conductance K^+ Channel (BK_{Ca2+})

Although calcium has a central role in controlling VSM constriction, cytosolic Ca^{2+} is not a uniform pool and spatially restricted areas with very high Ca^{2+} concentration occur inside VSM and, depending on its location, cytosolic Ca^{2+} can have opposite effects on VSM tone. As discussed previously, global increases in cytoplasmic Ca^{2+} cause vasoconstriction, but spatially restricted increases in cytosolic Ca^{2+} may cause vasodilation. Release of Ca^{2+} by the ryanodine receptor in SR causes a localized area of very high Ca^{2+} concentration that activates BK_{Ca2+} channels. The opening of these channels (Fig. 4.7) hyperpolarizes the cell membrane, thereby closing voltage-gated Ca^{2+} channels and relaxing the cell. In this manner, the constrictor action of several vasoconstrictors is buffered. Indeed, mice with gene deletion of one of the units of this channel develop hypertension. Moreover, as shown in Figure 4.7, several vasodilator factors that utilize the cAMP and the cGMP (and their respective kinases, PKA and PKG) pathways utilize activation of BK_{Ca2+} channels as a mechanism of vasodilation. NO, via its activation of guanylate cyclase and generation of cGMP, is among the ligands capable of activating BK_{Ca2+}. In addition, NO is capable of directly activating BK_{Ca2+} in the absence of cGMP. This novel mechanism of action, which depends on nitrosylation of thiol groups, is emerging as an important mechanism for regulating protein function. The importance of this channel in regulating vascular tone has been highlighted by the finding in humans that a gain-of-function mutation of one of its units protects against hypertension.

ATP-Regulated K^+ Channel (K_{ATP})

As its name indicates, ATP-sensitive potassium channels are regulated by intracellular ATP (or a function of it), H^+ cytoplasmic concentration, as well as several signal transduction pathways (Fig. 4.8). Activation of these channels, as detailed previously, hyperpolarizes the cell membrane and, by closure of voltage-gated Ca^{2+} channels, relaxes VSM. There are several endogenous activators of the K_{ATP} channel, all capable of profound vasodilation and lowering blood pressure: Calcitonin gene-related peptide (CGRP), vasoactive intestinal peptide (VIP), prostacyclin, and adenosine are among the most prominent. There are also several pharmacologic activators of this channel already available in clinical practice (e.g., diazoxide) that can induce profound hypotension. In addition, activation of the channel has been found to be a major contributor to the long described "metabolic inhibition" of sympathetic vasoconstriction in exer-

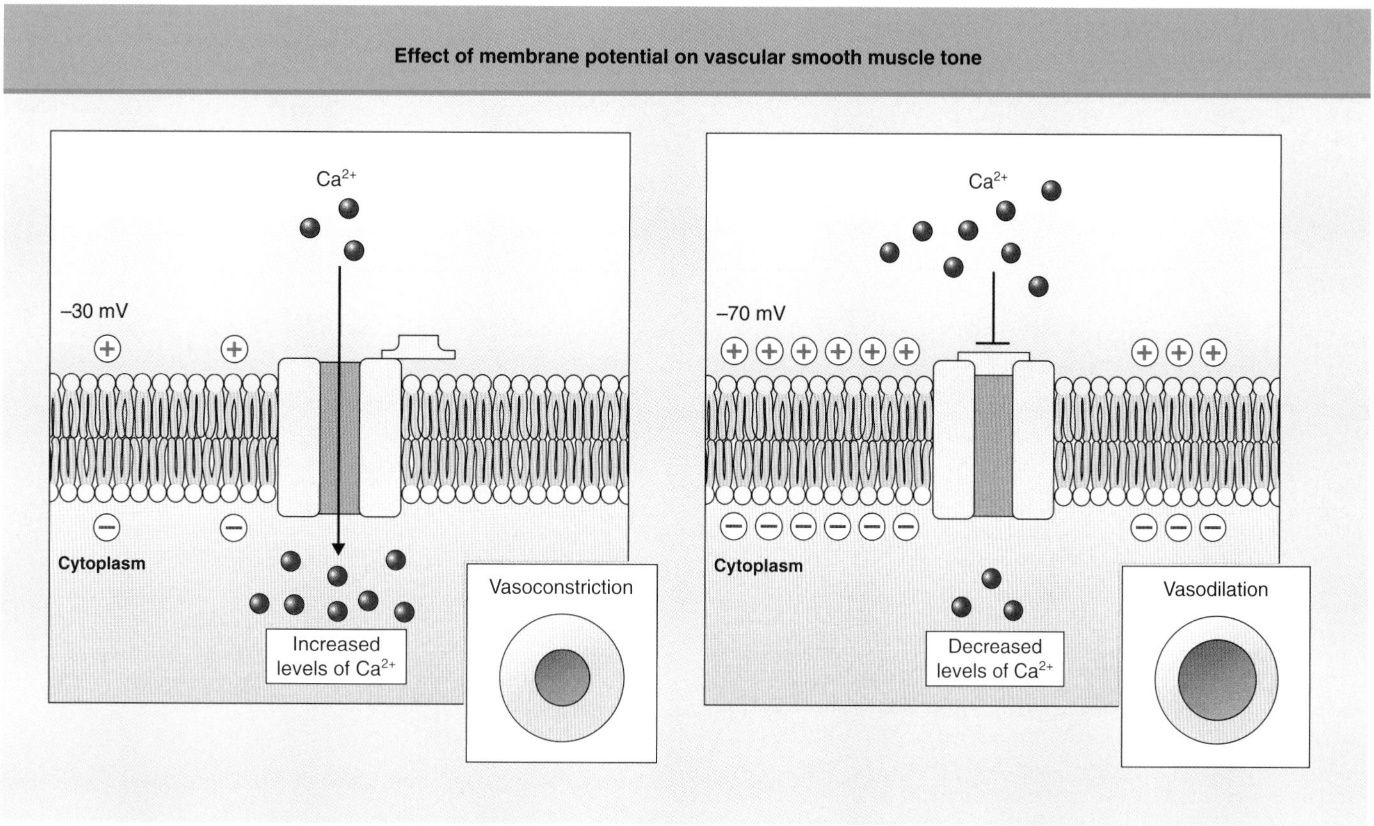

Effect of membrane potential on vascular smooth muscle tone

Figure 4.6. Effect of membrane potential on vascular smooth muscle tone. Because sustained vascular smooth muscle constriction is only possible if calcium enters the cell from the extracellular space via voltage-gated calcium channels, changes in membrane potential can determine the degree of vascular constriction/relaxation, even in the presence of ligands with opposite action.

cising skeletal muscle. Pathologic activation of the channel contributes to the vasodilation and hypotension of some types of distributive shock.

Voltage-Gated K⁺ Channel

These channels are regulated by voltage, so their activity increases with membrane depolarization. Thus, they may serve to limit the membrane depolarization that occurs in response to many vasoconstrictors. Several vasodilators that act via the cAMP–PKA pathway are believed to activate these channels. Likewise, several vasoconstrictors that activate PKC may inhibit these channels, thereby potentiating their effect.

Inner Rectifying K⁺ Channel (KIR)

These channels are so named because the K flow across them is more readily inward than outward ("inner rectification"). That is, they allow no or small outward K^+ currents because their intracellular domain is blocked by polyamines. What is remarkable about one of these channels, the KIR2.2 channel, is that extracellular K^+ concentration regulates the blocking by polyamines so that small increases in K^+ concentration open the channel, hyperpolarizing the membrane and relaxing the cell. This is of interest because it has long been known that whereas high concentrations of extracellular K^+ (>20 mM) depolarize the VSM membrane and trigger constriction, small increases in extracellular K^+ concentration (~6–8 mM) cause vasodilation.

Indeed, exercise causes muscle venous blood K^+ concentration to increase to ~7 mM, and potassium-depleted dogs do not increase their extracellular K^+ concentration during exercise, nor do they have the normally expected vasodilation. Finally, it is worth remembering that high intake of K^+ is almost always associated with lowering of blood pressure. The discovery of KIR channels has opened new avenues of research in this very important field.

CIRCULATING FACTORS THAT REGULATE VASCULAR TONE

Arterial blood pressure results from the interaction of the cardiac output and the resistance of the arterial side of the circulation. Vascular resistance is regulated by myriad neuronal and hormonal factors that engage the mechanisms reviewed previously. The physiological and/or clinical roles of many mechanisms have yet to be clearly defined, and only those demonstrated to be clinically important for regulation of vascular tone in health and disease are the focus of this discussion. Alpha-adrenergic agonists, angiotensin II, vasopressin, and endothelin are the clinically important vasoconstrictors (Table 4.1). The natriuretic peptides and nitric oxide are the most important vasodilators. Many of the factors that vasoconstrict upon binding to their receptors on VSM can also bind to alternative receptors on endothelium, thereby promoting NO

Basic Biology and Critical Care Medicine

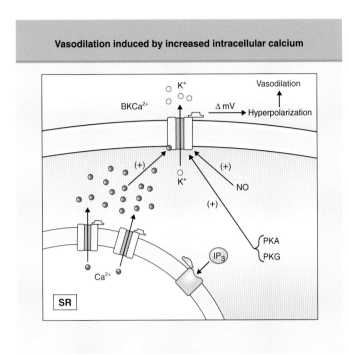

Figure 4.7. Vasodilation induced by increased intracellular calcium.
Because of the spatial relationships of sarcoplasmic reticulum (SR) located near the plasma membrane, released calcium can activate calcium-regulated large-conductance protein channel (BKCa^{2+}). Exit of K$^+$ hyperpolarizes the cell and causes relaxation. As shown, BKCa^{2+} is also under the influence of several vasodilator mechanisms such as nitric oxide (NO; which directly nitrosylates it) and ligands that activate protein kinase A (PKA) and protein kinase G (PKG); see Figure 4.3.

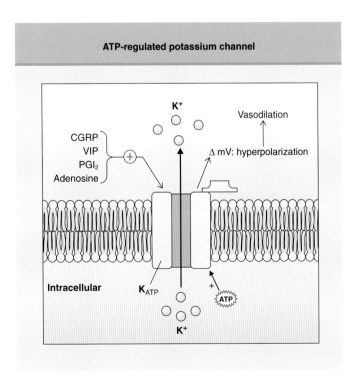

Figure 4.8. ATP-regulated potassium channel. This channel is gated by ATP and likely by other elements that reflect cellular metabolism, such as pH and lactate concentration. It can be directly activated by several vasodilator ligands.

Table 4.1 Circulating Vasoconstrictors

Vasoconstrictor	Receptor	Location
Norepinephrine	α_1	VSM
Epinephrine	α_1	VSM
Angiotensin	AT$_1$	VSM
Endothelin	ET-A	VSM
Vasopressin	V1a	VSM

Table 4.2 Selected Vasodilators

Vasodilator	Receptor	Location
Natriuretic peptides (ANP, BNP)	ANP-A	VSM
Nitric oxide	Soluble guanylate cylase	VSM
Epinephrine	β_2	VSM
Angiotensin	AT$_2$	Endothelium via NO
Endothelin	ET-B	Endothelium via NO
Vasopressin	V$_2$	Endothelium via NO

synthesis and vasodilation (Table 4.2). The clinical significance of this consistent vasodilatory motif for the vasoconstrictors remains to be fully elucidated.

Vasoconstrictors

The role of pressor catecholamines and the renin–angiotensin system in the regulation of arterial blood pressure is well understood and was outlined previously (see Fig. 4.2). The clinical syndromes associated with catecholamine excess (pheochromocytoma) and angiotensin II excess (renovascular hypertension and reninoma) emphasize the potency of both systems and their pharmacologic potential, but their relative importance in the regulation of vascular tone can be appreciated by comparing the effect of their blockade in upright and supine subjects. When an individual assumes an upright position, blood pools in the lower extremities, preload decreases, and cardiac output falls. Pharmacologically induced sympathectomy results in marked hypotension during upright tilt, indicating that sympathetic activation is needed for blood pressure maintenance during changes in posture in normal subjects. In contrast, inhibition of angiotensin II by converting enzyme inhibition (CEI) has no effect on blood pressure in normal subjects during upright tilt. However, during sodium depletion, administration of a CEI causes a precipitous decline during tilt. This marked sensitivity to the depressor effect of CEI or angiotensin AT1 receptor blockade is common to all states of arterial underfilling and is cause for particular caution in their administration in severe congestive heart failure.

Vasopressin

As the name implies, this hormone has a very potent vasoconstrictor effect, but its role in circulatory physiology has been overshadowed by its antidiuretic effect. Several distinct receptors are activated by vasopressin, including the V1a receptor on vascular smooth muscle and the V2 receptor on the renal collecting duct and on vascular endothelium. Vasopressin is released from the neurohypophysis in response to increased serum osmolality. Vasopressin binds V2 receptors in the kidney that mediate insertion of aquaporin water channels into the luminal membrane of the collecting duct and, thereby, the antidiuretic effect of the hormone. Vasopressin at a plasma concentration of 5 to 7 pg/mL is sufficient to maximally concentrate the urine.

Vasopressin is also secreted in response to a decrease in perfusion pressure, and plasma levels of several hundred picograms per milliliter are found in profound hypotension. The V1a receptor-mediated effects of vasopressin are more complex than the V2 effects, and only gradually has their clinical importance to the regulation of vascular tone been appreciated. V1a agonists are potent constrictors of vascular smooth muscle in vitro, with a dynamic range of 10 to several hundred pg/mL. On a molar basis, vasopressin is a 100-fold more potent vasoconstrictor than norepinephrine. V1a antagonists do not lower blood pressure in normal subjects, which is not surprising given that vasopressin secretion is fully suppressed in euvolemic, water-loaded subjects. Most unexpectedly, however, administration of vasopressin does not raise blood pressure significantly in normal subjects. Similarly, patients with the syndrome of inappropriate antidiuretic hormone and circulating levels greater than 40 pg/mL are not hypertensive. However, animal studies have provided compelling evidence for the role of vasopressin in maintaining blood pressure during states of arterial underfilling. The plasma concentration of vasopressin is moderately elevated in patients with extracellular fluid volume depletion or with decompensated heart failure (15–30 pg/mL), and blockade of V1a receptors causes a modest decrease in blood pressure, indicating that vasopressin contributes to the maintenance of pressure in these conditions. Furthermore, in vasopressin-deficient animals such as Brattleboro rats, hemorrhage volumes that are otherwise tolerated are rendered lethal.

The absence of a significant pressor effect in normal subjects but pressor effect in states of arterial underfilling suggests that vasopressin pressor sensitivity is regulated, just as is vasopressin secretion, by a baroreflex. In fact, the autonomic nervous system suppresses the pressor response to vasopressin, and in primary autonomic neuropathy a two- or three-order of magnitude increase in sensitivity is observed. This phenomenon, suggesting the loss of a heterologous desensitizer, may explain the markedly superior vasoconstrictor effect of vasopressin in vitro.

The importance of vasopressin in the regulation of vascular tone is further emphasized by our discovery of a syndrome of vasopressin deficiency that is characteristic of vasodilatory shock states. We found in vasodilatory septic shock, in vasodilatory shock after cardiopulmonary bypass, and in the late "irreversible phase" of hemorrhagic shock that vasopressin levels are unexpectedly low for the setting of shock, and that replacement of the hormone restores vascular tone, raises blood pressure, and reduces the requirement for catecholamine pressors.

Endothelin

Endothelin (ET-1) is the most potent endothelium-derived vasoconstrictor, but in contrast to the roles of the catecholamine, renin–angiotensin, and vasopressin systems, the role of endothelin in the regulation of vascular tone remains to be fully elucidated in man. Nonetheless, important, occasionally paradoxical, information is available from administration of ET-1, from ET-A and ET-B receptor knockout mice, and from studies of endothelin-converting enzyme (ECE) inhibitors and endothelin receptor antagonists.

$$\text{Prepro endothelin-1} \rightarrow \text{big endothelin-1} \rightarrow \text{ECE} \rightarrow \text{endothelin-1}$$

Endothelin-1 is synthesized as prepro ET-1, which is cleaved to "big" ET-1 and then via ECE to ET-1. ET-1 acts via the endothelin receptors ET-A and ET-B. ET-A receptors on vascular smooth muscle mediate vasoconstriction, whereas ET-B receptors on endothelium mediate vasodilatation via release of NO and also prostacyclin. The net effect of these opposing effects varies depending on the vascular bed.

Homozygous knockouts of ET-1, ET-A, and ET-B all develop lethal phenotypes. However, heterozygous knockouts have yielded insights into the role of ET-1 on vascular tone. The pressor effect of administered ET-1 and the depressor effect of inhibition of ECE notwithstanding, heterozygous knockout of ET-1 induces an elevation of basal mean arterial blood pressure (MAP). This paradoxical result may represent deranged central cardiovascular control. Heterozygous knockouts of either ET-A or ET-B receptors show a significantly reduced pressor response to systematically administered ET-1. Heterozygous knockouts of ET-A do not show significant change of MAP, but heterozygous knockouts of ET-B demonstrate a significantly higher MAP, perhaps due to a decrease in ET-B-mediated clearance of the hormone. Administration of an ET-A antagonist or a mixed ET-A/ET-B antagonist reduces MAP in ET-B knockout mice to normal levels. Finally, homozygous knockout of ET-B in endothelium results in hypertension. In the aggregate, these data suggest a role for ET-B in the regulation of basal vascular tone.

Natriuretic Peptides

Three natriuretic peptides have been identified: A type, B type, and C type. A type and B type function primarily in the cardiovascular system. Three receptors bind these natriuretic peptides: ANP-A, ANP-B, and ANP-C. Both ANP and BNP bind to the ANP-A receptor; ANP has the higher affinity. CNP binds to the ANP-B receptor. No BNP selective receptors have been found. ANP-C appears to be a regulatory receptor. ANP and BNP have both central and peripheral effects. Peripheral effects include natriuresis, vasodilation, and inhibition of the renin–angiotensin and aldosterone system (see Fig. 4.3).

Transgenic and knockout mice have been used to elucidate the role of natriuretic peptides in blood pressure regulation. Transgenic mice that constitutively express BNP develop chronic hypotension. Transgenic mice that overexpress either ANP or BNP have systolic blood pressure that is 20 to 30 mm Hg lower than that of wild-type littermates. ANP knockout mice show salt-sensitive hypertension due to a failure to suppress renin. BNP knockout mice do not develop salt-sensitive hypertension, but in the setting of ventricular pressure overload they do develop cardiac fibrosis. Receptor knockout mice have also been created, and selective vascular ANP-A knockout mice were found to be normotensive due to increased NO activity.

Nitric Oxide

NO is a potent vasodilator (see Fig. 4.3), and three NO synthase (NOS) enzymes are known: endothelial, neuronal, and inducible. Blockade of NOS raises MAP in normal subjects consistent with the constitutively active eNOS. Knockout mice have been created in which each of the three NOS genes is disrupted, and the eNOS knockout mice are notable for the development of moderate hypertension with basal blood pressure levels typically 20 mm Hg higher than those of control littermates. No data demonstrate unambiguously that underexpression of NOS is linked to human hypertension, but blockade of NOS rendered experimental animals susceptible to salt-sensitive hypertension; high-salt diet alone produced no increase in blood pressure.

AUTOREGULATION

The ability of an organ, independent of neuronal or hormonal factors, to maintain a constant blood flow despite changes in perfusion pressure, or to alter blood flow despite constant perfusion pressure, is described as autoregulation.

Autoregulation is believed to be achieved by two main mechanisms: myogenic control that maintains flow over a varying range of pressures and metabolic control that transduces varying metabolic demand to alter flow at a constant perfusion pressure. The degree of participation of these mechanisms varies in different vascular beds. Demand–flow coupling is best characterized in the coronary circulation and is beyond the scope of this chapter.

Myogenic Control
The myogenic response is characterized by a decrease in vessel diameter after an increase in transmural pressure and by an

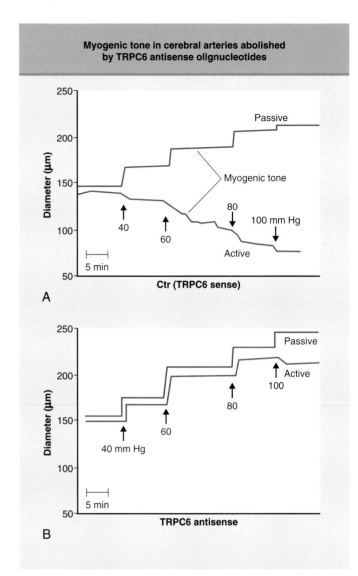

Figure 4.10. Myogenic tone in cerebral arteries abolished by TRPC6 antisense oligonucleotides. Cerebral arteries cultured with sense (A) or antisense TRPC6 oligonucleotide (B) and then stripped of endothelium were mounted in calcium containing buffer (active tracings) or zero Ca^{2+} buffer containing an opener of the voltage-gated Ca^{2+} channel (passive tracings) and then subjected to step increases in perfusion pressure for arteriograph measurement of the response of vessel diameter. (Data from Welsh DG, Morielli AD, Nelson MT, Brayden JE: Transient receptor potential channels regulate myogenic tone of resistance arteries. Circ Res 2002;90:248–250.)

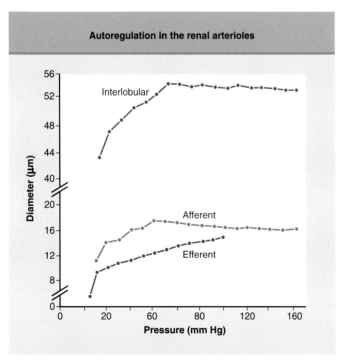

Figure 4.9. Autoregulation in the renal arterioles. The pressure–diameter characteristics of renal microvessels at increasing 10 mm Hg increments. (Data from Edwards RM: Segmental effects of norepinephrine and angiotensin II on isolated renal microvessels. Am J Physiol 1983;244:F526–F534.)

increase in vessel diameter after a decrease in this pressure. Myogenic control can be demonstrated in the autoregulation of the mesenteric, skeletal muscle, cerebral, renal, and coronary circulation. Strength of the myogenic response is greatest at the resistance vessels, and larger and very small vessels possess a relatively weak myogenic response. Strength varies in different vascular beds; for example, rat small mesenteric vessels have a weak myogenic response compared to that observed in similar-sized cerebral and skeletal muscle vessels. Different vessels within the same organ may respond differently, and the myogenic response of the afferent arteriole of kidney contrasts with the absent response of the efferent (Fig. 4.9).

The myogenic response appears to be initiated by a pressure-induced alteration of vessel wall tension rather than a change in cell length or pressure. Wall tension is reduced by vessel constriction, providing a negative feedback that limits myogenic vessel constriction.

Because neither the blocking of nerve endings in the adventitia nor the stripping of the endothelium fail to significantly alter the myogenic response, a mechanoelectrical coupling unit situated in the vascular smooth muscle is inferred. This unit can be characterized as a vascular wall stretch reflex with an afferent limb mechanoreceptor coupled to an efferent limb providing excitation–contraction. Stretch-activated cation channels, voltage-dependent calcium channels, and the extracellular matrix and cytoskeleton have all been postulated to participate in the myogenic response, but a transient receptor potential channel (TRPC6) homolog is the best documented mediator of the response.

Arteries pretreated with a sense oligonucleotide for a transient receptor potential channel (TRPC6) homolog and then stripped of endothelium showed active myogenic tone. Myogenic tone is evident as step increases in pressure result in step decreases in diameter, as illustrated in the "active" tracing in Figure 4.10*A*. The diameter–pressure relationship in the absence of myogenic tone was defined in the presence of a Ca channel opener in a zero Ca bath with step increases in pressure causing step increases in diameter, as illustrated in the passive tracings in Figure 4.10*A*. In contrast to the sense oligonucleotide, the TRPC6 antisense oligonucleotide largely abolishes myogenic tone—that is, the active tracing (Fig. 4.10*B*) approximates the passive.

SUGGESTED READING

Edwards RM: Segmental effects of norepinephrine and angiotensin II on isolated renal microvessels. Am J Physiol 1983;244:F526–F534.

Jackson WF: Ion channels and vascular tone. Hypertension 2000;35:173–178.

Landry DW, Oliver JA: The pathogenesis of vasodilatory shock. N Engl J Med 2001;345:588–595.

Landry DW, Levin HR, Gallant EM, et al: Vasopressin deficiency contributes to the vasodilation of septic shock. Circulation 1997;95:1122–1125.

Melo LG, Veress AT, Chong CK, Pang SC, Flynn TG, Sonnenberg H: Salt-sensitive hypertension in ANP knockout mice: Potential role of abnormal plasma renin activity. Am J Physiol 1998;274:R255–R261.

Quayle JM, Nelson MT, Standen NB: ATP-sensitive and inwardly rectifying potassium channels in smooth muscle. Physiol Rev 1997;77:1165–1232.

Standen NB, Quayle JM: K^+ channel modulation in arterial smooth muscle. Acta Physiol Scand 1998;164:549–557.

Sudoh T, Kangawa K, Minamino N, Matsuo H: A new natriuretic peptide in porcine brain. Nature 1988;332:78–81.

Surks HK, Mochizuki N, Kasai Y, et al: Regulation of myosin phosphatase by a specific interaction with cGMP-dependent protein kinase Ia. Science 1999;286:1583–1587.

Wagner HN Jr, Braunwald E: The pressor effect of the antidiuretic principle of the posterior pituitary in orthostatic hypotension. J Clin Invest 1956;35:1412–1418.

Welsh DG, Morielli AD, Nelson MT, Brayden JE: Transient receptor potential channels regulate myogenic tone of resistance arteries. Circ Res 2002;90:248–250.

REQUIREMENT FOR OXYGEN IN METABOLISM

Mammalian cells require molecular oxygen as a substrate for a variety of enzymatic reactions involved in biosynthesis, molecular modification, and bioenergetics. Some oxidases utilize oxygen in enzymatic reactions that involve the insertion of two oxygen atoms into metabolic substrates. Other cellular systems consume O_2 through the function of mixed function oxygenases, which hydroxylate substrates by inserting only one of the two oxygen atoms. These processes are critically important for cell metabolism, but they account for only a small fraction of the oxygen consumed. The majority of oxygen is utilized by the mitochondrial electron transport system in the generation of ATP. Failure to supply sufficient oxygen to maintain all of these processes endangers cell survival. A fundamental goal of the critical care physician is to ensure that the oxygen supply to all tissues remains sufficient to prevent the consequences that arise from oxygen deprivation.

Mitochondrial Respiration

The cells of the body produce the majority of their ATP through aerobic respiration in the mitochondria. These organelles are attached to the actin cytoskeleton in the cell and consist of an outer membrane that surrounds a highly impermeable inner membrane. The matrix compartment within the inner membrane contains the enzymes that participate in the Krebs cycle, as well as proteins involved in the electron transport chain. In glycolysis and the Krebs cycle, hydrogen atoms are sequentially removed from metabolic substrates. These reducing equivalents (electrons) are then delivered to the mitochondrial electron transport chain, which consists of a series of multisubunit complexes. Electrons travel from complex I & II → III → IV because these proteins exhibit increasingly positive standard reduction–oxidation (redox) potentials. This property is associated with a greater electron affinity in the later complexes compared to the earlier ones. As electrons are passed through complexes I, III, and IV, the release of free energy is conserved and utilized to extrude a proton from the matrix compartment to the intermembrane space. The pumping of protons out of the matrix creates an electrical potential and a pH gradient across the inner membrane, with the matrix highly negative (−180 mV) relative to the intermembrane space. Complex V is an ATP synthase embedded in the inner membrane. This complex is not directly involved in electron transport. Rather, it generates ATP from ADP + Pi, using free energy obtained by leaking protons back into the matrix compartment (Fig. 5.1).

The rate of mitochondrial oxygen consumption is largely regulated by the rate of ATP utilization by the cell. This coupling between electron transport and ATP synthesis is a consequence of the relationships among mitochondrial membrane potential (ΔΨm), electron transport/proton pumping, and ATP synthase activity. For example, when the cellular metabolic rate slows, the rate of ADP arrival at the ATP synthase decreases. This slows the activity of the ATP synthase, causing the ΔΨm to increase because fewer protons are reentering the matrix. The increase in ΔΨm inhibits proton pumping and electron transfer by increasing the gradient against which these complexes must extrude protons. The reduced rate of electron transport thereby decreases oxygen utilization at complex IV. If leaks develop in the inner membrane and permit proton entry, or if specialized proton channels in the inner membrane (uncoupling proteins) admit protons to the matrix, electron transport and oxygen consumption proceed without ATP generation. This process,

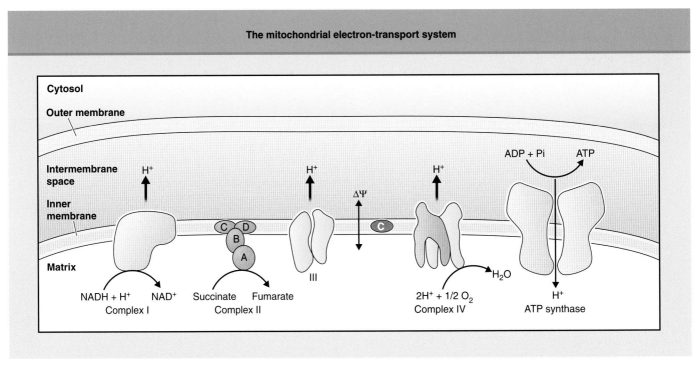

The mitochondrial electron-transport system

Figure 5.1. The mitochondrial electron-transport system. Functional structure of mitochondrial membranes and the electron transport system.

referred to as uncoupling, utilizes oxygen and generates heat without contributing to ATP production.

At mitochondrial complex IV, also known as cytochrome c oxidase, four electrons are transferred to O_2, which is reduced to H_2O. Studies of the enzyme kinetics of this complex reveal that it exhibits a very high affinity for O_2 (Wilson and coworkers, 1977). When removed from the cell and studied as an enzymatic complex in solution, its rate of activity remains high until the local oxygen tension decreases to less than 1 mm Hg. These properties allow mitochondrial respiration to continue until the oxygen tension at the mitochondria reaches levels approaching anoxia (Fig. 5.2).

OXYGEN DELIVERY AT THE CELLULAR LEVEL

As mitochondria consume O_2, the intracellular PO_2 decreases and a gradient in oxygen tension develops across the plasma membrane. Driven by that gradient, oxygen diffuses into the cell from the surrounding interstitial space. In steady-state conditions, the rate of oxygen diffusion into the cell exactly matches the rate of cellular oxygen utilization. This situation is illustrated in Figure 5.3, which depicts an isolated cell surrounded by a well-stirred environment. It is reasonable to ask what the normal intracellular PO_2 would be under these conditions. The answer to this question depends on the rate of O_2 consumption by the cell and on the extracellular PO_2. For a cell consuming oxygen, the mitochondrial PO_2 will be somewhat less than the extracellular PO_2, reflecting the gradient generated by the consumption of oxygen (Jones, 1986). Studies assessing the gradient in PO_2 between the cell surface and the mitochondria indicate that mitochondrial PO_2 is typically 2 to 4 mm Hg less than extracellular PO_2. If the extracellular PO_2 increases or decreases, the mitochondrial PO_2 will increase or decrease in parallel, with the

difference between cell surface and mitochondria always remaining the same under steady-state conditions (Fig. 5.4).

Oxygen Supply-Dependent Metabolism

When mitochondrial PO_2 falls below the critically low level needed to sustain oxygen consumption, the rate of electron transport and ATP production becomes limited by the arrival of

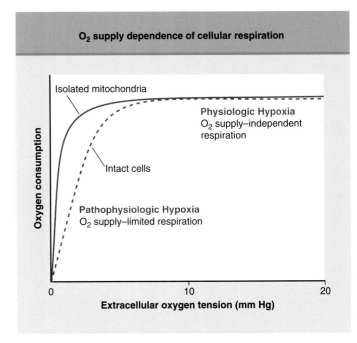

O_2 supply dependence of cellular respiration

Isolated mitochondria

Physiologic Hypoxia
O_2 supply–independent respiration

Intact cells

Pathophysiologic Hypoxia
O_2 supply–limited respiration

Oxygen consumption

Extracellular oxygen tension (mm Hg)

Figure 5.2. O_2 supply dependence of cellular respiration. Relationship between oxygen partial pressure (PO_2) and the rate of oxygen consumption by isolated mitochondria or intact cells.

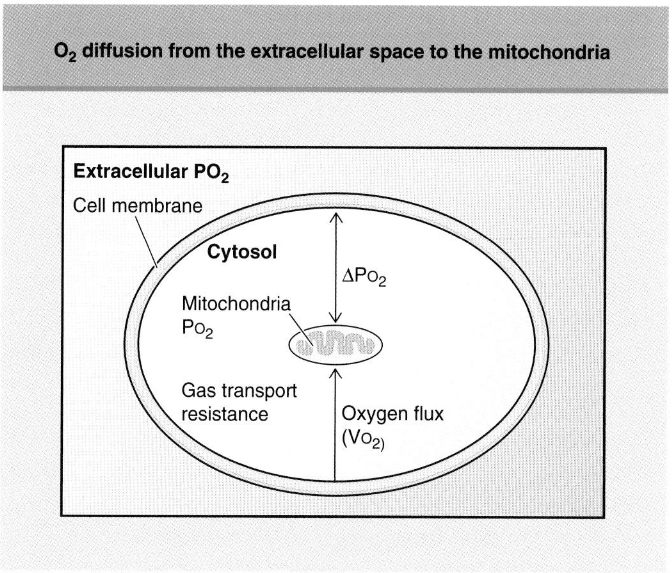

O₂ diffusion from the extracellular space to the mitochondria

Figure 5.3. O₂ diffusion from the extracellular space to the mitochondria. The consumption of O₂ by the mitochondria generates a gradient in PO₂. This gradient is proportional to the rate of oxygen consumption (O₂ flux) and the diffusive gas transport resistance in the cell.

O₂ at cytochrome c oxidase. Because a gradient in PO₂ normally exists between the cell membrane and the mitochondria, the extracellular PO₂ associated with the onset of supply-limited consumption at the mitochondria is typically 3 to 5 mm Hg greater than the critical mitochondrial PO₂. Hence, oxygen

Relationship between extracellular and mitochondrial Po₂

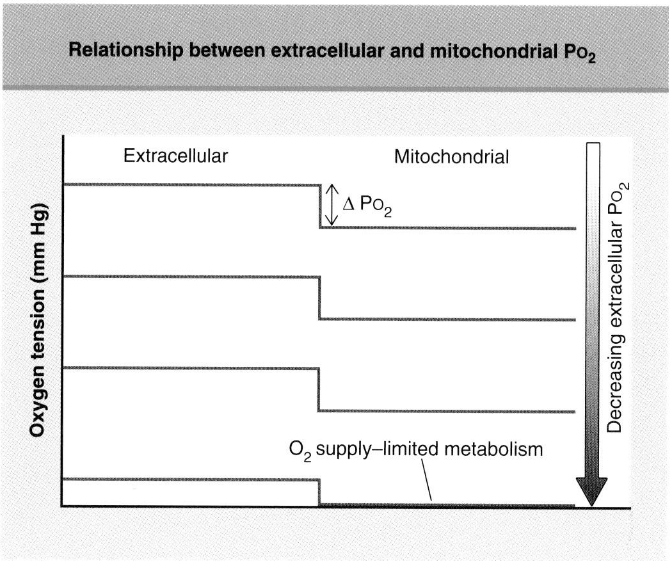

Figure 5.4. Relationship between extracellular and mitochondrial PO₂. The mitochondrial PO₂ is determined by extracellular PO₂ and the intracellular gradient in PO₂. When cellular O₂ uptake remains constant, changes in extracellular PO₂ will produce equal changes in mitochondrial PO₂. If extracellular PO₂ falls below a critical level, mitochondrial PO₂ will fall below its critical threshold and the rate of O₂ consumption of the cell will become O₂ supply limited.

consumption of most cells is adequate to sustain respiration as long as the oxygen tension surrounding the cell exceeds 5 or 6 mm Hg.

If the extracellular PO₂ decreases to a point at which mitochondrial PO₂ is below its critical point, the rate of electron transport and oxygen consumption becomes O₂-supply limited. If cellular ATP utilization continues, then the mitochondrial ΔΨm will decrease because entry of protons (via the ATP synthase) exceeds the rate of proton extrusion. Prolonged decreases in ΔΨm threaten cell survival because they can trigger swelling of the matrix compartment, which can lead to rupture of the outer mitochondrial membrane. The resulting leakage of cytochrome c from the intermembrane space to the cytosol then triggers apoptotic cell death. In situations in which mitochondrial potential decreases, the mitochondria can utilize ATP generated by anaerobic glycolysis to operate the ATP synthase in the reverse direction. In these conditions, the ATP synthase acts as a proton pump, extruding protons from the matrix compartment and helping to protect the ΔΨm at the expense of glycolytic ATP produced in the cytosol. However, the ability to sustain anaerobic glycolysis in tissues that do not receive blood flow is limited, so the protection afforded by this mechanism is relatively short-lived. If ATP production is completely halted, necrotic cell death will ensue because essential ATP-dependent processes cannot be sustained.

OXYGEN DELIVERY AT THE CAPILLARY LEVEL

The primary function of the vascular system is to continually provide an adequate supply of oxygen to every cell in the body. Oxygen diffuses from areas of higher partial pressure to lower partial pressure. Oxygen diffuses out of the capillaries because the oxygen tension in the surrounding tissue is less than the PO₂ in the capillary blood (Fig. 5.5). This situation was first described by August Krogh, a physiologist who was awarded a Nobel Prize for his work. Krogh envisioned each capillary as though it were

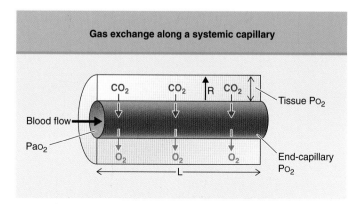

Figure 5.5. Gas exchange along a systemic capillary. Oxygen diffusion from capillary to tissue. Consumption of O₂ by the cells surrounding the capillary generates a gradient in PO₂ from blood to tissue.

surrounded by cells arranged in a cylinder. As oxygen leaves the blood, the hemoglobin saturation decreases and the PO_2 decreases accordingly. Hence, blood leaving the capillary has a lower oxygen tension and O_2 content than blood entering. According to the Fick relationship, the oxygen consumption by the cylinder can be calculated as the product of capillary blood flow and arteriovenous O_2 content difference:

$$Vo_2 = \text{blood flow} \times (CaO_2 - CvO_2) \qquad \text{(Equation 1)}$$

where VO_2 is the rate of O_2 uptake, and CaO_2 and CvO_2 are the arterial and end-capillary blood O_2 contents, respectively. Consequently, cells located farther from the capillary will typically experience lower PO_2 conditions than cells immediately adjacent to the capillary wall. Since the capillary PO_2 is lowest at the outflow end, the cells located farthest from the capillary at the venous end of the tissue cylinder would typically experience the lowest oxygen environment in the tissue.

Carbon Dioxide Elimination

Carbon dioxide produced by the cells is normally carried away in venous blood, and the Fick relationship can be applied to CO_2:

$$VCO_2 = \text{blood flow} \times (CvCO_2 - CaCO_2) \qquad \text{(Equation 2)}$$

where VCO_2 is the rate of CO_2 production, and $CvCO_2$ and $CaCO_2$ are the venous and arterial CO_2 contents, respectively. The arteriovenous PCO_2 difference across a capillary is typically smaller than the PO_2 difference because most tissues produce less CO_2 per unit time than they consume O_2. In addition, the slope of the relationship between CO_2 content and PCO_2 in blood is steeper than for the oxyhemoglobin dissociation curve. This allows the tissue to load a given volume of CO_2 into capillary blood without producing as large a change in partial pressure as for O_2.

THE CONCEPT OF TISSUE HYPOXIA

The oxygen delivery into a tissue cylinder will decrease if blood flow, arterial PO_2, or arterial hemoglobin concentration decreases. Classically, these conditions are referred to as stagnant hypoxia, hypoxemic hypoxia, and anemic hypoxia, respectively. These conditions rarely occur as singular events except under controlled experimental conditions, but it is useful to consider their effects on tissue oxygenation.

Stagnant Hypoxia

If blood flow into a capillary is decreased while the arterial PO_2 remains constant, the slower transit of red cells through the capillary will allow more time for O_2 to diffuse into the tissue (Schumacker and Samsel, 1989). Consequently, the end-capillary PO_2 and O_2 content will decrease (Fig. 5.6). This will lower the "average" capillary and tissue PO_2 values, although the mean level of tissue oxygenation is less important to consider than is the minimal level in the tissue. Cell survival is not threatened as long as the minimal extracellular PO_2 everywhere exceeds the critical cellular PO_2. This condition is referred to as "physiological hypoxia," indicating that the tissue PO_2 is decreased from its normal value but cell survival and function are not threatened. Physiological hypoxia can be detected by the cells, and it triggers adaptive responses including the upregulated expression of glycolytic enzymes and membrane glucose transporters. These responses are anticipatory in that they help to protect the cell in the event that the tissue hypoxia becomes more severe.

As blood flow into the cylinder decreases, CO_2 accumulates in the cells and the tissue PCO_2 increases. Driven by the increase in tissue PCO_2, CO_2 diffuses into the capillary blood, causing the end-capillary PCO_2 to increase. In steady-state conditions during stagnant hypoxia, CO_2 elimination from the tissue is maintained by increasing venous PCO_2 and $CvCO_2$. The decrease in capillary

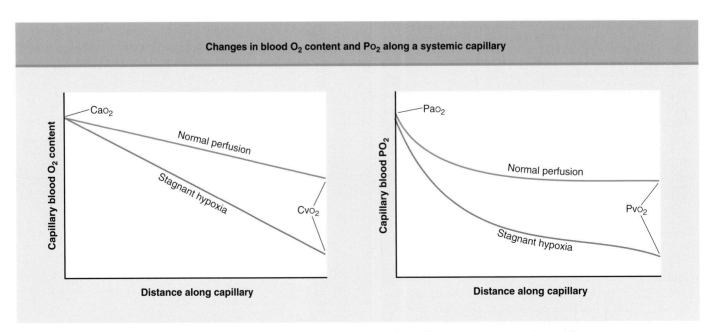

Figure 5.6. Changes in blood O_2 content and PO_2 along a systemic capillary. Oxygen consumption and the decrease in capillary PO_2 during physiological hypoxia produced by lowering blood flow.

O₂ supply–limited metabolism during pathophysiologic hypoxia

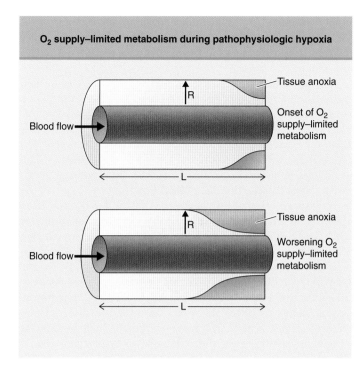

Figure 5.7. O₂ supply–limited metabolism during pathophysiological hypoxia. Pathological oxygen supply-limited metabolism during stagnant hypoxia. Regions of tissue anoxia do not consume oxygen, causing the overall O₂ uptake of the tissue to decline.

Critical capillary Po₂ during hypoxemic hypoxia

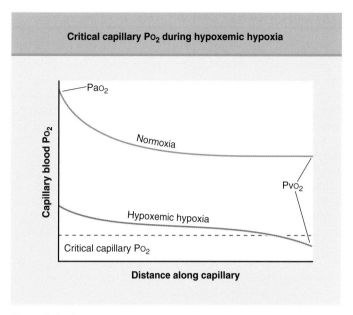

Figure 5.8. Critical capillary Po₂ during hypoxemic hypoxia. Pathophysiologic O₂ supply–limited metabolism during hypoxemic hypoxia.

pH caused by this hypercarbia will shift the oxyhemoglobin dissociation curve to the right, enhancing the unloading of oxygen at any given capillary P_{O_2}.

If blood flow into the cylinder is reduced to a critically low level, a state of pathophysiological hypoxia develops. In this situation, the P_{O_2} at the venous end of the cylinder farthest from the capillary falls below the critical threshold. This "lethal corner" is therefore the most vulnerable area of the tissue because it is the first to experience oxygen supply–dependent metabolism. If blood flow is reduced even further, more of the tissue cylinder becomes recruited into this anoxic region, which does not receive adequate oxygen to support normal metabolism (Fig. 5.7). When this happens, the overall O₂ consumption by the tissue cylinder decreases because only a subset of the cells is supplied with O₂. During pathophysiological stagnant hypoxia, the oxygen deprivation is severe enough to compromise tissue function and induce cellular injury.

Hypoxemic Hypoxia

If blood flow through a capillary is held constant while the oxyhemoglobin saturation is decreased, the oxygen transport into the tissue will decrease. This condition has been termed "hypoxemic hypoxia" because it normally results from a decrease in arterial oxygen tension. Hypoxemic hypoxia lowers the P_{O_2} at the capillary entrance and at every point along its length. Theoretically, this threatens oxygen supply to cells in the lethal corner because it lowers the end-capillary oxygen tension driving diffusion. When the O₂ tension along the capillary is no longer sufficient to supply tissue regions with adequate oxygen, O₂ consumption decreases in those regions where the P_{O_2} is less than the critical threshold. Further decreases in capillary P_{O_2} will recruit successively more of the tissue region into this supply-dependent state (Fig. 5.8).

In practice, true hypoxemic hypoxia rarely occurs because the decrease in tissue P_{O_2} triggers local vasodilation, resulting in an increase in capillary blood flow. Although the increase in blood flow does not restore P_{O_2} at the capillary entrance, it does lessen the decrease in P_{O_2} along the capillary. This response helps to sustain tissue oxygenation despite significant arterial hypoxemia.

In terms of CO₂ transport, hypoxemic hypoxia is not generally associated with an increase in tissue or end-capillary P_{CO_2}. Because capillary blood flow is maintained, CO₂ produced in the tissue can be adequately carried away without any increase in venous P_{CO_2}.

Anemic Hypoxia

When the arterial hemoglobin concentration (hematocrit) decreases, the delivery of oxygen to the capillary declines even if blood flow is maintained. Classically referred to as "anemic hypoxia," this condition is associated with a normal O₂ tension at the entrance of the capillary, but the lesser hemoglobin concentration produces a steeper decrease in saturation and P_{O_2} as blood moves through the capillary. This amplifies the decrease in end-capillary P_{O_2} and saturation compared to that seen with a normal hematocrit.

As is the case with hypoxemic hypoxia, anemic hypoxia is normally accompanied by an increase in capillary blood flow as a result of local vasodilation (a response to tissue hypoxia) and the decrease in blood viscosity (which tends to lower the vascular resistance). For this reason, anemic hypoxia is not associated with an increase in tissue or venous P_{CO_2}.

Basic Biology and Critical Care Medicine

OXYGEN TRANSPORT AT THE TISSUE LEVEL

In a simplistic sense, intact tissues can be thought of as collections of capillary tissue units arranged in parallel. However, video microscopic studies of the microcirculation reveal important differences between real tissues and this idealistic model. First, the various cells comprising a tissue often exhibit disparate requirements for O_2 based on differences in their contributions to tissue function. For example, tubular epithelial cells in the kidney exhibit high metabolic rates secondary to their ion transport activity compared to nearby fibroblasts. Therefore, not all capillaries require the same blood flow to meet the oxygen demands of the cells they support. Second, capillary blood flow is frequently intermittent such that at any instant only a fraction of the capillaries is being perfused. Thus, tissue hypoxia can develop if a given capillary is shut off for an excessive amount of time, even though its flow might be adequate during the times when it is perfused. Third, the distances between capillaries vary and capillary geometry is often tortuous. Hence, it is difficult to know which cells are served by a particular capillary, whether they are served by more than one capillary, and what distances oxygen must diffuse to supply them. Finally, it is difficult to measure the supply of oxygen to a given cell within an intact tissue. Collectively, these factors make it difficult to determine whether the cells of an intact tissue are adequately oxygenated. The following sections examine the factors that influence the ability of tissues to extract oxygen from a limited supply.

Assessing the Efficiency of Tissue Oxygen Extraction

In normal tissues, the relationship between oxygen delivery (DO_2) and consumption (VO_2) can be described by a bilinear relationship consisting of an O_2 supply-independent region and an O_2 supply-dependent region (Cain, 1977) (Fig. 5.9). At normal or high levels of oxygen delivery, VO_2 is set by metabolic demand and is relatively independent of oxygen supply. At O_2 deliveries below a critical DO_2, regions of tissue anoxia begin to develop and oxygen uptake becomes limited by the failure to

supply adequate O_2 to maintain consumption in some areas (Schumacker and Cain, 1987). As the delivery is further reduced, progressively more tissue volume is recruited into this undersupplied category.

It is important to note that the O_2 requirement of certain tissues is dependent on the level of blood flow. For example, as renal blood flow increases, the rate of glomerular filtration typically will increase, presenting an increased load for reabsorption along the renal tubules. Hence, the relationship between DO_2 and VO_2 for the kidney is characterized by a "plateau" region with a pronounced slope, reflecting the increased metabolic activity associated with a high blood flow.

A bilinear relationship between DO_2 and VO_2 has been observed in small tissue regions, whole organs, and even for whole body. Identification of the critical DO_2 at the intersection of these lines provides a useful measure of the minimum O_2 delivery necessary to adequately supply all the cells of the tissue. However, it is difficult to compare critical DO_2 values between organs, or between a single organ and whole body, because the oxygen demands differ in scale. For example, myocardium exhibits a higher critical DO_2 per gram of tissue than does resting skeletal muscle because the metabolic rates of these tissues differ. A more useful variable in comparing tissues or patients is the O_2 extraction ratio (ERO_2). The extraction ratio is defined as the ratio of VO_2/DO_2:

$$ERO_2 = VO_2/DO_2 = (CaO_2 - CvO_2)/CaO_2 \qquad \text{(Equation 3)}$$

As O_2 delivery to the tissue is reduced, increases in ERO_2 sustain oxygen consumption (Fig. 5.10). The ERO_2 provides information on the level of O_2 delivery relative to the O_2 consumption of the tissue, but it does not provide information on the adequacy of that O_2 supply relative to tissue oxygen demand. Hence, a low ERO_2 could result from a high O_2 delivery relative to tissue oxygen demand or from a normal oxygen delivery to a tissue whose ability to extract oxygen from blood is impaired. The O_2 extraction at the critical O_2 delivery (ERO_2crit) provides a normalized index of the ability of a tissue, an organ, or an organism to sustain VO_2 in the face of a reduction in DO_2. The ERO_2crit

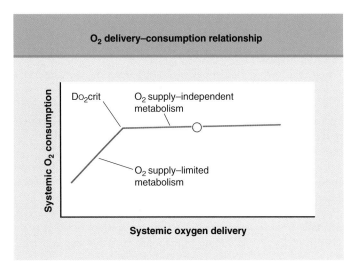

Figure 5.9. O_2 **delivery–consumption relationship.** Relationship between oxygen delivery (Do_2) and oxygen consumption (Vo_2) by a tissue, an organ, or the whole body.

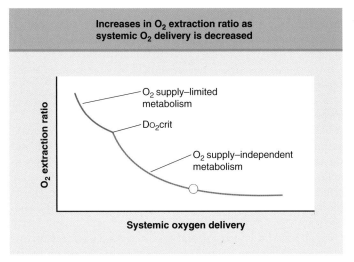

Figure 5.10. **Increases in O_2 extraction ratio as systemic O_2 delivery is decreased.**

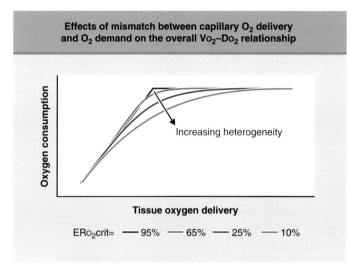

Figure 5.11. Effects of mismatch between capillary O₂ delivery and O₂ demand on the overall Vo₂–Do₂ relationship. Effects of heterogeneity in the matching of tissue oxygen delivery with respect to oxygen demand on the relationship between Do₂ and Vo₂ in a tissue.

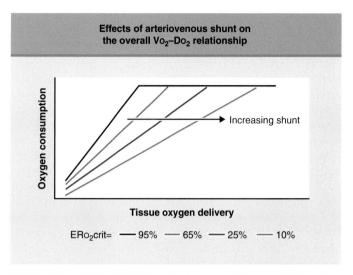

Figure 5.12. Effects of arteriovenous shunt on the overall Vo₂–Do₂ relationship. Effects of oxygen shunting on the relationship between Do₂ and Vo₂ in a tissue.

reflects the efficiency of O_2 extraction because it describes the ability of the tissue to take up O_2 from blood at the point where some tissue regions become O_2 supply dependent. If the ERO_2crit is low (e.g., 40%), this means that some tissue regions would become anoxic when less than half of the delivered O_2 is being extracted from blood. In contrast, a high ERO_2crit (75%) would reflect a more efficient use of a limited O_2 supply.

An empirical characteristic of the tissue DO_2–VO_2 relationship is that O_2 extraction continues to increase even after delivery falls below the critical point. The continued increase in extraction is not adequate to maintain VO_2, but it still increases. The ability to continue to increase ERO_2 below the critical point, due in part to further decreases in PO_2 in tissue regions that still consume O_2, may also reflect adjustments in microvascular blood flow that improve capillary O_2 delivery in relation to O_2 demand. These concepts are examined next.

Microvascular Matching of Capillary O₂ Delivery in Relation to Vo₂

Ideally, each capillary in a tissue should be supplied with a blood flow that is proportional to the O_2 demand of the cells it supports. Hence, tissue regions with greater metabolic demand receive relatively more blood flow than regions with low rates of ATP utilization. Ideally, localized increases or decreases in metabolic demand for O_2 within the tissue should be accompanied by a redistribution of capillary blood flow in accordance with the altered needs. However, the extent to which real tissues can achieve this efficiency of O_2 distribution is limited (Connolly and colleagues, 1997). Analogous to ventilation–perfusion inequality in the lung, heterogeneity of systemic capillary blood flow relative to oxygen demand will decrease the efficiency of oxygen extraction (ERO_2crit) by the tissue. Optimal matching of O_2 delivery in relation to O_2 demand is less important when oxygen delivery is high because all tissue regions receive O_2 in excess of that needed to maintain metabolism.

The importance of microvascular matching of DO_2 and VO_2 is illustrated by examining the consequences of a mismatch in DO_2 relative to O_2 demand as blood flow into a tissue is progressively decreased (Fig. 5.11). When some capillaries are overperfused and others are underperfused relative to the O_2 demands of the cells they support, tissue regions with low DO_2 relative to VO_2 will become O_2 supply limited at a point at which other regions are still excessively perfused. This will result in the onset of O_2 supply-limited metabolism at a point at which the O_2 extraction ratio is still low. If the extent of this mismatch is small, it can be difficult to detect by inspection of a DO_2–VO_2 plot, which is mostly affected near the critical point. In the face of experimental error, these subtle changes can be difficult to identify until the extent of heterogeneity is large.

Effects of O₂ Shunting within Tissues

In the lung, intrapulmonary shunt diminishes gas exchange efficiency by admixing desaturated venous blood with oxygenated blood leaving the alveolar capillaries. By analogy, transit of blood through nonnutrient channels will diminish the efficiency of tissue oxygen extraction. The consequences of systemic shunt on the DO_2–VO_2 relationship are shown in Figure 5.12. Theoretically, shunting may consist of blood flow in thoroughfare channels that bypass tissue capillaries, or it may occur by the countercurrent diffusion of oxygen between arterial and venous vessels in close proximity. One example of this occurs in the kidney, in which oxygen shunting between descending and ascending medullary capillaries may take place. In either case, decreases in ERO_2crit result, rendering tissue metabolism more vulnerable to decreases in tissue oxygen delivery.

FACTORS AND INTERVENTIONS THAT INFLUENCE TISSUE O₂ EXTRACTION EFFICIENCY

In experimental studies, a number of different interventions have been shown to affect tissue oxygen extraction ability, as reflected by changes in the ERO_2crit. A common characteristic of these interventions is their ability to influence or alter the microvascular control of blood flow distributions. These interventions include experimental sepsis, which induces hypotension and degrades ERO_2crit at the tissue and the whole body levels (Nelson and associates, 1988). Certain inhaled anesthetic agents also diminish tissue O_2 extraction ability, as does hypothermia, most likely by affecting vascular tone. Interestingly, the degree of sympathetic vasoconstrictor activity has a major effect on the ability of local tissues to extract O_2 from a limited supply (Maginniss and coworkers, 1994). This was illustrated in an experimental preparation in which blood flow to a small region of intestine or skeletal muscle was locally controlled with a pump, allowing it to be adjusted independent of the level of systemic delivery. These studies showed that very low ERO_2crit values in the isolated tissue were obtained if systemic blood pressure and cardiac output were bounding, whereas much higher efficiency of local extraction (i.e., a high ERO_2crit) was achieved if systemic blood pressure and cardiac output were lowered to the point that sympathetic tone was significantly increased. Hence, high sympathetic tone contributed to a high critical extraction in tissues, whereas low sympathetic activity undermined the local ability of tissues to efficiently extract oxygen. This response reflects the dual nature of microvascular control by extrinsic (neurohumorally mediated) and intrinsic tissue microvascular control mechanisms. When sympathetic vasomotor tone is low as a result of high cardiac output and blood pressure, tissue microvascular tone permits significant flow through nonnutrient pathways, resulting in a poor oxygen extraction ability within a small region of tissue in which DO_2 is lowered. In contrast, if cardiac output is lowered to the point where sympathetic activity is highly activated, the resulting increases in microvascular tone effectively limit blood flow to nonnutrient vessels, resulting in a high ERO_2crit at the tissue level.

ANAEROBIC METABOLISM AND LACTIC ACID PRODUCTION

When blood flow to a tissue decreases, the O_2 extraction ratio increases as the venous O_2 content decreases. At the same time, the venous CO_2 content increases because CO_2 produced by the tissue begins to accumulate. When tissue O_2 delivery falls below the critical threshold, anaerobic glycolysis occurs as cells attempt to maintain ATP production. The increased production of lactic acid causes a metabolic acidosis, which is buffered by various systems including bicarbonate. The buffering of lactic acid by bicarbonate creates a new source of CO_2 production, which adds to the CO_2 produced by tissue metabolic activity. Hence, at O_2 deliveries below the critical point there are two potential sources of CO_2 resulting from continued aerobic respiration and lactate buffering. Theoretically, one could detect the onset of O_2 supply-dependent metabolism by measuring the O_2 delivery where the arteriovenous CO_2 content difference increases as a result of lactate buffering. This is analogous to measuring the lactate threshold during exercise by detecting the additional CO_2 released by the buffering of lactic acid above the anaerobic threshold.

However, analysis has shown that most of the increase in tissue PCO_2 during hypoperfusion is due to the decrease in tissue blood flow (the Fick relationship), whereas only a small fraction

can be attributed to the release of CO_2 from the buffering of metabolic acidosis (Raza and Schlichtig, 2000). During hypoxemic hypoxia, when blood flow to the tissue remains constant while arterial O_2 saturation decreases, the small increase in tissue (or venous) PCO_2 below the critical DO_2 is technically difficult to measure. This problem in detecting the increase in $PvCO_2$ below the critical point arises because (1) the arteriovenous PCO_2 difference is already small because blood flow is high, and (2) increases in CO_2 due to lactate buffering tend to be offset by decreases in CO_2 production as tissue VO_2 decreases. Therefore, although it is theoretically possible to identify the critical DO_2 by measuring the arteriovenous PCO_2 difference, in practice this approach does not work.

Gastric Tonometry as an Assessment of Pathophysiological Hypoxia

Gastric tonometry, a relatively noninvasive method for assessing gastric mucosal tissue PCO_2, has been used by some investigators attempting to detect O_2 supply-dependent conditions in the gut (Gutierrez and colleagues, 1992). In this method, a drug is administered to inhibit acid secretion by gastric parietal cells, and a nasogastric tube fitted with a thin-walled balloon is advanced into the stomach and filled with saline. After allowing time for CO_2 in the balloon to equilibrate with gastric contents and the gastric mucosa, the saline is removed and its PCO_2 is measured. Simultaneously, an arterial blood gas sample is obtained to determine arterial PCO_2. An abnormally large arterial–gastric PCO_2 difference has been interpreted as an indicator of O_2 supply-dependent metabolism in the gut. However, as described previously, the Fick relationship predicts that tissue PCO_2 should increase when tissue blood flow is decreased, whether or not O_2 delivery is below the critical point. Moreover, increases in PCO_2 would not be expected during hypoxemic hypoxia, even when O_2 delivery is inadequate. Thus, although large increases in the arterial–gastric mucosa PCO_2 difference indicate the possibility of gastric hypoperfusion, the absence of a significantly increased PCO_2 difference is a poor indicator of whether oxygen delivery to the mucosa is adequate to prevent anaerobic metabolism.

DOES OXYGEN SUPPLY LIMIT CELLULAR METABOLIC ACTIVITY IN CRITICAL ILLNESS?

Early studies suggested that patients with acute respiratory distress syndrome or multiple organ failure exhibited profound O_2 supply dependency at the whole body level, even when systemic O_2 delivery was within the normal range (Powers and associates, 1973). This conclusion was based on the observation that whole body VO_2 varied significantly as systemic DO_2 was experimentally adjusted by altering the level of positive end-expiratory pressure. This failure to exhibit the expected plateau in oxygen consumption as DO_2 was adjusted can be interpreted three different ways. Some investigators believed that critical illness undermined the regulation of tissue oxygen supply, such that some tissue regions were severely hypoxic, whereas other regions were excessively perfused. A second interpretation was that cells in these patients were impaired in their ability to utilize oxygen even when normal levels of tissue PO_2 were present. This would represent a form of metabolic inhibition that presumably could be overcome by increasing tissue O_2 to "supranormal" levels. A third interpretation was that the findings reflected measurement artifacts due to the shared use of cardiac output in the DO_2 and VO_2 calculations (Archie, 1981).

Subsequent studies provided new information that has altered the interpretation of the early findings. First, it was noted that some of the apparent correlation between DO_2 and VO_2 could have resulted from the numerical interdependence between O_2 delivery (calculated from measured cardiac output and blood O_2 contents) and O_2 uptake (calculated from the Fick relationship using the same measured cardiac output and O_2 contents). The use of the measured cardiac output in DO_2 and VO_2 could conceivably create a spurious relationship between DO_2 and VO_2, manifested as the apparent slope in a plot of O_2 uptake as a function of delivery. Important insight came from studies of critically ill patients during termination of life support (Ronco and coworkers, 1991, 1993). In these studies, VO_2 and DO_2 were measured independently, allowing the relationship between VO_2 and DO_2 to be defined over the physiological and pathophysiological ranges of oxygen delivery and allowing the critical point to be defined in each patient. The patients demonstrated the expected plateau in VO_2 at higher levels of O_2 delivery and decreases in VO_2 below the critical point. At the critical delivery, O_2 extraction ratios of approximately 60% were observed—similar to the value typically observed in normal animals. These findings therefore contradicted earlier reports of pathophysiological O_2 supply dependency in critically ill patients, although this conclusion is limited to terminally ill patients during withdrawal of life support.

If O_2 consumption in some tissue regions becomes limited by O_2 supply during critical illness, and if this is a significant factor influencing the morbidity and/or mortality associated with the disease, then clinical management should be aimed at optimizing systemic O_2 delivery in order to maintain tissue metabolism. Prospective studies have tested this question by comparing outcomes in patients managed according to normal clinical practice relative to other patients who were managed by administration of fluids and/or inotropic agents so as to maintain oxygen delivery at a targeted high level. Prospective, randomized controlled clinical studies indicate that some patient groups benefit from such treatment, whereas others do not. In high-risk patients undergoing surgery, management aimed at maintaining O_2 delivery produced a significant reduction in mortality (Boyd and colleagues, 1993). On the other hand, groups of critically ill patients who were maintained at higher levels of O_2 delivery failed to demonstrate improved outcome, and in some cases this treatment may have been detrimental (Hayes and associates, 1994). One interpretation of these results is that periods of relative hypoperfusion associated with major surgery, which were presumably prevented by supporting systemic O_2 transport, represent an important contribution to the morbidity and mortality during the postoperative period. In contrast, patients who have already developed significant organ dysfunction do not appear to benefit from management aimed at optimizing systemic oxygen transport. Moreover, efforts to achieve excessive levels of DO_2 transport in critically ill patients may introduce complications that worsen the morbidity associated with the syndrome.

These findings cannot rule out the possibility that patients with multiple organ failure may still suffer from oxygen supply-limited metabolism in some tissues during their illness. If O_2

supply-dependent metabolism does develop, it seems likely that it is limited to relatively small regions of tissue, and that the supply-dependent state may only occur transiently. If so, then the changes in VO_2 at the whole body level would be very difficult to detect by conventional methods. Some insight may come from animal studies showing that severe sepsis is associated with a significant impairment in the ability of specific tissues such as gut to extract oxygen efficiently, whereas other tissues such as skeletal muscle do not become impaired. In animal studies, the decrement in oxygen extraction efficiency was evident at the level of the small intestine but more difficult to detect at the whole body level. It seems reasonable to conclude that patients with critical illness may exhibit impairment in the regulation of tissue oxygen delivery, manifested by an increase in the heterogeneity of oxygen delivery with respect to oxygen need. This may not be sufficient to create O_2 supply-dependent conditions when systemic oxygen delivery is normal because even relatively poorly supplied regions would receive adequate O_2 supply as long as the systemic delivery is within the normal range. However, these patients would be at increased risk for sustaining ischemic tissue injury in cases in which cardiac output declines because poorly perfused tissue regions could be forced into supply-dependent conditions when overall delivery declines. To the extent that patients with critical illness develop an increased heterogeneity in systemic O_2 delivery, it would be important to prevent the onset of systemic hypoperfusion states in order to preserve adequate O_2 supply to all tissue regions. Future progress in clarifying the adequacy of oxygen delivery in critically ill patients will require the development of novel methods capable of determining the existence of pathophysiological hypoxia within intact organs.

SUGGESTED READING

Archie JP Jr: Mathematic coupling of data: A common source of error. Ann Surg 1981;193:296–303.

Boyd O, Grounds RM, Bennett ED: A randomized clinical trial of the effect of deliberate perioperative increase of oxygen delivery on mortality in high-risk surgical patients. JAMA 1993;270(22):2699–2707.

Cain SM: Oxygen delivery and uptake in dogs during anemic and hypoxic hypoxia. J Appl Physiol 1977;42:228–234.

Connolly HV, Maginniss LA, Schumacker PT: Transit time heterogeneity in canine small intestine: Significance for oxygen transport. J Clin Invest 1997;99:228–238.

Gutierrez G, Palizas F, Doglio G, et al: Gastric intramucosal pH as a therapeutic index of tissue oxygenation in critically ill patients. Lancet 1992;339:195–199.

Hayes MA, Timmins AC, Yau EH, et al: Elevation of systemic oxygen delivery in the treatment of critically ill patients. N Engl J Med 1994;330:1717–1722.

Jones DP: Intracellular diffusion gradients of O_2 and ATP. Am J Physiol 1986;250:C663–C675.

Maginniss LA, et al: Adrenergic vasoconstriction augments tissue oxygen extraction during reductions in O_2 delivery. J Appl Physiol 1994;76(4):1454–1461.

Nelson DP, Samsel RW, Wood LD, Schumacker PT: Pathological supply dependence of systemic and intestinal O_2 uptake during endotoxemia. J Appl Physiol 1988;64:2410–2419.

Powers SR Jr, Mannal R, Neclerio M, et al: Physiologic consequences of positive end-expiratory pressure. Ann Surg 1973;3:265–271.

Raza O, Schlichtig R: Metabolic component of intestinal PCO(2) during dysoxia. J Appl Physiol 2000;89(6):2422–2429.

Ronco JJ, Fenwick JC, Phang PT, et al: O_2 delivery, O_2 consumption and the critical O_2 delivery threshold for anaerobic metabolism in septic and nonseptic dying patients. Am Rev Respir Dis 1991;143:A82.

Ronco JJ, Fenwick JC, Tweeddale, et al: Identification of the critical oxygen delivery for anaerobic metabolism in critically ill septic and nonseptic humans. JAMA 1993;270:1724–1730.

Schumacker PT, Cain SM: The concept of a critical oxygen delivery. Intensive Care Med 1987;13:223–229.

Schumacker PT, Samsel RW: Analysis of oxygen delivery and uptake relationships in the Krogh tissue model. J Appl Physiol 1989;67:1234–1244.

Wilson DF, Erecinska M, Drown C, Silver IA: Effect of oxygen tension on cellular energetics. Am J Physiol 1977;233:C135–C140.

Chapter 6

Monitoring and Treatment of Pain, Anxiety, and Delirium in the ICU

Margaret A. Pisani and E. Wesley Ely

KEY POINTS

- Pain may often be underrecognized and inadequately managed. Insufficient pain management can lead to emotional distress and depression, delirium, anxiety, sleep disturbances, and physical disabilities, as well as increased health costs.
- Pain in the intensive care unit (ICU) may come from many sources, such as the particular illness, surgery, trauma, or the associated medical care; an important source of pain in the ICU may be related to procedures.
- Preventing pain is more effective than treating established pain.
- There is evidence that agitation may have a deleterious effect on ICU patient outcomes.
- Not all anxious patients will exhibit agitation. Some may become withdrawn and fearful. In all patients with anxiety and agitation, the first priority is to identify and treat any precipitating physiological abnormality, such as pain, hypoxemia, hypercarbia, hypotension, hypoglycemia, and withdrawal from alcohol or drugs.
- Delirium is extremely common in the ICU due to many characteristics of ICU patients, including advanced age, critical illness, and multiple medical procedures and interventions, as well as the interaction between host factors, the acute illness, and iatrogenic or environmental factors.
- Clinical practice guidelines of the Society of Critical Care Medicine recommend routine daily monitoring of delirium in all mechanically ventilated patients.

Patients admitted to an intensive care unit (ICU) often experience agitation, anxiety, pain, and sleep deprivation. Delirium is a frequent contributor to ICU agitation, with an incidence that varies from 30% in open-heart surgery patients to 87% in medical ICU patients. More than 90% of critically ill patients receive medications for sedation and analgesia during their ICU stay. Both inadequate and excessive sedation and analgesia have a risk for adverse outcomes, including delirium, prolonged mechanical ventilation, increased ICU length of stay, and increased diagnostic testing. Finding a balance between patient comfort and oversedation can be difficult. This chapter reviews what is known about monitoring and treatment of pain, anxiety, and delirium in the ICU setting.

PAIN

Assessment

The International Association for the Study of Pain defines pain as "an unpleasant sensory and emotional experience associated with actual or potential tissue damage, or described in terms of such damage." Pain may often be underrecognized and inadequately managed. Insufficient pain management can lead to emotional distress and depression, delirium, anxiety, sleep disturbances, and physical disabilities, as well as increased health costs. The Joint Commission for the Accreditation of Health Organizations has mandated that pain assessment be the "fifth vital sign."

Pain in the ICU may come from many sources, such as the particular illness, surgery, trauma, or the associated medical care, including phlebotomy, chest tubes, dressing changes, endotracheal tubes, restraints, or suctioning. An important source of pain in the ICU is related to procedures, but research in this area has been limited. Procedural pain is described as "the unpleasant sensory and emotional experience that arises from actual or potential tissue damage associated with diagnostic or treatment procedures." Studies have shown that between 22% and 70% of patients remember having moderate to severe pain during their ICU stay. In a study of adult ICU patients receiving mechanical ventilation, two thirds remembered the ICU stay and the endotracheal tube and reported pain, fear, anxiety, lack of sleep, feeling tense, inability to communicate, lack of control, nightmares, and loneliness. For adult patients in the ICU, one of the most painful and distressing procedures was turning, a frequent procedure that is generally performed without premedication. Box 6.1 lists common behaviors that indicate pain in adults.

There is a limited literature addressing pain assessment in the ICU. In this setting, specific barriers that may interfere with effective pain management (e.g., mechanical ventilation, delirium, and the need for balancing hemodynamic stability) exist. Patient self-reporting has been the standard criterion for pain assessment. In the non-ICU setting, the recommendation is that three attempts should be made to elicit self-reporting of pain before assuming that a patient cannot provide such a report. This may be difficult in the ICU, where patients are critically ill, often intubated, and have altered levels of consciousness or

Adapted from the AGS Panel of Persistent Pain in Older Persons: The management of persistent pain in older persons. J Am Geriatr Soc 2002;50(6):S205–S224.

delirium. When patient self-reports are not available, behavioral indicators of pain, such as splinting and facial expression, as well as physiologic variables, such as heart rate, blood pressure, respiratory rate and pattern, and diaphoresis, can be used to guide analgesic needs and response to therapy.

Tools to evaluate pain should be specific to age, disease state, and site of pain. Assessment should evaluate the location, characteristics, aggravating and alleviating factors, and intensity of the pain. A number of tools that are quick and easy to use have been developed to quantify pain (Box 6.2).

The Visual Analogue Scale (VAS) consists of a 10-cm horizontal line with descriptions at either end, from "no pain" to "severe pain" to "worst pain ever." The VAS is reliable and valid in many patient populations, but it has not been tested in an ICU population and performs less well in the elderly. Effective use of the VAS requires motor responsiveness and the ability to understand and follow directions, so it may not be appropriate for many critically ill patients. In unresponsive patients, however, the VAS can be used by caregivers to estimate patient

Box 6.2 **Pain Rating Scales**

Visual Analogue Scale
Numeric Rating Scale
Faces Scale
McGill Pain Questionnaire

comfort. The Numeric Rating Scale (NRS) is a 0- to 10-point scale with 0 representing no pain and 10 representing the worst pain. If a patient complains of pain, he or she is asked, "On a scale of 0 to 10, with 0 being no pain, and 10 being the worst pain imaginable, how do you rank your pain?" The NRS is a valid instrument, correlates with the VAS, and is similarly easy to administer but also requires a cognitively intact patient. The NRS has been used in both cardiac and surgical patients and is useful in both young and older individuals.

The Faces Scale is a pain scale that consists of happy to frowning to grimacing faces and does not require verbal capacity to complete. This scale was developed as a self-reporting pain tool for children. There is moderate agreement between the Faces Scale and the VAS in adult patients. The McGill Pain Questionnaire is a multidimensional tool and has been validated for use with older adults and patients in ICUs. This tool uses descriptive words, such as throbbing, aching, and tiring, to rate the character and quality of the pain. It is designed to capture sensory and affective components of the pain.

Surrogates can be another source of information regarding pain in a critically ill patient. Both family members and other surrogates have been evaluated for their ability to assess pain in noncommunicative ICU patients. Seventy-three percent of the time, surrogates could accurately estimate the presence or absence of pain, but they were able to accurately describe the degree of pain in only 53% of patients.

Currently endorsed critical care clinical practice guidelines recommend that pain assessment and response to therapy should be performed on a regular basis using a scale appropriate to the patient population and systematically documented. Patient report should be obtained whenever possible and use of the NRS or VAS is recommended. For patients who cannot communicate, pain should be assessed through subjective observation of pain-related behaviors (see Box 6.1) and by physiological indicators, such as heart rate, blood pressure, and respiratory rate. Changes in these parameters should be monitored following analgesic therapy. Health care providers should also anticipate events that are painful, such as surgery, intubation, and other procedures, and provide appropriate preemptive pain treatment.

Pharmacologic Management

The pharmacologic management of pain is complex and includes nonsteroidal anti-inflammatory drugs (NSAIDs), acetaminophen, and opiates. Agents for pain control should be selected based on their pharmacology and potential for side effects (Table 6.1). Nonopioid analgesics, such as acetaminophen, may offer effective relief for musculoskeletal pain, back pain, and soft tissue injury pain. The role of acetaminophen in the ICU is limited to relieving mild pain or as an antipyretic. It should not be used in patients with liver dysfunction and maximum dosing should not exceed 4000 mg per day. In patients with a significant alcohol history or poor nutritional status, dosage of acetaminophen should not exceed 2000 mg per day.

NSAIDs may be used when acetaminophen is not effective. They provide analgesia via the nonselective, competitive inhibition of cyclooxygenase, an enzyme in the inflammatory cascade. Side effects from NSAIDs are common and include gastrointestinal bleeding, bleeding secondary to platelet inhibition, renal impairment, and sodium retention. NSAIDs may reduce opioid

Table 6.1 Pharmacology of Analgesics

Agent	Equianalgesic Dose (IV)	Half-Life (hr)	Metabolic Pathway	Active Metabolites	Adverse Effects
Morphine	10 mg	3–7	Oxidation	Yes	Histamine release
Fentanyl	200 µg	1.5–6	Glucuronidation	No, parent drug accumulates	Rigidity with high doses
Hydromorphone	1.5 mg	2–3	Glucuronidation	None	—
Acetaminophen	—	2	Conjugation	—	—
Ibuprofen	—	1.8–2.5	Oxidation	None	Bleeding, GI and renal adverse effects

requirements, however, and their use has not been well studied in the ICU setting.

Opioids are the preferred agents for pain control in the ICU. They induce analgesia by interacting with both central and peripheral opioid receptors. The agents most commonly used include morphine, fentanyl, and hydropmorphone. There are no comparative trials of opioids in critically ill patients. Morphine is an excellent pain reliever and also increases venous and arteriolar capacitance. Side effects include hypotension, nausea, mood disturbances, ileus, histamine production, and respiratory depression. Fentanyl is a synthetic opioid that has a faster onset of action than morphine and does not cause histamine release. Accordingly, it may be preferred over morphine in patients with hemodynamic instability. Hydromorphone is a semisynthetic opioid with minimal hemodynamic effects, but respiratory depression is more common. Opioids have an increased half-life in older patients and may possibly have a greater analgesic effect. A prophylactic bowel regimen to prevent constipation should be initiated in ICU patients requiring opioids.

Preventing pain is more effective than treating established pain. A pain management plan and goal of therapy should be established for each patient, and this plan should be reevaluated as the clinical condition of the patient changes. Analgesics should be administered on a continuous or scheduled intermittent basis, with supplemental bolus dosing as required. Intramuscular administration is not recommended in the ICU due to the possibility of altered perfusion and variable absorption. If a continuous infusion is used, daily awakening from analgesia should be considered to allow for more effective analgesic titration and lower total drug dose. Daily awakening is associated with a shorter duration of ventilation and a shorter ICU stay.

Psychological factors influence pain perception. Early control of depression may assist in effective pain management, especially for patients with a prolonged ICU stay when the likelihood of depression is increased.

ANXIETY AND AGITATION

Assessment

Causes of anxiety in ICU patients are multifactorial and include an inability to communicate, continuous noise, ambient lighting, and excessive stimulation due to frequent monitoring of vital signs, repositioning, lack of mobility, and inadequate analgesia. Sleep deprivation is reported in more than 50% of ICU patients and may also cause or increase anxiety. Anxiety may be reduced by frequent reorientation, along with maintaining patient comfort with both pharmacologic and nonpharmacologic means.

Agitation is common in ICU patients and can be caused by factors such as anxiety, pain, delirium, and adverse drug effects. Not all anxious patients will exhibit agitation; some may become withdrawn and fearful. In all patients with anxiety and agitation, the first priority is to identify and treat any precipitating physiologic abnormality, such as pain, hypoxemia, hypercarbia, hypotension, hypoglycemia, and withdrawal from alcohol or drugs.

There is evidence that agitation may have a deleterious effect on ICU patient outcomes. This effect may be secondary to patient ventilator dysynchrony, an increase in oxygen consumption, and inadvertent removal of catheters or other devices. Frequent assessment of the level of agitation and sedation is important in the ICU setting. Many scales have been developed and applied to patients in the ICU (Table 6.2).

The first scale to assess sedation in the ICU was developed by Ramsay in 1974. This scale is a 6-point system that ranges from 1 (anxious or agitated) to 6 (unarousable). This scale has excellent interrater agreement and good agreement with objective measures of sedation. The Ramsay Scale has no behavioral descriptors to help distinguish among the various levels, and it was used for many years with no real validation against neurological constructs or clinical outcomes.

The Riker Sedation–Agitation Scale (SAS) provides a symmetric approach to grading patient behavior. There are three

Table 6.2 Subjective Tools to Assess Sedation

Instrument	Description
Ramsay Scale	Six-point system ranging from 1 (anxious or agitated) to 6 (unarousable). No behavioral descriptors. Excellent interrater agreement ($\kappa = 0.88$).
Riker Sedation–Agitation Scale (SAS)	Seven-level scale with three severity levels each for sedation and agitation and one level for calm, awake patients. Excellent interrater reliability ($\kappa = 0.85$–0.93). Shown to detect changes in sedation over time.
Motor Activity Assessment Scale (MAAS)	Developed from the Riker SAS. Seven-level scale with three severity levels each for sedation and agitation and one level for calm, awake patients. Behavioral descriptors are provided at each level to assist in patient classification. Good interrater reliability ($\kappa = 0.83$).
Richmond Agitation–Sedation Scale (RASS)	Ten-level scale ranging from combative to unarousable. Four levels of agitation and five levels of sedation and one level for alert and calm. Uses the duration of eye contact following verbal stimulation as the principal means of titrating sedation. Excellent interrater reliability ($\kappa = 0.91$). Excellent discrimination between levels of consciousness compared to neuropsychiatric expert reference standard.

Table 6.3 The Richmond Agitation–Sedation Scale (RASS)			
Score	Term	Description	
+4	Combative	Overtly combative, violent, immediate danger to staff	
+3	Very agitated	Pulls or removes tubes or catheters; aggressive	
+2	Agitated	Frequent nonpurposeful movement, fights ventilator	
+1	Restless	Anxious but movements not aggressive or vigorous	
0	Alert and calm		
−1	Drowsy	Not fully alert but has sustained awakening; eye opening/eye contact to voice (>10 sec)	} Verbal stimulation
−2	Light sedation	Briefly awakens with eye contact to voice (<10 sec)	
−3	Moderate sedation	Movement or eye opening to voice but no eye contact	
−4	Deep sedation	No response to voice, but movement or eye opening to physical stimulation	} Physical stimulation
−5	Unarousable	No response to voice or physical stimulation	

Procedure for RASS assessment
1. Observe patient.
   Patient is alert, restless, or agitated.   Score 0 to +4
2. If not alert, state patient's name and say to open eyes and look at speaker.
   Patient awakens with sustained eye opening and eye contact.   Score −1
   Patient awakens with eye opening and eye contact, but it is not sustained.   Score −2
   Patient has any movement in response to voice but no eye contact.   Score −3
3. When no response to verbal stimulation, physically stimulate patient by shaking shoulder and/or rubbing sternum.
   Patient has any response to physical stimulation.   Score −4
   Patient has no response to any stimulation.   Score −5

levels of severity of sedation, three levels of agitation, and one level for calm, awake patients. The SAS also has excellent interrater reliability and has been validated against other subjective scales as well as against the bispectral index (BIS). The SAS is one of the most widely used sedation scales due to its ease of use and the nature of its validation studies. The Motor Activity Assessment Scale (MAAS) was developed from the SAS. It is a seven-level scale with behavioral descriptors for each level to help clinicians classify patients. MAAS has good interrater reliability and has been validated against the VAS and clinical parameters such as vital signs.

The Richmond Agitation–Sedation Scale (RASS) is a 10-point rating scale with four levels for agitation, five for sedation, and one for calm, awake patients. This scale was designed with the anchor centered at level 0, positive ratings for agitation, and negative ratings for sedation (Table 6.3). Unique features of the RASS are that it is the only scale with a published procedure for the assessment (which takes 10 sec), and it is also the only scale that completely separates ratings according to patient's response to verbal and then to physical stimulation. The RASS uses the duration of eye contact following verbal stimulation as the principal means of titrating sedation. This sedation scale has excellent interrater reliability and has been validated against neuropsychological reference standard raters (criterion validity) and five methods of construct validity, including an attention screening examination, quantity of psychoactive drugs, successful extubation, the Glasgow Coma Scale, and the BIS. It is the only sedation scale validated for use over time in patients in the ICU, which is exactly how these tools are intended to be used.

Computer-processed electroencephalographic (EEG) technology such as the BIS has also been developed to provide an objective assessment of the depth of sedation. The BIS incorporates several components of the processed EEG that change with varying depths of sedation. Extensive data suggest that BIS values are descriptive of patient wakefulness and responsiveness in the operating room. In ICU patients, BIS is associated with the degree of procedural recall and is correlated with subjective assessments. BIS may be useful when titrating sedation therapy, especially during neuromuscular blockade, although clinical trials demonstrating improvement in outcomes are still needed before such monitoring will become routine outside of the operating room.

Treatment

The use of sedatives is important in maintaining patient comfort and safety in the ICU. Sedatives should be administered to achieve predefined sedative goals for the patient. A common target level of sedation in the ICU is a calm patient who can be easily aroused while maintaining a normal sleep–wake cycle. Patients requiring mechanical ventilation may require deeper levels of sedation, but it is a common misconception that every mechanically ventilated patient should be sedated. The desired level of sedation should be defined on ICU admission and reevaluated on a daily basis as the patient's clinical condition changes.

Sedative–hypnotic medications are used to control of anxiety and sedation (Table 6.4). Benzodiazepines produce antegrade amnesia and block acquisition and encoding of new information and unpleasant experiences. They lack any analgesic properties and vary in their potency, onset, duration of action, volume of distribution, metabolism, and presence or absence of active metabolites. Patient-specific factors can affect the intensity and duration of activity of benzodiazepines. Careful attention must be paid to individual patient titration based on age, hepatic and renal function, alcohol abuse, and concurrent drug therapy. Titrating medications to specific and clinically determined "target" sedation scale levels (e.g., based on oxygenation and tolerance of mechanical ventilation) is the recommended method of choosing the quantity of sedatives, although this is far from objective. In addition, many suggest that when patients are "intolerant" of mechanical ventilation, the ventilator should be adjusted to achieve patient comfort rather than "adjusting" the patient with medications. Relief of anxiety and maintenance of

Table 6.4 Pharmacology of Selected Sedatives

Agent	Onset of Action (min)	Half-Life (hr)	Metabolic Pathway	Active Metabolite	Adverse Effects
Diazepam	2–5	20–120	Desmethylation and hydroxylation	Yes—prolonged sedation	Phlebitis
Lorazepam	5–20	8–15	Glucuronidation	None	Solvent-related acidosis/renal failure in high doses
Midazolam	2–5	3–11	Oxidation	Yes—prolonged sedation, worse with renal failure	
Propofol	1–2	26–32	Oxidation	None	Elevated triglycerides, pain at injection site

adequate sedation should be attempted with intermittent dosing of benzodiazepines. Patients who require frequent dosing to maintain the desired effect may benefit from a continuous infusion, but care should be taken to use the lowest effective infusion rate with continual reassessment of the dosing needs. Benzodiazepines can accumulate and may produce oversedation.

Diazepam has rapid onset and awakening after single doses of the drug. Its disadvantage is the presence of long-acting metabolites. It is not recommended for use in patients requiring extended anxiolysis or sedation in the ICU. Lorazepam has a slower onset of action, making it less useful for the treatment of acute agitation. It does have less drug–drug interactions due to its metabolism by glucuronidation. Polyethylene glycol and propylene glycol, which are the solvents used for lorazepam, have been implicated as the cause of reversible acute tubular necrosis, lactic acidosis, and hyperosmolar states after prolonged high-dose infusions (18–25 mg/hr). Lorazepam can be administered by bolus or continuous infusion. Midazolam has a rapid onset of action and a short duration when given as a bolus dose. The rapid onset makes midazolam the preferred drug for treating acutely agitated patients. Prolonged sedation may occur with continuous infusions due to an active metabolite.

Propofol is an intravenous anesthetic agent with sedative and hypnotic properties at lower doses than used for general anesthesia. Propofol produces a similar degree of anesthesia compared to benzodiazepines (and, indeed, both classes of agents have a similar mechanism of action as γ-aminobutyric acid (GABA)-mimetic agents acting primarily at the ventrolateral preoptic area in the anterior hypothalamus). Propofol has a rapid onset and short duration once it is discontinued. Adverse effects include hypotension, which may limit its use in septic patients, bradycardia, and hypertriglyceridemia and lactic acidosis with prolonged use. Propofol is usually reserved for situations in which a short duration (e.g., less than 48 hr) of sedation is anticipated. It is also useful for sedating patients with fulminant hepatic failure who are awaiting liver transplantation, in whom frequent assessment of the stage of hepatic encephalopathy is necessary.

DELIRIUM

The *Diagnostic and Statistical Manual of Mental Disorders, Fourth Edition* criteria for the diagnosis of delirium are summarized in Box 6.3.

The prevalence of delirium in ICU cohort studies ranges from 20% to 80% depending on the characteristics of the patient population and the instrument used. Patients with delirium can be hypoactive, hyperactive, or present a mixed picture with periods of hyperactive and hypoactive delirium. A study on delirium subtypes from a cohort of 613 ventilated and nonventilated ICU patients found that among patients who developed delirium, pure hyperactive delirium was rare (<5%), whereas hypoactive and mixed types of delirium were the predominant subtypes (~45% each). The hypoactive subtype was significantly more common in older patients than in the young. The risk factors for and clinical implications of these subtypes are the subject of ongoing investigations.

Pathophysiology

Delirium is thought to be related to imbalances in the synthesis, release, and inactivation of neurotransmitters modulating the control of cognitive function, behavior, and mood. Three neurotransmitter systems involved in the pathophysiology of delirium are dopamine, GABA, and acetylcholine. Whereas dopamine increases excitability of neurons, GABA and acetylcholine decrease neuronal excitability. An imbalance in one or multiple of these neurotransmitters results in neuronal instability and unpredictable neurotransmission. In general, an excess of dopamine and depletion of acetylcholine are two major physiological problems believed to be central to delirium. Other neurotransmitter systems thought to be involved in the development of delirium are serotonin imbalance, endorphin hyperfunction, and increased central noradrenergic activity.

Risk Factors

Several studies have assessed risk factors for developing delirium in postoperative patients, medical admissions, oncology patients, and patients with hip fractures. Very few studies have

---

Box 6.3 *Diagnostic and Statistical Manual of Mental Disorders, Fourth Edition* **Criteria for the Diagnosis of Delirium**

1. Disturbance of consciousness, with reduced ability to focus, sustain, or shift attention.
2. A change in cognition or the development of a perceptual disturbance that is not better accounted for by a preexisting dementia.
3. The disturbance develops after a short period of time and tends to fluctuate.
4. Evidence from history, physical examination, or laboratory findings that the disturbance is caused by the physiologic consequences of a general medical condition.

reported risk factors for developing delirium in ICU patients. Box 6.4 lists risk factors associated with delirium in a variety of settings. Delirium is extremely common in the ICU due to many characteristics of ICU patients, including advanced age, critical illness, and multiple medical procedures and interventions, as well as the interaction between host factors, the acute illness, and iatrogenic or environmental factors. Excessive noise may contribute to alterations in mental status in the ICU. The Environmental Protection Agency recommends that noise levels in a hospital be kept below 45 dB during the day and below 35 dB at night. Sound levels within an ICU average above 50 dB, with levels above 70 dB occurring every 9 minutes, even at night. Psychoactive drugs are the leading iatrogenic risk factor for complications in hospitalized patients. Benzodiazepines, narcotics, and other psychoactive drugs are associated with a 3- to 11-fold increased relative risk for the development of delirium.

Delirium and Outcomes

Delirium has been associated with poor outcomes in hospitalized patients, including increased length of stay (Fig. 6.1), institutionalization, and greater mortality (Fig. 6.2). Delirium has also consistently been associated with poor functional recovery after acute illness and surgery. Cognitive impairment interferes with weaning from mechanical ventilation, predisposes to the development of nosocomial pneumonia, and increases length of stay.

The development of delirium is associated with a threefold increased risk of death after controlling for preexisting comorbidities, severity of illness, coma, and the use of sedative and analgesic medications. These data also showed that delirium is

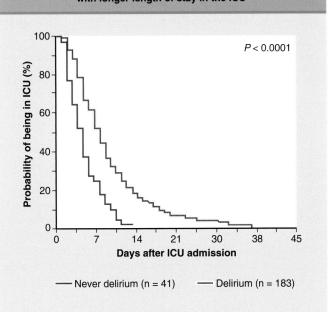

A

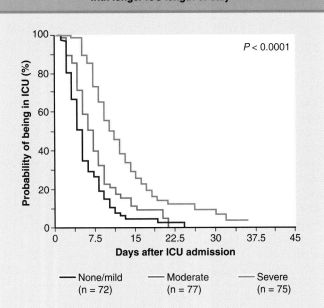

B

Figure 6.1. Delirium versus length of ICU stay. These Kaplan–Meier plots show the relationship between delirium and length of ICU stay. *A*, Never vs. ever delirium (according to whether or not the patient ever developed delirium in the ICU). *B*, Delirium severity. Patients who had severe delirium had the longest lengths of stay.

Box 6.4 Risk Factors for Delirium

Age over 70 years
BUN to creatinine ratio ≥ 18
Administration of psychoactive drugs
Transfer from a nursing home
Renal failure (creatinine > 2.0 mg/dL)
Total parental nutrition
Prior history of depression
Liver disease (bilirubin > 2.0 mg/dL)
Rectal or bladder catheters
Prior history of cognitive impairment or dementia
Hypo- or hypernatremia
Central venous catheters
History of stroke, epilepsy
Hypo- or hyperglycemia
Use of physical restraints or posey vest
Underlying comorbidities
Hypo- or hyperthyroidism
Sleep deprivation
Alcoholism
Hypothermia or fever
Cardiogenic or septic shock
Human immunodeficiency virus infection
Malnutrition
Acute respiratory distress syndrome
Hearing or vision impairment
Drug overdose or illicit drug use

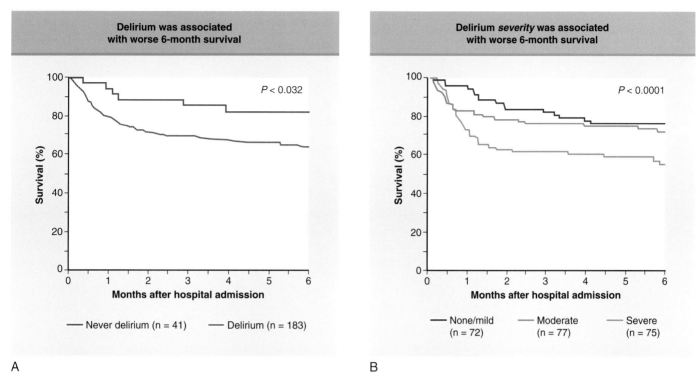

Figure 6.2. Delirium versus 6-month survival. These Kaplan–Meier plots show the relationship between delirium and 6-month survival. *A,* Never vs. ever delirium (according to whether or not the patient ever developed delirium in the ICU). *B,* Clinical severity. The never delirium group, composed of those who were always normal and those who were coma-normal (e.g., deeply sedated and then normal when drugs stopped), had higher survival rates than the ever delirium group, which was composed of those with delirium only and delirium-coma.

not simply a transition state from coma to normal because delirium occurred just as often among those who never developed coma as it did among those with coma and persisted in 11% of patients at the time of hospital discharge. Three prospective studies found that delirium was associated with an increased risk for development of dementia during the subsequent 2 or 3 years. In light of these findings, future studies should determine whether or not prevention or treatment of delirium changes clinical outcomes, including mortality, length of stay, cost of care, and long-term neuropsychological outcomes, among survivors of critical illness.

Assessment of Preexisting Cognitive Impairment and Delirium in the ICU

The most recent clinical practice guidelines of the Society of Critical Care Medicine recommend routine daily monitoring of delirium in all mechanically ventilated patients. Three guiding principles inform the recommended approach for cognitive assessment in the ICU. First, baseline cognitive status should be established, and ICU physicians should not assume a normal baseline cognitive status, especially in older patients. Second, the development and identification of new cognitive impairment and/or delirium in the ICU should be recognized and addressed. Third, all attempts should be made to diminish further insults to the brain.

Knowledge of a patient's preexisting cognitive status provides critical information that can affect the patient's health care at many levels, including (1) assessing decision-making capacity and ability to give informed consent for treatment, (2) provid-

ing a baseline for evaluating changes in mental status that occur commonly during acute hospitalization and ICU stay, (3) choosing treatment options that have the potential for mental status effects, and (4) identifying patients at high risk for decline in mental status during hospitalization who may benefit from preventive measures for delirium. The term *preexisting cognitive impairment* refers to either dementia or mild cognitive impairment that is present in chronic form prior to admission.

A study evaluating the prevalence of preexisting cognitive impairment in patients age 65 or older admitted to a medical ICU found a prevalence between 31% and 42%, depending on the instrument used. The study used two previously validated measures of proxy assessment of cognitive impairment: the Modified Blessed Dementia Rating Scale and the Informant Questionnaire on Cognitive Decline in the Elderly. Patients with preexisting cognitive impairment were significantly older, more likely to be female, less likely to be currently married, more likely to be admitted from a nursing home, and more likely to have higher APACHE II scores on ICU admission than those without preexisting cognitive impairment. Attending physicians and interns were unaware of 53% and 595 of cases of preexisting cognitive impairment, respectively. Both attending and intern recognition of preexisting cognitive impairment significantly increased as the severity of cognitive impairment increased.

After assessment of baseline cognitive status through interview with the family or ICU staff, the patient's level of consciousness/sedation is assessed using an objective sedation assessment. The recommended standard of care is to use

Practice of Critical Care

objective assessment scales in order to avoid oversedation and to promote earlier liberation from mechanical ventilation. Four frequently used sedation scales are described in Table 6.2. A comatose or deeply somnolent patient will be unable to perform the cognitive testing. Often, a second attempt at cognitive assessment is indicated later on in the day given the fluctuating nature of altered levels of consciousness. In addition, cognitive and delirium assessments should not be performed immediately following sedation for a procedure. All patients who are responsive to verbal stimuli should be assessed for delirium. Box 6.5 lists key points to consider in delirium assessment.

The first delirium assessment tools designed specifically for nonverbal, intubated ICU patients were published in 2001. The Intensive Care Delirium Screening Checklist has a high sensitivity (99%) but only a moderate specificity (64%) for delirium. The Confusion Assessment Method for the ICU (CAM-ICU) was validated in a large cohort study of ICU patients against delirium expert assessments and found to have a sensitivity of 95% to 100%, a specificity of 89% to 93%, and high interobserver reliability. The CAM-ICU was designed to be a serial

---

Box 6.5 Key Points in Delirium Assessment

- Requires accurate baseline assessment.
- Consider depression, psychiatric illness, dementia.
- Lethargy and decreased activity are more predominant features than agitation and hallucinations in older persons.
- Acute changes in mental status may represent a potential medical emergency that requires frequent reassessment of the patient.
- Lucid intervals are characteristic because of the fluctuating nature of delirium.

---

assessment tool for use by bedside clinicians (nurses or physicians). Thus, it is easy to use, taking an average of only 1 minute to complete and requiring minimal training. Using the CAM-ICU, the prevalence of delirium in the ICU has ranged from 70% to 87%.

Table 6.5 outlines the four key features of CAM-ICU, their description, and the methods used to determine each feature.

Table 6.5 CAM-ICU Features and Descriptions

	Absent	Present
1. Acute Onset or Fluctuating Course		

A. Is there evidence of an acute change in mental status from the baseline?

OR

B. Did the (abnormal) behavior fluctuate during the past 24 hours, that is, tend to come and go, or increase and decrease in severity as evidence by fluctuation on a sedation scale (e.g., RASS), GCS, or previous delirium assessment?

	Absent	Present
2. Inattention		

Did the patient have difficulty focusing attention as evidenced by **scores *less than 8*** on either the auditory or visual component of the **Attention Screening Examination (ASE)**? (Instructions on next page.)

	Absent	Present
3. Disorganized Thinking		

Is there evidence of disorganized or incoherent thinking as evidenced by **incorrect answers to 2 or more of the 4 questions and/or inability to follow the commands**?

Questions (Alternate Set A and Set B)

Set A	*Set B*
1. Will a stone float on water?	1. Will a leaf float on water?
2. Are there fish in the sea?	2. Are there elephants in the sea?
3. Does one pound weigh more than two pounds?	3. Do two pounds weigh more than one pound?
4. Can you use a hammer to pound a nail?	4. Can you use a hammer to cut wood?

Other

1. Are you having any unclear thinking?
2. Hold up this many fingers. (Examiner holds two fingers in front of patient)
3. Now do the same thing with the other hand. (Not repeating the number of fingers)

	Absent	Present
4. Altered Level of Consciousness		

Is the patient's level of consciousness anything *other than alert* such as vigilant, lethargic, or stuporous (e.g., RASS other than "0" at time of assessment)?

- **Alert**   Spontaneously fully aware of environment and interacts appropriately
- **Vigilant**   Hyperalert
- **Lethargic**   Drowsy but easily aroused, unaware of some elements in the environment, or not spontaneously interacting appropriately with the interviewer; becomes fully aware and appropriately interactive when prodded minimally
- **Stupor**   Becomes incompletely aware when prodded strongly; can be aroused only by vigorous and repeated stimuli, and as soon as the stimulus ceases, stuporous subject lapses back into the unresponsive state

	Yes	No
Overall CAM-ICU (Features 1 and 2 and either Feature 3 or 4):		

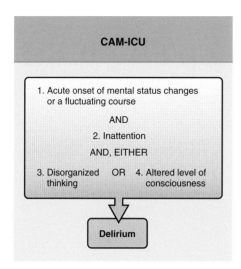

Figure 6.3. CAM-ICU. Algorithm used to detect delirium with the Confusion Assessment Method for the ICU (CAM-ICU). Delirium is defined as an acute onset of mental status changes *or* a fluctuating course *and* inattention *and either* disorganized thinking or an altered level of consciousness.

According to the CAM-ICU, delirium is considered to be present if both features one and two are found as well as one of the latter two features (Fig. 6.3). The CAM-ICU has been translated into numerous languages, and numerous aspects of neurologic monitoring are discussed and available for download via an educational Web site (www.icudelirium.org).

Pharmacologic Management of Delirium

Early diagnosis and correction of metabolic abnormalities, treatment of infections, and appropriate ventilator management should be a routine part of critical care that will often reveal and treat a variety of causes of delirium in the ICU population. Withdrawal from alcohol, benzodiazepines, or narcotics is a readily missed cause for delirium in the ICU and should be considered in all patients.

There have been no randomized studies assessing the utility of various medications used to treat delirium in the ICU. Practice guidelines list antipsychotics as the medication of choice. Antipsychotics seem to be particularly effective in treating symptoms of agitation and delusions, but they are also effective in hypoactive delirium. In the ICU, haloperidol is frequently used because it has fewer active metabolites, limited anticholinergic activity, and fewer sedative and hypotensive effects than thioridazine or chlorpromazine. Haloperidol does not suppress the respiratory drive and works as a dopamine receptor antagonist by blocking the D_2 receptor, which results in treatment of positive symptoms (e.g., hallucinations and unstructured thought patterns) and produces a variable sedative effect.

In the non-ICU setting, the recommended starting dose of haloperidol is 0.5 to 1.0 mg orally or parenterally, with repeated doses every 20 to 30 minutes until the desired effect is achieved. In the ICU setting, a recommended starting dose would be 5 mg every 12 hours (IV or PO), with maximal effective doses usually of approximately 20 mg/day. Because of the urgency of the situation in many ICU patients, much higher doses of haloperidol are often used. Unfortunately, there are few formal pharmacologic investigations to guide dosage recommendations in the ICU. Newer "atypical" antipsychotic agents (e.g., risperidone, ziprasidone, quetiapine, and olanzapine) may also prove helpful for delirium, but there have been no controlled trials of any of these agents. Adverse effects of typical and atypical antipsychotics include hypotension, acute dystonias, extrapyramidal signs, laryngeal spasm, malignant hyperthermia, glucose and lipid dysregulation, and anticholinergic effects such as dry mouth, constipation, and urinary retention. Perhaps the most immediately life-threatening adverse effect of antipsychotics is torsades de pointes, and these agents should not be given to patients with prolonged QT intervals.

Benzodiazepines, which are used most commonly in the ICU for sedation, are not recommended for the management of delirium because of the likelihood of oversedation, exacerbation of confusion, and respiratory suppression. However, they remain the drugs of choice for the treatment of delirium tremens and other withdrawal syndromes.

CONCLUSION

Pain, anxiety, and delirium are important aspects of critical illness. They should be assessed in every ICU patient by staff that have been adequately trained using standard scales. Research is needed to assess how treatment of pain, anxiety, and delirium affects ICU outcomes.

SUGGESTED READING

Desbiens NA, Wu AW: Pain and suffering in seriously ill hospitalized patients. J Am Geriatr Soc 2000;48(5 Suppl):S183–S186.

Ely EW, Gautam S, Margolin R, et al: The impact of delirium in the intensive care unit on hospital length of stay. Intensive Care Med 2001;27(12):1892–1900.

Ely EW, Margolin R, Francis J, et al: Evaluation of delirium in critically ill patients: Validation of the Confusion Assessment Method for the Intensive Care Unit (CAM-ICU). Crit Care Med 2001;29(7):1370–1379.

Ely EW, Shintani A, Truman B, et al: Delirium as a predictor of mortality in mechanically ventilated patients in the intensive care unit. JAMA 2004;291(14):1753–1762.

Ely EW, Truman B, Shintani A, et al: Monitoring sedation status over time in ICU patients: Reliability and validity of the Richmond Agitation–Sedation Scale (RASS). JAMA 2003;289(22):2983–2991.

Graf C, Puntillo K: Pain in the older adult in the intensive care unit. Crit Care Clin 2003;19(4):749–770.

Jacobi J, Fraser GL, Coursin DB, et al: Clinical practice guidelines for the sustained use of sedatives and analgesics in the critically ill adult. Crit Care Med 2002;30(1):119–141.

Kress JP, Pohlman AS, O'Connor MF, Hall JB: Daily interruption of sedative infusions in critically ill patients undergoing mechanical ventilation. N Engl J Med 2000;342(20):1471–1477.

Pisani MA, Redlich C, McNicoll L, Ely EW, Inouye SK: Underrecognition of preexisting cognitive impairment by physicians in older ICU patients. Chest 2003;124(6):2267–2274.

Ramsay MA, Savege TM, Simpson BR, Goodwin R: Controlled sedation with alphaxalone-alphadolone. Br Med J 1974;2:656–659.

Riker RR, Picard JT, Fraser GL: Prospective evaluation of the Sedation–Agitation Scale for adult critically ill patients. Crit Care Med 1999;27(7):1325–1329.

KEY POINTS

- To prevent emergence of antimicrobial resistance, pharmacokinetic/pharmacodynamic (PK/PD) determinants of antibiotics need to target rapid bacterial eradication and be of sufficient magnitude to eradicate resistant pathogens from colonized areas.
- Area under the inhibitory concentration–time curve (AUIC) can be used as a universal parameter for all classes of antibiotics when the dosing intervals are constrained within three or four half-lives. AUIC more than 125 and AUIC more than 250 are associated with optimal antimicrobial effect and maximal killing, respectively, whereas AUIC less than 100 risks the selection of resistance.
- There are many confounding factors in measurements of serum protein binding and its relation to antibiotic activity. Tissue homogenate levels reflect the composite of partitioned drug at a site. Although a few in vitro and animal studies have evaluated the impact of neutrophils on the pharmacodynamics of antibiotics, the influences of the host defense system on the effect of antimicrobials are, in general, poorly characterized. Further evaluation of these parameters and their relationship to serum concentrations should be a high priority.
- Monotherapy with fourth-generation cephalosporins or carbapenems for serious infections caused by *Pseudomonas aeruginosa* or extended-spectrum β-lactamase–producing *Klebsiella* in immunocompromised hosts is not considered to be safe from the perspective of prevention of resistance. Such patients should be treated with combination therapy, including an aminoglycoside (usually tobramycin) or an antipseudomonal fluoroquinolone such as ciprofloxacin.
- AUIC of fluoroquinolones needs to exceed 100 to 125 to obtain high rates of bacteriologic and clinical cure for both gram-positive and gram-negative bacteria. In general, combination therapy should be considered for the treatment of nosocomial infections due to *P. aeruginosa* when a fluoroquinolone is employed, although *P. aeruginosa* treated with ciprofloxacin at a minimum inhibitory concentration (MIC) of 0.25 or less will be killed at AUIC more than 157 with ciprofloxacin monotherapy.
- Clinical studies of vancomycin AUIC for clinical and microbiologic outcomes with methicillin-resistant *Staphylococcus aureus* show that high values closer to 400 and at least 866 are needed for positive clinical outcomes and microbiologic eradication, respectively, which may explain cases of nonresponsiveness to vancomycin even in *S. aureus* with vancomycin MIC less than 8.0 µg/mL. When the required concentration of vancomycin cannot be reached because of risk of complications or difficulty in administration, an alternative therapy with combination therapy such as quinupristin–dalfopristin plus vancomycin may be considered.

With the emergence and spread of antimicrobial resistance in major nosocomial pathogens, antibiotic treatment in the intensive care unit (ICU) is facing new challenges. Many standard treatment antibiotics in long-term use are no longer universally effective, and others are threatened with potential failure as resistance patterns evolve. Increasing methicillin resistance and the potential risk of rising vancomycin resistance in *Staphylococcus aureus* and growing prevalence of multidrug-resistant nonfermenters, such as *Pseudomonas aeruginosa* and *Acinetobacter* spp., are of special concern to those who must manage infections in the ICU.

Resistance may be considered a side effect of failure to eradicate a pathogen. Therefore, bacterial eradication should be one of the primary goals of antibiotic therapy. Eradication is the primary effect of the antibiotic, and it is at least as important as clinical improvement. The more rapid the bacterial eradication, the better the chances of not selecting resistance because "dead bugs don't mutate." Elimination of resistant pathogens from colonized areas in addition to the infection site must also be considered because these regions supply pathogens for the initiation of new infections. For example, eradication of resistant pathogens from nasopharynx may be necessary to prevent antibacterial resistance in respiratory tract infection.

Development of new antibiotics would be a solution to the ongoing problem of resistance. However, there are few new antimicrobials and no new classes of antimicrobial in late-stage development. Thus, we must focus on strategies to optimize the use of what we have. Appropriate use of available antibiotics based on pharmacokinetics (PK) and pharmacodynamics (PD) describes the interaction between antibiotic and bacteria and is an opportunity to both defeat preexisting resistance and address the development of resistance.

PHARMACOKINETICS/PHARMACODYNAMICS OF ANTIBIOTICS

Whereas PK of antibiotics deals with the time course of concentration of a drug, PD of antimicrobial agents expresses the relationship between serum concentration of antibiotics and their antimicrobial effect. Described in this manner, PD of antibiotics focuses on the time course of their antimicrobial activity, and it should be related to the time course of the antimicrobial concentration. Perhaps this is why the most useful parameters are area under the concentration versus time curve (AUC) as time-related change in concentration in relation to minimum inhibitory concentration (MIC), which is a measure of 24-hour exposure at a constant concentration.

In traditional studies, the MIC breakpoint is the most popular prediction tool for antimicrobial success. The MIC is derived from incubation of bacteria with antibiotic concentration for 18 to 24 hours. A MIC breakpoint is a number reflective of an organism subpopulation, and it may or may not predict killing of a particular infecting pathogen. It requires interpretation in the context of achieved antibiotic concentration and the particular MIC in the patient. Typically, the MIC susceptibility breakpoint is determined in clinical trials from the observed clinical response at usual doses of antibiotics. This is not a very precise endpoint, since many factors unrelated to antibiotic action on bacteria may influence clinical improvement. Clinical efficacy can be achieved without bacteriologic efficacy in many milder outpatient infections, such as acute bacterial exacerbations of chronic bronchitis, acute otitis media, and acute sinusitis. Antibacterial effect needs to be evaluated within the context of proven bacterial killing and known antimicrobial concentrations. Regardless of the clinical outcome, bacterial resistance is much more closely linked to the concentrations in the patient and the MIC. Low dosing may not result in clinical failure, but it can easily result in microbiologic failure and resistance in the organism.

There are problems in the interpretation of MIC. For example, the MIC, approximating a continuous exposure of the drug for 18 to 24 hours, may not expose the bacterial population long enough to fully select resistant subpopulations that usually exhibit regrowth only after 24 hours of incubation. An example is glycopeptide heteroresistant, methicillin-resistant *S. aureus*. Furthermore, MIC, as interpreted from a reading at 18 to 24 hours, does not provide useful information on the time course of antimicrobial activity during the test. For example, it does not distinguish concentration-dependent killing from time-dependent killing. The MIC measures only the end result of antibiotic concentration and time of continuous exposure.

Studies on PK/PD of antibiotics during the past 20 years have generated the necessary relationships to guide effective antimicrobial therapy. However, confusion regarding targets and endpoints has sometimes affected studies that seek breakpoints (both in vitro and in vivo). These studies demonstrate that maintaining serum concentration of antibiotics above their MIC is not the only important factor in achieving an antimicrobial effect. Some antibiotics enhance killing as concentration to MIC ratio increases, and some of these show prolonged antibiotic effect after concentration has decreased below MIC (postantibiotic effect). Based on these findings, three PK parameters, time above MIC ($T > $ MIC), peak level:MIC ratio (C_{max}:MIC), and

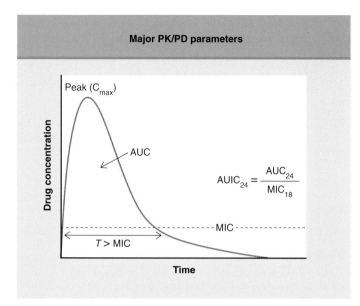

Figure 7.1. Major PK/PD parameters. Relationship between the concentration vs time curve. MIC, minimum inhibitory concentration against the organism; C_{max}, peak concentration; $T > $ MIC, time above MIC; AUC_{24}, area under the concentration versus time curve over 24 hours; AUIC, area under the inhibitory concentration–time curve.

AUC:MIC ratio have been suggested as major factors relating to antimicrobial efficacy. We prefer to use the term AUIC (area under the inhibitory concentration–time curve) to represent the 24-hour AUC:MIC ratio (Fig. 7.1). We prefer to link this to microbial killing rate in vivo and to resistance. In these cases, the target is at least 100. In non–seriously ill patients for whom the target is cure and the bacteria are not measured, it is probably sufficient to target lower values such as 30, but these may still select resistant pathogens at the site and elsewhere.

MAJOR PK/PD PARAMETERS THAT DETERMINE ANTIMICROBIAL EFFECTS

A number of in vitro studies and animal studies have shown that major PK/PD parameters determining antimicrobial effects are different among antibiotics, for example: $T > $ MIC for β-lactams, oxazolidinones, and macrolides; C_{max}:MIC for aminoglycosides; AUIC for vancomycin and fluoroquinolones. However, the three major PK/PD parameters are interrelated because each is linked to dose, concentration, and MIC. Higher dose produces not only a higher peak level:MIC and a higher AUIC but also a longer duration of $T > $ MIC. Especially within dosing intervals of three or four half-lives in humans, the importance and ability to differentiate between these parameters diminish. Antibiotics with low peak concentrations and long half-lives, such as fluoroquinolones, long-acting macrolides, and azalides, do not show definite differences between the three major PK/PD parameters in the degree of correlation to antimicrobial effect, at least when they are evaluated in settings similar to that of human PK. In this regard, AUIC (with the advantage of integrating both concentration and time factors) has been suggested as a good candidate for a universal parameter for all classes of antibiotics. Using the universal parameter also makes it easier to compare

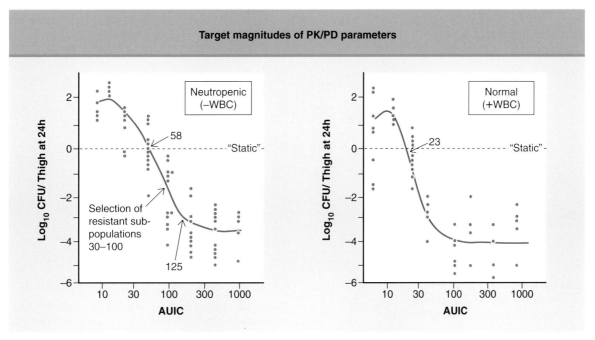

Figure 7.2. Target magnitudes of PK/PD parameters. Relationship between levofloxacin AUIC and the surviving inoculum of *Streptococcus pneumoniae* after 24 hours of treatment in a murine thigh model of infection. In neutropenic mice, the bacteriostatic AUIC in this model was 58, whereas mice with intact host defense required only an AUIC of 23 for bacteriostatic actions. A log kill in excess of 3 (i.e., bactericidal action) required AUIC values greater than 100 regardless of the state of host defense. (We added lines and interpretive callouts.) AUIC, area under the inhibitory concentration–time curve; MIC, minimum inhibitory concentration; WBC, white blood cell. (Data from Schentag JJ, Meagher AK, Forrest A: Fluoroquinolone AUIC break points and the link to bacterial killing rates. Part 1: In vitro and animal models. Ann Pharmacother 2003;37:1287–1298.)

antimicrobial activities across different classes and to evaluate the effect of antibiotics in combination. However, AUIC only applies accurately to both time-dependent and concentration-dependent antibiotics when the dosing intervals are constrained within three or four half-lives. Inattention to this latter condition has created controversy between animal and human models.

TARGET MAGNITUDES OF PK/PD PARAMETERS

Target magnitudes of PK/PD parameters necessary for treatment efficacy suggested by PK/PD studies may differ depending on the endpoint of efficacy used: bacteriostasis at 24 hours, 1 or 2 log killing at 24 hours, maximum killing at 24 hours, the dose protective of 50% of animals from death (PD_{50}), or maximal animal survival at 3 to 5 days. Discrepancies in the target magnitudes of PK/PD parameters for efficacy of antibiotics often occur in animal models when different endpoints of evaluation are applied to the analysis of the data (Fig. 7.2).

Because an antibiotic may need to eradicate pathogens from more than one site in the body, endpoints of more definite antibacterial action, such as maximal bactericidal effect in 24 hours (≥3 log killing), bacterial eradication to counts below the limit of detection, maximum killing effect, and/or maximal survival, should ordinarily be used as the target of efficacy. These do not directly test the human treatment strategy of short duration of treatment using antibiotics with rapid bactericidal action,

but the data do help to avoid artificially low targets and thereby decrease the risk of selecting resistant pathogens. It may also be beneficial to minimize toxicity in cases in which the toxicity is not related to short duration of exposure. Shorter duration of parenteral antibiotic therapy can save money by reducing the cost of hospital treatment.

Target Magnitudes of PK/PD Parameters Related to Killing Rate

There are relatively few human PK/PD studies of antibiotics that have focused attention on the magnitudes of PK/PD parameters associated with the rate of bacterial killing. In vitro and animal studies have used assessment points of 24 or 48 hours after dosing begins to determine the extent of bacterial killing, which is different than the rate at which killing occurs. Relatively early points of measurement have the built-in limitation of minimal bacterial killing that occurs with most relatively static drugs this early in the treatment period. Generally, clinical studies have evaluated microbiological efficacy after sufficient duration of treatment to kill organisms, such as 7 or 14 days or longer. In fact, the killing rates earlier in the period of treatment can be quite different even though antibiotics show the same extent of killing at the final evaluation points (Fig. 7.3). Particularly for concentration-dependent agents such as the fluoroquinolones, bactericidal endpoints need to be measured earlier in humans and probably serially to detect differences that occur between agents over the time of treatment.

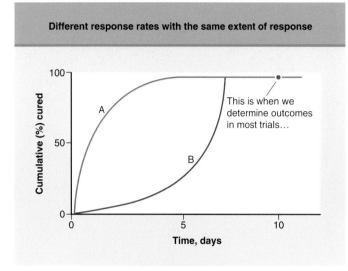

Figure 7.3. Different response rates with the same extent of response. Two antibiotics, A and B, are illustrated to have a different rate of approach to their maximum response of nearly 100%. This could illustrate time to bacterial eradication or time to clinical resolution. In either case, the difference between A and B cannot be differentiated because the only assessment point is day 10. This is a typical endpoint problem in registration trials and forces the conclusion of equivalence in final outcome, even when the rate of improvement differs greatly. (Data from Schentag JJ, Meagher AK, Forrest A: Fluoroquinolone AUIC break points and the link to bacterial killing rates. Part 2: Human trials. Ann Pharmacother 2003;37:1478–1488.)

Target Magnitudes of PK/PD Parameters for Repression of Resistance

Although target magnitudes of PK/PD parameters to prevent the emergence or selection of resistance have been evaluated in a few studies, almost all studies have focused on gram-negative organisms such as *P. aeruginosa* and a narrow spectrum of antibiotics, typically β-lactams and fluoroquinolones.

New in vitro parameters linked to resistance, such as mutant protective concentration (MPC) and mutant selection window (MSW), have been developed for *S. pneumoniae* and *S. aureus*. These new parameters are actively being investigated, especially with fluoroquinolones (Fig. 7.4). MPC is defined as an antibiotic concentration above which a microbe must acquire two concurrent resistance mutations for growth. It is measured experimentally as the lowest concentration that allows no colony growth when more than 10^9 to 10^{10} cells are applied to drug-containing agar plates. High inocula are used in these studies to ensure that there are some mutated organisms present at baseline in the sample.

Once the MPC is derived, then it must be interpreted in relationship to in vivo antibiotic concentrations over time. Dosing strategies that produce antimicrobial concentrations inside MSW (concentrations between MPC at the high end and MIC at the low end) are expected to enrich resistant mutant subpopulation selectively because, within this window, antibiotics suppress the predominantly susceptible organism population but there is selective enrichment of the minority resistant subpopulation. Concentrations of antibiotics above the MPC can restrict the selection of antibiotic-resistant mutants because a

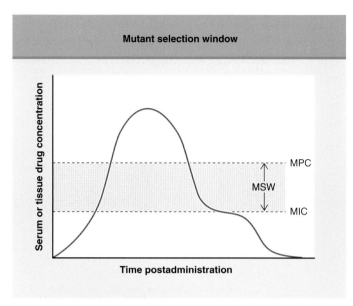

Figure 7.4. Mutant selection window. A hypothetical pharmacokinetic profile is shown in which minimum inhibitory concentration (MIC) and mutant prevention concentration (MPC) are arbitrarily indicated. The area between MPC and MIC represents the mutant selection window (MSW). (Data from Zhao X, Drlica K: Restricting the selection of antibiotic-resistant mutants: A general strategy derived from fluoroquinolone studies. Clin Infect Dis 2001;33(Suppl 3):S147–S156.)

second mutation is needed for bacteria to overcome this drug concentration, which occurs very rarely. The lower concentrations below MIC do not confer enough changes on the organism population to be selective of mutants because the susceptible population prevails at this level. According to this hypothesis, antibiotic regimens that place concentrations above MIC, but insufficient to reach MPC, are even more dangerous than very low AUICs, at least from the perspective of selecting resistance. This highlights the problem of AUICs between 30 and 100, which appear to select resistance in patients whose hose defense is compromised.

Although studies on MPC/MSW are actively being conducted for fluoroquinolones, there is debate about the relevance of extended application of MPC/MSW to other antibiotics. There is nothing unique about fluoroquinolones, and thus MPC/MSW should apply in general to antibiotics, but further investigation is needed on the general application of the MPC/MSW concept to antibiotics with mechanisms of resistance other than the point mutation.

On the other hand, MPC and MSW describe only concentration-dependent selection of resistance, whereas AUICs apply for either selection of resistance or killing rate. Using AUICs, windows can be established for optimal antimicrobial effect (AUIC > 125) and maximal killing rates (AUIC > 250) as well as for the risk of selecting resistance (AUIC < 100) (Table 7.1).

PROTEIN BINDING OF ANTIBIOTICS

Many investigators have advocated that protein binding and its related topic, tissue level of antibiotics, should be considered in assessing antibiotic effects. On the premise that only the free

Table 7.1 AUIC Window by Antimicrobial Effect[a]			
AUIC (Peak:MIC)	*In vitro* Time to Eradication (hr)	Murine 24-hr Eradication	Human Time to Eradication
30 (3:1)	8–24	Static	>10 days
125 (6:1)	4–8	2–4 log kill	3–5 days
>250 (15:1)	0.5–1	4+ log kill	1–2 hr

[a] AUIC, area under the inhibitory concentration–time curve; MIC, minimum inhibitory concentration. (Data from Schentag JJ, Meagher AK, Forrest A: Fluoroquinolone AUIC break points and the link to bacterial killing rates. Part 2: Human trials. Ann Pharmacother 2003;37:1478–1488.)

form of antibiotics in extravascular space is active against extracellular organisms, considerable effort has been devoted to assess the influence of static measures such as protein binding on the time course of antimicrobial effect. There have also been many efforts to measure the concentrations of antibiotics directly at infection sites.

The magnitude of the hindering effect of protein on the level of free antibiotics has been calculated by multiplication of the serum drug concentration by the percentage of protein binding measured in vitro. However, several points need to be considered before use of this method in the general consideration of antibiotic activity.

First, binding of drugs to serum protein is a continuing dynamic of association and dissociation. It is measured in a static system after equilibration across a membrane. Thus, the proportion of binding at steady state varies depending on association constant, drug concentration, and protein concentration. Even with a given association constant and protein concentration, the proportion of binding can change continuously with changing total drug level in vivo (Fig. 7.5). In this regard, calculating free in vivo drug concentrations with a single percentage of protein binding obtained in vitro at a fixed drug and protein concentration is unlikely to apply evenly over the entire interval between dosages.

Second, since the effect of protein binding is buffered by relatively large amounts of extravascular fluid, the percentage of protein binding in vitro measured at equilibrium does not contribute to the same extent in the in vivo situation. For a drug whose volume of distribution (VD) is 39 liters, 90% protein binding may lower the free drug level in extravascular fluid by only 40%. In the case of a drug with 9 liters of VD, the same protein binding lowers extravascular free drug by 60% (Fig. 7.6).

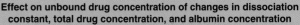

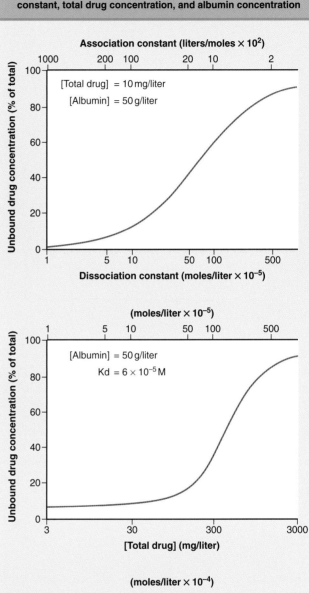

Effect on unbound drug concentration of changes in dissociation constant, total drug concentration, and albumin concentration

Figure 7.5. Effect on unbound drug concentration of changes in dissociation constant, total drug concentration, and albumin concentration. The free concentration of a drug (molecular weight of 300) rises with increasing dissociation constant, increasing total drug concentration, and decreasing albumin concentration. Even with very high binding affinity and normal albumin concentration, binding capacity becomes saturated at high drug concentrations, and the free drug concentration rises rapidly. (Data from Koch-Weser J, Sellers EM: Binding of drugs to serum albumin [first of two parts]. N Engl J Med 1976;294:311–316.)

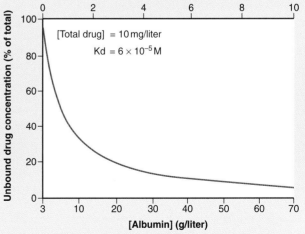

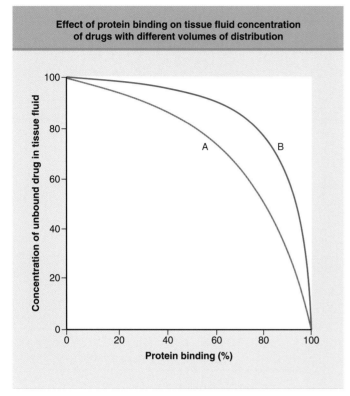

Effect of protein binding on tissue fluid concentration of drugs with different volumes of distribution

Figure 7.6. Effect of protein binding on tissue fluid concentration of drugs with different volumes of distribution. Drug A is lipid insoluble, unable to cross cell membranes, and restricted to the extracellular fluid; volume of distribution = 9 liters. Drug B is lipid soluble and can pass intracellularly; volume of distribution = 39 liters. For drug B, the 90% binding in plasma may lower the free concentration in plasma and tissue fluid by 40%. For drug A, 90% binding lowers the concentrations by 60%. (Data from Wise R: Protein binding of beta-lactams: The effects on activity and pharmacology particularly tissue penetration. I. J Antimicrob Chemother 1983;12:1–18.)

Finally, antibiotics bind to bacteria, interstitial and cellular associated proteins, and intracellular substances, and these binding sites may compete with serum albumin for antibiotic binding. In most cases, bacteria are better antibiotic binding sites than albumin molecules. Any of these can modulate the effects of in vitro serum albumin binding on actual drug distribution. Furthermore, inflammation of infected tissues is expected to alter passage of intravascular antibiotics into the tissues, which has neither been considered nor reasonably measured, and some antibiotics are believed to exert their antibiotic effect on bacteria even after binding to protein.

Considering these confounding factors, assessment of the effect of protein binding on antibiotic activity as a percentage of serum albumin binding at equilibrium should be approached with caution. Perhaps the most conservative approach is to assume that protein binding has no impact unless it is extremely high affinity (enough to keep the drug away from the bacteria) or extremely high capacity (>98%, again enough to keep the drug away from the bacteria). Such conditions are rare in antibiotics because if they occur, the antibiotics would fail and not reach the market.

TISSUE LEVEL OF ANTIBIOTICS

A variety of methods or specimens have been used to measure the tissue or extracellular fluid (ECF) level of antibiotics, including tissue homogenates, lymphatic drainage, tissue cage reservoirs, chemically or mechanically induced skin blisters, surgically implanted cotton threads, implanted fibrin clots, and microdialysis. The wide diversity of models with different conditions has confused the interpretation of the effective level of antibiotics at infection sites.

Tissue homogenate is a mixture of blood, ECF, and intracellular fluid (solids and water). Because intracellular tissue is a major constituent of that mixture (80% of the tissue by weight), measured concentrations of drugs in tissue homogenate may result in misinterpreting the ECF level due to their propensity to penetrate into cells. For β-lactams with negligible intracellular penetration, the concentration in tissue homogenate will be much lower than the true concentration in ECF because of dilution during homogenization, when cells are lysed (Table 7.2). The opposite phenomenon will occur for fluoroquinolones and macrolides because intracellular drug is freed when cells are lysed (Table 7.3). As another example, linezolid distributes evenly across tissue and ECF, so homogenization has no overall effect and the concentration remains approximately the same as ECF. Some models are hindered if extravascular penetration lags in equilibration due to a small surface area-to-volume ratio,

Table 7.2 Calculation of Tissue Drug Recovery and Tissue:Serum Ratio (Nonexcretory Organs) for β-Lactams[a]

Site	Tissue Mass (%)	Concentration (μg/g)	Recovery (μg)
Blood	4	40.00	0.960
ECF	16	40.00	6.400
Intracellular fluid (solids plus water)	80	0.01	0.008
Total recovery (%)	100		
Total recovery (μg)			7.360
Tissue:serum ratio			0.180

[a]Calculated at a postdistributive concentration in serum of 40 μg/mL in a 1.0-g tissue homogenate specimen from a person with a hematocrit of 40%. (Data from Nix DE, Goodwin SD, Peloquin CA, et al: Antibiotic tissue penetration and its relevance: Models of tissue penetration and their meaning. Antimicrob Agents Chemother 1991;35:1947–1952.)

Table 7.3 Calculation of Tissue Drug Recovery and Tissue:Serum Ratio (Nonexcretory Organs) for Quinolones[a]

Site	Tissue Mass (%)	Concentration (μg/g)	Recovery (μg)
Blood	4.0	4.0	0.16
ECF	16.0	4.0	0.64
Intracellular fluid (water)	53.6	4.0	2.14
Intracellular fluid (solids)	26.4	22.0	5.80
Total recovery (%)	100		
Total recovery (μg)			8.75
Tissue:serum ratio			2.20

[a]Calculated at a postdistributive concentration in serum of 40 μg/mL in a 1.0-g tissue homogenate specimen from a person with a hematocrit of 40%. (Data from Nix DE, Goodwin SD, Peloquin CA, et al: Antibiotic tissue penetration and its relevance: Models of tissue penetration and their meaning. Antimicrob Agents Chemother 1991;35:1947–1952.)

inflammation around devices, different protein content from ECF, drug adherence, evaporation of fluid, and so on.

Levels of antibiotics in epithelial lining fluid (ELF) and alveolar macrophage (AM) cells have been considered to represent the actual effective levels of antibiotics exerting antibiotic activity in lung infections. For this reason, antibiotics achieving higher concentrations in these sites than in serum, such as macrolides and fluoroquinolones, tend to be preferred in the treatment of pulmonary infection. However, it is not known what medium actually represents the lung site of infection—ELF or alveolar interstitial fluid. In addition, the inflammation created in association with bacterial infection results in increased vascular permeability. Therefore, ELF levels of antibiotics measured in healthy people would not reflect the actual antibiotic concentrations in lung infections. It may be better to view pulmonary penetration from the perspective of interstitial fluid penetration, and thus achievable serum concentrations. In general, ELF seems to be subject to most of the concentrations of tissue homogenizations and it probably provides similar information.

Assessment of free ECF level of antibiotics is not easy, especially when the many influencing factors relate to protein binding of drugs. Further evaluation is needed. We prefer to express AUIC values using the serum concentration of total drug because these values correlate with microbiologic killing outcomes in patients. Development of more relevant methods to measure the tissue level of antibiotics is also necessary to assess the real PK/PD of antibiotics at the infected site.

INFLUENCE OF HOST DEFENSES

The influences of the host defense system on the effect of antimicrobials are poorly characterized in PK/PD studies. In most models, they are neglected entirely. In human trials, they are part of the overall determination of target AUIC. Although a few in vitro and animal studies have evaluated the impact of neutrophils on PD of antibiotics, this factor has not been tested independently of serum concentration alone in human trials. Whereas the enhanced antibiotic activity by neutrophils was suggested to be different by organisms in an animal study, the impact of neutrophils and other immune system factors on antimicrobial activity in infections by different microorganisms and antibiotics needs to be quantified as part of the AUIC threshold action. Seldom has this been separated, although in animal models infected with *S. pneumoniae*, the impact of neutrophils on fluoroquinolone killing has served to lower the target bacteriostatic AUIC by approximately twofold (see Fig. 7.2).

PK/PD OF ANTIBIOTICS BYCLASS

PK/PD of β-Lactams

On the basis of animal infection models, the target magnitude of $T > \text{MIC}$ β-lactams for efficacy against gram-positive organisms has been suggested to be approximately 30% to 40% of the dosing interval. This magnitude was supported by the finding that 90% to 100% of mice infected with pneumococci survived when $T > \text{MIC}$ was above this threshold. Human studies conducted in patients with acute otitis media also provided similar

magnitude ($T > \text{MIC}$ of 60%) to achieve an 80% bacteriologic cure rate. However, in regard to eradication of nasopharyngeal carriage and prevention of emergence of resistance at the colonized area, serum concentrations above MIC for 80% to 100% of the dosing interval may be necessary.

On the other hand, it has been suggested, based on both animal models and human trials, that longer $T > \text{MIC}$ of β-lactams (>80 or 100%) is necessary to treat gram-negative organisms. Clinical studies performed in nosocomial pneumonia with gram-negative organisms demonstrated that 100% $T > \text{MIC}$ was needed to cure patients with cefmenoxime, which could only be achieved when AUIC was higher than 125.

Fourth-generation cephalosporins and carbapenems have been used as single-agent therapy for *P. aeruginosa* pneumonia. For a target endpoint of $T > \text{MIC}$ as at least 100% (which could be achieved when AUIC was higher than 125), monotherapy of fourth-generation cephalosporin in the case of serious infections by *P. aeruginosa* or extended-spectrum β-lactamase producing *Klebsiella* in immunocompromised hosts is not considered to be safe for the prevention of resistance. Such patients should be treated with combination therapy including an aminoglycoside or a fluoroquinolone, which are also active against the infecting pathogen.

The clinical and bacteriologic responses of imipenem for treatment of severe nosocomial pneumonia are lower than those of ciprofloxacin (56% vs 69% and 59% vs 69%, respectively). When *P. aeruginosa* is the offending pathogen, failure to achieve bacteriologic eradication and development of resistance during therapy are common. Imipenem shows more rapid eradication than typical β-lactams, which can be achieved with an AUIC higher than 250.

A high dose of infusing 2 g meropenem over 3 hours every 8 hours is recommended to lower the probability of resistance. When a susceptible *P. aeruginosa* has a subpopulation with MIC of 4 µg/mL against meropenem, the MIC can be increased to 16 µg/mL by oprD downregulation during treatment. A simulation analysis showed that the expected attainment of killing for *P. aeruginosa* with MIC of 16 µg/mL was more than 80% when the regimen of 2 g infusion over 3 hours was used. In other dosing settings, acceptable rates of maximal killing were not expected. Usually, *P. aeruginosa* increases its MIC to meropenem to 8- to 32-fold through a combination of oprD2 downregulation and stable derepression of the ampC enzyme. In these cases, the combination of meropenem with other antibiotics is required. Dosage-lowering strategies with carbapenems can easily foster resistance and should be approached with caution, especially when employing carbapenem monotherapy against *P. aeruginosa*.

PK/PD of Fluoroquinolones

There is an ongoing controversy regarding the target level of AUIC of fluoroquinolones for gram-positive bacteria. Animal models and most in vitro studies with a static endpoint have indicated that the threshold AUIC of fluoroquinolones against *S. pneumoniae* can be lower, ranging from 25 to 35. The same values in animals apply to gram-negative pathogens unless the endpoint is survival, where the target is at least 100. The low AUICs have usually derived from application of a bacteriostatic endpoint of antibacterial effect in animal models. The problem with extrapolation to humans is that there is an end point

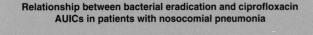

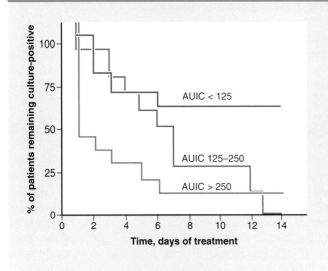

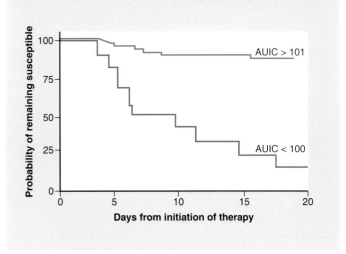

Figure 7.7. Relationship between the daily cultures and three groups of ciprofloxacin AUICs in 74 patients with nosocomial pneumonia. The patients with AUICs less than 125 had only 30% of the cultures become negative in 14 days. If the AUIC was 125 to 249, the cultures became negative in all patients, but more than half required 6 days to achieve organism eradication. The patients with AUICs greater than 250 had more than 60% of their cultures negative after 1 day of therapy. These data establish concentration dependence to the action of ciprofloxacin in patients. AUIC, area under the inhibitory concentration–time curve. (Data from Forrest A, Nix DE, Ballow CH, et al: Pharmacodynamics of intravenous ciprofloxacin in seriously ill patients. Antimicrob Agents Chemother 1993;37:1073–1081.)

Figure 7.8. Relationship between the initial AUIC and the time to onset of organisms' developing resistance. The selection of bacterial resistance in four nosocomial lower respiratory tract infection clinical trials was examined in 127 patients. When the initial AUIC was more than 100, only 8% of patients developed resistant organisms to the antibiotic responsible for the AUIC of more than 101. When the initial AUIC was less than 100, 93% of the patients developed resistance to the antibiotic started at that low AUIC value. AUIC, area under the inhibitory concentration–time curve. (Data from Schentag JJ, Gilliland KK, Paladino JA: What have we learned from pharmacokinetic and pharmacodynamic theories? Clin Infect Dis 2001;32(Suppl 1):S39–S46.)

mismatch. Low AUIC breakpoints target bacteriostatic effect obtainable with 24 hours of exposure to antibiotics, and these correlate with clinical cures since there is host defense and microbial endpoints are assumed and often not measured. When a bactericidal effect was the endpoint, an AUIC more than 100 to 125 was also necessary against pneumococci in most in vitro studies and animal studies (see Fig. 7.2). With respect to selection of bacterial resistance, in vitro PD studies based on the MPC and MSW hypothesis revealed that AUICs needed to protect resistance selection were more than 100 and more than 200 for *S. pneumoniae* and *S. aureus*, respectively.

Studies in animals and humans with gram-negative bacilli suggest that the AUIC of fluoroquinolones must exceed 100 to 125 to obtain high rates of bacteriologic and clinical cure. Values of more than 250 are associated with a very rapid eradication of gram-negative bacilli from endotracheal aspirates of patients with nosocomial pneumonia (Fig. 7.7). The PK/PD parameter predictive of the development of resistance in patients with nosocomial lower respiratory tract infection (LRTI), who were treated with multiple antibiotics including ciprofloxacin, was an AUIC less than 100 (Fig. 7.8).

Ciprofloxacin, a second-generation fluoroquinolone, remains the most potent antipseudomonal quinolone in terms of in vitro microbiological activity. Newer generation fluoroquinolones, such as gatifloxacin and moxifloxacin, armed with more potent antimicrobial effect against gram-positive pathogens, are considerably less active than ciprofloxacin against *P. aeruginosa*.

A study analyzed the target magnitude of AUIC to suppress amplification of fluoroquinolone resistance in *P. aeruginosa* using data derived from mice and a mathematical model. The AUIC value that would suppress the mutant subpopulation obtained by this method was 157, whereas the value of 52 readily amplified the resistant subpopulation. When a 10,000-subject Monte Carlo simulation was performed, none of the available fluoroquinolones were expected to achieve the target AUIC value (≥125 or 157) against *P. aeruginosa* at a rate of at least 90% with routinely used dosage regimens. This study suggested that combination therapy should be considered for the treatment of VAP due to *P. aeruginosa* when a quinolone is employed. However, this depends on the MIC of the *P. aeruginosa*; if the MIC to ciprofloxacin alone is less than or equal to 0.25, *P. aeruginosa* will be killed at an AUIC more than 157 with ciprofloxacin monotherapy. No other fluoroquinolone is active enough alone to achieve an AUIC of 157 vs *P. aeruginosa* in monotherapy regimens. Thus, local conditions must be tested before deciding between single-agent ciprofloxacin and its use in combination regimens.

PK/PD of Glycopeptides

Glycopeptides, such as vancomycin and teicoplanin, have been used mainly for treatment of nosocomial infections due to methicillin-resistant *S. aureus* (MRSA) and *Enterococcus fae-calis*. Although vancomycin demonstrates concentration-independent killing of gram-positive bacteria, AUIC is closely associated with clinical outcome.

A 24-hour AUC of approximately 393 can be obtained at a dose regimen of 750 mg q 12 hours of vancomycin. In the case of *Enterococcus faecium* (MIC = 4.0 μg/mL), the AUIC with the dosage regimen is just 98. When 1000 mg of vancomycin is given every 8 hours, the obtainable AUIC is 190, which may be enough to cover microorganisms with an MIC of 4.0. However, if the vancomycin MIC is 8 or 16 μg/mL, use of the new antibiotics or vancomycin in combination would be mandatory to achieve adequate AUICs.

In studies that evaluated a correlation between vancomycin AUIC and clinical and microbiological outcomes of MRSA infections, vancomycin treatment of *S. aureus* LRTIs with an AUIC less than 125 was clearly suboptimal. Values closer to 400 and 866 or higher were needed for positive clinical outcomes and microbiological eradication, respectively. It was not immediately clear why the high AUIC values were needed to eradicate *S. aureus* in LRTI. The study data suggest that nonresponsiveness to vancomycin may occur in *S. aureus* even when vancomycin MIC is less than 8.0 μg/mL. In fact, we have observed cases of clinical failure of vancomycin against infections due to *S. aureus* with susceptible MIC level ($\leq$4 μg/mL). The typical example is heterogeneous vancomycin-resistant staphylococci.

To combat the problem of declining responsiveness of MRSA strains to vancomycin and the threat of selecting vancomycin resistance in them, more refined dosing regimens based on PK/PD of vancomycin should be applied. The high AUIC level necessary for treatment of MRSA pneumonia should be evaluated with the target of 400 in mind. When the required amount of vancomycin cannot be reached because of risk of complications or difficulty in administration, alternative or combination therapy rather than high-dose vancomycin monotherapy must be considered.

PK/PD of Aminoglycosides

Because of their nephrotoxicity and ototoxicity, use of aminoglycosides is decreasing. They have a broad-spectrum antibacterial activity, especially against a variety of gram-negative pathogens including *P. aeruginosa*. They are frequently administered in combination with cell wall–active agents to provide synergy in the treatment of serious infections.

Aminoglycosides show a concentration-dependent killing, and the PK/PD parameters related to their efficacy are C_{max}:MIC, and AUIC. Target values of 8 to 10 and 80 to 100, respectively, have been suggested. Based on the PK/PD characteristics of aminoglycosides, once-daily dosing of aminoglycosides with very high peaks and a long time below MIC has become a common dosing practice. Although once-daily dosing of aminoglycosides has revealed trends for decreased toxicity relating to sustaining lower trough level, clinical improvement achieved by this method was trivial. The beneficial effects of aminoglycosides alone are clearly modest, and the clinical outcome of treated patients may be attributed to the universal use of concomitant antibiotics. Clinical usefulness of the once-daily dosing of aminoglycosides needs to be further evaluated because no studies have demonstrated PK/PD parameters while

using these regimens, and these need to be carefully evaluated as a determinant of outcome.

CONCLUSION

PK/PD studies have provided a more reasonable approach to antibiotic treatment of infectious diseases. In the era of antibiotic resistance, proper dosing of antibiotics according to PK/PD determinants has also been considered as a strategy to overcome this problem as well as a strategy toward the development of new antibiotics. However, further evaluations need to be performed on PK/PD parameters and their magnitudes in determining rapid eradication of pathogens and prevention of antibiotic resistance as well as the linkage to clinical effect. Issues concerning the influence of protein binding, measurement of tissue level of antibiotics, and the quantification of the impact of the host defense system need to be resolved. The strategy of targeting higher magnitudes of PK/PD parameters is considered preferable in order to achieve the goal of repressing antibiotic resistance in both the infected tissue and the colonized area. Furthermore, combinations of antibiotics or alternative, more active (higher AUIC) antibiotics need to be used when target magnitudes of PK/PD parameters are not expected to be achieved with monotherapy of an available antibiotic (Boxes 7.1 and 7.2).

Antibiotic regimen can be individualized based on both PK characteristics of patients and the MIC of the offending pathogen (dual individualization). With the dual individualization of antibiotic therapy, the effects of antibiotics can be optimized and development of antibiotic resistance can be oppressed. Early eradication of pathogens and rapid cure due to the optimized antibiotic therapy also offer potential economic benefits through shorter hospitalization and switch to oral therapy. Pharmacokinetic parameters can be reasonably estimated from computerized software without direct measurement when some determining factors, such as age, weight, and serum creatinine levels, are provided.

Box 7.1 Benefits

- Optimization of antimicrobial effect
- Oppression of developing antibiotic resistance
- Individualization of dose and interval of antibiotics
- Potential of economic benefits through early discharge and/or outpatient antibiotic therapy

---

Box 7.2 Risks

- Debates on pharmacokinetic/pharmacodynamic—major parameters determining antimicrobial effects, target magnitudes, influence of serum protein, tissue concentration of antibiotics, influence of host immunity, effect of combined therapy
- Unfamiliarity of software estimating pharmacokinetic parameters

SUGGESTED READING

Craig WA: Pharmacokinetic/pharmacodynamic parameters: Rationale for antibacterial dosing of mice and men. Clin Infect Dis 1998;26:1–10.

Dagan R, Klugman KP, Craig WA, et al: Evidence to support the rationale that bacterial eradication in respiratory tract infection is an important aim of antimicrobial therapy. J Antimicrob Chemother 2001;47: 129–140.

Forrest A, Nix DE, Ballow CH, et al: Pharmacodynamics of intravenous ciprofloxacin in seriously ill patients. Antimicrob Agents Chemother 1993;37:1073–1081.

Koch-Weser J, Sellers EM: Binding of drugs to serum albumin (first of two parts). N Engl J Med 1976;294:311–316.

Nix DE, Goodwin SD, Peloquin CA, et al: Antibiotic tissue penetration and its relevance: Models of tissue penetration and their meaning. Antimicrob Agents Chemother 1991;35:1947–1952.

Paladino JA, Zimmer GS, Schentag JJ: The economic potential of dual individualisation methodologies. Pharmacoeconomics 1996;10(6):539–545.

Schentag JJ: Antimicrobial management strategies for gram-positive bacterial resistance in the intensive care unit. Crit Care Med 2001;29: N100–N107.

Schentag JJ, Gilliland KK, Paladino JA: What have we learned from pharmacokinetic and pharmacodynamic theories? Clin Infect Dis 2001;32(Suppl 1):S39–S46.

Schentag JJ, Meagher AK, Forrest A: Fluoroquinolone AUIC break points and the link to bacterial killing rates. Part 1: In vitro and animal models. Ann Pharmacother 2003;37:1287–1298.

Schentag JJ, Meagher AK, Forrest A: Fluoroquinolone AUIC break points and the link to bacterial killing rates. Part 2: Human trials. Ann Pharmacother 2003;37:1478–1488.

Schentag JJ, Nix DE, Adelman MH: Mathematical examination of dual individualization principles (I): Relationships between AUC above MIC and area under the inhibitory curve for cefmenoxime, ciprofloxacin, and tobramycin. DICP Ann Pharmacother 1991;25:1050–1057.

Schentag JJ, Strenkoski-Nix LC, Nix DE, et al: Pharmacodynamic interactions of antibiotics alone and in combination. Clin Infect Dis 1998; 27:40–46.

Suh B, Craig WA: Protein binding. In Lorian V (ed): Antibiotics in laboratory medicine. Baltimore, Williams & Wilkins, 1996, pp 296–329.

Wise R: Protein binding of beta-lactams: The effects on activity and pharmacology particularly tissue penetration. I. J Antimicrob Chemother 1983;12:1–18.

Zhao X, Drlica K: Restricting the selection of antibiotic-resistant mutants: A general strategy derived from fluoroquinolone studies. Clin Infect Dis 2001;33(Suppl 3):S147–S156.

Chapter 8

Nonantimicrobial Measures to Prevent Infections in Critical Care

Didier Pittet, Ilker Uçkay, Philippe Eggimann, and Hugo Sax

KEY POINTS

- Nosocomial infections generally exceed 25% in intensive care units (ICUs) worldwide, and infections acquired in these units account for more than 20% of all nosocomial infections in general, although ICU beds account for only 5% of all hospital beds and ICUs care for less than 10% of patients admitted. The costs are equally tremendous.
- Catheter-related infections can be sharply reduced by prevention programs based on education and global prevention strategies. Further improvement of efficacy is theoretically possible by using new technologies such as coated catheters, but this approach is futile if the basic measures and educational activities have not been fully implemented.
- Prevention of ventilator-associated pneumonia is not easy and should be based on multimodal approaches.
- Despite the large body of evidence supporting the effectiveness of hand hygiene in preventing cross-transmission, health care workers' compliance with recommendations in the absence of promotion programs remains unacceptably low worldwide, usually 30% to 50%.
- Efforts to control antimicrobial resistance should focus on both antibiotic use and infection control practices.

All types of intensive care units (ICUs), with the exception of coronary units, have high incidence rates of nosocomial infection with a resulting important impact on clinical outcome and additional costs and length of stay. The prevalence of nosocomial infections generally exceeds 25% in ICU wards worldwide, and infections acquired in these units account for more than 20% of all nosocomial infections in general, although ICU beds account for only 5% of all hospital beds and ICUs care for less than 10% of patients admitted. The costs are equally tremendous. For example, at the medical ICU of the University of Geneva Hospitals, the costs for treatment, length of stay, and care for all nosocomially infected patients are equivalent to the costs for all noninfected patients, although the nosocomially infected patients only account for 26% of the entire ICU population (Fig. 8.1). Assessment of mortality attributable to nosocomial infections in the ICU setting is difficult because these infections and mortality attributable to the underlying disease

share common risk factors. Crude mortality rates are estimated to vary between 10% and 80%. Thus, in contrast to widespread belief, the attributable morbidity and mortality due to nosocomial infections in the ICU are in excess of the rates of morbidity and mortality for the infections that initially led to the patients' hospitalization.

Nosocomial infections in the ICU are not an inevitability of modern medicine. They can and should be prevented to decrease associated morbidity, mortality, prolonged ICU stay, costs, and antimicrobial resistance rates. This chapter discusses nonantimicrobial measures for infection control in the ICU in general, with a particular emphasis on hand hygiene, the single most important measure to prevent cross-transmission and decrease nosocomial infections. Problems of multiresistant organisms, antibiotic control, and prevention of some key ICU-specific infections are also discussed. Antibiotic therapy, diagnosis, antibiotic prophylaxis, and management of invasive fungal infections are addressed in other chapters of this book.

EPIDEMIOLOGY, PATHOPHYSIOLOGY, AND OVERALL RISK FACTORS

The type of ICU plays a role. It is obvious that ICUs harboring severe burn patients, neonates, or intubated patients have a higher incidence of infection than, for example, coronary care units (CCUs). Infection rates also tend to be higher in surgical than in medical ICUs, and they are higher in adult ICUs than in pediatric units. The distribution of infection occurring at different sites in the ICU differs from that encountered in general wards. Whereas urinary tract infection predominates in general wards, respiratory tract infection is the most common infection in most ICUs. In the European Prevalence of Infection in Intensive Care (EPIC) study conducted in 1992, the largest 1-day point prevalence study of nosocomial infections in critical care (Fig. 8.2), respiratory tract infection was estimated to account for approximately 65% of all nosocomial infections. The overall prevalence of ICU-acquired infection was 20.6%, with a country-to-country variation ranging from 9.7% to 31.6%. These differences were more likely to reflect clinical care practice and selection of patients than real differences in quality of care, highlighting the importance for correctly performed adjustment for case mix before any rate comparison could be evaluated. Trends toward higher acquisition rates paralleled trends toward higher mortality rates.

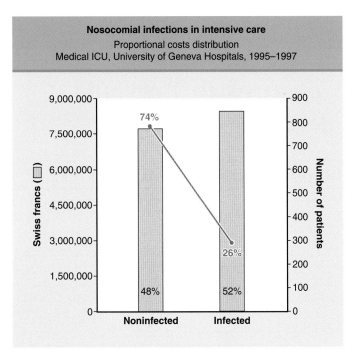

Figure 8.1. Nosocomial infections in intensive care. Proportional costs distribution, medical ICU, University of Geneva Hospitals, 1995–1997.

Host colonization is a prerequisite for the development of infection, particularly in critical care. Although factors favoring the progression from colonization to infection are not completely understood, it is estimated that almost 50% of infections acquired in the ICU are preceded by colonization with the same microorganism. Factors associated with colonization are similar to those associated with infection (duration of hospitalization, high exposure to devices, and prolonged antibiotic therapy). Several studies in the 1970s showed that severity of illness and ICU admission contributed to rapid colonization with gram-negative bacteria. Often, these are endemic in the ICU, which implies that the physiological flora of a given patient can be substituted by the local endemic flora after some days in the ICU.

Reasons for the high prevalence rates are many. One is the high workload. In general, the higher the workload, the lower the compliance with precaution measures and the higher the rate of nosocomial infection. Workload is inversely correlated with compliance in hand hygiene, and data from the medical ICU at the University of Geneva Hospitals have shown a parallel increase in nosocomial infection and the bed occupancy rate (Fig. 8.3). Other reasons include the selection pressure for resistant organisms induced by the high amount of antimicrobial use and the extensive exposure to medical devices. Furthermore, the patients' underlying conditions also play an important role. ICU patients normally have a seriously compromised ability to ward off infections due to impairment of natural host defense mechanisms by underlying diseases (malignancies and malnutrition) or as a result of severe medical and surgical interventions (increasing metabolic demand, injured tissue and wounds, major trauma, and perfusion deficits). Numerous studies have shown a correlation between the number of active comorbidities and the nosocomial infection rate and other medical complications. Moreover, natural chemical barriers in the stomach are often altered by H_2 blockers, and physiologic mechanisms for evacuating and cleansing hollow organs are disrupted or circumvented by the insertion of devices such as endotracheal tubes and urinary catheters. Almost all patients admitted to an ICU will

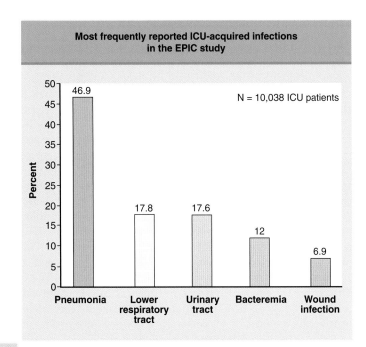

Figure 8.2. Most frequently reported ICU-acquired infections in the EPIC study.

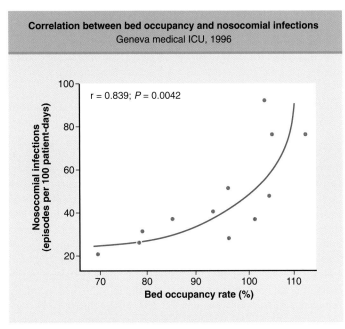

Figure 8.3. Correlation between bed occupancy and nosocomial infections, Geneva Medical ICU, 1996.

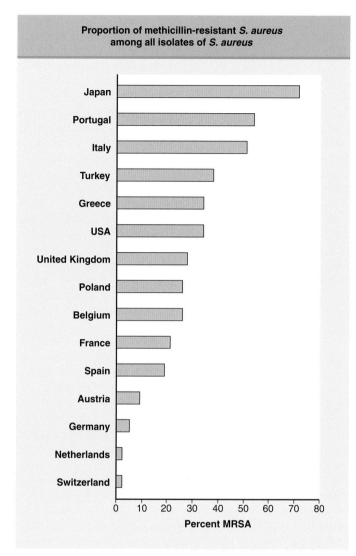

Figure 8.4. Proportion of methicillin-resistant *S. aureus* among all isolates of *S. aureus*.

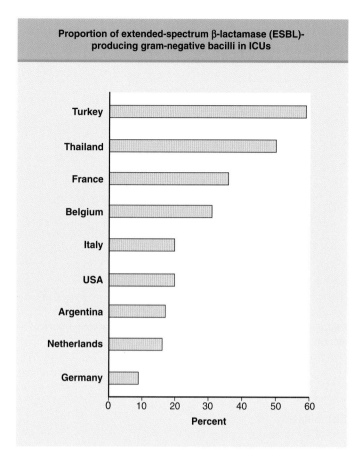

Figure 8.5. Proportion of extended-spectrum β-lactamase (ESBL) producing gram-negative bacilli in ICUs.

become a problem as, for example, in the case of a steady increase in nosocomial infections by nonalbicans *Candida* species. In summary, ICU-acquired infections and their control have become a major issue for hospital epidemiologists and infectious diseases and critical care physicians.

INFECTION CONTROL AND PREVENTION: A GENERAL OVERVIEW

The main strategy to combat nosocomial infections is to employ an infection control program. Infection control and prevention strategies are efficacious and contribute to substantial cost savings. The results of the pioneering Study on the Efficacy of Nosocomial Infection Control (SENIC), published in 1985, are illustrative. Hospitals were divided in two groups: One group of hospitals benefited from an infection control team/program and the other did not. Following an observation period of 5 years, the average rate of nosocomial infections increased by 18% in the group of hospitals without infection control, whereas a decrease of 32% was observed in the group of hospitals that benefited from an infection control program (Fig. 8.6). Although the study was scheduled for regular wards, other studies have confirmed the effectiveness of infection control in other settings, including the critical care setting. A general overview of the possible logistics in infection control is summarized in Figure 8.7.

have at least one vascular access or device breaking the normal skin barrier and enabling a direct connection to the external environment.

Nosocomial infections not only occur individually but also can develop as outbreaks. Epidemics are associated with specific organisms sometimes introduced from the exterior and remaining within the ICU because of the continuous selection pressure of antibiotics. These do not need to be virulent; it is sufficient to be resistant enough in order to persist. Leading pathogens are methicillin-resistant *Staphylococcus aureus* (MRSA) (Fig. 8.4) and multiresistant nonfermentative gram-negative rods such as *Pseudomonas* species, *Enterobacter* species, *Serratia* species, *Stenotrophomonas maltophilia*, and *Acinetobacter* species, all of which can become long-lasting problems. Pathogens producing extended-spectrum β-lactamases (ESBLs), such as *Klebsiella* species or *Escherichia coli*, are also a major concern in many countries (Fig. 8.5). To this list of pathogens, vancomycin-resistant enterococci (VRE) have been added in some areas of the world. In addition, pathogens other than bacteria can

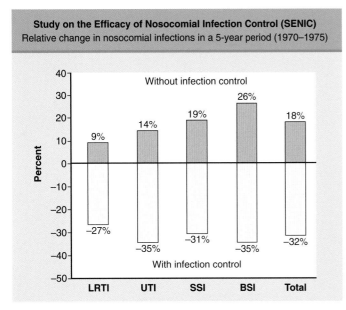

Figure 8.6. Study on the Efficacy of Nosocomial Infection Control (SENIC). Relative change in nosocomial infections during a 5-year period (1970–1975).

Surveillance

Although resource demanding, a correctly performed surveillance is a condition sine qua non for effective infection control. Surveillance may help to define and detect common or unusual sources of cross-infection or failure in patient care management. It summarizes rates and reports feedback for corrective actions, and it is best performed by dedicated, specifically trained infection control staff in close collaboration with the ICU team. Controversy exists regarding whether surveillance should be continued postdischarge. It is wise to prolong it for a brief period after the patient has left the ICU because many infections attributed to the ICU may become evident only in the days while the patient is on the general ward; this is particularly true for surgical site infections. Nevertheless, this approach is labor-intensive and may not always be justified. Hugonnet and associates assessed the added value of surveying discharged patients for 48 hours after discharge from a medical ICU. Only 5% of nosocomial infections were detected after discharge; thus, they concluded that postdischarge is resource demanding and allows the detection of only a few additional infections. However, target-oriented, postdischarge surveillance could be a rational alternative.

Surveillance can be passive—for example, a computer system reporting whenever certain key pathogens, such as MRSA, VRE, ESBL, *Serratia* spp., or resistant *Acinetobacter* spp., are detected in the microbiological laboratory. This kind of surveillance primarily collects data and resistance patterns. It has two disadvantages: a low sensitivity, since it does not detect nonmicrobiologically proven infections, and a low specificity because of the high prevalence of colonized, rather than infected, patients in ICUs.

Surveillance can also be active and target-oriented. The infection control team identifies and prioritizes specific objectives to be attained by surveillance and implementation of control measures (e.g., incidence and control of catheter-related blood-stream infection or active control of the spread of MRSA). In the ICU, where total surveillance requires one dedicated infection control nurse per 20 to 25 ICU beds, we recommend combining targeted and laboratory-oriented surveillance models because together they are more effective.

"Total surveillance" considers all types of nosocomial infections and attempts to correct problems as they arise but is labor-intensive and resource demanding. Daily active continuous surveillance by a full-time, dedicated infection control nurse enables the nurse to detect nosocomial infections as they arise, inform critical care colleagues about isolation precautions and specific control measures, and give immediate advice to ICU staff. This daily presence facilitates contact with ICU physicians and nurses and secures their active collaboration, thus contributing to a further reduction in nosocomial infections.

Acting

Surveillance implies the recognition and control of infections and cross-transmission. To decrease the incidence of infection, promotion and prevention programs and guidelines should be implemented. Prevention begins with the implementation of key basic rules, which are discussed briefly with a special emphasis on hand hygiene, the most important measure to prevent pathogen cross-transmission.

Basic Rules

Infection Transmission

The three major routes of infection transmission in hospitals are contact, droplet, and airborne transmission. Contact transmission is the major route of cross-transmission during health care in the hospital and occurs via physical contact with skin, most commonly from contaminated or colonized health-care workers' (HCWs) hands to patients. Physical contact also applies to contact with contaminated surfaces or instruments. Typical

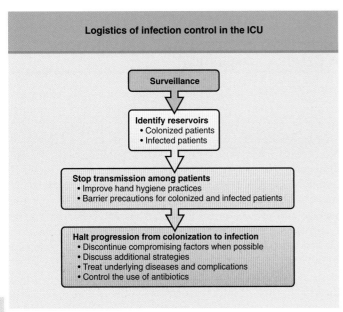

Figure 8.7. Logistics of infection control in the ICU.

examples of contact transmission include MRSA and VRE spread.

Droplet transmission occurs when large respiratory particles that contain infecting microorganisms (produced during coughing, sneezing, and talking or during invasive procedures such as bronchoscopy and suctioning) are subsequently deposited on the mucous membranes of the host's eye, nose, and mouth. Close contact, less than 1 m, increases the risk for transmission to occur since respiratory droplets do not last very long in the air and usually travel only short distances.

Airborne transmission occurs when infectious droplet nuclei or contaminated dust particles are inhaled. Droplet nuclei are less than 5 µm in size and can remain suspended in the air for long periods and travel long distances; therefore, special air handling and ventilation are required to prevent transmission.

Isolation Precautions

The Centers for Disease Control and Prevention and the Hospital Infection Control Practice Advisory Committee issued recommendations in 1996 defining two levels of transmission prevention: Standard precautions apply to all patients, and transmission-based precautions apply to patients with documented or suspected colonization and infection with specific microorganisms.

Standard precautions delineate the concept that all patients, irrespective of diagnosis, should be treated in a way that minimizes the risk of microorganism dissemination in the hospital. They protect both HCWs and patients. Standard precautions (Table 8.1) apply to blood, all body fluids (secretions and excretions) visibly bloody or not, and nonintact skin and mucous membranes. Transmission-based, specific precautions apply to selected patients having either a suspected or confirmed clinical syndrome or a specific diagnosis that predictably places others at risk of acquiring an infection. These patients are to be isolated accordingly.

ICUs should be equipped with at least one (ideally several) private room(s). A private room is mandatory for airborne-transmitted pathogens. It should be under negative pressure and equipped with HEPA filters. Patients with pulmonary and laryngeal tuberculosis, varicella and disseminated zoster, acute viral hemorrhagic fever, or severe measles should be placed in such a room with at least six air changes per hour and an appropriate discharge of air before it is circulated to other areas in the hospital. The door of the room should be kept closed and traffic should be reduced to an absolute minimum. An anteroom would be beneficial to allow air pressure differentials to be maintained at the time of door opening.

Patient care equipment in direct contact with intact skin may be colonized with epidemiologically important microorganisms. Sixty percent to 85% of stethoscope membranes were found to be colonized with high counts of pathogenic bacteria and, hence, should be considered a potential source of cross-transmission. Personal stethoscope membranes and the like should be disinfected between patient contacts.

Plants harbor potential pathogens and should be kept outside the rooms of severely immunocompromised patients. Neutropenic patients should be isolated in private rooms under specific contact and droplet precautions. We recommend that the rooms of all severely immunocompromised patients have anti-*Legionella* filters attached to water supplies, and regular microbiologic surveillance of *Legionella* sp. in circulating water systems is mandatory. In addition, the influence of construction work on possible *Aspergillus* sp. transmission should be recognized.

The risk of microorganism transmission by linen and eating utensils is negligible if they are handled according to any applicable hospital policy. The room and bedside equipment of patients on specific isolation are to be cleansed as routinely recommended for hospitals. Contaminated materials must be eliminated in a closed bag. For microorganisms capable of surviving for long periods in an inanimate environment, such as *Clostridium difficile*, special cleansing procedures are required according to hospital policy. Table 8.2 describes specific isolation techniques, and Box 8.1 gives examples of pathogen-specific transmission-based precautions.

Table 8.1 Standard Precautions	
Precaution	**Description**
Hand hygiene	After contact with blood, body fluids, secretions, excretions, contaminated items; after removing gloves; between patient contacts
Gloves	For anticipated contact with blood, body fluids, secretions, excretions, contaminated items; for anticipated contact with mucous membranes, nonintact skin
Mask, eye protection, face shield	To protect mucous membranes of the eyes, nose, and mouth during procedures and patient care activities likely to generate splashes or spray of blood, body fluids, secretions, and excretions
Gowns	To protect skin and prevent soiling of clothing during procedures and patient care activities likely to generate splashes or spray of blood, body fluids, secretions, and excretions
Patient care equipment handling	To ensure that skin, mucous membranes, and clothes are not exposed to equipment soiled with any body fluids; to ensure that reusable equipment is not reused until it has been appropriately reprocessed; to ensure that single-use items are discarded properly
Sharp object handling	Avoid recapping used needles; place used sharp objects and needles in puncture-resistant containers

Table 8.2 Practices of Specific Isolation	
Practice	**Description**
Contact	Private isolation if possible. Cohorting in case of an outbreak. Door can remain open. Skin and clothing protection; gloves, nonsterile, and gown. Changed after contact, followed by hand hygiene.
Droplet	Private isolation if possible. Cohorting in case of an outbreak. Maintain 1-m distance between infected and other patients. Door can remain open. Mucous membrane protection within 1 m of infected patient; within this distance, surgical mask necessary. Patient should wear surgical mask when exiting the room.
Airborne	Private isolation, strictly limited; negative air pressure (6–12 changes/hr, adequate air discharge). Door should remain closed. Respiratory protection; ultrafiltrant N-95 mask should be worn by health care workers entering the room and by patients exiting the room.

Hand Hygiene

HCWs' hands are the principal instruments in the course of complete nursing and highly invasive care in the ICU. Lack of or inadequate hand hygiene practice was the direct cause of cross-transmission in many endemic and epidemic situations. Since the days of Ignaz Semmelweis, hand hygiene was, is, and always will be the single most important measure to prevent cross-transmission and to reduce the rate of nosocomial colonization and infection. Indications for hand hygiene (also called opportunities) are listed in Box 8.2. Hand hygiene is the term used for hand cleansing methods and includes washing hands with water alone or water and nonantimicrobial/antimicrobial soap or hand rubbing with a waterless alcohol-based compound. Today, alcohol-based hand rubbing is considered the standard of care unless hands are visibly soiled. Alcohol-based hand rubbing consists of applying a small amount (3–5 mL) (i.e., a palmful)

of a fast-acting antiseptic preparation on both hands, covering all surfaces of the hands and fingers, and then rubbing hands together for 10 to 15 seconds; passive drying is obtained in 10 to 15 seconds, depending on the alcohol proportion of the solution and viscosity of the preparation.

Despite the large body of evidence supporting the effectiveness of hand hygiene in preventing cross-transmission, HCWs' compliance with recommendations in the absence of promotion programs remains unacceptably low worldwide, usually 30% to 50%. In intensive care, it is even lower. Explanations for such a low compliance include insufficient time due to high workload, inconvenient placement of hand cleansing facilities, inferior priority compared with other patient needs, lack of institutional priority for hand hygiene, lack of institutional safety climate, negative role models by opinion leaders, allergy or intolerance to hand hygiene solutions, and lack of role model of superiors and awareness of recommendations or skepticism toward their effect on nosocomial infection. Not surprisingly, high demand for hand hygiene is inversely correlated with the number of opportunities per hour of patient care (Fig. 8.8). The systematic recourse to hand rubbing bypasses this time constraint: It is efficacious with application times of only 15 to 20 seconds. Furthermore, it is also more efficacious compared to other antimicrobial agents (Fig. 8.9), acts faster (Fig. 8.10), and irritates skin less often. The hand rub solution can be carried in pockets, circumventing the need to go to a sink to wash and dry hands. Figure 8.11 shows an example from the University of Geneva Hospitals. To improve compliance with hand hygiene recommendations, a system change must be addressed in ICUs in which alcohol-based hand rubbing has not yet become a standard of care. However, this is not the only parameter of a suc-

Box 8.2 Indications for Hand Hygiene (Opportunities) during Patient Care

1. *Before* having direct contact with patients
2. *Before* donning sterile gloves when inserting a central intravascular catheter
3. *Before* inserting indwelling urinary catheters, peripheral venous catheters, or other invasive devices
4. *After* contact with a patient's intact skin (e.g., taking a pulse or blood pressure or lifting a patient)
5. *After* contact with body fluids or excretions, mucous membranes, nonintact skin, or wound dressings
6. *If moving* from a contaminated body site to a clean body site during patient care
7. *After* contact with inanimate objects (including medical equipment) in the immediate vicinity of the patient
8. *After* removing gloves

Adapted from Pittet D, Hugonnet S, Harbarth S, et al: Effectiveness of a hospital-wide programme to improve compliance with hand hygiene. Lancet 2000;356:1307–1312 and www.who.int/patientsafety/events/05/HH_en.pdf (accessed October 27, 2005).

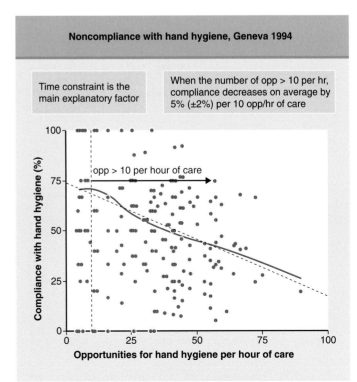

Figure 8.8. Noncompliance with hand hygiene, Geneva, 1994.

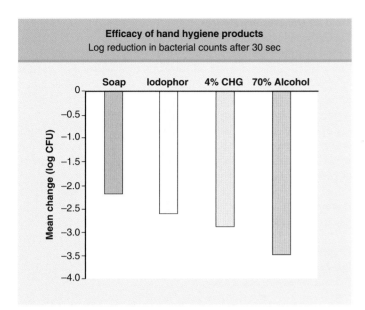

Figure 8.9. Efficacy of hand hygiene products. Log reduction in bacterial counts after 30 sec.

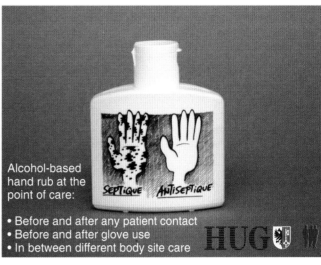

Figure 8.11. Hand rub solution.

cessful promotion program. Improving hand hygiene implies a multimodal approach at the individual and institutional levels. Education of HCWs, patients, and all hospital staff is a cornerstone and should be promoted at all levels of experience. Degree of knowledge does not predict appropriate behavior. Every HCW must be aware of the availability of guidelines and potential risk for cross-transmission to patient and acquisition from patient; recognize high-risk opportunities; and have knowledge of its impact on morbidity, mortality, and costs of nosocomial

infections. In addition, knowledge must be acquired on skin care and use of protection agents; evidence for the impact of improved hand hygiene on the reduction of infection rates and cross-transmission; and hand hygiene technique with the amount of solution to use, the duration of the procedure, and the reason for the choice of the agent.

Knowledge alone is not sufficient, however. Reminders in the workplace may help HCWs improve and maintain practices. We have used posters on hospital walls ("talking walls"; Fig. 8.12) and obtained active participation at the individual and institutional levels (i.e., hospital senior management). These actions possibly promoted an appropriate institutional safety climate and clearly illustrated the support from superiors in the hierarchic structure. Nurses and physicians should serve as positive role models. Within social groups, opinion leaders exert a significant amount of influence over others. Participatory decision making and the introduction of monitoring and regular feedback of hand hygiene performance complete the promotion campaign.

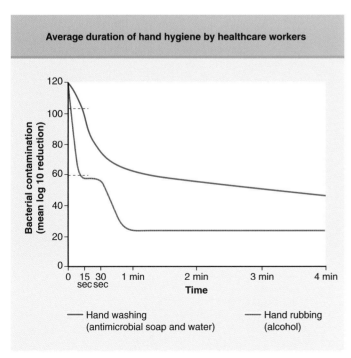

Figure 8.10. Average duration of hand hygiene by healthcare workers.

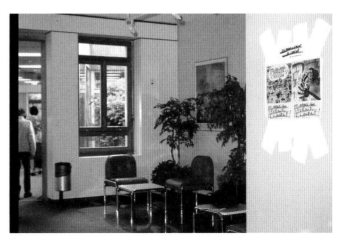

Figure 8.12. "Talking walls."

As shown in Box 8.3, the key for successful hand hygiene promotion is to implement a multimodal strategy. At the University of Geneva Hospitals, we implemented such a promotion program and showed significant reductions of MRSA cross-transmission and nosocomial infection hospitalwide over 4 years. During the study period, average compliance with hand hygiene increased from 48% to 66%. The costs of the entire program correspond to approximately 1% of the financial burden of nosocomial infections.

Vaccination

As for many infection prevention strategies, vaccination is an elegant solution for preventing nosocomial transmission of pathogens. The most important vaccinations in the ICU setting are for varicella-zoster virus if there is no anamnesis or serological confirmation of German measles during childhood, hepatitis B, and the combined vaccination for measles, rubella, and mumps, particularly in the pediatric ICU.

Nutrition

Deficiency in nutrition is one of the important risk factors for acquiring an infection; thus, the patient's nutritional status has to be routinely evaluated and deficiencies have to be substituted. Enteral feeding is preferred because it may prevent the intestinal translocation of pathogens, in contrast to parenteral nutrition, which is a risk factor for catheter-associated bloodstream infection.

Engineering and Administrative Control for Medical Equipment

The contribution of the design of critical care units to infection control is difficult to evaluate, and several well-designed studies failed to find improvement after the units were moved into modern structures; however, it seems prudent to consider some issues when remodeling or designing new units. Adequate space around beds is important. Clean function and storage should be physically separated from dirty function and waste disposal. Sinks should be located in convenient places. New diagnostic and therapeutic devices are constantly introduced into ICUs. Cleaning and reprocessing protocols for these devices should be provided, and HCWs should be sufficiently trained in their proper use.

Avoid All Unnecessary Devices

This basic rule cannot be emphasized enough. In an ICU setting, a good example is urinary catheters. The EPIC study highlighted the relative importance of all kinds of devices for nosocomial infections. Although there may be some reports of reduced urinary tract infections by the use of cranberry juice or acidification of the urine, urinary catheters have to be removed as soon as possible. In contrast to patients in regular wards, ICU patients often cannot be acidified, are more immunocompromised, and are often not able to indicate complications such as development of prostatitis.

Understaffing

Understaffing of HCWs should be avoided.

Prevention of Typical ICU-Related Infection/Colonization

Central Venous Access Lines

The incidence of catheter-related bloodstream infection (CRI) ranges from 2 to 14 episodes per 1000 catheter-days. On average, microbiologically documented, device-related bloodstream infections complicate the use of a central venous line in 3 to 5 per 100 cases. However, this represents only a small portion of cases, and most episodes of clinical sepsis are considered to be catheter related. Nearly 90% of all primary bloodstream infection in the ICU is due to catheters. Attributable morbidity of CRI is significant, with additional ICU stay and high attributable costs. Four distinct pathways may be identified in the infection process of CRIs (Fig. 8.13). External and internal catheter surface colonization pathways involve colonization

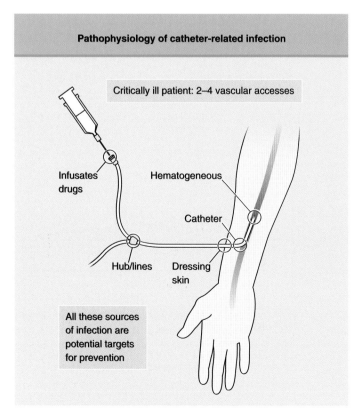

Pathophysiology of catheter-related infection

Critically ill patient: 2–4 vascular accesses

Infusates drugs

Hematogeneous

Catheter

Hub/lines

Dressing skin

All these sources of infection are potential targets for prevention

Figure 8.13. Pathophysiology of catheter-related infection.

of the skin insertion site and hub, respectively. Because the hub is opened up to five times per hour, its colonization can be a major source of infection. Additional pathways include microbial contamination of the infusate (so-called intrinsic contamination) and hematogenous seeding from a distant source. A large proportion of these infections are preventable, and this has been the objective of precise guidelines whose major issues are listed next.

Hand hygiene

Infection prevention is based mostly on the optimal adherence to the basic rules of hygiene. A strict adherence to hand hygiene measures (hand washing and/or hand antisepsis) and to aseptic techniques in caring for patients and handling devices is the key requirement of these precautions.

Technique of catheter insertion

Skin preparation should include hair cutting rather than shaving. Maximal sterile barrier precautions during insertion, including not only small fenestrated drapes and the use of sterile gloves but also gown, cap, mask, and a large drape, can minimize catheter colonization and further CRIs. Rigorous cleansing and disinfection of the insertion site are regarded as other key points. Povidone iodine (10%), aqueous chlorhexidine (2%), and alcohol (70%) are effective. We favor the use of a combination of isopropyl alcohol (75%) and chlorhexidine (0.5%).

Topical antimicrobial ointments have been proposed to prevent catheter colonization, but they favor colonization by resistant organisms and are no longer recommended.

Site of insertion

Central lines inserted in the jugular site are more likely to be colonized than those inserted via the subclavian route. This is due to factors favoring skin colonization, such as proximity of oropharyngeal secretions, higher skin temperature, and difficulties in immobilizing the catheter and maintaining an optimal dressing, particularly in men. Careful fixation of the catheter at the skin exit site may avoid complications such as leakage of the fixing device and movements in the intradermal portion. This technique allows the use of small dressings that are easier to secure.

Type of catheter

Whether catheters with multiple lumens are more prone to infection than single-lumen devices is a matter of debate. What is known is that the infection rate is higher with polyvinylchloride catheters than with polyurethane devices. A meta-analysis suggested that tunneled short-term CVCs are associated with a reduced rate of CRI, but this may be the case only for those inserted in the jugular site.

Dressing

Semipermeable transparent dressings are now widely used. Easy to place, they allow continuous observation of the skin insertion site and may reduce the risk of extrinsic contamination. However, they promote moisture and bacterial proliferation and have been repeatedly associated with higher CRI rates compared to traditional gauze dressings. Therefore, the systematic use of transparent dressings cannot be recommended in critically ill patients, particularly within the first 24 hours after insertion.

The precise duration that a gauze dressing can be safely left on a central line is unknown, but it should be systematically renewed every 48 to 72 hours if an earlier change is not clinically indicated.

Catheter handling, replacement, and/or guidewire exchange

Except for blood products and lipid emulsions, administration sets can be safely replaced every 72 hours. The duration of catheterization has been linked to the risk of CRIs, particularly after 7 days, but the efficacy of systematic routine replacement of central lines has not been proven with regard to decreasing the risk for infection. Guidewire exchange may increase the likelihood of infection of the new catheter, but it reduces the rate of complications associated with CVC placement in a new site, which may be technically difficult, particularly in severely ill patients. Randomized prospective studies failed to detect any preventive benefit associated with guidewire exchange compared to insertion at a new site. For many experts, guidewire exchange with systematic (semi)quantitative culture of the catheter tip is mandatory in any case of sepsis without clinical evidence of another source of infection. This allows removal of the exchanged catheter and mandates further insertion at a new site only if the culture of the removed material is positive.

Intraluminal antibiotic lock or flush

Intraluminal antibiotic lock, as well as flush with antibiotics, has been reported to reduce the rate of CRIs, but only a few studies have been conducted on ICU patients. Vancomycin has been proposed and used. However, the use of antimicrobial agents for this purpose may lead to the emergence of vancomycin-resistant, gram-positive organisms, which must be avoided because the glycopeptide antibiotics are the only drugs currently available for the treatment of infections due to methicillin-resistant staphylococci and resistant enterococci.

Antibiotic- and antiseptic-coated catheters

Several randomized clinical studies suggested that the use of catheters impregnated with either chlorhexidine and silver sulfadiazine or minocycline and rifampin was associated with a significant reduction of microbiologically documented CRIs of 30% to 45% and 65% to 80%, respectively. Compared to chlorhexidine–sulfadiazine-coated catheters, the minocycline–rifampin-impregnated catheters were reported to be associated with significantly lower colonization [relative risk, 0.35; confidence interval (CI), 0.24–0.55] and CRIs (relative risk, 0.08; CI, 0.01–0.63). The authors argue that this difference may be due, in part, to the absence of silver sulfadiazine in the intraluminal surface (Fig. 8.14). However, the duration of catheter placement may well have played a role. Impregnated catheters failed to prevent CRIs in neutropenic cancer patients with a mean catheterization time of 20 days compared to 6, 7, and 8.3 days for others. In a meta-analysis, we confirmed that the potential benefit of these devices may be lost after 7 to 10 days.

Educational programs

Sherertz and colleagues reported that an educational program of physicians-in-training can decrease the risk of CRIs. A 1-day course on infection control practices and procedures of vascular access insertion was shown to reduce the infection rate

Prevention effect of coated catheters		
Type of coating	**In vitro studies**	**Clinical studies**
Chlorhexidine-Si-sulfadiazine	⊕	⊕
Minocycline-rifampin	⊕	⊕
Liberation of silver	⊕	⊕

Figure 8.14. Prevention effect of coated catheters.

Table 8.3 Education-Based Prevention of Catheter-Related Infection: Guidelines Included in the Global Preventive Strategy[a]	
Method	**Description**
Material	Complete listing to avoid insertion interruptions
Insertion	Skin preparation: hair cutting instead of shaving
Antisepsis	Chlorhexidine 0.5% in alcohol 75%
	Max. barrier precautions: gown, cap, mask, drapes
Technique	Promotion of subclavian/wrist vein
Dressing	Dry gauze, occlusive adhesive band
Replacement	72-hr intervals: dress, sets, devices
	24-hr intervals: lipid or blood product lines
Removal	Peripheral lines after 72 hr
	Central lines over guidewire as clinically indicated
Hygiene	Hand antisepsis strongly emphasized for any care

[a]Adapted from Eggimann P, Harbarth S, Constantin MN, et al: Impact of a prevention strategy targeted at vascular-access care on incidence of infections acquired in Intensive care. Lancet 2000;355:1864–1868.

by almost 30%, from 4.5 to 2.9 per 1000 catheter-days. The educational program included a 1-hour introduction to basic infection control principles (hand hygiene, isolation and barrier use, and handling of patients with resistant organisms and varicella virus). Thereafter, these students and physicians rotated through a series of 1-hour stations, during which they received 5 to 15 minutes of didactic instruction followed by hands-on instruction overseen by faculty members. Training was provided in (1) blood draws through vascular lines, (2) arterial puncture, (3) insertion of arterial lines and catheters, (4) peripheral venous catheter insertion, (5) phlebotomy, and (6) urinary catheter insertion.

At the University of Geneva Hospitals, we performed a study targeted at the reduction of CRIs in 3154 patients admitted to a medical ICU. Specific guidelines included in the strategy and implemented through an educational program targeted at vascular access care are discussed in the preceding sections and summarized in Table 8.3. The program consisted of slide show-based educational sessions and the bedside training of the entire ICU staff, including nurses (Fig. 8.15). Following the introduction of the program, the incidence density of exit site catheter infection decreased by 64% and that of bloodstream infection by 67%. Although the overall exposure to catheters did not significantly differ between the control and the intervention periods (median duration, 4 days; $P = 0.94$), the infection rates decreased due to a reduced incidence of both microbiologically documented infection (from 6.6 to 2.3 episodes per 1000 CVC-days) and clinical sepsis (from 16.3 to 3.9 episodes per 1000 CVC-days). Overall, the incidence density of nosocomial infections was reduced by 35% (from 52.4 to 34.0 episodes per 1000 patient-days). Due to regular repetitions, the success of our

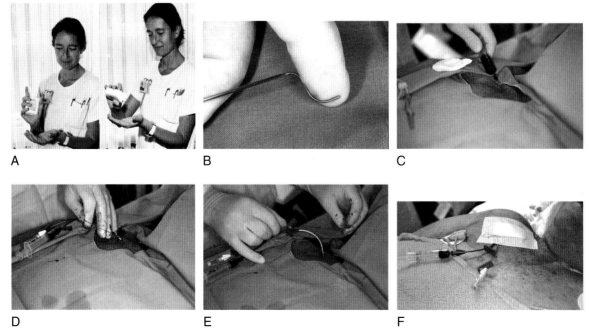

A B C

D E F

Figure 8.15. Examples of the educational slide show used at the University of Geneva Hospitals.

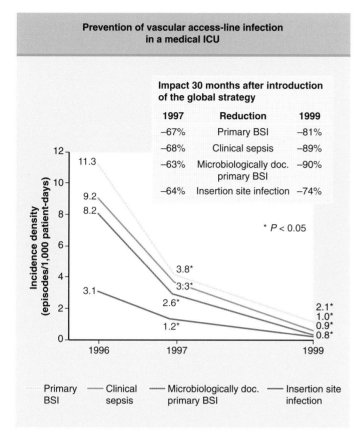

Figure 8.16. Prevention of vascular access line infection in the ICU.

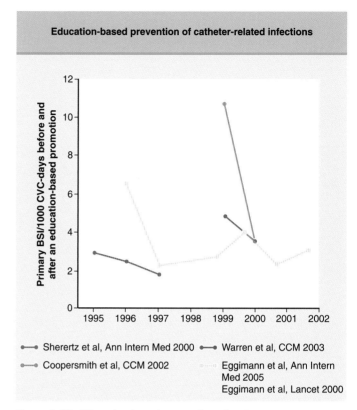

Figure 8.17. Education-based prevention of catheter-related infections.

program was maintained over several years (Fig. 8.16). Other experiences with prevention programs based on education and global prevention strategies are shown in Fig. 8.17. These observations indicate that educational programs are successful when based on multimodal and multidisciplinary approaches, including communication and education tools, active participation and positive feedback, and systematic involvement of institution leaders. Further improvement of efficacy is theoretically possible by implementation of new technologies such as coated catheters. Nevertheless, we consider that this approach is futile if the basic measures and educational activities have not been fully implemented (Fig. 8.18).

Ventilator-Associated Pneumonia

The prevalence of nosocomial pneumonia within the ICU setting ranges from 10% to 65%. Ventilator-associated pneumonia (VAP) is estimated to occur in approximately 25% of mechanically ventilated patients. Pneumonia incidence is constant during the first 8 to 10 days but develops in approximately 5% of patients with each additional day of mechanical ventilation. Nasotracheal intubation is associated with a significantly higher risk of infection than orotracheal intubation. Crude mortality of VAP ranges from 20% to 50% and attributable mortality from 8% to 27%. Impairment of reflexes protecting the airways is the most important risk factor for early onset VAP. Aspiration of oropharyngeal flora is the presumed mode of inoculation. In late-onset VAP, the main risk factors are the presence of the endotracheal tube, changes in endogenous flora, and

changes in the surrounding ICU environment and patient management. ICU length of stay is significantly longer for patients with early- and late-onset VAP (10.3 and 21.0 days, respectively) compared to patients without VAP (3.5 days). Data from the University of Geneva Hospitals are shown in Table 8.4.

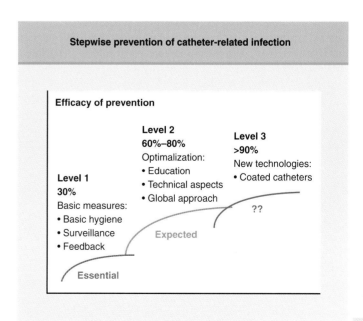

Figure 8.18. Stepwise prevention of catheter-related infection.

81

Table 8.4 Morbidity and Costs Associated with VAP: Medical ICU, University of Geneva Hospitals, 1995–1997[a]

	No. of Pairs	Cases	Controls	Attributable to VAP
Length of stay (days)				
Total population	97	15.0 (2–134)	10 (2–45)	5.0
Survivors	50	15.5 (4–63)	11 (3–45)	5.5
Duration of MV (days)				
Total population	97	10 (1–123)	7.0 (1–34)	3.0
Survivors	50	11 (2–61)	7.5 (1–34)	3.5
Costs (Swiss francs)				
Total population	97	32,145	22,670	9475
Survivors	50	33,819	24,048	9771

MV, mechanical ventilation.
[a]Data from Hugonnet 41th ICAAC 01.

Box 8.4 VAP Prevention Strategies

1. Place mechanically ventilated patients in a semirecumbent position by maintaining the head of the bed at approximately 30° or greater above the horizontal plane as tolerated by the patient.
2. Intubate the trachea orally whenever possible to minimize the risk of nosocomial sinusitis; avoid nasotracheal intubation because of the association between nosocomial sinusitis and ventilator-associated pneumonia.
3. Use oral gastric tubes rather than nasogastric tubes; nasogastric tubes may increase the possibility of nosocomial sinusitis.
4. Extubate patients and remove orogastric tubes as soon as clinically indicated.
5. Prevent accidental extubation; adequately secure the endotracheal tube to the patient and/or restrain the patient per hospital policy, if necessary, to prevent accidental self-extubation.
6. Provide adequate sedation to prevent unexpected extubation.
7. Avoid gastric overdistention; monitor gastric residual volumes before administering scheduled enteral feedings (gastric residual, 150–200 mL).
8. Provide oral hygiene at least once daily.
9. Drain condensate from ventilator circuits regularly with gloved hands; open ventilator circuit and carefully drain condensate into an open container, being careful not to touch the circuit tip to the container; reconnect tubing carefully to avoid contamination; empty container contents into hopper immediately; do not empty fluid into the trash can or onto the floor.
10. Use in-line valved T adapters or holding chambers for aerosolized medication delivery.
11. Use noninvasive mechanical ventilation via face mask when appropriate to minimize the need for tracheal intubation.
12. Avoid overuse of antibiotics.
13. Provide daily chlorhexidine oral rinse (only for patients undergoing cardiac surgery).
14. Provide immunizations for influenza and *Streptococcus pneumoniae*.
15. Clean hands as frequently as indicated during patient care (see also Box 8.2), including immediately after glove removal.
16. Change gloves as soon as necessary.

Adapted from Zack JE, Garrison T, Trovillion E, et al: Effect of an education program aimed at reducing the occurrence of ventilator-associated pneumonia. Crit Care Med 2002;30:2407–2412 and www.who.int/patientsafety/events/05/HH_en.pdf (accessed October 27, 2005).

Prevention is not simple and should be based on multimodal approaches (Box 8.4). A large proportion of VAP is related to the continuous aspiration of contaminated oropharyngeal secretions and/or possibly gastric content, and many preventive measures are targeted at interrupting this process (Fig. 8.19). Several randomized studies have found that sucralfate, which does not lower gastric pH, is associated with lower rates of VAP than histamine H_2 receptor antagonists, but data suggest that it may be less efficient in stress ulcer prophylaxis; however, this field remains controversial.

Selective digestive decontamination (SDD) is the most extensively studied method for the prevention of infection in ICU patients but remains a matter of debate. In most studies, SDD resulted in significant reductions in the incidence of VAP, but variations in definitions and case mix make comparisons hazardous. These reductions were generally not associated with improved patient survival or decreased morbidity. In addition, no formal cost–benefit analyses of SDD are available. Moreover, SDD is associated with the selection of microorganisms that are intrinsically resistant to the antimicrobial regimen used and may lead to antibiotic resistance acquisition. Accordingly, investigators have proposed that as long as the benefits of SDD are not firmly established, its routine use for mechanically ventilated patients is not advised. However, further investigation in the context of strictly controlled clinical trials is warranted.

Continuous subglottic aspiration of oropharyngeal secretions is an original concept first described by Vallès and coworkers. In a series of 190 mechanically ventilated patients, these authors observed a marked reduction in the incidence-density of nosocomial pneumonia from 39.6 episodes per 1000 ventilator-days in the control group to 19.9 episodes per 1000 ventilator-days in patients receiving continuous aspiration. This effect was confirmed in patients after cardiac surgery.

Noninvasive ventilation significantly reduces the risk of VAP in chronic obstructive pulmonary disease (COPD) as well as for immunocompromised and most other patient populations. It reduces the number of intubations, the use of respiratory antibiotics, as well as global mortality. Nourdine and colleagues proved that noninvasive ventilation may also have a positive impact on other nosocomial infections. In this study, the incidence-density of lower respiratory tract, urinary tract, and bloodstream infections was 14.2 episodes per 1000 patient-days in patients who

had undergone successful noninvasive ventilation compared to 30.3 episodes per 1000 patient-days in those who required mechanical ventilation. A matched case–control study in two groups of ICU patients confirmed that compared to mechanical ventilation, noninvasive ventilation significantly improved survival of critically ill patients requiring ventilator assistance, essentially by lowering the risk of both nosocomial infection and nosocomial pneumonia (18% vs. 60% and 8% vs. 22%; $P < 0.01$ and $P = 0.04$, respectively).

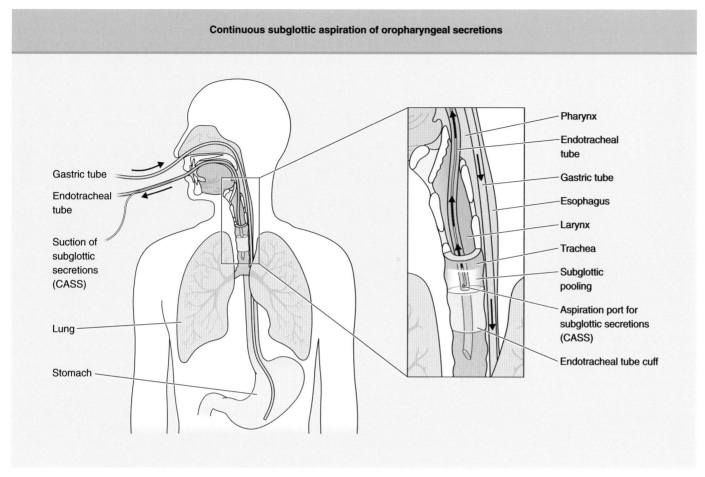

Figure 8.19. Continuous subglottic aspiration of oropharyngeal secretions. CASS, continuous aspiration of subglottic secretions.

Less continuous sedation, as well as the use of fewer invasive devices such as central venous access and urinary catheterization, may also have played an important role in the reduction of the observed infection rates. Continuous sedation is a significant risk factor for VAP. In a prospective study of 250 critically ill patients, Rello and associates reported that mechanical ventilation after cardiopulmonary resuscitation (odds ratio, 5.13; CI, 2.14–12.26) and continuous sedation (odds ratio, 4.40; CI, 1.83–10.59) were significant risk factors for the development of VAP.

Newer approaches to prevention are emerging. Repeated antibiotic oral solutions are effective but harbor the disadvantage of resistance selection. The use of antiseptics, such as chlorhexidine, may be beneficial and not associated with resistance acquisition. Short-chain antimicrobial peptides are being investigated on a preventive basis in phase III trials. They act successfully in vitro on bacteria as well as on fungi by selectively disrupting microbial membranes.

TARGETING ANTIBIOTIC RESISTANCE

In the ICU, where antibiotics are used more frequently and in larger amounts than in almost any other ward in the hospital, antibiotic resistance promotes and propagates the persistence of multiresistant nosocomial pathogens. The whole process induces

a fatal circuit inasmuch as these multiresistant pathogens have to be treated again with broader spectrum antibiotics, which in turn increases the resistance pattern. The result is virtually a panresistance for certain microorganisms, with a negative effect on patient outcome (Fig. 8.20). Moreover, the close proximity

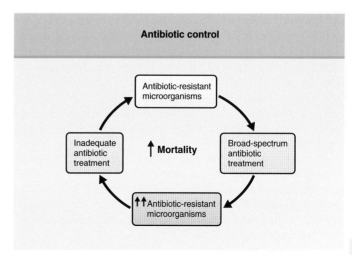

Figure 8.20. Antibiotic control.

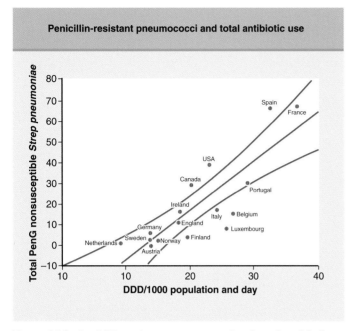

Penicillin-resistant pneumococci and total antibiotic use

Figure 8.21. Penicillin-resistant pneumococci and total antibiotic use. (Adapted from Albrich WC, Monnet DL, Harbarth S: Antibiotic selection pressure and resistance in Streptococcus pneumoniae and Streptococcus pyogenes. Emerg Infect Dis 2004;10:514–517.)

of patients and the high workload of HCWs facilitate transfer of resistant organisms from patient to patient. The relation between antibiotic resistance and antibiotic use in the ICU has been confirmed in a large, multicenter study—the Intensive Care Antimicrobial Resistance Epidemiology project conducted in 1994. The use of antimicrobials showed important variations between institutions with similar prevalence of resistant bacteria, confirming that efforts to control resistance should focus on both antibiotic use and infection control practices. This is not surprising since even population-based studies in much larger settings have shown a linear correlation between antibiotic use and resistance, for example, among pneumococci (Fig. 8.21).

Infection control strategies do reduce nosocomial infections and have proven their potential to save money by diminishing antibiotic use. It seems logical that by reducing antibiotic use and limiting the spread of resistance by cross-transmission, we would favorably change the ecology within the ICU and antibiotic resistance in the hope that multiresistant organisms would be replaced by more sensitive ones. Even if this change did not alter the rate of ICU-acquired infection, it would surely contribute to reducing the costs associated with antibiotic use and isolation measures and improve patient safety. Antibiotic control thus becomes another major objective for infection control professionals and critical care physicians.

Antibiotic control is not easy to implement. Antibiotic use in general is warranted by the clinical situation of individual patients. Critical care physicians tend to treat their patients with the best available drugs according to their beliefs. A coordinated strategy at the hospital or ward level faces this obstacle. However, there are ways to combat it.

First, guidelines for the duration of antibiotic prophylaxis and therapy must be implemented and their application controlled.

This is an issue of special importance. Unnecessary use of antimicrobials, especially broad-spectrum antibiotics, must be reduced to a minimum. The deescalation of antibiotics should not be forgotten either. As soon as the antibiogram is known, the antibiotic should be replaced with a narrower spectrum drug. Prestratification to identify patients with a high risk of colonization by multiresistant pathogens (prolonged hospitalization, high exposure to devices, and previous antibiotic therapy) would help to distinguish between those patients for whom broad-spectrum antibiotics should be started and those at low risk and for whom a narrower spectrum would be sufficient.

Second, antibiotic use can be restricted by directives. The experience reported in the literature is ambiguous. There are several studies with different methodologies. It is clear that restriction of antibiotics reduces costs, but is there evidence of a real efficacy in reducing resistance? This question cannot be clearly answered, and reducing the use and the resistance to one antibiotic (class) may promote resistance to another compound or class of compounds. Rahal and colleagues (1998) implemented a restriction for cephalosporins and reported a reduction of 44% of nosocomial infections by multiresistant organisms. However, due to an increase in the concomitant use of imipenem, there was a simultaneous 69% increase in the rate of *Pseudomonas aeruginosa* resistant to imipenem, showing a compensatory increase in resistance for nonrestricted antibiotics.

Third, sophisticated computer programs could help to guide the administration of antibiotics. An example has been developed at the Latter Day Saints Hospital in Salt Lake City by combining an antibiotics list with precise guidelines for their use. According to published data, it has at least contributed to reduce the incidence of side effects, the total number of antibiotics used, and their costs. However, guides for antibiotic use do not necessarily have to be computer programs. Consulting a hospital pharmacologist or infectious disease specialist has also proven its efficacy.

Finally, a programmed regular change or rotation in the empiric prescription of first-choice antibiotics is another option. The antibiotics changed should, but do not need to be, of different classes. Kollef and coworkers (1997) investigated the influence of a programmed change in first-choice antibiotics on the incidence of VAP and nosocomial bacteremia after cardiac surgery. During a 6-month period, they prescribed ceftazidime for the empiric treatment of suspected gram-negative bacterial infections. This was followed by a 6-month period during which ciprofloxacin was used in place of ceftazidime. The incidence of VAP decreased significantly in the second period ($P = 0.028$). This was primarily due to a significant reduction in the incidence of VAP attributed to antibiotic-resistant gram-negative bacteria ($P = 0.013$). They also observed a lower incidence of bacteremia attributed to antibiotic-resistant, gram-negative bacteria. Similar findings are confirmed by others. A prospective cohort study reported a decrease in mortality associated with infection (2.9 vs. 9.6 deaths/100 admissions, $P < 0.0001$) during rotation of antibiotics in a surgical ICU. The long-lasting impact of changes or rotations in empiric antibiotic prescription, however, remains unknown, and such programs are not routinely incorporated in most hospitals. The approach is challenging, and its value in delaying the emergence of resistance needs to be further studied.

ESBL-PRODUCING AND NONFERMENTATIVE GRAM-NEGATIVE RODS

ESBL-producing gram-negative rods are present in many ICUs worldwide and are reaching the threshold of a veritable pandemic. Their transferable plasmid-mediated antibiotic resistance emerges with the use of broad-spectrum antibiotics, especially third-generation cephalosporins and aminoglycosides, ensuring that the bacteria persist in the ICU. Large outbreaks, even involving several ICUs and spread to other hospital units, have been reported. Nonfermentative gram-negative rods share the same distribution pattern, selected by pressure of antibiotics to which the bacteria are resistant by acquisition or by nature.

Infection control has to focus on early detection and prompt containment of resistant gram-negative bacteria imported from outside the ICU setting. Once imported, it is often very difficult to control their spread. Sometimes, the entire ward may have to be closed temporarily. Simple contact isolation and alcohol-based hand rubbing are the most important measure and may already diminish horizontal transmission. In some circumstances, targeted surveillance cultures (screening of the perianal region) to identify asymptomatic carriers with chromosomal or plasmid-mediated ESBL strains may be indicated, especially in the case of patients transferred from epicenters of antimicrobial resistance. Microbiologic surveillance of all patients admitted to the ICU is only warranted in some outbreak situations.

CONCLUSION

Despite high workload, time constraints, and severe morbidity of patients in the ICU (Fig. 8.22), infection prevention and control are possible and effective and should be mandatory. A multimodal approach with the assistance of a specialist team and all HCWs involving surveillance, isolation, basic rules, and perhaps even antibiotic control will help to significantly reduce the rate of nosocomial infections (Box 8.5, Table 8.5, and Fig. 8.23).

Acknowledgment

We are indebted to Rosemary Sudan for expert and outstanding editorial assistance.

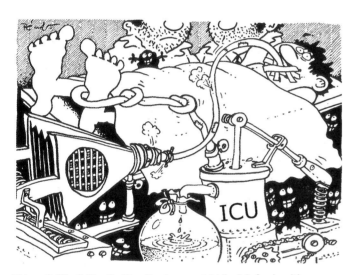

Figure 8.22. Critically ill patients are at high risk for health care–associated infection.

Box 8.5 Controversies in Nonantimicrobial Measurement to Prevent Infection in Critical Care

- Postdischarge surveillance
- Total surveillance
- Private room at disposal
- Understaffing, increased bed occupancy rate
- Multiple lumen catheters
- Guidewire exchange of catheters
- Coated catheters
- Targeting antibiotic resistance
- Restriction of antibiotic use
- Programmed rotation of antibiotics

Table 8.5 Risks and Benefits of Infection Control

Controversy	Risks	Benefits
Postdischarge surveillance	Costly, labor-intensive Detects essentially surgical site infections	Detects half of surgical site infections
Total surveillance	Labor-intensive; resource-demanding	Immediate detection of infections and dangers
Private room at disposal	Costly No evidence-based protection of neutropenic patients	Enables isolation of patients with airborne-transmitted pathogens
Understaffing; increased bed occupancy rate	Reduced personal costs	Increase in the incidence of nosocomial infections
Multiple lumen catheters	More prone to infection?	Concomitant administration of many products
Guidewire exchange of catheters	Reduced rate of CVC placement complications	Increases the likelihood of infection of the new catheter
Coated catheters	Reduction of catheter-related infections	Emergence of resistance; no benefit after 7–10 days and no benefit in neutropenic cancer patients
Sucralfate for prophylaxis of VAP	Lower rates of VAP than with H_2 receptor antagonists	Less efficient stress ulcer prophylaxis?
Selective digestive decontamination	Reduction in incidence of VAP	No improved survival; no decreased morbidity; no cost benefit analyses? Selection of resistant organisms
Targeting antibiotic resistance	Reduction in incidence of nosocomial infections?	Reduction in antibiotic resistance and antibiotic costs Improved patient safety
Restriction of antibiotic use	Reduced resistance in a global manner?	Reduced costs
Programmed rotation of antibiotics	Reduced mortality? Reduced VAP?	Long-term effects unknown

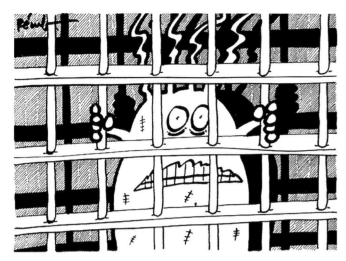

Figure 8.23. Appropriate infection control measures keep multiresistant bacteria away.

SUGGESTED READING

Boyce J, Pittet D: Guideline for hand hygiene in health-care settings: Recommendations of the CDC-HICPAC/SHEA/APIC/IDSA Hand Hygiene Task Force. MMWR 2002;51(RR16):1–44

Eggimann P, Harbarth S, Constantin MN, et al: Impact of a prevention strategy targeted at vascular-access care on incidence of infections acquired in intensive care. Lancet 2000;355:1864–1868.

Hugonnet S, Eggiman P, Borst F, et al: Impact of ventilator-associated pneumonia on resource utilization and patient outcome. Infect Control Hosp Epidemiol 2004;25:1090–1096.

Hugonnet S, Eggiman P, Sax H, et al: Intensive care unit–acquired infections: Is postdischarge surveillance useful? Crit Care Med 2002;30:2636–2638.

Kollef M, Vlasnik J, Sharpless L, et al: Scheduled change of antibiotic classes: A strategy to decrease the incidence of ventilator-associated pneumonia. Am J Respir Crit Care Med 1997;156:1040–1048.

Monnet D, Archibald L, Phillips L, et al: Antimicrobial use and resistance in eight US hospitals: Complexities of analysis and modeling. Intensive Care Antimicrobial Resistance Epidemiology Project and National Nosocomial Infections Surveillance System Hospitals. Infect Control Hosp Epidemiol 1998;19:388–394.

Nourdine K, Combes P, Carton MJ, et al: Does noninvasive ventilation reduce the ICU nosocomial infection risk? A prospective clinical survey. Intensive Care Med 1999;25:553–555.

Pittet D: Improving compliance with hand hygiene in hospitals. Infect Control Hosp Epidemiol 2000;21:381–386.

Pittet D, Boyce JM: Hand hygiene and patient care: Pursuing the Semmelweis legacy. Lancet Infect Dis 2001;April:9–20.

Pittet D, Harbarth S: The intensive care unit. In Bennett J, Brachman P (eds): Hospital infections 4th ed., Philadelphia, Lippincott-Raven, 1998, pp 381–402.

Pittet D, Hugonnet S, Harbarth S, et al: Effectiveness of a hospital-wide programme to improve compliance with hand hygiene. Lancet 2000; 356:1307–1312.

Rahal J, Urban C, Horn D, et al: Class restriction of cephalosporin use to control total cephalosporin resistance in nosocomial Klebsiella. JAMA 1998;280:1233–1237.

Rello J, Diaz E, Rocque M, Valles J: Risk factors for developing pneumonia within 48 hours of intubation. Am J Respir Crit Care Med 1999;159:1742–1746.

Sherertz RJ, Ely EW, Westbrook DM, et al: Education of physicians-in-training can decrease the risk for vascular catheter infection. Ann Intern Med 2000;132:641–648.

Valles J, Artigas A, Rello J, et al: Continuous aspiration of subglottic secretions in preventing ventilator-associated pneumonia. Ann Intern Med 1995;122:229–231.

Vincent J, Bihari D, Suter P, et al: The prevalence of nosocomial infection in intensive care units in Europe. Results of the European Prevalence of Infection in Intensive Care (EPIC) study. JAMA 1995;274:639–644.

Zack JE, Garrison T, Trovillion E, et al: Effect of an education program aimed at reducing the occurrence of ventilator-associated pneumonia. Crit Care Med 2002;30:2407–2412.

Antibiotic Prophylactic Strategies in the ICU

Miguel Sánchez

KEY POINTS

- The epidemiology of ICU-acquired infections and the importance of prevention
- The carrier state and the pathophysiology of ICU-acquired infections
- Patient populations at risk
- Systemic antibiotic prophylaxis
- Topical antibiotic prophylaxis

Intensive care unit (ICU)-acquired infections are a frequent complication of the practice of critical care, with their cumulative incidence varying considerably among different patient populations. Coronary care units report nosocomial infection rates of 2.7%, whereas up to 40% of medical and surgical critically ill patients may develop infections during their ICU stay. The risk of acquiring an infection in the ICU is also a function of the degree of severity of illness within a given subset of patients, and its cumulative incidence increases substantially and is associated with the use of certain devices. Nosocomial pneumonia, for example, is 21 times more frequent in endotracheally intubated patients under mechanical ventilation. Incidence rates of ventilator-associated pneumonia (VAP) ranging from 7% to more than 40% have been reported. In long-term ventilated surgical patients, VAP was suspected clinically and microbiologically confirmed in 48% of patients in one series, whereas up to 30% of medical ICU patients acquire VAP during their ICU stay.

The development of infection during ICU stay is associated with significant increases in morbidity and mortality. Patients who suffer an episode of VAP or nosocomial bloodstream infection have been shown to need prolonged hospital stays and to be at an increased risk of dying. In one series of patients admitted to a medical ICU, the occurrence of VAP was associated with a significant 27.1% attributable mortality and an increased length of ICU stay. Length of ICU stay was doubled in surgical ICU patients developing bloodstream infection and the attributable mortality was 35%; 50% of case patients died compared to 15% of matched controls. Most authors therefore agree that the development of nosocomial infection significantly impacts mortality of critically ill patients.

Another frequent consequence of ICU-acquired infection is the development of bacterial and fungal resistance. Resistant strains may be selected during correct systemic antibiotic therapy for adequately documented infection. Some studies suggest that infection with resistant strains is associated with increased mortality. This issue, however, remains controversial because it is not a universal finding in studies comparing outcomes of infections with sensitive and resistant strains of *Staphylococcus aureus* or gram-negative bacilli.

The importance of the prevention of infection in critically ill patients is therefore based on its potential to reduce both morbidity and mortality. It remains less clear whether the prevention of the development of resistance, although an objective of utmost importance, is followed by reductions in morbidity and/or mortality.

RISK FACTORS/RATIONALE FOR PROPHYLAXIS

Several aspects are important for the correct indication of prophylactic strategies. In individual patients, the presence of risk factors for infection has to be considered, the most important of which is an expected duration of endotracheal intubation of more than 48 hours. Patients who prior to endotracheal intubation have altered protective airway reflexes due to a decreased level of consciousness or other causes are at a particularly high risk of early onset VAP. Second, in order to choose the adequate preventive measure, one has to consider the mechanisms of development of the targeted type of infection.

Device-Related Risk

The frequent device utilization in intensive care is responsible for most nosocomial ICU-acquired infections. The most common risk factors in critically ill patients for infections of the respiratory tract, bloodstream, and urinary tract are endotracheal intubation with mechanical ventilation, central venous catheters, and urinary catheters, respectively. Compared to a conscious patient with a natural airway and spontaneous breathing, the presence of an endotracheal tube and mechanical ventilation in patients under sedation and muscle relaxation poses a 6- to 21-fold risk for development of nosocomial pneumonia. Several mechanisms contribute to the increased risk of respiratory tract infection. A decreased level of consciousness after head trauma or stroke or the need for reintubation, both requiring emergency endotracheal intubation, are associated with aspiration of contaminated oral and/or gastric contents due to the absence of upper airway reflexes. In the absence of systemic antibiotics, intubated stroke and head trauma patients have a 36% incidence of pneumonia developing soon after intubation. In a mixed ICU population without formal indication for systemic antibiotic therapy, which includes patients intubated for acute pulmonary edema, patients recovering from cardiac arrest, and patients in a coma due to drug overdose, head trauma, and stroke, the incidence of early onset pneumonia was 51.3% in the control group of a multicenter infection prevention study performed at ICUs with predominantly medical patients. Other risk factors for the development of VAP during prolonged endotracheal intubation that have been reported are the infusion of muscle relaxants and the absence of systemic antibiotic therapy.

Rationale for Prophylaxis

The presence of potentially pathogenic microorganisms (PPMs) in the digestive tract plays a central role in the pathophysiology of most nosocomial infections. The characteristics of this so-called digestive tract "carrier state" both explain the mechanisms of different types of infection and serve as a basis for the design of preventive strategies (Table 9.1).

Microbial colonization of the digestive tract begins soon after birth and remains relatively constant throughout life. The oropharyngeal cavity in healthy humans contains flora composed mainly of facultative anaerobes and a few potentially pathogenic "community" bacteria, such as *Streptococcus pneumoniae, Haemophilus influenzae, Moraxella cattharalis,* and *Streptococcus viridans.* Fifteen to 40% of the healthy population also carry *S. aureus* in their nose and throat. The esophagus, the stomach with its acid pH, and the small intestine are relatively germ free. The concentration of normal flora in the lumen of the gut increases toward the terminal ileum and reaches 40% of feces in the distal end of the colon, up to approximately 10^{12} colonies per gram of feces. Distal flora is composed of 99.9% anaerobic bacteria, which lines the intestinal epithelium, and 0.1% aerobic flora, mainly *Escherichia coli, Candida* spp., and a small number of other Enterobacteriaceae.

Infections caused by microorganisms that colonize the digestive tract of the patient on admission to the ICU are called "primary endogenous." Pneumonias of primary endogenous development, for example, are caused by the flora present in the oropharynx of patients at intubation. These microorganisms have either been aspirated before admission by a comatose patient or are aspirated or inoculated by the endotracheal tube during the procedure of intubation. Because most patients require endotracheal intubation within the first few days after hospital admission, the flora causing primary endogenous

infections is usually the "community flora" that colonizes the oropharynx of healthy individuals. Exceptions to this relatively sensitive bacterial etiology are patients who chronically carry hospital flora after recent discharge and patients admitted to the ICU from other wards after prolonged hospital stay, in whom the bacteria causing primary endogenous infections are nosocomial flora. Primary endogenous infections usually develop during the first few days after ICU admission but may develop as long as 9 days later, during the second week of ICU stay, if primary colonization persists.

After ICU admission, alterations of the control mechanisms of the oropharynx and the gut occur associated with disease and/or its therapy and lead to significant changes of the normal colonization pattern. Fibronectin covers the oropharyngeal mucosa and enhances the binding of gram-positive organisms, such as *S. aureus* and the members of the endogenous oropharyngeal flora. Polymorphonuclear elastase, present in saliva of critically ill intubated patients, is associated with loss of fibronectin, thereby leaving receptors for gram-negative bacteria uncovered. In the gut lumen, parenteral broad-spectrum antibiotics reduce the number of bacteria of the relatively sensitive resident flora. A concomitant increase in fungal species and resistant bacteria occurs because indigenous flora no longer competes for the same nutrients and for the same receptors on host cells or produces bacteriocins and volatile fatty acids. Within a few days of hospitalization, reductions in normal flora may occur, which is progressively replaced by resistant nosocomial PPMs, including *Pseudomonas aeruginosa, Acinetobacter* spp., resistant Enterobacteriaceae, resistant gram-positive cocci, and fungi. Infections caused by microorganisms that are acquired and begin colonizing the digestive tract after admission to the ICU are called secondary endogenous. The prevalence of abnormal digestive tract colonization increases with the severity of illness. In a severely ill population, characterized by a mean APACHE II score of 26.6, an abnormal colonization pattern was present in 50% of patients admitted to the ICU within 48 hours of hospital admission. Usually, nosocomial microorganisms are selected in the patient's own digestive tract, mainly after institution of systemic antibiotic therapy. Depending on the extent of antibiotic selection pressure, the prevalence of colonization of concomitant patients, and inanimate sources, breeches of hygiene may allow acquisition by cross-colonization of more or less resistant abnormal flora, which then starts colonizing the gastrointestinal tract. Strain identity studies have established that in most cases, the digestive tract is the most frequent reservoir of microorganisms for nosocomial infections. Prior digestive tract colonization has been reported for secondary endogenous gram-negative, gram-positive, and yeast infections.

Table 9.1 Pathophysiology of Infections: The Carrier State				
Type of Infection	**Prior Digestive Tract Carriage**	**Acquisition**	**Type of Flora**	**Comment**
Primary endogenous	Yes	Present on ICU admission	Community[a]	Not an ICU-acquired infection
Secondary endogenous	Yes	Acquired in ICU	Nosocomial	True ICU infections
Exogenous	No	Acquired in ICU	Nosocomial	True ICU infections

[a]In patients with prolonged hospital stay prior to ICU admission, colonizing flora may be nosocomial.

In order to eradicate PPMs from the digestive tract, Garlock proposed as early as 1939 the administration of enteral antimicrobials to prevent postoperative wound infection in patients undergoing colorectal surgery. Enteral antimicrobials have also been used in hematological patients since the early 1970s to prevent respiratory tract, urinary, and skin infections in granulopenic patients.

In the 1980s, Christiaan Stoutenbeek, Rick Van Saene, and Durk Zandstra introduced a technique of infection prophylaxis with nonabsorbable antimicrobials—that they called *selective decontamination of the digestive tract* (SDD)—into the critical care setting. After extensive laboratory and clinical research, they proposed an enteral antimicrobial regimen consisting of tobramycin, polymyxin E, and amphotericin B administered as an oropharyngeal paste as well as an oral solution through the nasogastric tube in long-term intubated patients. Several characteristics were considered key and indispensable for an antimicrobial drug to be effective in preventing infection through eradication of potentially pathogenic microorganisms from the digestive tract. Antimicrobial compounds selected for oral administration should not at all or only minimally be absorbed through the digestive tract mucosa in order to exert their effect within the gut lumen. As a consequence, high intraluminal concentrations can be achieved without the risk of systemic side effects or adverse events. At dosages of 100 mg every 6 hours, polymyxin and aminoglycoside concentrations in feces exceed 100 mg/g in most instances, whereas simultaneous plasma concentrations are below the level of detection, although in bone marrow transplant patients with mucositis, detectable serum levels of tobramycin have been reported. Similar gut lumen concentrations can be achieved with other nonabsorbable antimicrobials, such as oral vancomycin. At dosages of 125 mg every 6 hours, fecal concentrations exceed 100 mg/liter without concomitant detection in serum. If constant and high intraluminal antimicrobial concentrations can be achieved, well above the minimal inhibitory concentration and compensating for inhibition by fecal contents, the development of resistance is highly unlikely. However, with the use of drugs such as quinolones or erythromycin as enteral antimicrobials, which are readily absorbed, intraluminal concentrations decrease along the digestive tract and systemic effects occur. As with parenteral antibiotics, which are secreted via saliva, bile, and mucosa into the throat and gut and are present in the oropharynx and feces only in low concentrations, they fail to clear digestive tract carriage with PPMs. In addition, low fecal concentrations of antibiotics (i.e., below the minimal inhibitory concentration) constitute a milieu that favors the selection of resistant strains. The ideal enteral antimicrobial should also have a narrow antimicrobial spectrum to avoid reducing the indigenous intestinal flora, thus preserving the colonization resistance of the gut, while being active against all aerobic gram-negative PPMs such as *Pseudomonas* and *Acinetobacter* spp. Unlike parenteral broad-spectrum antimicrobials, oral polymyxin E has been shown to leave the resident anaerobic flora that lines the oropharyngeal and intestinal mucosa unaffected in healthy human volunteers. It has been recommended that the mechanism of action should preferably be bactericidal with a low minimal bactericidal concentration (MBC) for ICU-associated flora, the rationale being that there are no cellular and humoral mediators of acute inflammation, such as leukocytes and their products, in the lumen of the gut to assist the action of the antibiotic. The inactivation of amphotericin B, polymyxin E, tobramycin, nalidixic acid, pipemidic acid, norfloxacin, ciprofloxacin, and neomycin by fecal and food compounds increases as a function of the concentration of feces when tested against *P. aeruginosa*, *Acinetobacter calcoaceticus*, *E. coli*, *Klebsiella oxytoca*, *Enterobacter cloacae*, and *Proteus mirabilis*. The loss of activity of tobramycin against *P. aeruginosa* was significantly smaller than the loss observed with polymyxin E, neomycin, and aztreonam, and its MBC was even slightly lower than that of norfloxacin and ciprofloxacin at a 30% concentration of feces. Of clinical relevance is that tobramycin and polymyxin E retain a relatively low MBC for *Acinetobacter* spp. at increasing concentrations of feces, whereas the fluoroquinolones are largely inactivated.

REGIMEN

The decision to employ prophylactic antibiotics should be based on stratification of risk for infection, considering mainly the presence of endotracheal intubation and need for mechanical ventilation. Patients requiring prolonged intubation, defined as the need for endotracheal intubation and mechanical ventilation for more than 48 hours, constitute the principal target population for antibiotic prophylaxis (Tables 9.2 and 9.3). Not only are intubated patients at high risk for nosocomial pneumonia but also endotracheal intubation has been shown to be an excellent marker for severity and therefore characterizes a high-risk population for other nosocomial infections. The complete regimen of SDD antibiotic prophylaxis in intubated patients consists of a combination of a 3- to 5-day course of an intravenous antibiotic with a mixture of topical nonabsorbable antibiotics administered both as a sticky paste to the oral cavity and as a suspension through the nasogastric tube.

Table 9.2 Regimen and Dosages of Antibiotic Prophylaxis					
Type	**Systemic**		**Local/Topical**		
Route	Intravenous	Oropharynx		Oral (nasogastric tube)	
Preparation	IV solution	Methyl cellulose paste or gel		Suspension	
Antibiotic	Ceftriaxone[a]	Polymyxin E + amphotericin B + tobramycin	Polymyxin E	Amphotericin B	Tobramycin
Dose	2 g	2%	100 mg	500 mg	80 mg
Regimen	Once per day		qid		
Duration	3 days		While intubated		

[a]Cefotaxime is equally effective; has been used in a 4- or 5-day regimen.

Table 9.3 Indications for Antibiotic Prophylaxis

Patient Population	Antiobiotic Prophylaxis		
	Topical		Systemic IV
	Oropharynx (Paste, Gel, or Liquid)	Oral (Nasogastric Tube or Swallowed)	
Endotracheally intubated (>48 hours):			
Infected	Yes	Yes	No
Noninfected	Yes	Yes	Yes (3–5 days)
Severe acute pancreatitis	No	Yes	No
Digestive tract colonization with multiresistant gram-negative bacilli	Yes	Yes	No

Systemic Prophylaxis

A third-generation cephalosporin is administered intravenously for 4 or 5 days to prevent primary endogenous, mainly respiratory tract, infections. A double-blind randomized study showed that a 3-day course of ceftriaxone, 2 g IV once per day, reduced the incidence of primary endogenous pneumonia from 51.3% to 14.3% in noninfected patients requiring long-term intubation. This also implies that in approximately half of the patients, very early or so-called "preemptive" therapy is given. Even shorter durations of systemic prophylaxis may be effective, as has been demonstrated in stroke and head trauma patients receiving three doses of cefuroxime 12 hours apart. Intravenous antibiotic prophylaxis after endotracheal intubation for patients in whom no infection-specific antibiotic therapy is indicated may be viewed in analogy to short-term surgical infection prophylaxis. The two criteria of long-term intubation and no concomitant systemic antibiotic therapy select the subset of patients who may benefit from short-term systemic antibiotic prophylaxis:

1. Coma
   Structural (ischemic or hemorrhagic stroke, head trauma)
   Metabolic (hepatic, drug overdose)
2. Trauma, particularly severe abdominal and thoracic trauma
3. Primary respiratory disorders such as pulmonary embolism, acute pulmonary edema, and status asthmaticus

Topical Prophylaxis

Polymyxin E or colistin, as noted previously, meets the criteria for an effective enteral antimicrobial agent and is therefore the principal component of most regimens: It is nonabsorbable, selective, and bactericidal. It is moderately inactivated by fecal and food compounds and needs to be administered in relatively high doses (600 mg per day). It is usually administered with tobramycin to close the gap for *Proteus* and *Morganella* species and to take advantage of an in vitro synergistic effect that has been reported for *Acinetobacter* species and *E. coli*. Aminoglycosides, particularly tobramycin, meet most of the aforementioned criteria for an adequate enteral antimicrobial. Tobramycin is only minimally absorbed, although low serum concentrations may be detected in patients with multiple organ failure and hemodialysis. It acts effectively and selectively on the aerobic gram-negative, potentially pathogenic flora, with only minimal action on the anaerobic intestinal flora. Vancomycin is usually administered at 0.5 to 2 g per day in three or four divided doses for pseudomembranous colitis produced by *Clostridium difficile*. An oral dose of 500 mg vancomycin four times daily yields concentrations of 1000 to 9000 mg/L of stool, with only trace amounts found in serum. However, concentrations in the therapeutic range have occasionally been found in the serum of anuric patients given the drug orally for treatment of colitis. When 125 mg is given orally, stool concentrations range from 100 to 800 mg/L. Conversely, vancomycin given intravenously may be associated with concentrations of up to 100 mg/L in stools of some patients, although it remains undetectable in most. Amphotericin B is highly inactivated by feces, and a high daily oral dose of 2 g (500 mg qid) is required to prevent intestinal overgrowth with yeasts.

Enteral antimicrobials clear PPMs from the digestive tract of experimental animals and humans. In healthy human volunteers, a daily oral dose of 600 mg of polymyxin E suppresses Enterobacteriaceae in 89% of fecal samples. The eradication or profound suppression of gram-negatives, *S. aureus*, and yeasts with the usual regimen employed—a polymyxin, an aminoglycoside, and an antifungal agent—have been proven in all studies published to date. In a multicenter trial involving 271 intubated patients, the effect of enteral antimicrobials on gram-negative carriage was evident within 3 days of the beginning of the protocol and remained significantly lower at all time points (Fig. 9.1). A concomitant significant reduction of the incidence of *Candida* spp. in oropharyngeal and rectal samples has also been demonstrated. There is much less experience with eradication of gram-positive bacteria, and the results are less uniform than with gram-negatives and yeasts. Intestinal carriage with vancomycin-resistant *Enteroccus faecium* can be cleared with oral bacitracin alone or in combination with doxycycline. It appears that the effect of bacitracin and doxycycline on vancomycin-resistant *Enterococcus* (VRE) is one of profound suppression rather than complete eradication. Follow-up rectal cultures show recolonization with VRE in experimental animals as well as in humans within 2 weeks after stopping administration of the antibiotics. The use of oral vancomycin is not without risk for selecting vancomycin-resistant microorganisms, particularly in countries where VRE is prevalent. In clinical trials employing oral vancomycin as part of the regimen of selective decontamination of the digestive tract, however, no increase in colonization or infection with vancomycin-resistant bacteria was detected.

Antimicrobial peptides, an essential component of the innate humoral immune response, are present in leukocytes and epithelia to act as a first barrier against microbial invasion. These

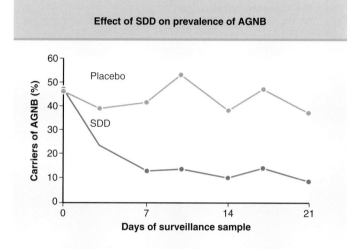

Figure 9.1. Prevalence of aerobic gram-negative bacilli (AGNB) at all sites (oropharynx, trachea, stomach, and rectum). SDD, selective decontamination of the digestive tract. (Redrawn with permission from Sànchez Garcia M, Cambronero Galache JA, Lopez Diaz, et al: Effectiveness and cost of selective decontamination of the digestive tract in critically ill intubated patients: A randomized, double-blind, placebo-controlled, multicenter trial. Am J Respir Crit Care Med 1998;158:906–908.)

compounds interact with anionic phospholipids of the outer bacterial membrane to produce pores and increase permeability. This mechanism of action seems to be the basis for their two most attractive features, namely broad-spectrum antimicrobial activity and low propensity for development of resistance. Antimicrobial peptides have a rapid bactericidal activity, and their antimicrobial spectrum includes multiresistant gram-positive cocci and gram-negative bacilli as well as yeasts. A synthetic analog of protegrin-1, iseganan, is undergoing phase II and III clinical trials to evaluate its use in preventing and/or eradicating abnormal oropharyngeal carriage for the prevention of VAP.

Clinical Experience
Prevention of Colonization and Infection
There is extensive experience with routine use of systemic and topical antimicrobials in ICUs, some of which have employed this method of infection prevention since the late 1980s. The concept of eradicating abnormal digestive tract colonization to prevent infection has been extensively investigated in more than 30 randomized clinical trials. The results of those trials evaluating SDD in critically ill patients unequivocally show a beneficial effect on the prevention of primary endogenous and secondary endogenous infections, particularly respiratory tract infections. In fact, antibiotic prophylaxis can be regarded as an evidence-based measure based on seven different meta-analyses performed in the past decade. One of the largest meta-analyses was performed by D'Amico and colleagues in 1998 on 5727 patients enrolled in 33 trials. Investigators provided these authors with data on 15 variables for each randomized patient so that an indi-

vidual patient meta-analysis could be performed. The use of the complete regimen of topical and systemic prophylaxis in this analysis is associated with a large protective effect, with an odds ratio of 0.35 and confidence interval of 0.29 to 041 for respiratory tract infections in endotracheally intubated patients. The combination of systemic and topical antimicrobials was also associated with a significant 20% reduction in mortality. Administration of only the topical component showed a less impressive but still major reduction in respiratory tract infection, with an odds ratio of 0.56 and a confidence interval of 0.46 to 0.68, and no significant effect on mortality. Liberati and associates updated D'Amico and colleagues' database, expanding the study of the effect of antibiotics on the cumulative incidence of respiratory tract infection and overall mortality. The database comprises the results from 36 randomized trials involving 6922 patients. The results of this meta-analysis confirm previous results for significant reduction in odds ratio of respiratory tract infection and mortality.

Outbreaks
High baseline prevalence and incidence of resistant strains of various species of bacteria causing clinically significant infections have been reported in surveys from ICUs throughout Europe and many other areas of the world. Apart from anecdotal reports of exogenous inanimate reservoirs, surveillance cultures of throat and gut consistently reveal that most PPMs, including multidrug-resistant gram-negatives and gram-positives, are carried in the digestive tract of the patients. Although barrier precautions certainly play an important role in reducing cross-transmission between colonized patients and in controlling outbreaks, Bonten and colleagues demonstrated that "colonization pressure" is the main determinant of the success of such measures. These authors observed that once the prevalence percentage of colonized patients exceeds a certain value, approximately 20% for vancomycin-resistant *Enterococcus*, even a high compliance with barrier precautions does not prevent the spread of microorganisms among patients. Given the fact that the main reservoir is the patient's orodigestive tract, several authors have shown that the administration of enteral antimicrobials effectively controls outbreaks with multiresistant strains that are refractory to all conventional measures. For example, Brun-Buisson and associates demonstrated that an outbreak of multiresistant Enterobacteriaceae could be controlled by administering enteral antimicrobials after all traditional control measures, mainly barrier precautions, had failed. Interestingly, the concomitant control group in this trial had a significantly reduced colonization and infection rate compared to the historical group that triggered the investigation. This observation supports the concept that enteral antimicrobials also reduce colonization pressure and thereby further contribute to the control of outbreaks. De Jonge and coworkers (2003) published the largest randomized trial to date evaluating a combined regimen of systemic and enteral antimicrobial prophylaxis specifically aimed at studying the incidence of resistant bacteria and ICU and hospital mortality. The antibiotics used were cefotaxime, colistin, tobramycin, and amphotericin B employed as a short-term systemic prophylaxis; topical oropharyngeal and enteral antimicrobials; inhaled colistin for tracheal colonization with gram-negative bacilli; and rectal enemas for patients with colostomy.

Specific Patient Populations

Martínez Pellús and associates evaluated the capacity of polymyxins to bind endotoxins in the gut lumen and showed that preoperative administration of polymyxin E with tobramycin and amphotericin B reduces endotoxin concentrations in feces and prevents endotoxemia as well as cytokinemia in patients undergoing cardiopulmonary bypass surgery. These results could not be reproduced by others employing polymyxin B and neomycin. In experimental peritonitis, prophylaxis with enteral antimicrobials prevents endotoxemia and bacterial translocation. An intriguing application of enteral antimicrobials is its use in the prevention of leakage of surgical upper gastrointestinal tract sutures. Contrary to the conventional concept, according to which anastomotic dehiscence is due to mechanical stress and/or local ischemia, the presence of potentially pathogenic bacteria in the leaking anastomosis was retrospectively identified as an independent risk factor for leakage of proximal digestive tract surgical sutures. Experimental data confirm that the intraluminal presence of *P. aeruginosa* results in an increased incidence of anastomotic leak, and in animals that had their anastomosis bathed by tobramycin, polymyxin B, and vancomycin, leak was almost completely prevented. A multicenter, double-blind, randomized, placebo-controlled study confirmed that anastomotic leak of an esophagojejunostomy after gastrectomy for gastric cancer can be prevented by disinfecting the luminal aspect of the surgical suture with enteral antimicrobials given through a tube with its tip proximal to the suture. In patients with severe acute pancreatitis, eradication of PPMs from the gut lumen by the administration of a short systemic course of cefotaxime and enteral antimicrobials, both oral and as an enema, is associated with a reduced incidence of secondary infections of pancreatic necrotic tissue. Reduction in secondary pancreatic infections in turn is associated with a significant reduction in morbidity and mortality. However, the recommendation of prolonged systemic antibiotic prophylaxis to prevent secondary pancreatic infections is still awaiting confirmation by appropriately designed trials. A double-blind, randomized, multicenter trial employing ciprofloxacin and metronidazole had to be prematurely interrupted after a scheduled interim analysis because of lack of effect on the incidence of secondary pancreatic infections, length of stay, need for surgical interventions, and mortality. Enteral antimicrobials have also been proven to reduce secondary endogenous gram-negative and yeast infections in liver transplant patients. Most protocols begin 1 to 3 days before the surgical intervention to achieve eradication of the target microorganisms. Improved surgical expertise has resulted in improved morbidity and mortality rates as low as 5%. The associated shortening of high-risk periods for infection, such as during endotracheal intubation and mechanical ventilation or ICU stay as a whole, has made the benefit of enteral antimicrobials less evident in this population, except possibly for a subset of patients requiring prolonged ICU stay.

CONTROVERSIES AND RISKS/BENEFITS

In certain circumstances, the efficacy of enteral antimicrobials may be reduced (Boxes 9.1 and 9.2). Inactivation of enteral antibiotics by fecal and food compounds has already been mentioned. In particular, the presence of divalent cations, such as Mg^{2+}, seems to interfere with the action of several antimi-

---

Box 9.1 Controversies

Resistance

- **Pro:** Topical antibiotics eradicate and prevent the acquisition of and colonization with resistant bacteria.
- **Con:** The generalized and prolonged use of systemic and topical antibiotics leads to selection of resistant strains.

Mortality

- **Pro:** A recently updated meta-analysis of 36 randomized control trials shows that the application of the complete regimen, topical and intravenous, of antibiotic prophylaxis is associated with a 22% reduction in mortality.
- **Con:** Only a minority of individual randomized trials have shown a significant reduction in mortality.

Workload

- **Pro/con:** The administration of enteral antimicrobials is cumbersome because it requires oral and nasogastric tube care every 6 hr. No commercial preparations are currently available. These have to be manufactured by the hospital pharmacist.

Clinical Relevance of Reducing Infections

- **Pro:** Nosocomial infections increase morbidity and mortality.
- **Con:** The occurrence of infection has no significant negative impact on outcome worth the effort, expense, and risks of antibiotic prophylaxis.

---

crobials on the outer membrane of *P. aeruginosa*. The frequent occurrence of prolonged ileus in critically ill patients may delay the action of enteral antimicrobials on distal gut flora for several days. Some researchers have employed antimicrobial enemas, whereas others suggest intravenous neostigmine to facilitate the access of enteral antimicrobials to the terminal digestive tract. Altered peristalsis may be the cause of varying fecal concentrations of antibiotics found by some.

Resistance

Experience in ICUs that have been employing enteral nonabsorbable antimicrobials for two decades confirms that the probability of the appearance of resistance or selection of resistant strains is low. Also, it has never been reported to occur in more than 30 randomized trials employing various different combinations of enteral antimicrobials. Since 1990, in our ICU at the University Hospital Príncipe de Asturias, high-risk intubated, mechanically ventilated patients have received enteral polymyxin E with gentamicin and amphotericin B while they remain intubated. We have detected neither the appearance of resistance in previously sensitive strains nor an increase in infections with intrinsically resistant bacteria, such as *Enterococcus* spp. or methicillin-resistant *S. aureus*, in clinical or surveillance samples. Studies specifically aimed at the detection of resistant microorganisms after prolonged administration of enteral antimicrobials have also not been able to detect an increase in the incidence of resistance. In fact, the previously mentioned large randomized SDD trial, with mortality and resistance as the two main outcome variables, reported significant reductions in mortality and resistance (Fig. 9.2).

Box 9.2 Risks and Benefits

Risk	Comment
Selection and increased colonization and infection with bacteria intrinsically resistant to the usual regimen of prophylactic antibiotics.	Nosocomial strains of enterococci, methicillin-resistant *Staphylococcus aureus*, and coagulase-negative staphylococci are resistant to aminoglycosides, and colonization is significantly increased in patients receiving topical prophylactic antibiotics.
Reduced compliance with barrier precautions	Reductions in the incidence of nosocomial ICU infections associated with antibiotic prophylaxis may cause a false sensation of reduced risk of infection and in turn lead to increases in exogenous infections. This type of infection cannot be prevented by antibiotic prophylaxis.

Benefit	Comment
Reduction of ICU-acquired infections	Particularly ventilator-associated pneumonia rates are significantly reduced (odds ratio, 0.35).
Reduction of resistance	Reduced incidence of gram-negative resistance: the reduction of gram-negative colonization and infection associated with the use of topical antibiotic prophylaxis also includes reduced rates of multiresistant gram-negative strains.
Reduction of ICU mortality	ICU mortality is significantly reduced (odds ratio, 0.78) when combined systemic and topical prophylaxis is administered.

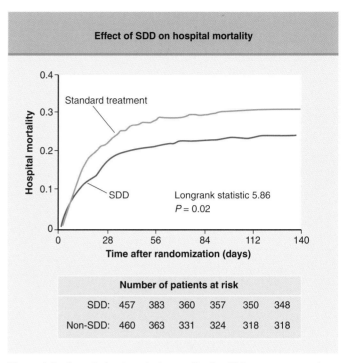

Figure 9.2. Cumulative hospital mortality for SDD treatment and standard treatment. (Redrawn with permission from de Jonge E, Schultz MJ, Spanjaard L, et al: Effects of selective decontamination of digestive tract of mortality and acquisition of resident bacteria in intensive care: A randomised controlled trial. Lancet 2003;362(9389):1011–1016.)

SUGGESTED READING

Bonten MJ, Slaughter S, Amberger AW, et al: The role of "colonization pressure" in the spread of vancomycin-resistant enterococci: An important infection control variable. Arch Intern Med 1998;158:1127–1132.

Brun-Buisson C, Legrand P, Rauss A, et al: Intestinal decontamination for control of nosocomial multiresistant gram-negative bacilli. Study of an outbreak in an intensive care unit. Ann Intern Med 1989;110:873–881.

D'Amico R, Pifferi S, Leonetti C, et al: Effectiveness of antibiotic prophylaxis in critically ill adult patients: systematic review of randomised controlled trials. BMJ 1998;316:1275–1285.

De Jonge E, Schultz MJ, Spanjaard L, et al: Effects of selective decontamination of digestive tract on mortality and acquisition of resistant bacteria in intensive care: A randomised controlled trial. Lancet 2003;362: 1011–1016.

Garrouste-Orgeas M, Chevret S, Arlet G, et al: Oropharyngeal or gastric colonization and nosocomial pneumonia in adult intensive care unit patients. A prospective study based on genomic DNA analysis. Am J Respir Crit Care Med 1997;156:1647–1655.

Hammond JM, Potgieter PD: Long-term effects of selective decontamination on antimicrobial resistance. Crit Care Med 1995;23:637–645.

Krueger WA, Lenhart FP, Neeser G, et al: Influence of combined intravenous and topical antibiotic prophylaxis on the incidence of infections, organ dysfunctions, and mortality in critically ill surgical patients: A prospective, stratified, randomized, double-blind, placebo-controlled clinical trial. Am J Respir Crit Care Med 2002;166:1029–1037.

Liberati A, D'Amico R, Pifferi S, Torri V, Brazzi L: Antibiotic prophylaxis to reduce respiratory tract infections and mortality in adults receiving intensive care. Cochrane Database Syst Rev 2004;CD000022.

Martínez-Pellús AE, Merino P, Bru M, et al: Endogenous endotoxemia of intestinal origin during cardiopulmonary bypass. Role of type of flow and protective effect of selective digestive decontamination. Intensive Care Med 1997;23:1251–1257.

Sánchez García M, Cambronero Galache JA, Lopez DJ, et al: Effectiveness and cost of selective decontamination of the digestive tract in critically ill intubated patients. A randomized, double-blind, placebo-controlled, multicenter trial. Am J Respir Crit Care Med 1998;158:908–916.

Silvestri L, Monti BC, Milanese M, et al: Are most ICU infections really nosocomial? A prospective observational cohort study in mechanically ventilated patients. J Hosp Infect 1999;42:125–133.

van Saene HK, Damjanovic V, Murray AE, de La Cal MA: How to classify infections in intensive care units—The carrier state, a criterion whose time has come? J Hosp Infect 1996;33:1–12.

Chapter 10

Severity of Illness Measures

Gordon D. Rubenfeld

KEY POINTS

- Severity of illness measures are confounder scores that combine multiple variables into a single measure that correlates with an outcome, usually hospital mortality.
- In addition to being accurate and robust, severity of illness measures should provide predictions independent of treatment, time, and diagnosis.
- The accuracy of severity of illness measures is assessed by their discrimination and calibration.
- Although useful to inform individual patient decisions, judgments based solely on objective predictions from severity of illness measures are problematic due to uncertainty and potential for bias.
- Severity of illness measures are useful to describe populations of critically ill patients and to control for confounding due to severity of illness, particularly in estimating risk-adjusted outcome as a measure of quality of care.

It is in my opinion a most excellent thing for the physician to practice forecasting. . . . For it is impossible to make all sick people well—that would indeed be better than fore-telling the course of their illness. But men do, as a matter of fact, die; some through the severity of their disease, before the doctor is called in—some immediately, some living on for a day, others a little longer. . . . Hence we must know the nature of these diseases, how far they are superior to the bodily powers. In this way one will justly gain a reputation and will be a good physician; one will indeed be better able to save those capable of cure if he has made up his mind long beforehand in each case, and no blame will attach to him if he has already foreseen and announced who is to die and who is to be preserved.

—Hippocrates, *Prognostica*, 5th century B.C.

Finally, no matter how sophisticated they become, objective probability estimates represent substantial simplifications of very complex systems. Opportunities to exercise human discretion must be kept open.

—Knaus and associates (1991, p. 389)

Interest in predicting outcome for critically ill patients dates to the beginning of critical care. In 1966, the prognostic significance of coagulation abnormalities in patients with shock was

described. In 1971, an index to predict the outcome of patients admitted to intensive care units (ICUs) who had taken an overdose of sedatives was published in the New England Journal of Medicine. In a 1977 publication, Cullen and colleagues studied the ability of 11 variables, including physiology, organ failure, and treatments, to predict survival at 1 year. These early efforts culminated in the first version of the Acute Physiology and Chronic Health Evaluation (APACHE) score published in 1981. Since then, numerous severity of illness measures have been developed for use in critically ill patients, including generic models that are intended for heterogeneous populations of critically ill patients as well as disease-specific models. This chapter focuses on severity of illness measures incorporating multiple variables that, taken together, correlate with a clinically important outcome, usually mortality or length of stay, in broad populations of critically ill patients.

As Hippocrates noted, separating those who are doomed to die from those with a chance at benefiting from therapy allows clinicians to devote resources to salvageable patients and make informed decisions about care for all patients. Severity of illness measures can inform decision making at the population level by providing descriptive data about groups of patients and allow intensivists to focus on specific factors that affect outcome after controlling for patients' severity of illness.

DEVELOPMENT AND VALIDATION OF SEVERITY OF ILLNESS MEASURES

Ideal Severity of Illness Measure

In addition to prognostic accuracy, there are several characteristics of an ideal severity of illness measure (Table 10.1). In fact, available severity of illness measures fail in one or several of these areas. The question is not whether there is a perfect severity of illness measure but whether available measures, despite their limitations, are sufficient to address the question they are being used to answer.

Development

The variables that are ultimately included in severity of illness measures are derived either subjectively (formally or informally from experts in the field) or objectively (by selecting the variables that are most strongly predictive of outcome from a wide range of possible variables). Frequently, a combination of both measures is used. The most common statistical method for modeling binary (live/die) outcomes is multivariate logistic regression. The logistic model yields a value between 0 and 1 that corresponds to the probability of the outcome being

Table 10.1 Characteristics of an Ideal Severity of Illness Measure	
Characteristic	**Explanation**
Time independent	
Severity of illness measures should account for the location and time spent prior to ICU admission.	Patients transferred from outside ICUs have a worse prognosis than patients admitted from within the referral institution even after accounting for other aspects of their severity of illness.
Treatment independent	
Severity of illness measures should not be affected by treatment decisions that may affect variables in the model and are highly variable across institutions.	Laboratory and physiologic variables are altered by treatment decisions (activated protein C, therapeutic hypothermia, vasopressors, renal replacement therapy, and permissive hypercapnia) that will alter the relationship of these variables with outcome.
Diagnosis independent	
Laboratory and physiologic derangement will have different significance in different diseases.	For any given set of laboratory and physiologic derangements, patients with trauma, diabetic ketoacidosis, and urosepsis are likely to have better outcomes than patients with coma, cirrhosis, and cancer.
Robust	
Severity of illness measures will be used in many different kinds of ICUs and should yield reliable predictions.	Coding problems, missing data, and diagnostic intensity can cause models to fail in different settings.

modeled, usually death. Some severity of illness models, such as the Study to Understand Prognoses and Preferences for Outcomes and Risks of Treatments (SUPPORT) model, predict survival time using the Cox survival model. A mathematical algorithm, called *stepwise regression*, that tests different combinations of variables by sequentially including different variables and testing the fit of the model is often used to select variables. Other approaches to selecting and weighting variables include classification and regression trees and neural networks, which rely less on assumptions about the mathematical relationship between predictors and outcome. Variable weighting (e.g., how much worse is a hematocrit of 27% than a mean arterial pressure of 70 mm Hg?) can also be derived either subjectively or objectively. A common objective method is to break the continuous variable into categories and assign each category an empiric "weight" based on its coefficient in a regression model. For example, if the odds ratio for mortality of a mean arterial pressure less than 70 mm Hg is 4.2 compared to a mean arterial pressure of 70 to 100 mm Hg, then it is assigned 4 points and the normal value is assigned 0 points.

Variables in generic critical illness severity of illness measures are classified into six categories: age, physiologic or laboratory measures of organ failure, acute diagnoses including reason for ICU admission, patient location prior to ICU admission, comorbidities, and treatments. Specialized severity of illness measures include variables specific for the population, such as burn extent and severity or anatomic injury scoring. Organ failure scores, such as the Multiple Organ Dysfunction Score, Sequential Organ Failure Assessment, and Logistic Organ Dysfunction System, assign points for increasing severity of organ dysfunction. Because organ failure is the principal predictor of death in critically ill patients, higher organ dysfunction scores are highly correlated with mortality and, therefore, are a type of severity of illness measure. Organ failure scores were, in part, developed to monitor the incidence and resolution of organ failures as surrogate endpoints in clinical trials. Unlike severity of illness measures such as APACHE, Simplified Acute Physiology Score

(SAPS), and Mortality Prediction Model (MPM), organ failure scores do not have published coefficients that allow a probability of death to be calculated. Organ failure scores also do not incorporate the other variables known to affect ICU outcome, including comorbidity and patient source.

The Medical Algorithms Project lists more than 30 severity of illness measures and organ failure scores applicable to critically ill patients. In addition to well-known measures, such as APACHE, SAPS, MPM, and the Pediatric Risk of Mortality, there are less well-known and disease-specific severity of illness measures, including the Physiologic and Operative Severity Score for the Enumeration of Mortality and Morbidity (POSSUM for surgical patients), the Postinjury Multiple Organ Failure Score (trauma), and models for predicting mortality in critically ill patients with neoplasms or cirrhosis.

The patient population used to derive the variables, weights, and overall model is essential. First, particularly if stepwise regression or some other objective, quantitative approach to variable selection is being used, the derivation population should be large enough to ensure that the model is not overfit. Some statisticians recommend 10 outcomes (e.g., deaths) for each variable that is considered for inclusion in the model. An intensivist considering 100 variables for inclusion in a model would need a population with at least 1000 deaths. These are probably minimum requirements, and some statisticians recommend 20 or even 50 outcomes for each variable that is being evaluated. Using smaller populations can lead to an overfit model that is so customized for the small training data set that it is unlikely to perform well in validation. The heterogeneity of the derivation population is as important as its size. A model's performance will depend a great deal on the patients used to derive it. If the derivation population lacks an important group of patients, specifically one in which the severity of illness measure performs poorly, then the measure will continue to perform poorly in that group of patients.

Several measures are used to assess the accuracy of severity of illness measures (Fig. 10.1). The easiest way to understand

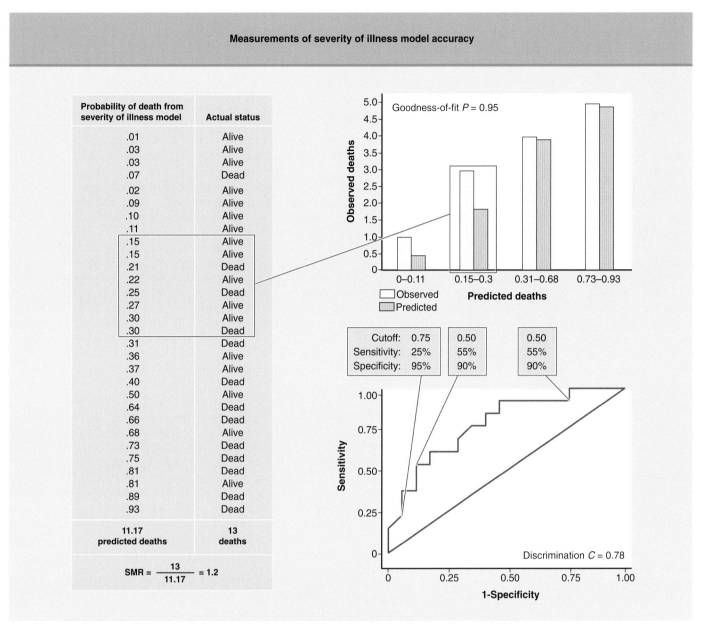

Figure 10.1. Measurements of severity of illness model accuracy. A hypothetical ICU database is evaluated for its calibration by comparing observed to predicted deaths across the range of probability of death *(top right)* and for its discrimination by plotting sensitivity and specificity at various cutoff points *(bottom right)*.

them is to think of a severity of illness measure as a diagnostic test that yields a continuous result (between 0 and 1 for logistic regression models and varying ranges for the different organ failure scores). Like a diagnostic test, for each measurement the patient will either die or live. Sensitivity, specificity, false-positive and false-negative rates, as well as predictive values of the severity of illness measure, can be calculated by choosing a specific cutoff. For example, if one assumes that everyone with a severity of illness measure predicted probability of death of 75% or greater dies, and those with a predicted probability of death of less than 75% live, then the sensitivity and specificity can be calculated by evaluating who actually lives and dies. The problem with this approach is that it only provides information on performance at a single cutoff. The area under the receiver operative curve (ROC) or the C statistic provides information

about the sensitivity and specificity across the entire range of test cutoffs. This measures the discrimination of the severity of illness measure—its ability to assign higher scores to people who die than those who live. Perfect discrimination is a C statistic of 1.0, indicating that the severity of illness essentially yields a binary result that assigns one value to everyone who dies and another value to everyone who lives. A poorly discriminating severity of illness measure that randomly assigns scores to survivors and nonsurvivors would have a C statistic of 0.5. A confidence interval can, and should, be generated around the C statistic, and tests for statistical significance between two C statistics can be calculated. Generic severity of illness measures in critical care have C statistics between 0.75 and 0.90. A limitation of the C statistic is also its benefit—namely, that it combines sensitivity and specificity into a single measure across cutoff values. At least when used for clinical decision making, there is usually a greater penalty for either a false-negative or a false-positive result. This information is not contained in the C statistic.

The other principal assessment of severity of illness measures is their calibration or fit. A perfect binary predictor might discriminate well but does not spread patient predictions out along a continuum or check to determine how well the assigned probabilities of death correspond to the actual risk of death. The common measure of calibration for logistic regression models is a goodness-of-fit test that groups patients into categories of predicted mortality (usually 10; Figure 10.1 uses 4 for simplicity). For example, in Figure 10.1, there are 8 patients whose predicted mortality is between 15% and 30%. Three of these patients died and the model predicted that only 1.8 would die. If the observed and predicted deaths are identical within each category, then the severity of illness measure has perfect calibration. The ratio of the overall observed to the predicted is called the *standardized mortality ratio* (SMR). When this ratio is greater than 1, it indicates that there are more deaths in the population than the model predicts; when it is less than 1, there are fewer deaths than predicted. The SMR can be 1 and the severity of illness measure can still have poor calibration if the model's underpredictions in one area exactly balance overpredictions in another. The statistical goodness-of-fit measure is a P value that is low when the model has poor calibration and the P value is greater than 0.5 when the model fits well. A limitation of this measure is that large data sets can yield poor measures of calibration when the actual deviations are quite small. There is disagreement in the statistical community about the best measure to use to quantitatively evaluate severity of illness measures. Some advocate measures such as the Brier score that incorporate aspects of calibration and discrimination. Others emphasize discrimination because models can be refit to improve their calibration. To some extent, severity of illness measures should be assessed based on the question that they are being used to address. For example, a severity of illness measure developed to guide the decision to withdraw life-sustaining treatment in bone marrow transplant patients would require high specificity (one would not want to withdraw life support in a patient who would otherwise survive), but its sensitivity (the number of patients who die for whom a prediction of death is made) and calibration are less important. Conversely, a severity of illness measure that is designed for population risk adjustment purposes would need to be well calibrated.

Validation

Regardless of the methods used to select and weight variables, to identify the derivation population, and to assess the statistical performance of the severity of illness measure, the ultimate test is validation in a new patient population. Some derivation techniques are more likely to yield severity of illness measures that validate than others. For example, both bootstrapping, which reestimates the model multiple times from random subsets of the derivation population, and a technique called *coefficient shrinkage*, which imposes a penalty on predictions at the extremes of the model, tend to yield predictors that perform better in new populations.

The critical care literature is replete with studies that have assessed the performance of generic ICU severity of illness measures in new populations showing that the models perform poorly. Frequently, authors conclude that their data uncover a flaw in the severity of illness model. In fact, all severity of illness models will perform less well in validation sets than in the derivation data. The greatest concern is that the severity of illness measure might be a biased estimator of outcome because an important component of risk has been omitted from the measure that is present in the validation data set. Generic critical care severity of illness measures are often based on specific patient subsets. This does not always have dire implications. Only when the subset of patients in whom the severity of illness measure is biased is relatively large, and when the degree of bias is large, is a biased model a likely explanation for poor model fit. Identifying this patient subset and proving that (1) the model fits the other patients well, (2) the subset is large, and (3) the model fit in the subset is particularly poor, strengthen this argument. It is not always the case that poor model fit indicates a biased model, and critical readers should know that there is a "differential diagnosis" for poor model fit (Table 10.2).

USING SEVERITY OF ILLNESS MEASURES

Individual Patient Assessments

Value

Perhaps the most controversial use of severity of illness measures is in making individual patient decisions. There is ample

---

	Table 10.2 Sources of Poor Model Fit in a Validation Study of a Severity of Illness Measure	
Source	**Definition**	**Comment**
Model	The model is biased by failing to account for some aspect of severity of illness that is present in the validation data that was not present in the derivation database	Current critical care severity of illness measures do not fully account for the poor prognosis of patients transferred to tertiary referral hospitals.
Care	Bad (or good) care will appear as poor model fit with either an excess or paucity of observed deaths compared to predicted.	The use of severity of illness measures to risk adjust outcomes and to benchmark ICUs is a cornerstone of quality improvement strategies.
Luck	Chance alone, particularly when patients are drawn from an unrepresentative or short period, can generate a validation data set that appears to deviate from good fit.	Most benchmarking strategies require a minimum number of patients sampled over a large period of time and also require that hospitals appear as outliers in consecutive years before deeming the care exceptional.
Data	Garbage in = garbage out. Variables for severity of illness measure must be recorded in the medical record and abstracted following the rules used in the derivation database.	Staff training, double data entry and abstraction of a sample of charts, and the use of computerized data entry improve reliability. Note that upcoding of severity of illness has been reported as a technique to falsely improve risk-adjusted mortality.

evidence that individual clinicians, like all decision makers, are influenced by recent cases and a host of cognitive factors that bias decisions away from rational choices based on data. In most studies, individual clinician prognosis adds independent information to the severity of illness prognosis. These, studies also demonstrate that objective probability estimates add independent information to physicians' predictions. Although most frequently discussed in the setting of withdrawing or withholding life support, objective probability estimates have been proposed to decide which patients to admit to, or discharge from, the ICU and how to allocate ICU nurses to patients. To some, objective information from severity of illness measures can greatly enhance patient care by providing prognoses that are independent of cognitive biases. To others, the idea of patient care being driven by an equation is problematic.

Limitations

Regardless of whether these tools should affect decisions, there is convincing evidence that, in practice, they do not. SUPPORT randomized patients and their providers receive detailed, accurate, objective prognostic data from a severity of illness mode. This information had no effect on clinical decision making. There are several potential problems with relying solely on objective probability estimates to guide clinical decisions. First, many of the prognoses provided by severity of illness measures are in a range that would not influence clinical decisions. For example, in the SUPPORT study, despite the fact that patients were selected specifically because they had a life-threatening diagnosis, only 2.7% of the 4301 study patients had a predicted 2-month survival of less than 1%. Objective prognostic information in the middle range may inform clinical decisions, but it is unlikely to determine them. Second, individual patient prognoses provided by severity of illness measures do not convey the uncertainty in the prognosis. For example, a predicted probability of death of 93% is different than a predicted probability of death of 93% ± 6%. Current measures only provide the prognosis, not its uncertainty. Prognoses provided by a severity of illness measure that has not been recalibrated for the ICU in which the patient is being cared for will reflect the patient's outcome in the average ICU from which the severity of illness measure was derived but may under- or overestimate the patient's prognosis in that ICU. Finally, all of the bad data and negative model issues that affect severity of illness model accuracy in populations can affect the predictions in individual patients.

In 1994, the mere suggestion that a computer program would be used to inform clinical intensive care decisions at a major London teaching hospital led to a public debate in which the severity of illness software was called a "doomsday machine" and an administrative decision was made to turn it off. This is not to say that objective prognostic information in critically ill patients is useless. Unfortunately, although there are ample data on the limitations of individual objective prognostic estimates in critically ill patients, there are equally persuasive data that decisions uninformed by objective outcome data are driven by factors that should not play a role, including patient race and age, physician age and training, and cognitive biases. Except in unusual scenarios in which the objective prognostic data indicate that the care is futile, it seems unlikely that clinicians or patients will ever rely solely on objective data to make decisions

to limit life-sustaining treatment because, even if perfectly accurate, this information does not incorporate patients', clinicians', or society's values for different outcomes or for handling uncertainty.

Population Assessments
Value

Severity of illness measures are essential to research and quality of care assessments in critical care. They serve two roles: to describe populations of critically ill patients and to control for confounding due to severity of illness. The results of severity of illness scoring or the predicted probability of death can be presented in research studies of critically ill patients to provide additional data so that readers can understand the patient population. More commonly, severity of illness measures are used to address the problem of confounding due to severity of illness. In clinical research in the ICU, investigators often must try to tease out the independent effect of a therapy, complication, or other factor from the multiple effects of organ failure, comorbidities, and treatments in critically ill patients. By combining these factors into a single confounder score and adjusting for this score in a regression model or stratified analysis, investigators attempt to focus on the independent and potentially causal effect of the exposure under study. Here, "exposure" is a generic term that applies to biologic exposures (infections, drugs, ventilator settings, inflammatory mediators, and genetic allele) as well as health services exposures (physician and nurse staffing patterns, time of ICU admission, and quality of care). Although they are methodologically equivalent, it is informative to consider three separate examples of using severity of illness measures to control for confounding in clinical trials, epidemiologic studies, and assessments of quality of care.

The randomized clinical trial is designed to address confounding by ensuring that the groups are randomly different and reducing questions of confounding to chance; therefore the roles of additional methods are not immediately clear. Severity of illness measures have three potential roles in clinical trials. Often, investigators are concerned that a trial of a therapy in the ICU will fail if the enrolled patients are either too well or too ill to benefit. Prior to randomization, a severity of illness measure can be used to establish the enrollment criteria for the study. On average, randomization balances severity of illness between arms of a trial; however, unequal randomizations do occur even in large trials. A severity of illness measure can be assessed prior to randomization and used as a stratification variable to guarantee that the arms of the trial are balanced on this variable. Finally, after completion of the trial, severity of illness measures can be used for subgroup analyses of the data and can be incorporated into multivariate models of the clinical trial data to improve the statistical power of the study by minimizing variance due to differences in severity of illness. Post hoc analyses of clinical trial data, including multivariate models of the treatment's efficacy, should be performed judiciously because they have yielded misleading results.

Epidemiologic studies, by definition, are not randomized experiments. Confounding is a major source of bias in these studies, and the use of multivariate confounding scores in stratified and multivariate analyses is routine. Many important exposures, including ICU complications, medical error, and organizational ICU changes, are difficult or impossible to randomize, and the only way to study them is with cohort studies that control for confounding using severity of illness measures.

Quality of care is an elusive concept in medicine that is well beyond the scope of this chapter. However, important proposed measures of quality of care include an ICU's risk-adjusted mortality, length of stay, or resource use. "Risk-adjusted" simply means controlling for patient severity of illness and other factors. If the risk adjustment is perfect, analyses will indicate which of the ICUs are outliers and have better or worse outcomes than the average ICU. These analyses are no different than epidemiologic studies except the exposure is the entire ICU, with an attempt to draw a causal inference between care in that ICU and its outcomes controlling for the patients' severity of illness. Much of the focus in this area is on benchmarking large numbers of ICUs in an attempt to identify and potentially steer patients away from or improve poorly performing ones. There is also value in sharing outcome data among hospitals, particularly if the hospitals are engaged in a collaborative quality improvement endeavor in which process improvement ideas can be disseminated. However, there is value in tracking risk-adjusted outcomes within a single ICU. Outcome outliers, low-risk patients who have poor outcomes and high-risk patients who do well, are excellent for reviewing at a critical care case conference. Tracking risk-adjusted outcome over time within the same institution provides useful data to share with frontline clinicians and can detect problems with care at an early phase. Of course, with the exception of the largest ICUs, the numbers in these analyses will be small and chance variation should be considered before transient improvements or declines in risk-adjusted outcome are overinterpreted.

Limitations

The principal limitations to using severity of illness measures in population analyses have already been described (see Table 10.2). One approach to dealing with the problem of a model that no longer fits the population is to recalibrate the model by rederiving the coefficients for the regression model. As new treatments become available, the relationship between severity of illness and mortality may change and recalibration is important. This is particularly useful for a group of ICUs that want to start collaborative benchmarking and wish to begin with a severity of illness model customized for their patients. However, an individual ICU that assesses its care with a severity of illness measure and identifies that its SMR is elevated should proceed cautiously in interpreting a recalibrated severity of illness measure. Mathematically, recalibration will almost certainly "fix" the SMR and make it a reassuring 1.0; however, this does not help the ICU distinguish between poor care and poor model fit.

The principal limitation of establishing causality in epidemiologic studies that use severity of illness measures to control for confounding is usually not the severity of illness measure. Frequently, there are biases that cannot be accounted for in the severity of illness measure. For example, studies that attempt to establish a causal link between a specific diagnostic test (e.g., the pulmonary artery catheter) and outcome are hampered by indication bias. Patients who are treated in a specific way may be different from those who are not. To the extent that this is driven purely by severity of illness, the study will be valid; however, other factors may be important that are not included in severity of illness measures. If this is the case, then the indication for treatment bias will not be completely addressed by controlling for severity of illness.

The literature on risk-adjusted outcome as a valid measure of quality of care is predominantly critical. Hospitals identified as having excellent risk-adjusted outcomes do not always have optimal processes of care. Hospitals identified as excellent or poor one year frequently do not appear in the same rank the next year, suggesting a role for random variation. Finally, publication of benchmarking data does not appear to direct health care decisions by patients or, in the United States, by purchasers. Despite these limitations, the Joint Commission on Accreditation of Healthcare Organizations has proposed risk-adjusted ICU length of stay and hospital mortality as candidate core measures of the quality of care for ICUs.

THE FUTURE OF SEVERITY OF ILLNESS MEASURES IN CRITICAL CARE

The electronic medical record will greatly facilitate the collection of large databases of critically ill patients from increasingly diverse patient populations. Genetic data, cytokine profiles, and detailed minute-to-minute physiologic information can be incorporated into severity of illness measures. More complex, computationally intensive modeling techniques, including neural networks and power spectral analyses of physiologic variables, will be incorporated. Although these tools can be expected to improve the calibration and discrimination of severity of illness measures, the fundamental challenges of decision making in individual patients, causal inferences from observational data, and definition of quality of care will remain.

SUGGESTED READING

Hadorn D, Keeler E, Rogers W, Brook R: Assessing the Performance of Mortality Prediction Models. Santa Monica, CA, Rand, 1993.

Harrell FE Jr, Lee KL, Mark DB: Multivariable prognostic models: Issues in developing models, evaluating assumptions and adequacy, and measuring and reducing errors. Stat Med 1996;15(4):361–387.

Iezzoni LI. Risk: Adjustment for Measuring Health Care Outcomes. Ann Arbor, MI, Health Administration Press, 1994.

Knaus WA, Wagner DP, Draper EA, et al: The APACHE III prognostic system. Risk prediction of hospital mortality for critically ill hospitalized adults. Chest 1991;100(6):1619–1636.

Knaus WA, Wagner DP, Lynn J: Short-term mortality predictions for critically ill hospitalized adults: science and ethics. Science 1991;254(5030): 389–394.

Le Gall JR, Lemeshow S, Saulnier F: A new Simplified Acute Physiology Score (SAPS II) based on a European/North American multicenter study. JAMA 1993;270(24):2957–2963.

Lemeshow S, Teres D, Klar J, et al: Mortality Probability Models (MPM II) based on an international cohort of intensive care unit patients. JAMA 1993;270(20):2478–2486.

Rubenfeld GD, Crawford SW: Withdrawing life support from mechanically ventilated recipients of bone marrow transplants: A case for evidence-based guidelines. Ann Intern Med 1996;125(8):625–633.

Thomas JW, Hofer TP: Research evidence on the validity of risk-adjusted mortality rate as a measure of hospital quality of care. Med Care Res Rev 1998;55(4):371–404.

Chapter 1

Hemodynamic Monitoring

Ognjen Gajic and Rolf D. Hubmayr

Restoring or maintaining tissue perfusion and oxygenation is thought to be central to the care of critically ill patients. The challenge at the bedside is to recognize the precision and accuracy of the monitored variables and to have some sense of if, and how, this information might contribute to the assessment of end organ perfusion and/or to the response to a specific therapy (e.g., a fluid bolus). In the absence of evidence from clinical trials that can be used to guide hemodynamic support in the intensive care unit (ICU), therapeutic decisions are based on the answers to the following questions:

1. Do the vital organs of this patient receive an adequate amount of blood and nutrients?
2. Would increasing systemic oxygen delivery benefit this patient?
3. If yes, what is the safest and the most effective way of increasing oxygen delivery to underperfused tissues?

Hemodynamic monitoring is often used to answer these questions. Common indications for hemodynamic monitoring are listed in Box 11.1. The following sections discuss the physiologic concepts behind hemodynamic monitoring and review methods and devices used to assess the adequacy of tissue perfusion.

PRINCIPLES OF HEMODYNAMIC MONITORING

Physiologic Concepts
Ensuring Sufficient Tissue Perfusion Has a Central Role in Resuscitation of Critically Ill Patients

An imbalance between delivery and need for nutrients such as oxygen in vital organs is thought to be common in all forms of shock. This imbalance is manifested by the accumulation of products of anaerobic metabolism and cellular dysfunction. Rapid restoration of systemic oxygen delivery is considered imperative if one is to prevent cell injury, systemic inflammation, and multiorgan failure. Although few would argue the merits of timely resuscitation of patients with shock, critical care practitioners must nevertheless be aware of certain limitations of hemodynamic monitoring in the care of critically ill patients:

- Temporal variability in metabolism from changes in the level of activity, pain, anxiety, and disease state is a common reason for short-term changes in cardiac output and oxygen delivery.
- Considering the large regional heterogeneity in blood flow and metabolic rate, indices of systemic oxygen delivery may be insensitive measures of local hypoperfusion.
- The type and timing of intervention, rather than a particular monitoring device, are the primary determinants of the successful outcome of resuscitation equipment.

In light of these caveats, it must be emphasized that the goal of this section is to highlight physiologic concepts and not to establish specific therapeutic guidelines based on numeric interpretation of monitored variables. The main determinants of global oxygen delivery and the relationship between oxygen delivery and consumption are expressed in the modified Fick equation:

Box 11.1 Common Indications for Hemodynamic Monitoring

Shock
Pulmonary edema
Perioperative high-risk surgery
Hypertensive emergencies
Increased intracranial pressure

$$DO_2 \text{ (mL/min)} = CO \text{ (L/min)} \times SaO_2 \text{ (\%)} \times Hb \text{ (g/L)}$$
$$\times 0.0134 \, VO_2 \text{ (mL/min)}$$

$$VO_2 \text{ (mL/min)} = CO \text{ (L/min)} \times (SaO_2 - SvO_2)$$
$$\times Hb \text{ (g/L)} \times 0.0134$$

where DO_2 is oxygen delivery; CO is cardiac output; SaO_2 and SvO_2 are arterial and mixed venous oxygen saturation, respectively; VO_2 is oxygen consumption; and Hb is hemoglobin.

As illustrated in Figure 11.1A, oxygen delivery is dependent on the performance of a pump (cardiac output) as well as the oxygen content of blood, which in turn is dependent on the amount and saturation of the oxygen carrier (i.e., hemoglobin). Cardiac output depends on preload, afterload, and contractility. Arterial and venous oxygen saturation depend on gas exchange in the lungs and in the peripheral tissues (oxygen uptake and consumption). All hemodynamic monitoring devices provide direct or indirect information about specific components of oxygen delivery and uptake (Fig. 11.1B).

Local versus Global Oxygen Delivery and Perfusion

In septic shock in particular, there may be a failure of autoregulation resulting in maldistribution of blood flow and severe local hypoperfusion despite normal or supranormal systemic oxygen delivery. This situation is proposed as a potential explanation for the fact that patients can generate lactic acidic (presumably indicating anaerobic metabolism) in the setting of a DO_2 that exceeds normal values. Current hemodynamic monitoring devices do not provide information about local hypoperfusion. Accordingly, lactic acidosis in a setting of adequate global oxygen delivery may alert a clinician about the possibility of local tissue hypoperfusion in certain conditions (e.g., ischemic bowel). Because of the complex kinetics and metabolism of lactic acid, however, the sensitivity and specificity of serum lactate as a measure of tissue hypoperfusion are low. The assessment of splanchnic oxygenation and perfusion via gastric tonometry has been evaluated in several clinical studies. Despite promising initial results, this technology has not been shown to improve the outcome of critically ill patients, and it has not found a place at the bedside outside a research setting. Alternatively, the appearance of lactic acid may represent the adverse effects of inflammatory cytokines on the electron transport system such that O_2 cannot be utilized despite being delivered in appropriate amounts.

Inaccuracy of Clinical Examination in the Hemodynamic Evaluation of Critically Ill Patients

Several studies have formally evaluated the accuracy of the physical exam in the hemodynamic assessment of critically ill patients. A large postural change in heart rate (>30 beats/min) is of diagnostic value in patients with severe blood loss, but it has poor sensitivity for moderate blood loss and in patients with hypovolemic shock due to dehydration. Accordingly, the accuracy and precision of physical exam may be disease specific.

In another study, clinicians were asked to predict hemodynamic data from 103 consecutive patients with either shock or hypoxemia who were undergoing simultaneous pulmonary artery catheterization (PAC). Accurate predictions with regard to cardiac output, pulmonary artery occlusion pressure (PAOP), central venous pressure (CVP), or systemic vascular resistance were made in less than 50% of cases and the information

obtained led to changes in therapy in 58% (that were not necessarily beneficial to the patients).

The Assessment of Cardiac Preload and Fluid Responsiveness

The major clinical question for patients with shock is whether they will increase their stroke volume in response to a fluid bolus. It is important to understand that this is a two-part question because the presence of inadequate tissue perfusion does not necessarily mean that the patient will benefit from fluid. If it is judged that improving cardiac output would be beneficial, it becomes important to understand the relationship between the preload and cardiac function. In patients, these relationships are extremely variable, emphasizing the importance of understanding concepts as opposed to using strict numeric recommendations. There is no single threshold in filling pressure.

According to the length–tension relationship of cardiac myofibrils (the Frank–Starling law of the heart), stretching the sarcomeres from their resting length brings actin and myosin filaments into a favorable geometric position (i.e., creating a larger overlap) that generates a more forceful contraction. Accordingly, increasing the length of sarcomere by increasing the end-diastolic volume (i.e., preload) will increase the stroke volume. This increase in stroke volume (the "steep" part of the curve in Figure 11.2) will continue until the maximum strength is achieved (the "flat" part of the curve in Figure 11.2). Further increase in end-diastolic volume then leads to overstretching, dilatation, and heart failure.

Venous return and, concurrently, cardiac preload may be increased by rapid infusion of intravenous fluids. Although an empiric "fluid challenge" is generally considered safe, there are theoretical consequences of unnecessary fluid administration. The effects of tissue edema on local perfusion have not been systematically studied, but avoiding unnecessary fluid administration may be beneficial in conditions characterized by increased vascular permeability. A large controlled clinical trial is under way to assess the effect of a fluid-liberal versus a fluid-conservative treatment strategy in patients with acute respiratory distress syndrome, as well as the effect of using PACs versus simply CVP monitoring, on mortality.

Because the physical examination does not allow accurate assessment of preload in critically ill patients, data generated by hemodynamic monitoring are required. Contrary to a long-standing belief, however, studies have demonstrated that the information generated by a PAC, and the measurement of PAOP in particular, has limited accuracy in assessing preload and fluid responsiveness. In fact, simple measures such as the analysis of respiratory variations in arterial pressure were found to be far superior to PAOP as markers of cardiac preload and fluid responsiveness in mechanically ventilated patients with septic shock.

Hemodynamic Monitoring and Outcome

PAC came under scrutiny after the publication of a large retrospective study that found an association between the use of the catheter and increased mortality. The controversy resulting from this finding led to multiple observational studies and several randomized clinical trials of the use of PACs that showed care providers had limited knowledge of cardiovascular physiology, did not know how to use the information derived from catheter, and were more likely to use the device in privately insured

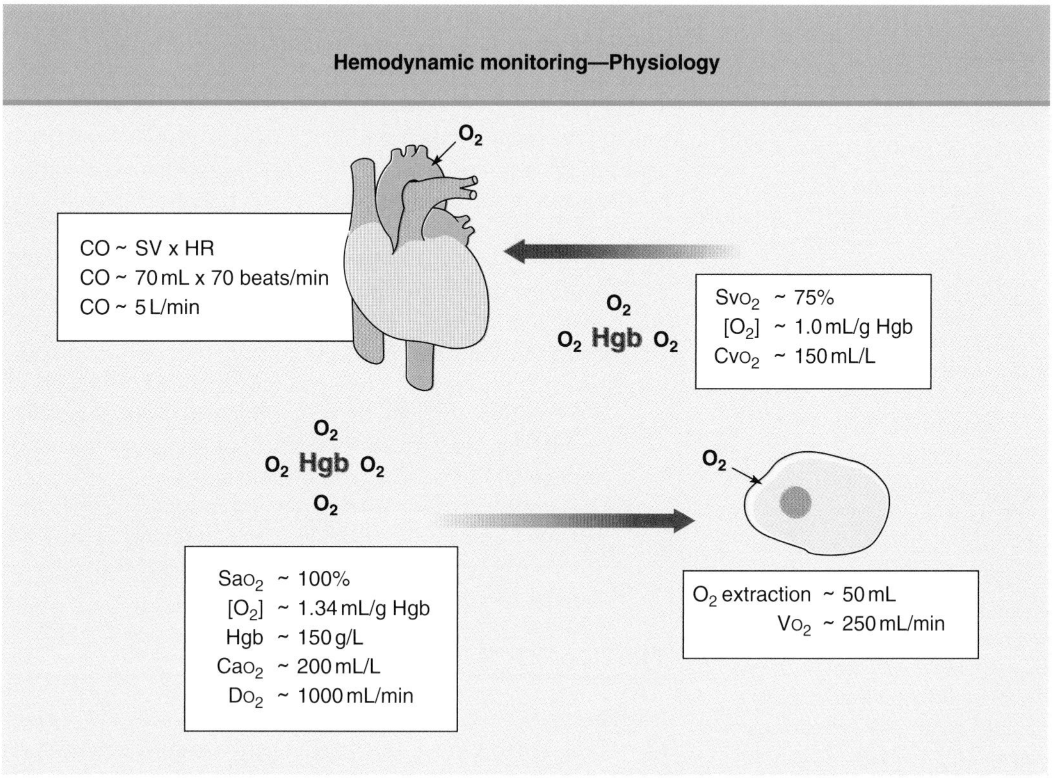

Figure 11.1. Hemodynamic monitoring. *A,* Hemodynamic monitoring: physiology. Simplified diagram of O_2 delivery and consumption. *B,* Hemodynamic monitoring: techniques. Target information obtained by hemodynamic monitoring devices. CO, cardiac output; Cao_2 and Cvo_2, arterial and venous O_2 content; Do_2, oxygen delivery; Hgb, hemoglobin; Sao_2 and Svo_2, arterial and venous O_2 saturation; Vo_2, oxygen consumption.

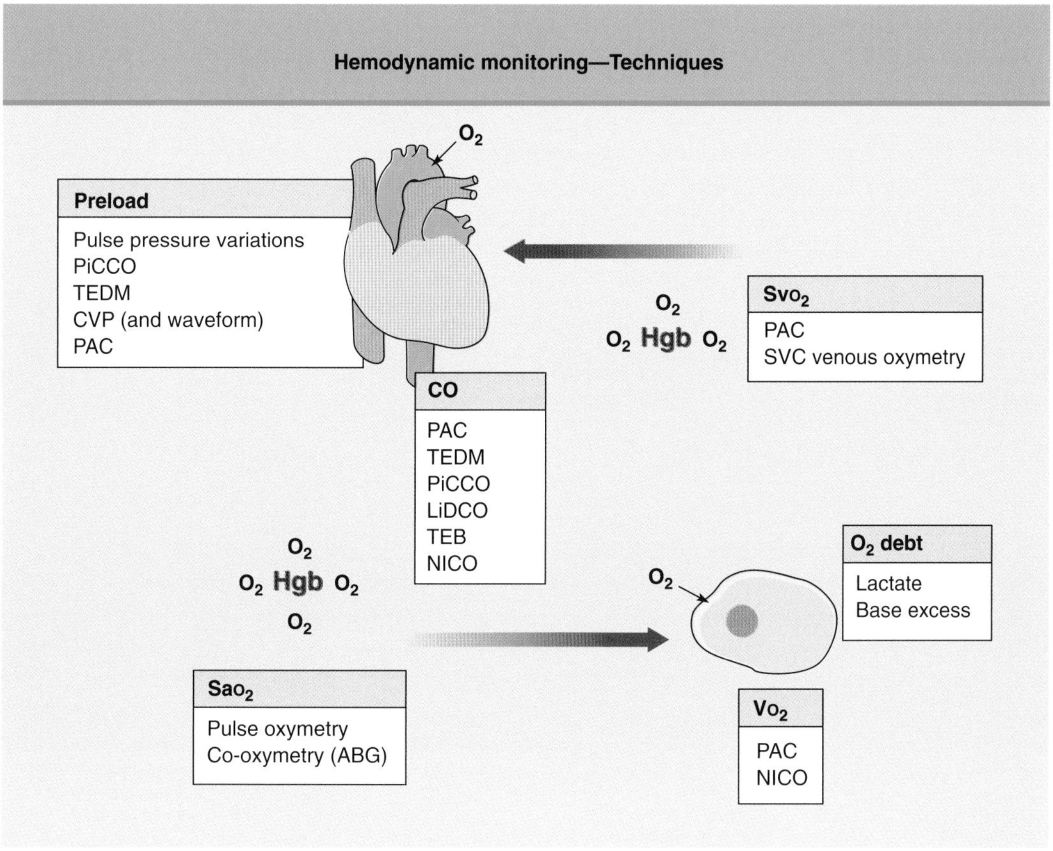

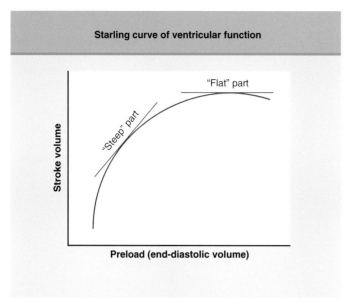

Starling curve of ventricular function

Figure 11.2. Starling curve of ventricular function. The relationship between ventricular end-diastolic volume (preload) and stroke volume. Under normal resting conditions and in hypovolemia, the increase in end-diastolic volume results in larger overlap in actin–myosin filaments and a more efficient contraction ("steep" part of the curve). Once the maximum strength is achieved, further increase in end-diastolic volume does not lead to an increase in stroke volume ("flat" part of the curve) and ultimately leads to cardiac dilatation and a decrease in efficacy of the cardiac contraction (heart failure).

patients. The main complications associated with the use of PAC and other hemodynamic monitoring devices are listed in Table 11.1.

The randomized trials, which tested the use of hemodynamic monitoring (mainly PAC) with and without protocolized intervention, are listed in Table 11.2. Three important conclusions can be made after a careful analysis of the study designs and outcomes:

1. Disease state and timing, type, and design of the intervention were more important determinants of outcome than hemodynamic monitoring per se.
2. Hemodynamic monitoring is unlikely to improve outcome unless it is coupled with a carefully planned, protocolized intervention. In fact, it is not known if hemodynamic monitoring has value beyond that of a protocolized approach.
3. Appropriate goal-oriented intervention, guided by hemodynamic monitoring, may improve outcome in patients with early septic shock and those undergoing high-risk surgery (preoperative optimization).

TECHNIQUES AND EQUIPMENT

It is necessary to emphasize the importance of technical expertise of the critical care team in adequate maintenance, calibration, troubleshooting, and quality assessment of devices used for

Table 11.1 Complications of Hemodynamic Monitoring

General complications associated with use of all hemodynamic monitoring devices	Errors in management resulting from an inaccurate measurement or interpretation of hemodynamic information
Complications associated with obtaining central venous access	Pneumothorax, internal bleeding, catheter-related infection, injury to the thoracic duct, pericardial tamponade
Complications associated with obtaining peripheral arterial access	Local hematoma, catheter-related infection, limb ischemia, retrograde embolization
Complications specific to the use of PAC	Pulmonary hemorrhage, pulmonary embolism
Complications associated with esophageal cannulation	Esophageal perforation, gastrointestinal bleeding

Table 11.2 Clinical Trials Testing the Efficacy of Hemodynamic Monitoring with and without a Goal-Oriented Therapeutic Intervention

Reference	Condition	Monitoring (Intervention Group/Control Group)	Intervention (Intervention Group/Control Group)	Outcome
Rivers et al (2001)	Early septic shock	CVPSVo2/routine	Fluid + red blood cells + inotrope or vasodilator routine	Improved survival in the intervention group
Boyd et al (1993)	Preoperative high-risk surgery	PAC both groups	Fluid and dopexamine/routine	Improved survival in the intervention group
Sandham et al (2003)	Intraoperative high-risk surgery	PAC/no PAC	Routine	No difference
Hayes et al (1994)	Heterogeneous ICU	PAC both groups	Dobutamine/routine	Worse survival in the intervention group
Gattinoni et al (1995)	Heterogeneous ICU	PAC both groups	Dobutamine/routine	No difference
Wilson et al (1999)	Preoperative high-risk surgery	PAC/no PAC	Dopexamine and fluid/routine	Improved survival in the intervention group
Rhodes et al (2002)	Established septic shock/acute lung injury (ALI)	PAC/no PAC	Routine	No difference
Richard et al (2003)	Established septic shock/ALI	PAC/no PAC	Routine	No difference

hemodynamic monitoring. Unless all technical requirements are fulfilled, the accuracy of the obtained measurements cannot be trusted.

Pulmonary Artery Catheter

PACs provide information about cardiac output, right and left heart filling pressures, and pulmonary arterial pressures and enable the measurement of the O_2 content in mixed venous blood. Intermittent measurements of cardiac output are thought to be helpful in assessing the response to therapy. Newer devices allow the continuous (beat-to-beat) trending of cardiac output, but their utility and cost-effectiveness have yet to be established. Mixed venous oxygen saturation varies with cardiac output and systemic oxygen delivery, and no single threshold defines adequacy of tissue oxygenation. In fact, mixed venous O_2 saturation is often elevated in situations in which the ability of tissues to utilize oxygen is thought to be impaired (e.g., mitochondrial dysfunction and possible maldistribution of blood flow in advanced sepsis). Nevertheless, venous oxygen saturation has been used successfully as one of the therapeutic end points of fluid resuscitation in early septic shock. PAOP is a surrogate measure of left atrial pressure and, in the absence of mitral valve disease, increased pulmonary venous resistance, or wedging of the catheter in smaller pulmonary arterioles, of left ventricular end-diastolic pressure. As such, it estimates the fluid filtration pressure in pulmonary vessels. Since compliance of the left heart is extremely variable, PAOP is not a good predictor of end-diastolic volume and hence stroke volume. Several studies have demonstrated the inaccuracy of PAOP as a measure of cardiac preload and fluid responsiveness. Unfortunately, many providers focus unduly on PAOP when managing patients with PACs. It is one possible explanation why, in some studies, PAC use was associated with adverse outcomes. Instead, a dynamic

approach that examines the changes in stroke volume and cardiac output in response to a particular intervention (fluid challenge) may be more informative as a guide to resuscitation of critically ill patients. The PAC can have a diagnostic use because it generally allows differentiation of specific types of shock (hypovolemic, distributive, and cardiogenic) and pulmonary edema (hydrostatic vs. permeability).

Minimally Invasive Hemodynamic Monitoring

The invasiveness of PAC and the recent controversy about its utility in the care of critically ill patients have renewed interest in alternative monitoring devices. Currently available, minimally invasive devices are listed in Box 11.2.

Arterial and Central Venous Pressure Waveform Analysis

Respiratory variations in systolic pressure and pulse pressure are reasonably accurate markers of cardiac preload and fluid responsiveness in sedated, mechanically ventilated patients with shock who have no spontaneous breathing. In a simplified view of heart lung interactions, Figure 11.3 demonstrates that unless the patient has a severe systolic dysfunction, any increase in pleural

---

Box 11.2 Minimally Invasive Hemodynamic Monitoring

Arterial and central venous pressure waveform analysis
Pulse contour analysis and transpulmonary thermodilution
Esophageal Doppler monitoring
Lithium dilution
Transthoracic bioimpedance
Indirect calorimetry

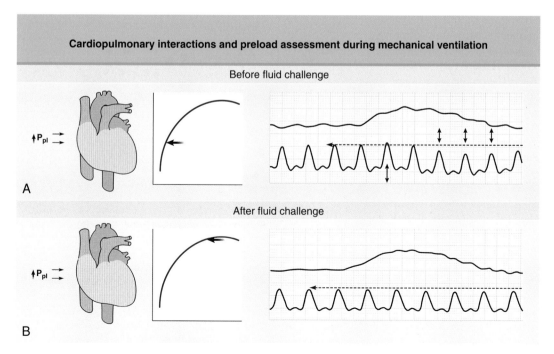

Cardiopulmonary interactions and preload assessment during mechanical ventilation

Before fluid challenge

A

After fluid challenge

B

Figure 11.3. Cardiopulmonary interactions and preload assessment during mechanical ventilation. Relation between the pleural pressure, venous return, Starling curve of cardiac function, and respiratory changes in arterial pulse pressure in the circumstances of positive pressure ventilation. A, Before fluid challenge. B, After fluid challenge. IVC, inferior vena cava; P_{pl}, pleural pressure; SV, stroke volume.

Practice of Critical Care

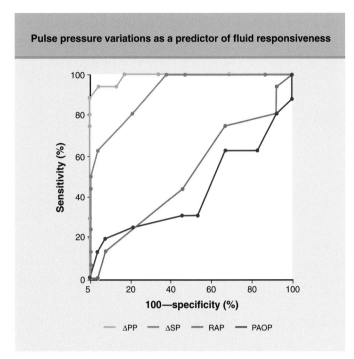

Figure 11.4. Pulse pressure variations as a predictor of fluid responsiveness. Receiver operating characteristic (ROC) curves that compare the ability of the respiratory changes in pulse pressure (ΔPP), the respiratory changes in systolic pressure (ΔSP), the right atrial pressure (RAP), and the pulmonary artery occlusion pressure (PAOP) to discriminate patients who respond (cardiac index increase = 15%) and do not respond to volume expansion. The area under the ROC curve for ΔPP was greater than those for ΔSP, RAP, and PAOP ($P < 0.01$) (Data from Michard F, Boussard S, Chemla D, et al: Relation between respiratory changes in arterial pulse pressure and fluid responsiveness in septic patients with acute circulatory failure. Am J Respir Crit Care Med 2000;162(1): 134–138.)

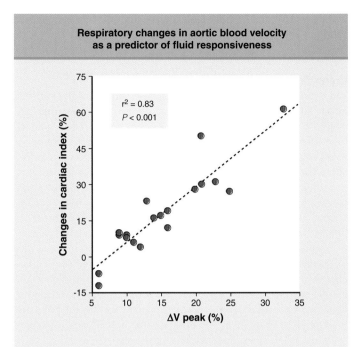

Figure 11.5. Respiratory changes in aortic blood velocity as a predictor of fluid responsiveness. Correlation between the changes of cardiac index after the fluid challenge and the respiratory variations in peak aortic blood flow velocities as determined by esophageal Doppler monitoring. (Data from Feissel M, Michard F, Mangin I, et al: Respiratory changes in aortic blood velocity as an indicator of fluid responsiveness in ventilated patients with septic shock. Chest 2001;119:867–873.)

pressure leads to a decrease in venous return and cardiac preload. In a patient who is already volume depleted, this causes hypotension (Fig. 11.3A). A fluid bolus ultimately improves venous return with the disappearance of respiratory variations (Fig. 11.3B). Pulse pressure variations of more than 12 mm had more than 90% sensitivity and specificity for an increase in cardiac output after a 500-mL fluid challenge—a far superior discrimination than either PAOP or CVP measurements (Fig. 11.4). Similarly, respiratory variations in aortic blood velocity (as assessed by transesophageal Doppler echocardiography; Fig. 11.5) were found to be an accurate marker of preload and fluid responsiveness in mechanically ventilated patients with septic shock. An increase in pulse pressure in response to passive leg raising may also give additional information with regard to cardiac preload and fluid responsiveness in critically ill patients receiving mechanical ventilation (Fig. 11.6).

Whereas a single measurement of CVP has a very low sensitivity for the assessment of preload, CVP waveform analysis may be more useful. In spontaneously breathing patients, the presence of respiratory variations in CVP suggests that the right ventricle can handle additional volume. A small study found good specificity and moderate sensitivity of the presence of respiratory variations in CVP as a measure of preload.

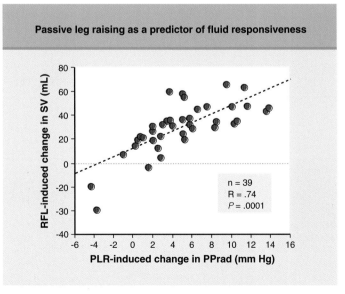

Figure 11.6. Passive leg raising as a predictor of fluid responsiveness. Correlation between the changes in pulse pressure waveform and the increase in stroke volume after passive leg raising (PLR) maneuver. (Data from Boulain T, Achard J-M, Teboul J-L, et al: Changes in BP induced by passive leg raising predict response to fluid loading in critically ill patients. Chest 2002;121:1245–1252.)

Two-Dimensional Echocardiography and Transesophageal Doppler Monitoring

Although in a strict sense echocardiography is a diagnostic test rather than a monitoring device, its availability in the ICU setting has contributed to the decrease in PAC use in recent years. Transesophageal and, to a lesser extent, transthoracic echocardiography allow a rapid differential diagnosis of shock with the assessment of the left and right ventricular function, estimation of preload from the measurement of left ventricular end-diastolic volume, and the inspiratory changes in the inferior vena cava diameter ("waterfall phenomenon").

Continuous esophageal Doppler is being used with increasing frequency to monitor stroke volume during anesthesia and surgery. Stroke volume is derived from the velocity of pulsatile blood flow through the descending aorta (derived from the changes in aortic diameter over time). It also provides an estimate of cardiac preload (i.e., systolic flow time corrected by the heart rate) and of fluid responsiveness based on respiratory variations in flow velocity (see Fig. 11.5). Figure 11.7 illustrates a Doppler signal of the descending aorta obtained from the esophageal probe. Although the initial studies performed in critically ill patients demonstrated good correlation of pulse Doppler echo with thermodilution cardiac output, the need for additional training limits its use in critically ill patients.

Pulse Contour Analysis and Transpulmonary Thermodilution

This technique provides a continuous estimate of the stroke volume using the pressure tracing obtained from a large (usually femoral) arterial catheter. The method requires calibration with another technique since the contour of the arterial pressure waveform also depends on vascular resistance. In one commercially available device, this calibration is accomplished using a transpulmonary thermodilution technique. Analogous to pulmonary artery thermodilution, cold injectate is infused into a central vein and a change in temperature is detected in a peripheral artery. The accuracy and precision of PCA are reasonable when compared to those of pulmonary artery thermodilution, unless there is a rapid change in vascular resistance. Transpulmonary thermodilution also allows estimation of intrathoracic blood volume, a determinant of left ventricular preload. The need to cannulate both a large artery and a central vein, however, limits the routine use of this technique.

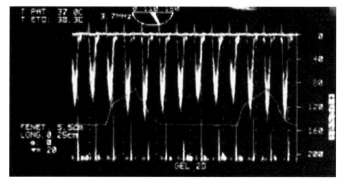

Figure 11.7. Transesophageal Doppler signal. Pulsatile Doppler signal obtained from the esophageal probe. (Used with permission from Feissel M, Michard F, Mangin I, et al: Respiratory changes in aortic blood velocity as an indicator of fluid responsiveness in ventilated patients with septic shock. Chest 2001;119:867–873.)

Lithium Dilution Cardiac Output

This noninvasive assessment of cardiac output utilizes the lithium dilution curve. A small amount of lithium is injected into a peripheral vein, and the concentration difference is measured in a blood sample obtained from a peripheral artery. Lithium dilution can then be used to calibrate a pulse contour analysis and enable continuous measurement of cardiac output. This method is less invasive (only peripheral arterial and venous cannulation is required) and correlates well with thermodilution cardiac output. However, it does not allow the estimation of cardiac preload. When coupled with pulse contour analysis and the analysis of respiratory variations in pulse pressure, lithium dilution can be an accurate, useful, minimally invasive monitoring technique.

Transthoracic Bioimpedance

Thoracic electrical bioimpedance measures the resistance of the thorax to a high-frequency, low-intensity electrical current flowing between the electrodes placed on the chest surface. As such, it is a function of intrathoracic fluid volume (i.e., the larger the amount of intrathoracic fluid, the higher the resistance to the flow of electrical current). Cardiac output can then be derived from cyclical changes in thoracic bioimpedance (thoracic fluid volume) resulting from cardiac contraction and aortic blood flow. The main shortcomings of this noninvasive technique are limited accuracy of measurements in patients with pleural effusions, pulmonary edema, and peripheral edema and an inability to assess cardiac preload.

Indirect Calorimetry (Indirect Fick Method)

In this technique, cardiac output is derived from CO_2 production based on a modified Fick equation:

$$CO = V_{CO_2}/(C_{VCO_2} - C_{aCO_2})$$

The partial rebreathing technique allows determination of cardiac output without the need for a direct measurement of venous CO_2 concentration. In patients without significant lung disease, cardiac output determined by indirect calorimetry correlates well with cardiac output obtained by PAC thermodilution. However, the dependence of exhaled CO_2 concentration on gas exchange in the lung (i.e., influenced by dead space, low ventilation-to-perfusion relationships, and shunt) limits its usefulness in critically ill patients, especially those on mechanical ventilation. In addition, this technique does not allow for the assessment of cardiac preload.

CONCLUSIONS

Hemodynamic monitoring is an essential component of the assessment and resuscitation of critically ill patients. Box 11.3

Box 11.3 Controversies in Hemodynamic Monitoring
Efficacy of goal-oriented resuscitation guided by hemodynamic monitoring
Utility of invasive hemodynamic monitoring (PAC) in critically ill patients
Accuracy and (cost) effectiveness of minimally invasive hemodynamic monitoring devices
Utility of techniques aimed at evaluating tissue oxygenation (gastric tonometry)

presents current controversies in hemodynamic monitoring of critically ill patients. Technical expertise is an essential component of accurate collection and interpretation of data. Emerging minimally invasive techniques may supplement or replace pulmonary artery catheterization in the hemodynamic monitoring of critically ill patients. However, prior to adopting the new technology at the bedside, careful assessment of efficacy as well as cost-effectiveness need to be performed.

SUGGESTED READING

Boulain T, Achard J-M, Teboul J-L, et al: Changes in BP induced by passive leg raising predict response to fluid loading in critically ill patients. Chest 2002;121:1245–1252.

Boyd O, Grounds RM, Bennett ED: A randomized clinical trial of the effect of deliberate perioperative increase of oxygen delivery on mortality in high-risk surgical patients. JAMA 1993;270:2699–2707.

Chaney JC, Derdak S: Minimally invasive hemodynamic monitoring for the intensivist: Current and emerging technology. Crit Care Med 2002;30:2338–2345.

Connors AF, Speroff T, Dawson NV, et al: The effectiveness of right heart catheterization in the initial care of critically ill patients. JAMA 1996;276:889–897.

Feissel M, Michard F, Mangin I, et al: Respiratory changes in aortic blood velocity as an indicator of fluid responsiveness in ventilated patients with septic shock. Chest 2001;119:867–868.

Gattinoni L, Brazzi L, Pelosi P, et al: A trial of goal-oriented hemodynamic therapy in critically ill patients. SvO$_2$ Collaborative Group. N Engl J Med 1995;333:1025–1032.

Hayes MA, Timmins AC, Yau E, et al: Elevation of systemic oxygen delivery in the treatment of critically ill patients. N Engl J Med 1994;330:1717–1722.

Magder S, Lagonidis D, Erice F: The use of respiratory variations in right atrial pressure to predict the cardiac output response to PEEP. J Crit Care 2001;16:108–114.

Michard F, Boussard S, Chemla D, et al: Relation between respiratory changes in arterial pulse pressure and fluid responsiveness in septic patients with acute circulatory failure. Am J Respir Crit Care Med 2000;162:134–138.

Rhodes A, Cusack RJ, Newman PJ, et al: A randomised, controlled trial of the pulmonary artery catheter in critically ill patients. Intensive Care Med 2002;28:256–264.

Richard C, Warszawski J, Anguel N, et al: Early use of the pulmonary artery catheter and outcomes in patients with shock and acute respiratory distress syndrome: A randomized controlled trial. JAMA 2003;290:2713–2720.

Rivers E, Nguyen B, Havstad S, et al: The Early Goal-Directed Therapy Collaborative Group: Early goal-directed therapy in the treatment of severe sepsis and septic shock. N Engl J Med 2001;345:1368–1377.

Sandham JD, Hull RD, Brant RF, et al: Canadian Critical Care Clinical Trials Group. A randomized, controlled trial of the use of pulmonary-artery catheters in high-risk surgical patients. N Engl J Med 2003;348:5–14.

Wilson J, Woods I, Fawcett J, et al: Reducing the risk of major elective surgery: Randomised controlled trial of preoperative optimisation of oxygen delivery. Br Med J 1999;318:1099–1103.

Modes of Mechanical Ventilation

Robert M. Kacmarek, Jesús Villar, and Atul Malhotra

KEY POINTS

- Our goal as clinicians is to always select the correct mode of ventilatory support for a given clinical setting that allows us to meet our ventilatory targets and to ensure patient ventilatory synchrony.
- Failure to achieve coinciding events of initiation, delivery, and termination of the patient's and the mechanical ventilator's breaths and to ensure that gas delivery during the inspiratory phase meets the demand of the patient has been referred to as patient–ventilator dyssynchrony or "fighting the ventilator."
- Classic modes of ventilation have been available on mechanical ventilators for more than 20 years and generally are the basic approaches to ventilatory support for the vast majority of patients; however, a number of new modes based on pressure ventilation format have been introduced since the 1990s.

One of the primary goals of ventilatory support is to ensure that the patient and mechanical ventilator are in synchrony; that is, to ensure that the initiation, delivery, and termination of the patient's and the mechanical ventilator's breaths coincide and that gas delivery during the inspiratory phase meets the demand of the patient. Failure to achieve this has been referred to as patient–ventilator dyssynchrony or "fighting the ventilator." Dyssynchrony results in increased patient effort and work of breathing, increased cardiovascular instability, and a heightened level of patient discomfort and anxiety. During the past several decades, ventilator manufacturers and clinicians have tried to develop the ideal mode of ventilatory support that would ensure perfect patient–ventilator synchrony. This has not been achieved; however, the overall response from various modes of ventilatory support today is much better than in the past. This chapter defines and illustrates the operation of the various modes of ventilatory support.

PRESSURE VERSUS VOLUME VENTILATION

The format for gas delivery in almost all ventilator modes is either pressure or volume targeting (Table 12.1). In volume-targeted ventilation (the original approach to ventilatory

support), a specific tidal volume is set by the clinician and the ventilator ensures that the volume is delivered regardless of pressure up to a clinician-set limit. In addition to tidal volume, flow waveform and peak flow or inspiratory time must be set. With this approach to ventilatory support, the focus is on ensuring that minute ventilation is maintained at a targeted level.

Pressure ventilation is essentially the complete opposite approach to gas delivery. A targeted peak airway and, as a result, a peak alveolar pressure are set. That is, with each breath, pressure increases to this level before the breath terminates. However, tidal volume and gas flow are allowed to vary from breath to breath, according to the mechanics of the respiratory system. During pressure ventilation, the clinician must set the targeted pressure and in some modes the inspiratory time. Flow is provided in a decelerating pattern in which the rate of deceleration is dependent on patient inspiratory demand and respiratory system mechanics. Essentially, the ventilator rapidly delivers flow to establish the targeted pressure but once the pressure target is met, flow must decrease to avoid exceeding the set pressure. This approach to ventilatory support focuses on ensuring a targeted alveolar pressure is met but never exceeded.

As noted in Table 12.2, pressure and volume ventilation respond differently to changes in impedance to gas delivery. With volume ventilation, pressure increases if it becomes more difficult to ventilate, whereas with pressure ventilation tidal volume decreases.

RANGE OF VENTILATOR MODES

In this chapter, ventilator modes are organized into two basic groups (Box 12.1): classic modes and new modes of ventilation.

Table 12.1 Pressure versus Volume-Targeted Ventilation[a]

	Pressure	Volume
Peak airway pressure	Constant	Variable
Peak alveolar pressure	Constant	Variable
Tidal volume	Variable	Constant
Peak flow	Variable	Constant
Flow pattern	Decelerating	Preset
Inspiratory time	Preset	Preset
Minimum rate	Preset	Preset

[a]Used with permission from Kacmarek RM, Dimas S, Mack C: Essentials of Respiratory Care, 4th ed. St. Louis, Mosby, 2005, p 690.

Table 12.2 Effect of Changing Compliance and Resistance during Pressure and Volume Ventilation[a]

	Pressure	Volume
Decreased compliance	↓ Volume	↑ Pressure
Increases compliance	↑ Volume	↓ Pressure
Increased auto-PEEP	↓ Volume	↑ Pressure
Decreased auto-PEEP	↑ Volume	↓ Pressure
Pneumothorax	↓ Volume	↑ Pressure
Bronchospasm	↓ Volume	↑ Pressure
Mucosal edema	↓ Volume	↑ Pressure
Secretions	↓ Volume	↑ Pressure
Pleural effusion	↓ Volume	↑ Pressure
Increased patient effort	↑ Volume	↓ Pressure
Decreased patient effort	↓ Volume	↑ Pressure

[a]Used with permission from Kacmarek RM, Dimas S, Mack C: Essentials of Respiratory Care, 4th ed. St. Louis, Mosby, 2005, p 691.

Box 12.1 Available Modes of Mechanical Ventilation

Classic Modes of Ventilation

Control
Assist/control
Assist/pressure support
Synchronized intermittent mandatory ventilation

New Modes of Ventilation

Within-breath adjustment	Between-breath adjustment
Automatic tube compensation	Pressure regulated volume control
Proportional assist ventilation	Volume support
Volume-assured pressure support	Adaptive support ventilation
	Airway pressure release ventilation
	Bilevel pressure ventilation

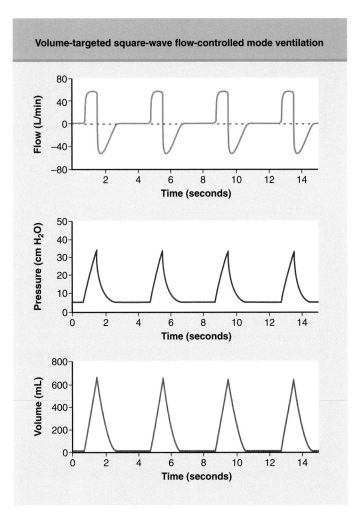

Figure 12.1. Volume-targeted square-wave flow-controlled mode ventilation. There is no negative deflection in airway pressure at the start of the breath. (Data from Hess D, McIntyre NR, Mishoe SC, et al: Respiratory Care: Principles and Practice. Philadelphia, Saunders, 2002, p 790.)

Classic modes comprise control, assist/control, assist (pressure support), and synchronized intermittent mandatory ventilation. All of these modes have been available on mechanical ventilators for more than 20 years and generally are the basic approaches to ventilatory support for the vast majority of patients. However, during the 1990s and continuing today, there has been an introduction of a number of new modes of ventilation, most of which are based on a pressure ventilation format. Many of these newer modes were designed to improve patient–ventilator synchrony by combining some of the advantageous aspects of pressure ventilation with volume ventilation. Individually, most of these modes can be classified as modes that adjust gas delivery within a given breath or those that adjust gas delivery between breaths. Essentially, most of these modes are based on some level of computerized control of gas delivery.

Control Mode

This is the original mode of ventilation available on mechanical ventilators. With this mode, the ventilator controls all aspects of gas delivery. That is, the patient is assumed to be a passive recipient of mechanical ventilation. With earlier ventilators,

patients were not able to trigger the ventilator to inspiration. However, with today's ventilators, even when sensitivity is adjusted to the most insensitive settings, patients with a strong ventilatory drive can still trigger the ventilator. Control mode is achieved today by sedation to apnea, and it is more commonly used in the operating room rather than in the intensive care unit. Controlled ventilation is available in both pressure and volume ventilation formats (Figs. 12.1 and 12.2).

Assist/Control Mode

This mode is essentially the control mode with the sensitivity set to allow easy patient triggering of a breath (Fig. 12.3). The patient determines the ventilatory rate; however, a backup rate is set to ensure a minimum level of ventilation. Box 12.2 lists the variables that must be set during both pressure- and volume-targeted assist/control. Worldwide, this is the most commonly used mode of ventilation.

Pressure Support

The closest mode to true assist ventilation available on today's ventilators is pressure support (Fig. 12.4). By "assist ventilation,"

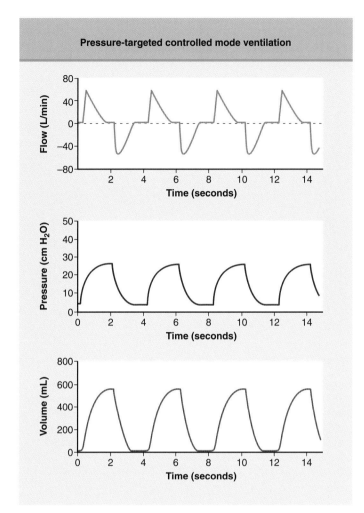

Figure 12.2. Pressure-targeted controlled mode ventilation. There is no negative deflection in airway pressure at the start of the breath. (Data from Hess D, McIntyre NR, Mishoe SC, et al: Respiratory Care: Principles and Practice. Philadelphia, Saunders, 2002, p 791.)

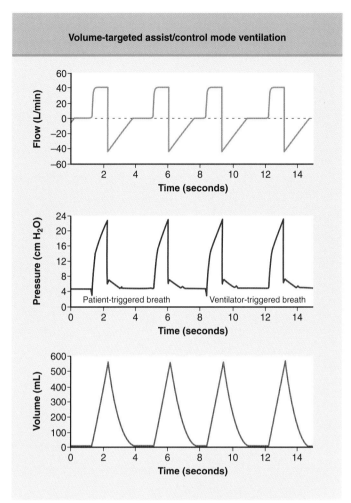

Figure 12.3. Volume-targeted assist/control mode ventilation. Each breath is patient triggered, as observed by the deflection in airway pressure at the onset of each breath. (Data from Hess D, McIntyre NR, Mishoe SC, et al: Respiratory Care: Principles and Practice. Philadelphia, Saunders, 2002, p 786.)

the implication is that there is no backup rate. In pressure support, alternate safety modes take over if patients are apneic for more than 20 seconds but no true backup rate is available. Pressure support is very similar to pressure assist/control. In addition to the backup rate available in the latter mode, the major feature of gas delivery that differs from pressure assist/control is the mechanism that terminates inspiration. With pressure assist/control, inspiration is always terminated by time, whereas with pressure support inspiration is usually terminated by flow. That is, when flow decreases to a specific level (usually 25% of the peak flow in that breath), the breath is terminated. However, there are two alternate methods of terminating inspiration in pressure support: pressure exceeding the set level after approximately 300 msec of inspiration or inspiratory time exceeding a set level (2–5 sec). Both of these secondary termination criteria are for patient safety or to prevent excessively lengthy inspiratory times (e.g., in the event of cuff leak or bronchopleural fistula).

Of the classic modes of ventilation, pressure support allows the patient the greatest control over the process of ventilation. Not only does the patient trigger the breath but also the ending

of the breath is based on patient demand. As with all pressure-targeted approaches to ventilation, pressure support allows the patient to vary the tidal volume on each breath. The only gas delivery variable set, other than sensitivity, is pressure level. Pressure support may be used on any patient who has a stable ventilatory drive.

Box 12.2 Parameters Adjusted during Assist/Control Ventilation[a]

Pressure Ventilation	Volume Ventilation
Target airway pressure	Tidal volume
Inspiratory time	Flow waveform
Backup rate	Backup rate
Sensitivity	Peak flow or inspiratory time
FIO_2	Sensitivity
PEEP	FIO_2
Rise time	PEEP

[a]With control mode all of the variables are set, and the backup rate becomes the actual patient ventilatory rate.

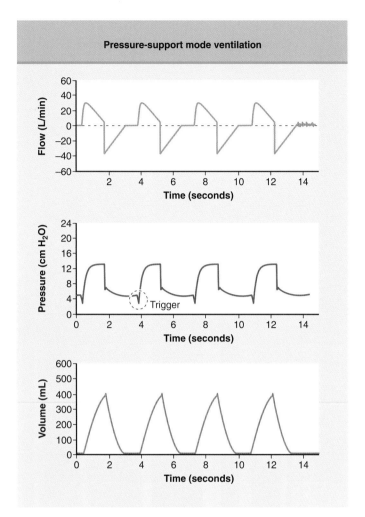

Figure 12.4. Pressure-support mode ventilation. (Data from Hess D, McIntyre NR, Mishoe SC, et al: Respiratory Care: Principles and Practice. Philadelphia, Saunders, 2002, p 787.)

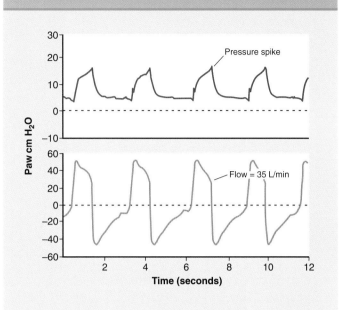

Figure 12.5. Pressure and flow tracings during pressure-support ventilation with the Nellcor Puritan Bennett 7200ae, demonstrating pressure cycling in pressure support. The pressure spike at the end of inspiration indicates that the patient desires to end the breath before the ventilator will allow exhalation. (Data from Branson RD, Campbell RS: Altering flow rate during maximum pressure support ventilation (PSVmax): Effects on cardiorespiratory function. Respir Care 1990;35:1056–1064.)

Inspiratory Termination Criteria

Also referred to as *E-senc*, expiratory sensitivity is available on many ventilators as a method to ensure the patient and ventilator end inspiration simultaneously. As illustrated in Figure 12.5, an increase in pressure at the end of a pressure support breath is not "normal" and does indicate that the patient has begun exhalation before the ventilator allows exhalation to occur. When this is observed, the patient is using accessory muscles of exhalation during the terminal aspect of the ventilator's inspiratory phase. This results in an increased ventilatory drive and ventilatory rate and also patient–ventilator dyssynchrony. E-senc allows adjustment of the percentage of peak flow terminating the breath. Whenever a spike at the end of a pressure support breath is present, a greater percentage of the peak flow should be set to terminate the breath. That is, whenever a spike is present, the E-senc percentage should be slowly increased until there is a smooth transition from inspiration to expiration. E-senc may be particularly useful in patients with heterogeneous time constants (e.g., emphysema patients will frequently experience ongoing flow into highly compliant lung units during late inspiration).

Rise Time

Synchrony at the onset of a pressure-targeted breath (pressure assist/control, pressure support, pressure regulated volume control, etc.) can be improved by adjusting the rise time. As shown in Figure 12.6, rise time varies the slope of the pressure increase at the onset of a breath by varying the time it takes flow to increase from zero to peak. Rise time, also known as *attack rate*, should be adjusted to ensure that airway pressure rises rapidly to peak level without any concavity during the initial airway pressure waveform. If the pressure waveform is concave, the rise time should be increased (more rapid); however, if peak pressure exceeds the set level at the onset of inspiration, rise time should be decreased. An increase in rise time results in an increase is peak flow and a decrease in inspiratory time (in pressure support). In most patients with a strong ventilatory drive, rise time should be set between the middle and most rapid level. Proper setting of rise time usually results in a decrease in ventilatory rate and improved patient comfort.

Synchronized Intermittent Mandatory Ventilation

This mode of ventilation combines spontaneous unsupported breathing with the assist/control mode. As with assist/control, the mandatory positive pressure breaths can be of a pressure- or volume-targeted format. Typical volume-targeted synchronized intermittent mandatory ventilation (SIMV) is illustrated in Figure 12.7. A mandatory rate is set, and in between mandatory

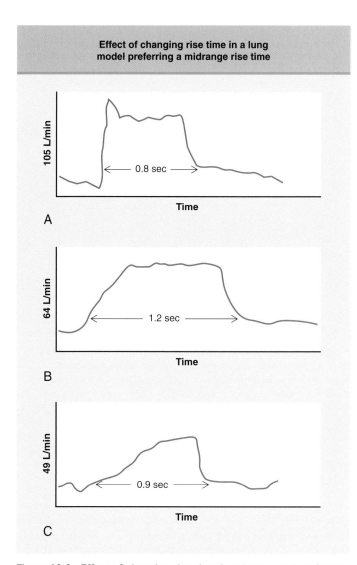

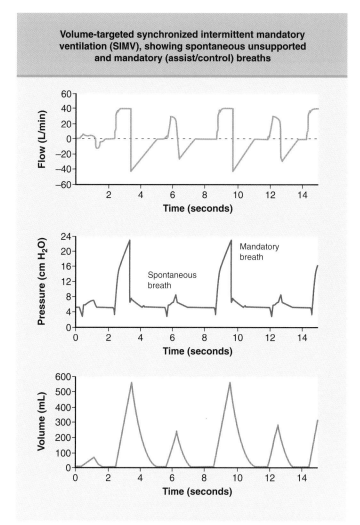

Figure 12.6. **Effect of changing rise time in a lung model preferring a midrange rise time.** *A,* Flow is in excess of demand, and a pressure spike is seen. *B,* As flow rate is decreased, inspiratory time (T₁) lengthens and the pressure spike is absent: Machine output matches demand. *C,* When flow rate is further reduced, demand exceeds machine flow rate and T₁ decreases. Deformation of the pressure waveform during the increase to the set pressure support ventilation level is also seen in *C.* (Data from Branson RD, Campbell RS: Pressure support ventilation, patient–ventilator synchrony, and ventilator algorithms. Respir Care 1998;43:1045.)

Figure 12.7. **Volume-targeted synchronized intermittent mandatory ventilation showing spontaneous unsupported and mandatory (assist/control) breaths.** (Data from Hess D, McIntyre NR, Mishoe SC, et al: Respiratory Care: Principles and Practice. Philadelphia, Saunders, 2002, p 786.)

breaths the patient can breathe spontaneously. An assist/control window is open at specific intervals based on the selected mandatory rate. Within each window, the patient is able to trigger a positive pressure breath; if the ventilator does not sense the patient's efforts during this time period, a control positive pressure breath is delivered. Ventilator adjustment is the same as with control mode except that the sensitivity must also be properly set.

Advocates of SIMV emphasize the benefits of spontaneous breathing between mandatory breaths. As shown in Figure 12.8, spontaneous breathing improves ventilation/perfusion matching (V̇/Q̇) because of better distribution of ventilation to dependent

lung. In addition, the negative intrathoracic pressure generated during spontaneous breaths decreases mean intrathoracic pressure, improving cardiac output. However, the work of breathing during SIMV can be excessive. As shown in Figure 12.9, as the mandatory rate decreases, the work of breathing for both mandatory and spontaneous breaths increases. The reason for this is that the respiratory center has difficulty rapidly changing outputs based on ventilatory mode as the mandatory rate decreases. Essentially, every breath is interpreted as the highest load requiring the higher output. This is illustrated in Figure 12.10. Note that the electromyogram activity of the diaphragm and the sternocleidomastoid muscles as well as the esophageal pressure changes is the same for mandatory and spontaneous breaths. In other words, patient effort is the same regardless of breath type, although the efficiency of gas delivery may be better during the mandatory breaths. Unfortunately, this set of circumstances increases ventilatory drive and increases the level of patient–ventilatory dyssynchrony.

Effect of spontaneous ventilation and positive-pressure ventilation on gas distribution in a supine subject

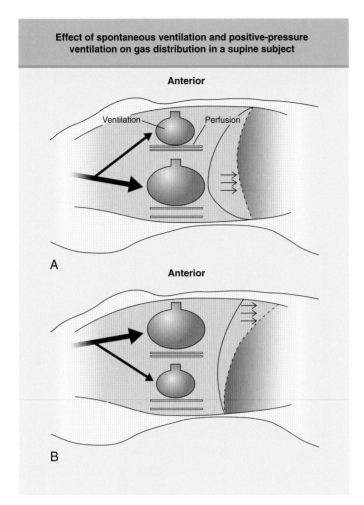

Figure 12.8. Effect of spontaneous ventilation and positive-pressure ventilation on gas distribution in a supine subject. During spontaneous ventilation *(A)*, diaphragmatic action distributes most ventilation to the dependent zones of the lungs, where perfusion is greatest. The result is good matching of ventilation to perfusion. During positive pressure ventilation *(B)*, because the diaphragm is doing little or no contraction, ventilation is primarily distributed to nondependent lung, increasing the level of ventilation-to-perfusion mismatch. (Data from Wilkens RL, Stoller JK, Scanlan CL: Egan's Fundamentals of Respiratory Care, 8th ed. St. Louis, Mosby, 2003, p 972.)

Inspiratory work per unit volume (work per liter, W/L) done by the patient during synchronized intermittent mandatory ventilation

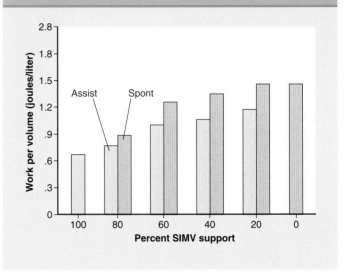

Figure 12.9. Inspiratory work per unit volume (work per liter, W/L) done by the patient during assisted cycles (green bars) and spontaneous cycles (purple bars) during synchronized intermittent mandatory ventilation. W/L increased with decreasing synchronized intermittent mandatory ventilation percentage for both types of breath. W/L for spontaneous breaths tended to exceed W/L for machine-assisted breaths. (Data from Marini JJ, Smith TC, Lamb VJ: External work output and force generation during synchronized intermittent mechanical ventilation. Am Rev Respir Dis 1988;138:1169.)

With most ventilators, pressure support can be applied during the spontaneous breaths; however, this negates the benefits of unassisted spontaneous breathing and increases the complexity of managing patients on ventilatory support and weaning patients from ventilatory support. In general, the lower the mandatory rate during SIMV, the greater the likelihood for patient effort to be excessive and dyssynchrony to be great.

Pressure-Regulated Volume Control

This mode of ventilatory support targets both a maximum airway pressure and a tidal volume and is a variation of pressure assist/control. It accomplishes both by varying the pressure applied on the subsequent breath based on the tidal volume achieved on the current breath. All ventilators that provide this mode of ventilation first deliver a test breath at a low level of pressure and, from the volume delivered, calculate the pressure

required to deliver the targeted tidal volume. The ventilator then automatically adjusts the pressure in one or two steps to the required pressure level needed to deliver the targeted tidal volume. During every subsequent breath, the tidal volume delivered is reassessed, and based on this assessment the pressure on the subsequent breath is adjusted 0 to 1+ cm H_2O to ensure that the targeted volume is delivered on the next breath. Pressure during pressure-regulated volume control (PRVC) can be increased to the maximum level selected and can be decreased with some ventilators to the continuous positive airway pressure (CPAP)/positive end-expiratory pressure (PEEP) level, allowing unassisted spontaneous breathing. The major concern with PRVC is that if a patient has a strong drive and the additional stimulus of hypoxemia, fever, sepsis, etc., the level of ventilatory support could decrease inappropriately to a very low level or no support. As a result, this mode should be applied cautiously in patients with a strong ventilatory drive. Adding a minimum pressure limit could result in a marked improvement in the operation of this mode—that is, setting a low pressure limit. As a result, this mode is most useful in patients essentially receiving control mode ventilation or those with limited ventilatory demand. All variables set during pressure assist/control are set during PRVC, with the addition of target tidal volume and maximum pressure limit.

Volume Support

Volume support essentially operates the same as PRVC but is based on a pressure support and not a pressure assist/control

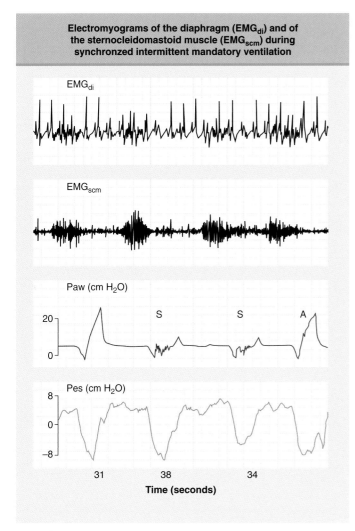

Figure 12.10. Electromyograms of the diaphragm (EMG$_{di}$) and of the sternocleidomastoid muscles (EMG$_{scm}$) in a representative patient, showing similar intensity and the duration of electrical activity in successive assisted (A) and spontaneous (S) breaths during synchronized intermittent mandatory ventilation. Esophageal pressure (Pes) changes are equal (equal effort) during A and S breaths. Paw, airway pressure. (Data from Imsand C, Feihl F, Perret C, Fitting JW: Regulation of inspiratory neuromuscular output during synchronized intermittent mechanical ventilation. Anesthesiology 1994;80:13–22.)

format. Ventilators go through the same assessment of pressure needed to deliver the tidal volume and provide breath-to-breath pressure adjustment to ensure targeted tidal volume is delivered. The same concern regarding a strong ventilatory demand exists with volume support as with PRVC, although some have recommended this mode as the weaning mode. The adjustments made to the ventilator during setup are the same as with pressure support except for the setting of a target volume and maximum pressure.

Adaptive Support Ventilation

This is a very unique new mode of ventilatory support that also operates on a pressure ventilation format. It attempts to adjust ventilator settings to ensure that an ideal ventilatory pattern is achieved. "Ideal" is defined as the pattern requiring the least

patient and ventilator work based on the patient's measured mechanical characteristics and breathing effort. The goal of adaptive support ventilation (ASV) is to provide a preset level of minute ventilation while minimizing the total work of breathing performed by the ventilator and the patient. ASV can be applied to patients requiring controlled ventilation and those actively breathing.

During setup, the clinician must indicate the patient's ideal body weight (IBW) and the percentage of minimal minute volume (% minimal MV) to be delivered. The % minimal MV can be adjusted between 25% and 350%. From the IBW and % minimal MV, the maximum rate is calculated as

$$22 \times \% \text{ min MV}/100 \text{ if IBW} > 15 \text{ kg or}$$

$$45 \times \% \text{ min MV}/100 \text{ if IBW} < 15 \text{ kg}$$

whereas maximum tidal volume delivered is the targeted MV/5. With this information, the ventilator determines the optimal breathing pattern that will minimize work of breathing—that is, a ventilatory pattern that results in minimum work based on the respiratory system mechanics of the patient.

With initial application of ASV, the ventilator provides a series of five pressure-limited test breaths at a rate of approximately 10/min with a maximum pressure of 15 cm H_2O. During these breaths, the ventilator measures dynamic compliance, the respiratory time constant, tidal volume, and patient rate. These measurements are used to determine the initial targets for breath rate and tidal volume. As ventilation continues, the ventilator recalculates these variables during each breath and determines new rate and tidal volume targets. Targets are based on the original work by Otis and colleagues (1950) that identified minimal ventilatory work.

Figure 12.11 illustrates the concept of ASV. In the center of the figure is the target tidal volume and rate, and around it are

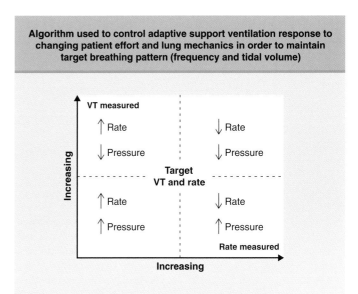

Figure 12.11. Algorithm used to control adaptive support ventilation response to changing patient effort and lung mechanics in order to maintain the target breathing pattern (frequency and tidal volume).

four quadrants identified by minimum rate and peak pressure increases or decreases. If a patient's ventilatory pattern falls into one of the four quadrants, a defined change in the frequency or pressure is initiated to move the ventilatory pattern back to the target.

This mode of ventilation is designed to ensure an ideal ventilatory pattern is maintained and can be used in all phases of ventilatory support. It continually adjusts ventilation as the patient status changes since it monitors patient lung mechanics on a breath-by-breath basis.

Automatic Tube Compensation

This mode of ventilation has been referred to as electronic extubation. Automatic tube compensation (ATC) is designed to provide sufficient ventilatory support during inspiration and sufficient decompression of the ventilatory circuit during expiration to maintain the tracheal pressure equal to baseline pressure.

The ventilator accomplishes this by having the resistance properties of all sizes of endotracheal and tracheostomy tubes programmed in its memory and continually measuring gas flow. From these data, the pressure needed to overcome resistance (resistance = change in pressure ÷ flow) of the endotracheal tube is continually calculated and applied.

Upon activation, the clinician must indicate the type and size of artificial airway and the percentage of automatic tube compensation desired (20%–100% on most ventilators). In addition, some ventilators only apply ACT during inspiration, whereas others apply it during both inspiration and expiration. The precise indications for ATC are not clear. Since this mode responds only to patient demand, if demand is low, ventilatory support is low. That is, if the patient generates a low inspiratory effort, little pressure is applied, whereas if the effort is great, the pressure is high (Fig. 12.12). ATC, like proportional assist ventilation (PAV), does not force a ventilatory pattern but is

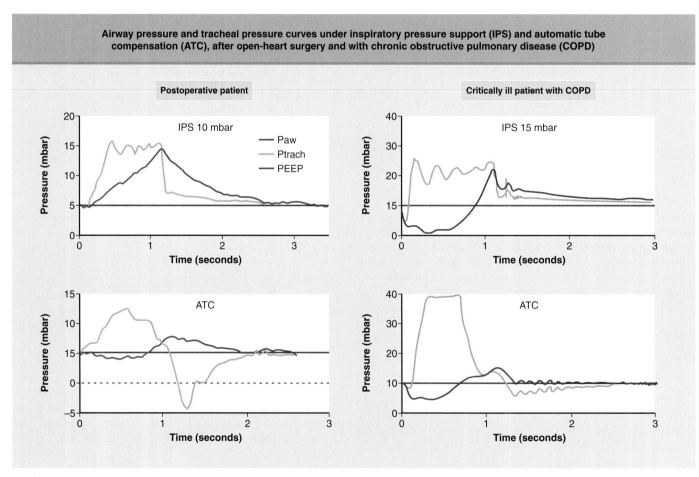

Figure 12.12. Airway pressure and tracheal pressure curves under inspiratory pressure support (IPS; top) and automatic tube compensation (ATC; bottom) in a patient after open-heart surgery (left) and a critically ill patient with chronic obstructive pulmonary disease (COPD; right). Although the ventilator decreases airway pressure (Paw) during expiration to subatmospheric pressure (bottom left), controlling the expiratory valve ensures that tracheal pressure (Ptrach) is above or equal to positive end-expiratory pressure (PEEP). The patient with acute respiratory insufficiency under ATC generates an inspiratory gas flow of > 2 L/sec (bottom right), which accounts for part of the deviation between Ptrach and PEEP. (Data from Fabry B, Haberthur C, Zappe D, et al: Breathing pattern and additional work of breathing in spontaneously breathing patients with different ventilatory demands during inspiratory pressure support and automatic tube compensation. Intensive Care Med 1997;23:545–552.)

designed only to unload the flow resistive properties of the artificial airway. The use of ATC has been recommended for those patients who are nearing readiness for liberation from mechanical ventilation. If the ATC pressure is stable at a low level (5–7 cm H_2O), extubation is indicated. ATC can also be used to determine the level of pressure support needed to satisfy patient demand. Note that in Figure 12.12 (right) a level of pressure support equal to the amount of ATC pressure would result in much lower effort by the patient and better patient–ventilator synchrony. Of note, postextubation upper airway resistance is frequently similar to the resistance imposed by the endotracheal tube. Therefore, some authors have questioned the use of ATC and other techniques to overcome airflow resistance during "weaning" since the mechanical load is likely to be similar following extubation.

The use of expiratory ATC does raise concerns in any patient with airways obstruction. The decompression of the airway during early exhalation may precipitate greater airways obstruction. As with many of these newer modes of ventilation, additional research is required before indications can be clearly defined.

Proportional Assist Ventilation

This mode of ventilation is similar to ATC but considers the mechanics of the total respiratory system plus the resistive properties of the artificial airway. That is, the ventilator delivers a pressure assist in proportion to the patient's desired tidal volume (volume assist) and instantaneous inspired flow (flow assist). The levels of these two aspects of ventilatory assist are automatically adjusted to meet changes in the patient's ongoing ventilatory demand. This adjustment works based on the law of motion applied to the respiratory system:

$$Pmus + Pappl = (volume \times E) + (flow \times R)$$

where Pmus is pressure generated by the respiratory muscles, Pappl is pressure applied by the ventilator, and E and R are elastic and resistance properties of the respiratory system, respectively. Assuming that R and E are linear during inspiration, the instantaneous flow and volume delivered are proportional to the resistive and elastic work of breathing, respectively. The ventilator measures the instantaneous flow and volume, whereas the clinician must measure and set values for E and R. Ideally, the ventilator should be able to measure on a breath-by-breath basis E and R and adjust gas delivery accordingly by estimating Pmus and assisting Pmus in a proportional manner. That is, the patient is the determinant of the ventilatory pattern. Patients have the freedom to select a ventilatory pattern that is rapid and shallow or slow and deep. The ventilator does not force any control variable except unloading of E and R in a proportional manner.

PAV is only useful in patients with a stable ventilatory drive who choose an acceptable ventilatory pattern. Of concern is the inability of most systems to reassess E and R on an ongoing basis. As a result, the level of unloading may not be appropriate if respiratory system mechanics are dynamically changing. A number of case series comparing the effects of PAV to those of pressure support have shown that PAV functions at least equivalently. However, PAV is not commercially available on ventilators in the United States.

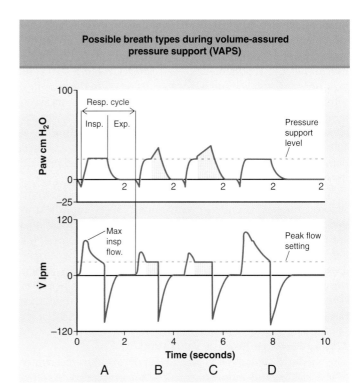

Figure 12.13. Possible breath types during volume-assured pressure support (VAPS). In breath A, the set tidal volume and delivered tidal volume are equal. This is a pressure-support breath (patient triggered, pressure limited, and flow cycled). Breath B represents a reduction in patient effort. As flow decelerates, the ventilator determines that delivered tidal volume will be less than the minimum set volume. In the shaded portion of the graph, the breath changes from a pressure—to a volume-limited (constant flow) breath. Breath C demonstrates a worsening of compliance and the possibility of extending inspiratory time to assure the minimum tidal volume delivery. Breath D represents a pressure support breath in which the tidal volume is greater than the set tidal volume. This kind of breath allowed during VAPS may aid in reducing work of breathing and dyspnea. (Data from Branson RD, David K: Dual control modes: Combining volume and pressure breaths. Respir Care Clin North Am 2001;7:397–408.)

Volume-Assured Pressure Support

Volume-assured pressure support (VAPS) is another within-breath adjustment mode of ventilatory support that is also referred to as pressure augmentation. These modes of ventilation are designed to combine the high initial flow of a pressure-limited breath with the constant volume delivery of a volume-targeted breath. Essentially, this mode adds flow at the beginning of the breath to meet the patient's demand for flow that exceeds the set peak flow. Similar to volume assist/control, the clinician sets a minimum tidal volume, a peak flow, and a pressure support level. The pressure support level should be sufficient to ensure tidal volume delivery, essentially equal to the plateau pressure needed to deliver the tidal volume with a volume-targeted breath. The peak flow should be set to ensure tidal volume is delivered in an appropriate inspiratory time. The basic control function of VAPS is illustrated in Figure 12.13. The delivered pressure and flow waveform vary based on the relationship between the tidal volume delivered and the minimum set tidal volume. If the two are equal, the breath is a typical pressure support breath. If the effort of the patient is minimized, the ventilator delivers a smaller volume at the set pressure support level, and when flow decreases to the peak flow setting the breath becomes a volume-targeted breath continuing until the minimum tidal volume is delivered. The lower the patient effort, the earlier in the breath is the change from pressure support to volume targeted. If the patient has a high demand, a volume greater than set will be delivered and the breath type remains a pressure-supported breath.

This mode differs considerably from PRVC and volume support since it maintains ventilatory support regardless of patient demand. This is a mode used to maintain ventilatory support, ensuring tidal volume and patient–ventilatory synchrony, and not to wean patients from it. Since the basic operation of VAPS is assist/control, it can be used with any patient for whom assist/control would be used, but it is most beneficial in those with varying ventilatory demand in whom a minimum target tidal volume is desired.

Airway Pressure Release Ventilation

This mode of ventilation is a combination of pressure-targeted SIMV and inverse ratio pressure control ventilation. As illustrated in Figure 12.14, airway pressure release ventilation (APRV) is essentially two levels of CPAP with spontaneous unassisted breathing allowed at each CPAP level. There are various approaches to setting APRV based on the belief that spontaneous breathing should be observed only during the high-level CPAP or during both levels of CPAP. If the clinician desires spontaneous breaths only at the high CPAP level, the time at the low level is very short, preventing complete exhalation; hence, there is an inverse ratio between high and low CPAP levels. In this setting, the high CPAP level is set to maintain oxygenation and the low level to assist ventilation by periodically decreasing lung volume.

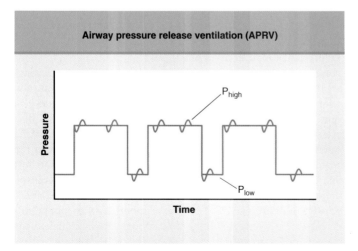

Figure 12.14. Airway pressure release ventilation (APRV). P_{high}, high continuous positive airway pressure (CPAP) level; P_{low}, low CPAP level. There are spontaneous breaths at both levels of CPAP. (Data from Kacmarek RM, Dimas S, Mack C: Essentials of Respiratory Care, 4th ed. St. Louis, Elsevier, 2005, p 713.)

The alternative approach is to set the low CPAP level to maintain oxygenation as if setting PEEP and the high level to provide a ventilatory assist as in SIMV. In this approach, the time at low CPAP is long enough to allow complete exhalation and spontaneous breathing at low CPAP levels. Proponents of APRV cite the benefits that spontaneous unsupported breathing has on ventilation–perfusion matching, cardiac output, and the need for sedation. However, as shown in Figure 12.15, the effort associated with spontaneous breathing under these conditions can result in very high esophageal pressure swings and high work of breathing, at least partially accounting for the greater cardiac output. In addition, dyssynchrony can be common with APRV. Dyssynchrony occurs at the mandatory transition from high to low or low to high CPAP levels. If the patient is exhaling when the ventilator increases pressure or inhaling when the pressure decreases, dyssynchrony results. This mode of ventilation has been most commonly used in the management of acute lung injury or acute respiratory distress syndrome (ARDS). However, it has not been shown to be more beneficial than the assist/control mode. Of concern is the fact that periodic release of airway pressure may allow collapse of unstable lung units in ARDS. This intermittent derecruitment of the lung may limit the ability to provide open lung protective ventilation, which many have advocated in ARDS. Thus, further work is clearly needed before APRV can be recommended.

Bilevel Pressure Ventilation

This is a modification of APRV. As shown in Figure 12.16, pressure support can be added to spontaneous breaths at the high or low CPAP level or both. This reduces the patient effort and esophageal pressure swings, but it also increases mean intrathoracic pressure, negating somewhat the increased cardiac output and beneficial ventilation to perfusion matching. In addition, the transition from high to low and low to high CPAP levels is coordinated with patient effort as in SIMV, markedly decreasing dyssynchrony. Like APRV, bilevel ventilation is used mostly in the management of acute lung injury and ARDS. Although the maintenance of spontaneous respiratory effort may help prevent lung collapse around the diaphragm, clinical trials showing beneficial effects on patient outcome are lacking.

SUMMARY

Very few data that identify the correct mode of ventilatory support for a given clinical setting exist. Our goal as clinicians applying these modes is to always select the approach to ventilatory support that allows us to meet our ventilatory targets and to ensure patient ventilatory synchrony. In addition, no data support the selection of a mode of ventilation to facilitate weaning from ventilatory support. The approach to weaning that minimizes time of ventilation is the spontaneous breathing trial, which can be performed from any mode of ventilatory support. During controlled ventilatory support, either volume-targeted or pressure-targeted modes can be used with equal efficacy. However, in the patient triggering the ventilator, patient–ventilator synchrony is clearly improved when pressure-targeted approaches to ventilatory support are used. Finally, it is the rare patient who cannot be appropriately managed with one of the classic modes of ventilatory support (control, assist/control, and pressure support).

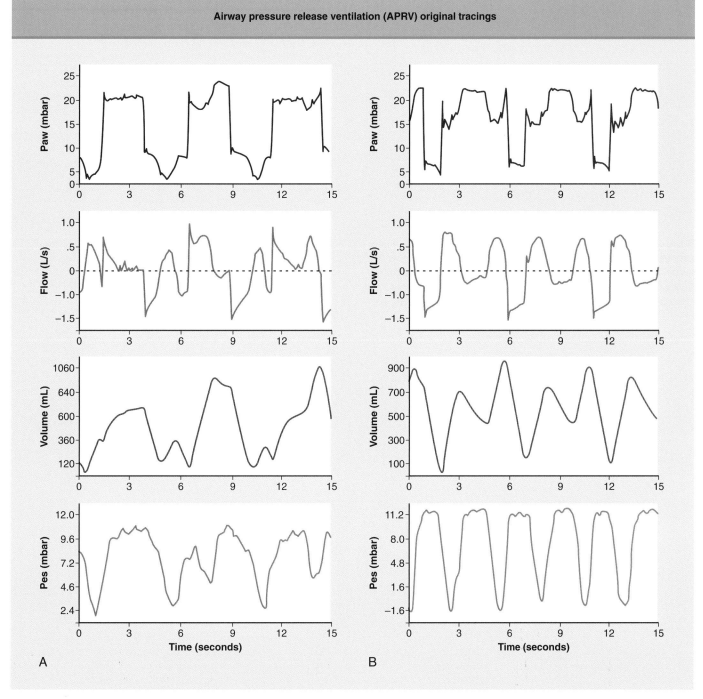

Figure 12.15. Airway pressure release ventilation original tracings. A synopsis of airway pressure (Paw), flow, volume, and esophageal pressure (Pes) is shown. *A,* Time intervals of the upper (P_{high}) and lower airway pressure (P_{low}) set to 2.5 seconds each, and *B,* time intervals of P_{high} = 4.0 seconds and P_{low} = 1.0 second in the same patient. Spontaneous breathing occurred on the upper and lower airway pressure in *A,* and tidal volumes varied considerably, depending on the pressure level from which an inspiration was started. When P_{low} was decreased to 1.0 second, as shown in *B,* spontaneous breaths occurred almost exclusively during P_{high}. This resulted in a more regular breathing pattern compared with *A.* Note, however, the large esophageal pressure swings (10–12 mbar or cm H_2O) per breath, indicating high patient effort on each spontaneous breath. Breaths were classified as follows: type A, spontaneous breath on the lower pressure level; type B, spontaneous breath on the upper pressure level; type C, the pressure increase from the lower to the upper pressure level triggered by an inspiratory effort of the patient; type D, mechanical breath; and type E, combined mechanical and spontaneous inspiration without a triggered pressure increase from P_{low} to P_{high}. (Data from Newman P, Golish W, Strohmeyer A: Influence of different release times on spontaneous breathing pattern during airway pressure release ventilation. Intensive Care Med 2002;28:1742.)

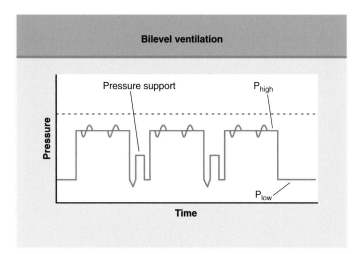

Figure 12.16. Bilevel ventilation. P$_{high}$, high continuous positive airway pressure (CPAP) level; P$_{low}$, low CPAP level. There are spontaneous breaths at both levels of CPAP, but in this case pressure support is applied to the breaths at P$_{low}$. Pressure support could also be applied to P$_{high}$. (Data from Kacmarek RM, Dimas S, Mack C: Essentials of Respiratory Care, 4th ed. St. Louis, Elsevier, 2005, p 714.)

SUGGESTED READING

Bransson RD, Davis K: Dual control modes: Combining volume and pressure breaths. Respir Care Clin North Am 2001;7:397–408.

Campbell RS, Branson RD, Johannigman JA: Adaptive support ventilation. Respir Care Clin North Am 2001;7:425–440.

Fabry B, Haberthur C, Zappe D, et al: Breathing pattern and additional work of breathing in spontaneously breathing patients with different ventilatory demands during inspiratory pressure support and automatic tube compensation. Intensive Care Med 1997;23:545–552.

Grasso S, Ranieri VM: Proportional assist ventilation. Respir Care Clin North Am 2001;7:465–474.

Hess D, Kacmarek RM: Essentials of Mechanical Ventilation, 2nd ed. New York, McGraw-Hill, 2002.

Kacmarek RM, Dimas S, Mack C: Essentials of Respiratory Care, 4th ed. St. Louis, Mosby, 2005.

Marini JJ, Wheeler AP: Critical Care Medicine: The Essentials. Baltimore, Williams & Wilkins, 1997.

Otis AB, Fenn WO, Rahn H: Mechanics of breathing in man. J Appl Physiol 1950;2:592–607.

Putensen C, Zech S, Wrigge H, et al: Long term effects of spontaneous breathing during ventilatory support in patients with acute lung injury. Am J Respir Crit Care Med 2001;164:43–49.

Tobin MJ: Principles and Practice of Mechanical Ventilation. New York, McGraw-Hill, 1994.

Chapter 13

Noninvasive Ventilation

B. Cabello and Jordi Mancebo

Noninvasive ventilation (NIV) for acute respiratory failure has been widely used in the intensive care unit (ICU), in the pneumology ward, and in the emergency department for the past two decades. There are several reasons to justify the increasing use of NIV. First, a number of studies have demonstrated the efficacy of this technique in various diseases and shown that com-plications related to invasive ventilation, such as pulmonary and nonpulmonary infections, can be markedly decreased. Furthermore, the clinical knowledge and experience of physicians and nurses has increased considerably, while at the same time interfaces are undergoing notable improvements and new devices are constantly appearing on the market.

During the past few years, new indications for the use of NIV and new devices for its application have been studied: ICU ventilators, domiciliary ventilators, masks with high-flow continuous positive airway pressure (CPAP), and, recently, a helmet interface. NIV has also been studied applying nonconventional gas mixtures, such as helium plus oxygen (heliox).

PRINCIPLES OF USE OF NIV

NIV for Acute Hypercapnic Respiratory Failure

Acute hypercapnic respiratory failure in chronic obstructive pulmonary disease (COPD) patients ensues after a period of rapid shallow breathing increasing dead space-to-tidal volume ratio, with consequent hypoventilation and respiratory acidosis. In these patients, the high respiratory center stimulation together with large negative intrathoracic pressure swings generated by the respiratory muscles are insufficient to generate adequate tidal volume. The rapid shallow breathing facilitates a further increase in pulmonary hyperinflation, which in turn jeopardizes respiratory muscle length–tension relationships. All these disturbances contribute to generate a vicious circle consisting of progressive hypercapnia and acidosis.

The increase in respiratory muscle effort may lead to respiratory pump failure and eventually to respiratory arrest. Mechanical ventilation is necessary for the respiratory muscles to rest until the cause of exacerbation is resolved. The combination of pressure support (increasing tidal volume with the same inspiratory effort) and positive end-expiratory pressure (PEEP) (helping to counterbalance the auto-PEEP) reduces the patient's effort to breathe and markedly modifies the breathing pattern. The increase in tidal volume and the decrease in respiratory rate improve alveolar ventilation, thus helping to decrease PCO_2.

In 1995, Brochard and colleagues published a prospective, randomized multicenter trial on the use of NIV as treatment in exacerbation of COPD patients admitted to an ICU. In this trial, 85 patients were enrolled; 43 patients were assigned to NIV and 42 to standard treatment. The rate of intubation was 11/43 (26%) in the NIV group and 31/42 (74%) in the standard group ($P < 0.001$). The frequency of complications was lower in the NIV group: 16% vs. 48% ($P = 0.001$). The mean hospital stay was shorter in patients with NIV: 23 ± 17 vs. 35 ± 33 days ($P = 0.005$). The in-hospital mortality rate was lower in patients with NIV: 4/43 (9%) vs. 12/42 (29%) ($P = 0.02$). They concluded that noninvasive ventilation could reduce the need for endotracheal intubation, the length of hospital stay, and the in-hospital mortality rate. It is important to emphasize that most patients who were enrolled in the protocol belonged to a select COPD population, which included only 31% of total patients with COPD.

Kramer and coworkers performed a randomized, prospective study to evaluate the possible benefits of NIV vs. standard therapy in patients with acute respiratory failure (ARF). The inclusion criteria were respiratory distress, evidenced by moderate to severe dyspnea, accessory muscle use, or abdominal paradox, and ARF, evidenced by pH less than 7.35, $PaCO_2$ greater than 45 mm Hg, and respiratory rate greater than 24 breaths/min. Severely unstable patients were excluded. A nasal mask was used in all patients. The primary outcome was the need for intubation. Secondary outcome measures included heart rate, arterial blood gases in spontaneous breathing, oxygen supplementation in semirecumbent patients, and self-assessment of dyspnea. Other secondary outcomes were duration of ventilator use, length of hospital stay, and mortality. The need for intubation was reduced from 73% in the standard therapy group (11 of 15 patients) to 31% in the NIV group (5 of 16 patients, $P < 0.05$). The reduction was even more striking in COPD patients, with 8 of 12 (67%) control patients requiring intubation compared with 1 of 11 (9%) NIV patients ($P < 0.05$). Heart and respiratory rates were significantly lower within 1 hour in the NIV group than in control patients. PaO_2 improved significantly in the NIV group in the first 6 hours. Dyspnea scores were better in the NIV than in control patients at 6 hours, and nurses and therapists spent similar amounts of time at the bedside for both groups. During the first 8 hours, respiratory therapists spent more time with the patients treated with NIV, but the difference was not statistically significant. In the second 8-hour period, a significant decrease in the amount of time that respiratory therapists spent with these patients was observed. The NIV did not significantly reduce duration of ventilator use, length of hospital stay, or mortality in comparison with standard therapy. The authors concluded that NIV reduces the need for intubation in patients with ARF who are stable, particularly COPD patients.

Plant and colleagues published the first prospective multicenter, randomized controlled study comparing NIV with standard therapy in medical wards outside the ICU environment. They enrolled 118 patients in each arm and the primary endpoint was "need for intubation." They excluded patients with a pH below 7.25, and the majority of the staff working in the wards (22/25) where the patients were treated had no experience in NIV. Some teaching in NIV, however, was given prior to the study. The median nurse:patient ratio was 1:11. The authors concluded that early use of NIV in COPD patients in the general ward leads to a faster improvement in physiologic variables (respiratory acidosis and respiratory rate). A decrease in the need for intubation, 32/118 (27%) in the standard group compared with 18/118 (15%) in the NIV group ($P = 0.02$), was observed. The in-hospital mortality was higher in the standard group: 24/118 (20%) compared with 12/118 (10%) in the NIV group ($P = 0.05$).

Attempts have been made to determine indicators of NIV success, and most studies have concluded that a lower baseline pH and the severity of underlying disease as evaluated with SAPS II or APACHE scores are predictors of NIV failure. The pH improvement (pH rising) in the first hours with NIV is a success predictor. Applying these factors, which may predict failure, can be helpful when deciding whether the patient should be transferred to a medical ward or to the ICU, thereby avoiding an unnecessary delay in endotracheal intubation.

NIV in Cardiogenic Pulmonary Edema

Congestive heart failure is a common cause of ARF. These patients usually have rapid clinical improvement with medical treatment, but in some cases they need mechanical ventilation. CPAP has been used to treat cardiogenic pulmonary edema, with several studies supporting its use (Figs. 13.1 and 13.2).

CPAP in cardiogenic pulmonary edema patients improves oxygenation as it increases functional residual capacity. In this scenario, favorable CPAP hemodynamic effects are decreases in right ventricular (RV) preload, which may increase RV afterload, decreases in left ventricular (LV) preload, decreases in LV transmural pressure, and decreases in LV afterload, thus improving overall cardiac performance. Patients with left heart failure present orthopnea. This is thought to reflect perivascular, peribronchiolar, and interstitial edemas, which compress airways and stimulate lung receptors, possibly provoking reflex bronchoconstriction.

Lenique and associates studied the effects of CPAP in patients with an acute exacerbation of chronic left heart failure. When they compared spontaneous breathing to CPAP 10 cm H_2O, they observed improvement in lung compliance, significant decreases in both the elastic and the resistive components of work of breathing, and significant reductions in inspiratory muscle effort during CPAP. Arterial PaO_2 significantly improved and breathing pattern remained essentially unchanged. Transmural filling pressures decreased with CPAP, which was interpreted as better cardiac performance.

Mehta and associates performed a randomized, controlled, double-blind trial to evaluate whether bilevel positive airway pressure vs. CPAP in patients with acute pulmonary edema improved ventilation, acidemia, and dyspnea. The study was carried out in the emergency department. Thirteen patients were randomized to the CPAP group and 14 received nasal bilevel positive airway pressure. After 30 minutes, significant reductions in breathing frequency, heart rate, blood pressure, and $PaCO_2$ were observed in the bilevel positive airway pressure group, as were significant improvements in arterial pH and dyspnea scores ($P < 0.05$ for all). Only breathing frequency improved significantly in the CPAP group (from 32 ± 4 to 28 ± 5 breaths/min, $P < 0.05$). At 30 minutes, the bilevel positive airway pressure group had greater reductions in $PaCO_2$ ($P = 0.057$), systolic blood pressure ($P = 0.005$), and mean arterial pressure ($P = 0.03$) than the CPAP group. Duration of ventilator use, ICU and hospital stays, and intubation and mortality rates were similar for the two groups. However, the myocardial infarction rate was higher in the bilevel positive airway pressure group (71%) compared to both the CPAP group (31%) and historically matched controls (38%) ($P = 0.05$). There were some marked differences in randomization. At the time of study entry, 10 bilevel positive airway pressure patients and 4 CPAP patients

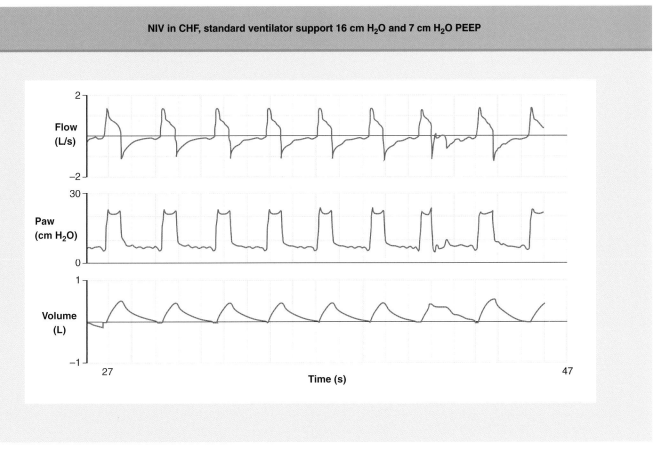

NIV in CHF, standard ventilator support 16 cm H₂O and 7 cm H₂O PEEP

Figure 13.1. Tracings of airflow (flow), airway pressure (Paw), and tidal volume. These tracings were obtained in a patient with congestive heart failure who was treated with NIV delivered via a standard ICU ventilator set at pressure support of 16 cm H_2O and 7 cm H_2O PEEP. The tidal volume was approximately 450 mL with a respiratory rate of 24 breaths per minute.

had chest pain ($P = 0.06$). Also in the NIV group, left bundle branch blocks were more common in the bilevel positive airway pressure group. This bias in randomization may be the cause of the higher incidence of the myocardial infarction in the group treated with NIV.

Masip and colleagues (2000) published the first randomized, prospective study using NIV for acute cardiogenic pulmonary edema. They compared patients with medical treatment plus oxygen versus medical treatment and NIV; the outcomes were intubation rate and resolution time, defined as clinical improvement with oxygen saturation of 96% or more and a respiratory rate less than 30 breaths/min. Thirty-seven patients were studied. Endotracheal intubation was required in 1/19 patients (5%) of the NIV group and in 6/18 (33%) of the conventional group ($P = 0.0037$). Resolution time was shorter in the NIV group: median, 105 hours vs. 30 minutes ($P = 0.002$). The authors concluded that NIV shortened the resolution time of acute cardiogenic pulmonary edema in comparison with oxygen therapy and decreased the intubation rate. No effect was found in terms of length of stay or mortality. They attributed this to the small size of the sample and did not find any significant difference in terms of acute myocardial infarction, such as the cause of acute pulmonary edema in the two groups: 6/18 patients (33%) in the NIV group vs. 5/19 patients (26%) in the NIV group.

A randomized, prospective, multicenter study by Nava and associates performed in an emergency department analyzed the role of NIV in cardiogenic pulmonary edema (CPE). One group was treated with medical treatment plus oxygen (control group) and the other with medical treatment plus NIV. Sixty-five patients were enrolled in each arm. The primary endpoint was need for intubation, and secondary endpoints were in-hospital mortality and changes in some physiological variables. The subgroups of patients with and without hypercapnia were analyzed separately. The authors thought these patients were more likely to benefit from the application of noninvasive pressure support. Patients with a $PaCO_2$ above or below 45 mm Hg were equally distributed between the two groups. Intubation was performed in 16/65 patients (25%) in the control group vs. 13/65 (20%) in the NIV group ($P = 0.530$). Mortality rate was 9/65 (14%) in the control group vs. 6/65 (8%) in the NIV group ($P = 0.410$). In the subgroup of patients with $PaCO_2$ above 45 mm Hg, the rate of intubation was 9/31 (29%) vs. 2/33 (6%) ($P = 0.015$). The logistic regression analysis did not confirm that a $PaCO_2$ level above 45 mm Hg was, per se, a determinant of intubation; they considered this could be due to the small size of the two subgroups of patients. There were no differences in total hospital stay, occurrence of a new acute myocardial infarction, or infectious and noninfectious complications. They concluded that NIV for treatment of CPE compared with

123

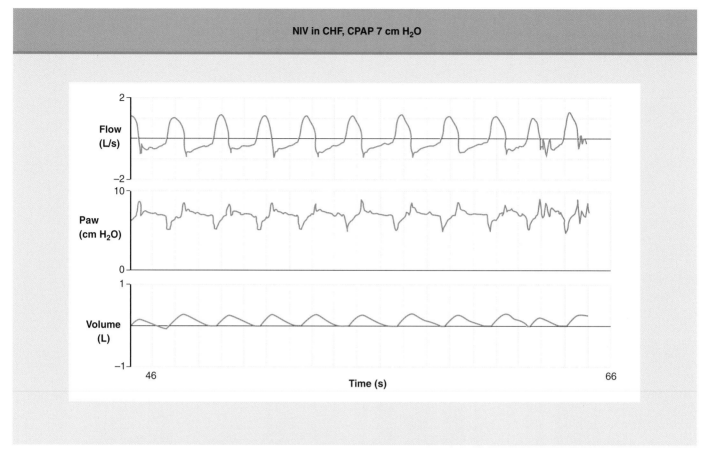

Figure 13.2. Tracings of airflow (flow), airway pressure (Paw), and tidal volume. These tracings were obtained in the same patient as in Figure 13.1 with CPAP 7 cm H_2O and the same ventilator. Tidal volume decreased to 266 mL and the respiratory rate increased up to 30 breaths per minute.

standard therapy produces faster gas exchange and dyspnea and respiratory rate improvements, but it does not affect survival or rate of intubation. The subgroup analysis showed that the need to intubate hypercapnic patients might be reduced by the use of NIV. They believed that the lack of a greater benefit in the NIV group could be related to the limited experience that most of the participating centers had in this study in terms of technique.

Patients with acute cardiogenic pulmonary edema may benefit from NIV. What is not clear is whether there are any differences between CPAP and NIV. The best time to initiate NIV treatment is as early as possible, at the same time as medical treatment. The ideal situation is a scenario in which caregivers are well prepared and skilled in the use of NIV. It is conceivable that hemodynamically unstable patients are not good candidates for NIV.

NIV for Acute Hypoxemic Respiratory Failure

Hypoxemic failure can be due to several underlying pathologies, such as acute lung injury, pneumonia, and CPE. CPAP in these pathologies may be useful because it increases functional residual capacity, improving the respiratory mechanics and gas exchange. The beneficial effects of PEEP in the redistribution of extravascular fluid, on alveolar recruitment, and in avoiding development of atelectasis can contribute to better oxygenation.

Pressure support can be effective in terms of decreasing the work of breathing.

Delclaux and associates (2000) studied the use of CPAP for the treatment of acute hypoxemic nonhypercapnic respiratory insufficiency. They compared CPAP vs. standard oxygen therapy. The main outcomes were improvement in oxygenation, rate of endotracheal intubation, adverse events, length of hospital stay, mortality, and duration of ventilatory assistance. No significant differences were found between the two groups for any of the clinical outcomes studied. After 1 hour of treatment, subjective response to treatment and median PaO_2/FIO_2 ratio were better with CPAP (203 vs. 151 mm Hg, $P = 0.002$). No differences in the rate of intubation were found in the CPAP group vs. the standard group [21/62 (34%) vs. 24/61 (39%), respectively]. The SAPS II scoring, an absence of cardiac disease, and PaO_2/FIO_2 ratio less than 200 mm Hg at 1 hour of treatment were independently associated with endotracheal intubation. A higher number of adverse events (cardiac arrest, gastric distention, nosocomial pneumonia, stress ulcer, pneumothorax, sinusitis, and facial skin necrosis) occurred with CPAP treatment (18 vs. 6, $P = 0.01$).

Antonelli and colleagues (1998) performed a randomized prospective trial to compare the role of NIV as an alternative to conventional mechanical ventilation with endotracheal intubation in patients with acute respiratory failure. The primary endpoints were the values for gas exchange and the frequency of mechanical ventilation complications, such as pneumonia, sepsis, and sinusitis. The secondary endpoints were survival, the duration of mechanical ventilation, and the duration of ICU stay. The baseline characteristics of the two groups were similar, except that in the conventional group (intubated patients) the mean arterial pH was significantly lower (7.37 vs. 7.45, $P = 0.002$) with an increase in PCO_2. They found the same short-term improvement in gas exchange with conventional ventilation [20/32 (62%)] and NIV [15/32 (47%)] ($P = 0.21$) in patients with acute hypoxemic respiratory failure. A decrease in the rate of complications related to intubation for the NIV group was observed (pneumonia and sinusitis) (31 vs. 3%, $P = 0.003$). Patients who did not require intubation after treatment with NIV had shorter stays in the ICU. They concluded that NIV was equally effective at improving gas exchange, and when endotracheal intubation was avoided ventilator-associated pneumonia was unlikely. They did not include patients receiving immunosuppressive therapy.

Antonelli and colleagues performed another investigation on immunocompromised patients (solid organ transplant recipients) who developed acute hypoxemic respiratory failure. They compared the NIV treatment vs. standard treatment. The primary outcome was the need for endotracheal intubation and mechanical ventilation. Secondary endpoints were complications not present on admission, duration of ventilatory assistance, length of hospital stay, and ICU mortality. Forty patients were enrolled, 20 in each group, with similar baseline characteristics. In the first hour of treatment, PaO_2/FIO_2 improved in 14/20 patients in the NIV group (70%) and 5/20 (25%) in the standard group. Over time, a sustained improvement in PaO_2/FIO_2 was noted in 12/20 (60%) in the NIV group vs. 5/20 (25%) in the standard group ($P = 0.002$). NIV was associated with a reduction in the rate of intubation (20 vs. 70%, $P = 0.002$), length of stay in the ICU (median days, 5.5 vs. 9, $P = 0.03$), and intensive care mortality (20 vs. 50%, $P = 0.05$). There was no difference in hospital mortality: 7/20 (35%) in the NIV group vs. 11/20 (55%) in the standard treatment group. Intubation was avoided in the subgroup of patients randomized to NIV with the diagnosis of pulmonary edema or pulmonary embolism (6 patients), whereas 5 of the 6 patients (83%) with the same diagnosis randomized to standard treatment required intubation ($P = 0.01$). The conclusion was that NIV should be considered in transplant recipients who develop acute hypoxemic respiratory failure.

In a prospective, randomized trial, Hilbert and coworkers (2001) compared intermittent NIV with standard treatment (oxygen therapy) in immunosuppressed patients. Patients were enrolled if they had pulmonary infiltrates, fever, and an early stage of hypoxemic ARF. They excluded patients with respiratory acidosis and a PaO_2/FIO_2 below 85 mm Hg; such patients were intubated. They hypothesized that intermittent use of NIV at an early stage of hypoxemic acute failure would reduce the need for endotracheal intubation and the incidence of complications. The primary outcome was the need for endotracheal intubation and mechanical ventilation at any time during the study. Secondary outcomes included the development of complications not present at admission, the length of stay in the ICU, the duration of ventilatory assistance, and death in the ICU or the hospital. All NIV patients showed significantly lower rates of endotracheal intubation (12/26 vs. 20/26, $P = 0.03$), serious complications (13/26 vs. 21/26, $P = 0.02$), death in the ICU (10/26 vs. 18/26, $P = 0.03$), and death in the hospital (13/26 vs. 21/26, $P = 0.02$).

Ferrer and associates studied the use of NIV to avoid intubation in patients with hypoxemic nonhypercapnic respiratory failure. They enrolled 51 patients in the NIV group and 54 in the oxygen therapy group. The primary endpoint was whether or not the use of NIV would prevent intubation. The intubation rate was 13/51 (25%) in the NIV group vs. 28/54 (52%) in the control group ($P = 0.01$). The incidence of septic shock was 12% vs. 31% ($P = 0.028$). The intensive care mortality was 9/51 (18%) in the NIV group vs. 21/54 (39%) in the control group ($P = 0.028$). There was a nonsignificant trend to decrease the incidence of hospital-acquired pneumonia in the NIV group. Multivariate analysis showed that NIV and pulmonary edema were independently associated with a decreased risk of intubation, and acute respiratory distress syndrome (ARDS) was independently associated with an increased risk of intubation. They concluded that the use of NIV prevented intubation in patients with hypoxemic respiratory failure, reduced the incidence of septic shock, and improved survival compared to patients receiving high-concentration oxygen therapy.

Most studies cited previously had heterogeneous populations with wide variability in the causes of hypoxemic respiratory failure. NIV may possibly avoid intubation while the underlying disease causing the hypoxia is being treated. Frequent causes of mortality in patients with acute hypoxemic failure are septic shock and multiple organ failure; they are closely related to invasive mechanical ventilation. This is especially relevant for immunocompromised patients because of their high mortality when they are intubated and placed on mechanical ventilation. On the other hand, delaying endotracheal intubation and using NIV instead may increase the possibility of respiratory and/or cardiac arrest in some patients.

A study on NIV failure predictors reported the following parameters as independent risk factors in hypoxemic ARF: age older than 40 years, SAPS II greater than 35, the presence of ARDS and community-acquired pneumonia, and PaO_2/FIO_2 less than 146 after 1 hour of NIV. It was concluded that use of NIV in acute hypoxemic respiratory failure could be useful in select populations. Risk of failure is higher in patients with a higher severity score, older age, ARDS or pneumonia, or failure to improve after 1 hour of treatment.

NIV and Pneumonia

The role of NIV in pneumonia has been analyzed with different results. COPD patients have the best outcomes. NIV may be useful because it helps to maintain oxygenation, decreasing the work of breathing while the antibiotic is effectively treating the underlying disease.

Confalioneri and associates designed the first prospective, randomized study comparing standard treatment plus NIV delivered through a face mask to standard treatment alone in patients with severe community-acquired pneumonia and ARF. Fifty-six patients (28 in each arm) were enrolled, and the two groups had similar baseline characteristics at inclusion. They observed a significant reduction in respiratory rate, need for endotracheal intubation [23/56 (21%) vs. 17/56 (50%), $P = 0.03$], and duration of ICU stay (1.8 ± 0.7 vs. 6 ± 1.8 days,

$P = 0.04$). The subgroup of patients with COPD and randomized to NIV had a lower intensity of nursing care workload ($P = 0.04$) and improved 2-month survival (88.9 vs. 37.5%, $P = 0.05$). They concluded that in selected patients with ARF caused by severe community-acquired pneumonia, the use of NIV was associated with a significant reduction in the rate of endotracheal intubation and duration of ICU stay.

Girou and colleagues (2000) performed a retrospective matched case–control study to compare outcomes in patients treated with NIV vs. invasive ventilation. The main outcomes were rates of nosocomial infections, antibiotic use, duration of ventilatory support, ICU stay, and ICU mortality. The population was COPD patients with acute exacerbation and CPE. They excluded patients with metastatic cancer, hematology malignancy with a poor short-term prognosis, and acute lung injury. Fifty were case patients and 50 were controls. All but two patients with CPE were hypercapnic on admission. Rates of nosocomial infections and nosocomial pneumonia were significantly lower in patients treated with NIV than in those treated with mechanical ventilation (18 vs. 60% and 8 vs. 26%; $P < 0.001$ and $P = 0.04$, respectively). The risk of acquiring an infection and the proportion of patients receiving antibiotics for nosocomial infections were also lower in the NIV group. ICU mortality was significantly lower in patients treated with NIV [2/50 (46%) vs. 13/50 (26%) in NIV patients]. Duration of ICU stay and ventilation were also shorter in NIV patients. It was concluded that use of NIV vs. mechanical ventilation is associated with a lower risk of nosocomial infections, less antibiotic use, shorter length of ICU stay, and lower mortality.

Jolliet and colleagues studied three aspects of NIV in ARF patients due to severe community-acquired pneumonia: the initial effect on respiratory rate, gas exchange, and hemodynamics; the clinical course and outcome during ICU and hospital stay; and the nursing workload as measured by the daily PRN 87 (Project Research in Nursing) score. Twenty-four patients were included. During the initial NIV trial, respiratory rate decreased from 34 ± 8 to 28 ± 10 breaths/min ($P < 0.001$) and PaO_2/FIO_2 improved from 104 ± 48 to 153 ± 49 ($P < 0.001$), whereas $PaCO_2$ remained unchanged. A total of 133 NIV trials were performed (median duration, 55 min; range, 30–540 min) over 1 ± 7 days. No complications occurred during NIV. Sixteen patients (66%) were intubated after inclusion. The patients who were subsequently intubated were older (55 ± 15 vs. 37 ± 12 years) and more severely hypoxemic (63 ± 11 vs. 80 ± 15 mm Hg; $P < 0.05$) than those not requiring intubation. Eight patients (33%) died, all in the intubated group. Median lengths of stay in the ICU and hospital were longer in intubated patients [ICU: 16 days (range, 3–64) vs. 6 days (range, 3–7), $P < 0.05$; hospital: 23 days (range, 9–77) vs. 9.5 days (range, 4–42), $P < 0.05$). PRN score was higher during the first 24 hours following intubation than during the first 24 hours of NIV (278 ± 55 vs. 228 ± 24 points, $P < 0.05$). The authors concluded that the intubation rate in patients with ARF due to severe community-acquired pneumonia is higher. The favorable outcome and shorter ICU and hospital stays when intubation is avoided warrant further studies in this population.

NIV during Liberation from Mechanical Ventilation

Several studies have evaluated the role of NIV during liberation from mechanical ventilation. In a prospective randomized trial,

Nava et al. found that patients with COPD who failed an initial spontaneous breathing test (SBT) and who were extubated and treated with NIV were liberated from ventilators more quickly (10.2 vs. 16.6 days, $P = 0.021$), spent less time in the ICU (15.1 vs. 24 days, $P = 0.021$), and were more likely to survive (92 vs. 72%, $P = 0.009$) than patients weaned by pressure support (PS) ventilation via the endotracheal tube. At 60 days, 88% of patients ventilated noninvasively were successfully weaned compared with 68% of patients ventilated invasively.

In another investigation, Girault and coworkers prospectively studied 33 COPD patients who failed a 2-hour T-piece trial. Sixteen patients were randomly assigned to conventional invasive PS weaning and 17 were randomly assigned to be weaned by noninvasive PS immediately after extubation. Although weaning with noninvasive PS significantly reduced the total duration of invasive mechanical ventilation and the probability of remaining intubated and mechanically ventilated compared to conventional PS, the total duration of ventilatory support related to weaning was greater in the noninvasive PS group. The lengths of ICU and hospital stay and the mortality rate at 3 months were similar for both groups. Differences with respect to Nava and colleagues's study may be due to differences in the severity of the disease, the selection of patients when deciding the moment for extubation, the settings in PS, and the experience of both teams in delivering PS.

The usefulness of NIV to facilitate early extubation has been reanalyzed in a randomized multicenter trial. This study was conducted on 43 mechanically ventilated patients with persistent weaning failure. A group of patients ($n = 21$) was extubated and received noninvasive ventilation with pressure support and a full-face mask. The other group ($n = 22$) remained intubated and followed a usual weaning strategy with daily SBT. Main results of this investigation were a shorter period of invasive ventilation, shorter ICU and hospital length of stay, and increased ICU and 90-day survival in patients extubated early and subsequently treated with NIV compared to the control group. This study, performed in a nonselected population of ICU patients who had criteria to proceed with weaning attempts, suggests that early use of NIV may be effective in skilled hands. Another interpretation, however, is that criteria to decide the failure of SBT were too strict and physicians were overzealous in interpreting clinical intolerance, or that some type of bias existed due to the unblinded nature of the study, and thus these patients remained under invasive mechanical ventilation for an unduly prolonged period of time.

Keenan and associates compared the use of NIV versus standard medical therapy (supplemental oxygen) in preventing the need for endotracheal reintubation in high-risk patients (cardiac or respiratory disease or who had required at least 2 days of ventilatory support) who developed respiratory distress during the first 48 hours after extubation. The main outcomes were rate of reintubation, duration of mechanical ventilation, lengths of ICU and hospital stay, and hospital mortality. Forty-two patients were randomized to the standard treatment group and 38 to the NIV group. There was no difference between the rates of reintubation (72% vs. 69%; relative risk, 1.04; 95% confidence interval, 0.78–1.38). No differences were found in hospital survival (31% for both groups). Neither were significant differences found in the ICU or hospital length of stay. They concluded that the addition of NIV to standard medical therapy does not improve outcome in a heterogeneous group of patients who develop respiratory distress during the first 48 hours after extubation.

Other Indications of NIV

There are studies using NIV during fiberoptic bronchoscopy (FOB) in hypoxemic respiratory failure in which avoidance of intubation is desirable. In a prospective randomized trial, Maitre and coworkers compared the delivery of CPAP as a technique for maintaining oxygenation during FOB vs. the delivery of oxygen only. They included 30 consecutive patients who needed FOB for diagnostic purposes with a PaO_2/FIO_2 ratio below 300 mm Hg. CPAP was delivered with a constant flow oxygen insufflation device open to atmosphere. During FOB and the 30 minutes after the technique, pulse oximetry (SpO_2) values were significantly higher in the CPAP group than in the oxygen group (95.7 vs. 92.6%, $P = 0.02$). In the latter group, 5 patients developed respiratory failure in the 6 hours after FOB requiring ventilatory assistance vs. no patients in the CPAP group ($P = 0.03$). The authors concluded that in hypoxemic patients, the use of a new CPAP device during FOB allowed minimal alterations in gas exchange and prevented respiratory failure after the use of this technique.

Antonelli and colleagues studied the efficacy of NIV as a technique to assist spontaneous breathing during FOB in hypoxemic patients with a PaO_2/FIO_2 ratio less than 200. Twenty-six patients with suspected pneumonia were enrolled. Thirteen patients were randomized to receive NIV during the FOB and 13 to receive conventional oxygen supplementation. The primary endpoints were changes in the PaO_2/FIO_2 ratio during FOB and within 60 minutes after the bronchoalveolar lavage. The mean PaO_2/FIO_2 ratio increased by 82% in the NIV group (261 ± 100 vs. 139 ± 38, $P < 0.001$) and decreased by 10% in the conventional oxygen supplementation group (155 ± 24 to 139 ± 38, $P = 0.23$). Sixty minutes after FOB, the NIV group had a higher mean PaO_2/FIO_2 ratio (176 ± 62 vs. 140 ± 38, $P = 0.09$) and a lower mean heart rate (91 ± 18 vs. 108 ± 15 beats/min, $P = 0.02$). No significant reduction in mean arterial pressure in comparison to controls was observed. One patient in the NPPV group and two patients in the control group were intubated. The authors concluded that in patients with severe hypoxemia, NIV is superior to oxygen supplementation in preventing hypoxemia during FOB with better hemodynamic tolerance.

NIV during acute asthma has been poorly studied. Meduri and associates reported their experience with NIV in 17 patients with acute asthma over a 3-year period. They initiated the ventilation with CPAP at 4 ± 2 cm H_2O and PS ventilation at 15 ± 5 cm H_2O to achieve a respiratory rate of less than 25 breaths/min and an exhaled tidal volume of 7 mL/kg or more. Pressure support was adjusted following the arterial blood gases results. From the beginning and up to 24 hours after initiation of NIV, the authors reported a significant increase in pH (from 7.25 ± 0.01 to 7.38 ± 0.02, $P < 0.0001$) and a significant decrease in $PaCO_2$ (from 65 ± 2 to 45 ± 4, $P < 0.0001$) and respiratory rate (from 29.1 ± 1 to 17 ± 1, $P < 0.0001$). The mean ($\pm SD$) peak inspiratory pressure to ventilate in the NIV-treated patients was 18 ± 5 cm H_2O and always less than 25 cm H_2O. Two patients required intubation for worsening $PaCO_2$. The duration of NIV was 16 ± 21 hours. All patients survived. The authors concluded that NIV for acute asthma via a face mask appears highly effective in correcting gas exchange abnormalities.

In a retrospective observational study, Fernandez and associates evaluated their clinical experience with the use of NIV in patients with an acute asthmatic attack. They documented clinical data, gas exchange, and outcome of these patients. Fifty-eight patients were included in the study. Twenty-five patients (43%) were not eligible for NIV—11 patients (19%) because of respiratory arrest on their arrival at the emergency room and 14 patients (24%) because of improvement with medical management. The remaining 33 patients were eligible for NIV (57%): 11 patients (33%) received invasive mechanical ventilation and 22 patients (67%) were treated with NIV. Three NIV patients (14%) needed intubation. The authors compared data at baseline, 30 minutes, 2 to 6 hours, and 6 to 12 hours after the onset of ventilatory support. Significant differences were observed in arterial blood gases on admission to the emergency room between mechanical ventilation and NIV groups: $PaCO_2$, 89 ± 29 vs. 53 ± 13 mm Hg ($P < 0.05$); pH, 7.05 ± 0.21 vs. 7.28 ± 0.008 ($P < 0.05$); and HCO_3^- level, 22 ± 5 vs. 26 ± 6 mmol/L ($P < 0.05$). No differences were found in the median length of ICU stay (4.5 vs. 3 days), median hospital stay (15 vs. 12 days), and mortality (0 vs. 4%). They concluded that face mask and NIV appears to be a suitable method for reducing the need for intubation in very select asthmatic patients.

INDICATIONS AND CONTRAINDICATIONS FOR NIV

Boxes 13.1 and 13.2 list indications and contraindications for NIV, respectively.

Box 13.1 Indications for NIV

Indications for NIV are
1. COPD exacerbations
2. Acute pulmonary edema
3. Selected populations of acute respiratory failure patients

Other indications for NIV are
1. Facilitation of weaning
2. Postoperative respiratory failure
3. Do-not-intubate patients
4. Community-acquired pneumonia
5. Obstructive sleep apnea and obesity hypoventilation syndrome

---

Box 13.2 Contraindications to NIV

Absolute contraindications to NIV are
1. Nonrespiratory organ failure: encephalopathy, severe gastrointestinal bleeding, and hemodynamic instability with or without cardiac ischemia
2. Facial surgery or trauma
3. Inability to protect the airway and/or high risk of aspiration
4. Patient intolerance or noncooperative patients
5. Claustrophobia

TECHNIQUES AND EQUIPMENT

The main difference between invasive and NIV is that with the latter, ventilation is delivered to the airway by a mask (nasal, oronasal, full-face, etc.) instead of an endotracheal tube. One disadvantage is that because the circuit is not well closed, there may be air leaks around the mask or through the mouth; this can make ventilation difficult, depending on the ventilatory mode used.

In a physiological study, Navalesi and colleagues analyzed the efficacy of NIV in improving breathing pattern and arterial blood gases (ABGs) in hypercapnic patients. Three different types of masks were used: nasal mask, nasal plugs, and full-face mask. Two modes of ventilation were delivered: pressure support and assisted control. Three 30-minute runs of NIV were performed in these patients, who were randomized to volume-assisted ventilation or pressure support with the three different masks for each patient. The main results were an improvement in ABGs during NIV compared to spontaneous breathing, a greater

decrease in $PaCO_2$ with full-face masks and nasal plugs than with nasal masks, a better acceptance of NIV with the use of nasal masks than with the other two interfaces, and the patients' tolerance was not significantly affected by the ventilatory mode. Also, no difference was found in the acute response to NIV between the two subgroups of patients studied—COPD and restrictive thoracic disease patients. All these patients were stable chronic hypercapnic subjects. The authors concluded that in patients with chronic hypercapnic respiratory failure, NIV outcome can be more affected by the type of interface than by the ventilatory mode.

The interfaces are the devices that connect the ventilator to the patients. Those most commonly used are oronasal models; other types of interface masks include the nasal interface and the helmet (Figs. 13.3 to 13.5). There are different kinds of nasal masks; they are mainly used for chronic indications of NIV, such as treatment of obstructive sleep apnea. Some nasal masks can be customized to suit each patient. The main disadvantages of nasal masks are air leaks and nasal dryness.

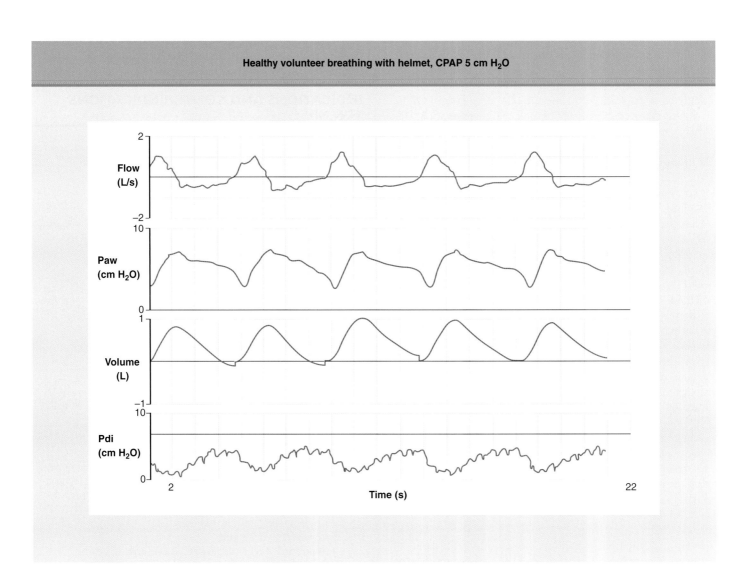

Figure 13.3. Tracings of airflow (flow), airway pressure (Paw), tidal volume, and transdiaphragmatic pressure (Pdi) obtained in a healthy volunteer breathing with a helmet with CPAP 5 cm H_2O. Tidal volume is approximately 850 mL and the respiratory rate is 16 breaths per minute.

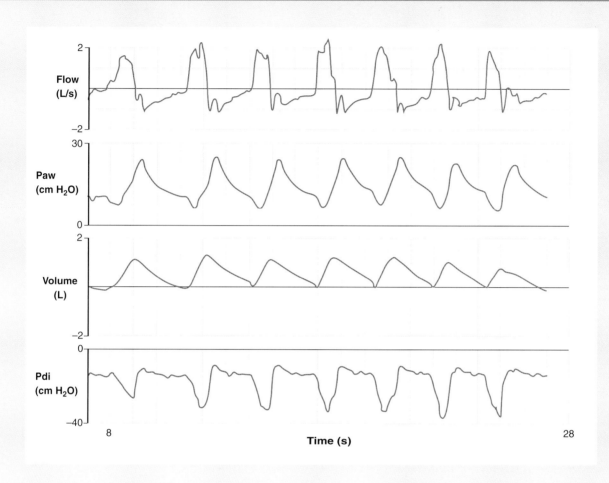

Healthy volunteer breathing with a helmet, pressure support 12 and PEEP 10 cm H₂O

Figure 13.4. Tracings of airflow (flow), airway pressure (Paw), tidal volume, and transdiaphragmatic pressure (Pdi) obtained in a healthy volunteer breathing with a helmet with pressure support of 12 cm H₂O and PEEP of 10 cm H₂O. Tidal volume is approximately 1200 mL and the respiratory rate is approximately 16 breaths per minute.

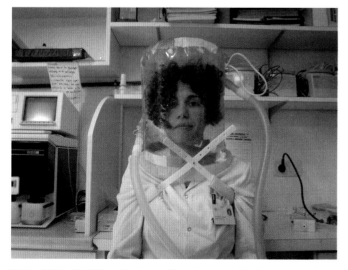

Figure 13.5. Healthy volunteer with a helmet interface connected to a standard ICU ventilator.

VENTILATOR MODES FOR NIV

NIV is usually delivered with pressure support ventilation and PEEP through an ICU ventilator with a full-face mask in most cases (Fig. 13.6). PS ventilation is a patient-triggered, pressure-limited, flow-cycled mode in which airway pressure is maintained constant during the whole inspiration, and when inspiratory flow reaches a certain threshold level the cycling from inspiration to expiration occurs. Pressure support allows the patient to retain relatively high control over respiratory rate and timing, inspiratory flow rate, and tidal volume. The level of external PEEP to be used in patients with clinically suspected dynamic hyperinflation and dynamic airway collapse should be adjusted with caution, since measurement of dynamic intrinsic PEEP in spontaneously breathing patients is not easy. It is recommended to start the NIV with a low level of pressure support (5–7 cm H₂O) and increase this progressively until an adequate tidal volume and a respiratory rate below 30 breaths

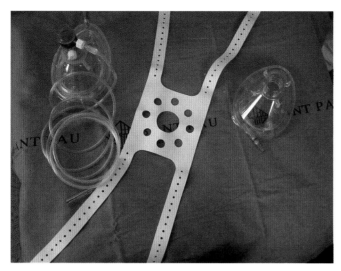

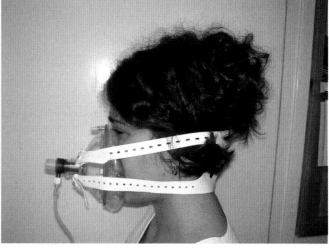

Figure 13.6. Two interfaces: *(left)* a high-flow CPAP mask and *(right)* a standard face mask.

Figure 13.7. Healthy volunteer with a high-flow CPAP mask.

per minute are reached. ABGs are needed to monitor the response to NIV. In case of air leakage, the modality can be switched to a pressure control mode with an imposed respiratory rate. Pressure control ventilation delivers time-cycled preset inspiratory and expiratory pressures at a controlled rate. The main advantage of this mode with respect to PS in the case of air leaks is that the ventilator will switch to expiration after a preset inspiratory time.

CPAP provides positive airway pressure during the entire spontaneous breath. This can be achieved with a ventilator or with a high-flow mask (Fig. 13.7). The main indication for the domiciliary use of CPAP is obstructive sleep apnea. In the emergency department and in the ICU, it is used mostly for treatment of acute cardiogenic pulmonary edema.

SUGGESTED READING

Antonelli M, Conti G, Rocco M, et al: A comparison of noninvasive positive-pressure ventilation and conventional mechanical ventilation in patients with acute respiratory failure. N Engl J Med 1998;339:429–435.

Brochard L, Mancebo J, Wysocki M, et al: Noninvasive ventilation for acute exacerbations of chronic obstructive pulmonary disease. N Engl J Med 1995;333:817–822.

Confalonieri M, Potena A, Carbone G, et al: Randomized trial of non invasive positive pressure ventilation in severe community acquired pneumonia. Am J Respir Crit Care Med 1999;160:1585–1591.

Delclaux C, L'Her E, Alberti C, et al: Treatment of acute hypoxemic non-hypercapnic respiratory insufficiency with continuous positive airway pressure delivered by a face mask. A randomized controlled trial. JAMA 2000;284:2352–2360.

Fernandez NM, Villagra A, Blanch L, Fernandez R: Non-invasive mechanical ventilation in status asthmaticus. Intensive Care Med 2001;27(3):486–492.

Ferrer M, Esquinas A, Leon M, et al: Noninvasive ventilation in severe hypoxemic respiratory failure: A randomized clinical trial. Am J Respir Crit Care Med 2003;168:1438–1444.

Girou E, Schortgen F, Delclaux C, et al: Association of noninvasive ventilation with nosocomial infections and survival in critically ill patients. JAMA 2000;284:2361–2367.

Hilbert G, Gruson D, Vargas F, et al: Noninvasive ventilation in immuno-suppressed patients with pulmonary infiltrates, fever, and acute respiratory failure. N Engl J Med 2001;344:481–487.

Keenan SP, Powers C, McCormack DG, Block G: Noninvasive positive-pressure ventilation for postextubation respiratory distress: a randomized controlled trial. JAMA 2002;26:287(24):3238–3244.

Kramer N, Meyer TJ, Meharg J, et al: Randomized, prospective trial of non-invasive positive pressure ventilation in acute respiratory failure. Am J Respir Crit Care Med 1995;151:1799–1806.

Jolliet P, Abajo P, Pasquina P, Chevrolet JC: Non-invasive pressure support ventilation in severe community-acquired pneumonia. Intensive Care Med 2001;27(5):812–821.

Masip J, Betbesé A, Paez J, et al: Non-invasive pressure support ventilation versus conventional oxygen therapy in acute cardiogenic pulmonary oedema: A randomised trial. Lancet 2000;356:2126–2132.

Mehta S, Gregory DJ, Kiihne S, et al: Randomized, prosective trial of bilevel versus continuous positive airway pressure in acute pulmonary edema. Crit Care Med 1997;25:620–628.

Nava S, Ambrosino N, Clini E, et al: Noninvasive mechanical ventilation in the weaning of patients with respiratory failure due to chronic obstructive pulmonary disease. A randomized, controlled trial. Ann Intern Med 1998;128:721–728.

Nava S, Carbone G, DiBattista N, et al: Noninvasive ventilation in cardiogenic pulmonary edema. Am J Respir Crit Care Med 2003;168:1432–1437.

Navalesi P, Fanfulla F, Frigiero P, et al: Physiologic evaluation of noninvasive mechanical ventilation delivered with three types of masks in patients with chronic hypercapnic respiratory failure. Crit Care Med 2000;28(6):1785–1790.

Plant PK, Owen JL, Elliott MW: Early use of non-invasive ventilation for acute exacerbations of chronic obstructive pulmonary disease on general respiratory wards: A multicentre randomised controlled trial. Lancet 2000;355:1931–1935.

Chapter 14

Tracheostomy

Bernard G. Fikkers, Graham Ramsay, and Christian Byhahn

KEY POINTS

- Percutaneous tracheostomy is the preferred technique for tracheostomy in the intensive care unit.
- It is impossible to give sound guidelines on the timing of tracheostomy because this depends on the clinical situation and prognosis of the patient. However, when ventilation is expected to last longer than 2 weeks, early tracheostomy compared to prolonged translaryngeal intubation is preferred.
- None of the techniques of percutaneous tracheostomy has significant advantages or disadvantages over another, and choice depends mainly on individual preference.
- Most contraindications for percutaneous tracheostomy are relative and depend on individual experience.
- In order to make meaningful comparisons in different studies, it is advisable to divide complications of percutaneous tracheostomy into major, intermediate, and minor groupings.

Tracheostomy has fascinated doctors since antiquity, but until the 19th century it was rarely performed and involved high mortality. The laryngologist Chevalier Jackson (1865–1958) described modern surgical tracheostomy in the early 1900s. The neurosurgeon C. Hunter Shelden (1907–2003) devised the first modern percutaneous kit in 1955. At approximately the same time, the Swedish radiologist Sven-Ivar Seldinger (1921–1998) described a technique to gain entrance to a hollow space, such as a blood vessel, by threading a flexible metal guidewire through a hollow needle. Pasquale Ciaglia (1912–2000), a thoracic surgeon from New York, popularized percutaneous tracheostomy in 1985 by using the Seldinger technique. Today, in modern intensive care practice most tracheostomies are done percutaneously.

PRACTICE OF PERCUTANEOUS TRACHEOSTOMY

Most methods for percutaneous tracheostomy rely on the Seldinger technique. Subsequently, dilation up to the degree required for the positioning of the tracheal cannula, with either a single- or a multiple-dilator technique, is necessary.

The preparation of this bedside procedure carried out in the intensive care unit (ICU) is very important. Nasogastric feeding is stopped at least 2 hours before the planned time of the pro-

cedure, and the stomach contents are emptied just before the actual procedure to prevent aspiration into the airway. Patients should be ventilated with pressure-controlled ventilation with a FIO_2 of 1.0. Pressure control avoids hypoventilation as a result of air leak during the procedure. Adequate analgesia, sedation, and muscle relaxation should be ensured. During the procedure, minimal monitoring should involve pulse oxymetry, electrocardiography, and capnography. The patient's head is positioned in retroflexion with a transverse pillow under the shoulder blades, if permitted. Employing a laryngoscope, the tube is withdrawn under direct vision so that the inflated cuff is placed between the vocal cords, facilitating reintubation if necessary. Simultaneously, the operation site is cleaned with chlorhexidine in 80% alcohol and draped. The landmark structures, such as the thyroid notch, cricoid cartilage, and tracheal rings, are palpated to define the proper location for the intended tracheostomy placement. It is prudent to check the intended puncture site for large vessels because these may sometimes cause profuse hemorrhaging.

Subsequently, a 1- or 2-cm transverse incision is made in the skin and subcutaneous tissues. In difficult cases, some blunt dissection, vertically down to the pretracheal fascia, may be done to more easily palpate and identify the tracheal cartilages with the tip of the finger. The trachea is punctured with a 14-Fr cannulated needle attached to a saline-filled syringe for continuous suction, aiming for the interspace between the first and second or second and third tracheal rings (although different studies have shown that accurate placement is achieved in less than half of the cases). The puncture should be guided by the fiberscopic view. It helps confirm the correct position of the puncture (i.e., in the midline of the anterior trachea) and ensures that the posterior wall is not injured. This is an important step in percutaneous tracheostomy. It should be kept in mind that continuous fiberscopy during percutaneous tracheostomy may contribute to early hypoventilation, hypercarbia, and respiratory acidosis. Therefore, if possible, fiberscopic time and suctioning during fiberscopy should be minimized during the procedure. This is particularly true in patients after neurotrauma with the possibility of increasing intracranial pressure due to hypercarbia. After threading the guidewire and proper dilation, the cannula can be inserted.

All five currently available techniques for percutaneous tracheostomy are based on Seldinger's technique. After threading a guidewire, the trachea is dilated in one or multiple steps in either antegrade or retrograde direction over the guidewire, and a cannula is inserted. The method of dilation and cannula insertion is mainly what distinguishes the different techniques.

131

Table 14.1 Techniques of Percutaneous Tracheostomy		
Technique	**Characteristics**	**Manufacturer**
Percutaneous dilational tracheostomy	Antegrade, multistep dilation with up to seven dilators	Cook Critical Care, Bloomington, IN, USA
Guidewire dilating forceps	Antegrade, two-step dilation with modified Howard–Kelly forceps	SIMS Portex Ltd., Hythe, Kent, UK
Translaryngeal tracheostomy	Retrograde, single-step dilation with the cannula	Tyco Healthcare, Athlone, Ireland
Ciaglia Blue Rhino	Antegrade, single-step dilation with a conically shaped, hydrophilically coated dilator	Cook Critical Care, Bloomington, IN, USA
PercuTwist	Antegrade stoma formation with a self-cutting plastic screw	Rüsch, Kernen, Germany

Table 14.1 gives an overview of the technical properties of the different systems in use, and Figure 14.1 illustrates these techniques.

INDICATIONS FOR PERCUTANEOUS TRACHEOSTOMY

Tracheostomy offers a number of practical advantages compared to translaryngeal intubation, such as a decrease in airway resistance, anatomical dead space, and work of breathing, thus facilitating weaning from mechanical ventilation in patients with marginal respiratory mechanics; better pulmonary toilet; improved patient comfort; the absence of laryngeal and vocal cord injuries; security of the airway; easier tube changes; and the possibility for oral nutrition and speech, which may in turn improve the patient's psychological status. Tracheostomy is an invasive procedure with a small but definite risk of operative mortality and morbidity. Translaryngeal intubation also has related problems. The tube is not easy to secure firmly, and the agitated patient may bite it, occluding the lumen. Oral hygiene is difficult to perform adequately and angular stomatitis may occur, usually related to the securing tapes. Long-term translaryngeal intubation may result in serious morbidity. However, in 1981, the conclusion of the first study to prospectively compare translaryngeal intubation to surgical tracheostomy was that the complications of tracheostomy were more severe than those of translaryngeal intubation, and tracheostomy was not advised in the first 3 weeks of ventilation. Recent studies, however, have established that a standard surgical tracheostomy can be performed with an acceptably low risk of perioperative complications.

Currently, tracheostomy is a standard procedure in critically ill patients. Indications for surgical and percutaneous tracheostomy are identical for patients in the ICU. These include relief of upper airway obstruction, protection of the tracheobronchial tree in patients at risk of aspiration, tracheal access for long-term positive pressure ventilation, and weaning from mechanical ventilation. Prolonged weaning from mechanical ventilation is the main indication for tracheostomy in the ICU. The reasons for the increasing popularity of percutaneous tracheostomy are its simple bedside application, ease of scheduling, avoidance of transporting critically ill patients, and its cost-effectiveness. Since in many institutions percutaneous tracheostomy is the method of choice, this means that the experience with surgical tracheostomy will decrease and it is likely to be carried out only in patients in whom percutaneous tracheostomy is contraindicated or has failed (i.e., in less optimal circumstances).

CONTRAINDICATIONS FOR PERCUTANEOUS TRACHEOSTOMY

Most contraindications are relative and depend on individual experience. Percutaneous tracheostomy is absolutely contraindicated in patients with an infection of the anterior neck, uncorrectable coagulation abnormalities, and known or expected difficult translaryngeal intubation. Relative contraindications are a large goiter, a history of neck surgery, a distance from the thyroid bone to the manubrium of less than 3 cm, elevated intracranial pressure, patients who need an emergency airway, patients who are younger than 16 years old and/or have a total body weight of less than 40 kg, patients with hypoxia despite intensive ventilatory support [positive end-expiratory pressure (PEEP) > 20 cm H_2O and/or FIO_2 > 70%], and obesity with inability to identify the proper landmarks. Patient selection is very important, particularly when sufficient expertise is not available.

The disadvantage of a percutaneous tracheostomy, although minimally invasive, is that it is still a procedure with the risk of complications. As with translaryngeal intubation, and after surgical tracheostomy, the upper airways are bypassed. Warming, humidification, and filtering of air do not take place before the inspired air reaches the lungs, although it is standard ICU practice to warm and humidify the inspired air at the ventilator. However, this problem may occur in ventilator-independent patients with tracheostomy, resulting in drying out of tracheal and bronchial epithelium. Another disadvantage is the loss of intrinsic PEEP ($PEEP_i$), normally mediated by glottic activity. This predisposes the patient to alveolar collapse or atelectasis. This is particularly significant in patients with chronic obstructive pulmonary disease, who utilize increased $PEEP_i$ as a compensatory strategy for pulmonary dysfunction.

TIMING OF TRACHEOSTOMY

The decision regarding when to perform a tracheostomy has always been controversial, although it is well known that the number of complications increases with an increasing duration of translaryngeal intubation. Much of this controversy originates from the difficulty of accurately predicting the length of time that patients require mechanical ventilation. It may well be impossible to give sound guidelines on the timing of tracheostomy because this depends on the clinical situation and prognosis of the patient, and not on a dogmatic time limit. The decision to convert a translaryngeal tube to a tracheostomy cannula in the ICU has to be individualized. This "anticipating approach" takes into consideration the potential benefits of the

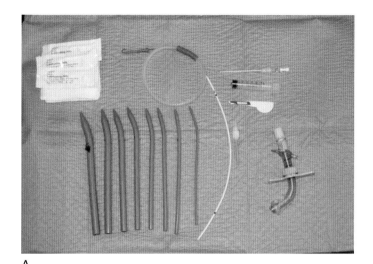

A

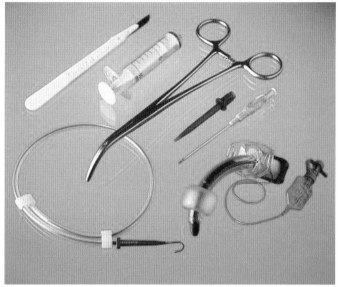

B

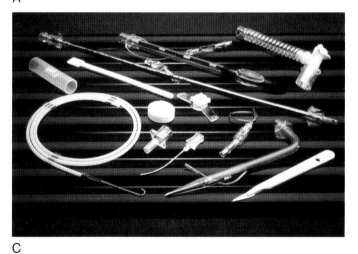

C

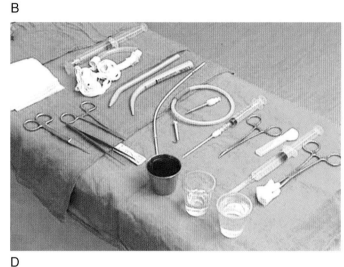

D

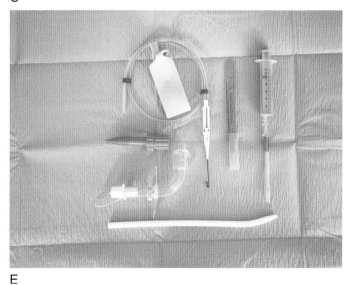

E

Figure 14.1. Techniques for percutaneous tracheostomy. *A,* Percutaneous dilational tracheostomy (Ciaglia); *B,* guidewire dilating forceps (Griggs); *C,* translaryngeal tracheostomy (Fantoni); *D,* Blue Rhino (Ciaglia); and *E,* PercuTwist (Frova).

procedure compared with prolonging translaryngeal intubation. Before the introduction of the percutaneous technique, the length of time of translaryngeal intubation tended to be longer. Since no data exist regarding the relative impact of tracheostomy in terms of patient outcome relative to prolonged translaryngeal intubation, recommendations for timing to achieve these benefits have been based on expert consensus. A consensus conference on artificial airways in 1989 recommended translaryngeal intubation as the method of choice for an artificial airway needed for up to 10 days, whereas tracheostomy is preferred when the need for an artificial airway exceeds 21 days. However, it is a misconception that a tracheostomy within 3 weeks is premature. This may result in a patient's undergoing a mandatory 2 or 3 weeks of translaryngeal intubation before tracheostomy is performed. In fact, tracheostomy should be secured as soon as it becomes apparent that sustained independent ventilation is not likely to happen within 2 or 3 weeks, such as in patients with irreversible neurological disorders or with major trauma. In patients with infratentorial lesions, it is proven that an aggressive policy toward early tracheostomy is justified based on the low frequency of successful extubations and high frequency of extubation failures. The decision should be made after 1 week of conventional ventilation. Early tracheostomy may be beneficial for ICU patients because it helps to reduce the number of days on the ventilator, ICU stay, and total hospital stay. Observational studies indicate that the absence of clear criteria for selecting patients for tracheostomy results in considerable variation in the timing of the procedure, with local preferences, rather than patient factors, guiding care. In 2004, the first study prospectively comparing the benefits of early and delayed tracheostomy was published. It showed that the benefits of early tracheostomy outweigh the risks of prolonged translaryngeal intubation, even in terms of mortality.

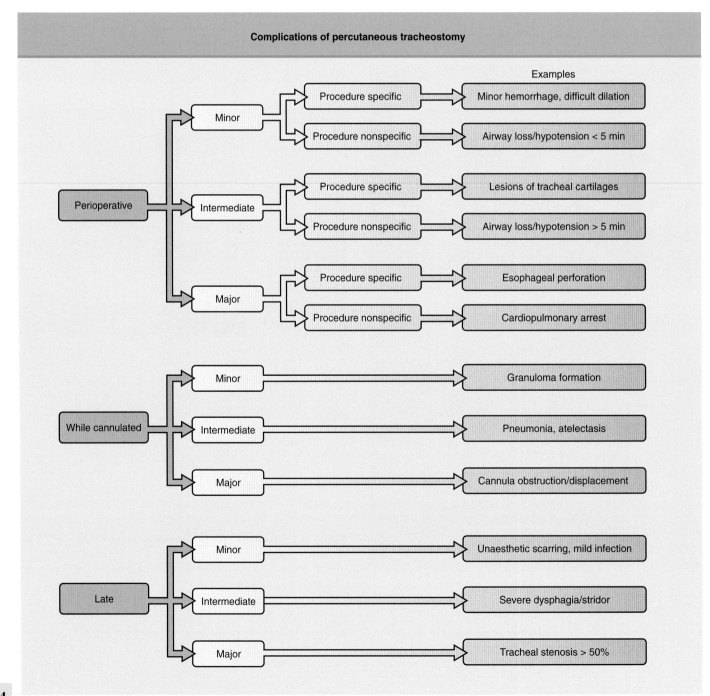

Figure 14.2. Complications of percutaneous tracheostomy.

COMPLICATIONS OF PERCUTANEOUS TRACHEOSTOMY

In 1992, a prospective study on percutaneous tracheostomy concluded that "(it) is a dangerous procedure with potential for catastrophic complications." Since then, the number of studies published in this field has been increasing each year. Unfortunately, these studies are difficult to compare because complication rates vary in different series depending on definitions and methods of detection. In addition, a learning curve exists for all of the techniques used in percutaneous tracheostomy. We have tried to make a sound classification of tracheostomy complications based on the available literature (Fig. 14.2).

"Perioperative complications" are procedure-related complications occurring within 24 hours of the procedure. "Postoperative complications" are divided into "complications while cannulated" and "late complications." "Complications while cannulated" are complications occurring after 24 hours until removal of the tracheostomy tube. "Late complications" occur after removal of the tracheostomy tube. According to the literature, major complications in percutaneous tracheostomy occur in approximately 3% of cases (range, 0–14%).

"Intermediate complications," when recognized and treated appropriately, should not result in serious morbidity. Intermediate complications in percutaneous tracheostomy occur in approximately 3% of cases (range, 0–26%). The incidence of minor complications is approximately 20%, but there is considerable study-to-study variability in reported complication incidence (range, 1%–58%). The procedure-related mortality may involve the perioperative period as well as during cannulation, and it is less than 0.5%.

CONCLUSION

Percutaneous tracheostomy has become an integral part of airway management in the critical care setting. Five different techniques are available and do not differ significantly in terms of overall complications. None of the techniques has significant advantages or disadvantages over another, not even in high-risk patients.

Regardless of the fact that percutaneous tracheostomy is a safe procedure, the tracheostomy team should include an experienced physician who is capable of handling eventual complications and an expert in airway management to further reduce both the incidence and adverse sequelae of perioperative complications.

SUGGESTED READING

Anon JM, Escuela MP, Gomez V, et al: Percutaneous tracheostomy: Ciaglia Blue Rhino versus Griggs' Guide Wire Dilating Forceps. A prospective randomized trial. Acta Anaesthesiol Scand 2004;48:451–456.

Freeman BD, Isabella K, Lin N, Buchman TG: A meta-analysis of prospective trials comparing percutaneous and surgical tracheostomy in critically ill patients. Chest 2000;118:1412–1418.

Heffner JE: Percutaneous dilatational vs standard tracheotomy: A meta-analysis but not the final analysis. Chest 2000;118:1236–1238.

Heffner JE: Tracheotomy application and timing. Clin Chest Med 2003;24:389–398.

Maziak DE, Meade MO, Todd TR: The timing of tracheotomy: A systematic review. Chest 1998;114:605–609.

Rumbak MJ, Newton M, Truncale T, et al: A prospective, randomized, study comparing early percutaneous dilational tracheotomy to prolonged translaryngeal intubation (delayed tracheotomy) in critically ill medical patients. Crit Care Med 2004;32:1689–1694.

Chapter 15

Monitoring Mechanical Ventilation

Salvatore Grasso and Vito Fanelli

KEY POINTS

- Mechanical ventilation is a valuable life support procedure that may lead to severe iatrogenic complications.
- Monitoring respiratory mechanics, gas exchange, and patient-ventilator interactions allows the risks to be minimized and facilitates weaning from ventilatory support.
- Continuous monitoring of the "stress index" may be useful in order to set up a lung protective ventilatory strategy.
- In the partially assisted ventilatory modes, delivered flow and volume depend on the interaction of the patient's effort, algorithm of positive pressure assistance, and mechanical characteristics of the respiratory system.
- Repeated measurements of arterial blood gases (ABGs) are mandatory in order to assess the efficacy of mechanical ventilation. Pulse oxymetry and capnography add useful information and are essential parts of basic monitoring in ventilated patients.

Mechanical ventilation is a valuable life-support procedure that may lead to severe iatrogenic complications. Monitoring respiratory mechanics, gas exchange, and patient–ventilator interactions allows the risks to be minimized and facilitates weaning from the ventilatory support.

MONITORING RESPIRATORY MECHANICS DURING CONTROLLED MECHANICAL VENTILATION

In modern ventilators, opening airway pressure (Pao) and flow are instantaneously measured through internal sensors (a pressure transducer and a pneumotachograph connected to a differential pressure transducer, respectively), and the relative tracings are displayed on a screen. Inspired and expired volumes are acquired through integration of the flow signal. Since the resistive and elastic characteristics of the ventilatory circuit may influence measurements, connecting external sensors distally to the Y piece of the ventilatory circuit allows a more accurate estimation of respiratory mechanics.

During controlled mechanical ventilation, at each breath the ventilator applies a constant flow or a constant pressure to the patient's airways for a fixed inspiratory time and allows passive expiration for a fixed expiratory time. Due to its peculiar char-

acteristics, the constant-flow mode is preferred for the assessment of respiratory mechanics. Indeed, from characteristics of the Pao versus time (Pao-t) tracing during constant-flow inflation, it is possible to infer the mechanical properties of the respiratory system (elastance, resistance, and inheritance). In a simple monocompartmental model of the respiratory system (Fig. 15.1) inflated with a perfectly constant flow, inspiratory Pao-t tracing is composed of the following:

1. The AB segment ("resistive" pressure increase) is a step increase in Pao that occurs at the beginning of inspiratory flow delivery. Point B depends on both inspiratory flow rate and airway resistances, according to Ohm's law:

$$\text{Resistance} = \text{driving pressure/flow rate} \quad \text{(Equation 1)}$$

where driving pressure (ΔP) is the resistive pressure applied to generate a given constant laminar flow.

2. The BC segment ("elastic" pressure increase) is a progressive increase in Pao that is generated by the progressive alveolus inflation. The slope of the BC segment may be quantitated as

$$C = \Delta V / \Delta P \quad \text{(Equation 2)}$$

where C is the compliance of the alveolus, ΔV is the delivered volume, and ΔP is the resulting increase in airway pressure.

3. Point C (Pao,peak) is the peak in Pao reached at end inspiration. For a given constant-flow rate and inspiratory time, Pao,peak includes both the "resistive" and the "elastic" pressure components.

4. The CD segment takes place if the ventilator performs an end inspiratory pause by closing both inspiratory and expiratory valves. As the inspiratory flow stops, the Pao value instantaneously decreases to the end-inspiratory static recoil pressure of the respiratory system (point E, the end-inspiratory plateau pressure, Pao, plat).

5. EF segment: after the end-inspiratory pause, the ventilator opens the expiratory valve, keeping the inspiratory valve closed. Depending on the position of the pressure transducer in the ventilatory circuit, it reads the atmospheric pressure. If an end-expiratory valve is added to the expiratory limb of the ventilatory circuit, the transducer reads the applied external positive end-expiratory pressure value (PEEPext).

The real Pao tracing in a patient receiving constant-flow mechanical ventilation shows several differences compared to

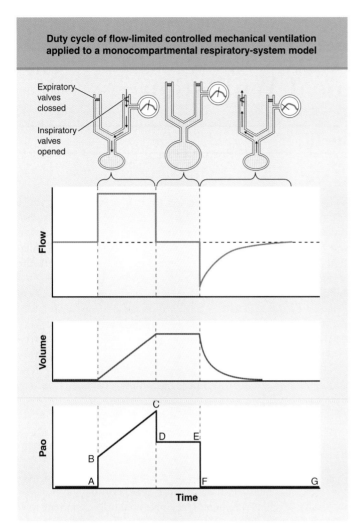

Duty cycle of flow-limited controlled mechanical ventilation applied to a monocompartmental respiratory-system model

Figure 15.1. Flow, volume, and Pao tracings recorded during constant-flow mechanical ventilation applied to a monocompartmental respiratory-system model. The dotted line refers to the theoretical value of alveolar pressure.

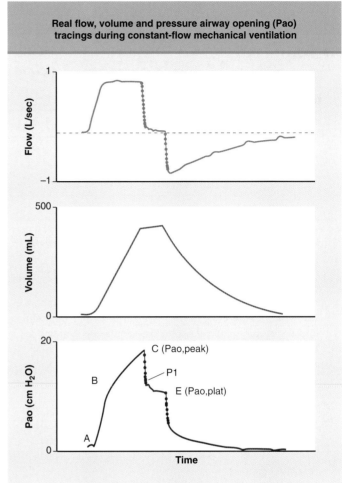

Real flow, volume and pressure airway opening (Pao) tracings during constant-flow mechanical ventilation

Figure 15.2. Flow, volume, and Pao tracings recorded during constant-flow mechanical ventilation applied to a patient.

the one obtained in the monocompartmental model (Fig. 15.2). Real mechanical ventilators are not able to generate a perfectly square inspiratory flow tracing such as in the model. In addition, the model does not take into account the respiratory system viscoelastic and inertial properties and the inhomogeneities in mechanical characteristics among different lung regions. Accordingly, the real Pao-t tracing is described as follows:

1. The AB tract (resistive pressure increase) is not perfectly perpendicular to the time axis but shows a discrete slope related to the inability of the ventilator to generate a perfectly square flow tracing.
2. A transient phase of pressure slope variation substitutes for the discrete B point. During this transient period, flow is delivered preferentially to lung areas with low resistances and high compliances.
3. The BC elastic pressure increase is not always linear compared to the model, but its profile may be curvilinear since respiratory system compliance and resistance may be nonlinear in the range of the delivered volume.

4. After the C point (Pao,peak), there is a sharp pressure drop to a point called P1, and subsequently Pao decays in 2 to 5 seconds to Pao,plat. The P1–Pao,plat pressure decay depends principally on the reequilibration of pressures among areas with different elastic and resistive characteristics (whose pressures at end inspiration are not in equilibrium).

Measurement of Respiratory Mechanics during Constant-Flow Ventilation

Resistance

Resistance is the expression of the opposition to gas flow through the respiratory system and is quantitated as the amount of pressure required to cause a unit rate of gas flow, according to Ohm's law:

$$\text{Resistance} = \text{driving pressure/flow rate} \qquad \text{(Equation 3)}$$

where driving pressure is the resistive pressure applied to generate a given constant laminar flow in the airways. Units of resistance are cm H_2O/liter/sec. The total respiratory system resistance is the sum of pulmonary resistance (airway resistance

+ lung tissutal resistance) and chest wall resistance (essentially tissutal resistances). Both lung and chest wall tissutal resistances are increased in some pathological conditions, such as in patients with severe chronic obstructive pulmonary disease (COPD) or in morbidly obese patients. Although several experimental methods have been proposed to measure resistance, in this chapter we focus on the rapid occlusion method originally proposed by Milic Emili and coworkers (1982). This technique is based on the sudden interruption of a constant flow previously applied to the respiratory system, a condition easily reproduced during constant-flow ventilation by applying an end-inspiratory pause (see Figs. 15.1 and 15.2). According to this method, the total resistance of the respiratory system (Rmax,rs) is proportional to the Ppeak − Pplat pressure decay when the constant flow is suddenly interrupted, according to the law

$$Rmax,rs = (Ppeak − Pplat)/flow \qquad \text{(Equation 4)}$$

Rmax,rs is further partitioned into the airway resistance (Rmin) and additional resistance (ΔR). The immediate decrease in pressure from Ppeak to P1 is proportional to the airway resistance (Rmin)

$$Rmin = (Ppeak − P1)/flow \qquad \text{(Equation 5)}$$

whereas the slower decay from P1 to Pplat is proportional to the additional resistance (ΔR):

$$ΔR = Rmax,rs − Rmin \qquad \text{(Equation 6)}$$

Partitioning between Rmin,rs and ΔR is useful in order to understand the clinical meaning of the increase in Rmax,rs (see Fig. 15.9). Rmin,rs is increased in several pathological conditions in which airway resistance is increased, such in as asthma, pulmonary edema, acute respiratory distress syndrome (ARDS), and COPD. However, since Rmin,rs is the sum of airway resistance and ventilatory circuit and endotracheal tube resistance, the hypothesis of an endotracheal tube obstruction should be ruled out. In case of doubt, the endotracheal tube should readily be changed, or tracheal pressure (Ptrach) should be measured through a subtle catheter advanced distally to the endotracheal tube.

Several limitations of the interrupter technique must be addressed. First, although inspiratory resistance is measured, extrapolating this value to expiratory resistances may be misleading. For example, in severe COPD patients, expiratory resistance is significantly higher than inspiratory resistance due to expiratory flow limitation (distal airways collapse during early expiration). Second, the measurement is influenced by the inspiratory flow rate and the lung volume at the moment of the inspiratory hold procedure. In normal subjects, the value of Rmin increases with flow and decreases with lung volume, probably due to the increase in airway diameter. In contrast, ΔR exponentially decreases with flow and increases with lung volume. Since the flow- and volume-induced variations in ΔR are more pronounced, overall Rmax,rs decreases with inspiratory flow and increases with lung volume. As a consequence, values of Rmax, Rmin, and ΔR should be referred to the lung volume and flow rate; in normal subjects, for a flow of 0.4 liters/sec and a tidal

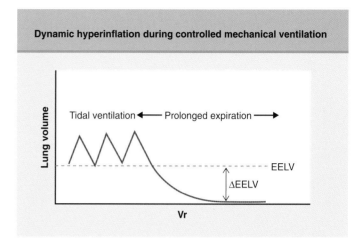

Dynamic hyperinflation during controlled mechanical ventilation

Figure 15.3. Difference (ΔEELV) between the end-expiratory lung volume (EELV) during mechanical ventilation and elastic equilibrium volume of the respiratory system (Vr) in a patient with dynamic hyperinflation. A complete lung emptying is obtained by disconnecting the patient from the ventilator at the end of mechanical expiratory time and allowing a prolonged (15–20 sec) passive exhalation to atmospheric pressure.

volume (VT) of 600 mL, Rmax,rs is 5 to 6 cm H_2O/liter/sec and Rmin is 2 to 3 cm H_2O/liter/sec.

Static Intrinsic Positive End-Expiratory Pressure

In normal subjects at rest, the end-expiratory lung volume (EELV) corresponds to the elastic equilibrium volume of the respiratory system (Vr) or functional residual capacity (FRC). When the time available for expiration is shorter than the time required for passive lung empty to Vr, air trapping develops and alveolar pressure remains positive at the end of expiration (dynamic hyperinflation). If the EELV during mechanical ventilation is higher than Vr, the amount of air trapping may be measured by allowing a prolonged passive lung empty to Vr (Fig. 15.3). Two different mechanisms leading to dynamic hyperinflation have been described.

First, dynamic hyperinflation without flow limitation occurs when expiratory time is shorter than the time required for passive lung empty to Vr. According to an empirical rule, this time may be estimated as three times the "time constant" of the respiratory system, expressed in milliseconds. The time constant of the respiratory system is proportional to both resistance and compliance (τ):

$$τ = resistance × compliance \qquad \text{(Equation 7)}$$

In a normal subject with a static compliance (Cst,rs) of 80 mL/cm H_2O and an expiratory resistance of 5 cm H_2O/liter/sec, passive lung empty takes 1.2 seconds, whereas in a patients with asthma, assuming an expiratory resistance of 30 cm H_2O/liter/sec, passive lung empty takes 7.2 seconds.

Second, dynamic hyperinflation due to flow limitation is generated by distal airway collapse at early expiration. Compared to normal subjects, in whom flow limitation occurs only during forced expiration, a distal airway collapse occurs during tidal exhalation in patients with severe emphysema.

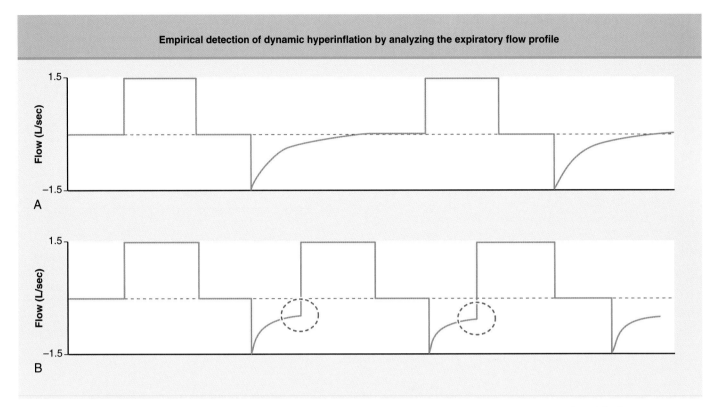

Empirical detection of dynamic hyperinflation by analyzing the expiratory flow profile

Figure 15.4. Flow tracing recorded during constant-flow mechanical ventilation. In a normal patient *(panel A)*, the end-expiratory flow is zero. In a patient with dynamic hyperinflation *(panel B)*, an ongoing flow at end expiration suggests incomplete lung emptying.

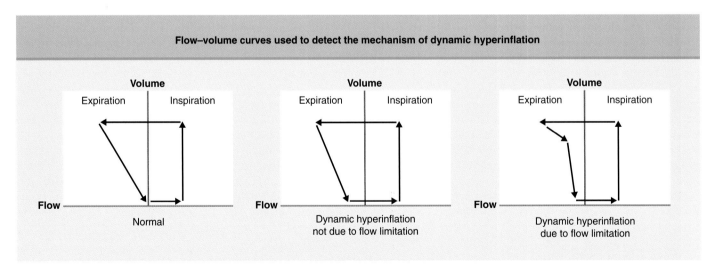

Flow–volume curves used to detect the mechanism of dynamic hyperinflation

Figure 15.5. Flow–volume curves obtained in a normal patient during constant-flow mechanical ventilation compared to flow–volume curves in patients with dynamic hyperinflation. When dynamic hyperinflation is due to flow limitation, the shape of the expiratory flow–volume profile shows an initial sharp decrease, abruptly followed by slope reduction, which makes the expiratory flow profile virtually linear.

During constant-flow mechanical ventilation, the occurrence of dynamic hyperinflation may be empirically detected if there is an ongoing flow at end expiration (Fig. 15.4). In addition, the shape of the expiratory flow profile during passive expiration is different, depending on whether air trapping is due to flow limi- tation or to mismatch between lung empty time and mechani- cal expiratory time. In flow-limited patients, the expiratory flow profile has an initial sharp decrease abruptly followed by a sudden slope reduction when the distal airway collapse occurs (Fig. 15.5).

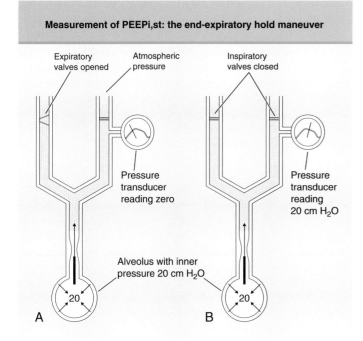

Measurement of PEEPi,st: the end-expiratory hold maneuver

Figure 15.6. Schematic representation of the respiratory system and a ventilatory circuit. *A,* During the expiratory phase, the ventilator opens the expiratory valve while the inspiratory valve is closed. Consequently, the pressure transducer reads atmospheric pressure. *B,* At end expiration, both inspiratory and expiratory valves are closed (end-expiratory hold maneuver). The pressure transducer now reads the end-expiratory alveolar pressure.

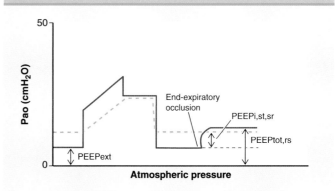

Measurement of PEEPi,st: through an end-expiratory hold maneuver

Figure 15.7. Recording of the Pao tracing obtained during a cycle of constant-flow mechanical ventilation followed by an end-expiratory hold maneuver. At the end of the maneuver, the PEEPtot value is obtained. The dotted line indicates the theoretical value of alveolar pressure.

Whenever dynamic hyperinflation is present, alveolar pressure remains positive at end expiration [static intrinsic PEEP (PEEPi,st)]. As shown in Figures 15.6 and 15.7, PEEPi,st may be measured through a 5- to 10-second end-expiratory hold maneuver consisting of the contemporary closure of both inspiratory and expiratory valves at end expiration. The pressure recorded at the end of the end-expiratory pause is the total respiratory system positive end-expiratory pressure (PEEPtot). In a normal subject submitted to a normal ventilatory pattern, PEEP$_{tot}$ is equal to zero or to the external positive end-expiratory pressure (PEEPext) if it is applied. In contrast, in a patient with dynamic hyperinflation, the value of PEEPtot is higher than the value of PEEPext. PEEPi,st is the difference between PEEPtot and PEEPext (see Fig. 15.7).

Static Compliance

Static compliance (Cst,rs) is measured as the change in respiratory system volume per unit change in applied pressure (with milliliters as volume units and centimeters of water as pressure units):

$$C_{st,rs} = V_T/(P_{ao,plat} - PEEP_{tot}) \qquad \text{(Equation 8)}$$

where Pao,plat is measured at the end of a 2- to 5-second end-inspiratory pause.

Elastance, the mathematical inverse of compliance, is expressed in cm H$_2$O/liters as

$$E_{st,rs} = (P_{ao,plat} - PEEP_{tot})/V_T \qquad \text{(Equation 9)}$$

PEEPtot is used instead of PEEPext for the calculation of Cst,rs in order to discriminate between an increase in Pao,plat due to dynamic hyperinflation (where PEEPtot is higher than PEEPext and Cst,rs is not affected) and an increase in Pao,plat due to reduction of Cst,rs (where PEEPtot is equal to PEEPext) (see Fig. 15.7).

Since the lung and the chest wall are structures "in series," Cst,rs is the sum of lung and chest wall compliance (Cst,L and Cst,cw, respectively). Similarly, Est,rs is the sum of lung and chest wall elastance (Est,L and Est,cw, respectively):

$$1/C_{st,rs} = 1/C_{st,L} + 1/C_{st,cw} \qquad \text{(Equation 10)}$$

and hence

$$E_{st,rs} = E_{st,L} + E_{st,cw} \qquad \text{(Equation 11)}$$

Here, Cst,cw and Est,cw are calculated as

$$C_{st,cw} = V_T/(P_{es}, \text{end inspiratory} - P_{es}, \text{end expiratory}) \qquad \text{(Equation 12)}$$

and

$$E_{st,cw} = (P_{es}, \text{end inspiratory} - P_{es}, \text{end expiratory})/V_T \qquad \text{(Equation 13)}$$

where Pes is the esophageal pressure. Normal values of Est,cw are between 3 and 5 cm H$_2$O/liter. From a theoretical standpoint, pleural pressure variations should be used instead of esophageal pressure to measure the lung surrounding pressure. However, pleural pressure measurements are virtually impossible in clinical practice, and esophageal pressure is commonly

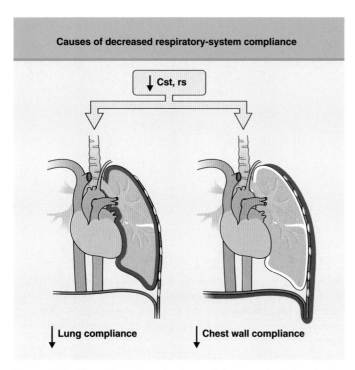

Causes of decreased respiratory-system compliance

$\downarrow$ Cst, rs

$\downarrow$ **Lung compliance** $\downarrow$ **Chest wall compliance**

Figure 15.8. The different mechanisms of decrease in Cst,rs due to decrease in lung compliance *(left)* or chest wall compliance *(right).* Partitioning between lung and chest wall mechanical impairment may require the measurement of esophageal pressure, and the definition of the cause of a decrease in chest wall compliance requires intra-abdominal pressure measurement.

used as a substitute. Pes is recorded with the patient in the semi-recumbent position through an air balloon-equipped catheter inserted in the lower third of the esophagus and connected to a pressure transducer. The balloon should be 10 cm long, with an internal volume of 10 mL and filled with 1 to 1.5 mL of air. For effective measurements, correct catheter positioning in the lower third of the esophagus should be checked using the occlusion test described by Baydur and coworkers. It consists of the simultaneous recording of Pao and Pes while the patient performs repeated inspiratory attempts against the occluded airway. If the esophageal balloon is correctly positioned, the negative deflections in Pes and Pao should be similar. Partitioning between lung and chest wall elastic properties may be useful in the differential diagnosis of the decrease in respiratory compliance (Figs. 15.8 and 15.9). Since the chest wall and abdomen are coupled through the diaphragm, increased abdominal pressure is one of the most important factors leading to chest wall stiffness. However, patients without abdominal hypertension may have chest wall mechanical impairment related to chest wall deformities, fluid overload, or pleural effusions.

Measurement of the Stress Index during Constant-Flow Ventilation

Several studies have shown that mechanical ventilation can worsen the preexisting lung injury in patients with ARDS. The hypothesis is that ventilator-induced cyclic tidal alveolar recruiting/derecruiting and/or overdistension induce worsening of the preexisting lung inflammation. Analyzing the Pao-t profile during

the period of constant-flow inflation (see the BC segment in Fig. 15.2) allows detection of the occurrence of tidal alveolar recruitment/derecruitment and/or overinflation. A downward Pao-t concavity indicates a progressive increase in compliance during tidal inflation, whereas an upward Pao-t concavity indicates a progressive decrease in compliance during tidal inflation (Fig. 15.10). The amount of mechanical stress due to recruitment/de-recruitment and/or overinflation may be quantified through a power equation fitting performed on the Pao-t profile during constant-flow inflation (stress index):

$$Pao = a \times t^b + c \qquad \text{(Equation 14)}$$

where the coefficients a and c are constants, and the coefficient b is a dimensionless number that describes the shape of the Pao-t profile. For a coefficient b that is less than 1, the Pao-t profile has a downward concavity (compliance increases with inflation), whereas for a coefficient b that is greater than 1 the Pao-t profile has an upward concavity (compliance decreases with inflation). Finally, when b equals 1, the Pao-t profile is straight and compliance remains constant during inflation. In intact animals with experimental ARDS, the stress index was able to predict the amount of lung tissue undergoing tidal alveolar recruiting/derecruiting and/or hyperinflation (as assessed through computed tomography analysis). Continuous monitoring of the stress index may be useful in order to develop a lung protective ventilatory strategy.

Measurement of Respiratory Mechanics through the Equation of Motion

Applying the equation of motion is an alternative approach to the measurement of respiratory mechanics in mechanically ventilated patients. At any instant during controlled mechanical ventilation, the total pressure applied to the respiratory system (Pappl) is equal to

$$\begin{aligned} Pappl = &\ (volume \times elastance) + (flow \times resistance) \\ &+ PEEPtot \qquad \text{(Equation 15)} \end{aligned}$$

Where Pappl is the positive pressure applied by the ventilator. From a mathematical standpoint, assuming that resistance and elastance are linear during the respiratory cycle and knowing the value of PEEPtot, the equation may be solved if three sets of Pao, flow, and volume values are known. However, due to the biological nature of the signals, several sets of data should be used in order to obtain a robust measurement. Drawbacks of the equation of motion method are related to the assumption of linearity of elastance and resistance during the entire respiratory cycle, which is not the case in several pathological conditions.

MONITORING RESPIRATORY MECHANICS DURING PARTIAL MECHANICAL SUPPORT

Critically ill patients are often capable of doing some work of breathing on their own. The basic form of partial mechanical support is assist-controlled mechanical ventilation (A/CMV), which consists of a constant flow or constant pressure breath triggered by patient inspiratory effort (patient-triggered controlled breath). In the other modes of partial ventilatory support, each spontaneous inspiratory effort is assisted by a

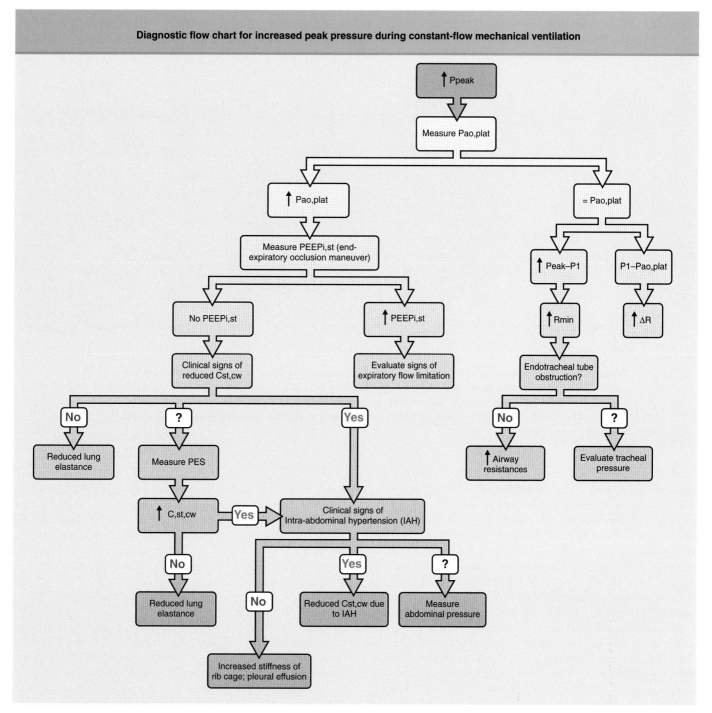

Figure 15.9. The differential diagnosis of a decreased respiratory system compliance requires the partitioning between lung and chest wall mechanical properties.

positive pressure applied by the ventilator. The level of pressure assist may be preset, such as in pressure support ventilation (PSV), or variable according to instantaneous estimation of the inspiratory effort, such as in proportional assist ventilation. A promising experimental mode of partial ventilatory support is based on measurement of the diaphragm's electromiographic signal through a set of electrodes positioned in the esophagus (neurally adjusted ventilatory assistance). In the partially assisted ventilatory modes, delivered flow and volume depend on the interaction between the patient's effort, the algorithm of positive pressure assistance, and mechanical characteristics of the respiratory system.

Static and Dynamic Intrinsic PEEP
During partial ventilatory assist mode, it is important to monitor intrinsic PEEP. A noninvasive measurement of PEEPtot may be obtained by recording the Pao tracing during a prolonged end-expiratory pause, while the patient makes some breathing

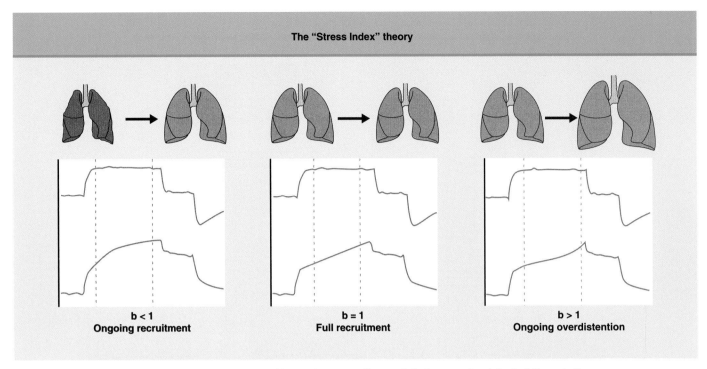

The "Stress Index" theory

b < 1
Ongoing recruitment

b = 1
Full recruitment

b > 1
Ongoing overdistention

Figure 15.10. Tidal alveolar recruitment/derecruitment and/or overinflation may be detected through the analysis of the Pao-t profile during the period of constant-flow inflation. A downward Pao-t concavity indicates a progressive increase in compliance during tidal inflation due to ongoing alveolar recruitment with inflation, whereas an upward Pao-t concavity indicates progressive decreases in compliance during tidal inflation due to ongoing alveolar overinflation with inflation.

attempts against the occluded airways (Fig. 15.11). Assuming that between two breathing attempts respiratory muscles are relaxed, in that moment the Pao value corresponds to PEEPtot. The accuracy of this method (originally proposed by Gottfried and coworkers) is critically dependent on the operator's experience: In some patients, the period of muscular relaxation may be too short to allow a correct PEEPtot measurement. In addition, if there is expiratory muscle activation during the end-expiratory occlusion, the measurement of PEEPtot is unreliable.

The gold standard in patients receiving partial ventilatory assistance is the invasive measurement of dynamic intrinsic PEEP (PEEPi,dyn). The method is based on the continuous measurement of flow, Pao, Pes, and eventually gastric pressure (Fig. 15.12). In order to generate an inspiratory flow, a dynamically hyperinflated patient must create a negative pleural pressure that is the opposite of intrinsic PEEP. Consequently, PEEPi,dyn is the value of Pes deflection from the beginning of the inspiratory effort to the point at which a positive inspiratory flow begins. An important prerequisite for this method is the correct identification of the inspiratory effort starting point on the Pes tracing. If the patient does not make any expiratory effort, the beginning of the inspiratory effort may be easily identified by an experienced operator, since Pes suddenly changes its slope at the beginning of the inspiratory muscle contraction (see Fig. 15.12). On the other hand, if the patient activates his or her expiratory muscles, the exact point at which inspiration begins cannot be identified from the Pes tracing alone since the sudden change in decay in Pes at the beginning of inspiration may depend on the termination of the expiratory effort and/or the start of the inspi-

ratory effort. Consequently, it is virtually impossible to identify the exact point at which inspiratory effort starts, unless expiratory muscle activity is measured. This may be done directly through electromyography of the transversus abdominis muscle or indirectly by recording the transdiaphragmatic pressure tracing (obtained from digital subtraction of esophageal to gastric pressure).

Work of Breathing

Work of breathing (WOB) may be partitioned into its physiological components: resistive, elastic and inertial, and additional "distorting" work, applied to move the chest wall and displace abdominal organs through the diaphragm.

WOB (expressed in joules) is performed whenever pressure (P) changes the volume (V) of the respiratory system:

$$WOB = P \times V \qquad \text{(Equation 16)}$$

WOB measurements may be referred to a single breath, but from a clinical standpoint it is useful to measure WOB per minute and WOB per liter of minute ventilation (WOB/liter = WOB per minute/minute ventilation). In a normal subject, the total WOB/liter at rest is between 0.3 and 0.6 J/liter. During invasive partial ventilatory support, the patient needs to perform additional "iatrogenic" work, which is wasted, to overcome the endotracheal tube and ventilatory circuit resistance and to trigger the ventilator.

Measurement of WOB during partial ventilatory support requires the recording of Pes and, eventually, gastric pressure. A

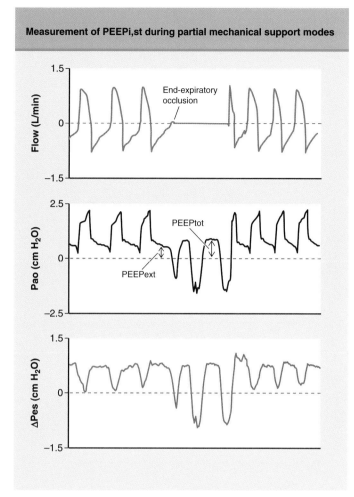

Measurement of PEEPi,st during partial mechanical support modes

Figure 15.11. Flow, Pao, and Pes tracings recorded during a prolonged end-expiratory pause. PEEPtot is measured as the Pao value read between two breathing attempts against the occluded airways.

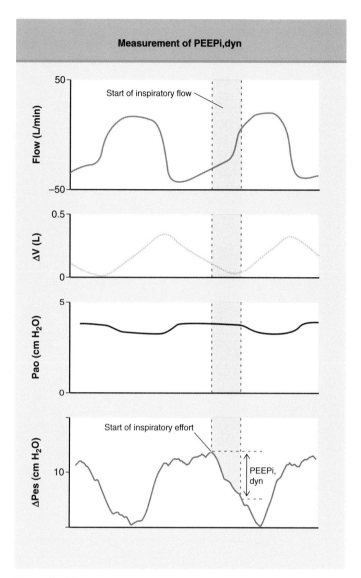

Measurement of PEEPi,dyn

Figure 15.12. Flow, volume, Pao, and Pes tracings recorded in a spontaneously breathing patient receiving positive continuous airway pressure. PEEPi,dyn is the value of Pes deflection from the beginning of the inspiratory effort to the point at which a positive inspiratory flow begins.

simple WOB estimation may be obtained by superimposing on the same pressure–time axes Pes tracings obtained during passive inflation (the static elastic recoil pressure of the chest wall) and during assisted breathing, respectively (Fig. 15.13). In fact, the area between these two tracings, measured as the difference between the time integral of each tracing [pressure–time integral (PTP)], has been proved to have a good correlation with the oxygen consumption of inspiratory muscles and hence may be used to estimate WOB. Knowing the Est,cw value (as estimated in a trial of CMV through the occlusion method) and assuming a linear Est,cw value in the tidal volume range, the static elastic recoil pressure of the chest wall is obtained by multiplying Est,cw for the instantaneous volume. Again, the correct identification of the inspiratory effort starting point is crucial for correct positioning of the static elastic recoil Pes tracing. As discussed previously, in patients with dynamic hyperinflation and/or expiratory muscle activation, it may be difficult or even impossible to determine this point. Jubran and coworkers (1995) proposed a brilliant solution to this problem by considering two separate hypotheses (Fig. 15.14). First, if dynamic hyperinflation is present, the sudden decrease in Pes that occurs

before the onset of positive flow depends on the inspiratory muscle contraction in order to overcome intrinsic PEEP and the static elastic recoil Pes tracing has to be superimposed on the spontaneous Pes tracing (upper bound of inspiratory PTP). Second, if dynamic hyperinflation is not present but the patient makes an active expiratory effort, the static chest wall recoil pressure should be superimposed on the spontaneous Pes tracing at a point corresponding to the onset of inspiratory flow (lower bound of inspiratory PTP).

Estimating WOB is useful to determine an optimal level of ventilatory support, which should normalize inspiratory muscle workloads and avoid excessive unloading (overassistance). The optimal PTP/min range during mechanically supported breathing is between 100 and 125 cm H_2O × sec/min.

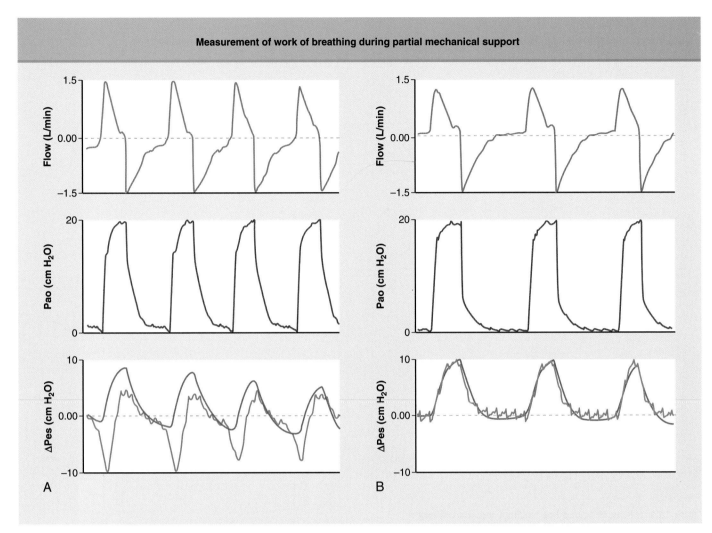

Measurement of work of breathing during partial mechanical support

A

B

Figure 15.13. Flow, Pao, and Pes tracings recorded during pressure support ventilation. In order to estimate the patient's work of breathing, the static elastic recoil pressure of the chest wall (blue line) has been superimposed on the Pes tracing measured during mechanically assisted breathing (orange line). The area between the two tracings is proportional to the spontaneous work of breathing. The patient performs a discrete work of breathing in panel A and is substantially passive (excluding a minimum effort wasted to trigger the ventilator) in panel B.

Respiratory Mechanics

Estimating the values of elastance and resistance during partial mechanical support is feasible by applying the equation of motion:

$$Pmus + Pappl = (volume \times E) + (flow \times R) + PEEPtot$$
$$\text{(Equation 17)}$$

where Pmus is the pressure generated by the patient's inspiratory muscles, and Pappl is the pressure applied by the ventilator. A reliable estimation of Pmus is commonly obtained through the measurement of transdiaphragmatic pressure (Pdi):

$$Pdi = Pes - Pga \qquad \text{(Equation 18)}$$

where Pdi is the deflection in pressure generated by diaphragm contraction, and gastric pressure (Pga) is measured through a balloon-tipped catheter similar to the one used for Pes mea-

surement, placed in the stomach. Due to its invasiveness and complexity, this method is limited almost exclusively to clinical research.

MONITORING GAS EXCHANGE DURING MECHANICAL VENTILATION

Repeated measurements of arterial blood gases (ABGs) are mandatory in order to assess the efficacy of mechanical ventilation. Pulse oxymetry and capnography add useful information and are essential parts of basic monitoring in ventilated patient.

ABGs are usually obtained at the beginning of mechanical ventilation and after any ventilatory setting change. Partial arterial oxygen pressure (PaO_2) variations in response to an inspired oxygen fraction (FIO_2) change are expected to occur within 10 minutes. Reaching a new equilibrium in gas exchange after variations in breathing pattern or PEEP levels may take longer (15–30 min). Instantaneous measurements of PaO_2 and

Estimation of "upper" and "lower" bounds of work of breathing

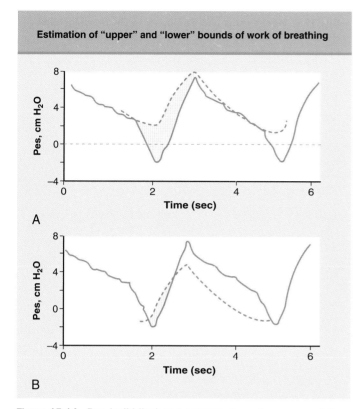

A

B

Figure 15.14. Pes (solid line) and estimated recoil pressure of the chest wall (Pes,cw, dashed line) tracings in a patient receiving PSV. *A,* Pressure tracings have been superimposed so that Pes,cw is equal to Pes at the onset of the inspiratory effort based on the hypothesis that the patient is dynamically hyperinflated. The integrated difference between the two tracings (hatched area) represents the upper bound inspiratory PTP. *B,* Pressure tracings have been superimposed so that Pes,cw is equal to Pes at the beginning of inspiratory flow, assuming that the patient is not hyperinflated. The integrated difference between the two tracings (hatched area) represents the lower bound inspiratory PTP. (Adapted from Jubran A, Van de Graaff WB, Tobin MJ: Variability of patient-ventilator interaction with pressure support ventilation in patients with COPD. Am J Respir Crit Care Med 1995;152:129–136.)

$PaCO_2$ are feasible through intraarterial devices. Baumgardner and coworkers (2002) used an ultra-fast response fiberoptic fluorescence-quenching PO_2 probe to measure the PaO_2 oscillations induced by mechanical ventilation in surfactant-depleted lungs. In their model, PaO_2 decreased at end expiration due to alveolar collapse and increased at end inspiration due to alveolar opening.

Pulse oximetry allows noninvasive measurement of arterial blood saturation in O_2 (SaO_2). Its working principle relies on the differences in light wave absorption spectra between oxyhemoglobin (O_2 Hb) and reduced hemoglobin (Hb). The red wavelengths (660 nm) are preferentially absorbed by Hb, whereas the infrared wavelengths (940 nm) are preferentially absorbed by O_2 Hb. In the presence of a pulsatile arterial blood flow, the ratio between 660 and 940 nm wavelengths absorbencies is measured and compared using a calibration algorithm based on measurements previously obtained in healthy volunteers. SaO_2 monitoring has paramount importance in the intensive care unit and anesthesia setting, but the method has some limitations: (1) accuracy deteriorates when SaO_2 falls to 80% or less; (2) motion

Phases of time capnogram during controlled mechanical ventilation

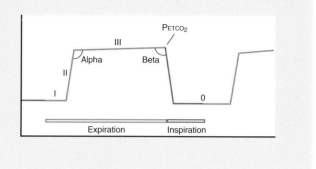

Figure 15.15. Morphologic pattern of the time capnogram in a patient receiving constant-flow mechanical ventilation.

artifacts may affect the measurement, although software for digital stabilization of the signal is available; (3) during low perfusion states, the pulsatile signal is lost and the SaO_2 reading is unavailable; (4) elevated carboxyhemoglobin and methemoglobin levels are not revealed and may cause inaccurate SaO_2 readings; (5) methylene blue and indocyanine administered as intravenous dyes can cause falsely low SaO_2 readings; (6) fluorescent and xenon arch surgical lamps may influence SaO_2 readings; and (7) in more pigmented patients, SaO_2 readings may be inaccurate.

Capnometry is the instantaneous measurement of CO_2 concentration and/or partial pressure at the airway opening. The majority of CO_2 analyzers are infrared (IR) spectrophotometers, and their working principle is based on the IR absorption pattern of CO_2 molecules since they specifically absorb the IR wavelengths of 4.3 μm. Time capnography is the graphic display of instantaneous CO_2 concentration versus time during the respiratory cycle. The time capnogram of a patient receiving constant flow mechanical ventilation has a typical morphologic pattern (Fig. 15.15):

Phase 0 is the inspiratory segment, whose normal value is zero, since the concentration of CO_2 in the inspired gas is negligible; values higher than zero suggest CO_2 rebreathing.

Phase I represents the CO_2-free gas coming from the anatomical dead space at the very beginning of expiration; this gas virtually does not participate in the alveolar gas exchange and therefore has a very low CO_2 concentration.

Phase II is a rapid, S-shaped upswing on the CO_2 tracing occurring as soon as the alveolar CO_2-rich gas reaches the spectrophotometer. Phase II slope is increased in the case of bronchospasm or endotracheal tube kinking.

Phase III depends on the ongoing outflow of alveolar CO_2-rich gas. In a normal subject, it shows a slightly positive slope, mainly due to differences in ventilation:perfusion ratio and time constants (τ) between different lung.

Alpha angle is the angle between phases II and III.

End tidal CO_2 is the partial pressure of CO_2 at the end of phase III (end of tidal expiration). The $PaCO_2$–$PETCO_2$ gradient is proportional to the alveolar dead space and its normal value is 1 to 5 mm Hg lower than $PaCO_2$.

147

Box 15.1 Mechanisms and Etiologies to Be Considered in the Differential Diagnosis of PETCO₂ Decrease during Mechanical Ventilation

$\downarrow$ **PETCO₂**

$\downarrow$ CO₂ output	$\downarrow$ Pulmonary perfusion
Hypothermia	Reduced cardiac output
Anesthesia	
Hypothyroidism	
	Hypovolemia
	Pulmonary embolism
	Cardiac arrest
$\uparrow$ Alveolar ventilation	Technical errors
Hyperventilation	Circuit disconnection
Apnea	
	Sampling tube leak
	Malfunction of ventilator
	Total airway obstruction
	Partial airway obstruction
	Accidental tracheal extubation

Box 15.2 Mechanisms and Etiologies to Be Considered in the Differential Diagnosis of PETCO₂ Increase during Mechanical Ventilation

$\uparrow$ **PETCO₂**

$\uparrow$ CO₂ output	$\uparrow$ Pulmonary perfusion
Light anesthesia	Increased cardiac output
Fever	
Malignant hyperthermia	
Hyperthyroidism	
Sodium bicarbonate	
Tourniquet release	
$\downarrow$ Alveolar ventilation	Technical errors/machine faults
Hypoventilation	Exhausted CO₂ absorber
Bronchial intubation	Inadequate fresh gas flows
Partial airway obstruction	Leaks in breathing system
Rebreathing	Faulty ventilator
	Faulty valves

Beta angle is a nearly 90° angle between phase III and phase 0 that occurs when fresh CO₂ free gas is delivered to the patient at the beginning of phase 0. Monitoring PETCO₂ gives important clinical information, that is summarized in Boxes 15.1 and 15.2.

SUGGESTED READING

Baumgardner JE, Markstakker K, Pfeiffer B, et al: Effects of respiratory rate, airway pressure and positive end expiratory pressure on PaO₂ oscillations after saline lavage. Am J Respir Crit Care Med 2002;166:1556–1562.

Baydur A, Behrakis PK, Zin WA, Jaeger M, Milic-Emili J: A simple method for assessing the validity of the esophageal balloon technique. Am Rev Respir Dis 1982;126:788–791.

Bhavani-Shankar Kodali: Capnography. A comprehensive educational website. www.capnography.com (accessed December 2004).

D'Angelo E, Calderini E, Torri G, et al: Respiratory mechanics in anesthetized–paralyzed humans: Effect of flow, volume and time. J Appl Physiol 1989;67:2556–2564.

Dreyfuss D, Saumon G: Ventilator induced lung injury: Lessons from experimental studies. Am J Respir Crit Care Med: 1998;157:294–323.

Gottfried SB, Reissman H, Ranieri VM: A simple method for the measurement of intrinsic positive end-expiratory pressure during controlled and assisted modes of mechanical ventilation. Crit Care Med 1992;20(5):621–629.

Grasso S, Terragni P, Mascia L, et al: Airway pressure–time curve profile (stress index) detects tidal recruitment/hyperinflation in experimental acute lung injury. Crit Care Med 2004;32(4):1018–1027.

Jubran A, Van de Graaff WB, Tobin MJ: Variability of patient–ventilator interaction with pressure support ventilation in patients with COPD. Am J Respir Crit Care Med 1995;152:129–136.

Malbrain ML: Abdominal pressure in the critically ill: Measurement and clinical relevance. Intensive Care Med 1999;25(12):1453–1458.

Maltais F, Reissmann H, Navalesi P: Comparison of static and dynamic measurements of intrinsic PEEP in mechanically ventilated patients. Am J Respir Crit Care Med 1994;150:1318–1324.

Ranieri VM, Grasso S, Fiore T, et al: Auto-positive end-expiratory pressure and dynamic hyperinflation. In Nahum A, Marini JJ (eds): Clinics in Chest Medicine-Recent Advances in Mechanical Ventilation. Vol 17.3 Philadelphia, WB Saunders, 1996, pp 379–394.

Tobin MJ, Van De Graaf WB. Monitoring of lung mechanics and work of breathing. In Tobin MJ (ed): Principles and Practice of Mechanical Ventilation. New York, McGraw-Hill, 1994, pp 967–1001.

Chapter 16

Patient–Ventilator Interaction and Weaning

Christian Putensen and Hermann Wrigge

KEY POINTS

- The physiologic rationale for spontaneous breathing in acute lung injury is explained.
- Criteria and an algorithm for weaning from ventilatory support are discussed; ventilator management of a patient who is recovering from acute respiratory failure must balance competing objectives.
- A systematic overview of different principles of partial ventilatory support is presented; ventilatory techniques are grouped according to the type of interaction between spontaneous breathing and mechanical ventilation.
- Although ventilatory modalities designed to support spontaneous breathing were initially developed with the aim of facilitating and accelerating the process of weaning from mechanical ventilation, they are increasingly being deployed as the primary modes of ventilation, even in patients in the acute phase of pulmonary dysfunction.
- Classification of different forms of patient–ventilator interactions is presented.

In recent years, developments in mechanical ventilation have resulted in a plethora of ventilatory modalities and techniques, all aimed at supporting spontaneous breathing. Many of these partial ventilatory support techniques differ only minimally from one another, both physically and physiologically, and cannot therefore be expected to produce significantly different treatment results. In the absence of large-scale comparative studies, the clinician is left to decide for him- or herself whether, when, and how to employ these ventilatory modalities to support a patient's inadequate attempts at spontaneous breathing.

Although the ventilation modes designed to support spontaneous breathing were initially developed with the aim of facilitating and accelerating the process of weaning from mechanical ventilation, they are increasingly being deployed as the primary modes of ventilation, even in patients in the acute phase of pulmonary dysfunction.

PRINCIPLES OF USE OF PARTIAL VENTILATORY SUPPORT

Patient ventilator interactions during partial ventilatory support can be described by different principles. To be able to use a ventilation mode that supports inadequate spontaneous breathing, it should be possible to infinitely vary the level of mechanical support between 0 and 100%. The following classification groups the ventilatory techniques according to the type of interaction between spontaneous breathing and mechanical ventilation:

Modulation of tidal volume (VT) through mechanical support of each breath-assisted ventilation: Every spontaneous attempt at inspiration should be mechanically supported by the ventilator. Although spontaneous inspiration is supported mechanically in different ways in different ventilation modes, an increase in the patient's respiratory rate, brought about by increased ventilatory demand, will always result in more mechanical support. Conversely, reduction in respiratory rate will lead to a reduction in ventilatory support, which in the case of apnea will be nil. Such ventilation modes thus do not permit infinitely variable support of spontaneous breathing. Stable spontaneous breathing and a sensitive synchronization mechanism are essential preconditions in these modes to ensure adequate alveolar ventilation and reduced work of breathing. This principle is applied during assist controlled ventilation (ACV), pressure support ventilation (PSV), proportional assist ventilation (PAV), and automatic tube compensation (ATC).

Modulation of the minute volume through the intermittent application of mechanical breaths in addition to nonassisted spontaneous breathing: In these modes, mechanical ventilatory support is constant and does not depend on the inspiratory efforts of the patient. Increased ventilatory demand does not result in any change in the level of mechanical support. However, by regulating the mechanical ventilatory rate, infinitely variable support of spontaneous breathing from 0% to 100% is possible. In the event of apnea, the set minute volume, at least, will be applied. However, since the patient can only breathe spontaneously between the mechanical breaths, normally at the set continuous positive airway pressure (CPAP) level, the opportunity for free spontaneous breathing decreases as the rate of mechanical ventilation increases. One example of the application of this method is intermittent mandatory ventilation (IMV).

149

Modulation of the minute volume by switching between two airway pressure levels with the opportunity for free spontaneous breathing at any time: Mechanical ventilation and spontaneous breathing are uncoupled. Changes in ventilatory demand do not result in any change in the level of mechanical support. By regulating the mechanical ventilation frequency and ventilation pressures, infinitely variable support of spontaneous breathing between 0% and 100% is possible. Because time-cycled switching between two CPAP levels supports spontaneous breathing, virtually unhindered spontaneous breathing is possible during any phase of the mechanical ventilatory cycle. This principle is applied during airway pressure release ventilation (APRV) and biphasic positive airway pressure (BIPAP).

Combinations of the techniques described previously: Many commercially available ventilators offer hybrid modes of ventilation, such as IMV + PSV, IMV + ATC, intermittent mandatory pressure release ventilation (IMPRV), BIPAP + PSV, BIPAP + ATC, and PAV + ATC. Although incorporated into many ventilators, very few of these ventilation modes that support spontaneous breathing have been shown to improve results in the treatment of patients. This is especially true of the increasingly popular combinations of different ventilation modalities that support spontaneous breathing and that, supposedly, utilize all the benefits of the individual ventilation methods for the patient. It remains doubtful, however, whether simply combining different methods of ventilation results in the addition of their positive effects. On the contrary, the possibility cannot be ruled out that the proven physiologic effects of one method of ventilation might be minimized or even abolished by combining it with another method. For instance, during IMPRV, a combination of APRV + PSV, overdistention of lung areas and an increase in dead-space ventilation with reduced CO_2 elimination may be produced by applying additional pressure support at the upper CPAP level. It appears to make more sense to use the currently available partial ventilatory support modalities selectively on the basis of the effects observed during their application, with the goal being to apply ventilation modes that support spontaneous breathing in accordance with their physiologic and pathophysiologic principles.

INDICATIONS AND CONTRAINDICATIONS

Traditionally, the first step toward combating acute respiratory failure is to apply controlled mechanical ventilation to ensure full alveolar ventilation and to perform the work of breathing on the patient's behalf until such time as the underlying respiratory function disorder (e.g., acute respiratory failure and chronic obstructive pulmonary disease) can be eliminated or improved. The criteria used to determine when to terminate mechanical ventilation are essentially based on the clinical and, often, subjective assessment of the attending intensive care physician or on standardized weaning protocols. The actual process of weaning the patient from mechanical ventilation is carried out by allowing spontaneous breathing attempts with a T-piece or CPAP or by gradually reducing mechanical assistance through the use of a ventilation mode that supports spontaneous breath-

ing. The benefit of this latter method of weaning, however, has only been demonstrated in patients unable to tolerate unassisted spontaneous breathing for a sufficiently long period.

Contraindications for Assisted Spontaneous Breathing

There is no conclusive evidence that controlled mechanical ventilation is more beneficial than a ventilation mode that supports spontaneous breathing, so long as the latter guarantees sufficient alveolar ventilation and reduces the work of breathing. Thus, controlled mechanical ventilation only appears to be indicated in patients with apnea or when apnea needs to be induced for therapeutic reasons (e.g., in the event of intracranial pressure increase or surgery).

Rationale for Maintained Spontaneous Breathing
Pulmonary Gas Exchange
Radiological studies demonstrate how ventilation is distributed differently during pure spontaneous breathing and controlled mechanical ventilation. During spontaneous breathing, the posterior muscular sections of the diaphragm move more than the anterior tendon plate. Consequently, in patients in the supine position, the dependent lung regions tend to be better ventilated, and better perfused, during spontaneous breathing. If, however, the diaphragm is relaxed, it will be pushed by the weight of the abdominal cavity toward the cranium, and the mechanical tidal volume will be distributed more to the anterior, less perfused lung regions. This leads to underventilation and atelectasis in the dorsal regions close to the diaphragm in patients who have healthy or abnormal lungs. This is coupled with an increase in venous admixture, an impaired ventilation–perfusion matching, and deterioration in arterial oxygenation. When spontaneous breathing is allowed during mechanical ventilation, it should increase ventilation to poorly or nonventilated areas of lung and so reduce the ventilation–perfusion mismatch.

In patients with acute respiratory distress syndrome (ARDS), unhindered spontaneous breathing during APRV/BIPAP leads to a considerable increase in arterial oxygenation by reduction flow of blood to nonventilated areas of the lung (shunt areas). Animal studies revealed comparable results regarding improvement in arterial oxygenation and suggested recruitment of previously nonaerated lung regions with improvement in end-expiratory lung volume as the main mechanism of improved gas exchange during spontaneous breathing with APRV/BIPAP (Fig. 16.1) Redistribution of aeration and ventilation to dependent lung regions close to the diaphragm by spontaneous breathing (Figs. 16.2 and 16.3) is also accompanied by improvement of perfusion of these regions. Clinical studies show, however, that spontaneous breathing during APRV/BIPAP does not necessarily lead to an instant improvement in gas exchange.

In contrast to controlled mechanical ventilation, assisted inspiration with PSV in patients with ARDS does not produce any significant improvement in gas exchange. Because spontaneous breathing can contribute to the recruitment of initially nonaerated lung areas, maintained spontaneous breathing with adequate mechanical support as per conventional ventilation strategies should, in terms of pulmonary gas exchange, be

Spontaneous breathing improves lung volume and oxygenation

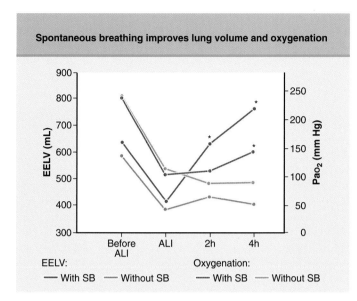

EELV:
— With SB   — Without SB

Oxygenation:
— With SB   — Without SB

Figure 16.1. Spontaneous breathing improves lung volume and oxygenation. Time course of arterial oxygenation and end-expiratory gas volume (EELV; measured by nitrogen washout) in 22 pigs with oleic acid-induced lung injury. Pigs were randomized to receive APRV with or without spontaneous breathing. Asterisks indicate a significant difference between APRV with and without spontaneous breathing (analysis of variance followed by Tukey's post hoc test). ALI, acute lung injury. (For details, see Wrigge H, Zinserling J, Neumann P, et al: Spontaneous breathing improves lung aeration in oleic acid-induced lung injury. Anesthesiology 2003;99:376–384.)

Redistribution of aeration and ventilation to dependent lung areas with spontaneous breathing

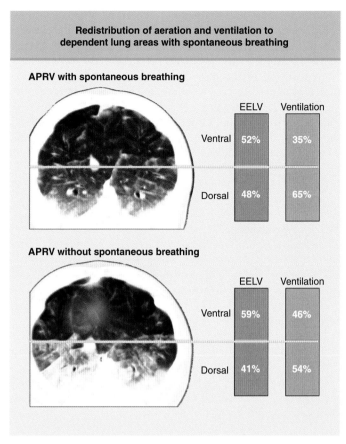

Figure 16.2. Redistribution of aeration and ventilation to dependent lung areas with spontaneous breathing. Transversal computed tomography scans of a pig with oleic acid-induced lung injury ventilated with airway pressure release ventilation (APRV) with (top) and without (bottom) spontaneous breathing. Percentages indicate relative distribution of end-expiratory lung volume (EELV) and ventilation (aeration difference between end-inspiratory and end-expiratory scan of dynamic scan series) of the dependent (dorsal) and nondependent (ventral) lung half of this slice.

Ventilation

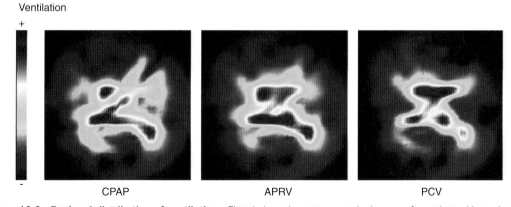

Figure 16.3. Regional distribution of ventilation. Electric impedance tomography images of a patient with moderate acute respiratory failure. The color-coded scale *(left)* indicates maximum impedance changes (red) to minimum impedance changes (blue) as surrogate for ventilation changes. Images show ventilatory modalities with an decreasing amount of spontaneous breathing from left to right [pure spontaneous breathing with continuous positive airway pressure (CPAP), partial support with airway pressure release ventilation (APRV), and full ventilatory support with pressure-controlled ventilation (PCV)]. Note that ventilation during spontaneous breathing with CPAP is less distributed to ventral lung regions, whereas during controlled ventilation impedance changes occur predominantly in ventral lung zones.

superior to controlled ventilation followed by weaning with respiratory support. Studies show that in polytraumatized patients who are at high risk of developing ARDS, maintained spontaneous breathing with APRV/BIPAP results in lower venous admixture and better arterial oxygenation over an observation period of more than 10 days compared to controlled ventilation with subsequent weaning. The incidence of atelectasis and pulmonary dysfunction is lower during maintained spontaneous breathing with APRV/BIPAP. These results clearly show that even in patients requiring mechanical ventilation, maintained and unhindered spontaneous breathing can counteract the progressive deterioration in pulmonary gas exchange as a result of alveolar collapse.

Work of Breathing

The aim in supporting spontaneous breathing mechanically is to reduce the work of breathing, which is increased as a result of pulmonary or extrapulmonary dysfunction, to a level that is normal or acceptable for the patient's general condition. This goal must be accorded the highest priority when respiratory failure is caused primarily by the insufficiency of the respiratory pump (i.e., the thoracic wall including respiratory muscles and the controlling respiratory neurons in the central nervous system).

None of the ventilation modes that control the minute volume by intermittently applying mechanical breaths (e.g., IMV and APRV/BIPAP) support the patient's spontaneous breathing activities. In such modes, spontaneous breathing normally takes place at a level of lung volume that is determined by the CPAP level. This enables lung volume to be recruited and the work of breathing to be decreased in patients who have a decreased functional residual capacity (FRC) as a consequence of expiratory alveolar collapse or atelectasis formation. When a patient with a reduced FRC breathes, a higher transpulmonary pressure is required to maintain a normal tidal volume. Increased transpulmonary pressure goes hand in hand with a rise in the elastic work of breathing. In such a situation, the patient will reduce the tidal volume, increase the respiratory rate, and recruit the auxiliary respiratory muscles. Attempts to reduce the work of breathing by employing mechanical ventilation are often made in this situation, although a more rational approach is to increase the FRC (e.g., by applying CPAP), which increases compliance and reduces the work of breathing. Clinical studies have demonstrated that oxygen consumption in patients with mild to severe ARDS and with recruitable lung areas does not increase as a result of spontaneous breathing with IMV or APRV/BIPAP. If, in such patients, nonassisted spontaneous breathing during APRV/BIPAP is compared with assisted ventilation with PSV, no significant differences in terms of oxygen consumption are apparent. A direct comparison of the work of breathing during APRV/BIPAP or IMV and during assisted ventilation with PSV is difficult for methodological and technical reasons. These forms of ventilation appear to be less well suited to patients primarily suffering from an inadequate respiratory pump who are experiencing problems weaning from mechanical ventilation due to muscle fatigue.

In patients suffering primarily from an inadequate respiratory pump, the overriding objective should be to apply an assisted form of ventilation that reduces the work of breathing for each spontaneous breath. In patients with chronic obstructive pul-

monary disease (COPD), several clinical studies have revealed a reduction in the work of breathing and oxygen consumption as pressure support with PSV is increased. A high degree of pressure support during PSV, however, can, as a result of the large applied V_T, lead to an increase in intrinsic positive end-expiratory pressure (PEEPi) in patients with COPD and expiratory gas flow limitation. In this case, patients cannot reduce the airway opening pressure or generate an inspiratory gas flow sufficient to trigger the ventilator, no matter how hard they try. Despite massive respiratory efforts, the patient receives no mechanical support for his or her respiratory activity ("missing breaths"), and oxygen consumption rises. Discrepancies between the respiratory rate apparent from the patient's breathing excursions and the rate displayed by the ventilator are a good indicator of missing breaths. During PSV, the inspiration termination criterion of 25% of the maximum inspiratory gas flow can lead to asynchrony between spontaneous breathing and mechanical ventilation, resulting in an increase in the work of breathing and oxygen demand. Exact adjustment of the PSV settings and clinical observation of the patient are essential at all times to avoid such deleterious interactions between spontaneous breathing and mechanical ventilation in PSV.

Cardiovascular Side Effects

The application of a mechanical ventilator breath generates an increase in airway and, therefore, intrathoracic pressure, which in turn reduces the venous return to the heart. In normo- and hypovolemic patients, this produces a reduction in right and left ventricular filling and results in decreased stroke volume, cardiac output, and O_2 transport capacity. In order to normalize the systemic blood flow during mechanical ventilation, blood volume often needs to be increased and/or the cardiovascular system needs pharmacological support. Reducing mechanical ventilation to a level that provides adequate support for existing spontaneous breathing should help to reduce the cardiovascular side effects of mechanical ventilation.

The periodic reduction of intrathoracic pressure resulting from maintained spontaneous breathing during mechanical ventilatory support promotes the venous return to the heart and right and left ventricular filling, thereby increasing cardiac output and O_2 transport capacity. During IMV and APRV/BIPAP, spontaneous breathing of 10% to 40% of the total minute ventilation increases cardiac output. A simultaneous rise in right ventricular end-diastolic volume during spontaneous breathing in APRV/BIPAP is an indication of improved venous return to the heart. Conversely, mechanical support of each individual inspiration with PSV produces no increase or very little increase in cardiac output.

Theoretically, augmentation of the venous return to the heart and increased left ventricular afterload as a result of reduced intrathoracic pressure should have a negative impact on cardiovascular function in patients with left ventricular dysfunction. Indeed, switching abruptly from CMV to PSV with a simultaneous reduction in ventilation pressures can lead to decompensation of existing cardiac insufficiency. However, provided that spontaneous breathing receives adequate support and sufficient CPAP is applied, the maintenance of spontaneous breathing should not prove disadvantageous and, therefore, is not contraindicated even in patients with acute myocardial infarction and cardiac failure.

Organ Perfusion

By reducing cardiac output and the venous return to the heart, mechanical ventilation can have a negative effect on the circulation of the blood and, therefore, on the functioning of other organ systems.

In the kidney, the reduction in cardiac output and venous return causes, via a sympathoadrenergic reaction, vasoconstriction of the afferent renal arterioles with reduction and redistribution of the renal blood flow from the cortical to the juxtaglomerular nephrons. This reduces the glomerular filtration rate and sodium excretion. The reduction in renal blood flow and increase in sodium content result at the macula densa, in conjunction with sympathoadrenergic stimulation, in activation of the renin–angiotensin aldosterone system, which increases renal vasoconstriction and further slows the glomerular filtration rate and sodium excretion. As a result of stimulation of baroreceptors in the aorta, a drop in transmural blood pressure and the number of stretch receptors in the left atrium, and lower intrathoracic blood volume, arginine vasopressin is released, causing vasoconstriction and the reabsorption of water at the distal tubules. At the same time, less atrial natriuretic peptide, an arginine vasopressin antagonist, is released because there is less expansion of the atria. The increase in venous return and cardiac output, brought about by a rhythmic reduction in intrathoracic pressure during maintained spontaneous breathing, should significantly improve kidney perfusion and function during ventilation.

In patients with ARDS, spontaneous breathing supported by IMV leads to an increase in glomerular filtration rate and sodium excretion. These results are corroborated by clinical data that show that there is an increase in kidney perfusion and glomerular filtration rate during spontaneous breathing with APRV/BIPAP in patients with ARDS compared to patients on pressure-limited ventilation.

Similarly, a reduction of cardiac output and venous return causes, via a sympathoadrenergic reaction, vasoconstriction and lower blood flow in the portal vein and, consequently, the liver. The same mechanism is responsible for a reduced perfusion of the splanchnic area.

TECHNIQUES AND EQUIPMENT

Analgosedation

In addition to ensuring sufficient pain relief and anxiolysis, the aim of analgosedation is to help the patient adapt to mechanical ventilation. Usually, the level of analgosedation required during controlled ventilation is equivalent to a Ramsay score of 5—that is, a deeply sedated patient who is unable to respond when spoken to and has no sensation of pain.

Conversely, when a ventilation mode is used that supports spontaneous breathing, a Ramsay score of 2 or 3 can be targeted (i.e., an awake, responsive, and cooperative patient). In a retrospective study of approximately 600 heart surgery patients, a reduction in consumption of analgesics and sedatives was observed when patients were allowed to breathe spontaneously from an early stage with APRV/BIPAP. Preliminary data show that maintaining spontaneous breathing with APRV/BIPAP in polytraumatized patients over an observation period of more than 10 days leads to significantly lower consumption of analgesics and sedatives than is the case with initially controlled

ventilation for 71 hours following by weaning. Obviously, a large part of analgosedation is used exclusively to adapt patients to controlled mechanical ventilation. Both from a medical and from an economic standpoint, it therefore appears sensible to provide mechanical support with spontaneous breathing.

Setting Ventilation Pressures and Tidal Volumes

Particularly in ARDS patients undergoing mechanical ventilation, which avoids end-expiratory alveolar collapse and end-inspiratory overdistention of the lung, clinical studies indicate less damage to the lung structure and lower mortality rates. In this context, it is important to stress that the improvement in pulmonary gas exchange is brought about by means of spontaneous breathing in APRV/BIPAP with a low CPAP level above the lower inflection point and a high CPAP level below the upper deflection point of the static pressure/volume curve of the respiratory system. Moreover, pulmonary compliance in this range of ventilatory pressures is greatest, which means that spontaneous breathing is efficient even with minimal respiratory effort. Maintained spontaneous breathing can improve gas exchange without any further increase in ventilation pressures, even when the mechanical ventilation is optimal in terms of lung–mechanics criteria. Although maintained spontaneous breathing in APRV/BIPAP, like controlled ventilation, is also able to maintain gas exchange when the ventilation pressure is reduced, it is not always possible to prevent atelectasis formation in the long term. In other words, maintained spontaneous breathing still requires optimal setting of the ventilation parameters.

Weaning and Discontinuation of Mechanical Ventilation

Whereas weaning from mechanical ventilation should start as early as possible (ideally with intubation), weaning in a stronger sense (also termed discontinuation of mechanical ventilation) was suggested to be considered only if the patient fulfills certain criteria (Box 16.1). Ventilator management of a patient who is recovering from acute respiratory failure must balance competing objectives. Discontinuing mechanical ventilation and removing the artificial airway as soon as possible reduces the risk of ventilator-induced lung injury, nosocomial pneumonia, airway

---

Box 16.1 Criteria for Discontinuing Mechanical Ventilation

1. Evidence of some reversal of the underlying cause of respiratory failure.
2. Adequate oxygenation: $PaO_2/FIO_2 \geq 150$ to 200 mm Hg, required PEEP ≤ 5 to 8 cm H_2O, $FIO_2 \leq 0.4$ to 0.5, and pH ≥ 7.25.
3. Hemodynamic stability as defined by the absence of clinically important hypotension and requiring no vasopressors or only low-dose vasopressors (e.g., dopamine or dobutamine < 5 $\mu g/kg/min$).
4. Patient is able to initiate an inspiratory effort.

PaO_2/FIO_2, ratio of arterial partial pressure of oxygen to fraction of inspired oxygen; PEEP, positive end-expiratory pressure.
These criteria refer to discontinuation of mechanical ventilation and not to using assisted spontaneous breathing. The decision to use these criteria must be individualized. Some patients who do not satisfy all the criteria may nevertheless be ready for an attempt to discontinue mechanical ventilation.

trauma from the endotracheal tube, and unnecessary sedation, but premature ventilator discontinuation or extubation can cause ventilatory muscle fatigue, gas exchange failure, and loss of airway protection. Before discontinuation of mechanical ventilation in a ventilated patient whose disease process has begun to stabilize and/or reverse can be considered, several major issues for patient management should be considered. First, it is necessary to understand all the reasons the patient continues to require mechanical ventilation (e.g., abnormal gas exchange, respiratory system mechanics, neuromuscular dysfunction, and/or cardiac compromise). Continued treatment of all the identified reasons is obviously integral to any ventilator discontinuation strategy. Second, the clinician needs to use assessment techniques to identify whether the patient can tolerate ventilator withdrawal. Third, if the patient continues to require ventilatory support, the appropriate ventilator management strategies must be employed. Fourth, for a patient who most likely will remain ventilator dependent for a longer period of time, an extended management plan is needed.

A task force of the American College of Chest Physicians, the Society for Critical Care Medicine, and the American Association for Respiratory Care that defined evidence-based medicine guidelines for weaning from mechanical ventilation provided recommendations that are given in brief in Box 16.2.

A key question is whether gradually lowering the level of support (weaning) offers advantage over providing a stable, unchanging level of support between spontaneous breathing trials (SBTs). The arguments for using gradual support reduction are that (1) that placing some ventilatory load on the patient may provide muscle conditioning and (2) that the transition to extubation or SBT may be easier from a low level of support than from a high level. Few data support either of these claims, however. On the other hand, maintaining a stable support level between SBTs reduces the risk of precipitating ventilatory muscle overload from overly aggressive support reduction. A stable support level also has the advantage of requiring far less practitioner time. A study by Esteban and colleagues (1995) partially addressed this issue; it compared daily SBTs (and a stable level of support for those who failed SBT) to two other approaches that used gradual support reductions (weaning with pressure support and intermittent mandatory ventilation). Daily SBT with stable support in between SBTs provided the most rapid ventilator discontinuation (see Box 16.2, recommendation 5). An example of an algorithm for discontinuation of mechanical ventilation is given in Figure 16.4. What has not been addressed is whether a strategy of gradual support reduction coupled with daily SBT offers any advantage. Other randomized trials that compared gradual reduction strategies using different modes but not daily SBTs found that the pressure support strategy was easier to reduce than the intermittent mandatory ventilation strategy. None of these studies offer evidence that a gradual support reduction strategy is superior to the strategy of stable support between SBTs, so the clinical focus during the 24 hours after a failed SBT should be on maintaining adequate muscle unloading, optimizing comfort (and thus sedation needs), and avoiding complications.

Ventilators and Ventilatory Modes

Modern standard ventilators designed to provide ventilatory support to patients in the intensive care unit (ICU) are often

---

> ### Box 16.2 Recommendations for Discontinuation of Mechanical Ventilatory Support
>
> **Recommendations for Patients Receiving Mechanical Ventilation for More Than 1 or 2 Days**
>
> 1. If the criteria given in Box 16.1 are satisfied, perform SBT and consider ventilator discontinuation if SBT is tolerated for 30 to 120 min.
> 2. Confirm patient's ability to protect the airway and assess airway patency before removing the artificial airway.
> 3. If the patient fails an SBT, determine and try to correct the reasons why the patient continues to require ventilatory support. Repeat SBT every 24 hr.
> 4. Patients who fail SBT should receive a stable, nonfatiguing, comfortable form of ventilatory support.
> 5. Weaning/discontinuation protocols designed for nonphysician clinicians should be developed and implemented by intensive care units. Protocols should aim to optimize sedation.
> 6. Patients who have failed several discontinuation attempts should be transferred to facilities that have demonstrated success and safety in accomplishing ventilator discontinuation.
> 7. Unless there is evidence of clearly irreversible disease (e.g., high spinal cord injury and advanced amyotrophic lateral sclerosis), a patient who requires prolonged ventilatory support for respiratory failure should not be considered permanently ventilator dependent until 3 months of weaning attempts have failed.
> 8. For a patient who requires prolonged ventilation, the weaning should be slow paced and should include gradually lengthening SBTs.

SBT, spontaneous breathing trial (preferably pure spontaneous breathing). For more details, see MacIntyre NR, Cook DJ, Ely EW Jr, et al: Evidence-based guidelines for weaning and discontinuing ventilator support. A collective task force facilitated by the American College of Chest Physicians; the American Association for Respiratory Care; and the American College of Critical Care Medicine. Chest 2001;120:375S–395S.

---

microprocessor controlled, have low internal resistance, have fast (demand flow) valves and response times, and offer extended monitoring facilities. The latter (e.g., visualized flow tracing, pressure volume loops, and the ability to perform occlusion maneuvers) can help to gain information concerning the pathophysiology of patients' respiratory failure and patient–ventilator interaction and may thereby help to set optimized ventilatory support. During SBTs, patients are either placed on CPAP with a low level of pressure support or disconnected from the ventilator and connected to a T-piece. Although there is no clear evidence favoring one or the other procedure, leaving the patient on the ventilator seems preferable since it allows continuous monitoring of spirometric variables and curves, including alarm routines.

Ventilatory support can be provided by setting either volume or pressure targets. Volume-targeted ventilation is advantageous if controlling minute ventilation is a priority (e.g., to control arterial CO_2 in patients with increased intracranial pressure). Especially in patients with inhomogeneous ventilatory units, decelerating flow characteristic during pressure-targeted ventilation should allow most efficient ventilation with respect to

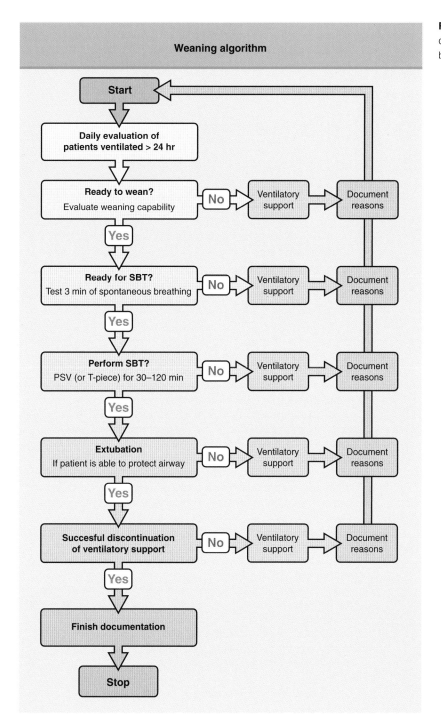

Figure 16.4. Weaning algorithm. Algorithm for discontinuation of ventilatory support. SBT, spontaneous breathing trial; PSV, pressure support ventilation.

maximum airway pressure and inspiratory time. In general, there is no striking evidence to prefer one or the other method with respect to patient outcome measures, and both principles are used worldwide with geographic preferences.

Important factors in achieving patient comfort and minimizing imposed loads include sensitive/responsive ventilator triggering systems, applied PEEP in the presence of a triggering threshold load from auto-PEEP, flow patterns matched to patient demand, and appropriate ventilator cycling to avoid air trapping.

A classification of different forms of patient–ventilator interactions has been presented. Table 16.1 summarizes specific

ventilatory modes for partial ventilatory support. Some newer ventilatory modes are briefly discussed.

Proportional Assist Ventilation and Automatic Tube Compensation

In contrast to PSV, the applied airway pressure is not constant during PAV. Instead, the level of pressure support is dynamically adjusted on a breath-by-breath basis to reflect the inspiratory efforts of the patient and the preset proportionality factors for the selective reduction of increased elastance and resistance. This is controlled by means of a positive feedback mechanism (Fig. 16.5). The fact that knowledge of the elastance and resis-

Table 16.1 Typical Ventilator Modalities for Partial Ventilatory Support[a]

Mode	Type of Support and Patient–Ventilator Interaction
Continuous positive airway pressure (CPAP)	Spontaneous breathing on a positive pressure without additional support
Pressure support ventilation (PSV)	Constant pressure support of each detected breath. Support level must be set.
Proportional assist ventilation (PAV)	Dynamic pressure support in linear proportion to actual flow and inspired volume of each single breath. Amount of resistance and elastance to be compensated must be set.
Automatic tube compensation (ATC)	Dynamic pressure support (or pressure decrease below CPAP during expiration) in nonlinear proportion to actual gas flow. Tube geometry data must be set.
Synchronized intermittent mandatory ventilation (SIMV)	Preset number of machine breaths (either volume or pressure controlled) that will be minimally applied and can be triggered in a time window. Additional spontaneous breaths are possible between machine breaths.
Airway pressure release ventilation (APRV) or biphasic positive airway pressure (BIPAP)	Time-cycled pressure-controlled ventilation (ventilator switches between two CPAP levels) during which spontaneous breathing is possible in any phase of the ventilatory cycle.

[a]Pressure or volume-controlled modes that allow only triggering by the patient are not listed. Some of the modes in this table can be combined (e.g., SIMV + PSV), or modifications of these modes ensure a certain tidal volume or minute ventilation, for example.

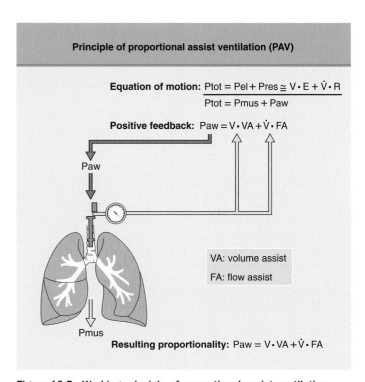

Principle of proportional assist ventilation (PAV)

Equation of motion: $\dfrac{Ptot = Pel + Pres \cong V \cdot E + \dot{V} \cdot R}{Ptot = Pmus + Paw}$

Positive feedback: $Paw = V \cdot VA + \dot{V} \cdot FA$

Paw

VA: volume assist
FA: flow assist

Pmus

Resulting proportionality: $Paw = V \cdot VA + \dot{V} \cdot FA$

Figure 16.5. Working principle of proportional-assist ventilation (PAV). The total driving pressure (Ptot) required for ventilation can be divided into two components: pressure dissipated against elastic forces of lungs and chest wall (Pel) and pressure dissipated against airway resistance (Pres). Pel is dependent on the elastance (E) of the respiratory system and increases with inspiratory volume (V). Pres is dependent on respiratory system resistance (R), which changes in proportion to gas flow ($\dot{V}$). During assisted spontaneous breathing, Ptot is delivered by patients' muscular driving pressure (Pmus) and pressure support by the ventilator (Paw). The equation of motion used here is simplified since linear relationships between changes in flow and volume with Pres and Pel are assumed. This is definitely not true for the pressure drop along the artificial airway but also not for some components of patients' R. During PAV, the idea is to separately compensate for both patients' increased elastic workload [by setting volume assist (VA)] and resistive workloads [by setting flow assist (FA)]. The resulting dynamic pressure support (Paw) is adjusted according to measured V and $\dot{V}$ in a positive feedback manner. If support is higher than the actual value of each component, this can result in overassist phenomena, during which the ventilator amplifies itself instead of the patient's effort.

tance during spontaneous ventilation is essential to be able to make the exact PAV settings limits the more widespread clinical use of this form of ventilation. In PAV, patients generally have the ability to modify their tidal volumes, resulting in higher tidal variation (Fig. 16.6) that is similar to physiological values measured in healthy volunteers. This may partially explain the higher ventilatory comfort observed during PAV. In addition, patients can respond to an increased ventilatory demand with an increase in tidal volumes, whereas during PSV, in which constant support is provided for each breath, ventilation is often not increased by increasing the V_T but by increasing the respiratory rate. In PSV, this leads to an increase in PEEPi and thus to more work of breathing and greater discomfort for the patient when compared with PAV. However, since routine measurements of respiratory mechanics during augmented spontaneous breathing are currently unavailable but would be necessary for setting the support level as a function of respiratory system mechanics during PAV, this mode cannot be generally recommended for routine clinical use. In addition, data from our group suggest that the basic assumption regarding the linear relationship between patient resistance and gas flow is not true.

During mechanically assisted spontaneous breathing, the endotracheal tube constitutes a significant resistive component—regardless of gas flow rate and tube diameter—that the patient must overcome with additional work of breathing. In this situation, the relationship of tube resistance to gas flow is nonlinear. Consequently, conventional PSV, which applies a constant airway pressure, over- or undercompensates for the respiratory effort, normally required to overcome tube resistance. To compensate for the tube resistance during ATC, the ventilator increases the airway pressure during the inspiratory phase and reduces it during the expiratory phase so that the tracheal pressure at the distal end of the tube is made independent of the tube resistance. If full compensation were provided by ATC, the patient would in effect be "electronically extubated." In patients with higher ventilatory demand, ATC has been found to compensate for the additional work caused by the tube better than pressure support up to 15 cm H_2O. This shows that the constant pressure support provided during PSV may not in itself be adequate when there is increased ventilatory demand to compensate for the additional work of breathing generated by the tube. In addition, ATC offered greater comfort than PSV. ATC was able to reduce the additional work created by the tube, especially in those modes that do not support every spontaneous breath taken by the patient. However, the first implementations

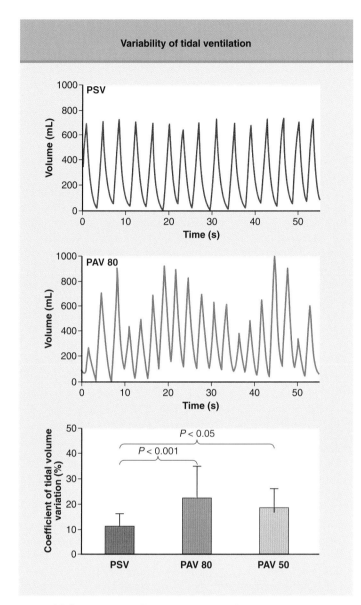

Figure 16.6. Variability of tidal ventilation. Original volume tracings of a patient supported with PSV *(top)* and equivalent support with PAV compensating 80% of measured resistance and elastance *(middle)*. *Bottom,* Coefficient of tidal volume variability of 13 patients with chronic obstructive pulmonary disease during PSV and two levels of support with PAV. Note that dynamic pressure support with PAV offers the patient the ability to modify tidal volume, as indicated by higher variability of tidal ventilation. (For details, see Wrigge H, Golisch W, Zinserling J, et al: Proportional assist versus pressure support ventilation: Effects on breathing pattern and respiratory work of patients with chronic obstructive pulmonary disease. Intensive Care Med 1999;25:790–798.)

of this mode in standard ICU ventilators failed to provide adequate compensation for the additional workload imposed by the artificial airway, mainly due to delayed pressure regulation and a modified algorithm compared with that originally described by Fabry and coworkers (2002). Thus, technical improvement is mandatory. In addition, a general recommendation to apply ATC in conjunction with various ventilation modes cannot be made due to a lack of data.

Several support modes (volume support, adaptive support ventilation, minimum minute ventilation, and a knowledge-based system for adjusting pressure support) were recently developed in an attempt to wean automatically by using feedback from one or more ventilator-measured variables. The minimum minute ventilation strategy (set at either 75% of measured minute ventilation or to a carbon dioxide target) and the knowledge-based system for adjusting pressure support can automatically reduce support safely with selected patients, but neither of these systems has been compared to the daily SBT approach described previously. Moreover, the premises underlying some of these feedback features (e.g., that an ideal volume can be set for volume support or that an ideal ventilatory pattern based on respiratory system mechanics can be set for adaptive support ventilation) may be flawed, especially in sick patients. Indeed, potentially flawed feedback logic may actually delay support reduction. Further research is needed on these automated approaches.

INTERPRETATIONS

Maintaining Spontaneous Breathing
In view of available data, it can be concluded that maintained spontaneous breathing during mechanical ventilation should not be suppressed, even in patients with severe pulmonary functional disorders. The improvements in pulmonary gas exchange, systemic blood flow, and oxygen supply to the tissue that have been observed when spontaneous breathing has been maintained during mechanical ventilation are reflected in the clinical improvement in the patient's condition. Compared to an initial period of controlled ventilation followed by weaning, maintained spontaneous breathing in APRV/BIPAP is associated with significantly fewer days of ventilation, earlier extubation, and shorter stays in the ICU. It should be noted that the positive effects of spontaneous breathing have only been documented for some of the clinically available ventilation modes that support spontaneous breathing. If one limits oneself to ventilation modes whose positive effects have been scientifically documented, then the modes of ventilation that support spontaneous breathing can be used even in patients with the most serious pulmonary functional disorders. Whereas controlled ventilation followed by weaning with modes that support spontaneous breathing used to be regarded as the standard in ventilation therapy, this approach should be reconsidered in view of the available data. Today, standard practice should be to apply mechanical support of spontaneous breathing as a primary mode, which is then continuously adapted to the patient's needs.

Discontinuation of Mechanical Ventilation
If the patient's pulmonary dysfunction is resolving, the clinical focus shifts to removing the ventilator as quickly as possible. Unnecessary delay in withdrawing mechanical ventilation increases the likelihood of complications, such as pneumonia, discomfort, and ventilator-associated lung injury, and it increases cost. However, the value of removing the ventilator as soon as possible must be balanced against the risks of premature withdrawal, which include difficulty in reestablishing an artificial airway, ventilatory muscle fatigue, and compromised gas exchange. The following principles for minimizing the length of invasive ventilatory support are considered evidence based:

1. Frequent assessment is required to determine whether ventilatory support and the artificial airway are still needed.
2. Patients who continue to require support should be continually reevaluated to ensure that all factors contributing to ventilator dependence are addressed.
3. With patients who continue to require support, the support strategy should maximize patient comfort and provide muscle unloading.
4. Patients who require prolonged ventilatory support beyond the ICU should go to specialized facilities that can provide more gradual support reduction strategies.
5. Ventilator discontinuation and weaning protocols can be effectively carried out by nonphysician clinicians.

The use of noninvasive mechanical ventilation to facilitate weaning should be considered, especially in patients with COPD.

PITFALLS AND CONTROVERSIES

Detecting Patients' Inspiratory Effort

To reduce effort markedly requires that the ventilator cycle be in unison with the patient's central respiratory rhythm. For perfect synchronization, the period of mechanical inflation must match the period of neural inspiratory time, and the period of mechanical inactivity must match the neural expiratory time. In current practice, ventilators provide positive pressure assistance to a patient's inspiratory effort when the pressure in the ventilator circuit decreases by a certain amount (usually 1 or 2 cm H_2O, pressure trigger) or inspiratory flow increases to, for example, 5 liters/min (flow trigger). Patients who struggle to reach the set sensitivity are unable to switch off their respiratory motor output immediately after successfully triggering the ventilator. Thus, considerable effort can be expended during the period of mechanical inflation following the trigger phase. Increased effort in this posttrigger phase may arise because of an inadequate level of positive pressure in the inspiratory limb during the period immediately before and during the milliseconds after opening of the inspiratory valve and may offset the prime objective of the ventilator—to unload the respiratory muscles.

Because modern ventilators always measure the result of the muscular effort distal to the patient (i.e., pressure/flow changes in the ventilator), discrepancies between indirect estimates of a patient's inspiratory time and the true value of inspiratory time may give rise to delay in triggering the ventilator and errors in estimating the duration of inspiratory time that may cause mechanical inflation to persist into expiration. Estimates of the duration of inspiration based on flow, esophageal pressure, and transdiaphragmatic pressures revealed substantial differences compared to the duration of inspiration measured with the diaphragmatic electromyogram. When inspiratory time measured by diaphragmatic electromyogram was taken as the reference standard, the inspiratory time estimated from the transdiaphragmatic pressure (from the initial deflection of the signal until the signal returns to baseline) had a mean difference of more than 50% from the reference value. Given the magnitude of these discrepancies, conclusions about patient–ventilator interactions based on indirect estimates of inspiratory time are susceptible to considerable error.

In addition, a delay in opening of the inspiratory valve may occur due to a decreased respiratory drive or increased PEEPi. This observation suggests that when elastic recoil pressure at the end of expiration is high, the subsequent inspiratory effort also needs to be proportionally increased if the ventilator is to be successfully triggered. Experimental approaches using the electromyogram of the diaphragm (e.g., measured with a specific esophageal catheter) may improve patient–ventilator interactions in future applications.

Some patients have a high elastic load, secondary to hyperinflation, and a low respiratory drive. As a result, inspiratory effort will be insufficient to successfully trigger the ventilator. The increased use of bedside displays of pressure and flow tracing has led to a growing awareness of the frequency with which patients fail to trigger a ventilator. When receiving high levels of pressure support or assist-control ventilation, one fourth to one third of a patient's inspiratory efforts may fail to trigger the machine. The number of ineffective triggering attempts increases in direct proportion to the level of ventilator assistance. Some authors have recommended reducing the level of pressure support as a means of decreasing the number of ineffective triggering attempts. Although this approach should decrease the number of failed triggering attempts, it is likely to be accompanied by a decrease in ventilator assistance. There are no rules for how best to achieve a good balance.

Weaning Failure

If a patient fails SBT, one should evaluate what caused the SBT failure and what reversible factors can be corrected. Although a failed SBT often reflects persistent respiratory system mechanical abnormalities, it should prompt a search for other causes or complicating factors, such as adequacy of pain control, appropriateness of sedation, fluid status, bronchodilator need, and control of myocardial ischemia and other disease processes that can affect discontinuation attempts. Assuming medical management is optimized, several lines of evidence support waiting 24 hours before reattempting SBT with a patient who has required ventilatory support for more than 1 or 2 days (see Box 16.1, recommendation 4). First, respiratory system abnormalities rarely recover over a period of hours, and thus frequent SBTs over a short period will probably not be helpful. Indeed, Jubran and Tobin found that SBT failure is often due to persistent respiratory system mechanical abnormalities that are unlikely to reverse rapidly. Furthermore, a failed SBT associated with severe respiratory muscle fatigue may cause structural inspiratory muscle damage, complete recovery from which may require 24 hours or more. Despite the need for increased ventilatory assistance in patients who do not tolerate unassisted spontaneous breathing (SBT), there is no need to suppress spontaneous breathing activity, but the respiratory muscles should be unloaded with assisted ventilation during recovery.

SUGGESTED READING

Brochard L, Rauss A, Benito S, et al: Comparison of three methods of gradual withdrawal from ventilatory support during weaning from mechanical ventilation. Am J Respir Crit Care Med 1994;150:896–903.

Esteban A, Frutos F, Tobin MJ, et al: A comparison of four methods of weaning patients from mechanical ventilation. Spanish Lung Failure Collaborative Group. N Engl J Med 1995;332:345–350.

Fabry B, Haberthür C, Zappe D, et al: Breathing pattern and additional work of breathing in spontaneously breathing patients with different ventilatory demands during inspiratory pressure support and automatic tube compensation. Intensive Care Med 1997;23:545–552.

Katz JA, Marks JD: Inspiratory work with and without continuous positive airway pressure in patients with acute respiratory failure. Anesthesiology 1985;63:598–607.

Kollef MH, Shapiro SD, Silver P, et al: A randomized, controlled trial of protocol-directed versus physician-directed weaning from mechanical ventilation. Crit Care Med 1997;25:567–574.

MacIntyre NR: Evidence-based ventilator weaning and discontinuation. Respir Care 2004;49:830–836.

MacIntyre NR, Cook DJ, Ely EW Jr, et al: Evidence-based guidelines for weaning and discontinuing ventilatory support: A collective task force facilitated by the American College of Chest Physicians; the American Association for Respiratory Care; and the American College of Critical Care Medicine. Chest 2001;120:375S–395S.

Putensen C, Zech S, Wrigge H, et al: Long-term effects of spontaneous breathing during ventilatory support in patients with acute lung injury. Am J Respir Crit Care Med 2001;164:43–49.

Wrigge H, Zinserling J, Neumann P, et al: Spontaneous breathing improves lung aeration in oleic acid-induced lung injury. Anesthesiology 2003;99:376–384.

Younes M, Puddy A, Roberts D, et al: Proportional assist ventilation. Results of an initial clinical trial. Am Rev Respir Dis 1992;145:121–129.

Chapter 17

Ventilator-Associated Lung Injury

Jesús Villar and Robert M. Kacmarek

KEY POINTS

- Unequivocal evidence from both experimental and clinical research shows that mechanical ventilation can damage the lungs and initiate an inflammatory response, possibly contributing to extrapulmonary organ dysfunction, referred to as *extrapulmonary organ trauma*.
- Overdistention of alveoli results in a loss of the lung's structural integrity, leading to alveolar flooding, disruption of epithelial fluid transport, worsening of the pulmonary and systemic inflammatory responses, and disorganization of epithelial repair with tissue fibrosis. This type of injury is referred to as *volutrauma*. This type of injury forms the basis for the use of small tidal volumes, 6 or 7 mL/kg of predicted body weight, during mechanical ventilation of patients with acute lung injury.
- Repetitive opening and collapse of unstable lung units causes injury similar to overdistention since the stress placed on the junctional tissue between collapsed and open lung units can reach 140 cm H_2O at a peak alveolar pressure of 30 cm H_2O. This injury is termed *atelectrauma*. As a result, sufficient positive end-expiratory pressure should be applied to maintain the lung open, on average 8 to 12 cm H_2O in acute lung injury and 12 to 16 cm H_2O in acute respiratory distress syndrome.
- Mechanical injuries caused by volutrauma and atelectrauma can trigger a complex array of pro- and anti-inflammatory mediators, resulting in a local and systemic inflammatory response. In addition, substances produced in the lung can be translocated into systemic circulation as a result of injury not only to the pulmonary epithelium but also to the capillary endothelium. This form of injury is referred to as *biotrauma*.
- Functional genomic approaches using gene array methodology to measure lung gene expression and address the contribution of mechanical stress to ventilator-associated lung injury (VALI) have identified genes differentially expressed in in vivo animal models of VALI. It is hoped that the rapidly evolving sciences of genomics, proteomics, and computational biology can be used to model VALI and to tailor mechanical ventilation strategies to create an ideal inflammatory environment for minimal injury, tissue repair, and cell regeneration.

Ventilation is an essential function of life and is also one of the first to be replicated by artificial means. Mechanical ventilators are used to provide life support for critically ill patients. Mechanical ventilation is the second most frequently performed therapeutic intervention after treatment of cardiac arrhythmias in intensive care units (ICUs), and it is the most important aspect of the supportive care of patients with respiratory failure. An average of 60% of ICU patients receive mechanical ventilation, and countless lives have been saved by its use. Ventilators are intended to deliver air/oxygen at tidal volumes sufficient to provide adequate alveolar ventilation, to reduce the work of breathing, and to enhance blood oxygenation. However, mechanical ventilation is a nonphysiologic process, and complications are associated with its use, including increased risk of pneumonia, impaired cardiac performance, and lung injury. During mechanical ventilation, pressures, gas volumes, ventilatory rates, and concentrations of inspired oxygen are applied beyond the levels that normal lungs usually experience. These patterns of ventilation may induce injury, referred to as ventilator-associated lung injury (VALI) or ventilator-associated trauma.

The possibility of VALI was first considered in the 1970s, although pathologists in the 1960s recognized a new severe pulmonary lesion that they called "respirator lung." There is now unequivocal evidence from both experimental and clinical data that mechanical ventilation can cause or aggravate acute lung injury (ALI) in the critically ill patient. This condition, VALI, resembles the syndromes of ALI and acute respiratory distress syndrome (ARDS); as a result, it is difficult to identify in humans because its appearance overlaps that of the underlying disease. The recognition of VALI has prompted a number of investigators to suggest that ALI/ARDS may in part be a product of our efforts to mechanically ventilate patients rather than the progression of the underlying disease. During the past 10 years, the concept of VALI has come more clearly into focus. A number of specific forms of injury caused by the trauma of mechanical ventilation have been identified: volutrauma, barotrauma, atelectrauma, biotrauma, and extrapulmonary organ trauma (Fig. 17.1). This chapter focuses on the evidence supporting these specific types of VALI but also, in brief, the clinical implications of these types of injury. Details on the clinical evidence linking ventilatory pattern to improved survival in ALI/ARDS are presented in other chapters.

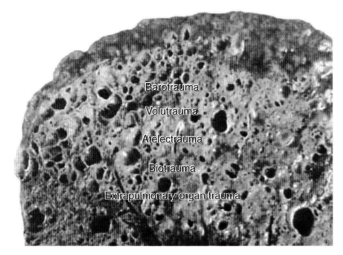

Figure 17.1. The five components of ventilator-associated trauma. The background represents a grossly "honeycomb" appearance of a fibrotic lung from a patient with recurrent aspiration who died in the early 1970s after a few weeks on mechanical ventilation at high tidal volumes.

PATHOPHYSIOLOGY AND RISK FACTORS FOR VALI

Alveolar Overdistention, Barotrauma, and Volutrauma

VALI characterized in animal models is manifested by increased permeability pulmonary edema, cell disruption, and diffuse pulmonary infiltrates (Fig. 17.2). The damage observed in VALI reflects the primary injurious stimuli and the secondary complex interactions of inflammatory mediators on alveolar epithelial and capillary endothelial cells. The pulmonary endothelium is a metabolically active surface that provides a regulatory interface for the continual processing of blood-borne vasoactive molecules, plays an active role in hemostasis and immunologic and inflammatory events, regulates vascular tone, and interacts with inflammatory cells and neighboring vascular cells. Experimental evidence indicates that VALI can be produced by ventilation with very large tidal volumes in normal lungs and by ventilation with moderate or even small tidal volumes in preinjured lungs. This type of injury has been referred to as volutrauma.

Alveolar overdistention results in the breakdown of the lung's structural architecture. The loss of epithelial integrity has several consequences: (1) alveolar flooding; (2) disruption of normal epithelial fluid transport, impairing the removal of edema from the alveolar space; (3) development or worsening of the pulmonary and systemic inflammatory responses; and (4) disorganization of epithelial repair and intense fibrosis. In patients who die from ARDS after being ventilated with high tidal volumes and high airway pressures, expanded pseudocysts identified around atelectatic areas suggest that traction forces exerted on the walls of collapsed alveoli by adjacent overexpanded lung units play an important role in the development of VALI. This regional overdistention can cause and/or worsen lung injury and affect outcome by altering cellular pathways that are important for the normal function of tissues and organs. Surprisingly, there is experimental evidence from the early 1970s supporting the contention that mechanical ventilation, at physiologic inspiratory pressures and volumes, does not cause lung injury. Normal lungs of dogs, baboons, and sheep ventilated with a peak alveolar pressure of less than 25 cm H_2O for periods of up to 48 hours do not experience changes in lung compliance or gas exchange. In contrast, during mechanical ventilation with higher peak alveolar pressures, lung compliance decreases and gas exchange abnormalities develop within hours due to an increase in alveolar surface tension and edema formation.

All mammals are similarly scaled with lung volumes when adjusted for size (Fig. 17.3). In all spontaneously breathing

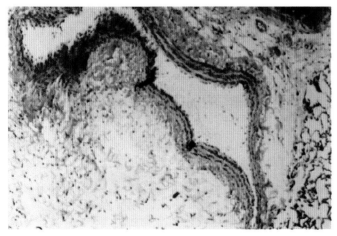

Figure 17.2. Perivascular and peribronchiolar edema, congestion, and inflammatory infiltrates in a normal lung of a healthy rat subjected to a VT of 20 mL/kg for 3 hours.

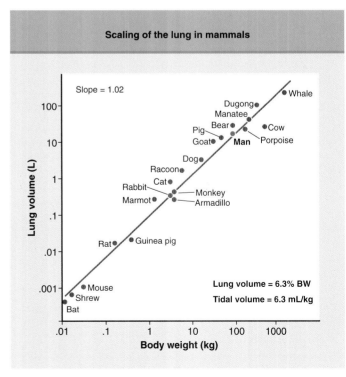

Figure 17.3. Scaling of the lung in mammals. (Adapted from Schmidt-Nielsen K: Body size and problems of scaling. In How Animals Work. New York, Cambridge University Press, 1972, pp 85–104.)

mammals, tidal volumes are approximately 6 or 7 mL/kg predicted body weight, yet historically tidal volumes of 12 to 15 mL/kg actual body weight were used in patients with acute respiratory failure, and peak alveolar pressures had been allowed to increase above 40 cm H_2O. In many patients, these volumes and pressures resulted in lung volume approaching the total lung capacity of healthy lungs. This one tidal volume fits all approach was formulated in the 1960s because anesthesiologists and critical care pioneers showed that small tidal volume-controlled ventilation resulted in a gradual loss of lung volume and hypoxemia. Large tidal volume ventilation was useful to prevent atelectasis.

The fact that alveolar epithelium can be disrupted by high alveolar pressure is evident when barotrauma develops. Pulmonary barotrauma is the accumulation of extraalveolar gas. Barotrauma in the form of pneumothorax, pneumomediastinum, or subcutaneous emphysema occurs in 5% to 15% of patients receiving mechanical ventilation. Cohort studies performed in the past decade showed that in mechanically ventilated patients in whom airway pressure and tidal volume were limited, barotrauma did not correlate to any ventilator parameter. However, barotrauma is more likely in patients ventilated with underlying lung disease (acute or chronic) and is also associated with an increased mortality and prolonged ICU stay.

In animals with healthy or injured lungs, large tidal volumes increase edema accumulation within the first few hours of initiating mechanical ventilation. It is likely that large tidal volume ventilation results in similar injury in patients with ALI, especially when alveolar flooding necessitates that the tidal volume delivered inflates fewer aerated alveoli. The high peak alveolar pressures also damage the endothelial barrier of the pulmonary circulation. The mechanical forces originating within the alveolus can cause hemorrhagic injury in the absence of preexisting inflammation. Microvascular disruption can be expected since the mechanical stress experienced by tidal inflation is greatly amplified at the interface of opened and closed lung units. When tissues are already atelectatic and the lung is exposed to 30 cm H_2O peak alveolar pressure, the traction force experienced by junctional tissues approximates 140 cm H_2O. Therefore, it is not difficult to envision vascular rupture under these conditions. Electron microscopy has demonstrated "capillary stress fractures" when microvascular pressures are markedly elevated. It is this "stress failure" of the alveolar capillary membrane that is responsible for the increased microvascular permeability edema seen with lung overinflation. Alveolar epithelial disruptions have also been demonstrated at normal and high capillary transmural pressures in healthy mammals. The dimensions of the elongated breaks in the epithelium have been estimated to be 4 µm (length) by 1 µm (width). At the same transmural pressure, stress failure of capillary walls occurs more frequently at high vs. low lung volumes (Fig. 17.4).

The cellular constituents of the lung change enormously during VALI. Alveolar overinflation elicits a well-coordinated response that contributes to cellular proliferation and inflammation. As the epithelium is progressively stretched, there is a nonreversible opening of water-filled channels between alveolar cells resulting in free diffusion of small solutes and even albumin across the epithelial barrier. The alveolar epithelium usually has extensive necrosis of type 1 cells, which causes the alveolar surface to be replaced by proteinaceous deposits (hyaline mem-

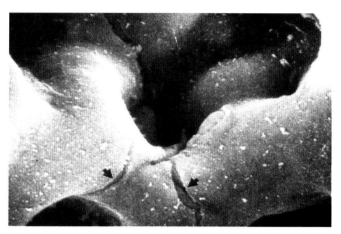

Figure 17.4. Scanning electron micrograph of a capillary at a transmural pressure of 52.5 cm H_2O. Note disruptions of the alveolar epithelial cells. (Fu Z, Costello ML, Tsukimoto K, et al: High lung volume increases stress failure in pulmonary capillaries. J Appl Physiol 1992;73:123–133.)

branes). Type 2 cells, in addition to secreting surfactant, provide a population of cells capable of replication and differentiation to replace type 1 cells. Overventilation alone can also produce surfactant abnormalities. Whereas short-term large tidal inflation can enhance surfactant secretion, prolonged large-volume ventilation results in decreased surfactant activity. In addition, due to damage of both the epithelial and the endothelial barrier, surfactant components may be lost into the bloodstream. Intraalveolar protein accumulation results in a dose-dependent inhibition of surfactant.

Atelectrauma and Positive End-Expiratory Pressure
Ventilation at low absolute lung volume (functional residual capacity) is an important contributor to VALI. Ventilation with high tidal volume and low or zero PEEP is more damaging than ventilation with low tidal volume and high PEEP, even when similar high levels of peak alveolar pressure are reached. Lung injury caused by the cyclic opening and closing of unstable lung units is termed atelectrauma. As discussed previously, the stress of opening a collapsed lung unit on the alveolar wall between open and collapsed lung can exceed 140 cm H_2O. PEEP has become an essential component of the care of critically ill patients who require ventilatory support. PEEP prevents alveolar collapse and improves oxygenation by maintaining functional residual capacity. Exposing alveolar epithelial cells in vitro to large cyclic deformation without PEEP leads to significantly reduced cell viability and fragmentation of the continuous alveolar surfactant film into less effective islands of surfactant. By limiting the deformation amplitude, a significant reduction in cell death at identical maximum stretch is obtained. In vivo, PEEP similarly attenuates VALI.

In healthy lungs, lung inflation occurs with modest increases in airway pressure. In the presence of pulmonary edema due to ALI, tidal volume has access to fewer alveoli as a result of airspace flooding. The compression of the same tidal volume into fewer alveoli causes a large increase in alveolar pressure. When a critical alveolar pressure is reached (inflection point), a sudden increment in volume occurs as alveoli are recruited and edema

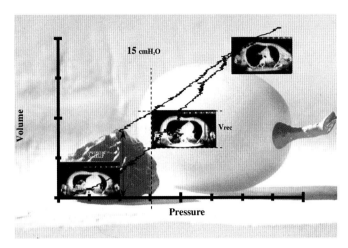

Figure 17.5. Pulmonary pressure–volume curve in a patient with severe acute lung injury. Specific protective ventilation strategies require that PEEP is set above the lower inflection to allow alveolar recruitment (V_{rec}) and the airway pressure below the upper inflection point to avoid overdistension. With this ventilatory strategy, both low (raisin) and high (swollen grape) lung volume injury can be avoided.

fluid is redistributed (Fig. 17.5). As airway pressure decreases to zero with deflation, alveoli close and reflooding occurs. The main effect of PEEP is keeping recruited alveolar units open. It is clear that in the initial phases of ALI, the lungs are edematous and show a reduced compliance with an inflection point on the ascending limb of the pressure–volume curve of the respiratory system. In general, the inflection point in acutely injured lungs is in the range of 8 to 16 cm H_2O. When PEEP is applied above the inflection point, a new recruited zone can be detected corresponding to the reduction in the disease zone (V_{rec} in Fig. 17.5). Because the presence of this new zone is a function of the underlying pathology, the same level of PEEP applied in different patients results in a different response in terms of gas exchange. This recruitment can be defined as the gas volume increase in poorly and nonaerated alveoli with the application of PEEP. Once this zone is fully recruited, it behaves as a relatively healthy lung in terms of gas exchange and mechanics. Therefore, since PEEP maintains recruitment of alveolar units that were previously collapsed, tidal volume will be distributed to more alveoli and peak alveolar pressure will be reduced and lung compliance increased.

There is no scientific evidence indicating that PEEP ruptures alveoli. Although some observations have shown that patients who are treated with PEEP have a higher incidence of alveolar rupture, they do not demonstrate that high PEEP is the cause. Patients who require the highest levels of PEEP are the sickest patients and those most prone to develop barotrauma. Since ALI is a nonhomogeneous process, overdistension of a given lung unit may be achieved at any PEEP level. However, there is plenty of experimental evidence indicating that PEEP is protective, attenuating VALI. The extensive alveolar edema developed after the application of high inspiratory pressures in animals with healthy lungs can be attenuated or prevented by the application of 10 cm H_2O or more of PEEP. It is well documented in surfactant-deficient or deactivated lung models that the application of moderate levels of PEEP decreases or reverses the formation of

hyaline membranes, promotes alveolar stability, and increases surfactant production.

Experimental, short-term, ex vivo or in vivo studies comparing several levels of PEEP (zero, low, below the lower inflection point, and above the lower inflection point) at low, normal, high, or extremely high tidal volumes in different animal models of ALI have shown significantly less pulmonary edema, a lower intrapulmonary shunt fraction, better oxygenation, and better outcome in those animals or lungs ventilated with a combination of low tidal volume and high PEEP. Injured lungs ventilated with any level of PEEP below the inflection point have decreased compliance and, in some instances, similar histological damage to those lungs ventilated with very low or no PEEP. From these observations, it can be concluded that to prevent VALI due to high shear forces between open and closed lung units (atelectrauma), ventilation should be provided with PEEP high enough to prevent end-expiratory collapse. In other words, open up the lung and keep it open.

Biotrauma: From Ventilator-Associated Lung Injury to Ventilator-Associated Trauma

Mechanical ventilation can trigger a complex array of pro- and anti-inflammatory mediators that may lead to enhanced lung healing and quicker restoration of pulmonary function. However, research on animals with healthy or preinjured lungs and on patients with ALI has demonstrated that some ventilatory strategies establish an imbalance in this normal stress response, altering lung cellular function and producing a local and systemic inflammatory response (Fig. 17.6). Ventilating normal lungs with large tidal volumes leading to VALI is accompanied by an inflammatory response with the release of cytokines from a variety of lung cells. This ventilator-induced inflammatory response (biotrauma) is the fourth component of ventilator-associated trauma and is the result of the mechanical activation of several intracellular signaling pathways in the lung. Biotrauma is a result of an imbalance in the delicate interplay between tissue deformation, interstitial and alveolar edema, inflammation, and lung mechanics. In general, ventilatory strategies that cause pulmonary epithelial or endothelial cell injury lead to impairments in the functional metabolic properties of these cells, resulting in alterations in hemodynamics, permeability, gas exchange, and inter/intracellular signaling.

Mechanical stress plays an important role in lung development and surfactant secretion. In addition, mechanical ventilation or cyclic mechanical stretch of lung cells play an important role in determining cellular function and gene expression, and the degree and pattern of the mechanical stimuli influence cellular response. Furthermore, cyclic mechanical stress has been shown to inhibit airway epithelial repair. It is well recognized that high alveolar pressures increase transit time and activation of leukocytes in the lungs. Cell deformation by mechanical forces directly causes conformational changes in molecules within the cell membrane, leading to activation of downstream messenger systems. Neutrophils and other leukocytes are considered central to the pathogenesis of most forms of ALI. Leukocytes do not cause damage while suspended in the bloodstream; however, a release of cytotoxic agents occurs when neutrophils adhere to endothelium, epithelium, or extracellular matrix proteins in the interstitium. Such neutrophil adherence is mediated predominantly through integrins (CD11/CD18) on

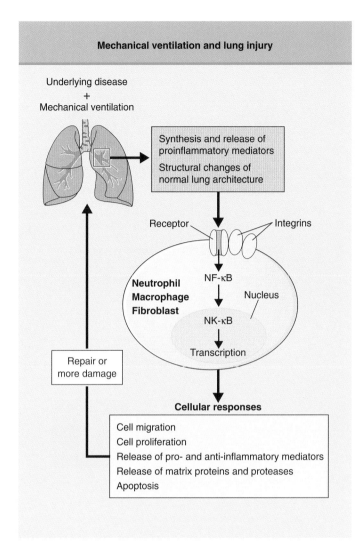

Figure 17.6. **Mechanical ventilation and lung injury.** Mechanical ventilation may lead to lung injury through the activation of various intracellular signaling pathways that in turn can initiate and/or enhance an inflammatory response. The course of this ventilator-induced lung injury will be influenced by the intensity of the cellular response.

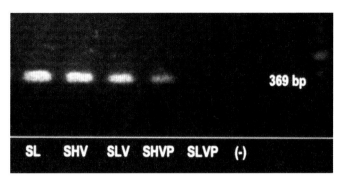

Figure 17.7. **Gene expression of tumor necrosis factor-α in the lungs of an in vivo animal model of sepsis-induced lung injury after 3 hours of mechanical ventilation using clinically relevant ventilatory strategies.** SL, sepsis, anesthetized, spontaneous breathing; SHV, sepsis, ventilated with high tidal volume (20 mL/kg) and PEEP of 0 to 2 cm H_2O; SLV, sepsis, ventilated with low tidal volume (6 mL/kg) and PEEP of 0 to 2 cm H_2O; SHVP, sepsis, ventilated with high tidal volume and PEEP above inflection point (8–10 cm H_2O); SLVP, sepsis, ventilated with low tidal volume and PEEP above inflection point. In general, the application of high PEEP, irrespective of the tidal volume, resulted in a marked attenuation of the pulmonary inflammatory response.

the cell surface (see Fig. 17.2). Activation of human neutrophils by integrin aggregation is mediated through the activation of the I-κB/nuclear factor-κB pathway. The fact that increased lung microvascular permeability induced by high tidal volume ventilation can be blocked with inhibitors of cation channels indicates that the extravascular lung water in VALI is in part due to the activation of specific cellular processes rather than simply due to the physical disruption of the alveolar–capillary membrane. In addition, it has been shown experimentally that lung damage can be attenuated by the administration of cytokine antagonists.

VALI not only increases lung permeability to small and large solutes but also decreases active Na^+ transport and lung edema clearance, and this impairment worsens with time of injurious ventilation. Alveolar liquid clearance occurs primarily by active ion transport across pulmonary epithelium. The clearance of pulmonary edema appears to be mainly controlled by Na^+ channels and Na,K-ATPases, but an intact epithelial barrier is critical for the resolution of alveolar edema. Cyclic mechanical stress

plays an important role in the regulation of extracellular matrix remodeling. Matrix metalloproteinases are a family of enzymes that degrade components of the extracellular matrix and are expressed by a number of cells, including neutrophils, alveolar macrophages, endothelial and epithelial cells, as well as stimulated connective tissue cells. These enzymes play an important role in the development of ALI since the administration of inhibitors in in vivo animal models suppresses high permeability pulmonary edema and protects the lung from oxidant-induced injury. It has been shown that high tidal volume ventilation causes upregulation, release, and activation of matrix metalloproteinase and plays an important role in the regulation of extracellular matrix remodeling.

Overinflation of the lungs causes overactivation of the immune system (Fig. 17.7). Healthy mice lungs ventilated with large tidal volumes evoke early inflammatory responses similar to those evoked by endotoxin (activation of nuclear factor-κB and cytokine release). These increased concentrations of cytokines are due to both tissue destruction and mechanotransduction. The highest levels of inflammatory mediators are seen with large tidal volumes or in the absence of PEEP. Experimentally, the combination of high tidal volume and zero PEEP has a synergistic effect on cytokine gene expression in preinjured lungs. Injurious ventilation of rats at very high tidal volumes with zero PEEP is associated with a 50-fold increase in some proinflammatory cytokines in bronchoalveolar lavage fluid, although this observation has been challenged by some studies that found no increase in certain cytokines in the bronchoalveolar lavage fluid during experimental VALI.

Functional genomic approaches using gene array methodology to measure lung gene expression and address the contribution of mechanical stress to VALI have identified genes differentially expressed in in vivo animal models of VALI. Despite a relatively brief period of ventilator challenge (30 min at a tidal volume of 25 mL/kg) as well as the absence of ultrastructural evidence of injury, significant upregulation of certain genes and suppression of other genes have been observed. Among the upregulated genes were transcription factors, stress proteins, and inflammatory mediators; the downregulated genes were associated with metabolic regulatory genes. The specific genetic determinants that render patients susceptible to the adverse effects of mechanical ventilation in the setting of ALI are unknown. The future delineation of genetic susceptibility loci for VALI is expected to lead to identification of the pathophysiologic mechanisms causing this injury.

The effects of VALI can be extended beyond the lung; the ventilator-induced cytokine storm may play a key role in initiating and propagating an inflammatory response not only in the lung but also in extrapulmonary organs by generating or amplifying multiple organ dysfunctions in the mechanically ventilated patient. This extrapulmonary organ trauma is the fifth component of ventilator-associated trauma (Fig. 17.8). It has been speculated that since the pulmonary endothelial barrier is damaged during ALI, lung cytokines can be trafficked from the alveoli and the interstitium into the systemic circulation. These mediators may stimulate dramatic changes in the architecture of other endothelial and epithelial cells in extrapulmonary organs and initiate or propagate a systemic inflammatory response. It has been postulated that the type of lung injury described in experimental models of VALI probably occurs in humans to a greater or lesser degree, and that the release of proinflammatory mediators into the circulation can influence the development of multiple organ dysfunction, the main cause of death in critically ill patients.

Similar to the postulated association of gut translocation of bacteria and their products leading to sepsis and multiple organ failure, injurious ventilatory strategies may be responsible for translocation of bacteria and their products from the alveoli into the bloodstream. Several studies have demonstrated that intratracheal instillation of gram-negative bacteria in experimental animals is accompanied by a reduced bacterial clearance, enhanced neutrophil response, and positive blood cultures after ventilation with airway pressures known to produce microvascular injury. These effects were diminished when PEEP was applied. Systemic dissemination of bacteria or endotoxin present in the lungs may promote distal organ swelling, infection, or dysfunction.

Oxygen, Respiratory Rate, and Inspiratory Time

In addition to tidal volume and PEEP, other factors are thought to influence the development of VALI: high inspired oxygen fraction, respiratory rate, inspiratory time, pulmonary perfusion, and body position. The exposure of animals or humans to a high inspired oxygen concentration for long periods can lead to lung damage through the increased generation of reactive oxygen species. Adults breathing 100% oxygen experience increased microvascular permeability to protein after 17 hours. Since ventilation with high oxygen content can also lead to absorption atelectasis and surfactant inactivation, the potential for parenchymal injury is increased when oxygen is associated with the mechanical stress of high distending pressures.

Although ventilation is the product of tidal volume and frequency, little attention has been directed at the role of ventilatory rate in the generation of VALI. It has been shown experimentally that increased respiratory frequency may augment lung injury through greater stress cycling or through

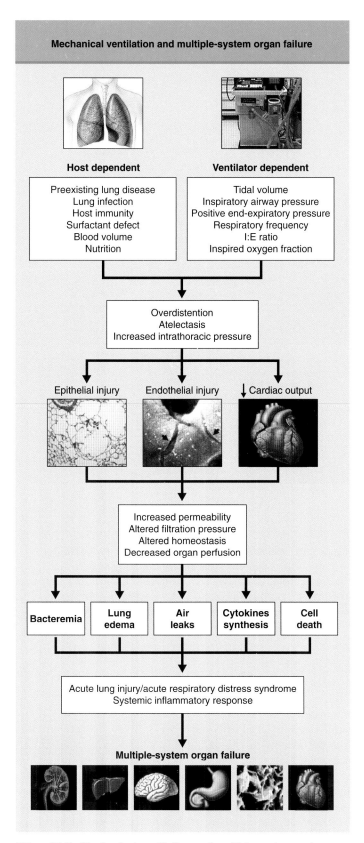

Figure 17.8. Mechanical ventilation and multiple-system organ failure. Postulated mechanism by which mechanical ventilation might contribute to multiple system organ failure.

Box 17.1 Monitoring for VALI during Mechanical Ventilation

Pulmonary Function Measurements

PaO_2/FiO_2
Plateau pressure
Tidal volume
Lung compliance
Intrapulmonary shunt
Extravascular lung water

Morphological Measurements

Computerized tomography scan
Electric impedance tomography

Biological Markers

Endothelium

Soluble intercellular adhesion molecule (sICAM)-1
Plasma von Willebrand factor antigen
TNF-α in bronchoalveolar lavage fluid
Angiostatin in bronchoalveolar lavage fluid

Epithelium

Type I alveolar epithelial cell-specific protein RT140
Purines

---

the deactivation of surfactant, but the clinical relevance of these findings is unclear. If cumulative damage plays a key role in the occurrence of VALI, then reducing respiratory rate and airway pressure amplitude may limit VALI. Reduced minute ventilation is generally associated with hypercapnic acidosis, which until recently was considered a necessary consequence of a noninjurious, protective ventilatory strategy. However, evidence indicates that the generation of hypercapnic acidosis may exert a protective effect on the severity of VALI.

Increasing inspiratory time during high-pressure/high-volume mechanical ventilation is associated with lung injury. When healthy animals were ventilated for 2 hours with pressure control ventilation at 45 cm H_2O, VALI was attenuated when a reduced inspiratory time (0.45 sec) was applied in conjunction with high levels of PEEP.

MONITORING FOR VALI DURING MECHANICAL VENTILATION

Critically ill patients are monitored extensively (Box 17.1). Pulmonary function measurements provide basic physiologic information on gas transport and exchange. The main goal of mechanical ventilation is to reverse and prevent hypoxemia. PaO_2/FiO_2 is the most reliable and routinely used tool to define the state of impairment in gas exchange of the lung. Peak inspiratory pressure provides a poor assessment of alveolar overdistention, since it is influenced by several factors independent of alveolar pressure. However, the end-expiratory plateau pressure is a good estimate of overdistention. Plateau pressures should be reduced as low as possible and always less than 30 cm H_2O. This means that tidal volume should always be less than 10 mL/kg and in most patients between 4 and 8 mL/kg predicted body

weight. To prevent repeated alveolar collapse and reexpansion, PEEP should be applied. PEEP levels sufficient to ensure that recruited lung is maintained open are essential. In general, 8 to 12 cm H_2O PEEP is required in ALI and 12 to 16 cm H_2O PEEP in ARDS.

Computerized tomography (CT) scanning is a useful tool for determining regional lung volumes during mechanical ventilation. However, CT is unlikely to become a routine clinical tool because of its cost, size, and the hazards associated with the transport of critically ill patients. Electric impedance tomography (EIT) does show promise as a routine monitoring method of lung volume in the ICU, but considerable work on EIT is required before it becomes a bedside reality.

In general, the goal of monitoring has been to measure the degree of injury rather than to prevent further injury and measure repair. Measures of further injury or repair have been limited to endpoints such as return of organ function. There is increasing interest in finding a biological marker that evaluates damage to the alveolar–capillary membrane. It is hoped that the rapidly evolving sciences of genomics, proteomics, and computational biology can be used to model VALI and to tailor mechanical ventilation strategies to create an ideal inflammatory environment for minimal injury, tissue repair, and cell regeneration.

Acknowledgment

This work was supported in part by grant 209/02 from the Dirección General de Universidades e Investigación, Canary Islands.

SUGGESTED READING

Dreyfuss D, Saumon G: Ventilator-induced lung injury: Lessons from experimental studies. Am J Respir Crit Care Med 1998;157:294–323.

Fu Z, Costello ML, Tsukimoto K, et al: High lung volume increases stress failure in pulmonary capillaries. J Appl Physiol 1992;73:123–133.

Herrera MT, Toledo C, Valladares F, et al: Positive end-expiratory pressure modulates local and systemic inflammatory responses in a sepsis-induced lung injury model. Intensive Care Med 2003;29:1345–1353.

Marini JJ, Hotchkiss JR, Broccard AF: Microvascular and airspace linkage in ventilator-induced lung injury. Crit Care 2003;7:435–444.

Parker JC, Hernandez LA, Peevy KJ: Mechanisms of ventilator-induced lung injury. Crit Care Med 1993;21:131–143.

Plötz FB, Slutsky AS, van Vught AJ, Heijnen CJ: Ventilator-induced lung injury and multiple system organ failure: A critical review of facts and hypotheses. Intensive Care Med 2004;30:1865–1872.

Ranieri VM, Suter PM, Tortorella C, et al: Effect of mechanical ventilation on inflammatory mediators in patients with acute respiratory distress syndrome: A randomized controlled trial. JAMA 1999;282:54–61.

Rouby JJ, Lhern T, Martin de Lassale E, et al: Histologic aspects of pulmonary barotrauma in critically ill patients with acute respiratory failure. Intensive Care Med 1993;19:383–389.

Tremblay L, Valenza F, Ribeiro SP, Li J, Slutsky AS: Injurious ventilatory strategies increase cytokines and c-fos m-RNA expression in an isolated rat lung model. J Clin Invest 1997;99:944–952.

Villar J, Kacmarek RM, Hedenstierna G: From ventilator-induced lung injury to physician-induced lung injury: Why the reluctance to use small tidal volumes? Acta Anaesthesiol Scand 2004;48:267–271.

Webb HH, Tierney DF: Experimental pulmonary edema due to intermittent positive pressure ventilation with high inflation pressures: Protection by positive end-expiratory pressure. Am Rev Respir Dis 1974;110:556–565.

Chapter 18

Weaning

Maureen Meade and Neill Adhikari

KEY POINTS

- Delayed weaning increases patient morbidity, mortality, and costs.
- Ideal weaning predictors are elusive: Tailor to your patient population and assess weaning potential on a daily basis.
- Evidence-based weaning protocols are the single most important proven method for safely reducing time on the ventilator.
- Sedation protocols with either daily cessation of sedatives or targeted sedation goals are integral adjuncts to weaning protocols.
- Pharmacologic interventions to facilitate weaning may cause more harm than good.

As patients recover from critical illness, clinicians strive carefully to wean them from life-supporting technology. Weaning from mechanical ventilation involves a multifaceted process (Fig. 18.1) consisting of reducing the rate of mandatory breaths from the ventilator and reducing the amount of mechanical support provided with each respiratory cycle. Ideally, these processes occur at the same rate at which a patient recovers the ability to initiate breaths spontaneously and to breathe without mechanical assistance. Patients may be weaned in a graded manner or, alternatively, they may progress immediately from full mechanical support to fully unassisted breathing. The latter approach occurs in the context of a formal clinical assessment commonly termed a spontaneous breathing trial or a trial of unassisted breathing. Either way, weaning generally includes a trial of unassisted breathing. The ability to breathe spontaneously and without mechanical support is commonly accepted as a necessary condition for the final phase of weaning—removal of the endotracheal tube.

Weaning is fundamental to the management of critically ill patients, who spend approximately 40% of their time on mechanical ventilation in the process of weaning (Esteban and colleagues, 1994). Meanwhile, mechanical ventilation poses known risks to patients, including increased susceptibility to airway trauma, ventilator-associated pneumonia, ventilator-induced lung injury, gastrointestinal bleeding, venous thromboembolism, and increased sedation use with all its attendant complications (American College of Chest Physicians Task Force, 2001). It follows that weaning should occur as quickly as possible. Overzealous attempts to wean, however, can lead to

respiratory muscle fatigue or cardiovascular instability, either of which may ultimately delay weaning. Premature extubation leading to reintubation carries additional risks of inability to reestablish the airway, pneumonia, and increased mortality. Because mechanical ventilation incurs significant morbidity, mortality, and costs, and because both premature weaning and delayed weaning can cause harm, weaning that is both expeditious and safe is highly desirable.

Aiming for an elusive threshold between weaning too slowly and too rapidly, the practice of weaning mechanical ventilation is further complicated by the distinct challenges of varied patient populations (Box 18.1). The course of weaning differs among patients with severe sepsis, elderly patients with an

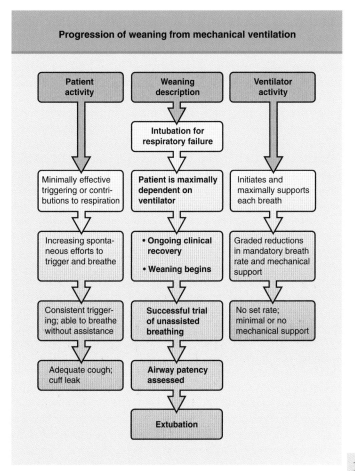

Figure 18.1. Progression of weaning from mechanical ventilation.

Practice of Critical Care

exacerbation of chronic obstructive pulmonary disease (COPD), patients with cervical spinal cord injuries, and healthy patients undergoing elective aortocoronary bypass.

REGIMENS

Weaning Predictors

The need for accurate prediction applies to all phases of weaning, whether clinicians are contemplating a graded reduction in mechanical support for a recovering patient, a trial of unassisted breathing, or a trial of extubation. From a pathophysiological perspective, conscious patients who fail in an attempt to wean do so most frequently as a result of impaired lung mechanics or impaired gas exchange, less frequently as a result of neuromuscular abnormalities or cardiovascular failure, and rarely as a result of central nervous system abnormalities. Clinicians have pursued weaning predictors that relate to each of these underlying processes. Candidates include an assortment of gas exchange variables (e.g., PaO_2 and $PaCO_2$), lung mechanics variables (respiratory rate, tidal volume, and compliance), hemodynamic variables (e.g., heart rate and blood pressure), and subjective signs (e.g., diaphoresis and agitation). Investigators have tested these and numerous other variables individually, as composite scores or derivations, and as complex systems (American College of Chest Physicians Task Force, 2001). Many potential predictors have been tested for their ability to predict success or failure at different phases of weaning and across a variety of patient populations.

Unfortunately, most plausible predictors of weaning and extubation success have been found, on balance, to have little predictive value in clinical investigations. The poor performance of candidate predictors in research settings may reflect inherent limitations of this type of research as much it reflects limitations of the predictors. Thus, clinicians are left to rely heavily on physiologic rationale in selecting weaning predictors for specific populations at particular junctures in weaning (Box 18.2).

Table 18.1 shows an abbreviated list of clinically accepted weaning predictors along with typical "threshold" values for these variables and their descriptions. Among these variables, those that most consistently appear to have predictive value include the rapid shallow breathing index (f/V_t; for all stages of weaning) and the ratio of 0.1-sec occlusion pressure to maximal inspiratory pressure ($P_{0.1}$/MIP; at extubation assessments). Like other putative weaning predictors, these are most useful in helping to identify patients who are likely to fail an attempt to wean and for whom weaning should therefore be delayed.

Table 18.1 Weaning Predictors (Abbreviated)[a]

Variables	Common Thresholds
Gas exchange	
Arterial oxygenation (PaO_2)	>50 to 60 mm Hg
Arterial carbon dioxide ($PaCO_2$)	<50 mm Hg
Arterial pH	>7.25 to 7.30
Lung mechanics	
Respiratory rate (RR)	<30 to 38 breaths/min
Tidal volume (V_t)	>4 to 6 mL/kg; >325 to 400 mL
Rapid shallow breathing index (f/V_t)	<60 to 105 breaths/liter/min
Minute ventilation (MV)	<10 to 15 L/min
Vital capacity (VC)*	>15 mL/kg; >1 to 1.5 L
Maximal inspiratory pressure (MIP)*	<−20 to −30 cm H_2O
Occlusion pressure at 0.1 second ($P_{0.1}$)	>4.5 to 5.0 cm H_2O
$P_{0.1}$/MIP*	>0.09 to 0.14
Hemodynamic	
Mean arterial blood pressure	Depends on baseline values or change from baseline values
Heart rate	Depends on baseline values or change from baseline values
Subjective	
Agitation	Persisting >5 min, despite encouragement and sedation as needed
Diaphoresis	Temporal relationship to initiation of attempt to wean

[a]Variables shown may be used to assess readiness for stepwise reductions in mechanical support, for trials of unassisted breathing, or for extubation. Those identified by an asterisk are used to assess readiness for extubation only; others have been used to identify patient readiness to start weaning, to undergo a trial of unassisted breathing, or to be extubated. Alternatively, predictors are employed to identify those patients likely to fail in an attempt at weaning.

Weaning Modes

When clinicians decide that a patient may tolerate a reduction of mechanical support, there are several ventilator modes that may facilitate this process, some of which may be more successful than others (Table 18.2). Historically, when using controlled mandatory ventilation, clinicians would reduce the rate of ventilator-initiated breaths in a stepwise fashion, allowing patients to initiate a greater proportion of their breaths autonomously. With this technique, each breath is of uniform volume regardless of whether it is patient triggered or ventilator initiated. Classic weaning modes, including synchronized intermittent mandatory ventilation (SIMV), pressure support,

Table 18.2 Ventilator Modes in Weaning		
Mode	**Weaning Description**	**Notes**
Reducing mechanical support		
Assist control	Reduce set rate on ventilator.	Patient-triggered breaths are of uniform set volume.
Synchronized intermittent mandatory ventilation	Reduce set rate on ventilator.	Patient-triggered tidal volume is determined by patient effort and ability only.
Pressure support	Reduce maximum pressure assisting each inspiration.	Patient triggers each breath; tidal volume is determined by patient effort and ability and level of pressure support.
Volume support	Reduce guaranteed minimal tidal volume.	Patient triggers each breath; pressure support level will vary according to patient effort and ability and set tidal volume.
Intermittent T-piece weans	Endotracheal tube is disconnected from ventilator circuit. Increase frequency and/or duration of periods of disconnect.	Patient triggers each breath; patient effort and ability determine each inspired volume.
Unassisted breathing trials		
T-piece	Endotracheal tube is disconnected from ventilator circuit.	Patient triggers each breath; patient effort and ability determine each inspired volume.
Pressure support	Ventilator augments each inspiration with minimal support only (5–8 cm H_2O).	Sufficient pressure support to overcome resistance of ventilator circuit.
Continuous positive airway pressure	Ventilator maintains minimal airway pressure throughout respiratory cycle (3–5 cm H_2O).	Sufficient pressure to replace loss of "physiologic" airway pressure that occurs with glottic closure.

and intermittent T-piece weans, offered some theoretical advantages to weaning with controlled mandatory ventilation. Using SIMV, clinicians reduce the set rate on the ventilator (as with controlled mandatory ventilation); however, the volume of each patient-triggered breath is determined solely by the effort of the patient, without assistance from the ventilator. Weaning in pressure support mode allows clinicians to gradually reduce the extent to which the ventilator will assist each patient-triggered inspiration. This mode is only used when patients can reliably trigger each breath. During T-piece weaning, for a discrete period of time patients initiate each inspiration autonomously and their efforts alone determine the inspired volume. Patients may undergo a T-piece wean once daily or several times daily to build up their endurance, just as an athlete might train for a marathon. On balance, current research suggests that pressure support weaning or multiple daily T-piece weans are superior to SIMV mode, but there is no definitive evidence to guide the choice between pressure support and multiple daily T-piece weans (American College of Chest Physicians Task Force, 2001).

Other options include combinations of the foregoing weaning modes. One example couples SIMV with pressure support to assist each patient-triggered breath. Newer ventilator modes that may also facilitate weaning include volume support and proportional assist ventilation (see Chapter 12), as well as noninvasive positive pressure ventilation (NPPV), which is described in the following section.

Whether or not patients wean in a graded fashion, clinicians generally conduct a trial of unassisted breathing prior to extubation. Classically, this refers to a T-piece trial, the duration of which will depend on the nature of the underlying respiratory insufficiency. For most patients, 30 minutes is sufficient; others require 2 hours or, rarely, much longer. There are several alternatives to classic T-piece trials, including supporting patients through a trial of spontaneous breathing with low-level continuous positive airway pressure (CPAP), pressure support, or both. Theoretically, low-level CPAP will overcome the loss of

physiologic airway pressure that occurs when an endotracheal tube crosses the glottis. In practice, monitoring during a trial of unassisted breathing is facilitated when patients continue to breathe through the ventilator circuit, allowing clinicians to observe changes in tidal volume and minute ventilation. When this is the case, the goal of low-level pressure support is to overcome the added work of breathing required to inspire through the resistance of the ventilator circuit.

Noninvasive Weaning

There may be substantial benefits to an approach of early extubation and implementation of noninvasive positive pressure ventilation for COPD patients who are alert, cooperative, and able to protect their airway (Burns and associates, 2003). Early trials suggest that noninvasive weaning can improve survival (a consistent finding), reduce patient morbidity, and conserve intensive care unit (ICU) resources (Fig. 18.2). Specifically, noninvasive weaning has been found to reduce the incidence of nosocomial pneumonia, the rate of tracheostomy, and the duration of mechanical support and ICU stay. Cautious skepticism may limit the integration of noninvasive weaning into routine clinical care. Because early trials did not uniformly report on reintubation and other adverse events, clinicians may be reticent to remove a secure airway from patients with limited respiratory reserve. Furthermore, because critically ill patients with diagnoses other than COPD were underrepresented in these trials, the role for noninvasive weaning among non-COPD patients is even more uncertain. As a final cautionary note, evidence suggests that there is no role for noninvasive ventilation among patients who fail a trial of extubation (Esteban and colleagues, 2004).

Weaning Protocols

Research suggests that the best way to determine when to start weaning is to develop a protocol, implemented by nurses and respiratory therapists, that begins testing for the opportunity to

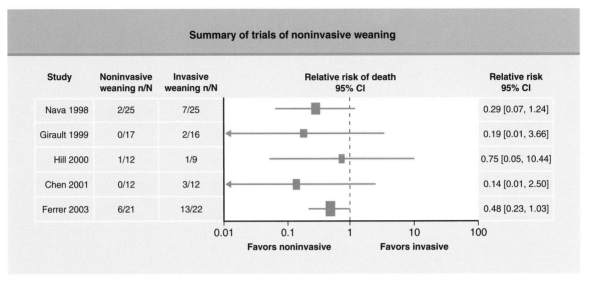

Figure 18.2. Summary of trials on noninvasive weaning. Data from five randomized trials comparing noninvasive weaning to invasive weaning are shown. The number of patients dying *(n)*, number of randomized to each group *(N)*, and relative risk not abbreviated of mortality and 95% confidence intervals (CIs) are presented for each trial. (Adapted with permission from Burns KEA, Adhikari NKJ, Meade MO: Noninvasive positive pressure ventilation as a weaning modality in patients with respiratory failure: a meta-analysis. Cochrane Database of Systematic Reviews 2003;4:CD004127.)

reduce support very soon after intubation and that reduces support at every opportunity (Ely and coworkers, 2001). A protocolized approach to the application of weaning predictors and weaning modes may have a greater effect on the rate and likelihood of successful weaning than the precise selection of predictors or the weaning mode.

Six randomized trials and several additional controlled studies have studied weaning protocols. Earlier trials consistently showed statistically significant and clinically important effects of weaning protocols, such as reduced duration of mechanical ventilation and increased rate of successful extubations (Table 18.3). Some of this research suggested that the cost of ICU care may decline significantly among those treated with a weaning protocol incorporating daily trials of unassisted breathing driven by respiratory care and nursing members of the ICU team, compared with those weaned without a protocol. The solid foundation of evidence in this area has prompted many multidisciplinary ICUs to incorporate weaning protocols into clinical practice. Recent studies that have not demonstrated benefits of weaning protocols may reflect changes in institutional practice to a more evidence-based approach to weaning.

Protocols for weaning from mechanical ventilation should be sufficiently flexible that the safety and comfort of patients assume primary importance. Detailed protocols generally may

Table 18.3 Randomized Trials Comparing Weaning Protocols to Physicians-Directed Weaning[a]

Study	Methods	Population	Intervention	Main Results
Strickland (1993)	Concealed randomization; analysis per protocol	N = 17, 1 center; multidisciplinary ICU	Computer protocol controlling SIMV/PS weans in patients passing screening criteria	Shorter duration of weaning
Ely et al (1996)	Concealed randomization; intention to treat analysis	N = 300, 1 center medical and coronary ICUs	Daily screening followed by TUB	Shorter duration of ventilation and weaning; trend to fewer tracheostomies
Kollef (1997)	Concealed randomization; intention to treat analysis	N = 357, 2 hospitals; medical–surgical ICUs	Protocol varied with ICU and applied to patients passing screening criteria	Shorter duration of ventilation; no change in length of stay
Marelich (2000)	Concealed randomization; analysis per protocol	N = 335, 1 center; medical and trauma ICUs	Daily TUB protocol and SIMV/PSV weans by protocol in patients passing screening criteria	Shorter duration of ventilation; tend to less pneumonia
Schultz (2001)	Concealed randomization; intention to treat analysis	N = 223 children, 1 center	SIMV/PSV weans by protocol in patients passing screening criteria	Shorter duration of weaning; no change in duration of ventilation or pneumonia
Randolph (2002)	Concealed randomization; intention to treat analysis	N = 182 children; 10 centers	Pressure support protocol or volume support protocol in patients failing unassisted breathing trial	No change in extubation failure rates or duration of weaning
Krishnan (2003)	Concealed randomization; intention to treat analysis	N = 299, 1 center; medical ICU; quasi-randomized	Daily screening followed by TUB	No change in duration of ventilation or extubation failure rate

[a]All trials included a no protocol control group and enrolled adults unless otherwise specified. Differences noted in "main results" were statistically significant and favored the protocol group. There were no mortality differences. SIMV, synchronized intermittent mechanical ventilation; PS, pressure support; TUB, trial of unassisted breathing.

Template for developing and implementing a weaning protocol

1. Convene a transdisciplinary team of stakeholders.
   - Respiratory therapists
   - Registered nurses
   - Physicians
   - Educators
   - Administrators

2. Describe your patient population and obtain baseline data (e.g. duration of mechanical ventilation).

3. Define criteria to assess, *on a daily basis*, readiness for a trial of unassisted breathing.
   Adapt existing evidence-based protocols to your setting.
   Include criteria for:
   - Clinical improvement
   - Current level of respiratory support
   - Gas exchange variables
   - Lung mechanics variables
   - Hemodynamic variables
   - Subjective variables

4. Define criteria to *pass* or *fail* a trial of unassisted breathing. Adapt existing evidence-based protocols to your setting. Include criteria from each of the categories outlined above. Include a time frame for observation.

5. Define additional criteria for extubation (e.g., cuff leak, cough effectiveness).

6. Describe explicit channels of communication, responsibility and accountability.

7. Create an education package.

8. Create an implementation package using effective behavior-changing strategies such as interactive education, opinion leaders, reminders, audit and feedback.

9. Measure the impact of the protocol in comparison to baseline data.

10. Amend the protocol or implemention package in response to performance measurements, feedback, and new literature.

Figure 18.3. Template for developing and implementing a weaning protocol.

not transfer smoothly from one ICU to another or from a research venue to general practice. Weaning protocols—the choice of weaning predictors and weaning modes—should be customized to each setting (Figs. 18.3 and 18.4).

Weaning and Sedation

The negative influence of excessive sedation on weaning is clearly established. Investigators have shown that a nursing-implemented protocol for targeted sedation can reduce sedation use, duration of ventilation, need for tracheostomy, and duration of ICU stay by nearly 2 days among patients with respiratory failure (Brook and coworkers, 1999). Others found that daily awakening of mechanically ventilated patients through interruption of sedation reduced the duration of ventilation and ICU stay by 3.5 days (Kress and associates, 2000).

Thus, the next major advance in the area of weaning from mechanical ventilation may arise from clinical trials of interventions focused on interactions between the lungs and the brain.

Cognitive impairment has been associated with increased rates of ventilator-associated pneumonia and failed extubation. Meanwhile, delirium may occur in up to 80% of mechanically ventilated patients. By altering the daily patterns and dosages of psychoactive drug delivery using sedation and weaning protocols, in combination with weaning protocols, significant improvements may be achieved in the outcomes of critically ill patients receiving mechanical ventilation, including long-term cognitive recovery.

Pharmacologic Interventions

Pharmacologic interventions geared to facilitate weaning have, in general, proved futile in research settings, including some interventions that remain in current use.

The catabolism of critical illness and the functional and structural neuromuscular abnormalities that develop in mechanically ventilated patients prompted research into the role of growth hormone in weaning from mechanical ventilation. In a randomized, double-blinded trial including 20 patients requiring ventilation for more that 7 days, growth hormone did not reduce the duration of weaning or the proportion of patients that remained dependent on mechanical ventilation after 12 days (Pichard and associates, 1996).

A similar rationale prompted investigations of anabolic steroids in weaning from mechanical ventilation. Oxandrolone is an anabolic steroid that attenuates loss of lean body mass and improves wound healing in burn patients. In a placebo-controlled trial of oxandrolone therapy for 41 surgical/trauma patients requiring more than 7 days of ventilation, patients receiving oxandrolone had a more prolonged course of mechanical ventilation, suggesting that oxandrolone may be detrimental in this circumstance (Bulger and colleagues, 2004).

Laryngeal edema is a relatively infrequent problem in adults following endotracheal intubation. Occasionally, however, airway compromise prevents extubation or necessitates reintubation. Corticosteroid administration may, in theory, ameliorate this problem as a result of anti-inflammatory effects. Three randomized trials of steroids in adults observed so few events that the collective results are essentially uninformative: They are consistent with both a large reduction in relative risk of reintubation and a large increase in relative risk of reintubation. Results among children differ. Two trials of dexamethasone prior to extubation in children have unequivocally demonstrated that steroids reduce postextubation stridor, although effects on reintubation were positive in one study and negative in the other. For clinicians who believe that preventing stridor is important, these results are compelling; for those who believe that dexamethasone is warranted only if it prevents reintubation, the question remains unanswered (Meade and colleagues, 2001) (Box 18.3).

Box 18.3 Controversies in Weaning

Which weaning predictors are most useful?
Is there a role for tracheostomy to facilitate weaning?
What is the optimal timing for tracheostomy?
Is there a role for noninvasive weaning?
What are acceptable rates of reintubation among varied ICU populations?

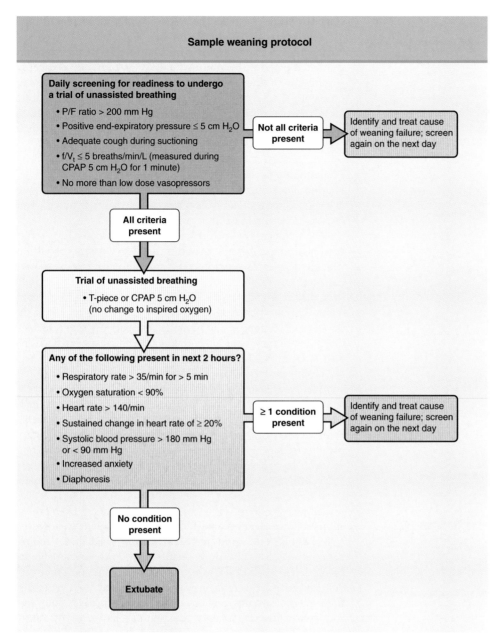

Figure 18.4. Sample weaning protocol.

Sample weaning protocol

Daily screening for readiness to undergo a trial of unassisted breathing

- P/F ratio > 200 mm Hg
- Positive end-expiratory pressure ≤ 5 cm H_2O
- Adequate cough during suctioning
- f/V_t ≤ 5 breaths/min/L (measured during CPAP 5 cm H_2O for 1 minute)
- No more than low dose vasopressors

Not all criteria present → Identify and treat cause of weaning failure; screen again on the next day

All criteria present

Trial of unassisted breathing

- T-piece or CPAP 5 cm H_2O (no change to inspired oxygen)

Any of the following present in next 2 hours?

- Respiratory rate > 35/min for > 5 min
- Oxygen saturation < 90%
- Heart rate > 140/min
- Sustained change in heart rate of ≥ 20%
- Systolic blood pressure > 180 mm Hg or < 90 mm Hg
- Increased anxiety
- Diaphoresis

≥ 1 condition present → Identify and treat cause of weaning failure; screen again on the next day

No condition present

Extubate

REFERENCES

American College of Chest Physicians, American Association for Respiratory Care, and American College of Critical Care Medicine Task Force: Evidence-based guidelines for weaning and discontinuing ventilatory support. Chest 2001;120(Suppl):375S–395S.

Brook AD, Ahrens TS, Schaiff R, et al: Effect of a nursing-implemented sedation protocol on the duration of mechanical ventilation. Crit Care Med 1999;27:2609–2615.

Bulger EM, Jurkovich GJ, Farver CL, Klotz P, Maier RV: Oxandrolone does not improve outcome of ventilator dependent surgical patients. Ann Surg 2004;240:472–480.

Burns KEA, Adhikari N, Meade MO: Noninvasive positive pressure ventilation as a weaning modality in patients with respiratory failure: A meta-analysis. Cochrane Database Syst Rev 2003;4:CD004127.

Ely EW, Baker AM, Dunagan DP, et al: Effect on the duration of mechanical ventilation of identifying patients capable of breathing spontaneously. N Engl J Med 1996;335:1864–1869.

Ely EW, Meade MO, Haponik EF, et al: Mechanical ventilator weaning protocols driven by non-physician health care professionals: Evidence-based clinical practice guidelines. Chest 2001;120(Suppl 6):454S–463S.

Esteban A, Alia I, Ibanez J, et al: Modes of mechanical ventilation and weaning: A national survey of Spanish hospitals; the Spanish Lung Failure Collaborative Group. Chest 1994;106:1188–1193.

Esteban A, Frutos-Vivar F, Ferguson ND, et al: Noninvasive positive-pressure ventilation for respiratory failure after extubation. N Engl J Med 2004;350:2452–2460.

Kress JP, Pohlman AS, O'Connor ME, et al: Daily interruption of sedative infusions in critically ill patients undergoing mechanical ventilation. N Engl J Med 2000;342:1471–1477.

Meade MO, Guyatt GH, Cook DJ, Sinuff T, Butler R: Trials of corticosteroids to prevent post-extubation airway complications. Chest 2001;120(Suppl):464S–468S.

Pichard C, Kyle U, Chrevrolet JC, et al: Lack of effects of recombinant growth hormone on muscle function in patients requiring prolonged mechanical ventilation: A prospective, randomized controlled study. Crit Care Med 1996;24:403–413.

Chapter 19

Ventilator-Associated Pneumonia

Antoni Torres, Amalia Alcón, and Neus Fábregas

The term ventilator-associated pneumonia (VAP) refers to pneumonia that arises more than 48 to 72 hours after intubation with no clinical evidence suggesting the presence or likely development of pneumonia at the time of intubation. VAP is a complication of intubation and ventilatory support and represents an important health problem that generates great controversy.

More than 50% of patients who are admitted to intensive care units (ICUs) already have been colonized at the time of admission with the microorganism responsible for subsequent infection. VAP occurs in 9% to 27% of all intubated patients and can be divided according to its presentation time as follows: (1) early onset VAP, which generally occurs within the first 5 to 7 days, depending on the study, generally carries a better prognosis, and is more likely to be caused by aspiration of antibiotic-sensitive bacteria colonizing the oropharynx, and (2) late-onset VAP, which is more likely to be caused by multidrug-resistant (MDR) pathogens and is associated with increased patient mortality and morbidity. However, patients who have received prior antibiotics or are at risk for health care-related pneumonia may also be colonized or become infected with these bacteria.

EPIDEMIOLOGY, PATHOGENESIS, AND RISK FACTORS

Epidemiology

Incidence/Prevalence

In mechanically ventilated patients, the incidence of VAP increases with duration of ventilation. The risk of VAP is highest early in the course of hospital stay, and it is estimated to be 3% per day during the first 5 days of ventilation, 2% per day during days 5 to 10 of ventilation, and 1% per day after day 10. Since most mechanical ventilation is short term, approximately half of all episodes of VAP occur within the first 5 days.

It is often difficult to define the exact incidence of VAP since there may be an overlap with other lower respiratory tract infections, such as infectious tracheobronchitis, and the exact incidence varies widely depending on the case definition of pneumonia and the population being evaluated.

In a report from an international multicenter cohort study by Alberti and colleagues (2002) conducted over a 1-year period that included 8353 patients (from 28 participating units) hospitalized longer than 24 hours in the ICU, the crude incidence of ICU infection-acquired episodes was 18.9%. The crude incidence of these infections ranged from 2.3% to 49.2% across ICUs and varied from 11.2% [95% confidence interval (CI), 9.2–13.1] in surgical units to 18.1% (95% CI, 16.4–19.8) in medical units and up to 20.7% (95% CI, 19.6–21.8) in mixed units. Respiratory tract infection (mainly pneumonia) was the most common site for both community- and hospital-acquired infections. The three main sources of ICU-acquired infection were the respiratory tract (with pneumonia comprising 75.6% of cases), primary bloodstream infection, and urinary tract infections, which together represented 83% of all reported sites. In studies including only patients with brain injury, the incidence of VAP ranges from 28% to 40%, demonstrating the high incidence of pulmonary infection in this particular pathology.

Morbidity/Mortality

VAP prolongs ICU length of stay and may increase the risk of death in critically ill patients, but the attributable risk of VAP appears to vary with patient population and causative organism. In a study by Heyland and associates, the attributable ICU length of stay in medical patients was longer and the attributable mortality was greater than in surgical patients. In this study, there was no difference between trauma and nontrauma patients or between those with early (<7 days) or late-onset pneumonia in attributable length of stay or mortality.

Papazian and coworkers' matched cohort study suggests that VAP is not linked to mortality, at least in surgical patients. These results agree with the conclusions of the Eole study. This study was conducted over 8 months in 230 study centers in France, and it included all patients with suspected pneumonia occurring during the fortnight after trauma or surgical procedure. VAP accounted for 36.2% of the pneumonia episodes. It was concluded that nosocomial pneumonia in surgical patients is characterized by a high frequency of early onset pneumonia, a high proportion of nosocomial organisms even in these early onset pneumonias, and moderate mortality rate. Pulmonary infections in surgical patients cannot be considered to be identical to other forms of nosocomial pneumonia; moreover, approximately 80% of these patients received antibiotic prophylaxis, a factor that could explain the incidence of gram-negative nosocomial pathogens and staphylococci.

Mortality in VAP is the result of combining the virulence of the pathogen, host defense, and adequacy of antibiotic treatment. The acute respiratory distress syndrome (ARDS) study group compared 134 patients with ARDS to 744 patients without ARDS on mechanical ventilation. VAP occurred in 36.5% of ARDS patients and 23% of patients without ARDS. VAP resulted in a considerable increase in attributable time on mechanical ventilation for both the overall population of ARDS patients and survivors. It was concluded that VAP considerably prolongs the time on mechanical ventilation without affecting survival.

The results of a multicenter study conducted during an 18-month period within the medical and surgical ICUs of four university-affiliated teaching hospitals in France suggested that in addition to severity scores, the underlying medical conditions, and the evolution of severity within the first 4 days in ICU, late-onset pneumonia independently contributed to ICU patient mortality when empirical antibiotic treatment was not appropriate. It is well known that the occurrence of late-onset VAP due to high-risk pathogens is the most important predictor of hospital mortality among patients developing VAP. Risk stratification should be used to identify those patients with antibiotic-resistant bacteria: prior treatment with antibiotics during hospitalization, prolonged length of stay in the hospital, and the

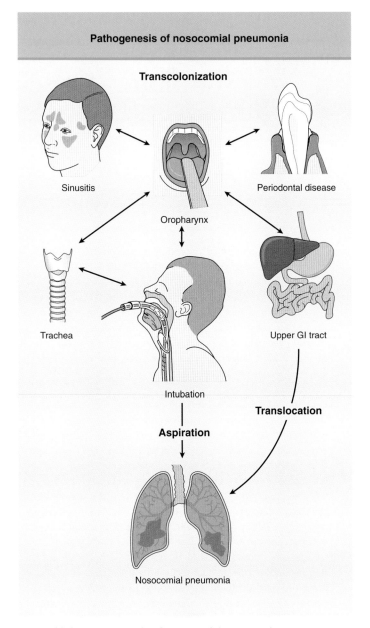

Figure 19.1. Pathogenesis of nosocomial pneumonia.
Etiopathogenesis of nosocomial pneumonia according to Estes and Meduri, 1995.

presence of invasive devices (central venous catheters, endotracheal tubes, and urinary catheters).

Pathogenesis

Nosocomial pneumonia requires the entry of microbial pathogens into the lower airway in large numbers or in smaller numbers of more virulent organisms (Fig. 19.1), which can overwhelm the host's mechanical (ciliated epithelium and mucus) and humoral (antibody and complement) components and cellular host defenses (polymorphonuclear leukocytes, macrophages, and lymphocytes and their respective cytokines). Aspiration of oropharyngeal pathogens or leakage of bacteria around the endotracheal tube cuff are the primary routes of bacterial entry into the trachea in mechanically ventilated patients. In addition, bacteria colonizing the endotracheal tube encased

Different potential routes of colonization and respiratory infection in mechanically ventilated patients

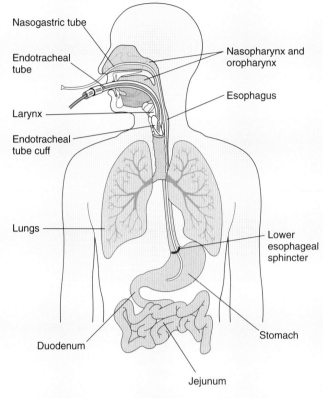

A

Schematic view of etiopathogenesis of ventilator-associated pneumonia

The mechanically ventilated patient

B

Figure 19.2. *A,* Potential routes of colonization and respiratory infection in mechanically ventilated patients. *B,* Schematic of the etiopathogenesis of VAP.

in biofilm may be embolized into the alveoli after suctioning or bronchoscopy. Inhalation of pathogens from contaminated aerosols, direct inoculation into the endotracheal tube, or bronchoscopic contamination are less common. Hematogenous spread from infected intravascular catheters or translocation is an uncommon route of pathogenesis. Bacterial colonization in the stomach and sinuses has been suggested as a potential reservoir for bacteria colonizing the oropharyngx and trachea. As depicted in Figure 19.2, several sources have been described that act as reservoirs for microorganisms that eventually reach the lungs. VAP is most commonly caused by aerobic gram-negative bacilli, such as *Pseudomonas aeruginosa, Escherichia coli, Klebsiella pneumoniae,* or *Acinetobacter* species, but infections due to gram-positive cocci, such as *Staphylococcus aureus* and particularly methicillin-resistant *S. aureus* (MRSA), have been rapidly emerging during the past decade. The frequency of specific MDR pathogens causing hospital-acquired pneumonia (HAP) may vary by hospital, patient population, and type of ICU patient, and it may often change with time, emphasizing the need for up-to-date local surveillance data on their prevalence. Infections due to anaerobic organisms may follow aspiration in nonintubated patients or within 24 hours of intubation, but otherwise they rarely cause VAP. Significant growth of oropharyngeal commensals (*Streptococcus viridans,* coagulase-negative staphylococci, *Neisseria* species, and *Corynebacterium*

species) from distal bronchial specimens is difficult to interpret but can produce infection in immunocompromised hosts and some immunocompetent patients. Rates of polymicrobial infection also vary widely but appear to be increasing and are especially high in patients with ARDS. The major VAP pathogens are shown in Table 19.1.

In early onset VAP, so-called core pathogens include community pathogens, such as methicillin-sensitive *S. aureus, Streptococcus pneumoniae,* and *Haemophilus influenzae,* as well as gram-negative enteric bacilli. The Eole study found that nosocomial pneumonia in surgical patients is characterized by a high frequency of early onset pneumonia, with a high proportion of nosocomial organisms even in the early onset pneumonias, and low mortality.

Late-onset pneumonia (>5–7 days) is usually diagnosed in patients who recently received antibiotic treatment and is most often caused by potentially resistant pathogens (MRSA, *P. aeruginosa, Acinetobacter baumanii,* and/or *Stenotrophomonas maltophilia*).

Risk Factors

For VAP to occur, the delicate balance between host defenses and microbial propensity for colonization and invasion must shift in favor of the pathogens' ability to establish tracheobronchitis and/or pneumonia. Risk factors for VAP are related to the health

Table 19.1 Major VAP Pathogens[a]

Pathogens	Frequency	Multidrug-Resistant Strains
Gram-negative pathogens		
Pseudomonas aeruginosa	+++	+++
Escherichia coli, Klebsiella pneumoniae (ESBL[+/−]), Enterobacter species, *Serratia marcescens*	++	+
Acinetobacter species	+	+++
Stenotrophomonas maltophilia	+	+++
Haemophilus influenzae	+	No
Legionella pneumophila	+	No
Gram-positive pathogens		
Staphylococcus aureus, methicillin-sensitive (MSSA) and methicillin-resistant (MRSA)	+++	+++
Streptococcus pneumoniae	+	++
Anaerobic pathogens	Rare	No
Fungal pathogens		
Candida species	Rare	+
Aspergillus fumigatus	Rare	No
Viruses (RSV, influenza, CMV)	Rare	No

[a]Abbreviations used: ESBL, extended spectrum β-lactamase; RSV, respiratory syncytial virus; CMV, cytomegalovirus; +, uncommon; ++, common; +++, frequent.

care environment, use of invasive devices, and a number of host- and treatment-related factors, such as prior surgery, exposure to antibiotics, other medications, and the presence and duration of exposure to invasive devices or respiratory therapy equipment. In Box 19.1, the independent risk factors for VAP are identified by multivariate analysis in different published studies.

Postsurgical patients are at high risk for VAP. Its development is closely associated with preoperative markers of severity of the underlying disease, a history of smoking, longer preoperative stays, longer surgical procedures, and thoracic or upper abdominal surgery. Box 19.2 describes the risk factors for antibiotic-resistant or MDR pathogens that cause VAP.

Box 19.1 Independent Risk Factors for VAP Identified by Multivariate Analysis in Different Published Studies

Host Factors	Intervention Factors
Pulmonary disease	Supine head position
ARDS	Muscle relaxants
Age > 60 years	Intubation
Impaired consciousness	Mechanical ventilation >2 days
Serum albumin < 2.2 g/dL	Positive end-expiratory pressure
Burns	Intracranial pressure monitoring
Head trauma	Reintubation
Organ failure	Frequent ventilatory circuit changes
Gastric colonization and pH	Nasogastric tube
Upper respiratory tract colonization	Transport out of the ICU
Sinusitis	Prior antibiotic or no antibiotic therapy
Severity of illness	H2 blockers ± antacids
Large-volume gastric aspiration	Continuous intravenous sedation

Box 19.2 Risk Factors for Antibiotic-Resistant or Multidrug-Resistant Pathogens Causing VAP

Prior antimicrobial therapy (90 days)
Prolonged hospitalization (≥5 days of hospitalization)
Local patterns of antibiotic resistance (in the community as well as within the hospital setting)
Risk factors for health care-acquired pneumonia are present
　Hospitalized in the preceding 60 days
　Nursing home/extended care facility resident
　Home infusion therapy (including antibiotics)
　Chronic dialysis
　Home wound care
　Family member with MDR pathogen
Immunosuppressive disease and/or therapy

CLINICAL FEATURES

Clinical criteria are generally qualified as performing poorly; they share a low specificity but there is an increasing trend toward the use of clinical scores for VAP diagnosis. The last published guidelines are those of the Health and Science Policy Committee of the American College of Chest Physicians. These guidelines state that a VAP episode should be suspected in patients receiving mechanical ventilation if two or more of the following clinical features are present: temperature of more than 38°C or less than 36°C, leukopenia or leukocytosis, purulent tracheal secretions, and decreased PaO_2. As a complement, the x-ray can help to define the severity of pneumonia (multilobar or not) and the presence of complications such as emphysema or cavitation (Fig. 19.3).

A diagnostic thoracentesis should be performed to rule out a complicating emphysema if the patient has a pleural effusion, especially if the effusion is greater than 10 mm on a lateral decubitus film or if the patient appears toxic. The routine examination of this fluid should include complete blood cell count and differential; measurement of protein, LDH, glucose (with comparison to serum values obtained at the time of thoracentesis), and pH; Gram stain and, in select patients, acid fast stain; and cultures for bacteria, fungi, and *Mycobacterium tuberculosis*. The clinical approach may be overly sensitive, and patients can be treated for pneumonia when another, noninfectious process is responsible for the clinical findings. These processes may include congestive heart failure, atelectasis, pulmonary thromboembolism, pulmonary drug reactions, pulmonary hemorrhage, or ARDS. Because of the imprecision of clinical diagnosis of VAP, reliance on this strategy may lead to the overuse of antibiotics. Tracheal colonization or purulent tracheobronchitis may mimic many of the clinical signs of VAP. For patients with ARDS, for whom it is difficult to demonstrate deterioration of radiological images, at least one of three clinical criteria should lead to more diagnostic testing, but other signs of pneumonia include hemodynamic instability or deterioration of blood gases.

In the early 1990s, Pugin and colleagues (1991) developed a clinical pulmonary infection score (CPIS) to diagnose pneumonia. Although it includes radiologic and microbiologic data, it can be applied when VAP is suspected. A modified score (Box 19.3) has shown its usefulness in two different studies from a research

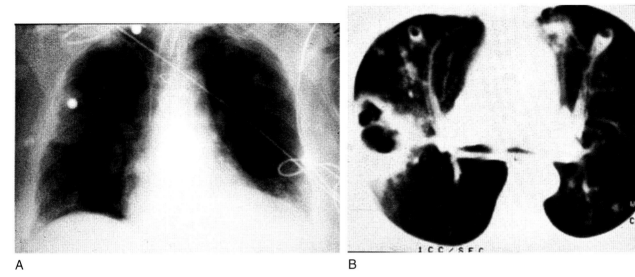

Figure 19.3. *A,* Cavitated VAP confirmed by CT scan. *B,* The image was not very apparent in the portable chest x-ray.

Box 19.3 Clinical Pulmonary Infection Score Calculation

Temperature (°C)
$\geq$36.5 and $\leq$38.4 = 0 points
$\geq$38.5 and $\leq$38.9 = 1 point
$\geq$39 and $\leq$36 = 2 points

Blood leukocyte (mm³)
$\geq$4000 and $\leq$110,000 = 0 points
<4000 or >11,000 = 1 point + band forms $\geq$ 50% = add 1 point

Tracheal secretions
Absence of tracheal secretions = 0 points
Presence of nonpurulent tracheal secretions = 1 point
Presence of purulent tracheal secretions = 2 points

Oxygenation: PaO$_2$/FIO$_2$ (mm Hg)
240 or ARDS (ARDS defined as PO$_2$/FIO$_2$, or equal to 200, pulmonary arterial wedge pressure $\leq$ 18 mm Hg and acute bilateral infiltrates) = 0 points
$\leq$240 and no ARDS = 2 points

Pulmonary radiography
No infiltrate = 0 points
Diffuse (or patchy) infiltrate = 1 point
Localized infiltrate = 2 points

Progression of pulmonary infiltrate
No radiographic progression = 0 points
Radiographic progression (after congestive heart failure and ARDS excluded) = 2 points

Culture of tracheal aspirate
Pathogenic bacteria cultured in rare or light quantity or no growth = 0 points
Pathogenic bacteria cultured in moderate or heavy quantity = 1 point
Same pathogenic bacteria seen on Gram stain, add 1 point

CPIS at baseline was assessed on the basis of the first five variables. CPIS at 72 hours was calculated based on all seven variables and took into consideration the progression of the infiltrate and culture results of the tracheal aspirate. A score > 6 at baseline or at 72 hours was considered suggestive of pneumonia.

---

group. The CPIS increased the specificity of the chest x-ray in the diagnosis of VAP. It was used in a prospective cohort study of 129 consecutive patients who developed pulmonary infiltrates in the surgical ICU to determine the predictors and outcome of pulmonary infiltrates. Overt community-acquired pneumonia (i.e., that occur <72 hr after hospitalization) was excluded. The most common etiologies of pulmonary infiltrates were pneumonia (responsible for only 30% of the pulmonary infiltrates), pulmonary edema (29%), acute lung injury (15%), and atelectasis (13%). A CPIS score higher than 6 virtually excluded acute lung injury, pulmonary edema, or atelectasis as etiologies of pulmonary infiltrates.

DIAGNOSIS

Recent studies have included different algorithms for improving VAP diagnosis and treatment. For example, the VAP diagnosis algorithm depicted in Figure 19.4 was proposed by the Health and Science Policy Committee of the American College of Chest Physicians. Blot and colleagues proposed a decisional tree for the early diagnosis and management of suspected VAP based on both plugged telescoping catheter (PTC), blind or fiberoptically guided, and endotracheal aspirate (EA) Gram stain analysis:

1. EA Gram stain is negative: VAP is very unlikely. No empiric antibiotic treatment for pneumonia is needed pending culture results of samples.
2. PTC Gram stain is positive: VAP is very likely. Early empiric antibiotic treatment choice is based on the results of the Gram staining of the PTC and/or the EA, as well as on epidemiological data. When culture results are obtained, the antibiotic treatment may be maintained, adapted, or stopped.
3. EA Gram stain is positive and PTC Gram stain negative: No satisfactory prediction is allowed before the culture results. The decision to start an empiric treatment

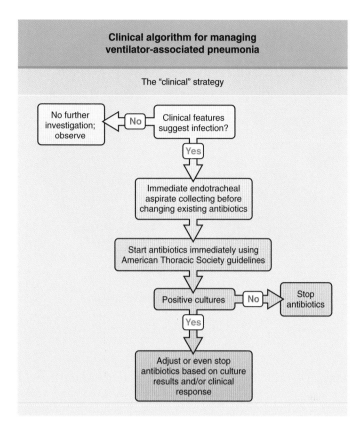

Figure 19.4. Clinical algorithm for managing VAP.

could depend on the severity of sepsis and underlying condition.

In the authors' experience, the main value of this diagnostic approach is to reduce the percentage of uncertainty to approximately one third of the episodes.

Singh and coworkers (2000) used the adaptation of the CPIS previously mentioned (see Box 19.2) to determine the "likelihood" of pneumonia. A CPIS of 6 implied that the patient was unlikely to have bacterial pneumonia. The CPIS was used not as a diagnostic tool as originally proposed by Pugin but, rather, as a screen for decision making regarding antibiotic therapy. In their study, 74% of patients with pulmonary infiltrates in the ICU had CPIS of 6. A 3-day duration for empiric ciprofloxacin monotherapy was selected because this time period allows microbiologic culture data to be obtained for assessing the need to continue antibiotics. Despite the short duration with monotherapy, the length of ICU stay or survival was not adversely affected. In 21% of patients in both groups, the CPIS increased to higher than 6 on day 3. Mortality at 14 or 30 days did not differ between the patients with CPIS higher than 6, who initially received monotherapy compared with standard therapy. The success of the experimental therapy includes the fact that patients with CPIS less than 6 did not have nosocomial pneumonia and thus CPIS accurately ruled out an infection. It is also conceivable that a proportion of patients with CPIS of 6 had a mild infection (tracheobronchitis or minimal pneumonitis) that was treatable with 3 days of monotherapy. Regardless of the precise explanation, the CPIS criteria were documented to be efficacious in minimizing antibiotic usage without compromising the clinical outcome. CPIS used as oper-

ational criteria in this study, regardless of the precise definition of pneumonia, was accurate in identifying patients with pulmonary infiltrates in the ICU for whom monotherapy with a shorter duration of antibiotics was appropriate. With regard to the use of antibiotics, in a study of 138 patients evaluated by collection of bronchoscopic specimens, Bonten and coworkers found that antibiotic therapy can be stopped in patients with negative quantitative cultures with no adverse effect on the recurrence of VAP or mortality.

Serologic studies are of little use in the initial evaluation of patients with HAP and should not be routinely performed. However, they may have epidemiologic value primarily for viral and *Legionella* infections.

Quantitative cultures can be performed on samples collected either bronchoscopically or nonbronchoscopically (Fig. 19.5), and each technique has its own diagnostic threshold and methodological limitations. Since all the methods have similar sensitivity and specificity for the presence of pneumonia and for the etiologic pathogen, the choice of method depends on local expertise, experience, availability, and cost.

TREATMENT

In selecting empiric therapy for patients who have recently received an antibiotic, an effort should be made to use an agent from a different antibiotic class, since recent therapy can predispose to resistance and inappropriate therapy if the same class is used again. Initial antibiotic therapy should be given promptly, since delays in administration may increase mortality in VAP. Initial empiric therapy is more likely to be appropriate if a protocol for antibiotic selection is developed based on algorithms such as those shown in Tables 19.3 and 19.4 but adapted to local patterns of antibiotic resistance, with each ICU collecting this information and updating it on a regular basis. If patients receive an initially appropriate antibiotic regimen, efforts should be made to shorten the duration of therapy from the traditional 14 to 21 days to as short as 7 days. Pharmacodynamic properties of specific antibiotics should also be considered in selecting an adequate dosing regimen. Monotherapy with selected agents can be used for patients with severe VAP in the absence of resistant pathogens, but patients in this risk group should initially receive combination therapy until the results of lower respiratory tract cultures are known and confirm that a single agent can be used. In Tables 19.5 and 19.6, intravenous antimicrobial treatments of some gram-negative bacilli and gram-positive cocci are detailed.

Aerosolized antibiotics have not been proven to have value in the therapy of VAP but may be considered as adjunctive therapy in patients with MDR gram-negative results who are not responding to systemic therapy.

Ibrahim and colleagues attempted to prove the usefulness of applying a clinical guideline for the antibiotic treatment of VAP in their medical ICU. Once the clinical diagnosis was made according to American Thoracic Society rules, they started treatment with vancomycin, imipenem, and ciprofloxacin. Treatment was modified after 24 to 48 hours based on the available culture results (EA or bronchoscopic BAL or nonbronchoscopic BAL), and a 7-day treatment was recommended. Although the use of this protocol did not reduce the hospital mortality or length of hospital stay, improving the effectiveness of prescribed antibiotic regimen and reducing the administration

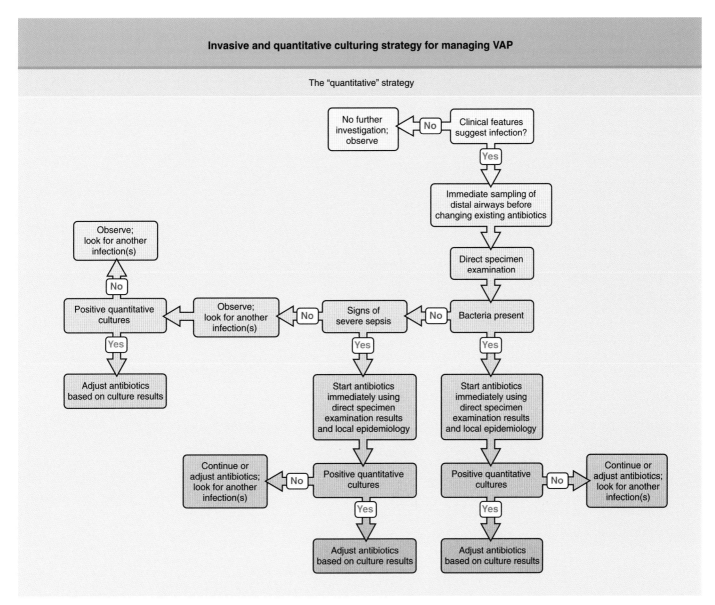

Figure 19.5. Invasive and quantitative culturing strategy for managing VAP.

of unnecessary antibiotic treatment seem to be worthwhile outcomes.

CLINICAL COURSE AND PREVENTION

Response to Therapy

Modification of Empiric Antibiotic Regimens

After the institution of empiric therapy, antibiotic choices may need to be modified once the results of blood or respiratory tract cultures become available, in conjunction with an assessment of the clinical response. This may be necessary when a resistant or unsuspected pathogen is found in a nonresponding patient, and therapy will need to be changed. Alternatively, therapy can be deescalated or narrowed because an anticipated organism (e.g., *P. aeruginosa* and *Acinetobacter* species) was not recovered or because the isolated organism is sensitive to an antibiotic that is less broad spectrum than that used in the initial regimen.

Critical to the routine use of any of the proposed empiric antibiotic regimens is the ability to recognize when a patient is not responding appropriately. Unfortunately, there is little information about the natural course of VAP resolution. In addition, because of the variability in diagnosing the infection, the natural history of presumed VAP may differ depending on the disease process present in a given patient. Clinical response may also be related to patient factors (e.g., age and comorbidity), bacterial factors (e.g., antimicrobial resistance patterns and virulence), and other events that may occur during the course of VAP.

A serial assessment of clinical parameters should be performed to define the response to initial empiric therapy, and modifications should be made based on this information, in conjunction with microbiologic data.

For the responding patient, antibiotics should be de-escalated and therapy should be narrowed to the most focused regimen, based on culture data. If lower respiratory tract cultures do not show highly resistant pathogens, then it is not necessary to continue therapy for these organisms.

Table 19.2 Initial Empiric Antibiotic Therapy for Patients with No Known Risk Factors for Multidrug Resistant Pathogens and Early Onset Hospital-Acquired Pneumoniae of All Severity and no Other Sites of Infection[a]

Potential Pathogens	Recommended Antibiotics

Streptococcus pneumoniae[b]
Haemophilus influenzae
Methicillin-sensitive Staphylococcus aureus
Antibiotic-sensitive enteric gram-negative bacilli
  Escherichia coli
  Klebsiella pneumoniae
  Enterobacter species
  Proteus species
  Serratia marcescens
	Second-/third-generation cephalosporin (cefotaxime, ceftriaxone)
	OR
	Third-/fourth-generation quinolone (levofloxacin, moxifloxacin)
	OR
	β-Lactam, β-lactamase inhibitor (ampicillin/sulbactam)

[a]Initial antibiotic therapy should be adjusted based on microbiologic data and clinical response to therapy.
[b]Frequency of penicillin-resistant S. pneumoniae and multdrug-resistant S. pneumoniae strains is increasing.

Table 19.3 Initial Empiric Antibiotic Therapy for Patients with Risk Factors for Multidrug-Resistant (MDR) Pathogens and Early or Late-Onset VAP of All Severity[a]

Potential MDR Pathogens	Combination Antibiotic Therapy[b]
Pseudomonas aeruginosa	Third-/fourth-generation anti-pseudomonal cephalosporin (cefepime, ceftazidime) OR
Klebsiella pneumoniae (ESBL+) Acinetobacter species	Carbepenem (anti-pseudomonal) (imipenem, meropenem) OR β-Lactam, β-lactamase inhibitor (pipercillin-tazobactam) PLUS Second-/third-generation fluoroquinolone (high-dose ciprofloxacin or levofloxacin) OR
Methicillin-resistant Staphylococcus aureus	Aminoglycoside (amikacin, gentamicin, tobramycin) PLUS Linezolid or vancomycin

[a]Initial antibiotic therapy should be adjusted or streamlined based on microbiologic data and clinical response to therapy.
[b]when extended spectrum β-lactamase (ESBL) microorganism is suspected, use a carbepenem. If Legionella pneumophila is suspected, the combination antibiotic regimen should include a fluoroquinolone rather than an aminoglycoside.

Table 19.4 Intravenous Antimicrobial Treatment of Some Gram-Negative Bacilli Causing VAP in Adults

Common Pathogens	Preferred Antimicrobial Agent	Example[a]	Comments
Pseudomonas aeruginosa	Third-/fourth-generation anti-pseudomonal cephalosporin OR Carbapenem OR β-Lactam, β-lactamase inhibitor PLUS Fluoroquinolone OR Aminoglycoside OR Monobactam	Cefepime 1.5 g 8hr q8hr Ceftazidime 2 g q8hr OR Imipenem 500 mg q6hr, meropenem 1 g q8hr OR Piperacillin-tazobactam 3 g q6hr PLUS Levofloxacin 750 mg qd Ciprofloxacin 400 mg q8hr OR Gentamicin 7 mg/kg/q24hr Tobramycin 7 mg/kg/24hr/q24hr Amikacin 20 mg/kg/q24hr OR Aztreonam	Some MDR strains may need therapy with aerosolized polymyxin or aerosolized aminoglycosides. Strains may persist after completing therapy. Adjust dose by serum peak and trough levels.
Escherichia coli Klebsiella spp. Serratia marcescens Enterobacter spp.	Cephalosporin	Cefazolin 2 g q8hr OR Fluoroquinolone (ciprofloxacin or levofloxacin)	Sensitivity of strains varies. See ESBL + MDR isolates of Klebsiella.
ESBL + isolates Klebsiella pneumoniae Escherichia coli Enterobacter spp.	Carbapenem	Imipenem + ciliastin 500 mg q6hr OR Meropenem 1 g q8hr	Sensitivity of strains varies.
Acinetobacter spp.	Ampicillin/sulbactam OR A carbapenem	Meropenem 1 g q8hr Ampicillin/sulbactam 3 g q6hr OR Imipenem 500 mg q6hr, meropenem 1 g q8hr	Sensitivity of strains varies.
Stenotrophomonas maltophilia	Trimethoprim (TMP)–sulfamethoxazole (SMX)	TMP SMX 3–5 mg/kg of TMP q8hr	

[a]All does listed are for patients with normal renal and hepatic function.

Table 19.5 Intravenous Antimicrobial Treatment of Some Gram-Positive Cocci Causing VAP in Adults

Common Pathogens	Preferred Antimicrobial agent	Example[a]	Comments
Staphylococcus aureus, methicillin susceptible (MSSA)	Penicillinase-resistant penicillin	Cefazolin OR Cefuroxime	Penicillinase-resistant penicillin or a cephalosporin preferred over vancomycin.
Staphylococcus aureus, methicillin-resistant (MRSA)	Vancomycin OR Linezolid	Vancomycin 10–15 mg/k q12hr OR Linezolid, 600 mg q12hr OR Vancomycin rifampin gentamicin	Vancomycin should be dosed to maintain high serum trough levels (10–13 µg/mL). Randomized trials comparing vancomycin to linezolid are in progress. Linezolid, bactrim, and rifampin may be given po. Dose of linezolid for adults <40 kg should be 10 mg/kg. Linezolid may be given orally,
Streptococcus pneumoniae	Second-/third-generation cephalosporin (cefriaxone or cefuroxime) OR Third-/fourth-generation fluoroquinolone OR β-Lactam, β-lactamase inhibitor	Ceftriaxone 2 g, cefuroxime 1.5 g q8hr OR Levofloxacin 750 mg Gatifloxacin Moxifloxacin OR Ampicillin/sulbactam 3 g q6hr	MDR strains should initially be treated with vancomycin or a third- or fourth-generation fluoroquinolone, Fluoroquinolones may be given orally when possible.

[a]All doses listed are for patients with normal renal and hepatic function.

The nonresponding patient should be evaluated for noninfectious mimics of pneumonia, unsuspected or drug-resistant organisms, extrapulmonary sites of infection, and complications of pneumonia and its therapy. Diagnostic testing should be directed to the most likely origin of treatment failure.

Prevention

The cornerstones of prevention of nosocomial pneumonia remain healthcare practitioners' hand washing, isolation of patients with multiresistant pathogens, and a judicious and restrictive use of antimicrobial treatment to prevent the selection of multiresistant pathogens. Therefore, measures to prevent VAP gain increasing importance. The relative role of different preventive measures is a matter of increasing interest, and this is particularly true for noninvasive ventilation, ventilator circuit, and secretion management strategies. The nonpharmacologic interventions for VAP are listed in Box 19.3.

Summary of Selected Evidence-Based Recommendations for Prevention of Modifiable Risk Factors for VAP

General

- Strict infection control measures, staff education, and compliance with alcohol-based hand disinfection are recommended to reduce cross-infection with MDR pathogens [Centers for Disease Control and Prevention (CDC)].
- Surveillance of ICU infections, such as VAP, is recommended to identify and quantify endemic and MDR pathogens. The information should be provided to the ICU staff in order to formulate appropriate antimicrobials for initial therapy in patients with suspected VAP or other nosocomial infections (CDC).
- Maintaining adequate staffing levels in the ICU is recommended to reduce length of stay, improve infection control practices, and reduce the risk of VAP.

- Careful monitoring and limited use and removal of all unnecessary invasive devices are recommended.
- An effective antibiotic control program, based on local microbiology and epidemiology, is recommended to reduce selective pressure for colonization and infection with MDR pathogens.
- Vaccination with pneumococcal and influenza vaccines is recommended, if indicated, before discharge from the hospital to prevent recurrent lower respiratory tract infections.

Antibiotics and Other Modifiable Medications

- Routine prophylaxis of VAP with oral antibiotics should be performed. Selective decontamination of the digestive tract (SDD), with or without systemic antibiotics, reduces

---

Box 19.4 Nonpharmacological Interventions for Ventilator-Associated Pneumonia Prevention

Noninvasive positive pressure ventilation
Isolation of patients with multiresistant pathogens
Hand washing
Gowns and gloves
Semirecumbent position
Chest physiotherapy and "kinetic" beds
Route of tracheal intubation
Subglottic aspiration tubes and cuff pressure level
Avoid biofilm formation
Avoid reintubation
Endotracheal suctioning system
Nasogastric tube type
Humidifiers
Ventilatory circuit changes
Tracheostomy
Early nutritional support

the incidence of VAP but is not recommended for routine use, especially in patients who may be colonized with MDR pathogens.

- Prior administration of systemic antibiotics may be beneficial in some patient groups, but it may increase the risk for colonization with MDR pathogens and subsequent infection.
- Prophylactic administration of cefuroxime at the time of intubation should be considered to prevent ICU-acquired HAP in patients with closed-head injury.
- Modulation of oropharyngeal colonization by the use of chlorhexidine prevents VAP.
- The routine combined use of sedative and paralytic agents depresses cough and pharyngeal reflexes, thereby increasing the risk of VAP, and is not recommended.
- Protocols to interrupt sedation are recommended.
- Data suggest a trend toward reduced VAP with sucralfate but slightly higher rates of clinically significant gastric bleeding. If needed, stress bleeding prophylaxis with either histamine type 2 or sucralfate is acceptable.

Patient Positioning and Enteral Feeding

- Patients should be kept in the semirecumbent position (30–45 degrees) rather than supine, especially when receiving enteral feeding (Fig. 19.6).
- Enteral nutrition is preferred over parenteral nutrition to reduce the risk of complications related to central intravenous catheters and to prevent villous atrophy of the intestinal mucosa that may increase the risk of bacterial translocation.
- Early enteral nutrition (day 1) benefits should be weighed against delayed enteral feeding to prevent VAP.
- Postpyloric feeding may decrease the risk of aspiration and ICU-acquired VAP, but it is not recommended for routine use. Intermittent or acidified enteral feeding is not recommended to prevent VAP.

Intubation and Mechanical Ventilation

- The use of an endotracheal tube increases the risk of VAP and therefore unnecessary intubation should be avoided.

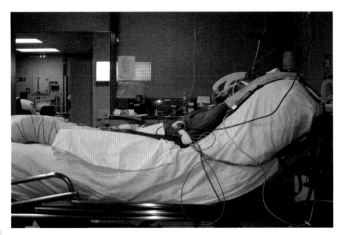

Figure 19.6. Semirecumbent position in mechanical and ventilated patients. This measure effectively reduces VAP.

Table 19.6 Impact of Noninvasive Ventilation on Rates of Nosocomial Infections, Pneumonia, and Defined Outcome Variables in Patients with Acute Exacerbations of Chronic Obstructive Pulmonary Disease and Hypercapnic Cardiogenic Edema Suitable for Noninvasive Ventilation[a]

Variable	Noninvasive Ventilation	Intubation and Mechanical Ventilation	P
Nosocomial infections rate	18%	60%	<0.001
Nosocomial pneumonia rate	8%	22%	0.04
Proportion of patients receiving antibiotics for nosocomial infection	8%	26%	0.01
Mean duration of ventilatory support (days) (SD)	6 (6)	10 (12)	0.01
Mean length of ICU stay (days) (SD)	9 (7)	15 (14)	0.02
Crude mortality	4%	26%	0.002

[a]Adopted from Girou E, Schortgen F, Delclaux C, et al: Association of non-invasive ventilation with nosocomial infections and survival in critically ill patients. JAMA 2000;284:2376–2378.

- Noninvasive positive pressure ventilation (NIPPV) using a face mask or helmet is recommended for use in certain patients with chronic obstructive pulmonary disease or congestive heart failure. Table 19.7 provides a comparison of pneumonia rates between patients under noninvasive ventilation and those under intubation and mechanical ventilation.
- Orotracheal intubation is preferred over nasotracheal intubation to prevent nosocomial sinusitis and to reduce the risk of VAP, although direct causality has not been proven.
- The endotracheal tube cuff pressure should be higher than 20 cm H_2O.
- Strategies to reduce the duration of intubation and mechanical ventilation by protocols to improve use of sedation and accelerated weaning are recommended.
- Continuous aspiration of subglottic secretions is recommended to reduce the risk of VAP (Fig. 19.7).

Respiratory Therapy Equipment

- Proper disinfection and sterilization of respiratory therapy equipment and bronchoscopes are strongly recommended to reduce cross-infection (CDC).
- Contaminated condensate in ventilator circuits should be eliminated and never flushed back into the airway or into on-line nebulizers.
- Use of passive humidifiers, with or without filtering capacity, is recommended to decrease ventilator circuit colonization, and these need not be changed more frequently than every 48 hours.
- Changing ventilator circuits is not recommended to prevent VAP.
- Controlled tidal volumes no greater than 6 mL/kg are recommended to reduce lung injury, especially in patients with ARDS.

Miscellaneous Modifiable Risk Factors

- Routine red blood cell transfusion and that of other allogenic blood products should be given in accord with a restricted transfusion trigger policy.

Subglottic aspiration using double lumen tubes for the prevention of VAP

Incorporated evacuation lumen

Large elliptical
dorsal opening

Subglottic area

A

B

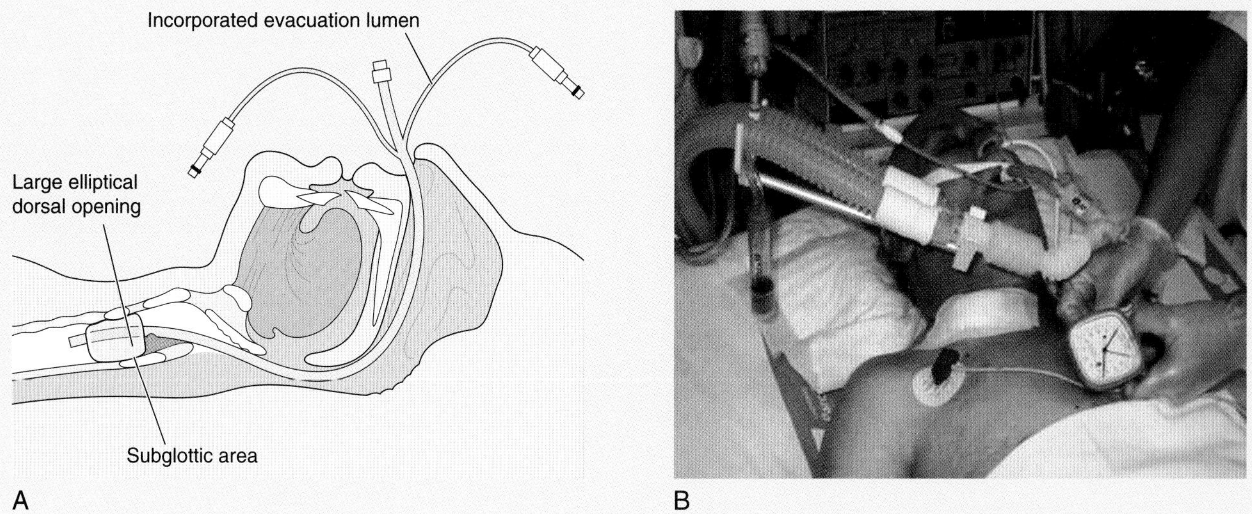

Figure 19.7. *A,* Subglottic aspiration using double lumen tubes for the prevention of VAP. *B,* Controlling the pressure of the cuff > 20 cm H_2O is an important goal in the prevention of VAP.

- Leukocyte-depleted red blood cell transfusions may reduce the incidence of pneumonia in select patient populations.
- Intensive insulin therapy is recommended to maintain serum glucose levels between 80 and 110 mg/dL in ICU patients to reduce the duration of mechanical ventilation, ICU stay, morbidity, and mortality.
- To improve future clinical trials analysis, the use of scores to stratify postoperative pneumonia, severity scores such as APACHE and the CPIS are recommended.

PITFALLS/COMPLICATIONS AND CONTROVERSIES

The following are controversies with regard to VAP (Table 19.8):

1. Diagnosis based on clinical scores only
2. Classification of VAP in early onset or late-onset according to hospitalization or ICU admission days
3. Endotracheal aspiration semiquantitative or quantitative for VAP microbial diagnosis
4. Usefulness of fibrobronchoscopically obtained respiratory samples
5. High dose of broad-spectrum antibiotics administered immediately after suspicion of VAP

CONCLUSIONS

The definition of VAP includes different entities that have different prognostics depending on the responsible microorganism and the patient's medical condition. Patients should be stratified according to type and disease severity, and an algorithm including clinical and microbiological analysis [as direct exami-

nation (Gram stain) of respiratory samples] is needed to improve diagnosis and treatment efficacy. We believe that the key point in clinical practice is to find a balance between the information provided by clinical judgment and the quantitative microbiology results of the lower airways. Giving prophylactic antibiotics may reduce early onset VAP but can result in late-onset VAP by high-risk antibiotic multiresistant microorganisms associated with high mortality. Guidelines for VAP treatment can increase the initial administration of adequate antimicrobial treatment and decrease the overall duration of antibiotic treatment. To develop these guidelines, local microbiological data should be used. Surveillance cultures may be useful in guiding the initial empirical treatment, but research focusing on outcome and cost is needed. Quantitative endotracheal aspirate secretion cultures and blind distal protected samples may be as useful as bronchoscope obtained respiratory samples.

Nevertheless, there is no gold standard diagnose for VAP, so clinical and microbiological features, together with the patient's

Table 19.7 Pitfalls and Complications of VAP

Pitfall	Complication
Direct Gram stain from respiratory sample negative	Decide not to start antibiotic treatment in an infected patient
General antibiotic guidelines for VAP treatment	Not full microbiological covering
Antibiotic treatment depending on onset time	Not full microbiological covering
Maintain antibiotic treatment for 2 weeks	Creating antibiotic resistances
Withdraw antibiotic treatment if negative cultures	Under treatment

185

disease evolution, continue to be the cornerstone guiding physicians' decisions. Broad-spectrum coverage followed by deescalation of antibiotic therapy can be thought of as a way to balance the need to provide adequate initial antibiotic treatment of high-risk patients with the avoidance of necessary antibiotic use that promotes resistance. High and individualized doses based on location and pharmacodynamic considerations with immediate initiation of antibiotic treatment (even when direct microscopy of stained samples is negative) and choice of antimicrobial based on (lung) penetration are essential. Empiric therapy should always be modified once the agent of infection is identified, or it should be discontinued if the diagnosis of infection becomes unlikely.

SUGGESTED READING

Alberti C, Brun-Buisson C, Burchardi H, et al: Epidemiology of sepsis and infection in ICU patients from an international multicentre cohort study. Intensive Care Med 2002;28:525–526.

American Thoracic Society: Hospital-acquired pneumonia in adults: Diagnosis, assessment of severity, initial antimicrobial therapy, and preventive strategies. A consensus statement, American Thoracic Society, November 1995. Am J Respir Crit Care Med 1996;153:1711–1725.

Bonten MJ, Bergmens D, Stobberingh EE, et al: Implementation of bronchoscopic techniques in the diagnosis of ventilator-associated pneumonia to reduce antibiotic use. Am J Respir Crit Care Med 1997;156:1820–1824.

Chastre J, Fagon JY: Ventilator-associated pneumonia. Am J Respir Crit Care Med 2002;165:867–903.

Combes A, Figliolini C, Trouillet JL, et al: Incidence and outcome of polymicrobial ventilator-associated pneumonia. Chest 2002;121:1618–1623.

Drakulovic MB, Torres A, Bauer TT, et al: Supine body position as a risk factor for nosocomial pneumonia in mechanically ventilated patients: A randomised trial. Lancet 1999;354:1851–1858.

Estes RJ, Meduri GU: The pathogenesis of ventilator-associated pneumonia: Mechanisms of bacterial transcolonization and airway inoculation. Intensive Care Med 1995;21:365–383.

Grossman RF, Fein A: Evidence-based assessment of diagnostic tests for ventilator-associated pneumonia. Executive summary. Chest 2000;117:177S–181S

Heyland DK, Cook DJ, Griffith L, et al: The attributable morbidity and mortality of ventilator-associated pneumonia in the critically ill patient. The Canadian Critical Trials Group. Am J Respir Crit Care Med 1999;159:1249–1256.

Hubmayr RD, Burchardi H, Elliot M, et al: Statement of the 4th International Consensus Conference in Critical Care on ICU-Acquired Pneumonia, Chicago, Illinois, May 2002. Intensive Care Med 2002;28:1521–1536.

Ibrahim EH, Ward S, Sherman G, et al: Experience with a clinical guideline for the treatment of ventilator associated pneumonia. Crit Care Med 2001;29:1109–1115.

Lambotte O, Timsit JF, Garrouste-Org, et al: The significance of distal bronchial samples with commensals in ventilator-associated pneumonia: Colonizer or pathogen? Chest 2002;122:1389–1399.

Montravers P, Veber B, Auboyer C, et al: Diagnostic and therapeutic management of nosocomial pneumonia in surgical patients: Results of the Eole study. Crit Care Med 2002;30:368–375.

Papazian L, Bregeon F, Thirion X, et al: Effect of ventilator-associated pneumonia on mortality and morbidity. Am J Respir Crit Care Med 1996;154:91–97.

Pingleton SK, Fagon JY, Leeper KV Jr: Patient selection for clinical investigation of ventilator-associated pneumonia. Criteria for evaluating diagnostic techniques. Chest 1992;102:553S–556S.

Pittet D, Hugonnet S, Harbarth S, et al: Effectiveness of a hospital-wide programme to improve compliance with hand hygiene. Infection Control Programme. Lancet 2000;356:1307–1312.

Pugin J, Auckenthaler R, Mili N, et al: Diagnosis of ventilator-associated pneumonia by bacteriologic analysis of bronchoscopic and non-bronchoscopic "blind" bronchoalveolar lavage fluid. Am Rev Respir Dis 1991;143:1121–1129.

Rello J, Diaz E: Optimal use of antibiotics for intubation-associated pneumonia. Intensive Care Med 2001;27:337–339.

Singh N, Rogers P, Atwood CW, et al: Short-course empiric antibiotic therapy for patients with pulmonary infiltrates in the intensive care unit. A proposed solution for indiscriminate antibiotic prescription. Am J Respir Crit Care Med 2000;162:505–511.

Souweine B, Mom T, Traore O, et al: Ventilator-associated sinusitis: Microbiological results of sinus aspirates in patients on antibiotics. Anesthesiology. 2000;93:1255–1260.

Torres A, Carlet J. Ventilator-associated pneumonia. European Task Force on ventilator-associated pneumonia. Eur Respir J 2001;17:1034–1045.

Torres A, Ewig S: Diagnosing ventilator-associated pneumonia. N Engl J Med 2004;350:433–435.

Value of Gram stain examination of lower respiratory tract secretions for early diagnosis of nosocomial pneumonia: Evaluations of outcome. Am J Respir Crit Care Med 2000;162:1731–1737.

Chapter 20

Clinical Assessment of the Acutely Unstable Patient

Jukka Takala

KEY POINTS

- Recognize actual or impending instability.
- Detect and start the treatment of those acute organ dysfunctions that have an immediate impact on survival: breathing, circulation, and central nervous system.
- Recognize a high risk of acute dysfunction of breathing, circulation, and central nervous system function.
- Set priorities for immediate therapeutic interventions and further diagnostic procedures to detect and treat the underlying cause and the organ dysfunctions that have a delayed impact on survival (metabolism, visceral organs, and immune system; these may also cause acute instability of breathing, circulation, and central nervous system function).
- Evaluate whether a discrepancy exists between the initial working diagnosis and the actual clinical condition and its evolution (including response to therapeutic interventions).

Every medical doctor should be able to recognize an acutely unstable patient and start the primary support of vital organ functions. This may sound self-evident and easy to achieve. Unfortunately, clinical experience and vast evidence in the literature clearly demonstrate that this is not the case. Patients who require emergency admission to intensive care frequently have evidence of prolonged instability of one or more vital organ functions or symptoms suggesting a high risk of acute instability. Failure to recognize an acutely unstable patient occurs at all levels of the health care system, from the general practitioner to the emergency department and hospital wards. The intensive care unit (ICU) is not immune to delayed diagnosis of impending instability either: Subtle signs preceding an acute deterioration may and do go unnoticed also in the most advanced intensive care environment. No sophisticated monitoring or diagnostic technology can replace clinical evaluation and judgment at the bedside. One of the most important advantages of intensive care is that it brings enough manpower close to the patient. This makes frequent clinical evaluation of the patient possible and helps to put into perspective the clinical course, response to interventions, and the information obtained from monitors and diagnostic tests.

WHY DO THINGS GO WRONG IN THE ACUTELY UNSTABLE PATIENT?

In comparison to the number of all hospitalized patients, the number of acutely unstable patients is relatively small outside of the ICU or specialized acute care/trauma centers. Hence, the exposure of individual health care practitioners to such patients is often relatively limited. Since the specialties in charge of the treatment of a specific disease or clinical condition usually are involved early in the management of the patient, the number of unstable patients seen by individual doctors is further diluted. For a representative example, in the author's institution (a 950-bed tertiary-care regional hospital center), approximately 60% (or 1800) of the approximately 3000 intensive care patients admitted annually are emergency admissions. Only approximately 20% (or 350–400) of these patients come directly from the emergency department. Another 20% come after emergency surgery, and approximately 12% (or 200) come after becoming acutely unstable in one of the many general hospital wards. Considering that the emergency department treats approximately 30,000 patients per year, acutely severely unstable patients clearly represent a very small minority of 1% or 2% of all admissions. Similarly, on average, less than one patient per day in all the hospital wards becomes acutely unstable enough to require intensive care. It is therefore not surprising that detecting these patients can be difficult and represents a major challenge.

The treatment of a patient anywhere outside the high-dependency care area (emergency department, intensive and intermediate care units, and recovery room) tends to increase the risk of delayed diagnosis of acute instability. Indeed, the vast majority of patients requiring emergency admission to the ICU from the hospital wards have characteristic signs of impending or actual instability for hours before admission.

There are several common causes of failure to detect the acutely unstable patient early (Box 20.1). First, evaluation of the function of vital organs is not consequently carried out in all patients, and the farther away the patient is from the acute care area, the higher risk that vital organ functions are not systematically evaluated. Second, even if a clinical evaluation is done, the findings are often not interpreted correctly. Also in this case, the risk of misinterpretation is high if the person or the unit/ward involved has limited experience in treating acutely unstable patients. Third, in today's highly specialized health care environment, focusing on a specific diagnosis is very common and may become a higher priority than evaluation of the vital organ functions—often merely because the people involved are highly competent in their specialty area and have limited competence and experience in evaluation of vital organ functions. Fourth, all doctors are quick in setting a working diagnosis; if the vital functions of the patient are not carefully and repeatedly evaluated, a discrepancy between the working diagnosis and the clinical status and its evolution can easily be missed. Classical examples of this include the patient with acute back pain who actually has aortic dissection; the patient with dyspnea who does not have a pulmonary embolism but, rather, septic shock; and the agitated patient who does not have delirium but, rather, severe sepsis. Fifth, "cookbook medicine" can be very helpful in defining diagnostic and therapeutic strategies for certain disease entities. Especially in the acute care area, in which relatively inexperienced personnel can be confronted with complex clinical problems, such approaches may obscure the importance of the evaluation and treatment of vital function disorders.

There is a potentially very important additional factor that contributes to the risk of missing relevant disorders of vital functions: It is common for younger and less experienced colleagues to be in charge of the front line of acute medicine.

The most important principle to keep in mind in order to avoid delays is that the acutely unstable patient always has abnormalities in airway patency, breathing, circulation, and consciousness, irrespective of the underlying diagnosis. Consequently, any abnormality in any of these functions signals that the patient is unstable and needs immediate evaluation and a strategy for therapeutic interventions and diagnostics; any diagnostics must not delay executing urgent therapeutic interventions to support the function of vital organs. In addition to evaluation of the immediate need to intervene and support vital organ functions, a primary evaluation should be performed to assess whether the patient needs immediate intensive care and where this can best be commenced.

The most important points to consider in evaluating an unstable patient and defining a treatment strategy are summarized in Box 20.2.

- The first step is to detect vital organ function instability or a high risk for the patient to become acutely unstable.
- Second, the immediate need for therapeutic or supportive interventions must be evaluated and the necessary interventions started.
- Third, the likely underlying cause for the acute instability should be defined. The most important issue in this primary evaluation is to consider the likelihood of causes

that can be specifically treated to stabilize the patient. A patient who is in acute hypovolemic shock due to a bleeding major blood vessel certainly needs to be treated for shock, but what this patient primarily needs is surgery to stop the bleeding, and indeed, aggressive volume resuscitation before surgical bleeding control may cause harm by aggravating the bleeding. On the other hand, a patient who is hypotensive due to septic peritonitis will profit from hemodynamic stabilization and antibiotics before surgery, whereas the unstable patient with acute coronary syndrome may be best stabilized by prompt angioplasty and stenting. These primary diagnostic considerations must not delay the necessary vital organ support: Primary interventions and diagnostics should proceed in parallel.

- Fourth, based on the likely etiology, the clinician needs to ask what can be expected from the clinical course. There is no sense in prolonging the treatment outside of the ICU if the patient will need transfer to the ICU anyway. However, if a primary intervention is likely to solve the problem, intensive care can be avoided. For example, severe dyspnea due to an acute attack of bronchial asthma may be promptly relieved, whereas severe dyspnea in a patient with pneumonia or decompensated chronic obstructive pulmonary disease is likely to require prolonged stabilization and treatment.
- Fifth, evaluate how the patient responds to primary treatment interventions. A discrepancy between the expected and actual response may reveal an erroneous working diagnosis. Evaluation of the response also helps in planning the further steps in treatment and diagnostics. A hypotensive patient who promptly responds to a volume challenge is unlikely to have ongoing major bleeding, whereas a poor response shifts the focus to searching for a source of ongoing major bleeding or other reasons for severe hypotension, such as septic shock. A hypoglycemic, unconscious patient not responding to glucose administration may have severe hepatic failure, a head injury in addition to hypoglycemia, and so on.
- Sixth, consider where further treatment and diagnostics should take place and how urgent the need is for further diagnostics. It may be better to admit the patient to the ICU before full diagnostics have been completed if the instability is very severe and there is a low probability of

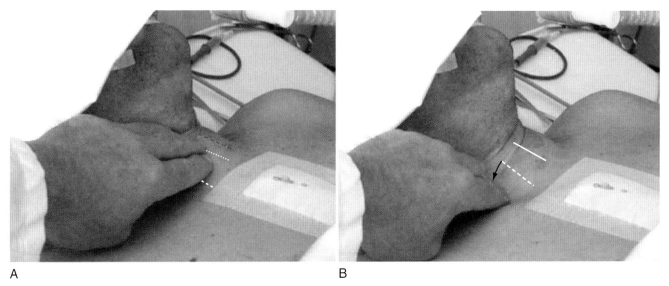

A   B

Figure 20.1. Checking the carotid pulse. Place the palpating fingers (forefinger to ring finger) on the midline of the trachea (white dotted line) *(A)* and displace the paratracheal tissues laterally while tracing the tracheal wall laterally and dorsally *(B)*. The carotid sheet (red dotted line) will then lie under the palmar side of your fingertips, and the carotid pulse should be evident.

a missed diagnosis necessitating immediate and specific intervention that cannot be performed in the ICU. It is possible that despite good acute care facilities, a specific treatment may not be readily available in the primary hospital and the patient may need to be transported without delay. Even if the primary team taking care of the patient has the capacity to provide excellent care, a transfer may need to be considered if such service will not be continuously available for the patient with an expected prolonged instability. A patient with severe pneumonia who can be treated with increased inspiratory oxygen should be transferred to the ICU rather than an intermediate care unit if he or she has a high risk of deterioration.

EVALUATION OF VITAL ORGAN FUNCTIONS

The first question to be asked is, "Is there a problem?" Doctors accustomed to highly specialized modern medicine are at high risk of forgetting this very basic and unscientific question. Does the patient look, behave, and give a general impression of being seriously ill? Often, this is so obvious that it cannot be missed, whereas at other times it is the patient's family members who realize that there is a clear deviation from the patient's normal condition and something must be seriously wrong.

If the patient is conscious and can be interviewed, it is worthwhile to perform a rapid anamnesis simultaneously with the primary evaluation. The primary evaluation of vital functions should be systematic and fast, and it should cover airway, breathing, circulation, and the central nervous system. The evaluation of metabolic and visceral organ functions usually requires more than just clinical evaluation, and it should primarily be covered to the extent that these may be the cause of the respiratory, circulatory, or central nervous system failure (a typical example is acute severe hypoglycemia). The primary evaluation should also include symptoms and signs of injury, even if the history does not indicate any physical injury. The systematic clinical assess-

ment includes components of different vital organ functions simultaneously and in parallel.

The evaluation of breathing, circulation, and the central nervous system is discussed separately for each organ system, and then a practical approach to including all these components in the rapid bedside assessment is summarized.

Is Cardiopulmonary Resuscitation Needed?

If the patient is unconscious, is not breathing, and has no palpable central arterial pulse, cardiopulmonary resuscitation (CPR) must be commenced unless there is a clear contraindication, such as a known living will, terminal illness, or a documented prolonged lack of circulation.

To determine whether CPR is necessary, simple assessment of level of consciousness (verbal and physical stimulation) can be done simultaneously while observing and checking respiratory movements and airflow and checking the carotid pulse (Fig. 20.1). When in doubt, CPR should be started until more comprehensive assessment is possible.

Evaluation of Airway and Breathing

Free flow of air during inspiration and expiration should first be evaluated (Box 20.3). In a conscious patient, this is normally obvious and can best be done by observing the patient when he or she speaks or attempts to speak. Any inspiratory or expiratory stridor is suggestive of airway obstruction and is usually associated with accentuated, forced breathing efforts as long as the patient is not fully exhausted. The cause of stridor should be immediately clarified in preparation for an emergency intervention for airway patency. In the extreme situation of complete airway obstruction, breathing efforts are fierce as long as the patient is conscious, and the motions of the thorax and abdomen are fully paradoxical; intercostal recession can be observed; and due to the lack of airflow, the patient cannot speak. Paradoxical respiratory movements can be easily observed visually; simultaneous palpation of the chest wall and abdomen helps to

---

evaluate the coordination of respiratory movements. Airway obstruction should always be included in the differential diagnosis when paradoxical breathing movements are present.

In the patient with a reduced level of consciousness, flow of air must be checked physically. This can best be done by placing a hand or ear close to the airway opening. The most common cause of airway obstruction in the patient with a decreased level of consciousness is the tongue. Raising the mandible forward and, if necessary, gently extending the neck will open the airway if the tongue was the sole reason for obstruction. If an open airway cannot be secured with this approach, laryngoscopy, clearing the larynx and the airway, and intubation are necessary. Although pharyngeal tubes are sometimes used to help keep the airway open and/or to help support ventilation, their placement should not delay intubation; if the patient tolerated a pharyngeal tube, sufficient airway protection is not present and the patient eventually needs to be intubated. Although laryngeal mask airways are increasingly being used also in emergency situations, intubation is clearly the method of choice for securing the airway.

Once free flow of air has been confirmed or secured by intubation, the adequacy of gas exchange, breathing pattern, and respiratory mechanics should be evaluated. A quick auscultation of both lungs at this stage gives a rough impression of potential gas exchange problems and the lack or presence of ventilation in certain lung areas. The auscultation should be accompanied by palpation of the thorax for the evaluation of chest wall stability and motion. The cooperative, conscious patient can be questioned regarding the presence of dyspnea, but clinical signs of dyspnea should also always be searched for. How does the patient breathe? Does it look effortless or is the patient visibly struggling? What are the breathing frequency and the depth of breathing? Increased breathing frequency and a rapid, shallow breathing pattern are classical symptoms of respiratory problems and impending exhaustion. Since all gas exchange problems tend to increase the respiratory drive, particularly useful information can be gained by observing how the patient inspires. Increased inspiratory effort is a very specific sign of increased respiratory drive; even when the patient is close to exhaustion and can no longer effectively perform the work of breathing, the inspiratory efforts remain increased as the patient gasps for air. Use of accessory muscles for breathing is also characteristic: In severe dyspnea, almost all muscles in the body may become accessory respiratory muscles. Special attention should be paid to the nares, jugulum, neck musculature, the intercostals, and the abdominal muscles.

Clinical signs of poor gas exchange are usually nonspecific. The presence of cyanosis should always be regarded as a sign of hypoxemia until blood gas analysis is available, whereas the absence of cyanosis does not exclude severe hypoxemia. If the peripheral circulation is severely vasoconstricted or the patient has low hemoglobin or high levels of carboxyhemoglobin (carbon monoxide intoxication), cyanosis will not be observed even in severe hypoxemia. Hypoxemia may cause a wide variety of symptoms in the central nervous system, ranging from mental alterations, agitation, and aggressiveness to unconsciousness (preterminal). Hence, the arterial blood oxygenation should first be checked by pulse oximetry and then confirmed by arterial blood gas analysis.

Pulse oximetry can be misleading if the peripheral circulation and consequently the signal quality are poor; hence, a blood gas sample should also be evaluated. Since the pulse oximeter evaluates the ratio of oxygenated to deoxygenated hemoglobin, high levels of abnormal hemoglobin will lead to falsely high saturation values; a classical example is carbon monoxide intoxication. Other nonspecific symptoms of hypoxemia include cardiovascular instability with tachycardia, hyper- or hypotension, myocardial ischemia, and arrhythmias. Carbon dioxide retention also causes a wide range of symptoms that can be very similar to those of hypoxemia. In addition, vasodilatation and perspiration may be present. Carbon dioxide retention also reduces the level of consciousness; CO_2 narcosis is unlikely if the arterial CO_2 level is less than 70 mm Hg (9.3 kPa), although individual variability is high. Pulse oximetry helps to evaluate whether hypoxemia is due to hypoventilation alone. If oxygenation is rapidly normalized by oxygen supplementation and the patient again rapidly desaturates when the oxygen is withdrawn, hypoventilation is likely the major problem. Only partial normalization with oxygen supplementation indicates the presence of ventilation/perfusion abnormalities.

As described previously, the coordination of respiratory movements is important. In addition to airway obstruction, incoordination of respiratory movements is an unspecific sign of increased loading of the respiratory muscles and can therefore be a warning sign of impending exhaustion. The patient may also alternate between breathing movements predominantly using the diaphragm and those emphasizing the rib cage. Such a strategy is always inefficient since more work per tidal volume is needed. Additional information on the respiratory mechanics can be gained by observation of the respiratory cycle: Does the patient expire to a relaxed end-expiratory volume or is the expiration incomplete? If the inspiration starts actively before a relaxed end-expiratory volume is reached, this suggests the presence of hyperinflation.

If the patient is conscious, has no dyspnea or tachypnea, and the respiratory movements are normal and coordinated, serious disturbances of respiratory function are very unlikely. Exceptions to this rule include intoxications, patients after general anesthesia, patients with chronic obstructive pulmonary disease (COPD), and the very early stages of hypoxemia. If respiratory dysfunction is present with other vital organ dysfunctions, the patient needs urgent vital organ function support and continuous monitoring.

Clinical Alarm Signs

Tachypnea and increased inspiratory efforts (drive)

Paradoxical or uncoordinated thoracoabdominal respiratory movements

Use of auxiliary respiratory muscles

Concomitant circulatory instability

Decreased level of consciousness (preterminal symptom in respiratory failure)

Hypoxemia and hypocapnia

Hypoxemia and acidosis

Hypoxemia and combined respiratory and metabolic acidosis (preterminal finding)

Probable Clinical Course of Respiratory Dysfunction

The expected clinical course is very relevant in planning the treatment strategy. Rapid recovery is possible in intoxications and respiratory depression, after general anesthesia, in an acute attack of bronchial asthma, in cardiogenic acute lung edema (depending on the etiology), and in pulmonary embolism. A prolonged recovery over days or even longer can be expected in acute lung injury and its most severe form, acute respiratory distress syndrome, in pneumonia-induced respiratory insufficiency, in lung contusion, and in unstable injuries of the chest wall.

Evaluation of Circulation

The initial assessment of circulation addresses the need for CPR, as described previously; that is, is the heart pumping blood to the aorta so that the central pulses are palpable? The following are the next questions to be answered: Is the cardiac output low? What is the volume status? Are there signs of tissue hypoperfusion? (Box 20.4 and Fig. 20.2). Clinical evaluation of cardiac output is notoriously inaccurate, but a rough estimation and differentiation between severe low flow state and normal or increased cardiac output is sufficient in the primary assessment. A rapid systematic assessment of circulation should primarily aim at detecting a low flow state and should evaluate whether this is associated with hypovolemia. If no signs of tissue hypoperfusion are present, this will allow time for a more detailed and precise evaluation of the circulation, including more diagnostics.

Very low cardiac output will eventually reduce the level of consciousness—this is a preterminal sign and necessitates immediate intervention. Decreasing cardiac output will progressively reduce tissue perfusion, first in the periphery and then in the more central vascular beds. Accordingly, the greater the number of central signs of insufficient circulation present, the more severe the disorder. Assessment of central and peripheral pulses and the heart rate gives a first indication of whether perfusion of the periphery is possible; in the next step, the skin temper-

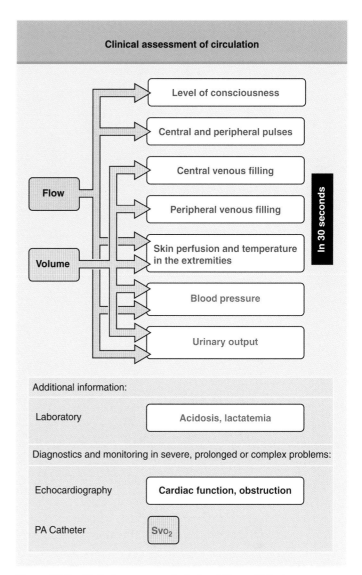

Figure 20.2. Clinical assessment of circulation. Clinical assessment of circulation consists of evaluation of blood flow and volume, first in the central vasculature and then peripherally. The primary evaluation can be done in 30 seconds and should be complemented by measurement of blood pressure and urinary output (requires 0.5–1 hr). Additional information can then be obtained through laboratory analysis of blood gases and lactate; in severe, prolonged, and complex problems, more diagnostics and monitoring are necessary.

ature and perfusion in the peripheral tissues should be evaluated. It is clear that external factors modify peripheral skin temperature and skin perfusion; nevertheless, changes in these variables provide useful information on the evolution of the clinical status and the response to treatment. Poor peripheral pulses, cold skin, and poor capillary perfusion are all indicative of a peripheral perfusion deficit and suggest low cardiac output. Peripheral capillary perfusion can best be assessed by evaluation of capillary refill rate in the fingers and toes: The nail bed and the tip of the finger/toe are compressed for 3 to 5 seconds in order to empty the capillaries (Fig. 20.3); when the compression is released, the capillaries should promptly refill, normally in less than 2 seconds. It is clear that no absolute references can

---

Box 20.4 Key Questions to Ask in the Evaluation of Circulation

1. Are central pulses present (i.e., does the heart pump blood into the aorta)?
2. Is the cardiac output low?
3. Is the circulating blood volume low, normal, or high?
4. Are there symptoms and signs of insufficient tissue perfusion?

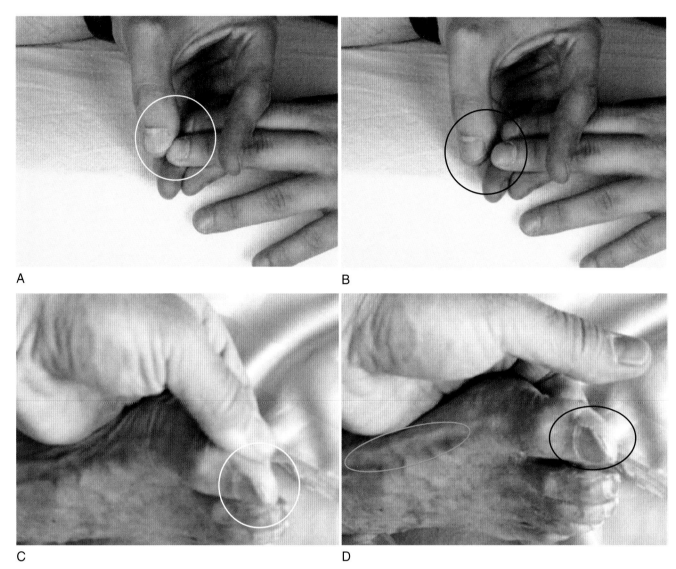

A

B

C

D

Figure 20.3. Capillary refill. Capillary circulation can be evaluated by compressing the nail bed or the skin next to it for 3 to 5 seconds so that the capillaries empty *(A)* and observing the time needed for capillary refill *(B)*. The normal refill time is less than 2 seconds; the investigator's own nail bed provides a reference. Normal refill is shown in *A* and *B*, whereas *C* and *D* demonstrate grossly abnormal capillary refill in a patient with sepsis; this patient had warm peripheral skin and normal venous filling (green oval) and also markedly delayed and patchy capillary refill.

be used for a "normal" capillary refill, and that environmental factors, such as exposure to cold, modify it. Nevertheless, it is a very useful objective indicator of peripheral perfusion, and the investigator's own capillary refill provides a readily available reference for evaluation. Abnormal capillary refill can also reveal a perfusion abnormality in the presence of normal peripheral skin temperature (e.g., in septic shock or in mild hypovolemia). If no clinical signs of peripheral vasoconstriction and hypoperfusion are present, the heart rate and blood pressure are normal, and the patient is conscious and not oliguric, an acute low flow state is unlikely.

Evaluation of the volume status includes evaluation of heart rate, central and peripheral venous filling, and the peripheral skin temperature and perfusion (see Fig. 20.3). In hypovolemia, capillary perfusion is normally one of the first clinical signs present, together with perhaps a slight increase in heart rate.

Since sympathetic stimulation is almost always present in acutely unstable patients, heart rate is an unspecific symptom, but even moderate tachycardia should be considered a potential symptom of hypovolemia. When hypovolemia becomes more severe, decreasing peripheral perfusion will lead to decreased peripheral venous filling and to progressive reduction of cutaneous blood flow and capillary perfusion, and central venous filling will also subsequently decrease. Venous filling is best tested by first observing whether the jugular veins are filled (Fig. 20.4). In the supine patient, this should normally be the case. In obese patients, the jugular veins may be poorly visible due to subcutaneous fat. If they are not visible spontaneously, digital compression horizontally at the base of the neck above the clavicle at the insertion of the posterior part of the sternocleidomastoid muscle will usually make the veins visible. Compression can then be applied more cranially and a vein can be emptied

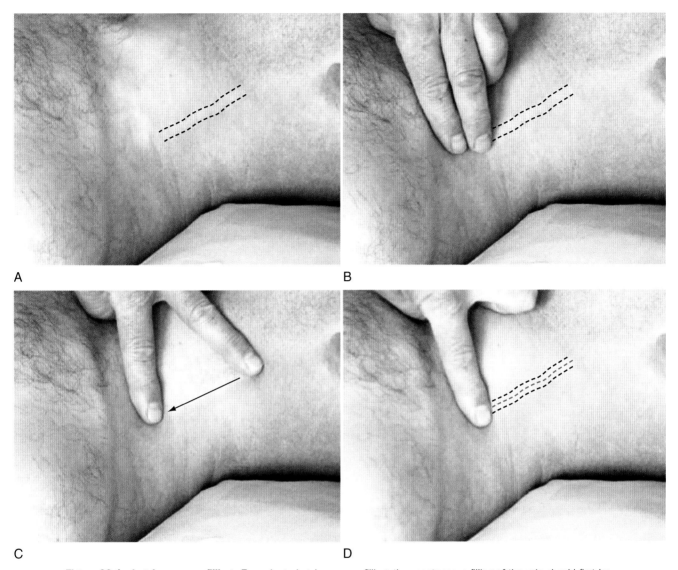

Figure 20.4. Jugular venous filling. To evaluate jugular venous filling, the spontaneous filling of the vein should first be observed (A). In the supine, normovolemic patient, the veins should be clearly visible and remain filled for at least part of the respiratory cycle up to a head elevation of 15 to 20°. The veins can be made visible by digital compression horizontally at the base of the neck above the clavicle at the insertion of the posterior part of the sternocleidomastoid muscle (B). Compression can then be applied more cranially, and a vein can be emptied using a second finger (C). The rate of filling after releasing the cranial compression gives a further indication of central venous return (D).

using a second finger. The rate of filling after releasing the cranial compression gives a further indication of central venous return. If time permits, venous filling can further be evaluated by elevating the upper half of the body gradually until the jugular veins remain empty throughout the respiratory cycle. Normally, this will happen with an elevation of only 10 to 15 degrees. The peripheral venous filling can be evaluated analogously, by visual observation, compression and emptying, and following the rate of refilling as the more distal compression is released.

With progressive volume loss, tachycardia becomes more severe and blood pressure is also likely to decrease (Box 20.5 and Table 20.1). The blood pressure response depends on the rate of volume loss and the compensatory mechanisms—blood pressure may be normal or only slightly reduced also in

---

Box 20.5 Symptoms and Signs of Acute Hypovolemia in the Order of Appearance

1. Tachycardia
2. Reduced capillary perfusion (slow recapillarization)
3. Reduced peripheral skin temperature (often a clearly detectable border between warm and cold skin)
4. Decreased venous filling (first in the periphery and then centrally)
5. Oliguria
6. Hypotension
7. Decreased level of consciousness

With successful treatment of hypovolemia, the symptoms and signs normalize in the reverse order.

Table 20.1 Severity of Acute Hypovolemia and Clinical Symptoms and Signs[a]	
Symptom/Sign	Blood Volume Lost (%)
Mild to moderate tachycardia	<15
Tachycardia (>120 bpm)	25–40
Hypotension (systolic blood pressure 80–100 mm Hg)	
Severe tachycardia	>50
Severe hypotension	
Decreased level of consciousness	

[a]These clinical findings are to be used as rough guidelines only and are best applicable to acute bleeding-induced hypovolemia.

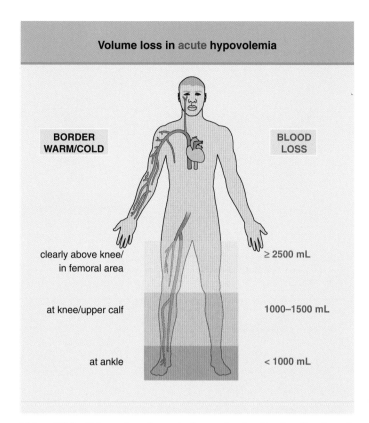

Volume loss in acute hypovolemia

BORDER WARM/COLD	BLOOD LOSS
clearly above knee/ in femoral area	≥ 2500 mL
at knee/upper calf	1000–1500 mL
at ankle	< 1000 mL

Figure 20.5. Volume loss in acute hypovolemia. Rough estimation of volume loss in acute hypovolemia can be based on observing the border between warm and cold skin. Vasoconstriction starts in the periphery and moves toward the central areas as hypovolemia progresses. This also helps to assess the amount of volume needed for resuscitation. A clear discrepancy between the estimated volume loss and the actual needs may be a sign of continuous volume loss or other undiagnosed problems.

moderate to severe hypovolemia. In preterminal hypovolemia, bradycardic rhythms may also occur before hypovolemic cardiac arrest. Severe acute hypovolemia is a common cause of pulseless electrical activity (PEA). If PEA occurs in a patient with empty neck veins, hypovolemia is the most likely explanation.

Clinical signs of low blood flow (impaired peripheral tissue perfusion) and hypovolemia (low venous filling) are easy to detect if systematically evaluated, and volume loading can be started and continued rapidly until central venous filling normalizes (Figs. 20.3, 20.4, and 20.5, Boxes 20.4 and 20.5, and Table 20.1). Simultaneously, an active search for the cause must be started.

If clinical signs of low blood flow are associated with distended neck veins, the cause of the circulatory failure is intrathoracic. Venous return can be impeded due to an elevated intrathoracic pressure (tension pneumothorax and hyperinflation), cardiac filling can be obstructed due to pericardial tamponade, and right ventricular outflow can be obstructed due to a pulmonary embolism. Acute right ventricular failure and left ventricular failure with subsequent right-sided congestion, as well as cardiac arrest, may also be reasons for low systemic blood flow and distended neck veins. This clinical presentation also necessitates a rapid search for the underlying cause since the patient is likely to acutely deteriorate unless the cause can be treated.

Poor tissue perfusion due to abnormally low vascular tone, typical for septic and anaphylactic shock, is perhaps the most difficult circulatory abnormality to evaluate clinically. In anaphylactic shock, the presence of accompanying cutaneous, mucosal, or respiratory symptoms and often a clear history help the evaluation, even if the cardiovascular symptoms and signs are complex. In contrast, in septic shock, signs of poor tissue perfusion and the overall impression of a seriously ill patient may be the only, very unspecific findings. Hence, a high degree of suspicion of sepsis is the key to detecting this abnormality early. The events leading to vasodilatory or distributive shock in sepsis are a combination of vasodilatation and loss of circulatory volume, often associated with temporary myocardial depression. Hence, the clinical presentation is highly dynamic, and the early hyperdynamic, hypotensive circulatory failure may rapidly convert to a low flow state once hypovolemia becomes more severe. The hypovolemia is in part relative due to vasodilatation, but it may rapidly become absolute when circulating volume is lost due to capillary leak. Before overt hypovolemia and after

volume resuscitation, the circulation is characteristically hyperdynamic unless myocardial depression is severe. The high blood flow may be apparent as a palpable peripheral capillary pulse and may coexist with heterogeneously perfused skin and in part poor capillary refill despite a warm periphery and normal venous filling (see Fig. 20.3). Since the condition is very dynamic and rapid changes do occur, frequent assessment and additional diagnostics, such as echocardiography and pulmonary artery catheterization, are often necessary to confirm the circulatory status. A hypotensive patient who responds poorly to volume loading and is seriously ill should be assumed to be septic unless shown otherwise.

Measurement of blood pressure and urinary output provides further information about the prerequisites of tissue perfusion (perfusion pressure) and the adequacy of renal perfusion. Urinary output decreases in all low cardiac output states, irrespective of the volume status. On the other hand, reduced urinary output is an early defense mechanism in hypovolemia. Accordingly, quantification of urinary output is useful for evaluation of both blood flow and volume status. Normal blood pressure in the presence of poorly perfused peripheral tissues can be misleading, and the severity of the circulatory status can be overlooked. Hence, blood pressure should always be put into context with the clinically assessed peripheral tissue perfusion.

As noted previously, many signs of inadequate tissue perfusion can be observed by clinical evaluation. In addition, laboratory tests are useful to assess the severity of the hypoperfusion and especially the response to treatment. The most useful laboratory tests in this respect are blood gas analysis to evaluate the severity of acidosis and measurement of lactate as a biochemical marker of the severity of shock. Increased blood lactate and metabolic acidosis due to hypoperfusion are signs of a severe and established perfusion problem; many of the clinical signs previously described are evident earlier. Hence, increased blood lactate and metabolic acidosis in a patient with circulatory problems are alarming signs. Treatment should be commenced promptly, and the adequacy of ongoing treatment should be evaluated. Moderate increases in blood lactate also occur in sepsis without shock; nevertheless, increased blood lactate should always be regarded as an indicator of severe acute illness, and it should decrease during successful treatment.

Clinical Alarm Signs
Hypotension
Large respiratory variations of pulse pressure
Hypotension and concomitant decreased level of consciousness

Probable Clinical Course of Circulatory Dysfunction
Rapid recovery is possible in circulatory dysfunction that is due to hypovolemia, provided that the underlying cause has also been successfully treated. Circulatory failure due to myocardial ischemia can be temporary and short-lived if the ischemia can be controlled pharmacologically or by invasive cardiologic interventions and if no extensive damage to the myocardium has occurred. Similarly, even severe circulatory failure due to pulmonary embolism may be rapidly reversible if pharmacologic, invasive angiologic, or surgical treatment can be commenced early. The most responsive reversible causes of acute circulatory failure are tension pneumothorax and cardiac tamponade.

If circulatory failure is due to pump failure secondary to prolonged ischemia, a basic disease that is not rapidly reversible (e.g., myocarditis, vasculitis, and acute or chronic heart failure), or septic shock, the duration is likely to be at least days.

Evaluation of the Central Nervous System
Systematic evaluation of central nervous system function starts by assessing the level of consciousness. Does the patient appear alert and are his or her eyes open? How big are the pupils? Are they symmetric, and do they react to light? Verbal and motor responses to verbal stimulation should be tested, and the adequacy of orientation should be checked by asking the patient for simple information, such as his or her name, where he or she is, time of day, date and year, why he or she is in the hospital, names of relatives, and so on. If the patient responds sufficiently and cooperates, proceed to testing major motor and sensory responses and searching for focal neurologic deficits. Even if the patient does not respond verbally to verbal stimulation, the motor response should be noted in order to observe potential focal deficits. The response to pain should be tested centrally in the innervation area of the cranial nerves (e.g., the supraorbital nerve) and peripherally in the limbs. The central testing for response to pain is important since spinal cord injuries or diseases affecting the spinal cord may lead to misinterpretation.

The first goal is to assess whether the level of consciousness is sufficient for protection of the airway and whether signs suggesting acute intracranial expansion are present. Airway patency, eye opening to stimuli, the size and symmetry of the pupils and their reaction to light, and the motor response to pain are the most important aspects to be checked in the primary assessment of the central nervous system.

There are several systems available for the classification of the level of consciousness. Perhaps the easiest to use in the primary assessment is the AVPU classification (A, awake; V, responds to voice; P, responds to painful stimuli; and U, unresponsive). A more comprehensive classification is the Glasgow Coma Scale (GCS) (Table 20.2). This scale gives a score (the lower the score, the more severe the abnormality) of 1 to 4 for eye opening, 1 to 5 for verbal response, and 1 to 6 for motor response, so that the maximum score (normal level of consciousness) is 15 and the lowest is 3 (no response). Patients with a GCS of less than 9 usually need to be intubated. These scales help clinicians to objectively evaluate the level of consciousness and to observe acute changes in the level of consciousness.

An acute worsening of the level of consciousness and the appearance of new focal signs are both alarming signals. Since circulatory instability, hypoxemia, and hypercapnia may interfere with the level of consciousness, a reevaluation should always be performed after the primary stabilization of circulation and gas exchange.

Since hypoglycemia and CO_2 retention rank high on the list of potentially fatal but rapidly reversible causes of unconsciousness, blood glucose testing and blood gases should be performed as soon as possible. If the patient needs to be intubated, capnometry will give a rapid semiquantitative evaluation of CO_2 retention.

Table 20.2 Glasgow Coma Scale[a]	
Reaction	**Score**
Eye opening	
Opens spontaneously	4
Opens to verbal command	3
Opens to painful stimulus	2
No response	1
Best verbal response	
Oriented and converses	5
Disoriented and converses	4
Inappropriate words	3
Incomprehensible sounds	2
No response	1
Best motor response	
Obeys verbal command	6
Localizes pain	5
Flexion withdrawal	4
Abnormal flexion (decorticate posturing)	3
Abnormal extension (decerebrate posturing)	2
No response	1

[a]GCS score: eye opening + best verbal response + best motor response (range, 3–15).

Since bacterial meningitis may also have a rapidly fatal course, the presence of meningismus (stiff neck) should be evaluated early. However, this should only be done if a reliable history or radiography excludes a cervical spine injury.

Any asymmetry of pupil size in a patient with a decreased level of consciousness suggests intracranial expansion and requires immediate further examination, usually by computed tomography scan. In particular, an epidural hematoma can be rapidly fatal. Since the history of unconscious patients is often unclear, patients should be carefully examined for signs of injuries. Intracranial bleeding may occur in conjunction with intoxications, and intoxicated patients may have spinal injuries as well.

Clinical Alarm Signs

Acute reduction in level of consciousness
New focal neurological findings
Stiff neck (meningismus)
Glasgow Coma Scale score of less than 9 (usually needs intubation for airway protection)

Probable Clinical Course of Acute Central Nervous System Dysfunction

Rapid recovery is possible, if the cause is promptly treated, for hypoglycemia-induced decreased level of consciousness, intoxications, epilepsy, mild brain injury (concussion), and some cerebrovascular problems, such as transient ischemia or promptly treated ischemic stroke, and less severe subarachnoidal bleeding. A prolonged clinical course lasting days can be expected for more severe injuries, ischemia, infections, and metabolic encephalopathies.

Dysfunction of Other Vital Organs

Dysfunction of vital organs from systems other than the respiratory, circulatory, or central nervous system is relevant in the assessment of the acutely unstable patient primarily to the extent that this dysfunction interferes with the respiratory, circulatory, or central nervous system, and to the extent that the dysfunction may require specific treatment in addition to the management of those systems. Hypo- and hyperglycemia, severe hypo- or hypernatremia, and acute hypo- and hyperkalemia are the most common such conditions.

Sepsis and Septic Shock

Sepsis and septic shock are briefly discussed separately since they produce a wide array of unspecific symptoms and signs that are often misinterpreted and that often precede acute instability of vital organs. A septic infection induces a systemic inflammatory response that is not specific to sepsis (several other conditions, such as severe injury, surgery, acute pancreatitis, and any other condition associated with the release of cytokines and other inflammatory mediators, may also cause some or several of the signs of the inflammatory response observed in sepsis). These symptoms include fever or hypothermia; tachycardia; hypotension and impaired capillary perfusion progressing to frank hypovolemia; changes in mental status (e.g., confusion and agitation) and level of consciousness; hyperventilation and dyspnea with hypocapnia and frequently hypoxemia; and peripheral tissue edema if substantial amounts of fluids have

been given. The laboratory findings include leukocytosis or leukopenia, thrombocytopenia, and an increase in inflammatory markers such as C-reactive protein. Increased levels of blood lactate and metabolic acidosis are also common. Since the symptoms change rapidly over time, the patient may be hypothermic, normothermic, or febrile. Early in sepsis, the periphery may be warm, with no overt signs of hypovolemia, but hypovolemia may develop rapidly.

A fundamental clinical feature is that the septic patient appears disproportionately sick for any other diagnosis associated with similar changes in many of the vital signs. Hence, sepsis should be suspected in any patient with an unknown diagnosis who appears sick and has signs of cardiovascular, respiratory, or mental instability. These patients should be monitored closely. Frequent clinical assessment and attention to the evolution of symptoms are likely to lead to the early diagnosis and treatment of sepsis.

Rapid Systematic Assessment at the Bedside

A protocol can be used to rapidly assess the unstable patient (Fig. 20.6). First, get an overall impression of the patient's appearance and behavior: Does he or she look ill? While standing at the patient's head, speak to the patient, check the airflow, observe the breathing movements and breath sounds, and check the carotid pulse and jugular venous filling. Check the control of eye opening, pupil size, and reaction, and if the level of consciousness is decreased, check the response to pain (supraorbital nerve compression). Second, move to the patient's side. Check breathing movements by palpation, get a first impression of the thorax and the abdomen by palpation and percussion, evaluate peripheral venous filling in the upper extremities, and check the skin temperature (border cold/warm) and peripheral capillary circulation. Check femoral pulses and pelvic stability (in trauma). Third, moving toward the feet, evaluate the peripheral venous filling in the lower extremities and check the skin temperature (border cold/warm) and peripheral capillary circulation. Throughout the assessment, pay attention to obvious signs of traumatic injuries. In trauma, the primary assessment of vital functions must be followed by a detailed search for injuries.

This first evaluation can be done in 30 to 60 seconds, and can be adapted and combined with immediate therapeutic interventions if a need is revealed in the systematic assessment (intubation, CPR, venous access, chest drainage, etc.). Depending on the circumstances, some components can be left out or performed in more detail after airway, breathing, and circulation have been secured: For example, if traumatic injuries can be excluded, assessment of thoracic and pelvic stability can be omitted; if neurological symptoms predominate, the level of consciousness should be assessed in more detail. If the circulatory status needs to be assessed repeatedly, these components can be assessed in less than 30 seconds.

The steps described here represent the author's own approach. You can adopt it or create your own. What is important is that you consistently and systematically evaluate your patients. By following the same basic procedure every time, you will find that the process of evaluation becomes automatic and you will not miss any of the information you need to identify and treat each clinically unstable patient who enters your ICU or whom you assess outside the ICU.

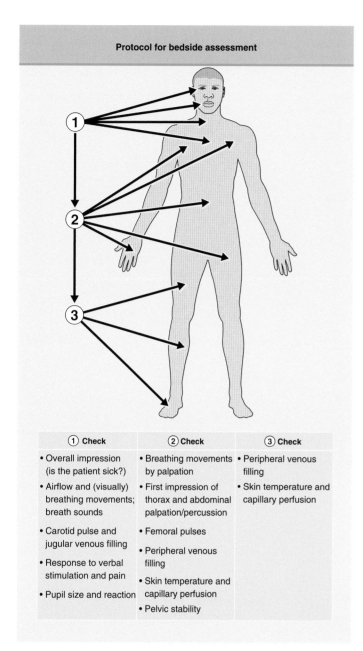

Protocol for bedside assessment

① Check	② Check	③ Check
• Overall impression (is the patient sick?)	• Breathing movements by palpation	• Peripheral venous filling
• Airflow and (visually) breathing movements; breath sounds	• First impression of thorax and abdominal palpation/percussion	• Skin temperature and capillary perfusion
• Carotid pulse and jugular venous filling	• Femoral pulses	
• Response to verbal stimulation and pain	• Peripheral venous filling	
• Pupil size and reaction	• Skin temperature and capillary perfusion	
	• Pelvic stability	

Figure 20.6. Protocol for bedside assessment. A practical approach for the rapid initial assessment of the unstable patient.

AVOIDING TYPICAL PITFALLS

Respiratory Problems

Increased inspiratory concentration of oxygen corrects hypoventilation-induced hypoxemia; a normal saturation value measured with pulse oximetry may therefore mask hypoventilation. Clinically assess the size of respiratory excursions, adequacy of airflow, and respiratory rate. Arterial blood gases are necessary for confirmation. In contrast, impending exhaustion cannot be revealed by arterial blood gas analysis, and repeated clinical assessment is necessary. In patients with COPD and chronic CO_2 retention, alleviation of the metabolic compensation signals a risk of acute decompensation. Acute respiratory failure may induce acute circulatory failure and vice versa. Sepsis is a common cause of dyspnea and is substantially more common in the acutely unstable patient than acute pulmonary embolism. Furthermore, the combination of dyspnea and a poor general condition is associated with pulmonary embolism only in a minority of cases, whereas this combination is typical of sepsis. A pulmonary embolism causes an acutely altered level of consciousness only as a terminal sign, whereas dyspnea and a decreased level of consciousness or altered mental state are typical signs of sepsis.

Circulatory Problems

Hypotension and decreased level of consciousness are preterminal findings in hypovolemic and cardiogenic shock (pump failure), whereas they are typical findings in septic shock. If a patient needs massive or continuous volume resuscitation to maintain circulatory stability, an untreated or undiagnosed hemorrhage should be suspected. An alternative explanation is septic shock with massive capillary leak. High doses of vasopressors and inotropes may worsen the circulatory problems by impairing the diastolic function of the heart ("stiff heart") due to too high afterload in severe systolic dysfunction. Use of these drugs in hypovolemia and ischemic myocardium predisposes to this problem. When in doubt, try reducing the vasopressors/inotropes and perform echocardiography. If a patient with a normal heart requires inotropes or vasopressors to stabilize the circulation, four conditions should be considered: hypovolemia (mismanagement: instead of vasoactive drugs, volume substitution is needed), septic shock (intensive care is urgently needed), intoxication (intensive care is urgently needed), and high tetraparesis.

Central Nervous System Problems

If the patient tolerates a pharyngeal or laryngeal airway due to unconsciousness, an intubation should be performed immediately. In a patient with a decreased level of consciousness and suspected meningitis, distinguishing between bacterial meningitis and meningococcal or pneumococcal sepsis is important because the risk of rapid circulatory collapse is very high in meningococcal/pneumococcal sepsis.

Metabolic Problems

Acute circulatory failure and sepsis are the most common causes of metabolic acidosis and hyperlactatemia in the acutely unstable patient.

CONCLUSION

Rapid, systematic evaluation of the key vital functions can be performed at the bedside to detect acute or impending instability. The clinical evaluation cannot be replaced by any laboratory tests or diagnostic techniques. Frequent repetition of this evaluation provides key information on the evolution of the clinical status and helps to avoid delayed treatment and misinterpretation of common clinical symptoms and findings.

SUGGESTED READING

Ball C, Kirkby M, Williams S: Effect of the critical care outreach team on patient survival to discharge from hospital and readmission to critical care: Non-randomised population based study. Br Med J 2003;327: 1014–1016.

Bellomo R, Goldsmith D, Uchino S, et al: Prospective controlled trial of effect of medical emergency team on postoperative morbidity and mortality rates. Crit Care Med 2004;32:916–921.

Bilkovski RN, Rivers EP, Horst HM: Targeted resuscitation strategies after injury. Curr Opin Crit Care 2004;10:529–538.

Committee on Trauma, American College of Surgeons: Advanced Trauma Life Support for Doctors, Student Course Manual. Chicago, American College of Surgeons, 2004.

Cook CJ, Smith GB: Do textbooks of clinical examination contain information regarding the assessment of critically ill patients? Resuscitation 2004;60:129–136.

Goldhill DR: Preventing surgical deaths: Critical care and intensive care outreach services in the postoperative period. Br J Anaesth 2005;95:88–94.

Goldhill DR, Worthington L, Mulcahy A, et al: The patient-at-risk team: Identifying and managing seriously ill ward patients. Anaesthesia 1999;54:853–860.

Hillman KM, Bristow PJ, Chey T, et al: Antecedents to hospital deaths. Intern Med J 2001;31:343–348.

Schein RM, Hazday N, Pena M, et al: Clinical antecedents to in-hospital cardiopulmonary arrest. Chest 1990;98:1388–1392.

Chapter 21

Nursing Issues in the Critically Ill

Sheila Adam

INTRODUCTION

The key features of nursing the critically ill patient can be summarized as skilled monitoring and assessment, delivery of therapies, maintenance of function, prevention of complications, and supportive care of normal physical and psychological needs (Table 21.1). Although many of these features are not directly associated with diagnosing and curing the patient, all are essential for the patient to survive to discharge and to achieve a relative quality of life. The majority of nursing time is taken up with direct patient care activities (Fig. 21.1).

The nursing ethos in critical care is to maintain the patient (and the patient's family) at the center of care. The goal is either to assist the patient to recovery or, where this is not appropriate, to ensure a peaceful and dignified death. The emphasis on caring has benefits for the patient, with a pattern of caring and concern being associated with early recognition of problems as well as being a key aspect in identification of complications that may reduce mortality (Minick, 1995).

Teamwork and interdisciplinary collaboration are essential features of caring for the critically ill patient. The typical intensive care patient requires intermittent support from many professionals and support workers, all of whom must work with the nurse, who provides a constant attendance day and night (Fig. 21.2). Effective collaboration between different professions has been shown to positively affect the outcomes of critically ill patients being transferred to the ward and is linked with improved mortality (Baggs and colleagues, 1999).

Stress in the Critically Ill Patient

The patient's physiological response to stress can cause considerable added strain on failing organs. Some nursing interventions may be able to reduce the patient's level of stress and attenuate some of its effects. Reported stressors from studies of critically ill patients following their discharge are outlined in Box 21.1.

The physiological response to stress involves the relay of emotional states via the limbic system to the endocrine system. Hypothalamic activation of sympathetic nervous activity occurs and adrenaline secretion is stimulated. This is highly effective as a short-term response, but if stimulation continues over long periods there may be severe detriment to the patient. The continued breakdown of protein stores will lead to muscle wasting and fatigue, the suppression of the inflammatory response will lead to secondary infection, the inhibition of tissue granulation will prevent healing, and the increased extracellular fluid volume will produce edema and fluid imbalance. The nursing focus should be on awareness of these extraneous stressors and interventions to relieve them.

Cross-Infection and Secondary Infection

Critically ill patients face significant risks from further nosocomial infection. Many of the necessary interventions have a

Table 21.1 Components of Nursing Skills

Exhibited Skill	Components
Assessment of the patient	Respiratory, cardiovascular, nutritional, renal, neurological, musculoskeletal, psychological
Interpretation of monitoring information	ECG, pulse oximetry, arterial waveforms, pulmonary artery waveforms, esophageal Doppler waveforms, arterial blood gases, electrolytes, BiS
Early recognition of problems	
Effective response to problems	
Technical skills and capability	Mechanical ventilation, infusion pumps, renal replacement therapy, intraaortic balloon pumps
Therapeutic interventions	Suctioning, repositioning, wound care, intravenous and arterial cannula dressings, tracheostomy care, placement of urethral catheters, placement of nasogastric catheters, gastric aspiration, initiation of weaning
Manipulation of drug therapy according to protocols and guidelines	Vasoactive infusions, sedative infusions, insulin, nitrates and other vasodilators, anticoagulant therapy, etc.
Communication with intubated patients	Lip reading, computerized communicators, Passy–Muir valves, alphabet boards, etc.

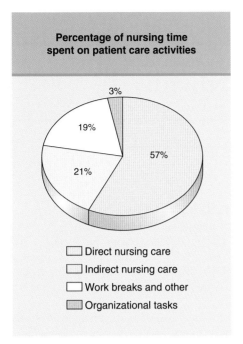

Figure 21.1. Percentage of nursing time spent on patient care activities. Breakdown of nursing activity by percentage of shift time spent on each category.

Box 21.1 Stressors Reported by Mechanically Ventilated Patients

Dyspnea/air hunger
Tension/anxiety/stress
Fear
Pain/discomfort
Agony/panic/frustration
Fatigue
Inability to talk
Confusion/bewilderment/altered level of consciousness
Anger/hostility
Depression
Insecurity/uncertainty
Mastery alterations
Sleeplessness
Hope alterations
Negative mood
Secretions
Self-efficacy alterations
Suctioning

From Thomas L: Clinical management of stressors perceived by patients on mechanical ventilation. AACN Clin Issues 2003;14:73–81.

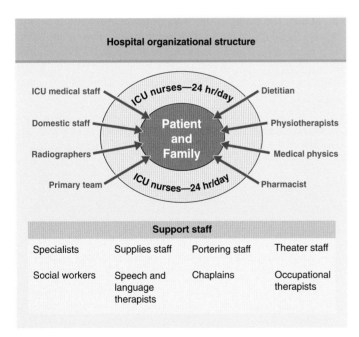

Figure 21.2. Hospital organizational structure. The patient in ICU model.

strong association with infection, such as mechanical ventilation (associated with 86% of pneumonias), urinary catheters (associated with 95% of urinary tract infections), and central venous catheters (associated with 87% of primary bloodstream infections).

Nursing care must emphasize preventive measures such as scrupulous hand washing, universal precautions, and any specific measures shown to reduce the incidence of nosocomial infection, such as 45-degree head-up positioning to reduce ventilator-associated pneumonia.

Sensory Imbalance and Delirium

Sensory imbalance or disorientation occurs when the level of sensory stimuli received by the individual is either too great or too minimal to be meaningful or recognizable. Nursing interventions focus on reduction of sensory overload, introduction of meaningful stimuli (therapeutic touch and orientation to time and place), and establishment of diurnal rhythms. Levels of noise in the critical care environment have been recorded that peak as high as 80 decibels and run continuously at a minimum of 50 decibels throughout the night (Topf and Davis, 1993). This requires vigorous management in order to prevent sensory disequilibrium.

Managing Sleep

Critically ill patients have very disturbed sleep, spending less than 6% of sleep time in rapid eye movement (REM) sleep and less time than healthy humans in stage 3 and 4 non-REM sleep. Polysomnography shows that they have an average of 19 arousals and 35 wakenings per hour. Proposed causes include the use of narcotics, disturbances in circadian rhythm, endotoxin release, and underlying disease. The intensive care unit (ICU) environment is not restful, but only 20% of arousals are associated with external auditory stimuli.

Nurses have used a number of different techniques to improve sleep in critically ill patients, including eliminating causes of discomfort before settling the patient (pain, feeling too cold or too hot, need for suctioning, and positioning), addressing any anxieties, massage, imagery, and relaxation. None have been shown to be effective in all patients, but many work for individual patients.

Managing Pain

Assessment of pain within an ICU setting is extremely difficult, particularly in situations in which the patient is unable to communicate verbally. Where nonverbal communication is impossible, the nurse must rely on physiological variables, such as tachycardia, raised blood pressure, and physical responses such as sweating, lacrimation, grimacing, and muscle tension. Unfortunately, these responses are subject to an enormous range of contributory factors that limit their interpretation. Nurses' assessment of the patient's pain has been shown to be influenced by a number of variables, including ventilatory status, length of time after surgery, and the patient's ability to communicate. Most nursing responses to patient pain are pharmacological in nature (combining use of analgesia and sedation); however, a small number of nonpharmacological interventions, including repositioning, reassurance, and other comfort measures such as massage, are also utilized. In up to 40% of cases, nurses do not reassess pain after analgesia, and patient's self-reported experience suggests that interventions are often inadequate. The use of standardized assessment tools such as the PAIN tool (Puntillo and associates, 2002) accompanied by a response algorithm is one method of improving the nursing response to pain.

Prevention of Complications from Immobility

Any critically ill patient will suffer considerable catabolism and loss of muscle mass due to the systemic inflammatory response. Multiple trauma patients have been shown to lose up to 17% of body mass after 21 days, two thirds of which was skeletal muscle. If the patient spends more than a couple of days in bed, this will be compounded by the effects of immobility. These include reduced functional residual capacity and $\dot{V}/\dot{Q}$ mismatch in the supine position, decreased cardiac output and perfusion, increased risk of deep vein thrombosis and peripheral edema, loss of bone density leading in the long term to hypercalcemia and hypercalciuria, urinary stasis and urinary tract infections, joint stiffness and contractures, and pressure (decubitus) ulcers.

Management hinges on regular turning and repositioning, knowledge of correct alignment and positioning of limbs to prevent joint injury, use of special support surfaces such as low-pressure mattresses and rotating beds, passive limb movements, physiotherapy, and, of course, mobilization as soon as the patient is stable.

NURSING SKILLS IN INTENSIVE CARE

Communication

The normal processes of communication in the critically ill are disrupted by sedation, opiates, endotracheal and tracheostomy tubes, fluctuating conscious levels, and fear. Communication with critically ill and ventilated patients is one of the greatest nursing skills. It requires patience, motivation, a perception of the patient as an individual, the use of eye contact, perseverance, and experience in order to provide the patient with an appropriate level of understanding and response. There are a number of techniques commonly utilized, including lip reading, mime/gesture/facial expression, pen/pencil and paper, alphabet or picture boards, computerized communicators, and use of one-way valves such as the Passy–Muir valve (Fig. 21.3) that allow redirection of exhaled air through the vocal cords to produce speech.

Eye Care and Oral Hygiene

Severe oral problems can cause considerable distress to patients as well as provide a reservoir of organisms such as *Candida albicans*, which can lead to systemic infection. Also, as many as 60% of critically ill patients who are sedated and on muscle relaxants may develop corneal ulceration (Imanaka and associates, 1997).

The healthy mouth has rapidly proliferating squamous epithelial cells lining from the inside of the lips to the oropharynx. These cells are highly vulnerable to the effects of poor blood flow, malnutrition, and drug toxicity and are therefore particularly at risk in the critically ill patient. Oral problems in the critically ill patient are related to the loss of normal cleaning mechanisms; the presence of an oral endotracheal tube, which causes pressure on the mucosa; a decreased or absent oral fluid intake; dehydration of the buccal mucosa related to inhaling dry

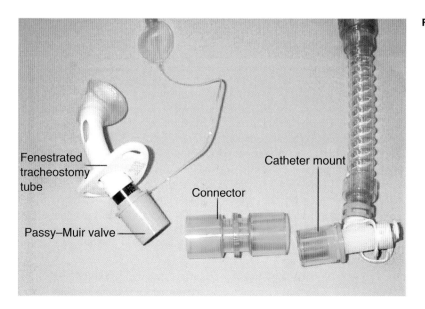

Figure 21.3. Passy–Muir valve.

Fenestrated tracheostomy tube

Catheter mount

Connector

Passy–Muir valve

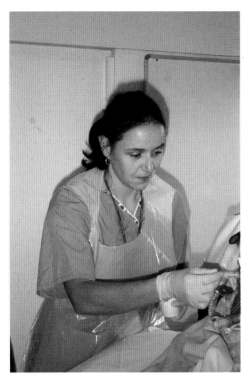

Figure 21.4. Oral or eye care.

Box 21.2 Factors Implicated in Diarrhea in the Critically Ill

- Antibiotic therapy
- Other drug therapy such as digoxin
- Use of sorbitol-containing linctuses
- Zinc deficiency
- Feed osmolality
- Low serum albumin levels
- Bacterial contamination of feeds
- Infection such as *Clostridium difficile*
- Fat malabsorption
- Lactose intolerance

gases, systemic dehydration, stress, and tachypnea (which increases mouth breathing); decreased salivary stimulation due to loss of food as a stimulating factor and increased sympathetic arousal; xerostomic drugs (e.g., atropine and catecholamines); and continued formation of plaque and debris on teeth with associated gingivitis (Fig. 21.4).

Ventilated and sedated patients are particularly susceptible to eye care problems due to their reduced/absent ability to blink, decreased tear production due to drugs such as phenothiazines and tricyclic antidepressants, decreased resistance to infection and increased risk of cross-infection from respiratory pathogens, increased likelihood of orbital edema with high positive intrathoracic pressures, and any systemic dehydration.

Patient Positioning

Although frequently unrecognized, the skill of positioning and repositioning the relatively immobile patient is an important nursing achievement that can have a major impact on recovery. The most obvious effects are seen with the use of prone positioning to improve oxygenation in acute respiratory distress syndrome patients, the use of specific lateral positioning to improve V̇/Q̇ matching, and the protective effects of ensuring maintenance of a 45-degree head-up position to prevent ventilator-associated pneumonia. However, the use of appropriate limb positioning and movement of the patient also reduce the likelihood of complications such as brachial plexus injury, contractures, and pressure (decubitus) sores.

Maintaining Nutritional Intake and Managing Bowel Dysfunction

Responsibility for the delivery of nutrition falls to the nurse caring for the patient, not only in ensuring that delivered feed matches prescribed feed but also in monitoring and evaluating the patient's ability to tolerate and assimilate the mode of nutritional delivery. Enteral nutrition is considered the most appropriate form of nutrition for the majority of patients but is also the mode most likely to cause problems with tolerance.

Despite a generally held belief to the contrary, patients are as likely to become constipated in critical care as they are to experience diarrhea. This is due to the use of opioids, low-residue feeds, and the effect of critical illness on gut motility. In a large study of critically ill patients (Montejo, 1999), there was a 15.7% incidence of constipation and a 14.7% incidence of diarrhea.

Many of the causes of diarrhea are not simply related to intolerance of enteral feed, although this may aggravate the situation. The patient should be investigated and treated for other likely causes of diarrhea prior to discontinuing enteral feeding (Box 21.2). Protocols are thought to improve the management of enteral nutrition and the complications associated with it (Fig. 21.5).

Weaning from Mechanical Ventilation

Weaning from the ventilator in the long-term ventilated patient or in patients who fail initial weaning attempts due to underlying chronic disease is commonly a difficult achievement (Fig. 21.6). No single ventilatory mode has been shown to be the most effective for every patient; however, whichever mode is chosen, it appears to work best in the context of a multiprofessional team approach and the use of weaning protocols (Ely, 2001). Nurses and physiotherapists are integral to this approach.

Psychological support and interaction with the weaning patient can be as important as optimizing the patient's physical condition, and the nurse must work with each patient to ensure that both are achieved. Logan and Jenny (1997) suggested that there are four themes of patient experience that have a positive impact on the patient's experience of weaning and that can be offered using specific nursing strategies (Table 21.2).

There is also evidence that the lack of frequent bedside presence by the nurse can delay weaning, particularly when nurses are caring for two or more patients simultaneously. This could be due to the fear and dependence that many patients feel during weaning and the need for constant support and reassurance.

Nursing the critically ill patient is a highly skilled and essential aspect of intensive care, requiring knowledge, technical and

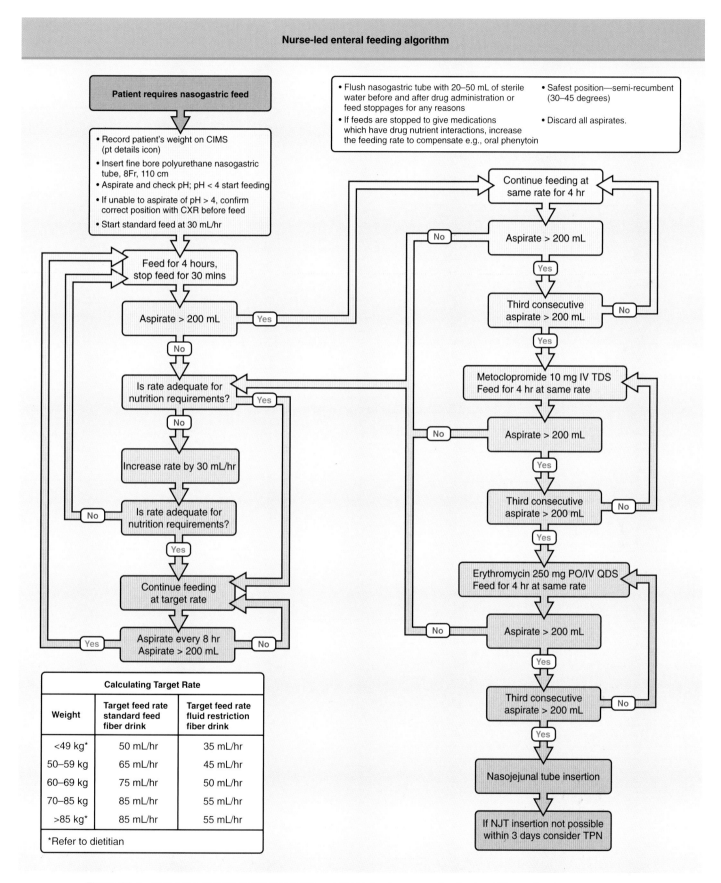

Figure 21.5. Nurse-led enteral feeding algorithm. UCLH intensive care unit enteral nutrition protocol.

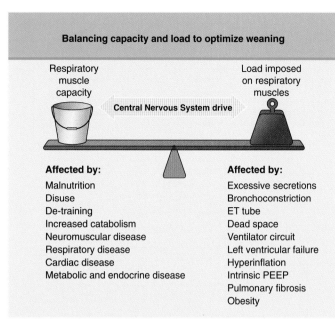

Figure 21.6. Balancing capacity and load to optimize weaning.

Theme	Definition	Nursing Strategy
Sense making	Cognitive activities related to self-orientation, threat perception, and understanding the situation	Visible presence, information, trustworthiness
Enduring	Physical, cognitive, and emotional activities involved in tolerating painful or frightening situations that persisted over time	Alleviation of discomfort, emotional support, feedback, encouragement, facilitation of family support
Preserving self	Cognitive and emotional activities aimed at sustaining personal integrity and overcoming feelings of alienation	Maintaining a caring attitude, personalizing communication, normalizing care
Controlling responses	Conscious efforts to cooperate with the treatment and achieve weaning goals, to control breathing, and to resist succumbing to negative emotions	Adjusting ventilator support, coaching, reducing patient activities, providing distraction

Table 21.2 Patient Experience during Weaning and Nursing Responses[a]

[a]From Logan J, Jenny J: Qualitative analysis of patients' work during mechanical ventilation and weaning. Heart Lung 1997;26:140–147.

behavioral skill, as well as compassion, caring, and commitment. Without this, the return to optimum physical and psychological recovery is unlikely to be possible for the patient.

SUGGESTED READING

Adam S, Osborne S: Critical Care Nursing: Science and Practice, 2nd ed. Oxford, Oxford University Press, 2005.

Baggs JG, Schmitt M, Mushlin A, et al: Association between nurse–physician collaboration and patient outcomes in three intensive care units. Crit Care Med 1999;27:1991–1998

Ely EW: Weaning from mechanical ventilation (part 1): Evidence supports the use of protocols. In Vincent JL (ed): Yearbook of Intensive Care and Emergency Medicine. Berlin, Springer-Verlag, 2001.

Imanaka H, Taenaka H, Nakamura J, et al: Ocular surface disorders in the critically ill. Anesth Analg 1997;85:343–346.

Logan J, Jenny J: Qualitative analysis of patients' work during mechanical ventilation and weaning. Heart Lung 1997;26:140–147.

Minick P: The power of human caring: Early recognition of patient problems. Scholarly Inquiry Nursing Practice 1995;9:303–317.

Montejo JC: Enteral nutrition-related gastrointestinal complications in critically ill patients: A multicenter study. The Nutritional and Metabolic Working Group of the Spanish Society of Intensive Care Medicine and Coronary Units. Crit Care Med 1999;27:1447–1453.

Parthasarathy S, Tobin MJ: Sleep in the intensive care unit. Intensive Care Med 2004;30:197–220.

Puntillo KA, Stannard D, Miaskowki C, Kehrle K, Gleeson S: Use of a pain assessment and intervention notation (P.A.I.N.) tool in critical care nursing practice: Nurses' evaluations. Heart Lung 2002;31:303–314.

Thomas L: Clinical management of stressors perceived by patients on mechanical ventilation. AACN Clin Issues 2003;14:73–81.

Topf M, Davis JE: Critical care unit noise and rapid eye movement (REM) sleep. Heart Lung 1993;22:252–258.

Chapter 22

Nutritional Support

René L. Chioléro, Ludivine Soguel, and Mette M. Berger

KEY POINTS

- Nutritional support is a life-saving therapy, but nutritional support alone cannot heal patients, nor can it completely reverse the catabolic process.
- Specialized nutrition support of vital organs is a new intervention. It is not directly related to the supply of nutrients and energy to the whole body but instead supports organ function or modulates the responses to injury.
- Clinical examination at intensive care unit (ICU) admission should systematically search for overt signs of malnutrition, such as muscle wasting or skin changes. Unfortunately, the usual anthropometric markers of malnutrition (skinfold thickness and skeletal muscle mass) are neither sensitive nor specific in critically ill patients due to fluid retention, which alters the anthropometric data.
- Providing nutrition to the critically ill patient is a complex process requiring special knowledge and skills. The ICU specialist should have a good understanding of the nutritional requirements of critically ill patients and should possess specialized training.

Malnutrition catastrophically influences the course of critical illness: A large body of evidence shows that it is associated with decreased survival, prolonged intensive care unit (ICU) and hospital stay, and increased septic and surgical complications. In critically ill patients, prevention of malnutrition therefore should be considered a high priority, and nutritional support is a life-saving therapy.

In parallel with significant progress in nutritional and metabolic support, other goals have emerged, such as specialized nutritional support of vital organs, prevention of infection, maintenance of the gastrointestinal (GI) integrity and function, enhancing immunity, maintaining the antioxidant defenses, reducing the initial inflammatory response, and restoring the inflammatory and immune responses when depressed. These new interventions are not directly related to the supply of nutrients and energy to the whole body but, rather, to the administration of specific nutrients to support organ function or modulate the responses to injury. For example, high doses of glucose and insulin provide metabolic support in patients with circulatory failure related to ischemic heart disease. Furthermore, improving glucose homeostasis has been shown to increase

survival and decrease the rate of clinical complications related to hyperglycemia and eventually to reduce both the hospital length of stay and costs for patients requiring prolonged ICU management.

The technical and practical aspects of this supportive therapy have become increasingly complex. Artificial nutrition started in the 1960s with total parenteral feeding, which may appear to be an easy feeding technique but actually has high potential for complications. Enteral feeding was introduced in the 1980s and required overcoming the pitfalls of the sick gut to ensure appropriate nutrition in critically ill patients. Indeed, enteral feeding may be very tricky, particularly in the sickest ICU patients, in whom GI failure is a consequence of the critical illness, and in those suffering from abdominal diseases. In such patients, the delivery of sufficient amounts of energy and nutrients solely by the enteral route may be difficult or even impossible. The proliferation of feeding solutions with "new nutrients" has considerably complicated the use of artificial nutrition, distracting the clinician from the main goal of nutritional support, which remains the provision of adequate quantities of energy and substrates.

This chapter focuses on some practical aspects and pitfalls of nutritional support in the critically ill. It does not include basic scientific knowledge supporting clinical nutrition.

NUTRITIONAL ASSESSMENT

Nutritional support in the ICU should start with nutritional history and assessment, as for any other patient requiring artificial nutrition. History should be focused on simple elements known to increase the nutritional risk:

- Diseases associated with progressive malnutrition, such as cancer and chronic GI or inflammatory diseases
- Recent anorexia
- Significant weight loss, defined as an unintentional weight loss greater than 10% of body weight in the 6 months before hospital treatment. Such weight loss has been shown to reflect clinical outcome in a general surgical population. A more sensitive criterion in the critically ill is a loss exceeding 5% within 2 months, which reflects the same severity and is more limited in time.

Biochemical signs of malnutrition detected before ICU admission, such as low predisease or preoperative plasma albumin (<30 g/liter) and prealbumin (<0.2 mg/liter), are also indicators of actual malnutrition. Clinical examination on ICU admission should systematically search for overt signs of

Practice of Critical Care

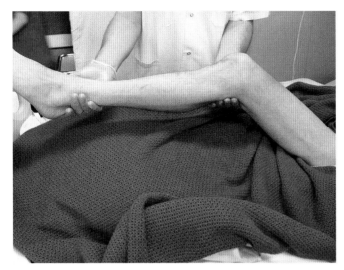

Figure 22.1. Loss of muscle mass due to malnutrition. Extreme muscle wasting in a previously healthy 50-year-old male who progressed to multiorgan failure after cardiogenic shock. This loss of muscle mass occurred in 4 weeks, despite adequate enteral and parenteral nutritional support. Such muscle wasting is a common result of prolonged hypermetabolic and catabolic state; critical illness polyneuropathy is also likely to contribute.

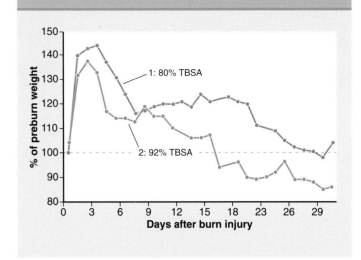

Figure 22.2. Typical weight curves of two patients with major burns (1: a 17-year-old with burns 80% TBSA; 2: a 23-year-old with burns 92% TBSA) during the initial edematous phase of fluid resuscitation, the progressive resolution of edema, and final weight loss due to loss of lean body mass. TBSA, total body surface area.

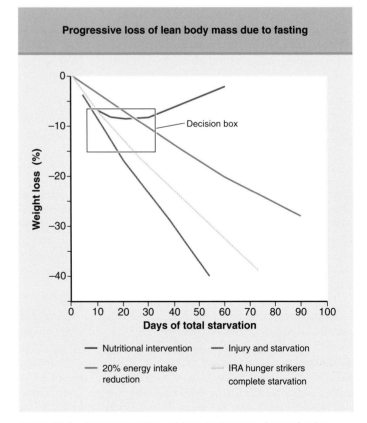

Figure 22.3. Progressive loss of lean body mass due to fasting. Effect of partial fasting achieved by a 20% restriction of energy intake, of complete fasting (IRA prisoners observed during their hunger strike), and of acute disease on weight loss. Added injury speeds the lean body mass loss process. (Data from Allison SP: The uses and limitations of nutritional support. Clin Nutr 1992;11:319–330.)

malnutrition, such as muscle wasting (Fig. 22.1) or skin changes. Unfortunately, the usual anthropometric markers of malnutrition (skinfold thickness and skeletal muscle mass) are neither sensitive nor specific in critically ill patients due to fluid retention, which alters the anthropometric data. Similarly, the previously mentioned classical biochemical markers of malnutrition have little diagnostic value in critically ill patients due to the development of the acute phase response, which modifies the turnover of most visceral proteins.

Nutritional assessment in the ICU should therefore be based on simple elements and aim to detect patients with actual malnutrition or those who are at risk of malnutrition requiring rapid nutritional support. In addition, the level of metabolic rate and protein catabolism, as well as the ability of the gut to cope with enteral feeding, should be assessed to determine the route and the timing of nutritional support when indicated. Although a large proportion of critically ill patients requiring artificial nutrition can be nourished by the enteral route, those patients in whom enteral feeding is limited or impossible, and who are indeed at highest risk, should be identified readily. This will avoid prolonged and unsuccessful attempts at exclusive enteral nutrition, which foster the development of accelerated malnutrition as well as nutritional complications.

The level of metabolic rate and of catabolism will determine the rapidity of development of malnutrition. Detection of hypercatabolic disease usually relies on a pure clinical approach based on the knowledge of defined conditions associated with rapid wasting, such as severe burns and trauma and severe sepsis. Patients with prolonged and complicated evolution are particularly prone to develop malnutrition during their stay. Body weight and composition change significantly over time in the most severe cases, with an initial edematous phase related to fluid accumulation (Fig. 22.2). This phase is followed by progressive loss of lean body mass, as schematically shown in Figure 22.3. In such patients, the detection of malnutrition can be

Table 22.1 Nutritional Support in Critically Ill Patients: Goals, Patients at Risk, and Tools

Objective	Patients at Risk	Tools
To detect actual malnutrition and patients at high risk on admission	ALL ICU patients	Medical history Clinical nutritional assessment Biochemical markers
To detect progressive malnutrition during the ICU stay	Patients with long ICU stay, particularly with sepsis	Repeated clinical nutritional assessment Body weight and prealbumin once weekly
To prevent malnutrition	Patients unable to resume rapid oral feeding Patients with long stay and hypercatabolic diseases	Targeted nutritional support Early enteral feeding Monitoring of nutrient supply and energy balance
To maintain gut integrity and functions	Patients with major burns Surgical patients with major stress Septic patients	Early enteral feeding Glutamine supplementation
To avoid hyperglycemia	Cardiac surgery patients with long ICU stay Other patients with long stay?	Intensive insulin therapy and glycemia monitoring
To modulate "immunity"	Cancer patients requiring major abdominal surgery	Immune-enhancing diets
To support the failing ischemic myocardium	Patients with acute myocardial infarction	Glucose–insulin–potassium
To reinforce antioxidant status	Patients exposed to major stress; ARDS, septic shock, major trauma, major burn, organ transplant, liver failure	Selenium 500 μg, zinc 10–20 mg, vitamins C (1 g) and E (100–300 mg; enteral)
To decrease protein catabolism	Patients with major burns	Beta-blockers Insulin Exercise–anabolic steroids

particularly difficult, and nutritional assessment should be performed one or two times per week. Some common risk factors favoring the development of malnutrition are summarized in Table 22.1.

Monitoring

Assessment should include body weight monitoring, muscle strength (if possible), and biochemical markers such as albumin and prealbumin plasma levels. The most important part of the daily assessment is the monitoring of daily energy delivery and of the progressing deficit. After day 5, the daily deficit should not exceed 500 kcal, or 20% of the energy target. Complications of acute malnutrition are likely to occur when the cumulative deficit exceeds 10,000 to 12,000 kcal. Body weight is another important indicator in patients who remain in the ICU for extended periods of time; the changes occurring early during the ICU stay are essentially related to fluid balance, whereas later changes also reflect protein catabolism and underfeeding. Figure 22.3 shows that the rapidity of weight loss is influenced both by the intensity of starving and by the basal condition: Partial or complete simple fasting causes increasing but slow weight loss, whereas added injury accelerates weight loss, with an increased risk of death.

TIMING AND TARGETS OF NUTRITIONAL SUPPORT

According to U.S. and European guidelines, all critically ill patients unable to resume efficacious oral feeding should receive artificial nutrition after no more than 5 days to prevent the development of malnutrition. In patients with current malnutrition, it is recommended to start feeding as soon as possible after ICU admission (i.e., after stabilization of vital functions). The catabolism is indeed proportional to the intensity of the acute condition, as shown by the proportionally higher urine nitrogen excretion (Fig. 22.4). If such patients are unable to feed orally, artificial enteral feeding should be started early after

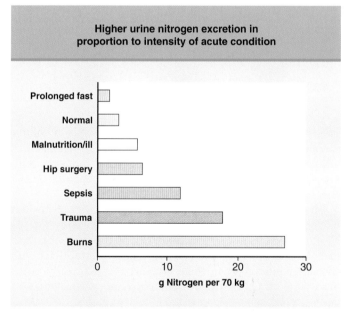

Higher urine nitrogen excretion in proportion to intensity of acute condition

Figure 22.4. Higher urine nitrogen excretion in proportion to intensity of acute condition. Effect of intensity of condition on protein catabolism reflected by mean daily nitrogen urinary excretion. (Data from Elwyn DH: Protein and energy requirements: Effects of clinical state. Clin Nutr 1993;12(Suppl 1):S44–S51.)

admission. The early start may improve the GI tolerance to nutrition.

Table 22.2 summarizes important practical aspects related to the timing of nutritional support. Numerous studies show that early enteral feeding is associated with a reduction of infections (incidence and number of infections) and length of ICU stay in patients with severe trauma and burns, but not of mortality, compared with parenteral feeding. Various meta-analyses have confirmed the benefit of early enteral feeding within 24 to 48 hours after major trauma. Many experts also recommend

Table 22.2 Timing, Route, and Type of Intervention According to Clinical Condition		
Time	**Clinical Condition**	**Intervention**
Admission	Critically ill patients—mechanical support of cardiac function, major trauma or burn injury, liver failure, severe sepsis or septic shock, liver–heart–lung transplantation, prior malnutrition	Antioxidant micronutrients
	Cardiac failure (← acute myocardial ischemia, etc.)	Glucose–insulin
	All patients admitted to ICU	Vitamin B ↑ (thiamine) to prevent neurological complications associated with glucose infusion
Day 1	Prior malnutrition–gut functional	Early enteral nutrition and progress stepwise over 4 days
	Major trauma or burn injury	
	Major cancer surgery	
Days 2–3	Patients likely to stay > 72 hr in the ICU and unable to feed themselves (invasive and noninvasive mechanical ventilation, neurological impairment)	Initiate enteral feeding, and progress stepwise
	Patients likely to stay > 72 hr in the ICU, not eating more than 500 kcal/day	Oral supplements
Days 3–5	Critically ill with nonfunctional gut	Parenteral nutrition
	Critically ill unable to feed themselves—gut okay	Full enteral nutrition support
Days 5–7	Growing energy deficit while on enteral nutrition (>10,000 kcal from admission)	Combine parenteral and enteral nutrition

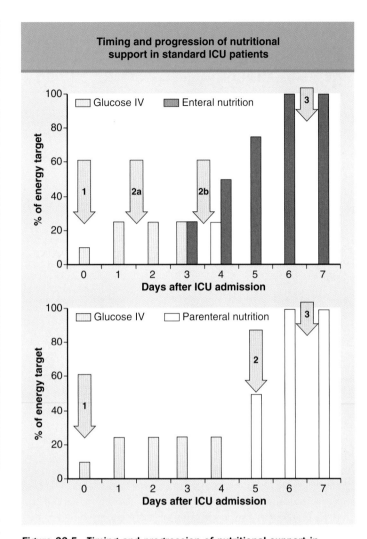

Figure 22.5. Timing and progression of nutritional support in standard ICU patients. (1) To provide organ support and antioxidant supplements—during this period glucose 5% to 10% provides some energy; (2) to prevent energy deficit by early (2a) or conventional (2b) enteral nutrition with a 4-day progression to energy target; and (3) full nutritional support. In the case of PN, support is started later (2) but progresses faster to target (3).

extending the use of early enteral feeding to those patients with major stress and with diseases of prolonged and complex evolution, although such practice is not entirely supported by the literature (Marik and Zaloga, 2001).

There is controversy regarding the energy targets of medical ICU patients (Rubinson and colleagues, 2004). Some authors have observed increased ventilator-associated pneumonia, diarrhea, and longer ICU and hospital length of stay (but with unchanged mortality) in those patients receiving early nutritional support. On the other hand, other authors have observed increased nosocomial bloodstream infections in medical patients receiving hypocaloric feeding. The value of early enteral support in medical ICU patients should therefore be reassessed in further studies, but it appears reasonable to set an energy target between 20 and 35 kcal/kg/day, according to body composition, type of illness, and gut capacity.

The most difficult question concerns the timing of parenteral nutrition (PN) in patients in whom enteral feeding is not possible (Fig. 22.5). Experimental and clinical data suggest that early PN may unfavorably reinforce acute phase and inflammatory responses. There are no data supporting the use of early parenteral feeding in ICU patients. We propose initiation of parenteral feeding after 4 or 5 days. In patients with overt malnutrition or in whom the cumulated energy deficit exceeds 10,000 kcal, parenteral support should be started earlier.

On initiation of feeding, the energy target can be set at approximately 20 to 25 kcal/kg/day in medical ICU patients and 25 to 30 kcal/kg/day in surgical patients. Feeding should progress stepwise to reach the set energy target (see Fig. 22.5): The time required to reach this objective should not exceed 4 days with enteral nutrition or 2 days with parenteral nutrition. Protein delivery progresses in parallel with energy delivery to reach a target of 1.3 to 1.5 g/kg/day.

Nutritional support may be required for prolonged periods, as shown in Figure 22.6 in the case of severe burns. The consequences of long-standing illness and repeated surgery on the lean body mass can only be partly counteracted by feeding, as shown by a weight loss of 12 kg (16% of initial weight) over 100 days in a severely burned patient (2 in Fig. 22.2), despite high energy and protein feeding.

METABOLIC ASPECTS: HYPERGLYCEMIA

Hyperglycemia is present in most critically ill patients. In Van den Berghe's study, among 1548 patients at ICU admission, plasma glucose exceeded 6.0 mmol/liter in more than 70%. In

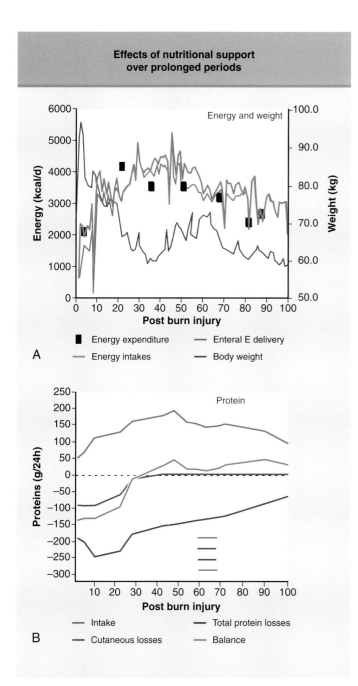

Figure 22.6. Effects of nutritional support over prolonged periods. Clinical case: A 23-year-old male with a 92% body surface burn injury who required a 110-day ICU stay. *A*, Evolution of weight and energy expenditure determined by indirect calorimetry, and energy delivery. *B*, Protein balance integrating the nutritional intakes, the cutaneous and enteral losses, and the urinary losses calculated from urinary urea. (Data from Chioléro R, Bracco D, Berger MM: Evaluation métabolique lors de la nutrition artificielle. In Nitemberg G, Chioléro R, Leverve X [eds]: Nutrition Artificielle de l'Adulte en Réanimation. Paris, SRLF-Elsevier, 2002, pp 47–66.)

this study, intensive insulin therapy was aimed at keeping plasma glucose between 4.4 and 6.1 mmol/liter. Impressive results were observed in patients with tight glycemic control, including reductions in ICU and hospital mortality, prolonged mechanical ventilation, septic morbidity, acute renal failure requiring extrarenal therapy, and critical illness polyneuropathy. Other studies have shown improved outcome in diabetics after acute myocardial infarction and reduced septic complications in burn and cardiac surgery patients.

A practical problem in prescribing insulin therapy in critically ill patients is related to the numerous factors that influence the sensitivity of tissues to insulin. In addition to preexisting diabetes and obesity, these factors include immobility, catecholamine and steroid administration (particularly epinephrine), and severe sepsis. In Van den Berghe's study, multiple regression analysis showed that history of diabetes, body mass index, blood glucose at admission, the level of energy intake, and diagnostic category were independent predictors of insulin requirements. It should be noted that insulin requirements change over time, decreasing with resolution of the acute condition. This often induces undesirable hyperglycemia and, less frequently, hypoglycemia (approximately 3%–5% in patients receiving intensive insulin therapy).

In practice, no predefined insulin rate can be proposed according to blood glucose level. Insulin therapy is adapted in a stepwise manner and is directed by four main factors: actual glucose level, change in glucose level over time, actual insulin infusion rate, and glucose target level, which can change according to the patient's diagnosis and condition. Our insulin therapy protocol, based on Van den Berghe's and Yale's insulin protocols, is shown in Table 22.3.

NUTRITIONAL SUPPORT IN ORGAN FAILURE

Since the 1990s, the concept of organ-specific nutritional and metabolic support has progressed rapidly. This concerns mainly the failing heart, lung, gut, and kidney (Table 22.4).

Cardiac Failure

The concept of administering glucose, insulin, and potassium (GIK) as metabolic support for the failing ischemic myocardium emerged in the 1960s. Since 1995, several well-controlled studies have been conducted in medical (acute myocardial infarction) and surgical (coronary artery bypass surgery) patients with ischemic heart disease and acute cardiac failure. They have provided sound evidence that glucose and insulin may rapidly improve the function of the failing myocardium and outcome in both diabetic and nondiabetic patients.

Several mechanisms explain the beneficial effects of this therapy. Glucose is an efficient substrate that can be oxidized by the ischemic myocardium, even when ischemia is profound. It activates the replenishment of citric acid intermediates depleted during ischemia. Glucose and insulin stimulate glycolytic ATP synthesis, thus providing energy for the membrane function; they decrease lipolysis and reduce free fatty acid oxidation in the myocardium. Several experimental and human studies suggest that insulin exerts a specific effect in myocardium metabolism or acts as a vasodilator, although its specific role remains controversial. It is interesting to note that GIK has little effect when there is no reperfusion by thrombolysis or percutaneous transluminal coronary angioplasty, suggesting that it may protect against ischemia–reperfusion injury or provide metabolic support during reperfusion.

Many regimens have been proposed using a wide range of glucose and insulin delivery rates. Basic practical aspects of glucose–insulin therapy are described in Table 22.4.

Table 22.3 Normogram for Blood Glucose Control in Critically III Patients[a]

3.1. General principles

Intravenous infusion of regular human insulin using a syringe infusion pump

Flushing 30 mL of insulin infusion through IV tubing before connecting it to decrease insulin loss by absorption

Regular monitoring of whole blood glucose every 1–4 hr according to BG and change over time

Determination of the blood glucose target (usually between 5 and 8 mmol/liter in cardiac surgery and septic patients)

3.2. Blood glucose monitoring

Check BG each hour until three consecutive values are in the BG target.

When three consecutive values are within target and nutritional delivery is unchanged, check BG every 2 hr until stable BG in target is achieved for three determinations, then every 4 hr.

Calculate rate of change in BG/hr.

Resume hourly BG determination under the following conditions: change in insulin IR, energy delivery (artificial nutrition), and catecholamine infusion rate.

3.3. Initial insulin infusion rate

Based on actual BG

Double in patients receiving epinephrine infusion

Glucose level (mmol/liter)	<8	8–9	9.1–10	>10
Insulin rate (U/hr)	0	2	4	6

3.4. Insulin infusion rate (IR)

Change in IR is determined according to BG level, ΔBG/hr, and actual IR rate.

Reduce IR when nutritional delivery is decreased. Shop insulin when feeding is interrupted.

In case of hypoglycemia: administer IV glucose (10–25 g) and stop insulin.

Determine change of IR from (1) K, coefficient related to the actual insulin IR (see 3.5), and (2) actual BG and ΔBG/hr (see 3.6)

This normogram may be inefficient in patients with marked insulin resistance and high glucose supply (i.e., cardiogenic shock + GIK therapy).

3.5. Determination of coefficient k

Insulin Infusion Rate (U/hr)	K = Rate Change (U/hr)
>15	3
10–15	2
6.1–9.9	1.5
3.0–6.0	1.0
<3.0	0.5

3.6. Determination of the change in insulin infusion rate (nc, no change)

	BG (mmol/liter) →				
BG change/hr (mmol/hr)	4–5.9	6–7.9	8–9.9	10–12	>12
↑ >2.8	nc	+k	+2k	+2k	+2k
↑ by 1.4–2.8	nc	+k	+k	+k	+2k
↑ by 0–1.3	nc	nc	+k	+k	+2k
Unchanged	–k	nc	+k	+k	+k
↓ by 0–1.3	–k	nc	nc	nc	+k
↓ by 1.4–2.8	Stop infusion	–k	nc	–k	nc
↓ by 2.9–4.0	Hypoglycemia	Stop infusion	–k	–2k	–k
↓ by 4.1–5.5	Hypoglycemia	Stop infusion	Stop infusion	Stop infusion	–2k

[a]BG, blood glucose concentration; IR, infusion rate.

Surgical and medical cardiac patients who exhibit persistent circulatory failure require nutritional support. Glucose–insulin is the first form of support and does indeed provide glucose in amounts that deliver significant quantities of energy. After this early 24- to 48-hour period, these patients eventually become candidates for complete nutritional support. Evidence shows that the gut may be used for partial feeding and should be used for this purpose with caution, despite the frequently published expert opinion not to use enteral feeding at all. In real life, it is difficult to deliver complete feeding through this route. In our hands, the usual maximum enteral energy delivery ranges between 750 and 1200 kcal/day in complex cases with severe hemodynamic failure requiring major support, such as intraaortic balloon pump (Fig. 22.7). Therefore, combined nutritional support should be considered after 4 to 7 days of hypocaloric enteral feeding in such patients, completing the enteral feeding with parenteral feeding to reach the energy target.

Modulating the Inflammatory Response

Several nutrients may downregulate acute and chronic inflammation, such as n-3 polyunsaturated fatty acids (derived from fish oil), γ-linolenic acid, and some micronutrients. Data from a Spanish multicenter prospective randomized controlled trial suggest that a combination of eicosapentaenoic and γ-linolenic acids, vitamins C and E, and β-carotene may favorably influence the clinical outcome of acute respiratory distress syndrome (ARDS) (Gadek and associates, 1999). A total of 142 patients meeting the European and U.S. criteria for ARDS were recruited. Nutritional goals (i.e., energy delivery > 75% of caloric goal during at least 4 days) were achieved in only 98 of the

		Table 22.4 Specialized Nutrition Support in the ICU[a]		
Patient Diagnosis	**Condition**	**Nutritional Intervention**	**Target**
Acute myocardial infarction	Thrombolysis, or primary angioplasty	Glucose 0.2–0.6 g/kg/hr + insulin continuous infusion	Blood glucose 5–8 mmol/liter
Coronary artery bypass surgery	Low cardiac output	Glucose 0.1–0.3 g/kg/hr + insulin continuous infusion	Blood glucose 5–8 mmol/liter
Severe trauma, multiple injury, brain injury	ICU, Injury Severity Score > 25	Early enteral nutrition, glutamine	Energy delivery > 80% REE by day 4 (or 20 kcal/kg), then increase to 1.3 REE
Severe burn	Burns > 30% body surface area	Early enteral nutrition (starting within 24 hr), glutamine	Energy delivery > 100% REE by day 4 (or > 30 kcal/kg), then by calorimetry Fat delivery < 20% energy supply
Acute renal failure	Continuous renal replacement therapy	Proteins Replacement flow < 2 liters/hr: 2 g/kg/day Replacement flow > 2 liters/hr: 2.5 g/kg/day	Metabolic homeostasis Prevent muscle wasting
Major stress/injury	Enteral nutrition possible	Early enteral feeding Enteral glutamine (0.5 g/kg/day) or ornithine α-ketoglutarate	Energy delivery > 80% REE by day 4 (20–25 kcal/kg) Enteral glutamine supply
Upper gastrointestinal intolerance + severe sepsis or multiple organ failure	Parenteral nutrition required	Parenteral glutamine ~0.35 g/kg/day	Parenteral nutrition > 5 days Prevention of glutamine depletion and gut failure
Obesity	Artificial nutrition	Hypocaloric nutrition: enteral or parenteral Protein: 2 g/kg ideal body weight Energy 15–20 kcal/kg or 60% of measured energy expenditure	Preventing visceral protein depletion and fostering wound healing

[a]REE, resting energy expenditure (measured or calculated by Harris–Benedict equation without correction for activity).

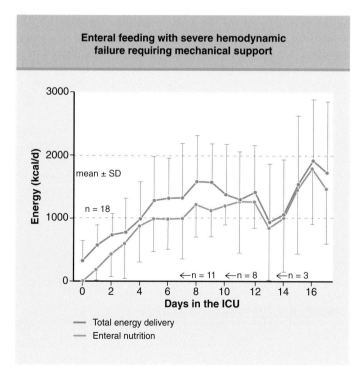

Figure 22.7. Enteral feeding with severe hemodynamic failure requiring mechanical support. Mean total energy delivery (solid line) with the detail of energy provided by enteral nutrition (dashed line) in 18 patients with intraaortic balloon pump. (Data from Berger MM, Revelly JP, Cayeux MC, Chioléro RL: Enteral nutrition in critically ill patients with severe hemodynamic failure after cardiopulmonary bypass. Clin Nutr 2005;24:124–132, Fig. 3.)

patients in whom statistical analysis was performed. The results showed significant improvement in pulmonary gas exchange, the dependence on oxygen, and shortening of ventilator time ($p = 0.027$) and also a trend toward improved survival ($p = 0.065$). Further studies are necessary to better delineate the role of specific nutritional support in such a condition.

Micronutrients

Several vitamins and trace elements have antioxidant (AOX) properties. The most important are selenium, zinc, vitamin C (ascorbic acid), and vitamin E (α-tocopherol). Critically ill patients are characterized by increased oxidative stress and low plasma concentrations of the AOX micronutrients (Berger and Chioléro, 2003). Therefore, the rationale for early supplementation during critical illness is strong. Trials providing only vitamins have shown no significant clinical benefits. Several small trials have shown clinical benefits in association with combined supplementation with selenium, zinc, and vitamin C in burn, trauma, septic, and inflammatory patients, but because they are underpowered, these trials do not support the systematic delivery of AOX micronutrients. Nevertheless, evidence is accumulating in favor of early large-dose (500 μg/day) selenium supplementation, with clinical benefits such as decreased incidence of acute renal failure, fewer infectious complications, shortening of ICU stay, and better outcome.

The best route for delivering this support has not been established. Evidence favors the intravenous route for achieving systemic effects due to its high bioavailability. Nevertheless, because the gut suffers from ischemia–reperfusion conditions, the direct intraluminal provision of AOX support is also rational. Trials are investigating the combined approach using simultaneous intravenous and enteral delivery: This is likely to be the future AOX option.

Gut Maintenance

Enteral feeding contributes to maintaining gut integrity and to improving function mainly through three mechanisms: mechanical stimulation, splanchnic vasodilatation, and provision of specific substrates to the intestinal mucosa (Fig. 22.8). Furthermore, it maintains GI motility, provides trophic stimulation of the intestinal mucosa, maintains microbial ecology, reduces infectious complications by stimulation of the GI-associated lymphoid tissue, maintains IgA production, and reduces costs.

Among the specific substrates, glutamine has gained a special place since it has gut-protective and immune-enhancing effects by both enteral and intravenous application (see Table 22.4). Several studies, including a meta-analysis, suggest that high-dose enteral glutamine (i.e., ~0.5 g/kg/day) is beneficial, whereas lower doses of enteral glutamine do not produce significant clinical benefit, suggesting a dose-dependent effect. High-dose intravenous glutamine administered with PN (i.e., ~0.35 g/kg/day) also exerts clinical benefits in very sick patients intolerant of enteral feeding; these consist of a reduction in the development of infection acquired in the ICU, particularly *Candida* infections, and improved survival.

Renal Failure

Several studies suggest that protein supply should be increased in patients on continuous renal replacement therapy. In addition to severe protein catabolism related to the critical illness, such patients lose amino acids and proteins through the renal replacement device membranes. This may exceed 25 g/day, particularly when hemofiltration flow exceeds 2 liters/hr. In such conditions, protein supply should be increased to 2.5 g/kg/day—that is, higher amounts than in critically ill patients without continuous renal replacement therapy and in patients without renal failure. In general, patients with acute renal failure are hypermetabolic and have increased requirements for all nutrients, which is in part explained by the demonstrated trace elements, vitamins, and glucose losses in the effluent.

ROUTES FOR ARTIFICIAL NUTRITIONAL SUPPORT: THE HIERARCHY

When artificial nutrition is required, the enteral route should be considered first. Gastric delivery of feeds is to be considered when access to the small intestine is not possible. In severely ill patients, gastric and pyloric motility are reduced, however, rendering gastric feeding difficult. In the case of persistent high gastric residues and overt regurgitation, or in the case of an incapacity to reach the energy target by the gastric route within 4 days, postpyloric access should be considered. Postpyloric placement of a feeding tube can be achieved using either self-migrating feeding tubes or endoscopic or radiological fluoroscopic placement. In the case of repeated abdominal surgery, surgeons may have the opportunity to place a percutaneous jejunal feeding tube.

Parenteral feeding is an alternative in the case of nonfunctional gut due to either complete or partial gut failure, reflected by the incapacity of the gut to accommodate the quantities of feeds required for complete energy delivery. PN has been reported to have higher complication rates, particularly infectious, to reinforce the inflammatory response, and to have higher costs. Many of the risks of indiscriminate and inappropriate use of PN have been recognized, and there is no doubt that PN increases the chance of iatrogenic complications. In the critically ill, the most important infectious complications are associated with a poor catheter care policy: Careful cannulation and maintenance of sterile techniques will prevent or minimize infections or sepsis. The placement of central venous catheters requires caution. Figure 22.9 shows a bilateral pleural effusion resulting from the paravenous intrapleural infusion of PN over 4 days. Techniques used in home PN, such as central venous catheter tunneling, or silicone catheters should not be used in the critically ill because they have no proven advantage and are costly: The effect of central venous catheter tunneling on infectious rates depends largely on indwelling time and quality of care.

DIFFICULT ENTERAL FEEDING

The main causes of difficult enteral feeding are summarized in Figure 22.10. The critically ill patient is characterized by impaired GI motility and particularly by pyloric closure, which may complicate enteral feeding. This is particularly true in patients with severe brain injury and elevated intracranial pressure, who always present with pyloric closure. In addition, patients 65 years or older, who constitute a large body of the ICU population, frequently suffer from cardiovascular disease, which requires use of vasoactive agents. The latter, particularly

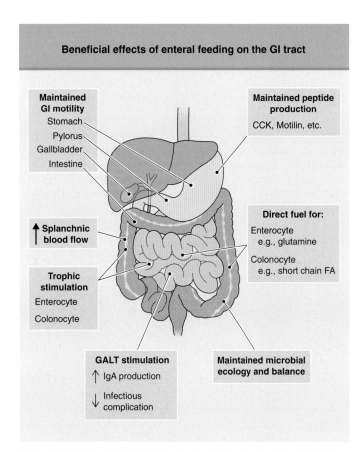

Beneficial effects of enteral feeding on the GI tract

Maintained GI motility
Stomach
Pylorus
Gallbladder
Intestine

Maintained peptide production
CCK, Motilin, etc.

↑ Splanchnic blood flow

Direct fuel for:
Enterocyte
e.g., glutamine
Colonocyte
e.g., short chain FA

Trophic stimulation
Enterocyte
Colonocyte

GALT stimulation
↑ IgA production
↓ Infectious complication

Maintained microbial ecology and balance

Figure 22.8. Beneficial effects of enteral feeding on the GI tract. Beneficial effects include mechanical stimulation, splanchnic vasodilation, and provision of specific substrates to the intestinal mucosa.

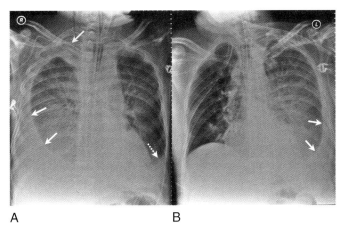

Figure 22.9. Bilateral pleural effusion resulting in acute respiratory failure caused by paravenous infusion of parenteral nutrition. *A,* Bilateral effusion; arrows show the limit of the pleural effusions and the tip of the initial subclavian venous catheter. *B,* The first right thoracic tube drained 2.8 liters of a latent solution and unmasked the left effusion of 1.7 liters.

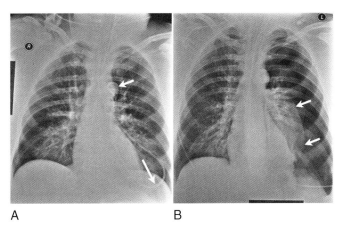

Figure 22.11. Pneumothorax caused by bronchial perforation by a feeding tube. *A,* Spiraled feeding tube loops in pleura and reverts to mediastinum. *B,* Collapse of the left lung. Note the left subclavian venous catheter on both x-rays.

catecholamines, are known to further reduce GI motility and to increase the pyloric sphincter tone. The most severely ill patients also receive various sedation regimens, including opiates, neuroleptics, and benzodiazepines, which also reduce GI motility. Finally, patients undergoing cardiac surgery are at increased risk of splanchnic ischemia, which is a relative con-

traindication to enteral feeding. Gastric feeding is therefore frequently difficult. Table 22.5 provides some tools.

Postpyloric feeding is one of these tools. Placing feeding tubes may result in significant complications, as shown in Figure 22.11. A major pneumothorax was caused by a feeding tube that was inserted through the trachea into the bronchus during the placement attempt, resulting in pleural perforation. This erroneous placement was not detected on air insufflation, demonstrating the importance of checking the position of the feeding tube tip before initiating feeding.

DIETS: FEEDING SOLUTIONS

Many types of diets are available from the nutrition industry, with a wide range of health claims (Table 22.6). The profusion of products is confusing to most clinicians. In the absence of GI pathology, the only important questions are how to provide energy and proteins (concentrated or not) and whether fibers are required. For such a purpose, only two or three polymeric diets are required in an ICU; disease-specific diets have not shown clear benefit. The elemental or semielemental diets also do not have any indication. Except in upper GI cancers, which benefit from immune-enhancing diets, the controversy is ongoing regarding the role of immune-enhancing diets in the critically ill. In contrast, the delivery of glutamine to the gut is based on strong evidence and can be accomplished by either the enteral provision of 0.5 g/kg of glutamine per day or a glutamine precursor provided as ornithine α-ketoglutarate boluses (20 g/day).

ORAL SUPPLEMENTS

Patients who do not strictly require artificial nutrition because they are nonintubated and apparently alert are often unable to eat efficiently (i.e., unable to meet their energy requirements): Anorexia is another characteristic of critical illness, as is taste disturbance. Such patients are at particularly high risk of malnutrition because they eat 300 to 700 kcal per day for prolonged periods while in the ICU and end up with a large energy deficit. Oral supplements, which contain 300 kcal/pack, are an efficient

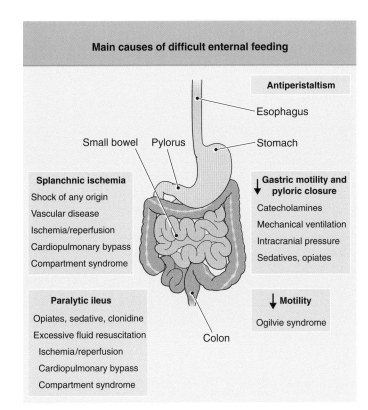

Main causes of difficult enteral feeding

Antiperistalsm

Esophagus

Small bowel Pylorus Stomach

Splanchnic ischemia

Shock of any origin
Vascular disease
Ischemia/reperfusion
Cardiopulmonary bypass
Compartment syndrome

↓ Gastric motility and pyloric closure

Catecholamines
Mechanical ventilation
Intracranial pressure
Sedatives, opiates

Paralytic ileus

Opiates, sedative, clonidine
Excessive fluid resuscitation
Ischemia/reperfusion
Cardiopulmonary bypass
Compartment syndrome

Colon

↓ Motility

Ogilvie syndrome

Figure 22.10. Main causes of difficult enteral feeding. Schematic diagram showing the main causes of difficult enteral feeding, characterized by impaired GI motility and pyloric closure.

Practice of Critical Care

Table 22.5 Troubleshooting: Common Technical Problems Encountered during Feeding after Cardiac Surgery, and Proposed Management[a]

Problem	Signs	Management/Prevention	Target

Gastroparesis	Gastric residue > 300 mL	Prevention: early enteral feeding
		Prokinetic drugs
		   Erythromycin (500 mg/day)
		   Metoclopramide (3 × 10 mg)
		   Cisapride (cave prolonged QT) (3 × 20 mg)
		Postpyloric feeding
			Gastric residue < 300 mL

Regurgitation of feeds during EN	Aspiration of GI juice in the pharynx, or worse in the trachea. Note: The blue dye of the feeds is no longer considered a diagnostic tool.	Prevention: position head of the patient at 30° or more Prokinetics Reduce EN Postpyloric access	Absence of suspect fluids in the pharynx
GI intolerance to EN	Large gastric residues, abdominal distention, ⇑ P_{IA}	Reduce EN and supplement with PN PN only if severe	Normal abdomen
Bowel ischemia	Abdominal distention, ⇑ (P_{IA}) Splanchnic acidosis: ⇓ pH_i ⇑ Arterial lactate	Improve hemodynamics Gastric decompression (aspiration)	Normal pH_i (>7.2) No distension Normal P_{IA}
Nonocclusive bowel necrosis	Abdominal distention	Stop EN (consider PN) Surgical resection	Normal abdomen
Small bowel perforation	As for any form of peritonitis (CT scan, clinical assessment)	Prevention: avoid delivery of pure distilled water into small bowel Surgery	
Abdominal compartment syndrome	⇑ P_{IA}	Reduce fluid loading Diuretics Gastric decompression	P_{IA} < 20 mm Hg
GI bleeding	Blood in nasogastric tube Endoscopic diagnosis	Prevention: anti-H_2 drugs Enteral nutrition (?) Treatment: proton pump inhibitors Endoscopic control of bleeding	No bleeding
Diarrhea	>5 liquid stools per day	Prevention: probiotics Fibers, probiotics Controlled continuous enteral feeding (pump controlled) Check hygienic manipulations of feeding tube and solution	<3 stools/day
Constipation	No stools for more than 5 days	Neostigmin (continuous or intermittent) Lactulose Fibers	1 stool/3 days
Pancreatitis	Ileus/subileus, pain Lab: ⇑ amylasemia and lipasemia Etiology after cardiac surgery: hypothermic cardiopulmonary bypass	Same as other pancreatitis Post-Treitz enteral feeding	No pain Normal transit
Acalculous cholecystitis	Abdominal ultrasound Lab: ⇑ alkaline phosphatase Nonspecific	Postpyloric feeding Interventional radiology Surgery	—
Insufficient energy delivery	Cumulated energy balance from admission shows deficit > 10,000 kcal	Prevention: daily assessment of energy balance and adequate prescription Avoid frequent and unnecessary interruptions of EN	Cumulative energy deficit 10,000 kcal

[a]EN, enteral nutrition; GI, gastrointestinal; PN, parenteral nutrition.

Table 22.6 Types of Diets

Condition	Solution	Caveat

No GI failure	First day: standard polymeric 1 kcal/mL
	Subsequent days
	   Standard polymeric 1.5 kcal/mL
	   Combined soluble and insoluble fiber diets
		Bronchoaspiration
		Energy deficit
		Diarrhea
		Bronchoaspiration

Cancer patient (upper GI tract)	Immune-enhancing diets	Sepsis
Diarrhea	Soluble fiber diets	Dehydration
Constipation	Soluble fiber diets initially followed by a mixture of soluble and insoluble fibers	Mechanical obstruction

way to reach the target. Two to four packs, delivered between meals, can be prescribed per day.

CONCLUSIONS

Nutritional support alone cannot heal patients, nor can it completely reverse the catabolic process. However, it can support organ function, reduce inflammation and the incidence of infection, and modulate the body's response to injury. Providing nutrition to the critically ill patient is a complex process requiring special knowledge and skills. In order to provide optimal care, the ICU specialist should have a good understanding of the nutritional requirements of critically ill patients and possess specialized training. Alternatively, the specialist should benefit from the support of a highly competent nutrition team.

SUGGESTED READING

Allison SP: The uses and limitations of nutritional support. Clin Nutr 1992;11:319–330.

Berger MM, Chioléro RL: Key vitamins and trace elements in the critically ill. In Cynober L, Moore F (eds): Nutrition and Critical Care Vol. 8, Nestlé Nutrition Workshops Series. Basel, Karger, 2003, pp 99–118.

Berger MM, Mustafa I: Metabolic and nutritional support in acute cardiac failure. Curr Opin Clin Nutrition Metab Care 2003;6:195–201.

Chioléro RL, Tappy L, Berger MM: Timing of nutritional support. Nestle Nutr Workshop Ser Clin Perform Programme 2002;7:151–164.

Elwyn DH: Protein and energy requirements: Effects of clinical state. Clin Nutr 1993;12(Suppl 1):S44–S51.

Gadek JE, DeMichele SJ, Karlstad MD, et al: Effect of enteral feeding with eicospentaenoic acid, γ-linolenic acid, and antioxidants in patients with acute respiratory distress syndrome. Crit Care Med 1999;27:1409–1420.

Goldberg PA, Siegel MD, Sherwin RS, et al: Implementation of a safe and effective insulin infusion protocol in a medical intensive care unit. Diabetes Care 2004;27:461–467.

Griffiths RD: Nutrition support in critically ill septic patients. Curr Opin Clin Nutrition Metab Care 2003;6:203–210.

Heyland DK, Novak F, Drover JW, et al: Should immunonutrition become routine in critically ill patients? A systematic review of the evidence. JAMA 2001;286:944–953.

Marik PE, Zaloga GP: Early enteral nutrition in acutely ill patients: A systematic review. Crit Care Med 2001;29:2264–2270.

Rubinson L, Diette GB, Song X, et al: Low caloric intake is associated with nosocomial bloodstream infections in patients in the medical intensive care unit. Crit Care Med 2004;32:350–357.

Van den Berghe G, Wouters PJ, Bouillon R, et al: Outcome benefit of intensive insulin therapy in the critically ill: Insulin dose versus glycemic control. Crit Care Med 2003;31:359–366.

Chapter 23

End-of-Life Care in the Intensive Care Unit

John M. Luce and Mitchell M. Levy

KEY POINTS

- Death is common in intensive care units (ICUs): 10% to 20% of Americans die in the ICU or soon after receiving ICU care.
- End-of-life care for ICU patients generally represents a transition from restorative treatment to the administration of palliative care and the withholding and withdrawal of life-sustaining therapy.
- The administration of palliative care and the withholding and withdrawal of life-sustaining therapy are ethically and legally justified.
- Proper end-of-life care includes providing an appropriate setting for dying patients, symptom management, and ensuring emotional and spiritual support for patients, families, and caregivers in addition to withholding or withdrawing life-sustaining therapy. It is important for critical care physicians to be trained in these palliative care skills.
- Endotracheal intubation and mechanical ventilation may be withdrawn rapidly or through a process called "terminal weaning," both of which are ethically appropriate.

Intensive care is costly, uncomfortable, potentially hazardous, and not always capable of sustaining life. Given these limitations, patients with progressive diseases such as chronic obstructive pulmonary disease, congestive heart failure, and cancer who recognize that death is imminent might prefer to die at home or in hospice, not in the intensive care unit (ICU). Similarly, patients with acute disorders such as severe burns and trauma should be allowed to die outside the ICU if they are beyond medical management. Ideally, only patients with reversible exacerbations of chronic disorders or with acute disorders that are amenable to treatment should want and receive ICU admission, and most, if not all, should leave the ICU alive.

However desirable this ideal might be, death is common in the ICU. In fact, many adult patients admitted to ICUs in the United States die there, and many more die after transfer to lower levels of care. In a study of deaths reported in six states in 1999, 38% occurred in hospitals and 22% occurred following admission to ICUs, leading Angus and colleagues to conclude that one fifth of all patients who die in the United States do so

after ICU admission. Some of these patients might have been expected to live because of intensive care, but most had a poor chance of survival. Furthermore, as shown in the Study to Understand Prognoses and Preferences for Outcomes and Risks of Treatment (SUPPORT), which was conducted more than 10 years ago, many patients with a limited life expectancy before admission have died with pain in less than optimal conditions in the ICU (Box 23.1).

The difference between ideal and actual ICU mortality rates described previously does not apply to underdeveloped countries with little or no heath care resources, let alone ICUs. The differences also are minimal in countries with limited ICU beds that restrict unit admission to patients with reversible disorders such as asthma and drug overdosage or explicitly ration admission by age and other criteria. In contrast, the United States and some other developed countries have ample ICU beds and rarely ration them in an overt fashion. Patients, families and other surrogates, and physicians and other caregivers in these developed countries tend to use intensive care to prolong life as long as possible, even when the likelihood of survival is extremely low. As a result, patients with advanced, severe, and possible irreversible disorders often expect and are granted a therapeutic trial of restorative treatment in the ICU. They undergo the administration of palliative care and the withholding and withdrawal of life-sustaining therapy only if the trial fails.

PREDICTING THE OUTCOME OF INTENSIVE CARE

Limiting ICU admission to patients likely to survive might be much simpler if one could predict who these patients might be. At the same time, "the transition from cure to comfort," as identified in the title of the first textbook on managing death in the ICU, might be facilitated by reliable prognostic information. Some of this information has been generated by single or multi-institutional studies of patients with disorders such as *Pneumocystis carinii* pneumonia and acute respiratory distress syndrome. Yet the outcome of these disorders changes over time, making it difficult for caregivers to decide in advance which patients will survive ICU admission or when they have failed a therapeutic trial.

Prognostic scoring systems, such as the Acute Physiology and Chronic Health Evaluation (APACHE) and SUPPORT, have been developed from large patient databases to overcome the

Box 23.1 Findings from SUPPORT of Hospitalized Adults with a 6-Month Mortality Rate of 47%

- Only 47% of physicians knew when their patients preferred to avoid CPR.
- 46% of DNR orders were written within 2 days of death.
- 38% of patients spent at least 10 days in an ICU.
- For 50% of conscious patients who died in the hospital, family members reported moderate to severe pain at least half the time.

CPR, cardiopulmonary resuscitation; DNR, do not resuscitate.
From the SUPPORT Principal Investigators: A controlled trial to improve care for seriously ill hospitalized patients: The study to understand prognoses and preferences for outcomes and risks of treatment (SUPPORT). JAMA 1995;274:1951–1958.

disadvantages of small outcome studies. These systems have been shown to be as accurate—or inaccurate—as prognoses made by physicians and nurses. The systems also have demonstrated good calibration in that the overall mortality predicted by them is comparable to that actually observed. However, they have not discriminated well between ICU survivors and nonsurvivors, and the systems cannot be used by themselves to decide who is too sick for ICU admission and who is certain to die there.

Because prognostication is so imprecise, medical decision making in the ICU, not to mention rationing of ICU beds, is difficult to objectify. Patients, surrogates, and caregivers must balance their desire to sustain life and avoid suffering, goals that may occasionally conflict, with a responsibility to use health care resources wisely. This responsibility perhaps is felt more keenly in countries in which ICU beds are limited and physicians are empowered to ration than it is in the United States, where access to beds is taken for granted and physicians have been urged by some ethicists to do everything possible for patients without regard to cost. Unfortunately, no country enjoys unlimited health care resources, rationing occurs to some degree in all countries, and end-of-life care in the ICU is challenging everywhere. As the costs of ICU care continue to increase, discussions about appropriate rationing will become more common.

ETHICAL AND LEGAL JUSTIFICATION FOR CARE AT THE END OF LIFE

The administration of palliative care, the withholding and withdrawal of life-sustaining therapy, and rationing are justified by four ethical principles (Table 23.1). The first three principles—

beneficence, nonmaleficence, and autonomy—are the basis of the fiduciary relationship through which physicians hold their patients' interests in trust. Although the relative importance of the three principles differs from country to country, the fiduciary relationship remains much the same.

The administration of palliative care is sanctioned in the United States by what has been interpreted as a constitutional right to die without undue pain and suffering. This right has been extended by the U.S. Supreme Court to include "terminal sedation," through which patients may be rendered unconscious and unwanted therapies, including fluid and nutrition, are forgone. According to the Court, terminal sedation and other forms of palliative treatment must comply with the ethical rule of double effect. Under this rule, acts such as the giving of sedatives and analgesics that lead to morally good effects, such as the relief of suffering, are permissible even if they produce morally bad effects, such as the hastening of death, provided that only the good effects are intended.

The rule of double effect is not necessarily followed in certain countries, such as Belgium and The Netherlands, where euthanasia and physician-assisted suicide are practiced. Furthermore, principles used to justify the withholding and withdrawal of life-sustaining therapy in the United States may not be embedded in the laws of other countries. In addition, although most U.S. ethicists draw no moral distinctions between withholding and withdrawing life-sustaining therapies, this distinction is drawn elsewhere. Indeed, countries differ not only in their ethical and legal traditions but also in the prevalence and manner by which life-sustaining therapies are forgone.

In the United States, the withholding and withdrawal of life-sustaining therapy is legally justified by the principles of informed consent and refusal, which have been applied in statutes and acknowledged in case law (Box 23.2). The right of adults with decision-making capacity to forgo treatment, including that which sustains life, has been accepted by court cases in many states and affirmed by the U.S. Supreme Court. The legal right of family members and other surrogates to make decisions for incapacitated adult patients also has been established by state courts under two standards: substituted judgment, in which surrogates may decide in accordance with patients' known wishes, and best interests, in which they decide with those interests in mind. Although the Supreme Court allows states to require strong evidence of patients' wishes before surrogates exercise

Table 23.1 Ethical Principles Governing End-of-Life Care

Principle	Definition
Beneficence	The obligation to do good for patients
Nonmaleficence	The obligation to avoid harm
Autonomy	Respect for the patient's right of self-determination
Distributive justice	The fair allocation of health care resources

Box 23.2 Legal Principles That Justify the Withholding and Withdrawal of Life-Sustaining Therapy in the United States

- Patients with the capacity to make medical decisions can refuse any and all treatment.
- Patients can designate family members and other surrogates to make decisions for them.
- Surrogates, formally designated or not, may make decisions for incapacitated patients.
- Decisions may be made on the basis of substituted judgment (what the patient wishes) or best interests (what is best for the patient).

substituted judgment, it does not mandate this requirement for states that choose to do otherwise.

To advance the substituted judgment standard, the U.S. Congress passed the Patient Self-Determination Act in 1990. This statute mandates that patients be asked on admission to medical facilities whether they have advance directives and that they be assisted in drawing up such directives if they have not already done so. Advance directives are of two types: instructional directives, which articulate what a patient would want done in a given situation, and proxy directives, which appoint a surrogate to make medical decisions in the event of the patient's incapacity. SUPPORT showed that in the early 1990s, most patients did not fill out advance directives, that many physicians were unaware of the directives when they were filled out, and that the directives had little impact on ICU decision making. Presumably, a similar situation exists today in the United States. Nevertheless, advance directives remain a potential way of reinforcing autonomy, even though that potential has not been realized.

Although the ethical principle of autonomy and the legal principles of informed consent and refusal are the most compelling justifications for withholding and withdrawing life-sustaining treatment in the United States, the concept of futility also has been used. This concept is invoked either to make decisions without consulting the patients or surrogates or on the relatively rare occasions when they request interventions—especially those that are costly, scarce, or both—that physicians believe they are unlikely to benefit from. Some interventions, such as attempted cardiopulmonary resuscitation in the setting of refractory septic shock, are physiologically futile in that they cannot be accomplished, and physicians are not obligated to offer them. Other interventions may sustain life, albeit only for a short time, and the legal status of denying them on the basis of futility is unclear.

PROPER END-OF-LIFE CARE IN THE INTENSIVE CARE UNIT

Proper end-of-life care in the ICU has several components (Box 23.3). One of these components is the provision of an adequate environment for dying patients. Assuming it is available, a private ICU room with enough space to accommodate visitors might be such an environment. Visiting hours should be relaxed, if necessary, to allow families and friends to spend as

---

Box 23.3 Components of Proper End-of-Life Care in the Intensive Care Unit

Providing an appropriate setting for dying patients
Symptom management
    Pain
    Anxiety
    Delirium
    Dyspnea
    Nausea and vomiting
    Hunger and thirst
Ensuring emotional and spiritual support
Withholding and withdrawing life-sustaining therapy

---

much time as they wish with their loved ones. Separate rooms for meeting with families may also be an important part of end-of-life care, providing a quiet, private space for difficult discussions. Some hospitals have separate palliative care units for patients and families; others offer palliative care teams or services that consult throughout the hospital.

Management of symptoms such as pain, anxiety, delirium, dyspnea, nausea and vomiting, and hunger and thirst is an essential component of end-of-life care. Pain can be managed indirectly by nonpharmacologic means. For example, placement of patients in a quiet environment in which friends and families may visit can diminish the sense of pain, as may the treatment of anxiety and depression. A direct approach to the management of pain generally centers on the use of opioids, and morphine is the opioid most commonly used, followed by fentanyl and hydromorphone. These drugs most often should be administered in anticipation of pain and not after its occurrence. In reports of ICU patients undergoing the withholding and withdrawal of life-sustaining therapy, opioids were titrated in doses that caregivers considered adequate to relieve pain, without shortening the time until death.

As is the case with pain, anxiety and its physical manifestation, agitation, can be managed nonpharmacologically. If drugs are required, benzodiazepines, such as lorazapam and midazolam, and propofol are preferred. Usually given by constant infusion in dying ICU patients, these drugs are comparable in the sedation they produce. There need be no limit to the doses of sedatives used for palliative care, although some patients, particularly those who are not having endotracheal intubation and mechanical ventilation withdrawn, may prefer to be conscious when they die. Delirium is best treated with orientation to the environment and the administration of haloperidol, a butyrophenone neuroleptic agent that is minimally sedating.

Depending on its cause, dyspnea is treated with oxygen, bronchodilators, corticosteroids, diuretics, and other interventions in patients undergoing restorative treatment inside and outside of the ICU. These interventions usually are forgone, however, when death is near. In this circumstance, opioids and sedatives, whose use in ameliorating dyspnea in outpatients is limited primarily by the hypotension and respiratory depression they produce, may be employed to treat breathlessness. Some physicians view noninvasive ventilation as a comfort measure that can relieve dyspnea. However, in some cases the use of noninvasive ventilation may lead to survival of patients for whom this is not a desired outcome.

Nausea and vomiting often respond to treatment of underlying disorders, including primary gastrointestinal diseases, or to the removal of drugs such as theophylline that cause these symptoms. Patients who do not respond to these measures may be given traditional antiemetic agents, including corticosteroids such as dexamethasone and butyrophenones such as droperidol, or newer agents, such as the serotonin receptor antagonists ondansetron and dolastron. Dying patients rarely perceive hunger and thirst, and the ketosis induced by starvation may actually be euphoric. In patients who are symptomatic from hunger and thirst, these symptoms can be alleviated with small amounts of food and fluids or by the application of ice chips and lubrication to the lips.

Administering drugs may be helpful in relieving suffering, but it is no substitute for providing emotional and spiritual support

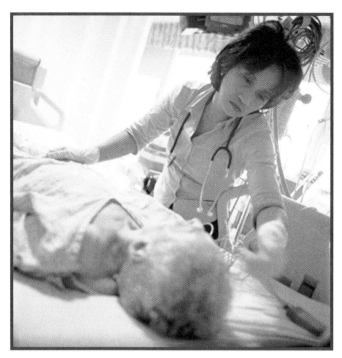

Figure 23.1. Compassionate care of a patient in the ICU.

Table 23.2 Approaches to Weaning Endotracheal Intubation and Mechanical Ventilation

Approach	Method	Potential Advantages	Potential Disadvantages
Rapid extubation	Patient given sedatives and analgesics; endotracheal tube and ventilator removed	Direct approach; family members may hold dying infant	Patient may be discomforted because of upper airway obstruction
Terminal weaning	Patient given sedatives and analgesics; inspired oxygen fraction, ventilator rate, and PEEP level reduced before ventilator removed	Patient may experience less discomfort	Death may be prolonged

PEEP, positive end-expiratory pressure.

to dying patients and their families. Physicians contribute to this support, of course, and their regular communications and presence at the bedside are greatly appreciated. Nurses, respiratory therapists, social workers, clergy, and other members of the health care team deliver most of the support, however (Fig. 23.1). Occasionally, patients or their families may request that friends, caregivers, and religious persons from outside a particular institution either provide consultations or participate in bedside rituals and observances. These should be allowed, if not encouraged.

Studies from ICUs throughout the world reveal that although any and all medical interventions may be withheld or withdrawn, variation exists in the type, number, and sequence of interventions. For example, in one investigation in an adult ICU in the United States, an average of five interventions were forgone per patient (Box 23.4). How endotracheal intubation and mechanical ventilation are withdrawn varies among ICUs. One approach is rapid extubation; the other is called "terminal weaning." Both approaches have potential advantages and disadvantages (Table 23.2).

Most patients die from their underlying diseases when endotracheal intubation and mechanical ventilation are withdrawn. Nonetheless, some survive, and at least in the United States, their survival should not be prevented by drugs that hasten death. At the same time, even patients who are too sick to survive should not receive drug agents that may interfere with observing tachypnea and other signs that may signal the need for symptom relief. For these reasons, although analgesics and sedatives may be given to relieve suffering, neuromuscular blocking agents should not be introduced to patients while intubation and mechanical ventilation are withdrawn. If patients are already receiving these agents, the agents should be discontinued if possible.

CONCLUSION

End-of-life care in the ICU can be delivered properly if clinicians follow an organized approach that emphasizes the comfort of patients, families, and caregivers. This kind of approach is both ethically and legally justified, and it works in most instances. That the approach is not always successful is due to two factors: The end of life cannot be predicted for all patients, and the transition from restorative to palliative treatment is not always seamless. Nevertheless, since the SUPPORT study was published, improvements have been made in the management of death in the ICU.

SUGGESTED READING

Angus DC, Barnato AE, Linde-Zwirble WT, et al: The use of intensive care at the end of life in the United States: An epidemiologic study. Crit Care Med 2004;32:638–643.

Cook D, Rocker G, Marshall J, et al: Withdrawal of mechanical ventilation in anticipation of death in the intensive care unit. N Engl J Med 2003; 349:1123–1132.

Curtis JR, Rubenfeld GD (eds.): Managing Care in the Intensive Care Unit: The Transition from Cure to Comfort. Oxford, Oxford University Press, 2001.

Knaus WA, Wagner DP, Draper EA, et al: APACHE II—A severity of disease classification system. Crit Care Med 1985;13:818–829.

Box 23.4 Therapies Frequently Withheld or Withdrawn

Cardiopulmonary resuscitation
Endotracheal intubation and mechanical ventilation
Renal dialysis
Vasopressors
Blood products
Antibiotics
Fluids and feedings

From Faber-Langendoen K, Bartels DM: Process of forgoing life-sustaining treatment in a university hospital: An empiric study. Crit Care Med 1992;20:570–577.

Levy MM: End-of-life care in the intensive care unit: Can we do better? Crit Care Med 2001;29:N56–N61.

Luce JM, Alpers A: Legal aspects of withholding and withdrawing life support from critically ill patients in the United States and administering palliative care to them. Am J Respir Crit Care Med 2000;162: 2029–2032.

Pochard F, Azoulay E, Chevret S, et al: French intensivists do not apply American recommendations regarding decisions to forgo life-sustaining therapy. Crit Care Med 2001;29:1887–1892.

SUPPORT Principal Investigators: A controlled trial to improve care for seriously ill hospitalized patients: The study to understand prognoses and preferences for outcomes and risks of treatment (SUPPORT). JAMA 1995;274:1951–1958.

Truog RD, Cist EFM, Brackett SE, et al: Recommendations for end-of-life care in the intensive care unit: The ethics committee of the Society of Critical Care Medicine. Crit Care Med 2001;29:2332–2348.

Vincent J-L: Forgoing life support in western European intensive care units: The results of an ethical questionnaire. Crit Care Med 1999;27: 1626–1633.

Chapter 24

Acute Exacerbations of Chronic Obstructive Pulmonary Disease and Asthma

Matthew T. Naughton and David V. Tuxen

KEY POINTS

- Hypercapnic chronic obstructive pulmonary disease (COPD) patients should be treated with noninvasive ventilation and supplemental oxygen sufficient to overcome hypoxemia but avoid hyperoxia.
- Intravenous or oral steroids in COPD should be limited to 3 to 10 days in most cases.
- In acute severe asthma, there is no proof that the intravenous administration of short-acting β-agonists has an advantage over adequate nebulized administration.
- In severe asthma, dynamic pulmonary hyperinflation due to mechanical ventilation can result in hypotension, pnemothoraces, and, in very severe asthma, circulatory collapse with pulseless electrical activity (i.e., electromechanical dissociation). This can be acutely relieved with a 60-second apnea test and thereafter prevented by a slow respiratory rate and a long expiratory time with permissive hypercapnia.
- Following acute severe exacerbations of COPD and asthma, precipitating factors should be sought and avoided or treated. Patient-orientated action plans should be instituted to avoid further acute deterioration.

EPIDEMIOLOGY

Worldwide, it has been estimated that 1.1 billion people have COPD, a prevalence expected to increase to 1.6 billion people by 2025. In the United Kingdom, 20% of men and 10% of women older than age 45 years report a chronic cough with sputum, with 4% of men and 2% of women meeting diagnostic criteria for COPD. In the United States, COPD is estimated to occur in up to 19% of the adult community and result in 16 million physician visits and 500,000 hospital admissions per year. COPD is the fourth most common cause of death worldwide, accounting for 5% of all deaths—an age-adjusted rate that has risen from 1965 to 1995, in comparison with those for cardiovascular disease and stroke, both of which have declined. The mortality of COPD patients admitted to the hospital is 15%, exceeding that for myocardial infarction. Risk factors for mortality in COPD are low body mass index, degree of airflow obstruction as measured by FEV_1, exercise limitation, and degree of dyspnea. Survival can also be predicted by the $PaCO_2$ (Fig. 24.1).

Asthma is estimated to occur in 20% of children and 8% of adults, with 5% to 10% of these having poorly controlled disease. Life-threatening episodes occur in 0.5% of patients. In the United States, asthma is responsible for 1.8 million emergency department visits per year, with 1 in 4 requiring overnight admission. New Zealand, Australia, and the United Kingdom have the greatest prevalence rates.

Chronic obstructive pulmonary disease (COPD) and asthma are conditions characterized by fixed and variable airflow obstruction, respectively. Increased use of inhaled steroids and exacerbation management plans have resulted in decreased hospital and intensive care admission rates for asthma. The same is not true for COPD. Although both can have common overlapping clinical presentations (Table 24.1) and are responsible for significant morbidity and mortality, with a demand on intensive care services, their etiology and management differ.

COPD is a condition in which permanent airflow obstruction occurs, associated with alveolar destruction (emphysema) and inflammation of the airway walls (chronic bronchitis). Asthma is defined by variable airflow obstruction that is reversible, completely or partially, spontaneously or with treatment, and is associated with airway inflammation and increased airway responsiveness to a variety of stimuli.

Table 24.1 Clinical Differences between COPD and Asthma		
	COPD	**Asthma**
Prevalence (% population)	5	10
Age	Older	Younger
Smoking history (pack year)	>20	<20
Allergic history	Rare	Common
Symptoms	Slowly progressive	Episodic
Cor pulmonale	Yes, when severe	Rare
Bronchodilator or steroid response (%)	<12	>12
Inflammation	Neutrophilic	Eosinophilic
High-resolution CT chest	Emphysema	Variable (normal or mucus-filled bronchi)

223

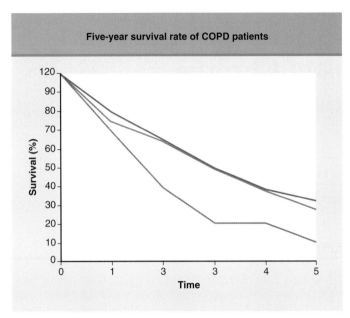

Figure 24.1. Five-year survival of COPD patients presenting with an acute exacerbation in relation to admission and discharge Paco$_2$ level. The best survival was in the group with normocapnia on admission and discharge (blue; mean Paco$_2$, 40 to 41 mm Hg), which was similar to the group with hypercapnia on admission and normocapnia on discharge (green; mean Paco$_2$, 59 to 44 mm Hg). The worst survival was in the group with hypercapnia on admission and discharge (red; mean Paco$_2$, 60 to 53 mm Hg). (Adapted from Costello R, Deegan P, Fitzpatrick M, McNicholas WT: Reversible hypercapnia in chronic obstructive pulmonary disease: a distinct pattern of respiratory failure with a favorable diagnosis. Am J Med 1997;102:239–244.)

RISK FACTORS

COPD

Ninety-five percent of patients with COPD have tobacco smoking as a risk factor. Other environmental factors include exposure to secondary tobacco smoke, air pollution, indoor fumes (e.g., indoor cooking with solid biomass fuel), and poor socioeconomic status. Host factors are also important but, with the exception of α_1-antitrypsin deficiency, are poorly understood.

Asthma

Although there is a clear familial prevalence of asthma, and several genes have been implicated, no single gene defined could allow for meaningful genetic planning. A number of other risk factors have been proposed, including (1) inadequate exposure to allergens due to excessive antibiotic use, (2) excessively clean dust-free environment (i.e., the hygiene hypothesis), (3) excessive exposure to common allergic (e.g., house dust mite, pollen, and animal dander) or nonallergic triggers (e.g., cold air, exercise, and atmospheric pollutants), and (4) exposure to medications that modulate airway control (e.g., aspirin and beta blockers). The increasing prevalence of asthma during the past 50 years has been attributed to increasing environmental exposures. Exposure to infections such as respiratory syncytial virus and parainfluenza (in children) and *Chlamydia* (in adults) has been implicated as a risk factor. Stress and socioeconomic status

have also been implicated. In 30% of patients, no precipitant can be identified.

PATHOGENESIS

COPD

Reduction in expiratory airflow occurs because of increased airway resistance and reduced lung elastic recoil. Airway resistance increases in the 4th- to 12th-generation airways as a result of mucosal inflammation, basement membrane thickening, edema, mucosal hypertrophy, secretions, and bronchospasm. Loss of lung elastic recoil is due to destruction of lung elastin and reduction in alveolar surface tension.

Reduced elastic recoil decreases expiratory airflow by reducing the alveolar pressure driving expiratory airflow. Forced expiration increases alveolar driving pressure but also causes dynamic airway compression, resulting in no improvement, or sometimes a reduction, in expiratory airflow. The importance of this factor is a function of the degree of emphysema in each individual patient.

Hypoxia and vascular wall changes lead to pulmonary vasoconstriction, pulmonary hypertension, cor pulmonale, and ventilation-to-perfusion heterogeneity. Most commonly, smoking-related COPD results in apical, rather than basal, disease (Fig. 24.2), whereas α_1 antitrypsin deficiency usually causes basal emphysema. Central respiratory drive may also be poorly responsive to the physiological trigger of hypercapnic acidosis, contributing to chronic hypercapnia. This may occur in the setting of sleep (i.e., obstructive sleep apnea), obesity, drugs (sedatives, antiepileptics, and alcohol), or metabolic disturbance (metabolic alkalosis).

Asthma

Postmortem studies indicate that small airway narrowing occurs as a result of bronchial wall edema, inflammatory cell infiltrates, smooth muscle hypertrophy and hyperplasia, collagen deposition beneath the basement membrane thickening, and intraluminal secretions of eosinophilic inflammatory cells. Eosinophils infiltrate the nerve bundles and release major basic protein, which antagonizes the inhibitory M_2 muscarinic receptor present on parasympathetic nerve endings.

The nocturnal (or circadian) exacerbation commonly seen in asthma is due to a combination of factors, including exposure to cool dry air, inhalation of excessive allergens related to bedding, and circadian changes in airway diameter and cortisol.

COPD and Asthma

In COPD and asthma, pulmonary hyperinflation has both static and dynamic components. The static component is the increase in functional residual capacity (FRC) that exists at the end of an exhalation that is long enough for all expiratory airflow to cease (i.e., 30–120 sec). This component of hyperinflation is primarily due to airway closure that occurs throughout exhalation. Dynamic hyperinflation is the further increase in hyperinflation that occurs because of failure to complete exhalation before beginning the inhalation associated with the next breath. The extent of dynamic hyperinflation depends on the severity of airflow obstruction, the amount inspired (i.e., the tidal volume), and the expiratory time. Thus, the degree of hyperinflation may vary with changes in tidal volume and/or respira-

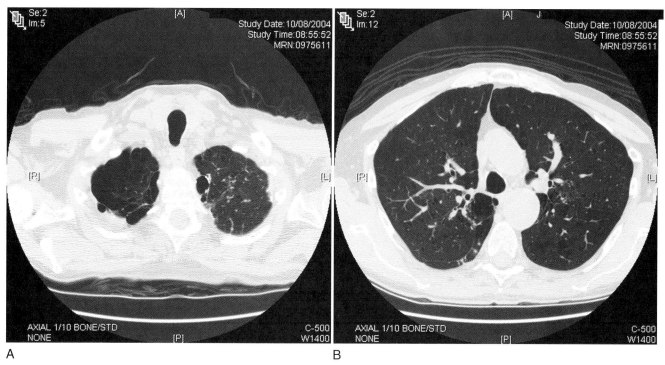

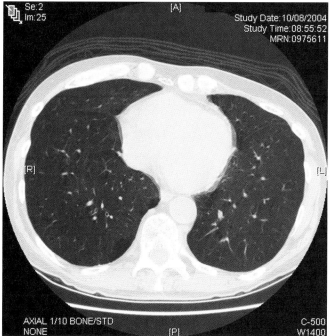

Figure 24.2. High-resolution CT scan of the chest of a patient with smoking-related COPD. Note the emphysematous changes in the apices (*A*) to a greater degree than in the midzones (*B*) and bases (*C*).

tory rate that occur in response to changes in CO_2 production (as a function of exercise, diet, fever, or the metabolic response to illness) or changes in dead space, as well as with changes in airflow obstruction that occur during an exacerbation.

Chest wall hyperinflation puts the inspiratory respiratory muscles at a mechanical disadvantage, increases the work of breathing, and predisposes patients to developing respiratory muscle fatigue. Chronic use of corticosteroids, electrolyte disturbances, and/or other medications may also contribute to this problem. In COPD, minor reductions in lung function due to infection, cardiac failure, or atelectasis increase the work of

breathing by increasing airway resistance, lung stiffness, and/or dead space. This may result in rapid decompensation with ventilatory failure, acute hypercapnia, and respiratory acidosis as the tidal volume falls as a result of the increased volume of trapped gas and diminished respiratory muscle strength.

CLINICAL FEATURES

COPD

Patients with severe airflow limitation who are normocapnic ($PaCO_2$, 35–45 mm Hg) are generally thin, may purse their lips

---

Box 24.1 Precipitants of Acute Respiratory Failure in COPD

Infective (pneumonia, bronchitis)
Left ventricular failure (systolic, diastolic failure, arrhythmias)
Uncontrolled oxygen
Medication—noncompliance or side effects
Sputum retention (postoperative, traumatic)
Sedation
Sleep disordered breathing
Pulmonary embolism
Nutritional (K, PO_4, Mg deficiency, CHO excess)
Pneumothoraces and bullae

---

during exhalation, use their accessory respiratory muscles for inhalation, are hyperinflated, and may develop right heart failure but only late in their course. In contrast, patients with a $PaCO_2$ greater than 45 mm Hg are generally more obese, have depression of their hypoxic and/or hypercarbic ventilatory drives (which can be worsened by excessive oxygen, alcohol, sedatives, or analgesics), have sleep-related hypoventilation, and are more likely to develop right heart failure early. Approximately 50% of patients with an acute exacerbation of COPD will be hypercapnic, a portion of them as a result of excessive oxygen administration.

Acute exacerbations of COPD seem to result from respiratory infections (~50%) or cardiac failure (~25%). The remaining 25% may have retained secretions, air pollution, coexistent medical problems (e.g., pulmonary embolus, gastroesophageal reflux, and medication compliance or side effects) or no cause can be identified (Box 24.1).

The most common bacterial isolates are *Streptococcus pneumoniae*, *Hemophilus influenzae*, *Streptococcus viridans*, and *Moraxella catarrhalis*. *Mycobacterium pneumonia* and *Pseudomonas aeruginosa* may also be found. Viruses have been isolated in 20% to 30% of exacerbations. These include rhinovirus, influenza and parainfluenza viruses, corona viruses, and, occasionally, adenovirus and respiratory syncitial virus have been isolated in 20% to 30% of exacerbations. Whether these organisms are pathogens or colonizers is often unclear. Pneumonia may account for 20% of those presentations requiring mechanical ventilation.

Left ventricular systolic failure may result from coexisting ischemic heart disease, fluid overload, or tachyarrhythmias.

Diastolic dysfunction may occur secondary to right ventricular dilation. Many of these patients have high levels of intrinsic positive end-expiratory pressure (PEEP) (or auto-PEEP), particularly during acute exacerbations, and this may decrease cardiac output by decreasing venous return. The increased work of breathing related to COPD will also contribute to heart failure because blood flow distributed to the respiratory muscles may increase by up to 10-fold. In the absence of roentgenographic evidence of pulmonary edema, left ventricular failure may be difficult to diagnose.

Uncontrolled oxygen administration may precipitate acute hypercapnia in patients with acute COPD exacerbations as a result of relaxing hypoxic vasoconstriction, thereby allowing increased perfusion to regions with reduced alveolar ventilation. Although a reduction in hypercarbic drive was previously thought to account for this problem, the contribution of abnormal drive is limited.

Asthma

An accurate and detailed history is needed to distinguish asthma from other causes of dyspnea. Classically, asthmatic patients will have wheeze, cough, and/or dyspnea occurring with exercise, at night, or with exposure to specific triggers. When asthma is mild, there is typically a prompt resolution following inhalation of short-acting β-agonists (SABAs).

The assessment of asthma severity (Table 24.2) and triage is crucial. Most commonly, patients with severe asthma have a history of previous hospitalizations for asthma (some that may be near fatal), low socioeconomic status, female gender, obesity, nighttime symptoms, FEV_1 less than 60% with optimal treatment, continual symptoms, reduced quality of life, use of oral or systemic steroids in the past 12 months, use of more than canister of SABA per month, elevated residual volume-to-total lung capacity (RV:TLC) ratio on pulmonary function testing, and a peak expiratory flow rate variability of more than 30% (i.e., variability- (best − worst)/best reading). A typical pattern is the progression over hours to days, occurring in the setting of a history of recurrent presentations. This form is associated with greater airway inflammation and generally responds poorly, or incompletely, to initial bronchodilator therapy but responds to steroid and bronchodilators over a few hours or days.

Less commonly, patients can present with hyperacute exacerbations, with the interval between the onset of symptoms and

Table 24.2 Assessment of Asthma Severity			
Symptom	**Mild**	**Severity Moderate**	**Severe and Life threatening**
Physical exhaustion	No	No	Yes
Speech	Sentences	Phrases	Words, or unable to speak
Pulse rate (bpm)	<100	100–120	>120 or <60
Pulsus paradox	Nil	May be palpable	Palpable
Wheeze intensity	Variable	Moderate to loud	May be quiet
Central cyanosis	Absent	May be present	Likely to be present without O_2
Peak exp flow (% predicted)	>75	50–75	<50 or <100 liters/minute
FEV_1 (% predicted)	>75	50–75	<50 or <1 liter
Oximetry (%)	>95	92–95	<92
$PaCO_2$ (mmHg)	38–42	35–44	>45
Arterial blood gas pH	7.35–7.45	7.35–7.50	<7.35
Conscious state	Normal	Normal	May be depressed

respiratory failure of less than 3 hours. This form of asthma occurs in younger patients, more commonly male, with intervening normal lung function but with highly sensitive bronchial reactivity to triggers, which is attributed to marked bronchial smooth muscle contraction. This form of asthma responds to SABA treatment within minutes to hours.

Physical examination should include assessment of speech (ability to speak in sentences, phrases, or words), oxygen saturation, heart rate, pulsus paradox, use of accessory muscles, chest auscultation, conscious state, and response to immediate inhaled bronchodilators. Pulse higher than 120 beats/min, respiratory rate higher than 30/min, and pulsus paradox more than 15 mm Hg indicate severe asthma. Auscultatory findings of a silent chest may indicate extremely severe bronchospasm or the presence of pneumothorax.

DIAGNOSIS

COPD

The diagnosis of COPD is usually established prior to patient presentation, with respiratory failure based on history, clinical examination, and investigations. Patients with COPD usually have a history of smoking more than 20 pack-years. In some settings, exposure to indoor solid fuel heating or cooking or a family history of α_1-antitrypsin deficiency may be causative or contributing factors. They may have a history of chronic cough and sputum production and describe exertional dyspnea and wheeze.

In patients with mild, stable disease, an expiratory wheeze on forced expiration and mild exertional dyspnea may be the only findings. In patients with moderate disease, modest to severe exertional dyspnea is associated with clinical signs of hyperinflation and increased work of breathing. In severe but stable disease, marked accessory muscle use is seen in association with tachypnea at rest, pursed lip breathing, hypoxemia, and signs of pulmonary hypertension [right ventricular heave, loud and palpable pulmonary second sound, and elevated "a" wave in jugular venous pressure (JVP)] and cor pulmonale (elevated JVP, hepatomegaly, and ankle swelling). In severe unstable COPD, there is marked tachypnea at rest, hypoxemia and tachycardia, and, in some cases, signs of hypercapnia (dilated cutaneous veins, blurred vision, headaches, obtunded mentation, and confusion).

Clinical examination may also identify associated medical conditions precipitating the exacerbation, such as pulmonary crepitations and bronchial breathing with pneumonia, crepitations and cardiomegaly related to heart failure, or mediastinal shift related to a pneumothorax.

The severity of COPD is best judged by assessing pulmonary function [i.e., peak expiratory flow rate (PEFR)] or FEV_1. The vital capacity (VC) is initially normal and decreases later in the course of the disease but to a lesser degree than the FEV_1. An FEV_1:VC ratio less than 70% with an FEV_1 50% to 80% of predicted without a bronchodilator response usually indicates mild COPD. A significant bronchodilator response (i.e., >12% or >200 mL increase in either FEV_1 or VC) implies a diagnosis of asthma. An FEV_1 30% to 50% predicted indicates moderately severe COPD, and an FEV_1 less than 30% predicted indicates severe disease.

Although the diagnosis may be based on spirometry alone, further lung function testing may be useful to characterize sever-

ity. Flow volume curves demonstrate reduced expiratory flow rates and show the characteristic "concave" expiratory flow pattern. Lung volumes measured either by helium dilution or by plethysmography show elevated TLC, FRC, and RV. The RV:TLC ratio is characteristically more than 40%, representing intrathoracic gas trapping. The diffusion capacity, a measurement of alveolar surface area, is usually less than 80% predicted and is reduced in proportion to the extent of emphysema.

Chest x-rays will commonly show hyperinflated lung fields as suggested by flattened diaphragms (best seen on lateral CXR), evidence of emphysematous bullae, and/or a paucity of lung markings. Pulmonary hypertension may be suggested by the presence of enlarged proximal pulmonary arteries, attenuated distal vascular markings, and right ventricular enlargement. High-resolution computed tomography (CT) scans show emphysema and can also confirm coexistent bronciectasis. Such scans are less sensitive than standard chest CT scans (1-cm slice) for detecting pulmonary lesions (e.g., neoplasms) (Fig. 24.3). Nuclear ventilation–perfusion scans show diffuse, well-matched, nonsegmental ventilation–perfusion abnormalities, with the degree of severity matching what is seen clinically.

Arterial blood gases are mandatory to assess the degree of hypoxia and hypercapnia and to determine the acid–base status. A serum bicarbonate level more than 30 mEq/liter indicates either renal compensation for a chronic respiratory acidosis or a primary metabolic alkalosis (e.g., diuretic therapy, high-dose steroids, or high-volume gastric fluid loss). Renal compensation for chronic hypercapnia will increase the serum bicarbonate by approximately 4 mEq/liter for each 10 mm Hg of chronic $PaCO_2$ rise above 40 mm Hg in order to return pH to the low normal range.

The electrocardiogram (ECG) is commonly normal but may show features of right atrial or right ventricular hypertrophy and strain, including P pulmonale, right axis deviation, dominant R waves in V1–V2, right bundle branch block, and ST depression and T wave flattening or inversion in V1–V3. These changes may be chronic or may develop acutely if there is a marked increase in pulmonary vascular resistance during the illness. The ECG may also show coexistent ischemic heart disease, tachycardia, and atrial fibrillation. Occasionally, continuous ECG monitoring is required to identify transient arrhythmias, which may also precipitate an acute deterioration.

Asthma

As with COPD, the diagnosis of asthma is usually apparent from history and examination. Tests of airflow obstruction are needed to assess severity. A PEFR of less than 100 L/min or an FEV_1 of less than 1 liter indicates a life-threatening asthma situation. These should be repeated to assess response to treatment.

In mild to moderate asthma, arterial blood gases show a respiratory alkalosis as ventilation generally increases. In severe asthma, hypoxemia is present and can be easily corrected with supplemental oxygen with normal pH and $PaCO_2$. In fulminant disease, hypercapnic respiratory acidosis develops with more severe hypoxemia. The respiratory acidosis may be compounded by lactic acidosis if intravenous SABAs (salbutamol, epinephrine, or isoprenaline) are used. Occasionally, continuously nebulized salbutamol can produce lactic acidosis.

The chest x-ray rarely shows consolidation but should be obtained regardless, seeking evidence of pneumothorax or

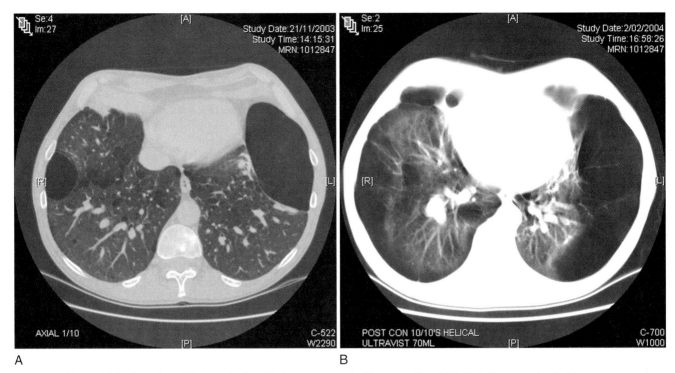

Figure 24.3. Benefits of high-resolution CT when compared with conventional CT. Note the more detailed lung parenchyma with high-resolution (1-mm thickness) CT of the chest (A) compared to the conventional (1-cm thickness) CT (B).

pneumomediastinum (Fig. 24.4). Importantly, a chest x-ray will also assist in excluding other differential diagnoses, such as left ventricular failure and possibly inhaled foreign bodies. If pulmonary infiltrates are found, the possibility of allergic bronchopulmonary aspergillosis should be considered. Serum IgE and eosinophil levels can be obtained in the acute setting. If either is elevated, the diagnosis of "extrinsic" asthma is established and even more attention should be paid to seeking out a specific allergen.

Other causes of "asthma" should always be considered (e.g., inhaled foreign body, aspiration, left ventricular failure, pulmonary embolus, and pneumothorax). A new asthma exacerbation in an already hospitalized patient is more likely to be due to these causes than due to the asthma.

TREATMENT

COPD

Oxygen

Oxygen given by low-flow intranasal cannulae (1–4 L/min) or 24% to 35% by Venturi mask should be initiated with the goal of achieving an arterial saturation ($SaCO_2$) of $90 \pm 2\%$ because this will limit O_2-induced increases in $PaCO_2$ (which occur most commonly in patients with initial $PaCO_2$ >50 mm Hg and pH <7.35). If the rise in $PaCO_2$ is excessive (>10 mm Hg), consider reducing the FIO_2 to a SaO_2 of 87% or 88% versus increasing the level of noninvasive positive pressure ventilatory support. Although high levels of O_2 should be avoided (SaO_2 >95%), reversal of hypoxia is important and O_2 should not be withheld in the presence of hypercapnia nor withdrawn if it worsens.

Inadequate improvement of hypoxia with oxygen suggests that an additional problem is present (e.g., pneumonia, pulmonary edema, pulmonary embolus, or pneumothorax) and the diagnostic investigation should be broadened. While this is occurring, however, additional O_2 should be administered to alleviate the hypoxemia.

Bronchodilators

Bronchodilators are routinely given in all exacerbations of COPD because a small reversible component of airflow obstruction is common, and bronchodilators may also improve mucociliary clearance of secretions.

Anticholinergic agents have a similar or greater bronchodilator action than β-agonists in COPD, and they also have fewer side effects and are not associated with the development of tachyphylaxis. Anticholinergic agents should be used routinely in COPD with acute respiratory failure, and many now believe them to be the agent of first choice. Ipratropium bromide, 0.5 mg in 2 mL, should be given either as a metered-dose inhaler (preferentially) or nebulized initially every 2 hours and then every 4 to 6 hours. Chronic use of a long-acting anticholinergic (i.e., tiotropium) reduces the incidence of exacerbations, but this agent should not be used in the intensive care setting.

Nebulized β-agonists are also effective bronchodilators in COPD, although they may cause tachycardia, tremor, mild reductions in potassium and PaO_2 (due to pulmonary vasodilatation), and tachyphylaxis. SABAs (e.g., salbutamol, terbutaline, or fenoterol) should be given by metered-dose inhaler or nebulizer every 2 to 4 hours in combination with ipratropium. The combination is more effective than either agent alone. Con-

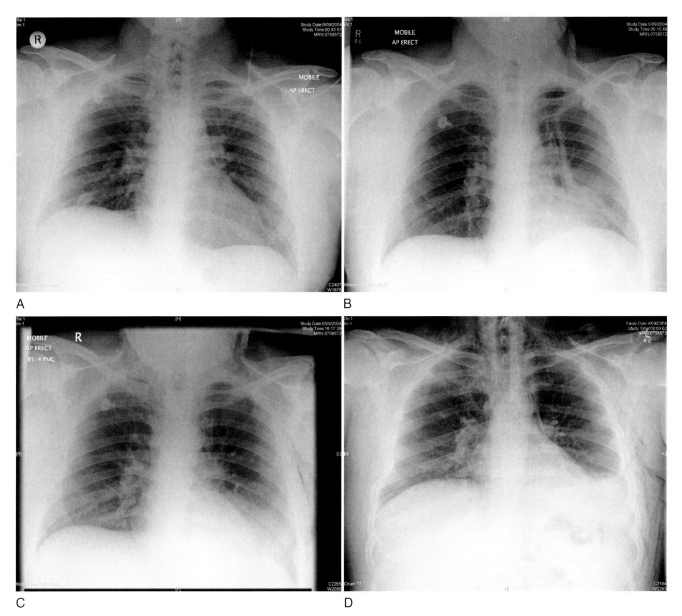

Figure 24.4. A series of chest x-rays of a 30-year-old male patient with asthma who presented with acute asthma and atypical chest pains. Note the initial "landscape" appearance suggesting obesity (A). Also note the irregular opacity adjacent to the left heart border and the suggestion of left-sided neck subcutaneous emphysema 4 hours later (B), more prominent left and early right-sided neck subcutaneous emphysema at 15 hours (C), and obvious widespread subcutaneous emphysema at 2 days (D).

tinuous inhalation is not recommended because this has been shown to increase side effects without augmenting the response to treatment. Parenteral administration is also not recommended. In stable patients, long-term use of β-agonists may improve symptoms of dyspnea, particularly in the subgroup of COPD with an objective bronchodilator response. Long-acting β-agonists (LABAs) may also have a beneficial effect on symptoms, quality of life, and exercise capacity.

Aminophylline is a weak bronchodilator in COPD. Although studies suggest that it improves diaphragm contractility, stimulates respiratory drive, improves mucociliary transport and right heart function, is anti-inflammatory, and is a weak diuretic, other studies have shown no or small benefits and frequent side effects when given to patients with acute COPD exacerbations. Accordingly, the literature does not support including this medication in the treatment of acute exacerbations.

Glucocorticoids
Short-term systemic corticosteroids improve the rate of airflow limitation in patients with acute COPD exacerbations. Current American Thoracic Society guidelines and Cochrane Reviews recommend a maximum dose equivalent to oral prednisolone at

229

0.5 mg/kg body weight for 3 to 10 days. Steroids should be avoided if the deterioration is clearly due to bacterial pneumonia without bronchospasm.

Long-term oral steroids in COPD are associated with a number of serious side effects (e.g., osteoporosis, diabetes, peptic ulcer, myopathy, systemic hypertension, fluid retention, and weight gain) that are likely to impair quality of life and precipitate readmission. Accordingly, long-term use should be avoided whenever possible. A small group of patients (no more than 15% of the COPD population) may have a more than 50% improvement in their FEV_1 following 2 or 3 weeks of systemic corticosteroids. In these patients, the dose should be tapered to the lowest possible that maintains this improvement, and alternate-day dosing and/or a trial of chronic inhaled steroids can be considered. In the majority of patients, long-term inhaled steroids do not improve lung function or survival (although a trial designed and supported by the pharmaceutical industry suggests they may improve quality of life and reduce hospital admissions).

Antibiotics

Antibiotics have an accepted role in the treatment of infection-induced exacerbations of COPD. Amoxicillin is a suitable first-line agent against *H. influenzae*, *S. pneumoniae*, and *M. catarrahalis*. If a chest x-ray suggests a component of pneumonia, then community-acquired pneumonia guidelines should be followed and treatment should include a tetracycline, macrolide, or fluoroquinolone.

Treatment of Associated Conditions

Treatment of associated medical conditions, such as fluid overload (diuretics), left heart failure (digoxin and vasodilators), pneumothorax (intercostal drainage), pulmonary embolus (anticoagulation), and electrolyte correction, should be undertaken as appropriate. Respiratory stimulants (e.g., acetazolamide, medroxyprogesterone, naloxone, doxapram, and almitrine) have no role because attempts to increase minute ventilation will increase dynamic hyperinflation and reduce muscle effectiveness and thereby increase work of breathing and fatigue. Narcotic- or benzodiazepine-induced respiratory depression is best managed with the appropriate antagonist—naloxone or flumazenil, respectively.

Excessive carbohydrate calories should be avoided because this increases CO_2 production and may worsen respiratory failure.

Noninvasive Ventilatory Support

Noninvasive ventilation (NIV), a technique in which ventilatory support is provided via a nasal, facial, total face, or oral mask (Fig. 24.5), should be considered in hypercapnic patients. Several randomized controlled trials have demonstrated improved respiratory physiology, reduced mortality, reduced iatrogenic complications, reduced need for intubation and mechanical ventilation, and reduced length of stay in hospital (Table 24.3 and Fig. 24.6). All studies have shown good tolerance of the technique (~80% of patients) with few side effects and improvements in both oxygenation and $PaCO_2$ compared with medically treated control patients. NIV unloads the inspiratory respiratory muscles, thereby reducing the work of breathing and the attendant CO_2 production. This immediately improves respiratory acidosis, even if alveolar ventilation is unchanged.

Indications for NIV to treat acute exacerbations of COPD are acute dyspnea, respiratory rate higher than 28 beats/min, or $PaCO_2$ higher than 45 mm Hg with a pH less than 7.35 despite optimal medical treatment. Although these indications include mild to moderate exacerbations, most randomized studies have used these as entry guidelines (Table 24.3). COPD patients liberated from invasive ventilatory support may also benefit from NIV, although studies have questioned the utility of its use in this setting. Side effects of NIV include discomfort, intolerance, skin necrosis (Fig. 24.7), gastric distention, barotrauma, and aspiration.

Choice of mask is extremely important. Face masks are generally preferred in the emergency setting, but if their use is complicated by air leaks, claustrophobia, discomfort, or nasal skin damage, then a larger face (head hood) may be better tolerated or more effective. Nasal masks are more suited to long-term support and usually not recommended for an acute exacerbation.

Table 24.3 Outcomes from Noninvasive Ventilation Studies in Acute COPD[a]							
Author, Year	*N*	**Setting**	**pH**	**ABG**	**ETI**	**LOS**	**Mortality**
Fernandez, 1993	12	ICU	7.19	↑	↓	↓	
Bott, 1993	60	Ward	7.35	↑	↓	↓	(↓)[b]
Brochard, 1995	85	ICU	7.28	↑	↓	↓	(↓)
Kramer, 1995	23	ICU	7.29	↑	↓	(↓)	(↓)
Confalonieri, 1996	48	Ward	7.29	↑	↓	↓	↓ (12 month)
Barbe, 1996	24	ED	7.33	↑	↓		
Angus, 1996	17	Ward	7.30	↑	↓		
Wood, 1998	6	ED	7.35	↑	↓		(↑)
Celikel, 1998	30	ICU	7.27	↑	↓		
Bardi, 1990	30	Ward	7.36	↑	↓		
Martin, 1900	23	ICU	7.27	↑	↓	(↓)	(↓)
Plant, 1900	236	Ward	7.32	↑	↓	↓	↓

[a]Indicate approaching but not statistically significant, ABG, arterial blood gases; ED, emergency department; ETI, need for endotracheal intubation; ICU, intensive care unit; LOS, length of stay.
[b]Arrows in parentheses.

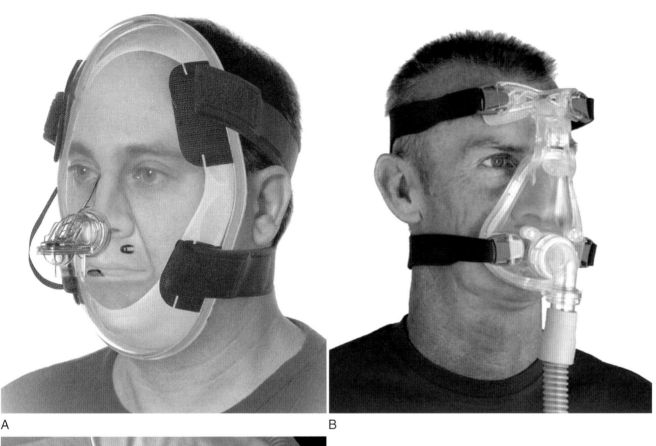

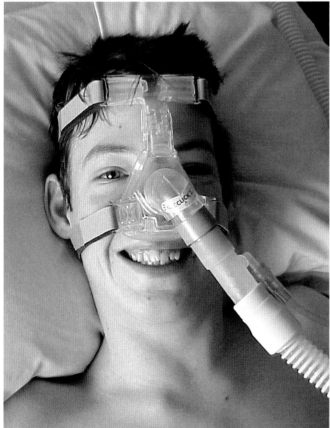

Figure 24.5. Masks used to deliver noninvasive ventilatory support.
(A) Full face mask, (B) face mask, and (C) nasal mask.

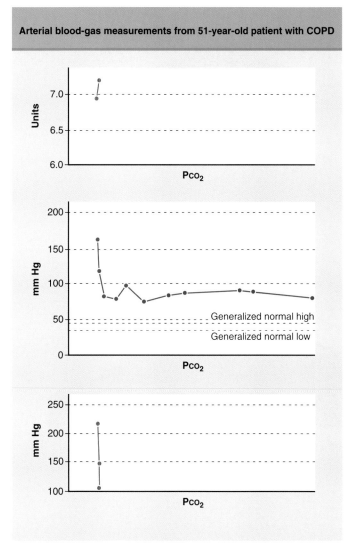

Arterial blood-gas measurements from 51-year-old patient with COPD

Generalized normal high

Generalized normal low

Figure 24.6. A series of arterial blood gases taken from a 51-year-old man with severe smoking-related COPD (FEV$_1$, 500 mL) over 84 hr who demonstrates acute hyperoxic-induced hypercapnia upon a background of chronic compensated hypercapnia. A reduction in inspired oxygen concentration and noninvasive ventilation prevented intubation and mechanical ventilation. Despite presenting with severe hypercapnic acidosis and altered conscious state, the patient was suitable for discharge 3 days later.

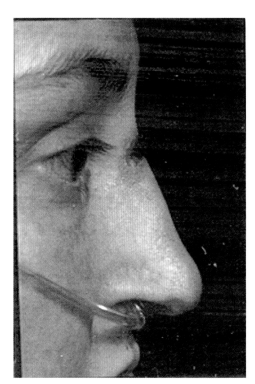

Figure 24.7. An ulcer on the bridge of the nose precipitated by an inappropriately fitting nasal mask.

Invasive Ventilatory Support

Invasive ventilatory support may be required if respiratory failure progresses despite the previously discussed measures or if the patient is drowsy, uncooperative, or in extremis. The decision to ventilate requires careful consideration in some patients who may have near end-stage lung disease and whose quality of life may not justify aggressive treatment. Obviously, this problem is markedly attenuated if primary care or outpatient specialty physicians appropriately address end-of-life issues with these patients prior to the acute exacerbation.

The goals of invasive ventilatory support in COPD are to allow respiratory muscles to rest and recover without causing them to atrophy from total inactivity and to minimize dynamic hyperinflation. A variety of approaches can be used, but pressure-support ventilation is frequently employed in milder exacerbations. Since auto-PEEP exists in virtually every patient during an acute exacerbation, however, continuous positive airway pressure (CPAP) should always be applied. The level of CPAP should be adjusted and readjusted empirically, observing the work of breathing associated with inspiration (or by observing the esophageal pressure trace if this is being monitored). It cannot be adjusted on the basis of the airway pressure trace. Pressure support should be titrated to achieve an adequate tidal volume (250–400 mL), adequate spontaneous rate (<30 breaths/min), and patient comfort without excessive minute ventilation (<115 mL/kg/min) or excessive correction of hypercapnia.

More severely affected patients need continuous ventilation or synchronized intermittent ventilation; dynamic hyperinflation should be avoided by using a low minute ventilation (115/mL/kg is a guide). This should be achieved by the use of a small tidal volume (8 mL/kg) and a ventilator rate less than 14 breaths/min. Plateau airway pressure (Pplat) should be measured by applying an end-inspiratory pause of 0.5 second following a single breath. This maneuver shortens expiratory time, and if it is applied to a series of breaths it will increase dynamic hyperinflation, increase the Pplat level, and increase the risk of volutrauma. If Pplat exceeds 25 cm H$_2$O, the ventilator rate should be reduced. If a higher minute ventilation is required for excessive hypercapnic acidosis, the degree of dynamic hyperinflation and its effects should be assessed using Pplat. Use of a high inspiratory flow rate is recommended because it results in a shorter inspiratory time and hence a longer expiratory time for a given ventilatory rate, which in turn reduces dynamic hyperinflation and alveolar pressure and improves gas exchange.

If dynamic hyperinflation is excessive (with attendant circulatory compromise and/or a risk of barotraumas), minute ventilation should be decreased, accepting the resulting hypercapnic acidosis. Muscle relaxants should be avoided unless essential. Normally, however, spontaneous ventilation should be encouraged to promote ongoing respiratory muscle activity and minimize wasting. Flow-by, pressure support, and low-level CPAP may all reduce the work of spontaneous breathing and promote a better ventilatory pattern. Care must be taken with all these supports because each can increase dynamic hyperinflation by a different mechanism, leading to circulatory compromise or risk of barotrauma. Flow-by increases resistance through the expiratory valve, pressure support increases tidal volume and may increase inspiratory time, and CPAP increases functional residual capacity.

Tracheostomy

Patients who have been invasively ventilated for 7 to 10 days and have failed a trial of extubation with noninvasive ventilatory support may benefit from the insertion of a tracheotomy tube. This may be done via dilational (Seldinger) or surgical techniques. Generally, the former is more convenient, can be done in the ICU, and heals more quickly upon removal. The advantages of a tracheostomy are that dead space is reduced; the endotracheal tube can be removed from the mouth or nose, thus reducing local irritation and sedation; and it facilitates suctioning. The disadvantages include nosocomial infection, local trauma, reduced capacity to cough effectively, and loss of natural humidification. Protection of the airway from secretions that accumulate above the tracheostomy is not 100% even with the tracheostomy cuff inflated. Appropriate reduction in time on ventilatory support with an awake cooperative patient, allowing for periods of some respiratory work to maintain muscle strength, is crucial before eventual cessation of ventilatory support and removal of tracheostomy. Usually, tracheostomies can be safely removed if suctioning occurs less frequently than every 2 hours and patients are capable of independent ventilation and coughing (i.e., adequate muscle strength and drive) and have no anatomic abnormality that would preclude natural ventilation.

Asthma

Response to treatment within the first 2 hours is an important predictor of outcome.

Oxygen

The patient should be allowed to sit upright and be given humidified oxygen at flow rates that keep the oxygen saturation higher than 90%. The development of oxygen-induced hypercapnia may indicate either underlying COPD with chronic hypercapnia or deteriorating progressive severe asthma.

β-Agonists

SABAs (salbutamol, albuterol, tertbutaline, and isoprenaline) are the cornerstone of acute asthma management. Salbutamol has β_2 selective bronchodilator properties with minimal β_1-mediated cardiac toxicity and is thus the first choice β-agonist. LABAs such as salmeterol or eformoterol should not be used in acute asthma management.

The mode of bronchodilator delivery is an important consideration. Multidose inhalers with spacer devices have the greatest penetration of drug into the lungs ($\sim30\%$), are inexpensive, and should be used in patients with mild to moderate severity who are cooperative. In severe asthma or in uncooperative patients, nebulizers should be used; however, only approximately 10% of the drug reaches the lungs. Nebulizers require 8 to 15 liters per minute gas flow to operate, and this can be achieved with an electric air pump or with pressurized oxygen or air. Nebulized particle size ranges from 1 to 3 μm. Intravenous delivery of β-agonist has no advantage over the inhaled route. In severe asthma, a standard approach is to initiate nebulized 5 mg salbutamol with 8 L/min oxygen every 30 minutes in severe cases and every 2 to 4 hours in mild to moderate asthma. The volume of salbutamol should be made up to 2 to 4 mL with saline or short-acting anticholinergics.

Side effects of the β_2-agonists include tachycardia, arrhythmias, hypertension, hypotension, tremor, hypokalemia, worsening of ventilation–perfusion matching, and hyperglycemia. Lactic acidosis (up to 10–12 mmol/liter) is a common, dose-related consequence of intravenous SABA, appearing in as many as 70% of patients approximately 2 to 4 hours after initiation of treatment.

When stable, SABAs should be replaced with LABAs in combination with inhaled steroid cover. LABAs should not be used as single treatments in asthma because there have been reported events of increased mortality, particularly in African Americans.

Anticholinergics

Anticholinergics should be used as an adjunct treatment to a SABA rather than a single first-line treatment. Again, metered dose inhalers are preferable, but the medication can also be administered via nebulizer (usual dosages are 250–500 μg every 4–6 hr). Blurred vision may occur due to local effects on the eye. Anticholinergic preservative-induced bronchospasm has been reported and should be considered in patients with persistent wheeze.

Corticosteroids

Systemic corticosteroids reduce hospitalization rates, mortality, and length of hospital stay in patients with asthma. Their mode of action is to primarily decrease the inflammatory response and the associated bronchospasm and mucus secretion, with an onset of action 6 to 12 hours after administration. Hydrocortisone (2–4 mg/kg) or methylprednisolone (0.5–1 mg/kg) is given intravenously, or prednisone or prednisolone (0.5–1.0 mg/kg) is given orally every 6 hours. These high doses are usually continued for 1 to 3 days or until clear clinical improvement is observed, after which they are tapered and replaced with inhaled steroids. Side effects of steroids include hyperglycemia, hypokalemia, hypertension, acute psychosis, myopathy, and gastritis. Longer term steroids are associated with additional problems, such as osteoporosis, cataracts, diabetes, oral thrush, and other secondary infections.

Aminophylline

Aminophylline has bronchodilatory and a variety of other anti-inflammatory properties due to its ability to inhibit phosphodiesterase. The role of theophylline in acute asthma is not clear due to conflicting results from clinical trials and its narrow

233

therapeutic window, and its side effects include vomiting, tachyarrhythmias, headaches, restlessness, and convulsions. It is a fourth-line agent following SABAs, anticholinergics, and steroids. A usual dosage regime is a loading dose of 3 mg/kg and infusion rate of 0.5 mg/kg. Serum levels need to be monitored.

Other Medical Treatments

Several alternative treatments have been proposed, such as methotrexate, intravenous γ-globulin, cyclosporine, colchicines, troleandomycoin, lignocaine, and magnesium sulfate, with either no or marginal effect. Helium gas mixture has been used, as has the sedative ketamine, with similar marginal degrees of success.

Noninvasive Ventilatory Support

Noninvasive ventilatory support has been used infrequently for several years in acute asthma, and only in recent years have reports confirmed its safety and efficacy. In addition to expiratory airway pressure countering the effects of auto-PEEP, inspiratory positive airway pressure may counter the increased inspiratory resistance. Potential complications with noninvasive ventilation are patient–ventilator asynchrony, gas trapping (pulmonary or gastric), and decreased cardiac output from decreased venous return. Careful monitoring, similar to that of an intubated patient, is required.

Invasive Ventilation

This should be considered in patients with severe and life-threatening asthma (Table 24.2) who have failed medical treatments as listed previously. As in COPD, the consequence of delayed expiratory airflow in asthma is that the inspired tidal volume cannot be completely exhaled to functional residual capacity and a proportion of each breath is trapped, impairing the arrival of each new breath. As lung volume increases, expiratory airflow also increases as a result of increasing small airway caliber and increasing elastic recoil pressure. This enables the lungs to inflate to an equilibrium point at which all the tidal volume is able to be exhaled during the expiratory time available. In mild airflow obstruction, this process is adaptive because it enables required minute ventilation to be achieved at a higher lung volume with only moderate loss of inspiratory muscle power. When airflow obstruction is severe, however, the equilibrium point may encroach on total lung capacity. The hyperinflation is the result of both airflow limitation and the increased minute ventilation required to provide a normal $PaCO_2$.

Complaints of needing ventilatory help, clinical appearance of exhaustion, deteriorating respiratory status, or reduced conscious state are more important indicators of the need for intubation than any specific $PaCO_2$.

The first 24 hours after intubation is the period of highest risk for ventilation-induced dynamic hyperinflation because airflow obstruction is often at its worst, CO_2 production and dead space are the highest, and hence the minute ventilation requirement is highest. At this time, patient respiratory distress and clinician desire to reduce hypercapnic acidosis can easily lead to a level of ventilation that results in excessive dynamic hyperinflation with risk of hypotension, pneumothoraces, and, uncommonly, circulatory collapse.

As in COPD, initial minute ventilation should be restricted to 115 mL/kg/min (8 liters/min for a 70-kg lean weight patient) or less, tidal volume 8 mL/kg (560 mL for a 70-kg lean weight

patient) or less, and respiratory rate 14 breaths/min or less. This should be delivered with a short inspiratory time ($VI \geq 80$ liters/min or $Ti \leq 0.5$ sec) to allow a long expiratory time ($Te \leq 3.5$ sec) to minimize dynamic hyperinflation. Either pressure or volume control mode can be used to achieve this. Volume control mode is more established, results in more reliable volume delivery, and is preferred by these authors. PEEP can be used to counter intrinsic PEEP, but the possibility of increasing lung volume further (as will occur if external PEEP exceeds intrinsic PEEP) must be kept in mind. External PEEP will only be necessary if the patient continues to have spontaneous ventilation and is unable to trigger the ventilation. Generally, these patients receive heavy sedation to suppress their normal response to hypercarbia when their bronchospasm is so severe that sufficient alveolar ventilation cannot be accomplished. Although some patients may require one or two bolus doses of neuromuscular blocking agents, these agents should be avoided if possible because of the concern for profound, long-term myopathy thought to occur more frequently in patients receiving the combination of neuromuscular blocking agents and corticosteroids.

Once initial ventilation is established, dynamic hyperinflation should be assessed by measuring Pplat and auto-PEEP and observing the response of central venous pressure and blood pressure to a transient period of reduced respiratory rate or ventilator disconnection. If Pplat is more than 25 cm H_2O or circulatory improvement occurs, respiratory rate should be reduced and ventilation reassessed. If Pplat is low (e.g., <20–22 cm H_2O) and hypercapnia is present, respiratory rate may be increased. Once asthma has improved, sedation may be reduced and spontaneous ventilation in CPAP mode with pressure support can occur. CPAP 5 to 10 cm H_2O can be introduced to match auto-PEEP and reduce work of breathing.

COMPLICATIONS OF INVASIVE VENTILATION

Hypotension can occur as a result of sedation, ventilation-induced dynamic hyperinflation, pneumothorax, hypovolemia, or arrhythmias. Pplat is commonly higher than 25 cm H_2O, but an equally important assessment for hypotension is the response of the blood pressure and central venous pressure to 60 sec of ventilator disconnection ("apnea test").

Circulatory arrest with apparent electromechanical dissociation is a recognized complication of severe asthma. It occurs usually within 10 minutes of intubation and can result in severe cerebral ischemic injury and death if not recognized and managed appropriately. Most patients can tolerate mechanical ventilation with 115 mL/kg/min ventilation; however, a small number of patients with unusually severe asthma can develop life-threatening levels of dynamic hyperinflation despite this restriction in minute ventilation. In these patients, a 60- to 90-second apnea test should be undertaken and ventilation resumed at the respiratory rate of 2 to 6 breaths/min. A common pitfall is the insertion of intravenous cannulae into the chest in the belief that this circulatory collapse is due to tension pneumothoraces. These procedures usually result in the complication they are seeking to relieve, and it is often difficult to know if a pneumothorax was initially present. Apnea testing should precede intercostal cannulae, and, if possible, incision with blunt insertion technique should be used.

Acute necrotizing myopathy is characterized by muscle weakness and histological evidence of myonecrosis, muscle cell vacuolization, and type II muscle atrophy. Myopathy ranges in severity from mild limb weakness to functional quadraparesis. Diagnosis is made by elevated creatine kinase levels and electromyography. Muscle biopsy is usually not required. There are no specific treatments and recovery is usually complete, but in severely affected patients significant weakness may still be present at 12 months.

PITFALLS, COMPLICATIONS, AND CONTROVERSIES

Boxes 24.2, 24.3, and 24.4 list the pitfalls, complications, and controversies.

Box 24.2 Controversies

Etiology of acute exacerbation of COPD and asthma
Dosage and duration of corticosteroids in acute COPD and asthma
Role of noninvasive ventilation and acute exacerbations of asthma
Role of intravenous short-acting β-agonists

Box 24.3 Pitfalls

Uncontrolled oxygen administration in COPD
Inadequate use of noninvasive ventilation in COPD
Excessive minute ventilation during mechanical ventilation
Circulatory collapse soon after intubation in patients with very severe asthma
Early intercostal cannula insertion during circulatory collapse
Development of myopathy due to prolonged muscle relaxation and steroids
High-resolution CT scans not contiguous and thus may miss pulmonary lesions
Inadequate post-ICU follow-up to recognize and treat precipitating factors

---

Box 24.4 Complications

Development of hyperoxic hypercapnia in COPD
Circulatory failure and pneumothoraces with mechanical ventilation
Myopathy
Lactic acidosis
Micro-macroaspiration of enteral feeds during sleep/supine position

---

SUGGESTED READING

Busse WW, Banks-Schlegel S, Wenzel SE: Pathophysiology of severe asthma. NHBLI workshop. J Allergy Clin Immunol 2000;106:1033–1042.

Hogg JC, Chu F, Utokaparch S, et al: The nature of small-airway obstruction in chronic obstructive pulmonary disease. N Engl J Med 2004;350: 2645–2653.

Malhotra A, White D: Treatment of oxygen induced hypercapnia (correspondence). Lancet 2001;357:883.

Manser R, Reid D, Abramson M: Glucocorticoid for acute severe asthma in hospitalized patients. Cochrane Database Systematic Rev. 2001 (January);CD001740.

Pauwels R, Buist AS, Calverley PMA, et al: Global strategy for the diagnosis, management, and prevention of chronic obstructive pulmonary disease. NHLBI/WHO Global Initiative for Chronic Obstructive Lung Disease (GOLD) workshop summary. Am J Respir Crit Care Med 2001:163(5):1256–1276.

Plant P, Owen J, Elliott M: Early use of noninvasive ventilation for acute exacerbations of chronic obstructive pulmonary disease on general respiratory wards: A multicentre randomised controlled trial. Lancet 2000;355:1931–1935.

Ram FSF, Picot J, Lightowler J, Wedzicha JA: Non-invasive positive pressure ventilation for treatment of respiratory failure due to exacerbations of chronic obstructive pulmonary disease. Cochrane Database Systematic Rev. 2004(January);CD004104.

Salmeterol Multicentre Asthma Research Trial (SMART): 2003 FDA safety alert. www.fda.gov/medwatch/SAFETY/2003/serevent.htm.

Sanders MH, Newman AB, Haggerty CL, et al: Sleep and sleep disordered breathing in adults with predominantly mild obstructive airway disease. Am J Respir Crit Care Med 2003;167:7–14.

Soroksky A, Stav D, Shpirer I: A pilot prospective randomized placebo controlled trial of bilevel positive airway pressure in acute asthmatic attacks. Chest 2003;123:1018–1025.

Acute Respiratory Distress Syndrome*

Luciano Gattinoni, Paolo Pelosi, Luca Brazzi, and Franco Valenza

KEY POINTS

- Due to differing definitions of acute respiratory distress syndrome (ARDS), there are wide variations in incidence estimates.
- It is important to differentiate between direct and indirect pathophysiologic pathways because the underlying pathologic processes are different and this may have an important effect on the approach to treatment.
- Symptomatic treatment is currently the cornerstone of ARDS therapy, but the search for etiology is as urgent and important as selecting the type of ventilatory support.
- Systematic daily assessment of etiology factors and their control, persistence, or development is mandatory, but pathophysiologic characterization must be repeated intermittently because lung lesions evolve and the approach to treatment must change during the course of the syndrome.

Since its first description more than 25 years ago, the acute respiratory distress syndrome (ARDS; originally known as adult respiratory distress syndrome) has received more attention than any single entity in critical care medicine. The syndrome consists of an acute, severe alteration in lung structure and function characterized by hypoxemia, low respiratory system compliance, low functional residual capacity, and diffuse radiographic infiltrates, along with increased lung endothelial and alveolar epithelial permeability.

EPIDEMIOLOGY, RISK FACTORS, AND PATHOPHYSIOLOGY

Epidemiology

As a consequence of the different definitions of ARDS, it has always been difficult to estimate the true incidence of this condition. The 1972 report of the National Heart, Lung, and Blood Institute of the National Institutes of Health (NIH) suggested that approximately 150,000 cases of ARDS occurred per year in the United States, which represents an incidence of 60/100,000 population per year. This figure has been challenged in a number of reports (Table 25.1), all of which give an incidence that is an order of magnitude lower than the NIH estimates. Two points must be stressed, however. First, different ARDS definitions play an obvious role when its incidence is estimated. Not surprisingly, defining ARDS according to more or less strict criteria results in incidence estimates that differ by more than 100%. Second, some studies suffer from substantial methodologic problems.

Risk Factors

The results of a systematic overview of the incidence and risk factors for ARDS (see Table 25.1) found that the strongest evidence to support a cause-and-effect relationship between ARDS and a risk factor was identified for sepsis, trauma, multiple transfusions, aspiration of gastric contents, pulmonary contusion, pneumonia, and smoke inhalation. The weakest evidence was identified for disseminated intravascular coagulation, fat embolism, and cardiopulmonary bypass. In some series, "pneumonia" is one of the most common associations, whereas in others sepsis, aspiration, and trauma are the major risk factors and none of the patients have pneumonia. Certainly, patients with fever, cough, pleuritic chest pain, pulmonary infiltrates, and blood cultures positive for *Streptococcus pneumoniae* qualify as having pneumonia as a risk factor for ARDS. Many of the acute, diffuse parenchymal lung diseases can, however, present with symptoms that are consistent with pneumonia (e.g., eosinophilic pneumonia, acute interstitial pneumonitis, hypersensitivity pneumonitis, and diffuse alveolar hemorrhage) and can meet the

		Incidence (100,000	
Author	Patient No.	Population/year)	Mortality Rate (%)
National Heart, Lung, and Blood Institute	—	60	—
Fowler	88	5.2	65
Webster	139	4.5	38
Evans	62	25	60
Villar	30/74	1.5/3.5	70/50
Thomsen	110/83	8.3/4.8	—
Lewandowski	17	3	58.8

Table 25.1 Incidence and Mortality of Acute Respiratory Distress Syndrome

*This chapter is adapted from Albert RK, Spiro SG, Jett JR: Clinical Respiratory Medicine, 2nd ed. Philadelphia, Mosby, 2004.

diagnostic criteria for ARDS. Whether these patients should be included under the rubric "ARDS" is debated.

Pathophysiology

Whenever an insult is applied to the lung, a host response is triggered that is characterized by a close interplay of cells and humoral factors and results in lung inflammation (Fig. 25.1; see also Chapter 1). Epithelium and endothelium are both involved, although injury to one or the other barrier may predominate. Some studies suggest it is useful to consider two different pathways by which this response may occur—the effect of the insult directly on the lung (direct insult) and pulmonary lesions that result from an acute systemic inflammatory response (indirect insult). This distinction may be important because the pathway affected may govern the expression of the pulmonary abnormalities.

Direct Insult

Lung injury has been reproduced in animal models by direct insult to the alveoli (e.g., intratracheal instillation of endotoxin or live bacteria, complement, and tumor necrosis factor). Pulmonary epithelium was thus subjected to the initial injury, with activation of alveolar macrophages. These, in turn, activate the inflammatory network, which leads to the pulmonary inflammation. The prevalent damage after the direct insult is intra-alveolar, with alveolar filling by edema, fibrin, collagen, neutrophilic aggregates, or blood, and often described as pulmonary consolidation.

Indirect Insult

Pulmonary lesions may originate indirectly through mediators that are released from extrapulmonary foci into the blood, as during peritonitis, pancreatitis, and various abdominal diseases. The primary target in such cases is the pulmonary

endothelial cell. The activation of the inflammatory network results in increased permeability of the endothelial barrier and recruitment of monocytes, polymorphonuclear neutrophil leukocytes, platelets, and other cells. Consequently, the prevalent damage is represented by microvessel congestion and interstitial edema, whereas intraalveolar spaces are relatively spared.

It is likely that direct and indirect insults can coexist. This may occur, for example, in patients who have pneumonia when one lung is initially directly affected, and the other is indirectly injured hours or days later as the inflammation spreads by means of loss of compartmentalization (indirect insult).

It may be important to differentiate between direct and indirect pathophysiologic pathways because the underlying pathologic process (i.e., predominantly consolidation versus interstitial edema and collapse) seems different in the two conditions, at least during the early phases, as confirmed in both pathologic and imaging studies. This may have an important effect on the approach to treatment. Figure 25.2, taken from the first report of the effect of positive end-expiratory pressure (PEEP) in ARDS studied using computed tomography (CT) scans, clearly emphasizes the point. Application of PEEP overdistended previously inflated lung regions in one patient and resulted in a remarkable recruitment in the second. Intuitively, the different responses of the respiratory system to the same perturbation suggest different underlying conditions.

Models of Acute Respiratory Distress Syndrome

Before the introduction of CT scan technology, imaging of ARDS was limited to chest radiographs, which showed (and this was part of the ARDS definition) a widespread and bilateral appearance of "pulmonary infiltrates." Thus, ARDS was considered to be a homogeneous alteration of the lung parenchyma, with reduced gas content, characterized by an abnormal stiffness. The CT scan completely changed this model because it has been consistently observed that the densities, which reflect the ratio of gas volume to the total lung volume, are primarily distributed in dependent lung regions such that nondependent lung regions are relatively normally inflated, whereas the intermediate regions are poorly inflated (Fig. 25.3). Typically, the normally inflated volume of lung tissue approximates 200 to 400 g in a lung that weighs as much as 2000 to 4000 g (compared with 1000–1200 g for a normal lung).

These observations led to the model of the so-called "baby lung" because the amount of residual, normally inflated lung had the volume of a lung of a 5- or 6-year-old child. The baby lung presents with the following characteristics:

- Small and a normal or near-normal compliance
- Normal and near-normal lung located in the nondependent lung regions
- Associated with a variable amount of abnormal lung, in part poorly inflated and in part collapsed or consolidated

Accordingly, the ARDS lung could be modeled as a mixture of three zones:

1. Normally inflated (the baby lung, nondependent)
2. Recruitable (i.e., collapsed lung that could be opened with adequate inflation pressure)
3. Consolidated lung (i.e., lung consists of alveolar filling such that it cannot be opened by increased alveolar pressure)

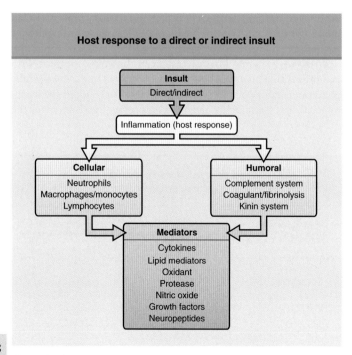

Figure 25.1. Host response to a direct or indirect insult.

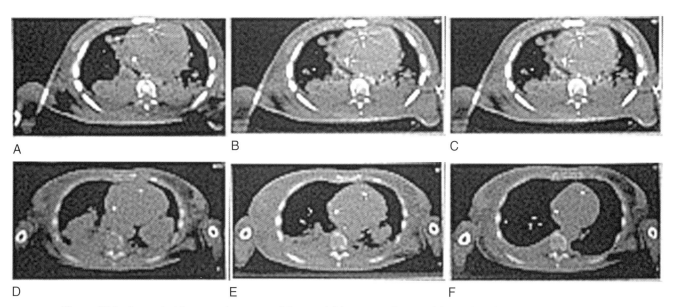

Figure 25.2. Computed tomography scans of the caudal lung at various positive end-expiratory pressures (PEEPs). *A–C,* Acute respiratory distress syndrome (ARDS) from bacterial pneumonia (direct insult). No changes in density (i.e., airspace collapse or parenchymal consolidation) and arterial partial pressure of oxygen (Pao_2) are observed with increasing levels of PEEP. *A,* At 5 cm H_2O, Pao_2 is 12.9 kPa (97 mm Hg), and density is 59%. *B,* At 10 cm H_2O, Pao_2 is 13.7 kPa (103 mm Hg), and density is 56%. *C,* At 15 cm H_2O, Pao_2 is 13.8 kPa (104 mm Hg), and density is 53%. *D–F,* ARDS from sepsis caused by peritonitis (indirect insult). There is substantial clearing of the densities (which, in this instance, seem to represent airspace collapse) with changes in PEEP. *D,* At 5 cm H_2O, Pao_2 is 4.5 kPa (34 mm Hg), and density is 70%. *E,* At 10 cm H_2O, Pao_2 is 6.5 kPa (49 mm Hg), and density is 52%. *F,* At 15 cm H_2O, Pao_2 is 16.1 kPa (121 mm Hg), and density is 32%. (10 cm H_2O = 1 kPa.)

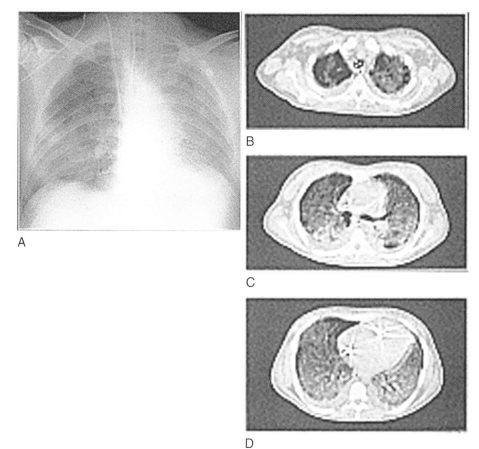

Figure 25.3. Acute respiratory distress syndrome in the early phase. *A,* Chest radiograph; *B,* computed tomography (CT) scan in the apical lung region; *C,* CT scan at hilum; *D,* and CT scan in the basilar lung region. All the images are at 10 cm H_2O positive end-expiratory pressure. Although the chest radiograph shows mainly a diffuse involvement, the CT scans clearly demonstrate a predominantly dependent distribution of the densities.

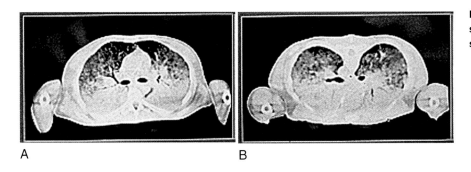

A   B

Figure 25.4. Redistribution of the lung densities shown in a patient lying supine (A) and in the same patient turned prone (B).

This model, however, implies that the lung in the nondependent regions is spared by the disease process. However, when patients are imaged in the prone position, densities can clear in the dorsal region and may develop (albeit to a lesser extent) in the ventral region (Fig. 25.4). Accordingly, the original baby lung model does not hold true because although the inflated tissue (the baby lung) is nondependent, the anatomic regions affected change.

The most important finding of regional chest CT analysis is that the excess tissue mass, which likely derives from edema, is not distributed according to gravity but is evenly distributed throughout the parenchyma, from ventral to dorsal in the supine position. Thus, the acute lung injury (ALI)/ARDS lung is characterized by diffuse, increased permeability (the whole lung is diseased), and its edema increases at each level, as a sponge soaks up water. The increased lung mass in a gravitational field, however, means increased lung weight, and the most dependent levels are compressed by the increased weight of the levels above. In other words, if it is assumed that the lung behaves as a fluid, each lung level from sternum to vertebra in the supine position is compressed by the pressure exerted by the levels above. This pressure, called superimposed pressure, equals, as in a fluid model, the density times the height of the superimposed lung. As shown in Figure 25.5, in the absence of gravity a lung outside the thorax would have pulmonary units of equal size, and each level would have the same gas/tissue ratio. In a gravitational field, on the contrary, the superimposed pressure causes size reduction (poorly inflated) and collapse (noninflated) of the pulmonary units of the dependent lung regions. Although this model accounts for the density redistribution seen in the supine position, it does not account for the more uniform distribution of densities seen in the prone position and indicates that other factors resulting from the forces generated by the need for the lung to fit within the thorax (e.g., the generally triangular shape of the lung, the effect of the weight of the heart and mediastinum on dorsal lung units, the effect of differences in ventral and dorsal aspects of the diaphragm with regard to the transmission of abdominal pressure to the lung, and/or regional differences in chest wall compliance) must play an important role.

The sponge model seems most appropriate when ARDS results from an indirect insult to the lung, such that the diffuse increase in permeability leads to widespread interstitial edema and collapse. This model, however, is less applicable to ARDS that results from a direct insult, in which the primary problem is consolidation with alveolar filling and the amount of recruitable lung (i.e., previously collapsed) is scarce.

The sponge model is also limited because many patients have little or no reversal of lung density on turning prone, which implies that other factors contribute to the extent of lung collapse. The lung sponge model theory has been challenged on the basis of previous experimental work in which regional volumes were measured by intraparenchymal markers. The newly proposed model is that in the edematous lung, increasing airspace pressure first causes the air–fluid interface to penetrate into the mouth of the alveolus (airway pressure approximately 20 cm H_2O), after which the air–fluid interface is inside the alveoli and the lung becomes compliant. The basic difference between the two views is that in the sponge model the edema is believed to be predominantly in the interstitium (causing alveolar collapse by compression), whereas in the air–fluid interface model the edema is predominantly in the alveoli. In both models, the total lung volume is near normal; however, the air–fluid interface model reasons that "recruitment" of airspaces results from displacement of fluid from the airspace to the interstitium, whereas the sponge model attributes this to opening of regions that are previously collapsed.

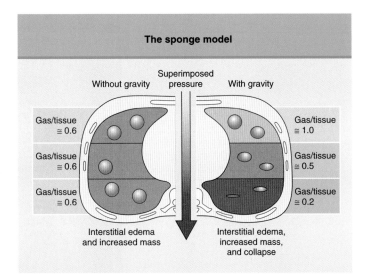

Figure 25.5. The sponge model. The edema is homogeneously distributed throughout the lung. In the absence of gravity, the lung would have pulmonary units of equal size (i.e., same gas/tissue ratio). In the presence of gravity, the superimposed pressure causes a size reduction and collapse of the dependent lung regions.

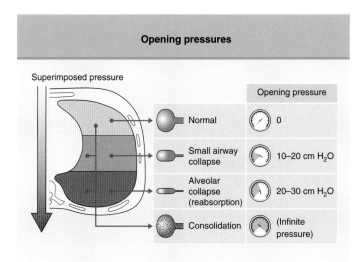

Figure 25.6. Opening pressures. The lung with acute respiratory distress syndrome is composed of normally inflated lung regions, consolidated lung regions, and collapsed (atelectatic) lung regions. Atelectasis may be caused by both compression atelectasis (needing up to 10–20 cm H_2O of transpulmonary pressure to reopen) and reabsorption atelectasis (which needs up to 20–30 cm H_2O of transpulmonary pressure to reopen). (10 cm H_2O = 1 kPa.)

Mechanisms of Positive Pressure

Mechanisms of lung opening (inspiration)

When a tidal volume (V_T) is delivered in ARDS, two phenomena may occur—inflation and recruitment. Recruitment is defined as the inflation of previously noninflated regions, and the pressures required to open the lung are known to be greater than those required to keep the lung open. Two kinds of collapse may coexist: One is collapse of the small airways, and the other is alveolar collapse from complete reabsorption of gases.

When the small airways collapse, some gas remains trapped behind the region of closure. If small airway collapse persists, it evolves into alveolar collapse as the alveolar gas is absorbed. The distinction between small airway and alveolar collapse is important because the pressures required for opening may be greatly different—10 to 20 cm H_2O to open small airways and 30 to 35 cm H_2O to reexpand alveoli that have collapsed because of gas reabsorption. Consequently, as shown in Figure 25.6, a complete range of opening pressures is found in ARDS, from 0 to 1 cm H_2O to inflate open units (not exactly an opening pressure) to 10 to 20 cm H_2O to counteract the small airway collapse (a pressure normally reached during normal tidal ventilation) and up to 30 to 35 cm H_2O transmural pressure to open areas of alveolar collapse (pressures not normally generated during normal tidal ventilation). At the end of the spectrum is the area of consolidation in which opening is impossible because the airspaces are occupied with inflammatory exudate and cells.

Indeed, it has been shown both in experimental animals and in humans with ARDS that lung opening (i.e., recruitment) is an inspiratory phenomenon that occurs, to a different extent, along a wide airway pressure range.

Keeping the lung open (exhalation)

The primary role of PEEP in ARDS is to keep pulmonary units open at end exhalation when they would otherwise collapse. For years, the "best PEEP" has been sought on the assumption that for each ARDS lung there is an ideal level of PEEP. That such a level does not exist is clearly shown by CT scans, and PEEP is always a compromise between lung stretching and lung recruitment (at least when patients are supine). Indeed, in a study of a series of supine patients using PEEP levels from 0 to 20 cm H_2O, regional quantitative analysis of the gas/tissue ratio showed, as expected from the sponge model, that the various levels of the same lung, from sternum to vertebra, require different levels of PEEP to stay open.

According to the sponge model, the superimposed pressure over a given lung level is a function of density of the levels above times their height. It follows that the level of PEEP required to keep ventral regions open (in the supine position) is 0 cm H_2O (no compression, no atelectasis). In the middle of the lung, the PEEP needed to counteract the superimposed pressure is higher, and it is highest in the most dependent lung regions. It follows that to keep the most dorsal regions open, the most ventral regions must be overexpanded, and consequently the PEEP used is not best but always a compromise (Fig. 25.7).

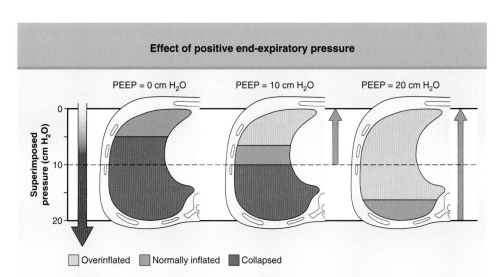

Figure 25.7. Effect of positive end-expiratory pressure (PEEP). Because PEEP acts as a counterforce to the superimposed pressure over a given lung level (indicated by arrows), at zero end-expiratory pressure the superimposed pressure is 0 in the ventral regions and 20 cm H_2O in the dorsal ones. To counterbalance 20 cm H_2O of superimposed pressure (dependent lung regions), a PEEP of 20 cm H_2O is necessary. However, while dependent lung regions are kept open, the nondependent ones become overinflated. (10 cm H_2O = 1 kPa.)

In the sponge model, the superimposed pressure causes compression atelectasis as a function of density and lung height, and accordingly

- Body size (the larger body has a larger lung) is an important variable to consider when deciding what PEEP level is appropriate to counteract superimposed pressure.
- Baseline lung density decreases with age, such that in neonates the baseline density is almost twice that of adults (thus, high levels of PEEP are sometimes required to keep the lung open in a small child who has ALI/ARDS).

Redistribution of ventilation–perfusion

Although explaining the effect of PEEP on lung inflation is quite straightforward using the sponge model, to explain its beneficial effects on oxygenation is more difficult. Compression atelectasis is much less prevalent in late-phase ARDS and in ARDS that results from primary lung injury. Accordingly, the ability to obtain recruitment with PEEP is limited. Although not proved, we believe that the mechanism of PEEP in this setting is not the prevention of airspace closure and end exhalation, but possibly involves redistributing ventilation from ventral to dorsal regions. In fact, overstretching the nondependent regions using PEEP decreases the compliance of these regions such that ventilation may be diverted toward the middle and dependent regions, and it increases the ventilation–perfusion ($\dot{V}/\dot{Q}$) ratio of the poorly inflated regions. Unfortunately, no data are available on regional distribution of blood flow in humans, and thus a real understanding of the ventilation and perfusion redistribution phenomena is not possible.

Mechanisms of Distribution of Tidal Volume

Distribution of the insufflated volume is a function of two factors—airway resistance and regional respiratory system compliance. The CT scan, taken in static conditions, enables inferences to be made regarding variations in regional compliance. The authors found that, in ARDS, the distribution of insufflated VT is a function of PEEP. In fact, on increasing PEEP from 0 to 20 cm H_2O, the fraction of VT that was distributed to nondependent lung compared with that which was distributed to dependent lung decreased from 2.5:1 to approximately 1:1 (i.e., the ventilation became more homogeneous). This phenomenon has always been associated with better oxygenation. The mechanism by which the VT is redistributed with PEEP is as follows: In the most ventral regions, which are already open, increasing PEEP causes a progressive stretching of the lung with a decrease of the regional compliance. In the most dorsal regions, PEEP maintains recruitment of otherwise collapsing lung and thereby increases the compliance of this region as more pulmonary units become available for inflation. The final effect depends on the balance between the overstretching and recruitment phenomena (Fig. 25.8).

Positioning

An important maneuver that is increasingly being used in ARDS is to place the patients in the prone position. In Figure 25.4, the effects on density redistribution from dorsal to ventral are shown. This effect does not arise from a variable distribution of edema. In ARDS, the interstitial edema, rich in proteins, is not "free" to move throughout the lung parenchyma. Instead, the density redistribution, according to the sponge model, results

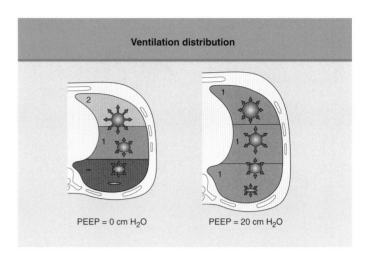

Figure 25.8. Effects of positive end-expiratory pressure (PEEP) on distribution of ventilation. At zero end-expiratory pressure, ventilation is preferentially distributed to the nondependent lung region (2:1:0) because the dependent regions are partially collapsed at end expiration. At high PEEP, the distribution of ventilation is more homogeneous (1:1:1) because of overstretching of nondependent units and recruitment of the dependent ones. (10 cm H_2O = 1 kPa.)

from "squeezing out" the gas from the dependent lung regions because of the superimposed pressure. According to the mandate that the lung fit within the thorax, density redistribution on turning indicates that the lung fits better within the thorax when patients are prone compared with when they are supine.

The redistribution of lung density induced by the prone position may be more pronounced in ARDS that results from extrapulmonary disease. In ARDS caused by pulmonary disease, densities change much less on going from the supine to the prone position (Fig. 25.9). The prone position, in approximately 60% to 70% of patients with ARDS, is associated with increased oxygenation. Several mechanisms are likely to be involved, and important differences may arise when ARDS occurs as a result of pulmonary versus extrapulmonary disease. In the latter, because atelectasis depends on lung density and height, a larger volume of lung opens in the prone position. In ARDS that results from pulmonary disease, the authors found that changes in thoracic compliance play a substantial role. In the prone position, for anatomic reasons, the dorsal component of the chest wall is stiffer than the anterior wall, and the VT is distributed more toward the ventral and abdominal regions, where the higher lung densities predominate (Fig. 25.10). Indeed, human and animal studies conclude that more homogeneous inflation or ventilation is the main mechanism of oxygenation improvement in the prone position.

Although prone positioning improves the gas exchange in most patients with ARDS, its positive effects on outcome are unproved. Although experimental work has shown that the prone position may protect against ventilator-induced lung injury, a randomized clinical trial on the use of the prone position for 6 hours per day for 10 days failed to show improvement in survival. The study, however, was criticized because of treatment rules, limited hours in the prone position, and late enrollment of some of the patients. Indeed, the prone position is still

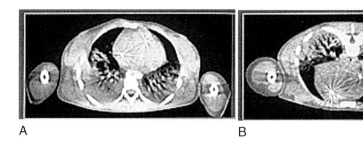

Figure 25.9. Distribution of lung densities that arise from consolidation, not collapse. Change of position from supine (A) to prone (B) does not affect the distribution of lung densities. Compare with Figure 25.4.

A   B

widely used and recommended for gas exchange problems, whereas further studies are recommended to establish its effect on outcome.

Chest Wall Compliance

Most of the available data on respiratory mechanics in ARDS relate to the respiratory system as a whole (i.e., the lung and the chest wall). The mechanical alterations observed were mainly attributed to the lung because chest wall compliance was considered to be normal. The few studies that investigated chest wall compliance per se found it to be decreased. Recently, it has become clear that in ARDS caused by pulmonary disease, chest wall compliance is normal, whereas in that from extrapulmonary disease, it is greatly decreased. It is more convenient to use the elastance (the reciprocal of compliance) to discuss the partitioning of compliance between chest and lung because the elastance of the respiratory system is the sum of chest wall and lung elastances.

Elastance is the pressure required to keep the respiratory system inflated. Part of this pressure is spent to keep the lung inflated and part to keep the thoracic cage (which includes the abdominal wall) expanded. Normally, lung and chest wall elastances are similar, such that half of the applied pressure keeps

the lung inflated and half expands the thoracic cage when inflated. In ARDS caused by extrapulmonary disease, however, more pressure is required to expand the thorax. The reverse is true for ARDS that results from pulmonary disease. Thus, although the total respiratory system elastance is similar in ARDS from pulmonary and that from extrapulmonary disease, its partitioning is different. This explains, for instance, why in ARDS from pulmonary disease, heart size tends to remain normal when PEEP is increased (i.e., low pleural pressure around the heart), whereas it decreases in ARDS caused by extrapulmonary disease (i.e., progressively higher pleural pressure because of the relative stiffness of the thorax; see Fig. 25.10). Accordingly, PEEP may have different hemodynamic consequences in ARDS that results from direct or indirect insults.

Normally, intraabdominal pressure measured through the bladder is in the range 5 to 10 cm H_2O. In ARDS caused by extrapulmonary diseases (most of which occur mainly in the abdominal compartment), intraabdominal pressure can be greatly increased. The authors found a strict correlation between abdominal pressure and chest wall elastance (i.e., increasing the abdominal pressure increases chest wall elastance, which reflects an increased stiffness of the thoracic cage). Because the importance of chest wall elastance is becoming increasingly clear, the authors believe that the measurement of intraabdominal pressure must be part of the assessment of patients with ARDS (both for respiratory treatment and for hemodynamic consequences). In fact, many patients admitted to the intensive care unit present with an abdominal pressure greater than 12 mm Hg, a condition that is not detectable on a clinical basis and requires objective measurement (bladder pressure).

Pulmonary Circulation

The ARDS lung is usually characterized by increased pulmonary artery pressure and increased pulmonary vascular resistances. A mean pulmonary artery pressure of 4 kPa (30 mm Hg) or greater is a universal hallmark of ARDS, regardless of etiology. A single mechanism is unlikely to explain the increased resistance. Moreover, the causes of the pulmonary hypertension may change over time. Indirect evidence suggests that a generalized vasoconstriction exists in ARDS and that this can be modulated with vasodilatation. Moreover, inhaled nitric oxide may selectively dilate vessels in ventilated areas, which suggests that hypoxemia (arterial and mixed venous) is not the cause of the observed functional vasoconstriction. Eicosanoids and other mediators are likely to be responsible. A second possible mechanism is vessel compression by the increased lung weight and superimposed perivascular pressure. The authors found, in vivo, that every increase of 0.13 kPa (1 mm Hg) of pulmonary artery pressure is

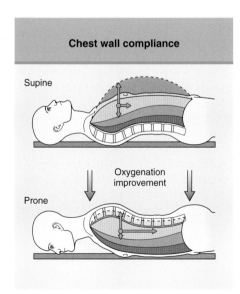

Figure 25.10. Effect of prone position on ventilation distribution. In the supine position, the distribution of ventilation is preferentially distributed to the ventral regions. When the patient is prone, the stiffness of the dorsal chest wall favors the distribution of ventilation to the dorsal regions, facilitating reinflation in this area.

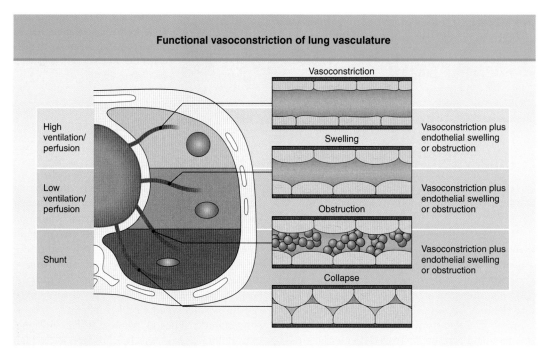

Figure 25.11. Functional vasoconstriction of lung vasculature. All the lung vasculature is functionally vasoconstricted. Moreover, endothelial swelling and obliteration may further increase pulmonary vascular resistance. In the dependent lung regions, vessel compression may also be present.

associated with a 14% increase in the original lung weight. Unfortunately, it is not possible to determine an independent variable because if it is possible that edema causes vessel compression, it is also possible that increased pulmonary artery pressure increases the interstitial edema through increased microfiltration. Anatomic alterations in the vascular wall have also been described, such as swelling of the endothelial cells and, with time, a medial hypertrophy. Finally, evidence of fibrin clot and cellular obstruction in the capillaries is found in 20% to 30% of patients with ARDS. With time, the collapsed or obstructed vessels undergo remodeling or become completely obliterated by fibrotic processes, which leads to microvascular destruction. A summary of pulmonary circulation alterations is presented in Figure 25.11.

In considering the overall circulatory function, however, it is noteworthy that in ARDS, despite the generalized vasoconstriction, collapsed lung regions are appropriately underperfused compared with the inflated regions. Indeed, it is not rare to find 50% to 60% of collapsed lung associated with a shunt fraction (i.e., the flow through the collapsed regions) of 20% to 30% of the cardiac output, which suggests that a somewhat appropriate flow diversion is still occurring.

The pathophysiologic consequences of elevated pulmonary vascular resistances depend on the cardiac reserve of each patient. If the right ventricle is able to increase its work, the hemodynamic consequences are nil. If right ventricular dysfunction is present, numerous systemic consequences arise.

Gas Exchange Alterations

The main alteration of gas exchange in ARDS is hypoxemia because of shunt and is usually associated with normocapnia or hypocapnia, at the expense of an increased minute ventilation.

If the minute ventilation were maintained constant, $PaCO_2$ would be increased as a function of the shunt, low ventilation–perfusion ratios, and dead space. Gas exchange is the final result of the match between ventilation and perfusion, which in turn depends on the anatomic structure of the lung (which changes with time and with the prevalent underlying pathologic process). An attempt to correlate lung structure with gas exchange alterations is given in Table 25.2.

Early acute lung injury/acute respiratory distress syndrome, indirect insult

In early ALI/ARDS caused by an indirect insult, the lung architecture is preserved and the primary pathophysiologic abnormality is edema with consequent collapse of dependent regions. The pulmonary blood flow through these regions is the main cause of shunt. The midlung regions are poorly inflated and, if perfused, could contribute to hypoxemia because of low $\dot{V}/\dot{Q}$. The nondependent regions are open and likely to be hyperventilated. The application of PEEP may keep open the otherwise collapsed regions and increase ventilation of the poorly inflated regions to the extent that shunt decreases and low $\dot{V}/\dot{Q}$ is improved. If the PEEP level is excessive, however, the upper regions are overstretched, with less capability of ventilation. Oxygen may be exchanged (a kind of "regional apneic oxygenation"), but CO_2 clearance is impaired. This is one possible explanation why, with excessive PEEP, shunt decreases but $PaCO_2$ may increase.

Early acute respiratory distress syndrome, direct insult

In early ARDS caused by a direct insult, the overall lung architecture is preserved but the prevalent damage is intraalveolar, with edema and collapse being secondary phenomena and quan-

Table 25.2 Gas Exchange

Acute Respiratory Distress Syndrome	Lung Injury	Lung Structure	Pulmonary Circulation	Mechanism of Gas Exchange	Corrections (Other Than Fraction of Inspired Oxygen)
Early	Direct	Collapse in the dependent regions	Vasoconstriction and partial collapse	Shunt	Positive end-expiratory pressure (PEEP, reexpansion)
		Poorly inflated in middle regions	Vasoconstriction	Low ventilation, perfusion ($\dot{V}/\dot{Q}$)?	PEEP (normalizing inflation)
		Inflated in upper regions	Vasoconstriction	High $\dot{V}/\dot{Q}$	Nitric oxide (increasing perfusion)
		Consolidation and collapse in dependent regions	Vasoconstriction plus possible collapse	Shunt	Inhaled prostaglandin PEEP (reexpansion)
	Indirect	Possible consolidation foci in middle regions	Vasoconstriction and low $\dot{V}/\dot{Q}$?	Shunt in consolidated area and low $\dot{V}/\dot{Q}$?	PEEP (?)
		Possible consolidation foci in nondependent regions	Vasoconstriction and high $\dot{V}/\dot{Q}$	Shunt in consolidated area	PEEP [ventilation redistribution to lower regions (?) by stretching upper regions?] plus nitric oxide–prostaglandins
		Consolidation	Vasoconstriction	Shunt	PEEP (ventilation redistribution to lower regions?)
Late	Widespread lesions	Fibrosis	Microvessel destruction and obliteration	Diffusion impairment?	No recruitment evident
		Bullae and emphysema-like alterations	—	Increased dead space	Nitric oxide?

titatively less important than in ARDS that results from indirect insult. The consolidated regions, if perfused, cause shunt just as if they were collapsed. It is likely that PEEP works by keeping the otherwise collapsed regions open. It is possible, however, that PEEP also works by redistributing VT from nondependent to dependent regions, thus improving the ventilation of low $\dot{V}/\dot{Q}$ regions.

Late-phase acute lung injury/acute respiratory distress syndrome

The situation is likely to be different in the late stage of ALI/ARDS, in which the lung architecture is markedly altered because of fibrosis, capillary destruction, and emphysema-like lesions. In such conditions, PEEP is still required to maintain oxygenation, but it does not work by "keeping open" the recruited units because collapse is scarce, if it occurs at all. Redistribution of ventilation or perfusion is a possible mechanism. Moreover, the structural changes of the lung may contribute to hypoxemia by some impairment of oxygen diffusion (fibrosis and interstitial thickening), whereas the emphysema-like lesions are likely to be the anatomic basis for carbon dioxide retention.

CLINICAL FEATURES

Originally, ARDS was defined as the presence of severe dyspnea, tachypnea, hypoxemia refractory to oxygen therapy, reduced lung compliance, and diffuse alveolar infiltration seen on chest radiographs. Subsequent authors used a PaO_2/fraction of inspired oxygen (FIO_2) ratio of less than 150 to characterize ARDS. In 1979, the National Heart, Lung, and Blood Institute introduced criteria based on time (fast and slow) and threshold oxygenation values at defined levels of FIO_2 and positive expiratory pressure. The explicit exclusion of cardiogenic pulmonary edema was introduced next with suggestions for a quantitative threshold for pulmonary wedge capillary pressure, and this was followed by the introduction of a quantitative measurement of

respiratory system compliance. In 1988, a new approach was proposed that involved a "lung injury score" to quantify, albeit roughly, the presence, severity, and evolution of acute and chronic damage involving lung parenchyma.

Recently, the American–European Consensus Conference on ARDS recommended that ARDS be described as a particularly severe subset of ALI, the latter of which was defined as a "syndrome of inflammation and increased permeability that is associated with a constellation of clinical, radiologic, and physiologic abnormalities that cannot be explained by, but may coexist with, left arterial or pulmonary capillary hypertension." A summary of ALI/ARDS definitions is presented in Table 25.3.

The definitions of ALI/ARDS are not of merely academic interest because testing new treatments requires trials in which the homogeneity of the study population plays a substantial role. Interestingly, considering the evolution of ARDS definitions, it is clear that more extensive and quantitative criteria were added over the years to define a more homogeneous population, but the recent American–European conference almost represents a return to the original, very simple definition. The dilemma is still unsolved—simple criteria mean that a large trial with a very inhomogeneous population is feasible; strict criteria result in a homogeneous population and a large trial becomes unfeasible. In the authors' opinion, work is still required to find the best compromise between these opposing needs.

DIAGNOSIS

The diagnosis of ALI/ARDS is simple, according to its current definition, because it requires only a known predisposing factor, bilateral pulmonary infiltrates on the chest radiograph, and a threshold PaO_2 value normalized for the FIO_2 in use.

An accurate patient history is of paramount importance to infer the etiology and pathogenesis of ALI/ARDS, and assessment of traditional signs must be carried out despite the availability of newer technology. Respiratory frequency, dyspnea,

Table 25.3 Acute Respiratory Distress Syndrome Definitions					
Reference	Clinical	Oxygenation Threshold	Bilateral Infiltrates	Respiratory System Compliance	Threshold Wedge Pressure
Ashbaugh et al	1	None	Yes	None	Clinical judgment
Bone et al	1	Partial pressure of arterial oxygen (Pao_2)/fraction of inspired oxygen (Fio_2) 21 kPa (150 mm Hg)	Yes	None	Clinical judgment
Zapol et al	1	$Pao_2 < 6.6$ kPa (<50 mm Hg) 100% Fio_2 after 2 hr 60% Fio_2 after 24 hr Positive end-expiratory pressure (PEEP) 5 cm H_2O	Yes	None	Clinical judgment
Pepe et al	1	$Pao_2 < 10.0$ kPa (<75 mm Hg) Fio_2 50%	Yes	None	>2.4 kPa (>18 mm Hg)
Bell et al and Fein et al	1	Pao_2 6.6 kPa (50 mm Hg) Fio_2 50%	Yes	None	>2.0 kPa (>15 mm Hg)
Fowler et al	1	Pao_2/alveolar $Po_2 < 0.2$	Yes	>50 mL/cm H_2O	>1.6 kPa (>12 mm Hg)
Murray et al	1	Pao_2/Fio_2 score 0–4 PEEP score 0–4	Chest radiograph score 0–4	Compliance score 0–4	Clinical judgment
Bernard et al	1	$Pao_2/Fio_2 < 26.6$ kPa (<200 mm Hg), acute respiratory distress syndrome $Pao_2/Fio_2 < 40$ kPa (>300 mm Hg), acute lung injury	Yes	None	Clinical judgment

symmetry or asymmetry of thoracic movements, percussion, and auscultation may provide insights into the etiology, prevalent underlying pathologic process, and the patient's ability to deal with the respiratory distress (e.g., signs of muscle fatigue must be carefully investigated so as not to delay initiating mechanical ventilatory support).

Etiologic Diagnosis
In most instances, the etiology that leads to ALI/ARDS is clear, as in aspiration or lung contusion. In some patients, however, the etiology is not apparent. In patients who have ALI/ARDS and signs of sepsis, a systematic search for all possible infection foci must be carried out, using all the available facilities.

Pathogenic Diagnosis
The authors suggest that ALI/ARDS be distinguished according to pulmonary and extrapulmonary causes. In most circumstances, this is an easy distinction based on an accurate history and clinical assessment. Such a distinction is more useful in the early phases of ALI/ARDS. With time, and with the structural changes that occur in the lung, the two processes are likely to overlap.

Pathophysiologic Characterization
Together with etiologic and pathogenic screening, the authors believe that every patient who has ALI/ARDS must be carefully investigated to define specific pathophysiologic characteristics because this enables treatment to be tailored more precisely.

Gas Exchange
Characterization of the degree of gas exchange impairment is the most common way of defining the severity of ALI/ARDS. To infer the underlying pathophysiologic process, it is always useful to observe the oxygenation response at different Fio_2 values (the authors believe a brief test with an Fio_2 of 1.0 is

useful) and to conduct a formal PEEP trial (e.g., 5, 10, and 15 cm H_2O). Changes in Fio_2 may markedly affect the Pao_2/Fio_2 ratio, and the response may help to estimate a possible $\dot{V}/\dot{Q}$ mismatch. The PEEP trial (in which hemodynamic status is controlled) may enable effective recruitment maneuvers to be inferred. The $Paco_2$ response during the PEEP trial (in which minute ventilation is kept constant) may also be informative. An increase in Pao_2 with a decrease in $Paco_2$ indicates effective recruitment. An increase in Pao_2 with an increase in $Paco_2$ could indicate overstretching of the nondependent lung (in addition to recruitment).

In some circumstances, it may be necessary to measure mixed venous (or central venous) blood gases. This is particularly true when cardiac output is low because the fraction of shunt flow is directly related to the cardiac output. In some cases, an increase in Pao_2 occurs simply because of a decrease in cardiac output, with no improvement in lung function.

Imaging
Although not proven to alter outcomes, we believe that chest CT scans should be obtained in all patients with ALI/ARDS. In a series of 74 patients with ALI/ARDS, 24 had pneumothoraces, and in 37% of these the pneumothorax was ventral in location and detected only by CT scan. Although this has not been well studied, cross-table lateral films may have discovered many of these. Moreover, in 60% of the cases the CT scan provided additional clinical information compared with conventional radiology, and in 22% the findings resulted in a change in the clinical management. These and other data emphasize the importance of this technology in routine clinical management. Also, CT scans are the best tool with which to discriminate between recruitment and consolidation, and the authors routinely perform a PEEP trial during the CT scan, taking images at different pressures. This may be of great help when tailoring the respiratory support because the potential for recruitment in a

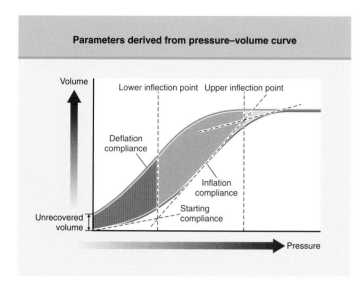

Figure 25.12. Parameters derived from the pressure–volume curve of the total respiratory system.

given patient is assessed precisely. Unfortunately, the pathology and physiology of ALI/ARDS evolve over time, which renders the findings less useful the longer the patient requires support.

Respiratory Mechanics

Lung volume

The authors believe that measurements of respiratory mechanics may be better interpreted if the starting lung volume is known. Accordingly, a simplified helium method is routinely used to determine the lung gas volume. The accuracy of the technique in a lung with edema in the airspaces has not been established, however.

Pressure–volume relationship

Another way to characterize the underlying pathologic process is the pressure–volume (PV) curve of the total respiratory system, from which several inferences may be derived (Fig. 25.12). The initial slope of the PV curve (also called the starting compliance) was thought to give an idea of the dimensions of the "baby lung" at atmospheric pressure. In adult men, starting compliances of 20, 30, and 40 cm H_2O roughly correspond to baby lung volumes of 20%, 30%, and 40%, respectively, of the original healthy lung. The inflection point (or, more precisely, the inflection zone) has been thought to suggest a potential for recruitment and indicates the pressures over which most of the recruitment may occur. The slope of the PV curve after the inflection point (inflation compliance) was thought to give some estimate of the amount of recruitment (the steeper the PV curve, the greater the recruitment). Finally, the upper inflection point indicates the pressure at which the stretching of pulmonary units becomes the prevalent phenomenon.

Recent theoretical and experimental data have challenged these views, however, because it has been shown that recruitment occurs along the entire PV curve. Indeed, to date, we know that the lower inflection point, more than the recruitment zone, may indicate the "start" of recruitment, that recruitment occurs along the entire PV curve, that it may occur even above the upper inflection point, and that the PV curve is also a

"recruitment curve." Unfortunately, it gives the fraction of the recruitment occurring at different pressures, but not the absolute amount of total recruitment actually occurring.

The gravitational gradient in pleural pressure (which is magnified in the supine vs. the prone position, and further magnified in injured compared with normal lungs) indicates that it would never be possible to find a single airway pressure at which all airspaces are open unless the pressure exceeds the transpulmonary pressure at which airspaces open in the most dependent lung regions. Of necessity, this mandates that the transpulmonary pressures in the most nondependent lung regions are increased by a factor governed by the gravitational pleural pressure gradient (generally found to be approximately 0.5 cm H_2O/cm height).

Partitioning: Respiratory system mechanics

The authors believe that this measurement should also be included in the routine assessment of patients with ALI/ARDS because the same applied pressure may result in completely different transpulmonary pressure, depending on the relative elastance of the lung and chest wall, and because these may be considerably different in ALI/ARDS that results from pulmonary and extrapulmonary diseases. Although the utility of this information has not been determined with regard to outcomes, the authors believe that this information is of great importance for the prevention of barotrauma and hemodynamic impairment. In this context, the intraabdominal pressure, because of its profound effect on the elastance of the thoracic cage, should also be measured.

Hemodynamics

In addition to a clinical assessment of cardiac output (e.g., skin perfusion, pulse volume, skin and mucous membrane color, extremity temperature, and urine output), invasive monitoring, including central venous pressure and arterial lines, is usually routine and safe in these patients. The utility of pulmonary artery catheters and other invasive means of monitoring the cardiac output is unclear (see Chapter 11). Quantitative assessment of hemodynamics has been deleted from the definition of ALI/ARDS. In some circumstances, however, measurement of cardiac output or pulmonary vascular pressures may still be necessary.

TREATMENT

Etiologic Treatment

A summary of most of the risk factors that lead to ALI/ARDS is given in Table 25.4. The search for etiology is as urgent and important as selecting the type of ventilatory support. The results of treatment strongly depend on the specific problem that leads to the episode of ALI/ARDS, whereas the type of ventilatory support may only "buy time" for the correct treatment to work.

In some instances, the etiology of the injury occurred in the past (e.g., trauma with lung contusion, an episode of smoke inhalation, or near drowning). In these, only symptomatic, and possibly pathogenic, treatments are possible. In other instances, however, ARDS results from etiologic factors present while patients are treated (e.g., pneumonia sepsis). Two rules must be followed:

Table 25.4 Distribution of Risk Factors for Acute Respiratory Distress Syndrome							
	Pepe et al	Fowler et al	Mancebo and Artigas	Villar and Slutsky	Suchyta et al	Hudson et al	Milberg et al	Heffner et al
Total patients who had ARDS/total patients in study (%)	46/136 (34)	68/936 (7)	35/35 (100)	74/1997 (4)	215/215 (100)	179/695 (26)	918/918 (100)	50/50 (100)
Cardiopulmonary bypass	—	4/237 (2)	—	—	—	—	—	—
Burn	—	2/87 (2)	—	—	—	—	—	—
Bacteremia	—	9/239 (4)	—	—	—	—	—	—
Massive blood transfusion	19/42 (45)	9/197 (5)	—	—	—	28/77 (36)	48/918 (5)	4/50 (8)
Bone fractures	15/34 (44)	2/38 (5)	—	—	—	7/63 (11)	—	—
Pneumonia	—	10/84 (12)	9/35 (25)	5/74 (7)	76/215 (35)	—	—	20/50 (40)
Disseminated intravascular coagulation	—	2/9 (22)	—	—	—	—	—	—
Pulmonary aspiration	10/32 (31)	16/45 (36)	—	9/74 (12)	25/215 (11)	13/59 (22)	85/918 (9)	5/50 (10)
Sepsis	9/19 (47)	—	6/35 (17)	30/74 (41)	31/215 (14)	56/136 (41)	340/918 (37)	9/50 (18)
Major trauma	—	—	4/35 (11)	14/74 (19)	20/215 (9)	—	230/918 (25)	6/50 (12)
Drug overdose	—	—	1/35 (2)	3/74 (4)	—	14/164 (8)	54/918 (6)	—
Near drowning	3/4 (75)	—	—	1/74 (1)	—	2/6 (33)	—	1/50 (2)
Pulmonary contusion	19/50 (38)	—	—	—	—	12/55 (22)	—	—
Abdominal surgery	—	—	—	4/74 (5)	—	—	—	—
Thoracic surgery	—	—	—	2/74 (3)	—	—	—	—
Postanoxic coma	—	—	—	2/74 (3)	—	—	—	—
Cerebral hemorrhage	—	—	—	2/74 (3)	—	—	—	—
Pancreatitis	1/1 (100)	—	5/35 (14)	—	—	—	—	—
Prolonged hypotension	2/4 (50)	—	—	—	—	—	—	—
Shock	—	—	2/35 (5)	—	—	—	—	3/50 (6)
Fat embolism	—	—	—	—	—	—	—	1/50 (2)
Smoke inhalation	—	—	—	—	—	—	—	1/50 (2)
Peritonitis	—	—	7/35 (20)	—	43/215 (20)	—	—	—
Systemic lupus	—	—	1/35 (2)	—	—	—	—	—
Others	—	—	—	—	20/215 (9)	—	—	—

1. Any etiologic factor found must be treated aggressively (be it surgical or medical treatment).
2. If a microorganism is suspected, no antibiotic, antifungal, or antiviral agent should be given until the appropriate sampling (e.g., bronchoalveolar lavage and blood, urine) has been carried out.

Pathogenic Treatment

One animal model commonly chosen to study lung injury that resembles ALI/ARDS is lipopolysaccharide (LPS) administration, which can cause a direct injury when instilled into the trachea or an indirect injury when given intravenously. Both the complement system and alveolar macrophages can be activated by LPS. Both events trigger a complex cytokine network that recruits cells and releases numerous humoral mediators. A simplified theoretical sequence of events is outlined in Figure 25.13. Although incomplete, it indicates the pathogenic targets of a number of clinical trials that have been conducted on patients who have ALI/ARDS or sepsis. Some strategies were based on blocking the trigger of the inflammatory response (e.g., anti-LPS antibodies) or focused on single elements of the inflammatory network (e.g., anti-tumor necrosis factor antibodies, soluble tumor necrosis factor receptors, and interleukin-1 receptor antagonist) or modified neutrophil function (liposomal prostaglandin E_1 and antioxidants); yet others addressed the consequences of inflammation, such as hemodynamic imbalances (e.g., inhibitors of nitric oxide synthase and prostaglandin E_1). A summary of these is given in Table 25.5. Almost all the studies found either no major benefit or that the intervention was actu-

ally harmful. Given the complexity of the network, perhaps multiple sites should be blocked or potentiated simultaneously as opposed to selectively blocking single events or mediators of the overall process.

In septic patients (most of whom present with ALI/ARDS) 4 days of treatment with activated protein C improves survival. Activated protein C, compared with other molecules tested in sepsis treatment, presents the widest range of actions on the complex network of coagulation/inflammation. In fact, it has anticoagulant, anti-inflammatory, and profibrinolytic effects.

Other positive results have been reported in septic patients given low-dose corticosteroid replacement. It is important to emphasize, however, that the positive effects are present when patients are characterized by relative adrenal insufficiency.

Symptomatic Treatment

Symptomatic (i.e., supportive) treatment is currently the cornerstone of ARDS therapy. The possible changes in mortality of ALI/ARDS over time that have been reported by some groups may result from differences in supportive treatment or from differences in the iatrogenic nature of the treatments.

Blood Gas Targets

Although it may be reasonable to accept a high $PaCO_2$, the authors believe that PaO_2 should be maintained at approximately 10.6 kPa (80 mm Hg) instead of 8.0 kPa (60 mm Hg), as suggested by other investigators, to avoid the risk of sudden deterioration of oxygen saturation. Recent literature suggests that the academia resulting from high $PaCO_2$ may be beneficial in

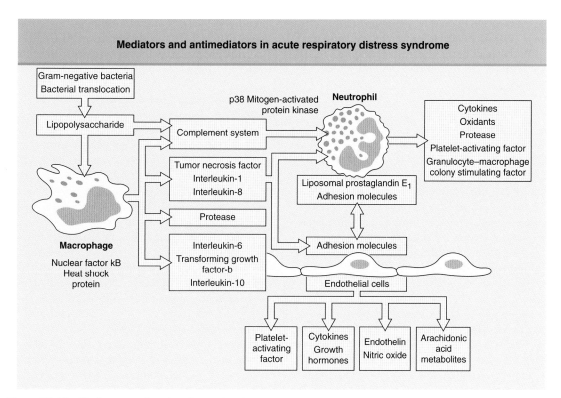

Figure 25.13. Mediators and antimediators involved in the inflammatory response in acute respiratory distress syndrome. The mediators against which pathogenic therapy has been tested in clinical trials are indicated in bold.

		Study Characteristics Present						No.		Results	
Strategy	Author	p	r	d1	d2	c	m	Patients	Diagnosis	Overall	Stratified
Antilipopolysaccharide	McCloskey et al	No	Yes	Yes	No	Yes	No	2199	Sepsis	=	na
	Ziegler et al	No	Yes	Yes	No	No	No	543	Sepsis	=	+
Interleukin-1 receptor antagonist	Fisher et al	Yes	No	No	Yes	Yes	No	99	Sepsis/shock	+	na
	Fisher et al	No	No	Yes	No	No	No	893	Sepsis	=	+
	Opal et al	Yes	Yes	Yes	No	Yes	No	696	Sepsis stratified	=	na
Antibodies against tumor necrosis factor (TNF)-α	Abraham et al	No	No	No	Yes	No	No	994	>50% acute lung injury	=	+
	Cohen and Carlet	Yes	Yes	No	Yes	Yes	Yes	553	Sepsis/shock	=	+
	Reinhart et al	Yes	Yes	No	Yes	Yes	Yes	122	Sepsis/shock	=	+
Antibodies against soluble TNF receptor	Abraham et al	Yes	Yes	Yes	Yes	Yes	Yes	498	Sepsis/shock	=	+
Cortisone	Bernard et al	Yes	Yes	Yes	No	No	No	99	Acute respiratory distress syndrome (ARDS)	=	na
	Bone et al	Yes	Yes	Yes	No	Yes	No	382	ARDS	=	na
	Luce et al	Yes	Yes	Yes	No	No	No	87	ARDS	=	na
	Meduri et al	Yes	Yes	Yes	No	Yes	No	24	ARDS (late)	+	na
Liposomal prostaglandin E₁	Abraham et al	Yes	Yes	Yes	No	Yes	No	25	ARDS	=	na
Prostaglandin E₁	Bone et al	Yes	Yes	Yes	No	No	No	100	ARDS	=	na
	Holcroft et al	Yes	Yes	Yes	No	No	No	41	ARDS	+	na
Antioxidants	Jepsen et al	Yes	Yes	Yes	No	No	No	66	ARDS	=	na
	Suter et al	No	No	No	Yes	No	No	61	ARDS	=	na
	Bemard et al	Yes	Yes	Yes	No	Yes	No	48	ARDS	=	na
Inducible nitric oxide synthase	Petros et al	No	Yes	Yes	No	No	No	12	Sepsis	=	na
Anticyclooxygenase	Haupt et al	No	Yes	Yes	No	Yes	No	29	Sepsis	=	na
	Yu and Tomasa	Yes	Yes	Yes	No	No	No	54	Sepsis	+	na

Table 25.5 Clinical Trials Directed at the Pathogenesis

c, multicenter; d1, double-blind; d2, dose ranging (more than one dose tested); m, multinational; na, not available; p, prospective; r, randomized; =, no positive result; +, positive result.

animal models of ALI/ARDS. Whether the approach of "permissive hypercapnia" translates into improvements in outcomes is unknown. The $PaCO_2$ may become elevated when low tidal volume ventilation is employed but, at the present time, should not be a primary blood gas target.

Lung Opening

Regardless of the prevalent damage that underlies ALI/ARDS, some degree of lung collapse is always present when the patient is referred to the intensive care unit. For hours or days before admission to the intensive care unit, most patients are likely to have secretions, high respiratory frequency, or low V_T, which are all risk factors for atelectasis. To reach the goal of an open, expanded lung, airway patency must be ensured (consider bronchoscopy) and atelectasis reversed if possible. Although formal rules to recruit the lung are not established, transmural pressure and respiratory system compliance must be considered.

Transmural pressure

The airspace opening pressure is the transpulmonary pressure (i.e., the difference between intraalveolar and pleural pressures). Transpulmonary pressure is a function of the pressure applied to the airways and of the elastances of the lung and chest wall, according to the following equation, in which Paw is the applied airway pressure, E_L is the elastance of the lung, and E_W is the elastance of the chest wall:

$$\text{Transpulmonary pressure} = \text{Paw} \times [E_L/(E_L + E_W)]$$

Normally, E_L equals E_W, and the transmural pressure, as an average, would be approximately half of the pressure applied to the airways. However, as previously discussed, in ALI/ARDS caused by direct or indirect insult, the $E_L/(E_L + E_W)$ value may be very different. For example, in ARDS that results from direct insult, the ratio is less than 1 for patients who have extrapulmonary disease. It follows that to achieve the same opening transmural pressure, a higher Paw is required in ARDS that arises from extrapulmonary problems than in ARDS that results from pulmonary conditions.

Respiratory system compliance

The recruitment maneuver may be difficult when respiratory system compliance is relatively good (as in moderate ALI) or when one lung has a good compliance compared with the other. In such conditions, it is difficult to achieve the adequate transmural pressure unless volumes up to 2 liters or more are insufflated. Artificially reducing the total respiratory system compliance (by applying external compression or turning prone) may help to reach the required transmural pressure without insufflating excessive volumes.

Once opened, the lung must be kept open, and PEEP is the leading strategy used to prevent lung collapse. The level of PEEP is a compromise between that required to keep the lung open and that which results in overstretching, as noted previously.

Iatrogenic Cost of Mechanical Ventilation

Inspired oxygen fraction

The suggestion that a high FIO_2 (>0.6) causes lung damage is based on experimental studies carried out on normal animals in which, in most cases, the inspired air was not appropriately humidified. In the authors' opinion, no consistent evidence shows that high FIO_2 is dangerous in ALI/ARDS because there is worldwide experience with patients treated for days or weeks with 100% oxygen who ultimately survive.

Plateau pressures and pressure swings

It has been suggested that 35 cm H_2O of plateau airway pressure is the safe upper threshold for mechanical ventilation. However, pressure per se is not dangerous (e.g., a diver may have an alveolar pressure of several atmospheres). What is important is the transpulmonary pressure, and possibly the difference in pressure between end expiration and end inhalation. A plateau pressure of 35 cm H_2O may be associated with a wide range of transpulmonary pressures, depending on the relationship between the lung and chest wall elastances and, in nonparalyzed patients, on the action of respiratory muscles.

The effect of high inflation pressures differs markedly, depending on the starting inflation pressure or, more specifically, the lung volume present at end exhalation.

Intratidal collapse and decollapse

The process of intratidal collapse and decollapse is thought to be one of the causes of ventilator-induced lung injury and may be more likely when compression atelectasis is the primary type of lung damage. In fact, during inspiration even low plateau pressures (20–25 cm H_2O) are sufficient to open the dependent lung regions in which "loose" compression atelectases, probably caused by small airway collapse, are recruited. However, if the PEEP level is not adequate, at end expiration the dependent lung regions collapse again. To avoid this phenomenon, a PEEP level sufficient to counteract the lung weight is required.

Ventilation Strategies

The authors believe that a single best mode and strategy of ventilatory support does not exist for all patients who have ALI/ARDS. To clarify and understand the differences between the various strategies, it is useful to start from the equation of motion for the respiratory system:

$$\text{Muscle pressure} + \text{ventilator pressure} = (V_T \times E) + (\text{resistance} \times \text{flow})$$

Respiratory support may thus be applied in three ways:
1. Driving pressure needed to overcome the elastic and resistive load of the respiratory system is furnished by the ventilator (i.e., the muscle pressure equals zero).
2. Driving pressure is furnished by a combination of muscle pressure and ventilator pressure.
3. Driving pressure is totally furnished by the respiratory muscles (i.e., the ventilator pressure equals zero).

Driving pressure provided by the ventilator only (controlled mechanical ventilation)

The mode chosen to deliver the ventilation may be volume- or pressure-targeted. In the volume preset modes, V_T is delivered with a predefined inspiratory flow-time profile. As seen from the equation for motion for the respiratory system, the pressure that the ventilator must generate depends on the mechanics of the respiratory system: The higher the elastance, the higher the ventilation pressure. During pressure preset ventilation, the ventilator applies a predefined pressure to the airways. In this case, the higher the elastance, the lower the V$_T$.

Driving pressure furnished by both respiratory muscles and ventilator

In general, ventilators deliver a positive-pressure breath at a preset T (assisted ventilation) or a preset pressure (pressure support), and the muscles of respiration activate the ventilator-delivered breath. A combination of pressure–volume targets is synchronized with intermittent mandatory ventilation, usually given along with pressure support, in which a low-rate, volume-targeted V$_T$ is associated with pressure-supported spontaneous ventilation. Some types of combined modality support may be delivered without intubation (i.e., noninvasive positive-pressure ventilation).

Driving pressure furnished exclusively by respiratory muscles

Driving pressure furnished exclusively by respiratory muscles is more a respiratory support than a ventilatory support because the respiratory muscles are sufficiently strong to overcome the impedance of the respiratory system.

Choice of ventilation strategy

Three studies compared 7 mL V$_T$/kg with 10 to 10.5 mL V$_T$/kg ideal body weight and were not able to show any difference in outcome. One compared two ventilatory strategies, high PEEP/low V$_T$ versus low PEEP/high V$_T$, and found impressive differences in mortality. The study was criticized, however, because of reporting an extremely high and early mortality rate (70%) in the high V$_T$/low PEEP group. The last study of this series is the NIH ARDS Network trial, which was the only study adequately powered. A 9% absolute reduction in mortality rate was observed in patients treated with 6 mL V$_T$/kg as opposed to 12 mL V$_T$/kg. In most of these studies, a "safety limit" for plateau pressure was set at 35 cm H$_2$O.

When patients begin to improve, we begin weaning by lowering the FIO$_2$. Once the FIO$_2$ reaches 0.4, we slowly start to wean mean airway pressure (1 or 2 cm H$_2$O/hr lower). At this point, we switch to a mixed form of ventilatory support (e.g., synchronized intermittent mandatory ventilation and pressure support). Spontaneous breathing is tested using continuous positive airway pressure when the patient maintains target blood gases with 5 to 10 cm H$_2$O PEEP and 5 to 10 cm H$_2$O pressure support. In less severe ALI/ARDS, noninvasive ventilation or continuous positive airway pressure may be the first approach. Whichever approach is selected, the first principle is *primum non nocere* with regard to the iatrogenic factors discussed previously.

With regard to fluids, the authors believe that the risks of fluid restriction to hemodynamics and kidney function outweigh any limited potential advantage relative to reducing lung edema. The edema in ALI/ARDS has a high protein concentration and, as such, is not easily removed unless the permeability defects are solved. Similarly, "normal" hemodynamic values are sought because studies have not shown any advantages in achieving supranormal values. Finally, we suggest that enteral nutrition be instituted as soon as possible (although there are no randomized controlled trials indicating that this intervention improves outcomes and one study suggests early enteral feeding results in a greater incidence of ventilator-associated pneumonia). If parenteral nutrition is used, the authors limit the caloric intake to 20 to 25 kcal/kg to avoid increasing the carbon dioxide load in a respiratory system that is already compromised, particularly during the weaning process.

Other Experimental Strategies

Strategies able regionally to redistribute V$_T$ may allow recruitment while preserving pressures within a safe range. Prone ventilation seems to redistribute V$_T$ more homogeneously. Other strategies include extracorporeal membrane oxygenation, high-frequency ventilation, and (more recently) ventilation with perfluorocarbons (i.e., liquid ventilation) and extracorporeal carbon dioxide removal along with low frequency, positive pressure ventilation. Intratracheal ventilation has been used to facilitate decreasing dead space while using low V$_T$ ventilation. Aside from prone positioning, only centers with the required experience and equipment should attempt these more complicated interventions, and then perhaps only in selected patients with ARDS using prospectively designed research protocols, because all these interventions remain experimental and, again with the exception of prone ventilation, carry high risks of complication.

Lung inflammation and epithelial cell injury result in a quantitative and qualitative surfactant deficiency in ALI/ARDS. Unfortunately, inhalation of synthetic surfactant has not been shown to be beneficial. Inhaled pulmonary vasodilators have also been tested, but a controlled trial of nitric oxide indicated that its beneficial effect on oxygenation is small and is limited to the first 24 hours of treatment.

CLINICAL COURSE AND PREVENTION

Independent of the initial etiology, other insults may occur during the course of the basic disease [i.e., nosocomial pneumonia, iatrogenic barotraumas (or better "volutrauma," as suggested by some authors), and the appearance of new foci of infection on heart valves or liver]. Accordingly, a systematic daily consideration of possible complications and their control is mandatory.

Pathophysiologic characterization must also be repeated intermittently during the course of the syndrome because lung lesions evolve and the pathophysiologic process, and therefore the approach to treatment, changes.

Intraalveolar (direct insult) or interstitial (indirect insult) edema characterizes the "early" phases of ARDS, with neutrophilic exudate at first, followed by monocytic and lymphocytic cell recruitment, which further contribute to the epithelial and endothelial injury. Although several proinflammatory and anti-inflammatory mediators and neutrophil markers have been found in patients with ARDS, the complexity of the defense mechanism is such that their importance is difficult to evaluate. The response may be homeostatic, which allows recovery to occur, or overwhelming, which perpetuates the lung injury and limits the repair process.

After approximately 1 week, during the so-called "intermediate" phase of ARDS, death of type I cells together with dysfunction of the remaining type II cells, which are unable to produce sufficient surfactant and actively transport sodium, contribute to maintaining lung edema and thus further distort lung mechanical properties. Endothelial dysfunction and death contribute to plasma and cell transfer from the vascular com-

251

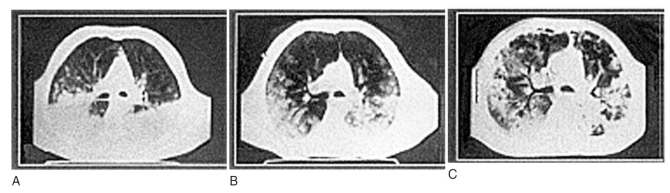

Figure 25.14. Evolution of the acute respiratory distress syndrome (ARDS) lung with time. *A,* Early ARDS (acute phase, week 1). *B,* Intermediate ARDS (week 2). *C,* Late ARDS (week > 3). Note the presence of dependent lung densities in the acute phase. In the late phase, lung densities disappeared while emphysema-like lesions appeared throughout the lung.

partment to the lung, whereas basement membrane collagen exposed to platelets leads to intravascular coagulation, which further compromises lung function.

Meanwhile, under the influence of a set of newly synthesized growth factors, interstitial fibroblasts differentiate into myofibroblasts and migrate into alveolar clots, thus initiating a fibroproliferative response that progressively leads to a fibrous, noncompliant lung. Thus, so-called "late" phase ARDS (>2 weeks) develops, in which several functional and structural modifications occur, such as resorption of the edema, widespread development of fibrosis, microvascular destruction, and development of emphysema-like lesions in the parenchyma (Fig. 25.14). The sponge lung model is not applicable in these conditions because the transmission of superimposed pressures is prevented by fibrosis. These differences in pathologic process imply that the approach to treatment of late-phase ARDS must also differ.

The value of $PaCO_2$ has not been used in classifying ALI/ARDS severity. The authors believe, however, that change in $PaCO_2$ (at a constant minute ventilation) is more informative than changes in oxygenation during the course of ALI/ARDS because this may predict the development of emphysema-like lesions that result from ongoing injury or repair.

The mortality rate of ALI/ARDS in its first description was 7 of 12 patients. Despite nearly three decades of progress in the supportive care of patients who have ARDS, recent studies and reviews continue to report mortality rates that range between 40% and 70%. A recent study that evaluated changes in outcome and severity of ALI/ARDS (as indicated by PaO_2/FIO_2 ratio or lung injury scores) during the past three decades showed that the mortality rate of patients with ARDS remained constant throughout the period studied. Different conclusions were reached in another review, which concluded that in the past 10 years the mortality rate decreased by approximately 20%. In the authors' opinion, a discussion on differences of outcome over the years is academic only. Differences in technology, patient populations, and overall treatments make comparisons extremely difficult.

Although the ability to prevent the development of ALI/ARDS is limited if aspiration pneumonia, pulmonary emboli, or indwelling catheters are considered as a source of sepsis in hospitalized patients, it is clear that careful attention to risk factors that may predispose to ALI/ARDS may be useful. In this context, for example, the efficacy of selective digestive decontamination to prevent secondary lung infection may be useful. In addition, if ventilatory-induced lung injury is a substantial cause of ALI/ARDS, minimization of those factors thought to contribute to this phenomenon (e.g., overstretching, repetitive airspace opening and closing, and surfactant inactivation) may be helpful.

SUGGESTED READINGS

Albert RK, Spiro SG, Jett JR: Clinical Respiratory Medicine, 2nd ed. Philadelphia, Mosby, 2004.

ARDS Network: Ventilation with lower tidal volumes as compared with traditional tidal volumes for acute lung injury and the acute respiratory distress syndrome. The Acute Respiratory Distress Syndrome Network. N Engl J Med 2000;342:1301–1308.

Bernard GR, Vincent JL, Laterre PF, et al: The Recombinant Human Protein C Worldwide Evaluation in Severe Sepsis (PROWESS) Study Group. Efficacy and safety of recombinant human activated protein C for severe sepsis. N Engl J Med 2001;344:699–709.

Gattinoni L, Caironi P, Pelosi P, Goodman LR: What has computed tomography taught us about the acute respiratory distress syndrome? Am J Respir Crit Care Med 2001;164:1701–1711.

Gattinoni L, Tognoni G, Pesenti A, et al: The Prone-Supine Study Group: Effect of prone positioning on the survival of patients with acute respiratory failure. N Engl J Med 2001;345:568–573.

Gattinoni L, Vagginelli F, Chiumello D, et al: Physiologic rationale for ventilator setting in acute lung injury/acute respiratory distress syndrome patients. Crit Care Med 2003;31(4 Suppl):S300–S304.

Goss CH, Brower RG, Hudson LD, et al: Incidence of acute lung injury in the United States. Crit Care Med 2003;31:1607–1611.

Vincent JL, Sakr Y, Ranieri VM: Epidemiology and outcome of acute respiratory failure in intensive care unit patients. Crit Care Med 31(4 Suppl):S296–S299.

Chapter 26

Pulmonary Embolism

C. William Hargett and Victor F. Tapson

Syndromes characterized by embolization of material into the pulmonary venous circulation may lead to marked cardiopulmonary dysfunction and are of special interest to the critical care practitioner. This chapter focuses primarily on thrombotic pulmonary embolism (PE), which is the most common and important syndrome. Pulmonary emboli of nonthrombotic material (e.g., fat, amniotic fluid, air, septic, and tumor) are briefly discussed in the context of the thrombotic paradigm.

Despite advances in the prevention, diagnosis, and treatment of venous thromboembolism (VTE), PE remains a sequela that is frequently missed and often fatal. PE can be the primary reason for admission to the intensive care unit (ICU) or arise as a complication of critical illness. Most frequently, PE results from proximal deep venous thrombosis (DVT) from the legs, but upper extremity thrombi (particularly common in patients with central venous catheters) may also embolize. Patients may present with a wide range of symptoms, including dyspnea, acute chest pain, cough, hemoptysis, and syncope. Identifying the presence of risk factors for VTE is key in suspecting the diagnosis and identifying prophylactic needs. Accurate diagnosis followed by effective therapy unequivocally reduces the morbidity and mortality of PE.

EPIDEMIOLOGY, RISK FACTORS, AND PATHOPHYSIOLOGY

Epidemiology

PE is one of the most common cardiovascular disorders. Measures of the frequency of VTE and PE are confounded by the nonspecific clinical findings and high rate of undiagnosed events. In the United States, the incidence of PE is estimated at 600,000 cases per year, resulting in approximately 100,000 to 200,000 deaths. Adjusting for patients with concomitant terminal illnesses, acute PE may account for as many as 100,000 deaths per year in the United States in patients with an otherwise good prognosis. Existing data suggest that the rate of VTE is particularly high in the critical care setting, where patients often have multiple identifiable risk factors.

Risk Factors

Recognizing the presence of risk factors for VTE (and thus PE) is key in suspecting the diagnosis and identifying prophylactic needs. Virtually every risk factor for VTE can be derived from Virchow's triad of stasis, venous injury, and hypercoagulability described nearly 150 years ago (Box 26.1). The incidence of VTE increases correspondingly with the severity of illness and number of risk factors.

Patients in the ICU are at especially high risk due to severe underlying disease, immobility, and venoinvasive catheters and devices. It is estimated that thrombosis follows 35% to 67% of long-term invasive venous catheterization. Specific risk factors for thrombotic complications of central venous catheters (CVCs) include femoral vein site, cannulation for more than 6 days, multiple lines, and nighttime placement.

Pathogenesis

PE can result in shunt, ventilation/perfusion ($\dot{V}/\dot{Q}$) mismatch, and/or low mixed venous oxygen content (in part as a function of time with shunt and low mixed venous oxygen content occurring early) as the principal physiologic effects. This pathophysiology leads to hypoxemia in approximately 85% of patients. The hemodynamic response to PE is variable, depending on the degree of occlusion of the pulmonary arterial bed and on underlying cardiovascular disease. Physiologically, the resultant decrease in the cross-sectional area of the pulmonary arterial bed causes an increase in the pulmonary vascular resistance (PVR). The increase in PVR impedes right ventricular outflow and reduces left ventricular preload, and thus cardiac output is diminished. Increasing levels of vascular obstruction produce worsening hypoxemia, which stimulates vasoconstriction and a

Box 26.1 Major Risk Factors for Venous Thromboembolism

Clinical Factor	Inherited Factor	Acquired Factor
Age (>40 years, especially > 70 years)	Factor V Leiden (APC resistance)	Anti-phospholipid antibody syndrome
Prior history of VTE	Antithrombin deficiency	Lupus anticoagulant
Major surgery (within 3 months)	Protein C deficiency	Anti-cardiolipin antibodies
Trauma	Protein S deficiency	Hyperhomocysteinemia
Immobilization/paralysis	Prothrombin gene (G20210A) defect	
Central venous catheterization	Heparin cofactor-2 deficiency	
Malignancy	Dysfibrinogenemia	
Myeloproliferative disease	Disorders of plasminogen	
Systolic heart failure	Elevated factor VIII levels	
Myocardial infarction	Elevated factor XI levels	
Stroke	Hyperhomocystinemia	
Obesity		
Pregnancy/postpartum		
Oral contraception		
Inflammatory bowel disease		
Nephrotic syndrome		
Paroxysmal nocturnal hemoglobinuria		
Sickle cell anemia		

APC, activated protein C; VTE, venous thromboembolism.

further rise in pulmonary artery pressure (PAP). The right ventricle eventually fails when it cannot generate a systolic pressure to overcome the increasing PAP and preserve pulmonary perfusion. In patients without underlying cardiopulmonary disease, more than 50% obstruction of the pulmonary circulation is generally required for a significant increase in the mean PAP. It follows that patients with underlying cardiopulmonary disease have less physiologic reserve compared to normal individuals and may suffer right-sided heart failure with a lesser degree of pulmonary vascular occlusion.

CLINICAL FEATURES

Multiple studies have shown that clinical evaluation alone is inadequate in diagnosing and excluding PE. The clinical manifestations of PE are nonspecific (Box 26.2), so careful attention to symptoms is critical in raising the possibility of the disease. Critical care patients with PE often have comorbid cardiopulmonary disease, and their presentations may be quite varied. The large majority of patients with proven acute PE present with at least one of the following factors: dyspnea, pleuritic chest pain, or tachypnea. Pleuritic chest pain and hemoptysis occur more commonly with pulmonary infarction due to smaller, peripheral emboli. Syncope suggests massive PE. PE should always be considered in cases of unexplained dyspnea, syncope, or sudden hypotension.

DIAGNOSIS

The most critical step in diagnosing PE is having a clinical suspicion of the problem. Given the varied presentations, suspicion should be based on the constellation of risk factors, symptoms, signs, electrocardiogram, biochemical labs, and chest radiographic findings (Figs. 26.1 and 26.2). Although clinical assessment alone cannot reliably diagnose or exclude PE, both clinical impression and clinical prediction rules are useful in establishing a pretest probability of PE. These estimates are at the root of systematic strategies for diagnosing PE.

The diagnosis of VTE in the critically ill patient is particularly challenging for several reasons. First, underlying systemic illnesses may mimic or mask the common signs and symptoms of VTE, and it follows that the clinical predictive models may not be valid in the ICU patient. Also, definitive testing may be limited by relative contraindications, such as mechanical ventilation, shock, and renal failure.

Physical Examination

Tachypnea is the most common physical finding of PE. Other signs include tachycardia, augmented pulmonic component of the second heart sound, fever, crackles, pleural rub, wheezing, and leg tenderness or swelling (see Box 26.2). These findings are nonspecific, may frequently be seen in patients with other types of cardiopulmonary disease (e.g., heart failure and chronic obstructive pulmonary disease), and may be due to the underlying disease or the superimposed acute PE. As with the clini-

Box 26.2 Common Symptoms and Signs of Acute
Pulmonary Embolism from the PIOPED Study

Symptoms	Signs
Dyspnea (78%)	Tachypnea (73%)
Pleuritic chest pain (59%)	Crackles (55%)
Cough (43%)	Leg swelling (31%)
Leg pain (27%)	Tachycardia (30%)
Hemoptysis (16%)	Loud pulmonic component of
Wheezing (14%)	second heart sound (23%)
Palpitations (13%)	Wheezes (11%)
Angina-like pain (6%)	Diaphoresis (10%)
	Fever (7%)

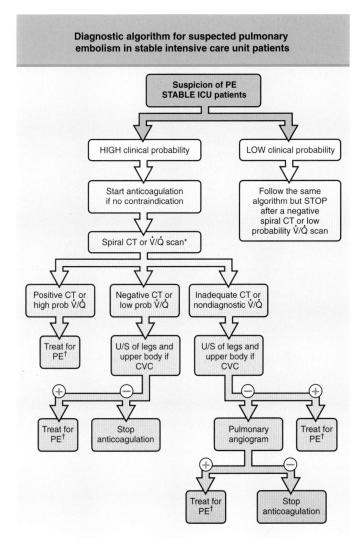

Figure 26.1. Diagnostic algorithm for suspected pulmonary embolism in stable ICU patients. *$\dot{V}/\dot{Q}$ scan is most useful when the chest radiograph is normal or near normal. †Treatment may include consideration of thrombolytics even in stable patients, depending on clot burden; consider echocardiography to help stratify patients. CT, computed tomography; CVC, central venous catheter; PE, pulmonary embolus; U/S, ultrasound; $\dot{V}/\dot{Q}$, ventilation–perfusion.

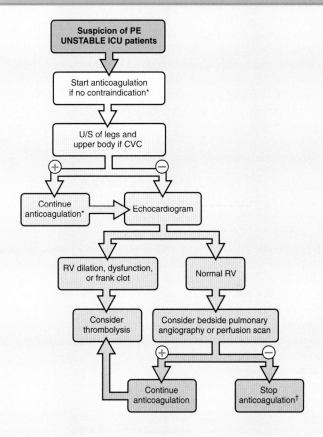

Figure 26.2. Diagnostic algorithm for suspected pulmonary embolism in unstable ICU patients. *Consider inferior vena cava filter if DVT is present and anticoagulation is contraindicated or also in the setting of massive pulmonary embolism with DVT when it is believed that any further emboli might be lethal and thrombolytic use is prohibited. †Stop anticoagulation after a negative pulmonary angiogram or a normal or low-probability perfusion scan. CVC, central venous catheter; PE, pulmonary embolus; RV, right ventricle; U/S, ultrasound.

cal symptoms, signs of PE should be particularly heeded when found in patients who have risk factors for VTE.

Chest Radiography

Chest radiography can only rarely be used for the conclusive diagnosis or exclusion of PE. Although the chest radiograph is often abnormal in patients with PE, the abnormalities are nearly always nonspecific. Common findings include atelectasis, pleural effusion, pulmonary infiltrates, and mild elevation of a hemidiaphragm. Classic findings such as Hampton's hump (i.e., a juxtapleural wedge-shaped opacity at the costophrenic angle indicating pulmonary infarction) or Westermark's sign (i.e., focally decreased vascularity distal to the occlusion) are suggestive of the diagnosis of PE but are only rarely observed. A normal chest radiograph in the setting of dyspnea and hypoxemia without evidence of bronchospasm or anatomic cardiac shunt is

strongly suggestive of PE. The presence of a pleural effusion increases the likelihood of PE in young patients who present with acute pleuritic chest pain. Although chest radiography may help diagnose other processes (e.g., pneumonia, pneumothorax, and rib fracture) that may cause symptoms similar to PE, it is important to remember that PE may frequently coexist with other underlying heart or lung diseases.

Electrocardiography

Similar to chest radiography, electrocardiography in patients with acute PE most often produces abnormal but nonspecific findings. These include T-wave changes, ST-segment changes, and right or left axis deviation. The classic patterns of S1Q3T3, right ventricular strain, and new incomplete right bundle branch block are infrequent in PE but may be common in the patient with massive PE and cor pulmonale. The presence of T wave inversion in the precordial leads may correlate with more severe right ventricular dysfunction.

Arterial Blood Gas Analysis

Approximately 85% to 90% of patients with PE have hypoxemia and an increased alveolar–arterial difference. A reduced carbon dioxide tension (hypocarbia) is also frequently present. Abnormalities in gas exchange are variable, however, particularly in young patients and those without underlying lung or heart disease. It follows that PE cannot be excluded based on a normal partial pressure of oxygen (PaO_2), normal alveolar–arterial difference, or normal or elevated partial pressure of carbon dioxide ($PaCO_2$). Hypoxemia is almost uniformly present, however, when there is a hemodynamically significant PE.

D-dimer

D-dimer, a specific by-product of cross-linked fibrin, has been extensively evaluated in the setting of suspected acute DVT and PE. Multiple rapid and inexpensive D-dimer assays are very sensitive and have a high negative predictive value for excluding the presence of VTE when used in concert with a low pretest probability in an outpatient setting. The low specificity of the D-dimer (i.e., many conditions are associated with elevated levels) makes it less useful in the complex, critically ill patient. Accordingly, the positive predictive value of a positive assay is low and should not be used in isolation to initiate further workup.

Cardiac Troponin

Patients with right ventricular strain secondary to acute PE may sometimes have elevated troponin T and I levels due to cardiac myocyte damage. Positive troponins are more common with large clot burdens and may be associated with a poorer prognosis. It follows that patients with PE and elevated troponins are more likely to have elevated right ventricular systolic pressures and right ventricular dilation/hypokinesis, and they are at increased risk for cardiogenic shock. Although a positive troponin may serve as a clue to the potential diagnosis of PE in the appropriate clinical context, a negative value is not sufficiently sensitive to rule out PE.

Brain Natriuretic Peptide

Plasma brain natriuretic peptide levels may be a supplementary tool for evaluating right ventricular function in patients with acute PE, but their exact utility is unclear and currently under evaluation.

Ventilation–Perfusion Scanning

Although the $\dot{V}/\dot{Q}$ scan is still often the initial diagnostic test for suspected PE, its use has decreased during the past decade in favor of contrast spiral computed tomography (CT). Lung scanning cannot be performed on ventilated patients in the ICU, and the availability of bedside perfusion imaging has decreased. Lung scanning also has the best predictive value when used in patients with normal or near normal chest radiographs. These factors notwithstanding, $\dot{V}/\dot{Q}$ scanning is still frequently employed in the diagnostic algorithm for acute PE. When abnormal, $\dot{V}/\dot{Q}$ scans are conventionally read as showing low, intermediate, or high probability of PE (Fig. 26.3).

The $\dot{V}/\dot{Q}$ scan is most useful when the result is concordant with the clinical likelihood of PE (e.g., in the setting of high clin-

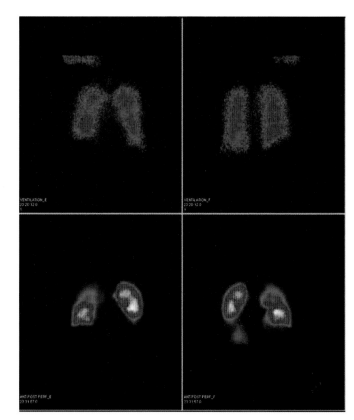

Figure 26.3. High probability ventilation–perfusion scan. High probability ventilation–perfusion scan (anteroposterior views) demonstrating normal ventilation bilaterally with multiple large segmental perfusion abnormalities within both lungs. The corresponding chest radiograph had no focal parenchymal opacities.

ical suspicion, a high-probability $\dot{V}/\dot{Q}$ scan is diagnostic for PE). With a high pretest probability for PE, any reading other than normal or high warrants further evaluation, as indicated by the results of the Prospective Investigation of Pulmonary Embolism Diagnosis (PIOPED) study in which 66% of patients with a high clinical pretest probability for PE and intermediate-probability scans and 40% of patients with low-probability scans were definitively diagnosed with PE by pulmonary angiography. This emphasizes the importance of continuing the evaluation for PE in patients in whom there is a high clinical suspicion even after a low- or intermediate-probability lung scan. Alternatively, in the setting of low clinical pretest probability of PE, a normal or low-probability $\dot{V}/\dot{Q}$ scan excludes significant PE in more than 95% of cases.

Spiral Chest Computed Tomography Scanning

Contrast-enhanced spiral CT of the chest may reveal emboli in the main, lobar, or segmental pulmonary arteries with more than 90% sensitivity and specificity (Fig. 26.4). Although some studies have been less encouraging, the aggregate data suggest that spiral CT with experienced readers is unlikely to miss large emboli. The clinical importance of the spiral CT having a lower sensitivity for small, subsegmental PE is under study. It seems reasonable that in the setting of high clinical suspicion for PE and a negative chest CT, studies of the deep veins of the legs should be pursued. An added benefit of spiral CT for suspected PE is that it provides visualization of potential nonvascular

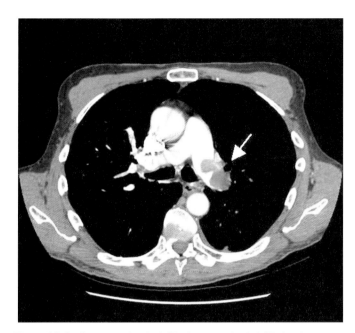

Figure 26.4. Contrasted spiral CT. Contrasted spiral CT showing a large embolus *(arrow)* in the left pulmonary artery.

pathology such as musculoskeletal or airway abnormalities, lymphadenopathy, pleural or pericardial disease, or parenchymal lesions such as consolidation or a lung tumor. The rate of non-diagnostic spiral CT scans is approximately 10%.

Magnetic Resonance Imaging

Magnetic resonance imaging (MRI) has excellent sensitivity and specificity for the diagnosis of DVT, and it may allow the simultaneous detection of DVT and PE. Disadvantages of MRI include difficulty in employing in the critically ill or ventilated patient.

Echocardiography

Echocardiography is best utilized as an ancillary rather than a primary diagnostic modality for PE because it is less sensitive and specific than many other techniques. However, as many as 80% of patients with documented PE have echocardiographic evidence of right ventricular enlargement or dysfunction, which may suggest the diagnosis (Fig. 26.5). McConnell's sign (regional wall motion abnormalities that spare the right ventricular apex) may be a more specific finding, and occasionally direct visualization of frank clot may guarantee the diagnosis. Echocardiography is often rapidly available and may more quickly lead to a presumptive diagnosis and give reason for subsequent thrombolysis in some cases of massive or hemodynamically significant PE. Echocardiography also affords serial cardiac evaluation for interval change, and it may be useful in identifying other causes of shock, such as aortic dissection and cardiac tamponade.

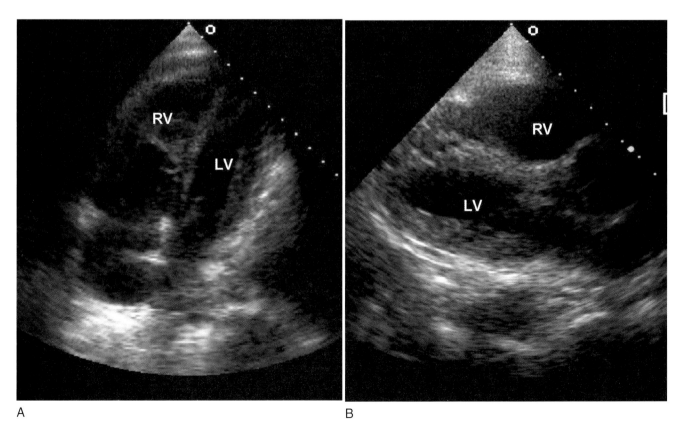

A

B

Figure 26.5. Transthoracic echocardiogram. Transthoracic echocardiogram in a patient with pulmonary embolus leading to a dilated right ventricle (RV) and compression of the left ventricle (LV) by septal flattening and bowing during diastole. *A,* Apical four-chamber view; *B,* parasternal long-axis view.

Pulmonary Angiography

Pulmonary artery angiography is extremely sensitive and specific in confirming or excluding acute PE and remains the "gold standard" diagnostic technique. Angiography is generally quite safe, with morbidity and mortality rates of 1% and 0.5%, respectively. Serious complications include respiratory failure, hemorrhage, and renal failure. Pulmonary angiography is frequently reserved for patients in whom preliminary noninvasive testing has been nondiagnostic.

Special Diagnostic Considerations

Massive Pulmonary Embolism

Patients with suspected massive PE may present with extreme hypoxemia and/or critical hypotension. Diagnostic evaluation must be performed rapidly, but severe illness may limit the patient's ability to undergo transport or testing. Spiral CT is unlikely to be negative in the setting of massive PE. Similarly, portable perfusion scans are more likely diagnostic (i.e., "high probability") when the clot burden is high. Right ventricular dilation and dysfunction are also more likely to be seen by echocardiography in the setting of massive PE.

Acute Deep Venous Thrombosis

In the critical care setting, the search for DVT can be especially useful in that it may establish a presumptive diagnosis and direct toward treatment. Compression ultrasound has a greater than 90% sensitivity and specificity for symptomatic proximal DVT, and it has replaced impedance plethysmography as the most common diagnostic test used in the setting of suspected acute DVT. Sensitivity is much lower in patients who are asymptomatic or morbidly obese and in distinguishing acute from chronic thrombosis. Contrast venography remains the gold standard for the diagnosis of DVT, but MRI and spiral CT (CT venography) are accurate noninvasive alternatives when available.

TREATMENT

Options for treatment of acute PE include anticoagulation, thrombolytic therapy, inferior vena cava (IVC) filter placement, and surgical embolectomy. Each approach has specific indications as well as advantages and disadvantages.

Anticoagulation

Anticoagulation reduces the mortality in patients with acute PE, and it should be immediately instituted unless contraindications are present. Although anticoagulants do not directly dissolve the thrombus or embolus, they prevent thrombus extension and indirectly decrease clot burden by allowing the natural fibrinolytic system to proceed unopposed. In the setting of a high clinical suspicion for PE, empiric anticoagulation is appropriate while diagnostic testing is under way, as long as the risk of anticoagulation is not excessive.

Unfractionated Heparin

Achieving a therapeutic activated partial thromboplastin time (aPTT) within 24 hours after the initiation of therapy with standard, unfractionated continuously infused intravenous heparin reduces the PE recurrence rate in patients with PE. "Traditional" heparin dosing with a 5000-unit bolus and 1000 U/hr is inadequate in many patients, and a more aggressive approach

decreases the risk of subtherapeutic anticoagulation. Heparin should be administered as an intravenous bolus of 5000 units followed by a maintenance dose of at least 30,000 to 40,000 units per 24 hours by continuous infusion (the lower dose being used if the patient is considered at risk for bleeding). A bolus of 80 U/kg followed by 18 U/kg/hr is an alternative recommendation. Following initiation, the aPTT should be measured at 6-hour intervals until it is consistently in the therapeutic range of 1.5 to 2.0 times control values. Further adjusting of the heparin dose should be weight-based.

Low-Molecular-Weight Heparin

A number of clinical trials have demonstrated the efficacy and safety of low-molecular-weight heparin (LMWH) for the treatment of acute VTE. Although they are more expensive than unfractionated heparin, LMWH preparations have some advantages, including greater bioavailability, more predictable dosing, and a decreased risk of heparin-induced thrombocytopenia (HIT). These preparations can be administered once or twice per day subcutaneously and do not require monitoring of the aPTT. Monitoring of anti-factor Xa levels is reasonable in certain settings, such as morbid obesity, very small patients (<40 kg), pregnancy, and renal insufficiency. LMWHs are renally metabolized and should be used with caution when the creatinine clearance is less than 30 mL/min. Some have suggested an upper weight limit of approximately 120 to 150 kg for LMWH use, with intravenous standard heparin being used in larger patients.

Warfarin

Warfarin therapy is less frequently utilized in ICU patients because of the frequent need for procedures and increased risk of bleeding in this population. However, when warfarin is employed, therapy should overlap with adequate anticoagulation with a heparin preparation for two reasons. First, the initiation of warfarin may cause a transient hypercoagulable state due to the abrupt decline in protein C anticoagulant activity. Second, warfarin produces a rapid decline in factor VII levels, resulting in an initial prolongation of the international normalized ratio (INR) before the other vitamin K-dependent factors have been depleted (i.e., elevation of the INR prior to true anticoagulation). It is recommended that a heparin preparation be employed for at least 5 days and maintained at a therapeutic level until two consecutive INR values of 2.0 to 3.0 have been documented at least 24 hours apart.

Newer Agents

Lepirudin, argatroban, and ximelagatran are direct thrombin inhibitors that have several advantages over heparin, including efficacy against fibrin clot-bound thrombin. The first two are Food and Drug Administration-approved parenteral drugs used for the treatment of HIT, and the third is an oral agent that has been studied extensively. A disadvantage of the direct thrombin inhibitors is lack of reversibility.

Special Case: Upper Extremity DVT

Upper extremity thrombosis is common in the critically ill and is most frequently related to a central venous catheter. Complications from upper extremity DVT are less frequent than from lower extremity DVT, but they should not be overlooked. CVC-related thrombosis should generally be treated similarly to uncomplicated DVTs but with an added emphasis on prompt CVC removal once the diagnosis is established. The risk of clot embolization with catheter removal is outweighed by the risk of chronic thrombotic complications and potential infection.

Complications of Anticoagulation

Bleeding and HIT are the major complications of anticoagulation. The rates of major bleeding in trials using heparin by continuous infusion or high-dose subcutaneous injection are less than 5%. Approximately 10% to 20% of patients receiving unfractionated heparin for at least 4 to 10 days will have a decrease in platelet count below the normal range or a 50% decrease in platelet count within the normal range. Most of these cases represent nonimmune (type I) disease. Immune-mediated HIT probably occurs 5 or more days after the initiation of heparin in approximately 0.3% to 3% of patients. If a patient is placed on heparin for VTE and the platelet count progressively decreases to $100,000/mm^3$ or less, all heparin therapy should be discontinued in lieu of an appropriate alternative therapy, such as argatroban or lepirudin.

Thrombolytic Therapy

Thrombolytic agents cause the direct acceleration of clot lysis and a reduction in clot burden by activating plasminogen to form plasmin, which then results in fibrinolysis as well as fibrinogenolysis. Defining those patients in whom the benefit of a rapid reduction in clot burden outweighs the increased hemorrhagic risk of thrombolytic therapy may be difficult. The case for thrombolytic use is strongest in patients with massive PE complicated by shock, which occurs in approximately 10% of patients with a mortality rate as high as 25%. Thrombolysis in these patients results in a more rapid resolution of abnormal right ventricular function. Emerging data suggest that patients with acute submassive embolism (extensive clot burden without shock or severe hypoxemia) may also benefit from thrombolysis. A prospective randomized clinical trial suggested that patients with acute PE without hypotension but with right ventricular dysfunction on echocardiogram may have had an improved clinical course when given thrombolytic therapy plus heparin versus heparin alone in that thrombolysis seemed to prevent clinical deterioration and the need for escalation of care. The subjective nature of the end points studied in this trial limits the interpretation of the results.

No clear data indicate that any one thrombolytic agent is superior to another, although shorter regimens and even bolus dosing may be favored in the case of massive PE. Each of the approved regimens is administered at a fixed dose, making measurements of coagulation unnecessary during infusion (Table 26.1). The aPTT should be measured after the thrombolytic infusion is completed and repeated at 4-hour intervals until the aPTT is less than twice the upper limit of normal. At this point, continuous intravenous unfractionated heparin should be administered without a loading bolus dose.

Thrombolytic therapy is contraindicated in patients at high risk for hemorrhage because both the lysis of hemostatic fibrin plugs and fibrinogenolysis can lead to severe bleeding (Box 26.3). Intracranial hemorrhage is the most devastating (and often fatal) complication of thrombolytic therapy and is generally stated to occur in approximately 2% of patients. Invasive procedures should be minimized because bleeding commonly occurs at sites

---

Table 26.1 FDA-Approved Thrombolytic Therapy Regimens for Acute Pulmonary Embolism

Agent	Regimen
Streptokinase	250,000 U IV (loading dose over 30 min), then 100,000 U/hr for 24 hr
t-PA	100 mg IV over 2 hr

t-PA, tissue-type plasminogen activator.

Box 26.3 Contraindications to Thrombolytic Therapy in Pulmonary Embolism

Absolute	Relative
Previous hemorrhagic stroke	Bleeding diathesis (e.g., severe liver dysfunction, anticoagulant use)
Intracranial surgery or pathology, including trauma	Uncontrolled severe hypertension (systolic BP > 180 or diastolic BP > 110)
Active internal bleeding (does not include menses)	Cardiopulmonary resuscitation
	Major surgery within the previous 10 days[a]
	Thrombocytopenia (platelets < 100,000/mm^3)
	Recent major trauma, internal bleeding, or nonhemorrhagic stroke
	Pregnancy

[a]This time frame may depend on the type of surgery and the level of critical illness.

---

of catheter placement. Retroperitoneal hemorrhage may result from a vascular puncture above the inguinal ligament and is often initially silent but may be life-threatening. The decision to use thrombolysis should be made on a case-by-case basis because there should be a lower threshold to administer therapy in the setting of a contraindication when a patient is extremely unstable from life-threatening PE.

Vena Cava Interruption

IVC filter placement can be performed to minimize the risk of PE from lower extremity thrombi. The primary indications for IVC filter placement include contraindications to anticoagulation, recurrent embolism while on adequate therapy, and significant bleeding during anticoagulation. Filters are sometimes also placed in the setting of massive PE when it is believed that any further emboli might be lethal. A number of filter designs exist, and they can be inserted via the jugular or femoral veins. Rare complications include insertion-related problems, filter migration, direct thrombus extension through the filter, and IVC thrombosis. Temporary filters have been utilized in patients in whom the risk of bleeding appears to be short term.

Surgical Embolectomy

Although surgical embolectomy is most commonly performed for chronic thromboembolic pulmonary hypertension, rare circumstances warrant its consideration in acute PE. A candidate

259

for acute embolectomy should have a documented massive PE with refractory shock, failure of or contraindication to thrombolytic therapy, and an available experienced surgical team.

Special Treatment Considerations: Massive PE

Once massive PE with hypotension and/or severe hypoxemia is suspected, supportive treatment should be initiated immediately. Cautious infusion of intravenous saline may augment preload and improve impaired right ventricular function. Dopamine and norepinephrine are the favored vasopressors if hypotension remains. Although dobutamine may boost right ventricular output, it may worsen hypotension. Supplemental oxygen, intubation, and mechanical ventilation are instituted as needed to support respiratory failure. Anticoagulation and thrombolytic therapy should be considered as described previously. Pulmonary embolectomy may be appropriate in patients with massive embolism in whom thrombolytic therapy is contraindicated.

CLINICAL COURSE AND PREVENTION

Course

Mean 1-month mortality rates of treated and untreated PE have been estimated to be 8% and 30%, respectively. In the International Cooperative Pulmonary Embolism Registry of 2454 consecutive patients, PE was the principal cause of death, with the 3-month mortality being 17.5%. In the PIOPED study, the mortality rate was approximately 15%, but only 10% of deaths occurring during the first year of follow-up were attributed to PE.

Most patients who survive an acute episode of PE have no long-term pulmonary sequelae. Only a small percentage of patients will develop chronic dyspnea and hypoxemia due to chronic thromboembolic pulmonary hypertension. Chronic leg pain and swelling from DVT (postphlebitic syndrome) may result in considerable morbidity.

Prevention

Prophylaxis for VTE substantially decreases the incidence for those at risk of the disease, but such measures appear to be grossly underutilized. In general medical patients at risk for venous thrombosis, either LMWH (enoxaparin 40 mg subcutaneously once daily) or subcutaneous heparin (5000 units every 8 hr) is generally adequate. Although 5000 units of heparin every 12 hours has been commonly used, there are fewer data to support this preventive regimen. LMWH may offer superior prophylaxis to subcutaneous heparin in some populations (e.g., after total hip or knee replacement), but there are insufficient data to generalize this to all critically ill patients. Abundant data now support either no increase or a small increase in the absolute rate of major bleeding with the use of subcutaneous low-dose unfractionated heparin or LMWH. Heparin-induced thrombocytopenia remains another possible complication.

Intermittent pneumatic compression (IPC) devices should be utilized when prophylactic doses of LMWH or heparin are contraindicated. Both methods combined (IPCs and heparin) would be reasonable in patients deemed to be at exceptionally high risk for VTE, but an additional reduction in risk in such patients has not been well substantiated. Every hospitalized patient should be assessed for the need for such prophylactic measures.

Box 26.4 Pitfalls and Complications of PE

Despite better understanding of the epidemiology of PE and improvements in diagnosis, therapy, and prevention, PE still is associated with a high mortality rate.

Diagnostic modalities such as CT scanning are not 100% sensitive.

Prophylaxis for VTE appears to be greatly underutilized.

Anticoagulation may have serious adverse effects, such as bleeding and HIT.

Box 26.5 Controversies in PE

Although consensus guidelines exist for the standard diagnostic approach to PE, there is no single, best approach that is uniformly accepted.

Defining which patients in whom the benefit of thrombolysis outweighs the hemorrhagic risk may be difficult.

Guidelines for prophylaxis are clear in some settings, but they remain controversial in others.

PITFALLS/COMPLICATIONS AND CONTROVERSIES

Boxes 26.4 and 26.5 indicate the pitfalls/complications and controversies.

NONTHROMBOTIC PULMONARY EMBOLI

Nonthrombotic pulmonary emboli may occur in certain clinical settings, such as fat embolism within 24 hours of traumatic fractures of the long bones and/or after various orthopedic procedures. Characteristic symptoms include dyspnea, petechiae, and confusion resulting from venous obstruction by neutral fat and from a vasculitis and capillary leak syndrome caused by free fatty acids. The diagnosis is clinical, therapy is generally supportive, and the prognosis is often good.

Amniotic fluid embolism is uncommon but represents one of the leading causes of maternal death in the United States. There are no identifiable risk factors, and the condition may occur during or soon after either spontaneous or cesarean delivery. The major clinical findings include hypoxemia with respiratory failure, disseminated intravascular coagulation, and cardiogenic shock. The primary therapy is supportive, but the condition is frequently fatal.

Air embolism may occur during invasive procedures, barotrauma, or related to the use of indwelling catheters. The most common passage for air into the arterial system is by incomplete filtering of a large air embolus by the pulmonary capillaries or via paradoxical embolization through a patent foramen ovale. The upright position is particularly hazardous for the admission of air into the venous circulation since, in this setting, venous pressure is below atmospheric pressure. Signs and symptoms of air embolism range from minimal to death, depending on the amount of air that embolizes. Immediate positioning in Trendelenburg and left lateral decubitus may open an obstructed right ventricular outflow tract. Administration of 100% oxygen aids in air reabsorption via nitrogen washout. Air aspiration should be attempted if there is a central venous catheter in the right atrium. Hyperbaric oxygen therapy may also be beneficial.

Other nonthrombotic causes of pulmonary vascular obstruction include septic material, cancer cells, and schistosomal disease.

SUGGESTED READING

Fedullo PF, Tapson VF: The evaluation of suspected pulmonary embolism. N Engl J Med 2003;349:1247–1256.

Goldhaber SZ: Echocardiography in the management of pulmonary embolism. Ann Intern Med 2002;136:691–700.

Hyers TM, Agnelli G, Hull RD, et al: Antithrombotic therapy for venous thromboembolic disease. Chest 2001;119:176S–193S.

Konstantinides S, Geibel A, Heusel G, et al: Heparin plus alteplase compared with heparin alone in patients with submassive pulmonary embolism. N Engl J Med 2002;347:1143–1150.

PIOPED Investigators: Value of the ventilation/perfusion scan in acute pulmonary embolism: Results of the Prospective Investigation of Pulmonary Embolism Diagnosis (PIOPED). JAMA 1990;263:2753–2759.

Rocha AT, Tapson VF: Venous thromboembolism in intensive care patients. Clin Chest Med 2003;24:103–122.

Tapson VF, Carroll BA, Davidson BL, et al: The diagnostic approach to acute venous thromboembolism: Clinical practice guideline. Am J Respir Crit Care Med 1999;160:1043–1066.

A Physiologically Based Approach to Perioperative Management of Obese Patients

Paolo Pelosi, Thomas Luecke, Pietro Caironi, and Davide Chiumello

KEY POINTS

- The influence of body mass on the respiratory function produces only mild effects in simple obesity, but in morbid obesity respiratory function is characterized by alterations of the pulmonary volumes, both static and dynamic.
- The influence of body mass in the perioperative period poses a number of problems to ventilatory management, particularly regarding administration of drugs for sedation and drug interactions.
- Intensive care unit admission in the postoperative period may help to reduce the incidence of postoperative pulmonary complications and morbidity.

Obesity is a metabolic disease in which adipose tissue represents a proportion of body mass tissue greater than normal. Up to 35% of the population in North America and 15% to 20% in Europe can be considered obese. Many etiologic factors may be implicated in determining obesity, including genetic, environmental, socioeconomic, and individual factors such as age and sex. In the absence of further pathologic conditions, adipose tissue represents 15% to 18% of body weight in males and approximately 25% in females.

New surgical techniques have been developed for the treatment of obesity, such as ileojejunal bypass or gastric binding. Moreover, laparoscopic surgery has been increasingly applied to obese patients. Since these patients are characterized by several systemic physiopathologic alterations, the perioperative management may present some problems, mainly related to their respiratory alterations.

This chapter discusses (1) the influence of body mass on the respiratory function and on the ventilatory management in the perioperative period and (2) the possible role of intensive care in reducing pulmonary complications and, likely, morbidity in the postoperative period.

DEFINITION OF OBESITY

In clinical practice, several criteria have been proposed to define the obesity condition:

1. Height/weight indexes: The advantage of using these is that one does not have to look up ideal body weight in a table.
2. Calculation of the ratio between the actual and "ideal" weight of the patient: The ideal weight in kilograms is computed by subtracting 100 (in men) and 105 (in women) from the patient's height in centimeters. A person who weighs more than 120% of ideal weight may be considered obese, and a person who weighs more than 200% of ideal weight may be considered pathologically obese.
3. Calculation of the body mass index (BMI; or Quetelet's index): This index is computed as the ratio between the weight (expressed in kilograms) and the height squared (expressed in meters). On the bases of BMI, it is possible to divide the population into several classes: (1) underweight with a BMI lower than $20 \, kg/m^2$, (2) normal weight with a BMI between 20 and $25 \, kg/m^2$, (3) overweight with a BMI between 25 and $30 \, kg/m^2$, (4) obese with a BMI between 30 and $40 \, kg/m^2$, and (5) morbidly obese with a BMI greater than $40 \, kg/m^2$. BMI is commonly used when dealing with obesity because it is simple to compute and correlates well with the risk of death. Values for obesity hypoventilation syndrome are nearly identical for those of simple obesity. However, it may be that there is relatively more fat and less muscle in obesity hypoventilation syndrome because these patients are sicker and less active. Typical examples of morbidly obese patients are shown in Figure 27.1.

RESPIRATORY FUNCTION IN THE PREOPERATIVE PERIOD

Simple obesity (i.e., uncomplicated by upper or lower airway obstruction leading to hypoventilation syndrome) generally produces only mild effects on respiratory function (Rochester, 1995). The deficits tend to be more severe in obesity hypoventilation syndrome. Forced vital capacity (FVC), functional residual capacity (FRC), total lung capacity (TLC), and maximal voluntary ventilation (MVV) are within normal values in most obese patients. In fact, in obese patients FVC is reduced by approximately 10% to 15%. On the contrary, in morbid obesity, the respiratory function is characterized by alterations of the

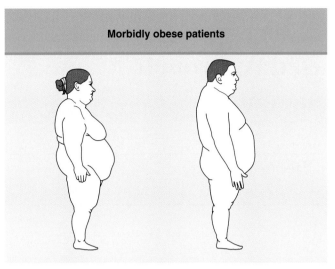

Morbidly obese patients

Figure 27.1. Representative morbidly obese patients. The increases in the abdominal mass and the face boundary suggest likely difficult intubation.

pulmonary volumes, both static and dynamic. A morbidly obese patient appears to have a reduction of FVC, FRC, and TLC with a decreased expiratory reserve volume (ERV), which is a typical restrictive pattern. In obese patients with BMI greater than 40 kg/m², FVC is reduced by 25% to 50% and MVV by approximately 30%, without any significant alteration in FRC or TLC. ERV is generally compromised, 35% to 60% predicted, because the obese abdomen displaces the diaphragm into the chest. In obesity hypoventilation syndrome, TLC is approximately 20% smaller, and FVC and MVV are approximately 40% smaller, than in simple obesity. ERV in obesity hypoventilation syndrome is equivalent to that in the most morbid obesity. FRC is 75% to 80% predicted in obesity hypoventilation syndrome.

Carbon dioxide production increases as a function of body weight, but the rate of increase per kilogram is 40% higher in normal than in obese subjects. The respiratory exchange ratio (Vco_2/Vo_2) is normal. Obese subjects at rest consume approximately 25% more oxygen than nonobese subjects. Morbidly obese patients are often hypoxemic, with a wide alveolar–arterial oxygen tension gradient (A–aPo_2), but hypoxemia may be mild or absent. Pao_2 is most likely to be abnormal when obese subjects are supine, even if it is normal when they are sitting. Interestingly, alveolar Po_2 decreases much more rapidly in obese subjects than in normals during voluntary breath-holding; the magnitude of the decrease in 15 seconds correlates with the severity of obesity, the reduction in FRC, and oxygen consumption.

Also, ventilation and perfusion are mismatched. The lung bases are well perfused, but they are hypoventilated due to airway closure and even alveolar collapse (up to 5% during spontaneous breathing). This effect is obviously more pronounced in obese patients with small lung volumes and in the supine position. On the other hand, the physiological dead space (V_D) and the ratio of dead space to tidal volume (V_D/V_T), as judged from nitrogen washout, are normal.

Most patients with severe obesity are eucapnic, even if obesity produces a greater demand on the ventilatory system to maintain a normal $Paco_2$. Patients with obesity hypoventilation

syndrome are hypercapnic, and they have a lower Pao_2 than patients with simpler obesity. The lower Pao_2 in obesity hypoventilation syndrome results mainly from an increase in $Paco_2$, but A–aPo_2 is also higher in obesity hypoventilation syndrome. Patients with obesity hypoventilation syndrome uncomplicated by obstructive airway disease can attain normal $Paco_2$ by voluntary hyperventilation. This is taken as evidence of abnormal ventilatory control in that patients with obesity hypoventilation syndrome can achieve eucapnia but choose not to. The magnitude of decrease in $Paco_2$ with hyperventilation is related to forced expiratory volume in 1 second (FEV₁), so mechanical impediments to breathing also contribute to hypercapnia in obesity hypoventilation syndrome (Rochester, 1995).

It is generally held that the compliance of the respiratory system is low in obesity, mainly because of the effect of obesity on the chest wall. Indeed, many investigators have found relatively large reductions in chest wall or total respiratory system compliance. An obese patient is characterized by a decrease in the compliance of the respiratory system (35% lower than expected values) because of a reduction of either lung or chest wall compliance. These alterations are directly due to the increase and the distribution of adipose tissue, and their importance in determining the inefficiency of respiratory function parallels the increase in abdominal mass. Variation in values for compliance of the chest wall may be a function of the technique and the degree of muscular relaxation. Researchers found that compliance of the chest wall and total respiratory system in simple obesity was 92% and 80%, respectively, of the values obtained in normal subjects. In patients with obesity hypoventilation syndrome, compliance of the chest wall and total respiratory system was 37% and 44% of normal, respectively, substantially lower than in simple obesity. Part of the decrement in respiratory system compliance resulted from a decline in lung compliance. Compliance of the lung is decreased by approximately 25% in simple obesity and 40% in obesity hypoventilation syndrome. Some of the reduction is likely due to increased pulmonary blood volume and some to increased closure of dependent airways.

Moreover, these patients are characterized by an increase in respiratory resistances; however, this increase is not likely due to airway obstruction but, rather, to reduced lung volume. In fact, the specific resistances (i.e., the resistances related to the lung volume) are relatively normal. The difference between airway and respiratory system resistance is little affected by increasing BMI, whereas there is a high degree of correlation between airway conductance and FRC. Thus, it has been concluded that the major reason for increased lung and respiratory resistance in obesity is the reduction in lung volume. The lung resistance in obesity hypoventilation syndrome is the same as in simple obesity, but chest wall and total respiratory system resistance are higher. The FEV₁/FVC ratio is normal in obese patients without underlying lung disease, even when their lung resistance is high. The same holds true in obesity hypoventilation syndrome. This can be interpreted to mean that the source of the increased resistance lies in lung tissue and small airways rather than in large airways. A minority of these patients can present various degrees of flow limitation, but this finding is not specific for obesity.

During quiet breathing at rest, the respiratory rate of eucapnic obese subjects is approximately 40% higher than in normal subjects. The duration of inspiration (T_i) as a fraction of total breath duration (T_i/T_{tot}) is normal. The tidal volume is normal in simple obesity both at rest and at maximal exercise. On the contrary, patients with obesity hypoventilation syndrome have a 25% higher response rate and a 25% lower tidal volume than subjects with simple obesity, but T_i/T_{tot} remains normal. The mean inspiratory flow (V_T/T_i) is normal in uncomplicated obesity, whereas the respiratory drive ($P_{0.1}$) is twice normal and it increases normally with CO_2 inhalation. The $P_{0.1}$ in former obesity hypoventilation syndrome patients is the same as in obesity, but values for $P_{0.1}$ in overt obesity hypoventilation syndrome are scanty. Accordingly, the diaphragmatic response to inhalation of CO_2 is elevated in uncomplicated obesity but lies in the normal range in obesity hypoventilation syndrome. The ventilatory response to inhalation of carbon dioxide is generally reduced by approximately 40% in simple obesity and 65% in obesity hypoventilation syndrome. In contrast, the ventilatory response to hypoxemia may be normal or higher than normal in simple obesity, even though the obese subjects have a reduced CO_2 response.

Because of the reduced compliance of the respiratory system and the increase in airway resistances, work of breathing is greater compared to that of normal patients (Rochester, 1995). When the inefficiency of respiratory function is not paralleled by an increase in ventilation, because of the simultaneous increased work of breathing, a hypercapnic syndrome associated with moderate hypoxemia can occur. Patients with simple obesity have a near normal capacity for physical exercise. The slopes of the heart rate blood pressure, minute volume, tidal volume, and respiratory rate responses of healthy young obese subjects to exercise are very similar to those of young normal subjects. At exercise, as at rest, obese subjects breathe faster with a smaller tidal volume. At the onset of exercise, obese subjects tend to have transient hypoventilation and desaturation.

The performance of obese subjects at exercise varies with the type of exercise. Obese subjects do less work for a given oxygen consumption, and for the same increased intensity of exercise the oxygen consumption is higher. Overall, the gap between obese and normal subjects remains relatively constant as work rate increases. Maximal cycle ergometer work rate and maximal exercise minute ventilation are approximately similar to those of normal subjects.

One important issue is to define the role of preoperative pulmonary function tests to predict postoperative pulmonary complications. In general, pulmonary function tests have not been reported to be extremely sensitive to predict postoperative pulmonary complications (Smetana, 1999). We performed preoperative pulmonary functional tests in 58 morbidly obese patients (BMI > 40 kg/m^2) undergoing abdominal surgery to identify which preoperative pulmonary functional test was better at predicting postoperative pulmonary complications. We found that 14 patients showed flow limitation as detected by application of negative expiratory pressure during expiration. Furthermore, FEV$_1$, FVC, and FEV$_1$/FVC were only partially decreased in patients with flow limitation compared to those without flow limitation. On the contrary, patients with flow limitation showed a marked reduction in inspiratory capacity. No difference in end-expiratory volume was detected between patients with or without flow limitation. More interestingly, patients with flow limitation and reduced inspiratory capacity

were characterized by an increased rate of respiratory complications (12% vs. 35%), alterations in chest x-ray after 24 hours (10% vs. 55%), and prolonged intensive care unit (ICU) stay (1.2 vs. 6.4 days) in the postoperative period. Several studies have reported that, at least in patients with chronic obstructive pulmonary disease, commonly used pulmonary functional tests (i.e., FEV$_1$, FVC and FEV$_1$/FVC) are not related to exercise capability, whereas inspiratory capacity is related. Moreover, we should expect that the presence of intrinsic positive end-expiratory pressure (PEEP$_i$) is a major determinant of respiratory failure in the postoperative period, promoting an increase in the work of breathing, rapid shallow breathing, and consequent reduction in lung volume and atelectasis. This was explained by the fact that patients with increased PEEP$_i$ are more likely to show a reduction in inspiratory capacity, due to increased end-expiratory volume, than in other expiratory functional parameters (Fig. 27.2). In other words, the inspiratory capacity is more representative than expiratory parameters to detect the presence of PEEP$_i$, which is likely the major determinant of respiratory failure in the postoperative period. Thus, we hypothesize that morbidly obese patients are characterized by the presence or absence of flow limitation. Patients with flow limitation are more likely to present PEEP$_i$, but both flow limitation and PEEP$_i$ are not easily detected by common pulmonary functional tests.

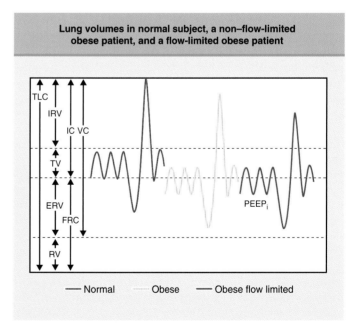

Lung volumes in normal subject, a non–flow-limited obese patient, and a flow-limited obese patient

— Normal   Obese   — Obese flow limited

Figure 27.2. Lung volumes in a normal subject, a non–flow-limited obese patient, and a flow-limited obese patient. The flow-limited obese patient maintains his or her own functional residual capacity (FRC) due to the presence of PEEP$_i$. In the absence of PEEP$_i$, the FRC would have further decreased, severely impairing respiratory function. PEEP$_i$ is likely one of the determinant of postoperative muscular fatigue and consequently may promote postoperative pulmonary complications. Patients with apparently normal FRC but decreased inspiratory capacity likely have elevated PEEP$_i$ and are at higher risk of postoperative pulmonary complications. ERV, expiratory reserve volume; IC, inspiratory capacity; IRV, inspiratory reserve volume; RV, residual volume; TLC, total lung capacity; TV, tidal volume.

Pulmonary Problems

We suggest that more attention should be given to inspiratory capacity as an easily available parameter able to detect indirectly the presence of flow limitation and PEEP$_i$. Inspiratory capacity, being related to PEEP$_i$, is likely very useful for predicting which patients will develop postoperative pulmonary complications.

RESPIRATORY FUNCTION IN THE INTRAOPERATIVE PERIOD

Body mass is an important determinant of respiratory function during anesthesia and paralysis not only in morbidly obese but also in moderately obese patients. Since obese patients have a respiratory condition that is physiologically poor, the morphological and functional variations of the respiratory system due to the induction and the maintenance of anesthesia and paralysis are more pronounced than in normal subjects.

Lung Volumes

The reduction in lung volumes is well associated with the increase in body mass. In morbidly obese patients, FRC decreases after induction of anesthesia to approximately 50% of preanesthesia levels (Damia and colleagues, 1988). Also, in healthy subjects the induction of anesthesia and paralysis leads to a decrease in FRC, and the magnitude of this reduction has been related to several individual factors, such as age, weight, and height. However, the mechanisms leading to FRC decrease during anesthesia are not completely understood. It is accepted that the main causes of the reduction in FRC during anesthesia and paralysis are atelectasis formation and blood shift from abdomen to thorax. The occurrence of atelectasis can be due to changes in the shape and motion of the diaphragm, the rib cage, or both, but it has been mainly ascribed to a decreased distribution of ventilation in the dependent lung regions during anesthesia and mechanical ventilation (i.e., the paravertebral regions in the supine position). The loss of diaphragmatic tone induced by anesthetics makes the diaphragm movement passively dependent. Because of a gravitational pressure gradient in the abdomen due to the presence of abdominal viscera, the distribution of ventilation is preferentially directed toward the nondependent lung regions. With an enhancement of body mass, an increase in intraabdominal pressure can occur (Pelosi and associates, 1997). The increased intra-abdominal pressure is mainly directed toward the most dependent lung regions with a more important cephalad displacement. This results in decreased movement of the dependent part of the diaphragm, where atelectasis is more likely to occur. When active, the ventilatory muscles counteract the intraabdominal pressure load toward the dependent diaphragm, limiting the negative effects on respiratory function. Therefore, removal of ventilatory muscle tone by anesthesia and muscle paralysis likely plays an important role in determining the reduction in FRC (Fig. 27.3). This preferential alteration of the diaphragm favors greater development of atelectasis in the dependent lung regions of the obese compared to in healthy subjects (Fig. 27.4).

Respiratory Mechanics

The alterations of respiratory mechanics that occur during anesthesia and paralysis are related to the extent of body mass. The decrease in compliance of the respiratory system with the

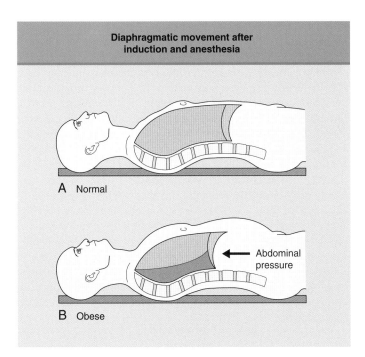

Figure 27.3. Diaphragmatic movement in a normal subject and an obese patient after induction of anesthesia. In the obese patient, the increase in intraabdominal pressure promotes a major cranial shift of the diaphragm associated with a marked reduction in the movement of the dependent part during ventilation favoring atelectasis formation.

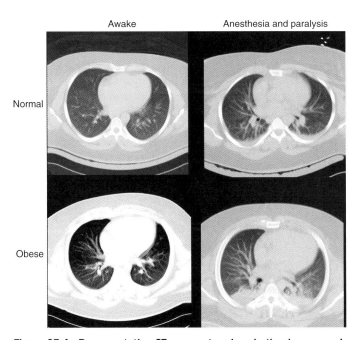

Figure 27.4. Representative CT scans at end-expiration in a normal subject and in an obese patient while awake and after anesthesia and paralysis. Note the impressive increase in atelectasis in the dependent lung regions in the obese patient.

increase of body mass is mainly determined by the reduction in lung compliance rather than in chest wall compliance. The more important factor for the decreased lung compliance is probably the reduction in FRC, since the intrinsic mechanic characteristic of lung parenchyma ("specific compliance") is nearly unchanged. Also, respiratory resistances are influenced by body mass mainly because of an increase in lung resistances. This is due to an increase in the airway resistance component, whereas the "viscoelastic" component is only weakly affected by body mass. However, the increase in airway resistance is mainly attributable to the reduction in lung volume since the specific resistances are relatively normal.

Gas Exchange

Oxygenation decreases with the increase in body mass. In fact, arterial hypoxemia, which characterizes awake obese patients, is worsened during anesthesia and paralysis. As previously discussed, these patients, different from normal subjects, are more predisposed with the induction of anesthesia to (1) the occurrence of pulmonary atelectasis and consequent shunt and (2) to an alteration of ventilation/perfusion ratio. The lung bases are underventilated because of airway closure and atelectasis, thus producing pulmonary "shunt" and hypoxemia. Even in obese patients without hypoventilation syndrome, the physiological dead space is increased compared to normal subjects during anesthesia (Hedenstierna and Svensson, 1976). Again, the severe reduction in FRC and an altered ventilation–perfusion mismatch may play a relevant role in determining the increased physiological dead space.

Respiratory Function and Prone Position

During surgery, the prone position is commonly used to expose the dorsal surface of the body for specific surgical indications. In anesthetized and paralyzed patients, the prone position ensuring free abdominal movements is not associated with adverse effects on respiratory function. However, as previously discussed, anesthesia and paralysis in obese patients may negatively affect respiratory function more than in normal subjects. Thus, it is generally recommended to avoid the prone position in obese patients when possible or to exercise extreme caution. We demonstrated that the prone position, in which the abdomen is free to move, increases FRC, lung compliance, and oxygenation. Thus, contrary to a common belief, the prone position in obese patients does not seem to have any adverse effects on pulmonary function. The increase in FRC in the prone position may be explained by a reduction of the cephalad displacement of the diaphragm and/or reopening of atelectatic segments. The prone position likely causes an unloading of the abdominal viscera, thus reducing the pressure on the diaphragm. The increase in FRC was paralleled by an increase in lung compliance and oxygenation.

The mechanisms by which the prone position improves oxygenation have not been fully elucidated. Proposed explanations include a prone position-induced increase in FRC, a change in regional diaphragm movements and a consequent change in regional ventilation, and a redistribution of perfusion along a gravitational gradient toward less atelectatic lung regions. However, as for normal subjects, we did not find any significant correlation between changes in FRC and oxygenation. Thus, the increase in FRC alone may not fully explain the improvement in oxygenation in the prone position. On the contrary, we found a good relationship between changes in chest wall compliance and variations in oxygenation: The greater the reduction in chest wall compliance between supine and prone, the greater the improvement in oxygenation. These findings suggest that the changes in regional mechanical properties of the chest wall, as previously reported also in patients with respiratory failure, may play a relevant role in determining a more homogeneous distribution of ventilation and improvement in oxygenation.

Intubating Obese Patients

A high degree of difficulty, requiring multiple attempts to obtain endotracheal intubation, is observed in a small number of patients. In 1% to 4% of patients, it is not possible to view the vocal cords, and failed intubation occurs in approximately 0.05% to 0.35% of patients. The highest incidence of intubation-related problems was found in obstetric and obese patients. Many factors can indicate difficulty of endotracheal intubation, such as dental configuration, extension of the atlanto-occipital joint, maxillary length and height, or limited mandible movements. Morbidly obese patients may present additional risk factors, such as an increased amount of soft tissue in the upper airways (leading to an increase in upper airway resistance), increased tongue size, large breasts (increasing the difficulty of direct laryngoscopy because there is little room between the breasts and the mouth for the handle of a conventional laryngoscope), and an increased neck circumference.

Moreover, as discussed previously, obese patients are characterized by an increased difficulty in oxygenation and mask ventilation. This is mainly due to a sharp decrease in lung volume with the induction of anesthesia, reduced compliance, and increased resistance (Damia and coworkers, 1988; Pelosi and coworkers, 1997). An additional difficulty in morbidly obese patients is the presence of an increased volume of gastric content, even after overnight fasting, which may favor pulmonary aspiration. On the basis of all these considerations, we believe that an endotracheal tube should be positioned when the patient is awake and in the reverse Trendelenburg position.

There are several reasons to choose this option:

1. Patients maintain patency of the natural airways and spontaneous breathing.
2. FRC is not reduced by anesthetics and muscle relaxants; thus, oxygenation is preserved.
3. Muscle tone maintains upper airway structures in the usual position so that they are much easier to identify.
4. Mask ventilation is not necessary.
5. The reverse Trendelenburg position allows maintenance of approximately physiological values of FRC, closing volumes, and gas exchange during the procedure. Moreover, this position improves the visual setting during intubation compared to the supine position.

Several techniques have been proposed for performing an awake intubation:

1. Blind nasal
2. Blind oral
3. Conventional direct laringoscopy
4. Fiberoptic intubation

One of the most popular methods of tracheal intubation of an awake patient is the blind nasotracheal route. This method has the advantage of being independent from visualization of the glottis and it has a good chance of success in a wide variety of patients of different age and body size. Unfortunately, in approximately 20% of patients it may cause upper airway bleeding, which could compromise subsequent fiberoptic efforts and is very uncomfortable. Similar techniques are described to perform blind orotracheal intubation: Under local anesthesia, a laryngeal mask airway is positioned and then a tracheal tube can be advanced possibly with the support of a gum elastic guide. Among the intubation techniques, conventional direct laryngoscopy is perhaps the most distressing for patients and requires a high level of cooperation. Fiberoptic intubation can be performed using either the oral or the nasal route, and the only major impediment is the presence of a significant amount of blood or secretions that can interfere with the visualization of vocal cords. Briefly, in this technique, a well-lubricated flexible fiberoptic laryngoscope is inserted into an endotracheal tube and then advanced through the nose or the mouth. Once the fiberoptic laryngoscope has been passed into the trachea, the endotracheal tube can be railroaded over the fiberoscope and properly positioned under direct vision with the tip above the tracheal carine. The fiberoptic laryngoscope can be withdrawn, the endotracheal tube connected to the breathing circuit, and general anesthesia induced. Numerous devices have been proposed to aid fiberoptic intubation through the mouth; all of them are designed to bring the tip of the instrument close to the laryngeal aperture without requiring much skill. The patient should be in the anti-Trendelenburg position to avoid the possible negative effects of the supine position on respiratory function.

Our experience related to fiberoptic intubation in morbidly obese patients (Croci and Pelosi) refers to 115 patients (29 male; age, 34 ± 8 years; BMI, 47 ± 5 kg/m^2) receiving general anesthesia for elective surgery (gastroplasty or jejunal bypass) in the Policlinico Hospital. The patients were intubated using a flexible fiberoptic laryngoscope. We decided to use small endotracheal tubes (7-mm ID in female and 7.5-mm ID in male patients), although if the anesthetist decides to position a larger

tube, it is possible to use a flexible, spiral wound endotracheal tube. The average time to perform intubation was 65 ± 30 seconds. No major complications were observed, such as hypoxemia (defined as oxygen saturation lower than 90%), hypotension (defined as systolic pressure lower than 90 mm Hg), aspiration of gastric content, or failed intubation (defined as required change of technique). Unfortunately, this technique is referred to as unpleasant by 17% of patients. However, fiberoptic intubation attenuates or abolishes the hypertensive response usually observed during conventional laryngoscopy.

Fiberoptic intubation was performed under local anesthesia and a slight sedation (benzodiazepines and opioids) that did not result in unconsciousness (the patients were always able to spontaneously breathe and obey simple orders). However, comparative studies between conventional intubation techniques and fiberoptic laryngoscopy are lacking.

We conducted a prospective controlled trial to compare conventional intubation techniques with fiberoptic intubation in morbidly obese patients. The study was performed at three different hospitals: Policlinico Hospital, Milan (Croci and Pelosi); S. Orsola Policlinico Hospital, Bologna (Fusari); and Gemelli Policlinico Hospital, Rome (Sollazzi). We investigated 30 patients (4 males; age, 40.3 ± 11.8 years; BMI, 48.8 ± 6.8 kg/m^2) divided into three groups of 10 patients each: group 1, conventional intubation using propofol and a depolarizing neuromuscular blocker (succinylcholine); group 2, conventional intubation using propofol and a nondepolarizing neuromuscular blocker (vecuronium bromide); and group 3, fiberoptic intubation as described previously. The main results are shown in Table 27.1. We found that

1. The time required to perform intubation was slightly longer in the fiberoptic group compared to conventional groups (100.9 ± 43.9 vs. 31.9 ± 26.2 and 75.0 ± 35.9 sec, respectively).
2. The frequency of attempted intubations (more than one and requiring a new complete sequence of intubation) was greater in the conventional groups than in the fiberoptic one (5/10 and 6/10 vs. 0/10, respectively).
3. The presence of at least one episode of artery saturation lower than 90% during induction procedure was more

Table 27.1 Comparison between Fiberoptic Intubation and Conventional Intubation Techniques (Succinylcholine and Vecuronium) in Morbidly Obese Patients[a]

Parameter	Group 1 (Fiberoptic)	Group 2 (Succinylcholine)	Group 3 (Vecuronium)	P
No. of patients	10	10	10	
Sex (male/female)	2/8	0/10	2/8	n.s.
Age (years)	42.7 ± 9.7	35.2 ± 10.3	43.0 ± 14.5	n.s.
BMI (kg/m^2)	48.4 ± 7.0	49.7 ± 7.6	48.3 ± 6.4	n.s.
Intubation time (sec)	100.9 ± 43.9	31.9 ± 26.2	75.0 ± 35.9	<0.01
Attempts > 1	0/10	5/10	6/10	<0.01
Sato$_2$ ≤ 90%	0/10	3/10	4/10	<0.01
Pao$_2$ < 100 mm Hg	0/10	3/10	6/10	<0.01
Pao$_2$ > 45 mm Hg	0/10	5/10	6/10	<0.01
PA$_{max}$ − PA$_{basal}$ (mm Hg)	14.9 ± 3.0	52.0 ± 23.2	43.5 ± 26.9	<0.01
HR$_{max}$ − HR$_{basal}$ (bpm)	11.6 ± 4.7	23.1 ± 7.4	28.8 ± 14.2	<0.01

[a]Data expressed as mean ± SD or as the ratio of the number of patients with the events and the total number of patients.
HR, heart rate; n.s., not significant.

frequent in the conventional groups compared to the fiberoptic one (3/10 and 4/10 vs. 0/10, respectively).

4. Oxygenation levels lower than 100 mm Hg immediately after intubation were more frequent in the conventional groups compared to the fiberoptic one (3/10 and 6/10 vs. 0/10, respectively).

5. The frequency of $PaCO_2$ levels higher than 45 mm Hg at the moment of intubation was greater in the conventional groups compared to the fiberoptic one (5/10 and 6/10 vs. 0/10, respectively).

6. The ranges of arterial pressures and heart rate changes were greater in the conventional groups compared to the fiberoptic one (52.0 ± 23.2 and 43.5 ± 26.9 vs. 14.9 ± 3.0 mm Hg, respectively, and 23.1 ± 7.4 and 28.8 ± 14.2 vs. 11.6 ± 4.7 bpm, respectively).

From this study, we concluded that fiberoptic intubation may be superior for maintaining respiratory function compared to conventional intubation with depolarizing or nondepolarizing neuromuscular blockers.

Thus, awake fiberoptic intubation is a safe and useful technique in morbidly obese patients receiving general anesthesia. However, more prospective controlled or randomized trials are warranted to better define the specific role of awake fiberoptic intubation in morbidly obese patients.

The use of videolaryngoscope has been proposed as an intubation technique in morbidly obese subjects. The videolaryngoscope is a conventional laryngoscope that is equipped with a fiberoptic at the tip of the laryngoscope, which allows a better view of the larynx, with consequent improvement in the intubation technique. In general, with a videolaryngoscope it is possible to gain at least 1 or 2 points on the Cormack scale in the intubation view. A study was conducted to evaluate the effectiveness of the videolaryngoscope technique to improve intubation in morbidly obese patients. In this study, 80 morbidly obese patients were evaluated and randomized to conventional or videolaryngoscopic technique. It was found that the use of videolaryngoscope resulted in a reduction in the time required for intubation and the number of intubation attempts. Furthermore, with videolaryngoscope better oxygenation was maintained during intubation. When encountering difficulties with intubation, some physicians apply the Fast-Trach intubating laryngeal mask, which has a rigid handle over which a special endotracheal tube can be placed. Frequently, this is very easy and it is associated with high success rates (Langeron and colleagues, 2000). When "blind" placement of the tube over the laryngeal mask is not feasible, the tube can be put on the fiberscope and directed through the vocal cords.

Another technical improvement with regard to intubation of morbidly obese patients is the use of continuous positive airway pressure (CPAP) during the preoxygenation period and induction of anesthesia (Coussa and associates, 2004). It has been shown that the use of CPAP (10 cm H_2O) prevented atelectasis formation and prolonged the "apnea" time (i.e., the time required to reach a saturation of 90% after induction of anesthesia and paralysis with 100% oxygen).

Thus, the combination of CPAP in the peri-intubation period and the use of the videolaryngoscope may be the easiest and most comfortable alternative technique to fiberoptic intubation in morbidly obese patients.

Ventilating Obese Patients

Increased intra-abdominal pressure seems to play a relevant role in the reduction of FRC, which seems to be the prevalent phenomenon in obese patients, resulting in a decrease in respiratory compliance and oxygenation. This suggests the occurrence of relevant collapse and lung-dependent atelectasis.

To approach the respiratory system alterations that occur in these patients, different modalities of ventilation have been proposed:

1. High inspiratory oxygen fractions
2. Ventilation using tidal volumes as high as 15 to 20 mL/kg ideal body weight
3. Inclusion of large, manually or automatically performed lung inflations (sighs)
4. Application of PEEP after a recruitment maneuver (Pelosi and coworkers, 1999)

The superiority of one or more of these different ventilatory settings in comparative studies has not been investigated.

As a consequence of respiratory modifications induced by general anesthesia and paralysis, the main aim of mechanical ventilation in obese patients is to "keep the lung open" during the entire respiratory circle. This counteracts negative effects induced by the increased body mass and the high intraabdominal pressure (airway closure, atelectasis, and impaired respiratory mechanics and oxygenation) that occur in the intraoperative period but that can persist for a few days in the postoperative period.

The use of low tidal volumes (and, as a consequence, low alveolar ventilation) and high inspired oxygen fraction (FIO_2) greater than 0.8 should be avoided since it has been clearly shown that this may lead to the formation of progressive reabsorption atelectasis.

The use of continuously high tidal volumes (>13 mL/kg ideal body weight) seems to be ineffective to further improve oxygenation, whereas it can induce hypocapnia if respiratory rate is not decreased. Moreover, the continuous use of high tidal volumes even during anesthesia can be deleterious to the lung structure and hemodynamics.

To ventilate a lung with a tendency to collapse, one must provide inspiratory pressure to open the collapsed lung regions (recruitment pressure), a PEEP high enough to keep the lung open at end expiration associated with low tidal volumes, and FIO_2 lower than 0.8.

Adequate opening pressure can be obtained by applying periodic large, manually performed lung inflations (recruitment maneuvers) (Pelosi and associates, 1999). Since morbidly obese patients are characterized by an increased intraabdominal pressure and reduced chest wall compliance, only 60% of the pressure applied at the airways is transmitted as transpulmonary pressure to inflate the lung (increasing the pressure needed to inflate the chest wall). Thus, to achieve a transpulmonary pressure sufficient to reopen collapsed alveoli, airway pressures up to 60 cm H_2O are necessary. On the other hand, an increased airway pressure application for a relatively short period of time (6 sec) is recommended to avoid negative effects on hemodynamics as much as possible. The recruitment maneuver should be performed only when volemic and hemodynamic stabilization is reached after induction of anesthesia. The recruitment maneuver should be repeated every 30 minutes in the absence of PEEP. The application of periodic hyperinflations (sighs) may also be beneficial, providing sufficient inspiratory pressures to reopen the lung and sufficient alveolar ventilation to avoid the formation of reabsorption atelectasis.

The role of PEEP in anesthesia is controversial: In fact, different studies report different results in oxygenation response in different patient populations and clinical conditions. This is likely due to the opposite effects induced by PEEP on oxygenation in different patients. PEEP can resolve atelectasis, if present, and prevent small airways collapse, improving ventilation–perfusion matching and oxygenation. On the other hand, increasing PEEP may lead to negative effects on ventilation–perfusion ratio and pulmonary shunt if alveolar overstretching and cardiac output reduction or redistribution become the prevalent phenomena. The final effect on oxygenation of PEEP application depends on the balance between positive and negative effects in any given patient. We found that applying 10 cm H_2O of PEEP during anesthesia and paralysis induced an oxygenation improvement in morbidly obese patients but not in normal subjects (Pelosi and coworkers, 1999). Moreover, we found that the partitioned pressure–volume curves measured at a PEEP of 0 and 10 cm H_2O roughly followed the same pattern in normal subjects, whereas in obese patients the pressure–volume curves at 10 cm H_2O PEEP were shifted upward and to the left, suggesting the occurrence of alveolar recruitment. The amount of alveolar recruitment was also related to the improvement in oxygenation.

Thus, we believe that during general anesthesia, morbidly obese patients should be ventilated with physiologic tidal volumes (6–10 mL per ideal body weight) and a respiratory rate to maintain normocapnia. In addition, an application of 10 cm H_2O PEEP after a recruitment maneuver associated with an FIO_2 between 0.4 and 0.8 is recommended. Further studies are needed to define the optimal levels of PEEP and tidal volume during general anesthesia in obese patients, to open and keep open the lung, improving oxygenation and respiratory mechanics.

MANAGING PREANESTHESIA AND ANESTHESIA

Obese patients pose a number of problems in the perioperative period relative to drug administration. Possible interactions of medications used to treat obesity with drugs used during anesthesia must be considered. Furthermore, the volume of distribution of drugs may be altered since fat contains less water than other tissues, leading to decreases in total body water content in obese patients. Premedication is characterized by drugs aimed at slightly sedating the patient to achieve better comfort and improve efficiency during anesthesia induction, obtaining an antisialagogue effect to improve clinical condition at the moment of intubation, and reducing the risk of inhalation of gastric contents at the moment of intubation by using prokinetics and antiacid drugs. Several drugs have been suggested to sedate obese patients preoperatively, among which midazolam and morphine have been found to be similarly effective. In particular, midazolam can be effectively given by different routes, such as oral, sublingual, or intramuscular, with comparable effects. Midazolam has been reported to be more effective than diazepam. However, midazolam can cause intraoperative

hypothermia, but the combination with atropine prevents midazolam-induced core hypothermia. It is evident that a combination with benzodiazepine and atropine as premedication is the most recommended choice. Obese patients have an increased incidence of gastroesophageal reflux and hiatal hernia. Furthermore, gastric acidity, gastric fluid volume, and intragastric pressure are increased. However, some studies have reported normal pH in obesity. Gastric emptying has been reported to be delayed in some studies but normal in others. Preoperative administration of an H_2 receptor antagonist can be used to increase gastric fluid pH; however, it has been associated with an increase in bacterial colonization but not infections. Also, the efficacy of metoclopramide to improve gastric emptying has been questioned. In general, it appears that administration of anti-H_2 and/or metoclopramide is not generally recommended in premedication.

The best drugs or technique for maintenance of anesthesia in obese patients have not been defined. The high incidence of fatty liver infiltration must be appreciated when selecting volatile anesthetics. The possibility of prolonged responses to drugs stored in fat, including volatile anesthetics, opioids, and barbiturates, should be considered in obese patients. Different techniques have been proposed, such as total intravenous anesthesia with propofol and opioids (alfentanil, fentanil, and remifentanil); inhalation anesthesia with isoflurane, desflurane or sevoflurane; and balanced anesthesia (intravenous associated with inhalation anesthesia). In general, it has been suggested that a balanced anesthesia with sevoflurane or desflurane associated with remifentanil and cisatracurium as paralyzing agent is the combination of choice to achieve a better depth of anesthesia, better hemodynamics, more rapid wash-in and wash-out (recovery), more rapid patient movements, and better oxygenation in the postoperative period.

Spinal and epidural anesthesia may be technically difficult in obese patients because bony landmarks are obscured. Increased epidural pressure secondary to engorged epidural veins makes predictability of anesthetic level difficult. It is prudent to reduce initial doses of local anesthetics used for regional anesthesia when body weight is greatly increased due to excess adipose tissue.

RESPIRATORY FUNCTION IN THE POSTOPERATIVE PERIOD

Respiratory function is dramatically altered in the postoperative period. Both upper abdominal and thoracic surgery result in a postoperative pulmonary restrictive syndrome. This restriction of pulmonary function may persist for several days, leading to a high incidence of postoperative pulmonary complications such as sputum retention, atelectasis, and bronchopulmonary infection, even in the absence of a previous demonstrable intrinsic lung disease. These complications produce further worsening of pulmonary function and cause secondary hypoxemia. Several factors may be involved in modifying ventilatory function during the postoperative period, such as reflex inhibition of the phrenic nerve, anesthesia, and postoperative pain.

In a group of morbidly obese patients, respiratory function was compared to that of normal subjects in the immediate postoperative period after abdominal intervention. In this series of patients, we found a pronounced reduction in FRC compared to that in normal subjects; FRC was approximately one-third the normal value. Considering the compliance of the respiratory system partitioned into its lung and chest wall components, we found that the reduction in respiratory system compliance was caused by a decrease in both lung and chest wall compliance.

Reduced chest wall compliance may be due to an increased adiposity around the ribs, diaphragm, and abdomen, limited movements of the ribs caused by thoracic kyphosis, and lumbar hyperlordosis from excessive abdominal fat content. Another possible cause is that the decreased total thoracic and pulmonary volume may pull the chest wall below its resting level and therefore to a flatter portion of its pressure–volume curve. However, the most likely cause of the reduction in chest wall compliance during the postoperative period is the increased intraabdominal pressure, which prevents, at least in part, the diaphragm from freely moving and affects the shape of the upper and lower thorax. Other abnormalities in respiratory function during the postoperative period are a reduction in the effectiveness of gas exchange, strictly dependent on the decreased lung volumes, and an increase in work of breathing, mainly resulting from a reduction in lung and chest wall compliance and high pulmonary resistances.

Particular attention should be given to the late phase of anesthesia, before extubation. Three main factors can lead to a progressive reduction of lung volumes and atelectasis formation during the extubation period: the supine position, aspiration inside the tube before and during extubation, and the use of a high oxygen fraction (1.0). Some studies have reported that aspiration inside the endotracheal tube associated with high oxygen fraction can lead to atelectasis formation and bronchoconstriction. Furthermore, these atelectases are present and maintained even in the postoperative period (Eichenberger and colleagues, 2002). Thus, we suggest that 10 minutes before planned extubation the patient should be positioned in the reverse Trendelenburg position (35°) and secretions from the airways should be aspirated; immediately after extubation, a recruitment maneuver should be performed to reduce the FIO_2 to 0.4 to 0.6. PEEP should be maintained until extubation, whereas no aspiration should be performed inside the tube during extubation.

Based on the previously discussed data, we support the hypothesis that marked derangement in FRC, elastic (reduction in lung and chest wall compliance), and resistive (increase in lung resistance) components of the respiratory system may account for the significant respiratory dysfunction and arterial hypoxemia that occur in the postoperative period. Figure 27.5 presents the physiologic determinants of postoperative impairment in respiratory function in morbidly obese patients. It is evident that both intraoperative and postoperative atelectasis play a crucial role in promoting postoperative pulmonary complications.

Managing Obese Patients in the Postoperative Period

All these alterations can explain the higher incidence of postoperative pulmonary complications in obese compared to nonobese patients. To reduce postoperative pulmonary complications, different techniques and treatments have been proposed, such as chest physiotherapy, incentive spirometry, and intermittent positive pressure breathing. Some authors have

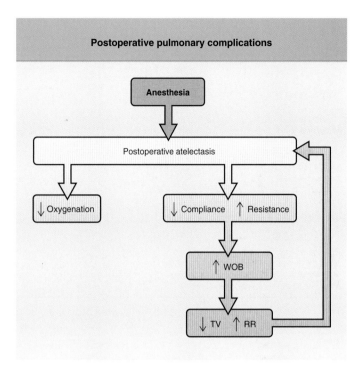

Figure 27.5. Postoperative pulmonary complications. Atelectasis during surgery and in the postoperative period is a major determinant of impairment in respiratory function. RR, respiratory rate; TV, tidal volume; WOB, work of breathing.

proposed the use of CPAP or bilevel positive airway pressure administered by noninvasive techniques during the first 24 hours of the postoperative period.

We believe that CPAP is the easiest method of respiratory assistance compared to ventilation, especially if performed in the ward or in the surgical department. CPAP should be administered in the postoperative period when the PaO_2/FIO_2 ratio falls below 300, and it should be maintained for a prolonged period during the day. The use of the helmet instead of the mask can improve the efficacy of the treatment and the comfort of the patient. The aim is to give a ventilatory support to more rapidly restore lung volumes to the preoperative values, improving oxygenation and reducing work of breathing. Moreover, for several days after surgery, patients should remain in a semirecumbent position (30–45°) to reduce the abdominal pressure on the diaphragm. Thus, a more physiological approach to respiratory treatment in the postoperative period may be useful for improving respiratory outcome.

The role of preventive admission of morbidly obese patients undergoing abdominal surgery into ICUs during the postoperative period is not yet defined (Marik and Varon, 1988). Some advantages of ICU admission are a gentler weaning from the ventilator, chest physiotherapy and noninvasive ventilatory treatment can be easily performed, optimized fluid treatment, and more careful pain control. On the other hand, there are increased costs and more difficulties in organizing the schedule of the surgical operations.

To define the role of preventive ICU admission in the postoperative morbidly obese patients, we compared the incidence of postoperative pulmonary complications and mortality in 38

Table 27.2 Postoperative Pulmonary Complications and Mortality in Obese Patients Admitted or Not Admitted to the ICU

	No. of Patients	BMI (kg/m²)	Age (years)	PPC (%)	Mortality (%)
No ICU admission					
Vaughan (1975)	70	—	—	—	5.7
Postlethwait (1972)	46	142[a]	34	0	—
Vaughan (1974)	17	147[a]	36	47	0
Fox (1981)	110	135[a]	35	21.8	0
Hall (1991)	102	>25.0	54	26.5	0
Brooks-Brunn (1997)	181	28.5	58	29.3	0
Total	**526**	—	**48**	**24.6**	**0.8**
ICU admission					
Our experience	**38**	**48.5**	**37**	**7.9**[b]	**0**

[a]Weight (kg).
[b]$P < 0.05$ vs no ICU admission.
PPC, postoperative pulmonary complications.

morbidly obese patients (18 males; age, 37.5 ± 9.9 years; BMI, 48.5 ± 6.6 kg/m²) admitted to our ICU after abdominal surgery between 1993 and 1998 to historical controls who were not admitted to the ICU in the postoperative period. The mean age, BMI, and abdominal surgery were comparable between groups.

After the surgical procedures (20 gastric binding and 18 jejunoileal bypass), all patients were admitted to the ICU for the postoperative treatment, intubated, and mechanically ventilated. The fluid treatment was titrated to achieve a diuresis higher than 0.5 mL/hr/kg ideal body weight, and antibiotic treatment was given for 2 or 3 days after surgery. Patients were mechanically ventilated with synchronized intermittent mechanical ventilation and pressure support to achieve a tidal volume of 13 mL/kg of ideal body weight and $PaCO_2$ within normal range, with a PEEP level set to give the "best oxygenation" (a PaO_2 increase of at least 10 mm Hg). Patients were successively weaned from the ventilator at first by reducing FIO_2 to obtain a PaO_2 of 90 to 100 mm Hg at FIO_2 40% and then by progressively reducing PEEP and ventilatory support. We performed extubation when the following criteria were satisfied: (1) FVC higher than 1 liter, (2) spontaneous unassisted tidal volume higher than 400 mL, (3) spontaneous respiratory rate lower than 25 breaths per minute, (4) PaO_2 higher than 80 mm Hg at 30% FIO_2 during spontaneous breathing and hemodynamic stability, and (5) no clinical or laboratory signs of infection.

In this population of morbidly obese patients, we evaluated the incidence of postoperative pulmonary complications, defined as the new occurrence of three or more of the following signs or symptoms: cough, positive sputum culture, dyspnea, chest pain or discomfort, fever (temperature higher than 38°C), tachycardia (more than 100 bpm), and positive chest x-ray (atelectasis, abnormal hemidiaphragm elevation, new pleural effusion, and new infiltrate).

As reported in Table 27.2, the incidence of postoperative pulmonary complications was significantly lower in obese patients admitted to the ICU compared to the population of historical controls who were not admitted to the ICU in the immediate postoperative period. Prospective randomized studies are needed to better define the role of the ICU in the treatment of morbidly obese patients in the postoperative period.

Box 27.1 Perioperative Ventilatory and Anesthesia Management in Morbidly Obese Patients

Premedication

Midazolam oral or sublingual
Atropine intramuscular

Intubation

Fiberoptic intubation, with light associated sedation with remifentanil if necessary
Conventional intubation by using a videolaryngoscope, with continuous PEEP of 10 cm H_2O and FIO_2 of 1.0

Mechanical Ventilation during Surgery

Tidal volume 6 to 10 mL/kg IBW and respiratory rate to maintain normocapnia
Recruitment maneuver (40–60 cm H_2O, 6 sec, three times in pressure or volume control) once hemodynamic stability has been obtained and volemia is stable after induction of anesthesia
Application of PEEP 10 cm H_2O, always after a recruitment maneuver
Reverse Trendelenburg position (35°) when possible
FIO_2 between 0.4 and 0.8

Ten minutes before planned extubation

Keep the patient in reverse Trendelenburg position.
Reduce FIO_2 to 0.4, if possible.
Aspirate airways secretions.
Perform a recruitment maneuver as described previously.
Keep 10 cm H_2O PEEP until extubation.
Do not aspirate inside the endotracheal tube during extubation.

Anesthesia and Paralysis

Anesthesia should be maintained with desflurane or sevoflurane in association with remifentanil.
Muscle paralysis should be maintained with cisatracurium.

Postoperative Period

Keep seated position as early as possible.
Perform chest physiotherapy aggressively.
Apply CPAP by helmet or mask if PaO_2/FIO_2 falls below 300.

Box 27.1 summarizes the overall management of ventilation in the perioperative period, as well as that of anesthesia, to avoid as much as possible atelectasis formation and postoperative pulmonary complications.

CONCLUSION

The important alterations in the respiratory function of morbidly obese patients in the perioperative period may play a significant role in determining pulmonary complications in the intra- and postoperative period. In morbidly obese patients, adequate ventilatory settings aimed at keeping the lung open during surgery and in the postoperative period associated with ICU admission may help to reduce the incidence of postoperative pulmonary complications.

Acknowledgments

We are indebted to the daily clinical work on obese patients performed by physicians and nurses in the ICU at Policlinico Hospital of Milan. We thank Dr. M. Croci, who was involved in the treatment of these patients for many years, and Dr. M. Fusari (S. Orsola Policlinico Hospital, Bologna) and Dr. L. Sollazzi (Gemelli Policlinico Hospital, Rome) for their active participation in the prospective controlled trial on fiberoptic intubation in obese patients. We are also indebted to Prof. G. Hedenstierna and the anesthesiological team (Drs. F. Henrick and F. Reinius) from the University of Uppsala, Sweden, for valuable discussions about atelectasis formation in obese patients and for permission to present the CT scan images.

SUGGESTED READING

Brooks-Brunn JA: Predictors of postoperative pulmonary complications following abdominal surgery. Chest 1997;111:564–571.

Coussa M, Proietti S, Schnyder P, et al: Prevention of atelectasis formation during the induction of general anesthesia in morbidly obese patients. Anesth Analg 2004;98:1491–1497.

Damia G, Mascheroni D, Croci M, Tarenzi L: Perioperative changes in functional residual capacity in morbidly obese patients. Br J Anesth 1988;60:574–578.

Eichenberger A, Proietti S, Wicky S, et al: Morbid obesity and postoperative pulmonary atelectasis: An underestimated problem. Anesth Analg 2002;95:1788–1792.

Fox GS, Whalley DG, Bevan DR: Anesthesia for the morbidly obese. Experience with 110 patients. Br J Anaesth 1981;53:811–816.

Hall JC, Torala RA, Hall JL, Mauder J: A multivariate analysis of the risk of pulmonary complications after laparotomy. Chest 1991;99:923–927.

Hedenstierna G, Svensson J: Breathing mechanics, dead space and gas exchange in the extremely obese, breathing spontaneously and during anesthesia with intermittent positive pressure ventilation. Acta Anaesth Scand 1976;20:248–254.

Langeron O, Masso E, Huraux C, et al:. Prediction of difficult mask intubation. Anesthesiology. 2000;92:1229–1236.

Marik P, Varon J: The obese patients in the ICU. Chest 1988;113:492–498.

Pelosi P, Croci M, Ravagnan I, et al: Respiratory system mechanics in anesthetized, paralyzed, morbidly obese patients. J Appl Physiol 1997;82: 811–818.

Pelosi P, Ravagnan I, Giurati G, et al:. Positive end-expiratory pressure improves respiratory function in obese patients but not in normal subjects during anesthesia and paralysis. Anesthesiology 1999;91:1221–1231.

Postlethwait RW, Johnson WD: Complications following surgery for duodenal ulcer in obese patients. Arch Surg 1972;105:438–440.

Rochester DF. Obesity and abdominal distention. In Roussos C (ed): The Thorax, Part C: Disease, 2nd ed. New York, Dekker, pp 1951–1973, 1995.

Smetana GM: Preoperative pulmonary evaluation. N Engl J Med 1999;340: 937–940.

Vaughan RW: Anesthetic considerations in jejunoileal small bowel bypass for morbid obesity. Anesth Analg 1974;53:421–429.

Vaughan RW, Wise L: Postoperative arterial blood gas measurement in obese patients: Effect of position on gas exchange. Ann Surg 1975;182: 705–709.

Chapter 28
Neuromuscular Respiratory Failure

Theodoros Vassilakopoulos and Charis Roussos

KEY POINTS

- Neuromuscular respiratory failure is more common than recognized and may result in substantial morbidity, mortality, and costs.
- In ICU patients, neuromuscular dysfunction may be reduced by avoiding neuromuscular blocking agents and by scheduling frequent drug "holidays" with clear evidence of recovery from neuromuscular blockade.
- Limiting the use of controlled mechanical ventilation will reduce ventilator-induced diaphragmatic dysfunction (VIDD).

INTRODUCTION

Neuromuscular diseases may affect the respiratory muscles. When they do, they cause hypercapnic and/or hypoxemic respiratory failure. Neuromuscular respiratory failure is a potentially fatal situation. Despite medical therapy, which is available in some but not all disorders leading to neuromuscular respiratory failure, mechanical ventilation is inevitable on many occasions. In fact, in many situations where no therapy exists, mechanical ventilation is the only solution until the natural repair processes "cure" the underlying disease.

EPIDEMIOLOGY, RISK FACTORS, AND PATHOPHYSIOLOGY

Epidemiology

Neuromuscular diseases, particularly poliomyelitis in the early 1950s, were the major reason for the development of mechanical ventilation and, indeed, of intensive care units (ICUs). Although poliomyelitis has been largely eliminated by immunization, a large number of neuromuscular disorders may lead to respiratory failure. The magnitude of the clinical problem of patients with neuromuscular disease and respiratory dysfunction is truly unknown. Neuromuscular dysfunction is associated with difficulty in separating from mechanical ventilation, increased hospital costs, and increased mortality.

Risk Factors

Given the vast number of diseases that can lead to neuromuscular respiratory failure, the risk factors are not common to all but are those of the specific underlying disorder.

Pathophysiology

Weakness of any of three muscle groups—inspiratory, expiratory, and bulbar—can lead to neuromuscular respiratory failure. Inspiratory muscle weakness can result in hypoventilation, respiratory acidosis, coma, and death from carbon dioxide narcosis. Expiratory muscle weakness results in inability to generate effective cough flows and in the accumulation of airway secretions. This most often occurs during intercurrent upper respiratory tract infections and results in atelectasis, pneumonia, and acute hypoxemic respiratory failure. Apart from loss of phonation and the ability to swallow, bulbar muscle weakness can cause the loss of the ability to protect the airway from aspiration of oral secretions and can result in airway collapse during breathing or coughing. Aspiration of secretions or food and airway collapse result in pneumonia and hypoxemic respiratory failure. Quite often neuromuscular diseases can simultaneously affect all three muscle groups, leading to both hypercapnic and hypoxemic respiratory failure.

Inspiratory Muscle Dysfunction

To take a spontaneous breath, the inspiratory muscles must generate sufficient force to overcome the elastance of the lungs and the chest wall (lung and chest wall elastic loads) as well as the airway and tissue resistance (resistive load). This requires an adequate output by the centers controlling the muscles, anatomic and functional nerve integrity, unimpaired neuromuscular transmission, an intact chest wall, and adequate muscle strength. This can be schematically represented by considering the ability to take a breath as a balance between inspiratory load and neuromuscular competence (Fig. 28.1). Under normal conditions, this system is polarized in favor of neuromuscular competence, i.e., there are reserves that permit a considerable increase in load. However, for a human to breathe spontaneously, the inspiratory muscles should be able to sustain the above-mentioned load over time and also adjust the minute ventilation in such a way that there is adequate gas exchange. The ability of the respiratory muscles to sustain this load without the appearance of fatigue is called "endurance" and is determined by the balance between energy supplies (Us) and energy demands (Ud) (Fig. 28.2). Energy supplies depend on the inspiratory muscle blood flow, the blood substrate (fuel) concentration and arterial oxygen content, the muscle's ability to extract and utilize energy sources, and the muscle's energy stores. Under normal circumstances, energy supplies are adequate to meet the demands and a large recruitable reserve exists. Energy demands increase proportionally with the mean tidal pressure developed by the inspiratory muscles (P_I), expressed as a

Pulmonary Problems

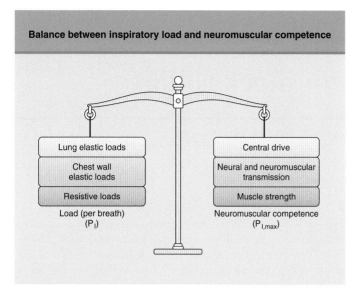

Figure 28.1. Balance between inspiratory load and neuromuscular competence. The ability to take a spontaneous breath is determined by the balance between the load imposed upon the respiratory system (pressure developed by the inspiratory muscles; P_I) and the neuromuscular competence of the ventilatory pump (maximum inspiratory pressure; $P_{I,max}$). Normally, this balance weighs in favor of competence, permitting significant increases in load. However, if the competence is, for whatever reason, reduced below a critical point (e.g., drug overdose, myasthenia gravis), the balance may then weigh in favor of load, rendering the ventilatory pump insufficient to inflate the lungs and chest wall.

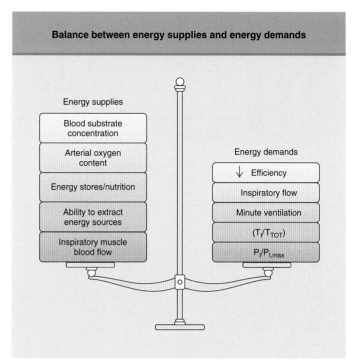

Figure 28.2. Balance between energy supplies and energy demands. Respiratory muscle endurance is determined by the balance between energy supplies and demands. Normally, the supplies meet the demands and a large reserve exists. Whenever this balance weighs in favour of demands, the respiratory muscles ultimately become fatigued, leading to inability to sustain spontaneous breathing decreased; VT/tI: mean inspiratory flow (tidal volume/inspiratory time); tI/ttot: duty cycle (fraction of inspiration to total breathing cycle duration); PI/PI,max, inspiratory pressure/maximum inspiratory pressure ratio; V'E, minute ventilation.

fraction of maximum inspiratory pressure ($P_I/P_{I,max}$), the minute ventilation (V'E), the inspiratory duty cycle (T_I/T_{TOT}), and the mean inspiratory flow rate (V_T/T_I), and are inversely related to the efficiency of the muscles. "Fatigue" develops when the mean rate of energy demands (Ud) exceeds the mean rate of energy supply (Us) (i.e., when the balance is polarized in favor of demands).

$$Ud > Us \Rightarrow W/E > Us$$

where W is the mean muscle power and E is the efficiency.

The product of T_I/T_{tot} and the mean transdiaphragmatic pressure expressed as a fraction of maximal transdiaphragmatic pressure (Pdi/Pdi,max) defines a useful "tension time index" (TTIdi) that is related to the endurance time (i.e., the time that the diaphragm can sustain the load imposed on it). Whenever TTIdi is smaller than the critical value of 0.15, the load can be sustained indefinitely; but when TTIdi exceeds the critical zone of 0.15–0.18, the load can be sustained for only a limited time period, in other words, the endurance time. This was found to be inversely related to TTIdi. The TTI concept is assumed to be applicable not only to the diaphragm but to the respiratory muscles as a whole:

$$TTI = P_I/P_{I,max} \times T_I/T_{TOT}$$

Because, as we have stated, the balance between energy supply and demand determines endurance, TTI of the inspiratory muscles has to be in accordance with the energy balance

view. $P_I/P_{I,max}$ and T_I/T_{TOT}, which constitute the TTI, are among the determinants of energy demands; an increase in either that will increase the TTI value will also increase the demands. The energy balance may then weigh in favor of demands, leading to fatigue.

But what determines the ratio $P_I/P_{I,max}$? The nominator, the mean inspiratory pressure, is determined by the elastic and resistive loads imposed on the inspiratory muscles. The denominator, the maximum inspiratory pressure, is determined by the neuromuscular competence, that is, the maximum inspiratory muscle activation that can be achieved. It follows, then, that the value of $P_I/P_{I,max}$ is determined by the balance between load and competence. But $P_I/P_{I,max}$ is also one of the determinants of energy demands; therefore, the two balances, that is, between load and competence and energy supply and demand, are in essence linked, creating a system (Fig. 28.3). Schematically, when the central hinge of the system moves upward, or is at least at the horizontal level, a balance between ventilatory needs and neurorespiratory capacity exists and spontaneous ventilation can be sustained indefinitely.

One can see that the ability of a subject to breathe spontaneously depends on the fine interplay of many different factors. Normally, this interplay moves the central hinge far upward and creates a great ventilatory reserve for the healthy individual.

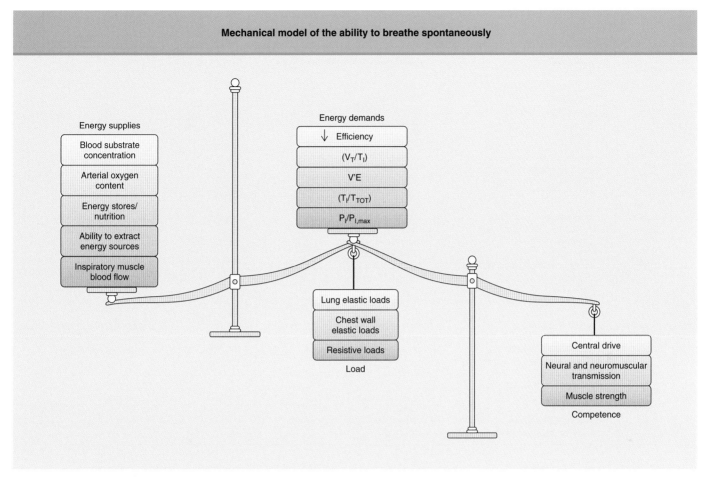

Figure 28.3. Mechanical model of the ability to breathe spontaneously. The system of two balances, incorporating the various determinants of load, competence, energy supplies, and demands is represented schematically. The PI/PI,max, one of the determinants of energy demands (see Fig. 28.2) is replaced by its equivalent: the balance between load and neuromuscular competence (see Fig. 28.1). In fact, this is the reason the two balances are linked. When the central hinge of the system moves upward or is at least at the horizontal level, a balance exists between ventilatory needs and neurorespiratory capacity and spontaneous ventilation can be sustained. In healthy persons, the hinge moves far upward, creating a large reserve. For abbreviations, see legends to Figures 28.1 and 28.2.

When the central hinge of the system, for whatever reason, moves downward, an imbalance develops between ventilatory needs and neurorespiratory capacity, and spontaneous ventilation cannot be sustained, leading to hypercapnic respiratory failure.

In neuromuscular respiratory failure, neuromuscular competence is significantly compromised. However, when expiratory or bulbar muscles are also affected, the development of pneumonia due to inability to clear secretions or aspiration will also increase the load of the inspiratory muscles. Neuromuscular diseases, such as bilateral diaphragmatic paralysis and tetraplegia (C5 transection) or flail chest that cause marked distortion of the chest wall during inspiration, greatly augment the chest wall elastic load. In addition, patients with chronic neuromuscular disorders have a chest wall compliance diminished by about two thirds the normal value. This is caused by the stiffening of tendons and ligaments and ankylosis of costosternal and costovertebral articulations that develop as a consequence of chronic restriction. At the same time, the endurance of the respiratory muscles is also decreased owing to muscle atrophy or

the underlying disease process. Thus, a variety of mechanisms may interact and lead to respiratory failure in patients with neuromuscular diseases.

CLINICAL FEATURES

Neuromuscular respiratory failure usually manifests as one of the following clinical appearances:

1. Hypercapnia due to suppression of the respiratory centers. Usually, this is a result of drug overdose and is characterized by bradypnea and a respiratory pattern of shallow breathing. The drugs associated are opioids and benzodiazepines. Typical patients are drug addicts, suicidal patients, and ICU patients receiving sedation and analgesia. The risk increases with age.
2. Hypercapnia due to neuromuscular weakness. Breathing is rapid and shallow, usually without signs of respiratory distress. In the clinical examination, abdominal paradox may be present. Normally, during inspiration the abdominal wall expands as a result of the contraction and

277

Table 28.1 Disorders of Respiratory Neuromuscular Function

Level	Examples	Associated Clinical Characteristics	Nerve Conduction	EMG
Upper motor neuron	Hemiplegia Quadriplegia Extrapyramidal disorders	Weakness Hyperreflexia Increased muscle tone Possible sensory and autonomic changes	Normal	Normal
Lower motor neuron	Paralytic poliomyelitis Amyotrophic lateral sclerosis Werdnig-Hoffmann disease Spinal muscular atrophies Postpolio syndrome	Weakness Atrophy Flaccidity Hyperreflexia Fasciculations Bulbar involvement No sensory changes	Normal	Deinnervation potentials Giant motor units

Peripheral neurons	Landry-Guillain-Barré syndrome
	Acute intermittent porphyria
	Diphtheria
	Lyme disease
	Toxins (lead, thallium triorthocresyl
	   phosphate)
	Saxitoxin
	Polyneuropathies associated with lupus
	   or polyarteritis
		Weakness
		Flaccidity
		Hyporeflexia
		Bulbar involvement
		Sensory and autonomic changes
			Reduced	Deinnervation potentials
				   in axonal neuropathies

Myoneural junction	Myasthenia gravis
	Botulism
	Eaton-Lambert syndrome
	Organophosphate poisoning
	Tick paralysis
	Black widow spider bite
		Fluctuating weakness
		Fatigability
		Ocular and bulbar involvement
		Normal reflexes
		No sensory changes
			Normal	Changes in the amplitude of the
				   muscle response to repetitive
				   nerve stimulation

Muscle	Muscular dystrophies Polymyositis Acid maltase deficieny Carnitine palmityltransferase deficiency	Weakness, usually proximal Normal reflexes No sensory or autonomic changes Often pain	Normal	Small motor units

downward movement of the diaphragm. However, in cases of diaphragmatic weakness, the diaphragm is unable to descend during inspiration in the supine position. Thus, the negative intrathoracic pressure, developed by the rest of the respiratory muscles, is transmitted toward the abdomen and reduces the abdominal pressure, causing an inward shift of the abdominal wall, which is called abdominal paradox. When the accessory inspiratory muscles (the sternocleidomastoids and the scalenes) are spared by the underlying disease, their intense contraction becomes evident on clinical examination. Dyspnea is the main symptom of respiratory muscle weakness. However, in cases of reduced mobility due to the underlying illness, dyspnea may be absent.

3. Hypoxemic respiratory failure. The clinical presentation is typical of either aspiration or classical pneumonia with tachypnea, fever, and usually copious secretions. Cough is either absent or weak, and the patient may have swallowing difficulties depending on the relative involvement of expiratory or bulbar muscles. Hypoxemic respiratory failure and, in severe cases, cyanosis are usually present.

A detailed description of the various diseases that could lead to neuromuscular respiratory failure is impossible in the context of this chapter. Table 28.1 summarizes the clinical characteristics of some common disorders according to the anatomic location of the lesion within the pathway from the respiratory controllers in the central nervous system to the respiratory muscles (Fig. 28.4). Neuromuscular diseases can be either

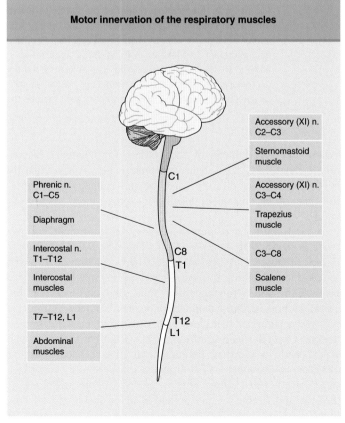

Motor innervation of the respiratory muscles

Accessory (XI) n.
C2–C3

Sternomastoid
muscle

Accessory (XI) n.
C3–C4

Trapezius
muscle

C3–C8

Scalene
muscle

Phrenic n.
C1–C5

Diaphragm

Intercostal n.
T1–T12

Intercostal
muscles

T7–T12, L1

Abdominal
muscles

C1

C8
T1

T12
L1

Figure 28.4. Motor innervation of the respiratory muscles. The motor innervation of the respiratory muscle group.

relentless and destructive, such as many forms of muscular dystrophy or amyotrophic lateral sclerosis, or totally or partially reversible. Some relatively frequent causes of reversible neuromuscular respiratory failure as well as some disorders specifically related to the ICU are presented in more detail.

Guillain-Barré Syndrome

A commonly reported abnormality associated with neuromuscular respiratory failure is Guillain-Barré syndrome (GBS). GBS is a demyelinating polyneuropathy with prolonged conduction time, whereas action potential may be reduced or normal in amplitude. Its onset is usually a few weeks after surgery, a flu vaccination, infection, pregnancy, or malignancy. An ascending neuropathy occurs, advancing fast and affecting all limbs at once. Unlike other neuropathies, proximal muscles are more affected, and trunk, respiratory, and cranial nerves may be affected as well. Mild sensory changes, such as distal paresthesias, and autonomic abnormalities, such as tachycardia, arrhythmias, and hypotension, may also be present.

Although not all patients with GBS develop respiratory failure, respiratory muscle involvement is a major complication, frequently leading to the need for mechanical ventilation. A useful index of the adequacy of respiratory muscle strength in GBS is vital capacity (VC). In fact, a fall in VC precedes the requirement for mechanical ventilation, which on average occurs when the VC falls below 15 mL/kg body weight. Thus, frequent measurement of VC is useful. Other predictors of the need for ventilatory support include cranial nerve involvement, history of infection 8 days before the onset of GBS, and a greatly increased cerebrospinal fluid (CSF) protein level.

Myasthenia Gravis

Myasthenia gravis (MG) is an antibody-mediated autoimmune disease leading to muscle weakness. It results from antibodies directed against acetylcholine receptors in the myoneural junction. Cell-mediated immunity, involving sensitized lymphocytes and the thymus gland, is also involved. Usually, myasthenia gravis presents in young adults with easy muscle fatigability. The most common presenting symptom is weakness of the eye muscles, manifesting as diplopia or ptosis. Dysarthria and dysphagia are also common, as is proximal weakness of the upper and lower extremities. It may progress to permanent weakness. A rapid decline in muscle action potentials on repetitive stimulation is seen on electromyography (EMG). VC is a poor predictor of the need for mechanical ventilation in MG patients. This can, probably, be ascribed to the erratic nature of MG, a disease whose course is largely influenced by many parameters.

Organophosphate Poisoning

Organophosphate insecticides, commonly used in agriculture, are a gradually increasing cause of accidental and suicidal poisoning, leading to respiratory failure, with high morbidity and mortality. Organophosphates inhibit acetylcholinesterase at the cholinergic synapses, as a result of the covalent binding of phosphate radicals to the active site of cholinesterases. Therefore, acetylcholine accumulates at the synapses first, causing overstimulation and then disruption of the impulse transmission at the neuromuscular junctions. Sweating, muscle fasciculations, coma, and respiratory distress can be observed.

Botulism

Botulism is caused by the toxin of *Clostridium botulinum*, which produces a presynaptic blockade of neuromuscular transmission, with reduced release of acetylcholine. Neuromuscular symptoms follow exposure to the neurotoxin within 2 to 24 hours. The bulbar musculature is affected first, with resultant diplopia and dysphagia. Ptosis, extraocular muscle weakness, and diminution of the gag reflex are also common. Because the neurotoxin also involves the autonomic nervous system, gastrointestinal symptoms such as nausea, vomiting, and ileus may also occur, and the pupils may be dilated. Mentation remains normal, and fever is absent. Severe respiratory muscle involvement is paralleled by decreases in VC and total lung capacity and an increase in residual volume (RV), reflected in hypercapnia, hypoxemia, and the need for mechanical ventilation.

ICU-related Neuromuscular Respiratory Failure

A usual cause of neuromuscular respiratory failure in the ICU is *critical illness polyneuropathy and myopathy* (CIPNM). This is a syndrome of acquired peripheral neuropathy characterized by failure to wean from mechanical ventilation, muscle atrophy, and diminished reflexes. Despite the high incidence of CIPNM, clinical risk factors are still unclear. Sepsis and multiorgan dysfunction increase the risk of CIPNM, as shown in both retrospective and prospective series. Thus, CIPNM likely represents an aspect of organ failure of sepsis and systemic inflammatory response syndrome (SIRS), presumably as a result of the same basic mechanisms that lead to multiple organ dysfunction such as inflammation, apoptosis, thrombosis, and oxidant injury. Hyperglycemia has been associated with an increased risk of CIPNM. The link between hyperglycemia and CIPNM may be related to a combination of the toxic effects of hyperglycemia and the antiinflammatory and neuroprotective effects of administered insulin that have been demonstrated experimentally. Other disease-specific factors associated with CIPNM in multiple studies include severity of illness, duration of ICU stay, female sex, and increased age. Observational studies have identified possible additional risk factors such as corticosteroids, neuromuscular blocking agents, aminoglycoside antibiotics, catecholamines/vasopressors, parenteral nutrition, and renal replacement therapy. However, the causal relationship of these factors to CIPNM is unclear.

Acute quadriplegic myopathy (AQM) is a cause of neuromuscular respiratory failure initially described during treatment of severe asthma. Weakness in AQM affects both proximal and distal muscles, including the diaphragm, and can be profound. Reflexes may be present or absent, but sensation remains intact. Initial reports of acute myopathy in individuals with asthma focused on the role of corticosteroids. Later, it became clear that the use of prolonged neuromuscular blockade was also associated with the development of acute myopathy. The syndrome has been reported in association with respiratory failure of various causes, including the acute respiratory distress syndrome, sepsis, and transplantation of heart, lung, and liver. The pathogenesis of AQM is not clear.

Prolonged neuromuscular blockade in the ICU is a cause of neuromuscular respiratory failure. Nondepolarizing neuromuscular blocking drugs (NMBDs) are competitive inhibitors of neuromuscular transmission. NMBDs are sometimes administered to critically ill patients in conjunction with sedation in

279

an effort to facilitate mechanical ventilation, reduce oxygen consumption, and control intracranial pressure. Most NMBDs rely to various degrees on hepatic metabolism and renal elimination for termination of effect. Thus, large doses of NMBDs in the setting of renal failure can result in prolonged neuromuscular blockade after only a few hours of administration. Additional risk factors for prolonged neuromuscular blockade include hypermagnesemia, metabolic acidosis, female sex, and the concomitant use of various antibiotics. However, none of these factors is as important as renal failure. Corticosteroids are also recognized to cause a proximal myopathy, and some groups consider the respiratory muscles to be vulnerable to these drugs.

A rapidly accumulating body of experimental evidence suggests that mechanical ventilation, with its attendant diaphragm muscle inactivity and unloading, is an important cause of diaphragmatic dysfunction. This phenomenon is referred to as *ventilator-induced diaphragmatic dysfunction* (VIDD). VIDD is associated with muscle atrophy, oxidative stress, myofibrillar disruption, and various remodeling responses within diaphragm muscle fibers. However, the precise involvement of each of these factors in the loss of diaphragmatic force-generating capacity is still unclear. Furthermore, the major cellular targets of damage within muscle fibers, and the associated mechanisms of interference with the contractile process (e.g., excitation-contraction coupling, cross-bridge cycling, force transmission by cytoskeletal elements), need to be defined in greater detail. Animal studies suggest that the onset of VIDD during controlled mechanical ventilation (CMV) is rapid. The "typical" clinical scenario in which to suspect VIDD is a patient who fails to wean after a period of controlled mechanical ventilation.

In the clinical setting, VIDD should be a diagnosis of exclusion based on an appropriate clinical history of having undergone a period of CMV, other possible causes of diaphragmatic weakness having been sought and ruled out. For example, prolonged neuromuscular blockade can be excluded by the lack of an abnormal response to train-of four stimulation, CIPNM by the absence of neuropathic changes on electrophysiologic testing, and AQM by the lack of corticosteroid exposure history (or by muscle biopsy in indeterminate cases).

DIAGNOSIS

The diagnosis of the specific disorders that lead to neuromuscular respiratory failure depends on the underlying disease. Arterial blood gas analysis demonstrates hypercapnia and/or hypoxemia.

The diagnostic approach to neuromuscular respiratory failure depends on the clinical presentation. In the setting of pneumonia and hypoxemic respiratory failure, bulbar and/or expiratory muscle involvement should be investigated. Absence of gag reflex and difficulties in phonation and swallowing point to bulbar muscle involvement. Inability to generate sufficient cough flows points to expiratory muscle involvement. Measurement of maximum expiratory pressure confirms the decrease in the force-generating capacity of the expiratory muscles. If the patient is uncooperative, magnetic stimulation of the expiratory muscles can be tried.

In the setting of hypercapnic respiratory failure, the first step is to exclude suppression of the respiratory centers. A valuable

diagnostic test is the measurement of $P_{0.1}$. $P_{0.1}$ is the airway pressure developed during the first 100 msec, after the onset of the inspiration, against an occluded airway. A reduced $P_{0.1}$ implies a decrease in respiratory drive and should raise the suspicion of drug overdose.

When the respiratory drive is adequate, inspiratory muscle weakness is likely present and should be documented. VC is an easily obtained measurement that, when decreased, points to respiratory muscle weakness. The VC averages approximately 50 mL/kg in normal adults. However, VC is not specific and may be decreased because of both inspiratory and expiratory muscle weakness as well as restrictive lung and chest wall diseases. Determination of maximal inspiratory pressure (MIP) is a more specific way to quantitate inspiratory muscle weakness.

When inspiratory muscle weakness is confirmed, the next diagnostic step is to unravel whether it is caused by diaphragmatic weakness, since the diaphragm is the most important inspiratory muscle. This is accomplished by the measurement of maximum transdiaphragmatic pressure (Pdi,max). Pdi,max is measured as the difference between gastric pressure and esophageal pressure upon a maximum inspiratory effort after the insertion of appropriate balloon catheters in the esophagus and the stomach, respectively.

The next diagnostic step consists of determining whether weakness is due to muscle, nerve, or neuromuscular transmission impairment. This requires the measurement of Pdi in response to bilateral supramaximal phrenic nerve electrical or magnetic stimulation, the so-called "twitch Pdi," with concurrent recording of the electromyogram of the diaphragm by either surface or esophageal electrodes (Fig. 28.5). Although technically demanding, this approach has the great advantage of being independent of patient effort-motivation. It allows for the measurement of phrenic nerve conduction time or phrenic latency, i.e., the time between the onset of the stimulus and the onset of compound muscle action potential (M wave) on the diaphragmatic EMG. A prolonged conduction time suggests nerve involvement. However, electrophysiologic testing has shortcomings. Although the conduction time or latency is prolonged in neuropathies that are predominantly demyelinating, it may be preserved in neuropathies that are predominantly axonal despite substantial diaphragm weakness. Moreover, when the above technique is used, it is important that costimulation of the brachial plexus be avoided; otherwise the action potential recorded from surface electrodes may originate from muscles other than the diaphragm. This problem is compounded if the phrenic nerve is stimulated by means of magnetic stimulators. Classically, an axonal neuropathy is characterized by the finding of preserved latencies with diminished action potentials (M wave). Fibrillation potentials and positive sharp waves may also be observed. However, these features can also occur in myopathic processes, and the distinction between axonal neuropathy and myopathy may be difficult. The diagnosis of myopathy is supported by histologic and biochemical data as well as by the observation that some patients have muscle that is inexcitable even by direct stimulation.

Lack of M wave after nerve stimulation is an indication of paralysis with the lesion located proximal to or at the neuromuscular junction. Decreased twitch Pdi in the face of normal M wave is characteristic of contractile dysfunction that resides within the muscle.

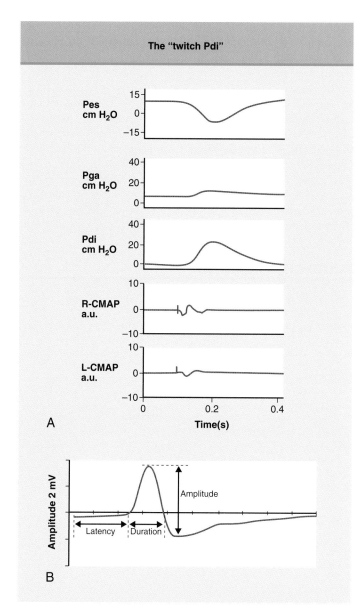

Figure 28.5. The "twitch Pdi." *A,* The twitch transdiaphragmatic pressure (Pdi) after magnetic/electrical stimulation. *B,* A detailed (enlarged) view of a compound muscle action potential (M wave), where the latency (time from stimulus to muscle depolarization), the duration, and the amplitude of the electromyogram are evident. a.u., arbitrary units; L-CMAP, left compound motor action potential; Pes, esophageal pressure; Pga, gastric pressure; R-CMAP, right compound motor action potential.

In special circumstances such as muscle weakness after mechanical ventilation with neuromuscular blocking drug use, simple tests such as the train-of-four (TOF) stimulation can be diagnostic. TOF consists of peripheral nerve stimulation with measurement of the response to four equal pulses over 2 seconds. Prolonged neuromuscular blockade is diagnosed by documentation of lack or attenuated response to TOF stimulation.

Clues to Diagnosis of Specific Diseases

Clues to the diagnosis of GBS are a characteristic "ascending paralysis" and a CSF protein that is elevated in the face of a CSF cell count of 10 or fewer mononuclear leukocytes/mm^3. A history of previous infection further supports the diagnosis of GBS.

Myasthenia gravis is confirmed by demonstrating fluctuating weakness that improves after the injection of acetylcholinesterase inhibitors such as edrophonium (Tensilon) and by the finding of a decremental response of the amplitude of the motor response to repetitive nerve stimulation.

The diagnosis of organophosphate poisoning is based essentially on a history of exposure to organophosphates and a decreased serum acetylcholinesterase level (<50% of the laboratory minimum normal value of 4.65 U/mL).

Botulism is verified by demonstrating neurotoxin in serum, stool, or contaminated food. Diagnosis is supported by repetitive nerve stimulation showing small amplitude motor responses that increase in amplitude at high rates of stimulation.

The diagnosis of AQM should be suspected by the presence of quadriplegia in patients with history of corticosteroid or NMBD use. Serum creatine phosphokinase levels can be normal or elevated during the acute phase of myopathy, and significant elevations may identify patients at risk of rhabdomyolysis. Muscle pathology appears to take at least two forms. One major variant appears as selective thick (myosin) filament loss and the second as widespread myonecrosis. Electromyography reveals reduced muscle membrane excitability.

TREATMENT

Precipitating factors are often the immediate cause for ICU admission of patients with neuromuscular disease. The identification of such factors is essential because they may be more amenable to therapy than the disease itself. Upper airway obstruction and aspiration should be suspected in patients with bulbar dysfunction, whereas microatelectasis and lower respiratory tract infections are common among all patients with generalized weakness. In addition, electrolyte and endocrine disorders may exacerbate respiratory dysfunction. Phosphate, potassium, magnesium, and calcium are all important for healthy neuromuscular function and should be kept within the normal range. Thyroid and growth hormone disorders should be corrected, and acid-base balance should be optimized.

Specific therapy can be applied, though, in many of the above mentioned diseases. In the case of drug overdose, there are specific antidotes that antagonize the action of the drugs, such as naloxone for the opioids and flumazenil for the benzodiazepines.

The treatment of prolonged neuromuscular blockade consists primarily of waiting for clearance of NMBD. Pharmacologic reversal of neuromuscular blockade may also be useful, but recovery will be incomplete in the presence of high concentrations of NMBDs or their metabolites.

Plasmapheresis has been shown to shorten the duration of the hospital and ICU stay for GBS patients if begun within 14 days of onset of symptoms. Immunoglobulin can also be used and is as good as plasma exchange and more convenient. A large percentage of patients (85%) exhibits complete or nearly complete recovery.

In myasthenia gravis, the treatment consists of symptomatic control with anticholinesterase agents, such as pyridostigmine, at a dosage that improves muscle weakness with a minimum of cholinergic side effects. Prednisolone can also be used. Plasmapheresis, which presumably removes antireceptor antibodies, may improve motor function for longer periods. If thymoma is the cause of myasthenia gravis, thymectomy gives remission in 30% of patients and worthwhile benefit in another 40%. Approximately 10% of patients with generalized disease will require mechanical ventilation.

Botulism therapy involves elimination of unabsorbed neurotoxin from the gut by means of enemas and gastric lavage, administration of trivalent antitoxin (against neurotoxins A, B, and E) to neutralize circulating neurotoxin in the serum, administration of high-dose penicillin to kill C. *botulinum* organisms if present, and surgical débridement of offending wounds.

Organophosphate poisoning requires full atropinization to control cholinergic symptomatology (e.g., salivary and tracheal hypersecretion). Intermittent dosing is performed using 2 mg atropine every 15 minutes until secretions are controlled. Up to 3 days of treatment may be needed. Oximes (pralidoxime, obidoxime) are cholinesterase reactivators and are approved as antidotes for the reactivation of inhibited acetylcholinesterase in organophosphate poisoning. Oximes have a beneficial response when administered within 24 hours after exposure.

CLINICAL COURSE AND PREVENTION

Neuromuscular respiratory failure is more common than recognized and may result in substantial morbidity, mortality, and costs.

In ICU patients, neuromuscular dysfunction may be reduced by avoiding neuromuscular blocking agents and by scheduling frequent drug "holidays" with clear evidence of recovery from neuromuscular blockade. Limiting corticosteroids to patients with clear indications and treating hyperglycemia have been shown to reduce the incidence of AQM and CIPNM, respectively. Efforts to prevent and aggressively treat sepsis will likely reduce the incidence of CIPNM. In the ICU, measures that reduce the length of stay may also decrease CIPNM. These measures include prevention of ventilator-associated pneumonia through use of semirecumbent positioning, reduction of ventilator-induced lung injury in patients with acute lung injury through use of low tidal volume mechanical ventilation, and limitation of sedative infusions through protocols that provide daily interruptions of sedative infusions. Limiting the use of controlled mechanical ventilation reduces VIDD.

SUGGESTED READING

ATS/ERS Statement on Respiratory Muscle Testing. Am J Respir Crit Care Med 2002;166:518–624.

Fanburg BL, Sicilian L (eds): Respiratory dysfunction in neuromuscular disease. Clin Chest Med 1994;15:607–810.

Kelly BJ, Luce JM: The diagnosis and management of neuromuscular diseases causing respiratory failure. Chest 1991;99:1485–1494.

Laghi F, Tobin MJ: Disorders of the respiratory muscles. Am J Respir Crit Care Med 2003;168:10–48.

Vassilakopoulos T, Zakynthinos S, Roussos C: Muscle function: basic concepts. In Marini JJ, Slutsky A (eds): Physiologic Basis of Ventilator Support. New York, Marcel Dekker, 1998, pp 103–152.

Vassilakopoulos T, Zakynthinos S, Roussos C: Respiratory muscles and weaning failure. Eur Respir J 1996;9:2383–2400.

Chapter 29
Pathophysiology of Cardiovascular Failure

Sheldon Magder

KEY POINTS

- Management of cardiovascular failure requires a good understanding of the underlying physiologic and pathophysiologic processes, but the macrophysiologic process has direct implications for the management of critically ill patients.
- The use of a physiologically based approach to management can allow rapid and directed management.
- The first question that should be asked when assessing a patient with cardiovascular failure and hypotension is, "What is the cardiac output?" The next step is to consider the differential diagnosis of a low systemic vascular resistance (SVR). All can be assessed by simple tests or clinical examination, and when a cause is not readily found, the likely cause of the decrease in SVR is sepsis or systemic inflammatory response syndrome (SIRS; septic signs without infection).
- Failure of the cardiovascular system has widespread consequences and likely contributes to the multiorgan failure seen in critically ill patients.
- It is important to consider the mechanisms of acute coronary ischemia when planning therapy for a critically ill patient.

The cardiovascular system is essential for the supply of nutrients to tissues, removal of metabolic waste products, and maintenance of normal volume status. Thus, failure of the cardiovascular system has widespread consequences and likely contributes to the multiorgan failure seen in critically ill patients. As multiorgan dysfunction increases, progressive cardiovascular dysfunction leads to greater deterioration of the overall organism, including further deterioration of the cardiovascular system and a downward spiral to death. Management of cardiovascular failure requires a good understanding of the underlying physiologic and pathophysiologic processes. Knowledge of basic cellular process involved in cardiovascular failure has increased tremendously in the past two decades, but this chapter emphasizes the macrophysiologic processes. This subject alone is extensive and has direct implications for the management of critically ill patients.

It is useful to consider failure of the cardiovascular system as forward failure and backward failure. The actual processes that produce forward and backward failure are generally the same,

but the distinction identifies the primary clinical problem that needs to be corrected for symptomatic improvement, and the therapeutic approaches can be quite different. Forward failure results in inadequate tissue perfusion and thus inadequate supply of nutrients and oxygen as well as inadequate clearance of waste. This is manifested clinically by symptoms of inadequate perfusion, including fatigue, weakness, or, if more severe, altered sensorium, cool clammy skin, and signs of organ dysfunction such as oliguric renal failure. Backward failure results in congestion of tissues. Backward failure of the left ventricle results in pulmonary congestion and symptoms including shortness of breath on exertion, orthopnea, paroxysmal nocturnal dyspnea, and frank respiratory failure. Backward failure of the right ventricle is associated with edema of dependent portions of the body.

GENERAL LOGIC OF THE CARDIOVASCULAR SYSTEM

Discussions of the pathophysiology of cardiovascular failure generally emphasize the role of the heart and its ability to generate cardiac output. However, there is also an important vascular component to cardiovascular failure for, as will be discussed in detail, cardiac output is determined by the interaction of cardiac function and function of the vasculature. We begin with a discussion of the general logic behind the physiology of the vascular system. The cardiovascular system works as a constant pressure system. Regional flows are produced by decreasing the resistance in local vascular beds. An analogy that helps understand the advantage of this strategy is the supply of water to a local community. A water tower provides a pressure head, and flow is provided to individual residences by opening the faucets at individual sites. Opening the faucets is the equivalent of decreasing regional resistances. Since pressure work is much more demanding for cardiac muscle than work related to muscle shortening and the ejection of volume, a relatively constant arterial pressure has the advantage of keeping the load on the heart constant.

POISEUILLE'S LAW AND ARTERIAL PRESSURE

Based on Poiseuille's law, the upstream arterial pressure (Part) minus the downstream pressure in the vasculature is equal to the product of cardiac output (Q) and the systemic vascular resistance (SVR). Since the downstream pressure is a relatively constant value, and low, it can be largely ignored, and as an approximation:

Cardiovascular Problems

Box 29.1 Cause of a Low SVR

- Sepsis (SIRS)
- Drugs
- Arteriovenous shunts
- Spinal/epidural injections
- Spinal injury
- Cirrhosis
- Thyroid disease
- Anaphylaxis
- Corticosteroid deficiency
- Anemia
- Beriberi

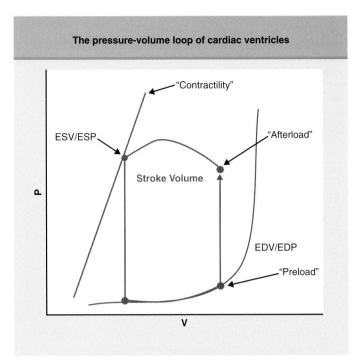

The pressure-volume loop of cardiac ventricles

Figure 29.1. The pressure-volume loop of cardiac ventricles. The blue curve at bottom is the passive filling curve of the ventricle. The heart fills to EDV/EDP, which gives the preload of the ventricle. It then contracts isovolumetrically until the aortic valve opens, which gives a good approximation of ventricular afterload. Volume is then ejected (stroke volume) until the end-systolic pressure-volume line is reached. The slope of this line is a good approximation of contractility. The ventricle then relaxes, giving an isovolumetric relaxation phase, and fills during diastole along the passive filling curve. EDP, end-diastolic pressure; EDV, end-diastolic volume; ESP, end-systolic pressure; ESV, end-systolic volume.

$$Part = Q \times SVR \qquad (Equation\ 1)$$

This simple relationship has major implications for the approach to cardiovascular failure. It indicates that an inadequate arterial pressure must be due to a dominant effect of either inadequate cardiac output (Q) or a low systemic vascular resistance (SVR). The word dominant is used because often both problems are present, but it is still worth considering which component dominates the clinical problem. Thus, the first question that should be asked when assessing a patient with cardiovascular failure and hypotension is, what is the cardiac output?

Decreased SVR

Based on Poiseuille's law (Equation 1), if cardiac output is normal or elevated, the hypotension is primarily due to a decrease in systemic vascular tone. The next step is to consider the differential diagnosis of a low SVR, which is listed in Box 29.1. All these can be assessed by simple tests or clinical examination, and when a cause is not readily found, the likely cause of the decrease in SVR is sepsis or SIRS (septic signs without infection).

Decreased Cardiac Output

If the cardiac output is decreased, the next step is to determine whether it is decreased because of a decrease in cardiac function or because of a decrease in the return of blood to the heart. Understanding of the rationale behind this approach requires an understanding of how cardiac output is determined. Cardiac output often is considered simply in terms of heart rate and stroke volume, but an equally important component is the return of blood to the heart. The following sections review the determinants of cardiac function followed by the determinants of the return of blood to the heart (return function) and then the importance to their interaction.

Determinants of Cardiac Function

As described by Otto Frank and Ernest Starling at the turn of the century, cardiac function can be well explained by the pressure-volume relationship of the ventricles (Fig. 29.1). The pressure-volume relationship also provides a useful graphic representation of the three determinants of stroke volume: preload, afterload, and contractility. During diastole, filling of the ventricles stretches the elastic structures of the ventricular walls and increases intraluminal pressure. This is represented by the passive-filling curve of the ventricle. At the end of diastole,

the final ventricular pressure determines the final end-diastolic volume and thus represents the preload for cardiac contraction (see Fig. 29.1). The slope of a line on a pressure-volume plot is elastance, or the inverse of compliance. Thus, the magnitude of the end-diastolic pressure needed to distend the ventricles depends upon the compliance of the ventricular wall. At low ventricular volumes, the curve has a gentle slope and the compliance is high. At higher volumes, the compliance abruptly becomes extremely low and there is a marked increase in pressure for small to minimal changes in volume. In the intact heart, this marked rise in pressure for a change in volume is largely due to constraint by the pericardium. However, even without an intact pericardium, collagen in the myocardium limits the increase in volume with increasing pressure. Excessive filling of one of the two ventricles can also impede filling of the other ventricle because the two ventricles are in a common space that is limited by the pericardium and mediastinal structure. Furthermore, excessive distention of either ventricle alters the normal curvature of the septum, which will affect the compliance of the other chamber. The limit to right ventricular filling as expressed by the steep part of the passive ventricular pressure-volume curve has the important function of preventing overfilling of the heart. Since limitation first occurs in the right heart, overfilling of the left heart and pulmonary congestion are avoided. As a corollary to this, it is difficult to produce pul-

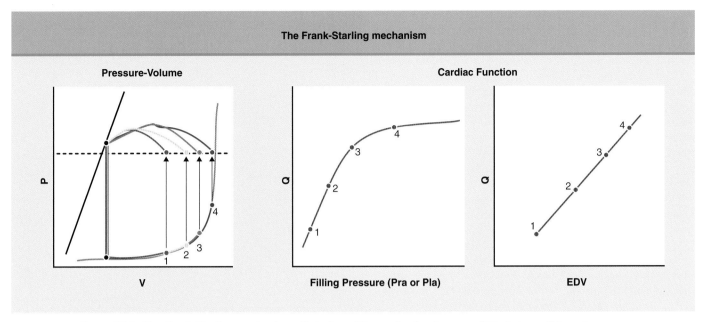

Figure 29.2. The Frank-Starling mechanism. Derivation of the cardiac function curve ("Starling curve") from the ventricular pressure-volume relationship. Because of the steep portion of the passive filling curve of the ventricle, at higher end-diastolic volume (EDV) there is a steep rise in pressure, which produces the plateau of the cardiac function curve when filling pressures are plotted on the x-axis. However, when EDV is plotted on the x-axis there is a linear relationship between EDV and cardiac output (Q) (assuming a constant heart rate). The implication is for any change in EDV there is the same change in cardiac output.

monary edema by giving excess volume to someone with a normal heart. The production of pulmonary edema by excessive fluid administration requires increased pulmonary capillary leak or left ventricular dysfunction. Under pathologic conditions, cardiac filling can also be limited by processes that compress the mediastinum such as blood or swelling of the mediastinum, a pneumothorax, or greatly inflated lungs.

As described by Sagawa, the heart ejects blood by becoming stiffer. In other words, myocardial contraction can be represented by the heart moving through a series of increasing elastance curves during systole so that contraction and cardiac ejection can be expressed as a time varying elastance. In the early phase of systole, the stiffening of ventricular muscle produces a marked rise in ventricular pressure at a constant volume. When the pressure in the left ventricular rises above the aortic pressure or the right ventricular pressure rises above the pulmonary artery pressure, the aortic and pulmonary valves, respectively, open and blood is ejected. During this phase, the pressure rises and the volume decreases so that there is little change in wall stress and the pressure at which the valve opens represents a good approximation of ventricular afterload (see Fig. 29.1). Ejection continues until it reaches the end-systolic pressure-volume line, which represents the highest elastance (lowest compliance) the ventricle can achieve in a cycle before relaxation begins. The difference between end-diastolic volume and end-systolic volume represents the stroke volume. Points on the end-systolic pressure-volume line represent the maximum possible values of end-systolic pressure and volume that the ventricle can achieve in a cycle at a given contractile state. The final slope of this line, and thus maximal elastance, is determined by the length of the cardiac action potential because the action

potential dictates the period of calcium entry into the myocytes, and by the speed with which the slope increases, for this determines how steep the line can become in a cardiac cycle. Thus, the slope of the end systolic pressure volume line is a good measure of the contractile status of the ventricle. The slope increases with agents that increase contractility and decreases with factors that decrease cardiac function, including disease states.

Examination of the effect of a change in preload on the stroke volume demonstrates the role of the Frank-Starling mechanism (Fig. 29.2). An increase in end-diastolic volume will result in exactly the same increase in stroke volume and cardiac output, assuming that heart rate, contractility, and afterload are constant. This means that whatever goes into the heart will be ejected. Consider what would happen if this did not occur. If the stroke volume of the right heart was 101 mL and that of the left heart was 100 mL, and the heart rate was 60 beats/min, in approximately one and a half hours total blood volume would be in the lungs. Thus, even very small differences in right and left ventricular outputs cannot be tolerated for more than a few beats. The Frank-Starling mechanism provides the "fine" tuning to cardiac output, whereas changes in heart rate and contractility provide the large, "coarse" changes.

Although the ventricular pressure-volume relationship gives a comprehensive view of factors that affect cardiac function and is a useful analytic tool, volume is a difficult parameter to obtain, especially in clinical situations. For this reason, the cardiac function curve, which is based only on cardiac filling pressures and cardiac output, is more often used (see Fig. 29.2). The cardiac function curve also has the advantage of allowing analysis of the interaction of cardiac function and return function, as discussed below. Overall cardiac function can be represented by the change in cardiac output for a change in right atrial pressure, which represents the preload for the whole heart. This relationship gives the function of the heart as a unit and includes right and left ventricular function, as well as the effects of changes in the pulmonary circulation on the right heart. Each curve assumes that afterload, contractility, and heart rate are constant. An increase in heart rate or contractility or a decrease in afterload shifts the curve upward, so that for any given preload there is a higher cardiac output. A decrease in heart rate or contractility and an increase in afterload shift the curve upward so that for any given preload there is a lower cardiac output. The cardiac function curve also is affected by changes in diastolic compliance; a decrease in diastolic compliance shifts the curve upward and an increase in compliance shifts the curve downward. Changes in compliance can be due to intrinsic changes in the properties of the myocardium or due to compressive forces around the heart. Based on all these variations, it should be clear that the cardiac function curve gives less specific information about the specific cause of a change in cardiac function than the pressure-volume relationship, but this plot is very practical because of the ease of measuring cardiac filling pressure.

An important feature of the cardiac function curve is that the relationship has a plateau. The plateau is related to the steep part of the passive filling curve, where an increase in ventriculated volume is very limited. In the plateau phase, sarcomere stretch, the ultimate determinant of the Frank-Starling mechanism, does not increase, despite large increases in pressure. The important point is that when the heart is functioning on the flat part of the cardiac function curve, further changes in preload do not affect cardiac output and the increase in the filling pressure only increases tension in the walls of the heart. This can compromise coronary flow, distort the ventricles, and produce peripheral edema.

Determinants of Return Function

An obvious point, but one that is often ignored in analysis of circulatory function, is that the heart can only pump out what it receives. Thus, the return of blood determines the capacity of the heart to pump blood. An initial naïve thought may be that the return of blood to the heart is simply due to blood that the heart pushes around the circuit, but this is not what happens. As will be shown in this section, the arterial pressure generated by the heart does not determine the total flow (cardiac output). As argued by Guyton, the heart increases cardiac output by lowering right atrial pressure, for this allows an increase in the return of blood to the heart. It does not regulate cardiac output by increasing blood pressure, for this does not determine cardiac output.

To understand Guyton's model, it is worth considering the emptying of a bathtub (Fig. 29.3). Flow out of a bathtub is determined by the height of the water above the hole at the bottom of the tub, the size of the hole and pipe draining the tub, and the downstream pressure in the pipe that drains the tub. The force of the water coming in through the taps does not affect outflow from the tub. The only way inflow from the tap can alter outflow is by increasing the height of water in the tub. The tub has a large surface area relative to the height (i.e., large compliance) so that large volume changes are needed to

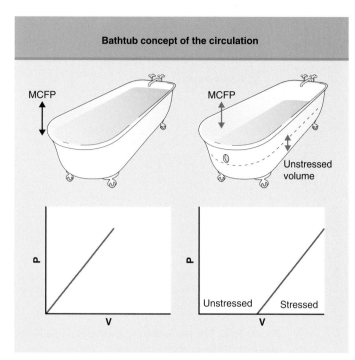

Figure 29.3. Bathtub concept of the circulation. Emptying of a bathtub depends on the height of the water above the bottom, the size of the drain, and the pressure at the end of the drain, but it does not depend on the pressure coming out of the tap. The tap only affects outflow by increasing the volume and therefore the height of water in the tub. Mean circulatory filling pressure (MCFP) is the pressure filling the compliant veins and is equivalent to the height of water filling the tub. At bottom is shown the pressure-volume relationship of the tub. In the tub on the right, the opening is on the side of the tub. Only the volume above the opening produces a force that drives the volume out. This is the stressed volume. The volume below this is necessary to get to the hole but does not contribute to outflow. This is the unstressed volume.

produce changes in the height of water, and thus the driving pressure, for emptying of the tub. The large surface area relative to the inflow means that, over the short run, flow from the tap has no effect on flow out of the tub. The circulatory system has many similarities to the bathtub. Approximately 70% of blood volume is located in small venules and veins at a low pressure so that veins and venules have a large compliance, much like a bathtub. The pressure generated by this volume was called the *mean circulatory filling pressure* (MCFP) by Guyton, and it represents the pressure that exists throughout the vasculature when there is no flow. MCFP is determined by the vascular volume and total compliance of the vascular system. The total compliance of a system with compliances in series or parallel at a constant pressure is simply the sum of the compliances of the individual parts. Since the compliance of the venules and veins is much larger than that of any other region in the vascular tree by a ratio of greater than 30:1, MCFP is largely determined by the compliance of the venules and veins. Just as the force from the tap has no effect on the outflow from the tub, arterial pressure has no effect on the outflow from the veins and venules. The arterial pressure can only affect venous outflow by providing volume and raising MCFP. However, it is important to remember where arterial flow comes from. It comes from the heart, which gets the volume from the veins and venules, since that is where most of the volume is located. There are only very small stores of blood elsewhere in the circulation that the heart can recruit to the veins and venules to change outflow. In fact, as the flow increases, arterial pressure rises, which means that the arterial volume actually increases. This would lower MCFP except that the decrease in pressure in the larger veins allows volume to be transferred to the arteries. Thus, volume and pressure in the small veins and venules remain relatively constant.

For the bathtub to empty, the pressure at the bottom of the drain must be lower than the pressure in the bathtub. Similarly, if the pressure in the right atrium is the same as the pressure in the veins and venules (i.e., equal to MCFP), there will be no flow back to the heart. Flow occurs only when right atrial pressure is lower than MCFP. This is accomplished by the pumping action of the heart. Thus, to repeat what was stated earlier, the role of the heart in generating cardiac output is not to generate an arterial pressure but rather to lower right atrial pressure. Note that the full 5 L/min of normal cardiac output flows from the right ventricle through the pulmonary vasculature with a systolic pressure of less than 20 mm Hg. This occurs because the pulmonary vascular resistance is very low. If the systemic vascular resistance was as low as pulmonary vascular resistance, total systemic blood flow could occur with a very low arterial pressure, but as discussed below there are advantages to having a much higher arterial pressure.

The lower the right atrial pressure the greater is the flow back to the heart. However, there is a limit to the increase in the return of blood to the right heart that can occur owing to an improvement in right heart function and lowering of right atrial pressure. When the pressure in the great veins returning blood to the heart falls below atmospheric pressure, the soft walled veins collapse. This limits the effect of lowering right atrial pressure further. The phenomenon has been called a vascular waterfall. When there is a waterfall in a river, the characteristics of the river below the waterfall do not affect the flow over the falls. Only the properties of the river above the falls and the source of water affect flow over the falls. Similarly, when the great veins collapse, further lowering of right atrial pressure does not increase flow. Thus, the flow that occurs when veins collapse is the maximal possible flow in the system because, as already noted, the heart can only pump out what it receives. This means that if the great veins were allowed to drain to atmosphere pressure, for that brief instant the flow in the system would be maximal even though there is no heart. The flow would end quickly because the volume is not returned to the venules and veins and MCFP would fall, but this still demonstrates that maximal flow does not require the heart. The heart actually gets in the way, for right atrial pressures greater than atmospheric pressure impede venous return. Thus, just as there is a limit to cardiac function, collapse of the great veins produces a limit to the return function.

Another factor that affects the return function is the resistance in the veins draining the compliant venules and veins. A decrease in venous resistance (Rv) allows greater outflow from veins and venules and an increase in Rv reduces the flow out of venules and veins. It is important to appreciate that the compliant region of the vasculature is largely upstream from the major venous resistance so that it is possible for there to be independent changes in venous resistance and venous compliance, although often they change together.

So far in this discussion, MCFP has been considered to be dependent upon all the volume in the vasculature. However, under baseline conditions, approximately 70% of total blood volume does not stretch the walls of vessels but simply fills the space required to make the vessels round. This volume is unstressed in that it does not contribute to vascular pressure (except for the gravitational component), and only the 30% of volume that actually stretches the walls, the stressed volume, produces the pressure in the vessels and MCFP. The analogy in the bathtub model is the equivalent of having the opening on the side of the tub instead of the bottom (see Fig. 29.3). Only the water above the opening contributes to outflow, but the volume below the hole is still necessary to get to the level of the hole. The water below the hole is thus the equivalent of unstressed volume, and the volume above the hole is stressed volume. An important homeoregulatory process is the regulation of the distribution of unstressed volume and stressed volume. This occurs by the contraction of vascular smooth muscle, which regulates the cross-sectional area of the venules and veins. Since elastin in vessel walls largely determines the compliance, contraction of smooth muscle produces a parallel shift in the pressure volume curve, at least in the physiologic range. The total volume for a given pressure, which includes stressed and unstressed volume, is called *capacitance*. This term should not be confused with compliance, which is the change in volume for a change in pressure. Capacitance is very difficult to measure, even in animals. However, it is a very important determinant of vascular function for it determines the actual MCFP for any given volume. It needs to be appreciated that anything that decreases vascular tone such as α-blockers and narcotics increases capacitance and decreases MCFP.

In summary, the four determinants of the return function are stressed vascular volume, venous compliance (Cv), venous resistance (Rv), and the right atrial pressure (Pra), for Pra is the downstream pressure for venous return. Guyton produced an equation for the determinants of venous return, which is again based on Poiseuille's law:

$$VR = (MCFP - Pra)/Rv \qquad \text{(Equation 2)}$$

Since MCFP = stressed volume/Cv (Equation 3), by substituting Equation 3 into Equation 2, one gets

$$VR = (\text{stressed volume} - Pra \times Cv)/RvCv \qquad \text{(Equation 4)}$$

and since maximum VR occurs when Pra = 0,

$$VRmax = \text{Stressed volume}/RvCv \qquad \text{(Equation 5)}$$

This last equation means that the maximum possible venous return in the cardiovascular system, and thus the maximum possible cardiac output, is determined by the stressed vascular volume, Rv and Cv, and does not require a heart except, of course, to allow the blood to go around again! The physiologic principle is that the heart handles whatever comes back to it and when it does not, the heart impedes the flow in the circulation by allowing a right atrial pressure greater than zero.

Guyton provided a useful graphic analysis of the circulation (Fig. 29.4). Because he identified right atrial pressure as the factor regulated by the heart, he made right atrial pressure the

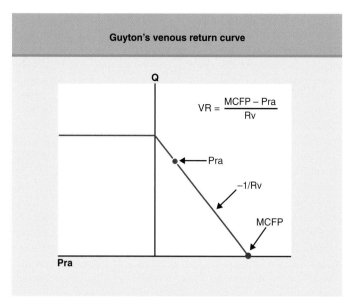

Figure 29.4. Guyton's venous return curve. The venous return curve plateaus when the pressure inside the veins is less than the outside pressure, which in this case is zero (atmospheric pressure). MCFP, mean circulatory filling pressure; Pra, right atrial pressure; Q, flow (cardiac output or venous return [VR]; Rv, resistance to venous return.

independent variable and put it on the x-axis and he put flow on the y-axis. When right atrial pressure equals MCFP, the flow is zero so that the x-intercept on this plot is MCFP. When right atrial pressure is lowered below the MCFP, flow increases. The slope of the relationship is –1/Rv. When right atrial pressure is below zero, lowering right atrial pressure further does not increase flow because of the vascular waterfall effect and the relationship is flat. This is the limit of the return function.

Interaction of Cardiac and Return Function

From Guyton's analysis it is evident that the actual cardiac output and right atrial pressure in the intact organism are determined by the interaction of pump function and return function. Since both of these functions share the same x- and y-axis, they

can be plotted together and the effects of changes in the individual functions can be analyzed (Fig. 29.5). An increase in pump function without a change in return function will result in an increase in cardiac output with a decrease in right atrial pressure. An increase in return function without a change in cardiac function will result in a rise in cardiac output with an increase in right atrial pressure. Changes in both cardiac and return functions to similar degrees result in a rise or fall in cardiac output with no change in right atrial pressure. This allows for some generalizations that can be useful guides for therapy. If a fall in arterial pressure is associated with a fall in cardiac output, the next question to ask is what happened to the right atrial pressure. If right atrial pressure rose, the primary problem is a pump problem. If right atrial pressure fell, the primary problem is the return function. Note that the right atrial and not the left atrial pressure is the key for this analysis, for the right atrium is where the heart and circuit interact for the determination of cardiac output. The left heart interacts with the arterial pressure, but this is already taken into account by the cardiac afterload, which affects the position and shape of the cardiac function curve.

Failure of Return Function

Once again, the four determinants of the return function are stressed vascular volume, venous resistance, venous compliance, and right atrial pressure. Since right atrial pressure is determined by the interaction of the return function and cardiac function and failure of the return function is identified by a low right atrial pressure, right atrial pressure is not really an independent factor in the return function. Of the remaining three factors of the return function, inadequate stressed vascular volume is by far the most important. This can be due to any factor that reduces blood volume, including hemorrhage, gastrointestinal losses, diuresis, severe diaphoresis, and failure to replace fluid losses. The treatment for all of these is obvious—replace the lost volume. What is not so obvious is the role of capacitance. Recruitment of unstressed volume into stressed volume allows maintenance of MCFP and thus maintenance of cardiac output and blood pressure. However, there is a limit to the reserve of unstressed volume. Normally this is in the range of 10 to perhaps as high as 15 mL/kg. Once this reserve is used up, a further loss

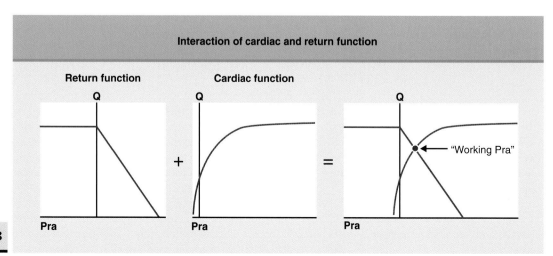

Figure 29.5. Interaction of cardiac and return function. The return function (venous return curve) and cardiac function curve are both plotted with right atrial pressure (Pra) on the x-axis and flow (Q) on the y-axis. They can thus be put on the same graph. The intersection of the two gives the Pra—cardiac output and venous return for the two functions.

of volume will result in a precipitous fall in cardiac output and blood pressure. This explains why arterial blood pressure can precipitously fall without warning in a previously stable, critically ill patient. What likely happens is that recruitment of unstressed volume into stressed volume has occurred to maintain MCFP. This allows the return function to remain normal, and thus cardiac output and blood pressure remain normal. At some point, however, the homeostatic reserve of unstressed volume is used up and the further loss of volume produces a marked fall in MCFP and thus in venous return and cardiac output (Fig. 29.6). Unfortunately, no simple clinical test can be used to assess the reserves in capacitance, and the reserves can only be surmised by considering the patient's volume history. One must ask whether the person has been loosing volume and whether sympathetic tone is increased or being supported by

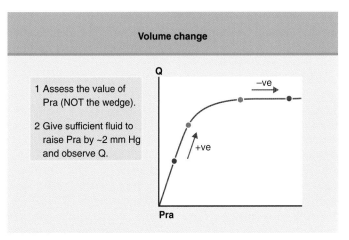

Figure 29.7. Volume change. A rise in cardiac output (Q) with a rise in right atrial pressure (Pra) indicates that the heart is functioning on the steep part of the cardiac function curve, and the increase in Pra without a change in cardiac output indicates that the heart is on the flat part of the function curve. −ve, negative response; +ve, positive response.

exogenous catecholamines. In situations where capacitance is thought to be decreased, agents that decrease venous tone such as α-adrenergic blockers and narcotics must be used very carefully for they will increase capacitance and result in a marked fall in MCFP and cardiac output. In sepsis, besides the loss of arterial tone, there also is a loss of venous tone. This increases capacitance, and more volume is needed to maintain MCFP and cardiac output. Exogenous catecholamines can help restore venous tone, but it is likely that the venous response to catecholamines is diminished as it is in the arterial tree.

Another abnormality in the return function can be a change in venous resistance. A rise in venous resistance lowers the slope of the venous return curve, and thus the return curve intersects the cardiac function curve at a lower cardiac output and lower right atrial pressure. This is the potential problem with the use of pure α-adrenergic agonists such as phenylephrine to increase SVR. Venous resistance is also increased by the inhibition of nitric oxide synthetase, and this could have contributed to the failure of nitric oxide synthetase inhibitors in the treatment of septic shock. Venous resistance can also decrease, and a decrease in venous resistance is likely an important factor in the high output state of sepsis (Fig. 29.7).

Venous compliance is determined by intrinsic properties of the vessel wall and is not normally regulated by neuroendocrine substances or pharmacologic agents. However, it has been shown that a large volume resuscitation in endotoxic animals can lead to a decrease in venous compliance in splanchnic vessels, which would also contribute to an increase in cardiac output in sepsis. This decrease in venous compliance presumably occurs via compression of capacitance vessels by the edema.

Failure of Cardiac Function

The four determinants of cardiac function are heart rate, preload, afterload, and contractility. A primary cardiac problem is defined as a low cardiac output and elevated right atrial pressure, and right atrial pressure is determined by the interaction of cardiac function and return function. Analysis of the

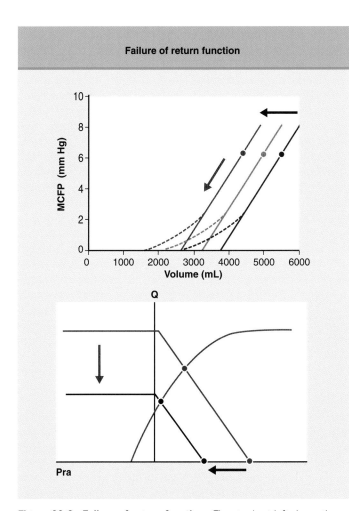

Figure 29.6. Failure of return function. The graph at left shows the pressure-volume relationship of the compliant region of the vasculature. A volume loss can be compensated by a leftward shift of the pressure volume relationship and thus maintain MCFP. However, eventually its capacitance cannot be decreased further, and a loss of volume results in a precipitous fall in MCFP. The bottom shows the consequence for the venous return curve. Initially there is no change in Pra and Q because there is no change in MCFP, but when MCFP falls there is a fall in venous return and cardiac output. Importantly, there is a fall in maximum cardiac output.

independent component of the role of cardiac dysfunction revolves around the remaining three factors. The identification of a decrease in cardiac output as being due to cardiac dysfunction based on an elevated right atrial pressure with decreased cardiac output is valid whether the primary cardiac problem is in the left or right heart. Even a pure left heart process can result in a decrease in cardiac output only by increasing right atrial pressure, for that is where the pressures that indicate the interaction of the cardiac and return function intersect. Left heart dysfunction results in an increase in pulmonary venous pressure, which increases pulmonary arterial pressure, which increases right ventricular afterload, which in turn increases right atrial pressure and that is what decreases venous return. The cardiac function curve analysis treats the heart as a unit, but once the problem is determined to be a primary cardiac problem, the next step is to determine if the problem is in the left heart, is in the right heart, or is global. This is done by comparing right and left atrial pressures. If left atrial pressure as determined by a pulmonary artery occlusion technique (Ppao) or echocardiography is elevated, and right atrial pressure is much less increased, the primary problem is in the left heart. If the right atrial pressure is elevated more than the Ppao, the problem is primarily in the right heart, and if they are both elevated, the problem is likely global, although this can also occur by great overdistention of the right ventricle with a primary right heart problem.

RIGHT HEART DYSFUNCTION

Importance of the Plateau of the Cardiac Function Curve

Right ventricular dysfunction is very common in critically ill patients. A key step in the management of critically ill patients is thus to determine whether or not the patient has reached the limit of the cardiac function curve, for once the plateau of the cardiac function curve is reached, further volume loading cannot increase cardiac output. The increase in volume above the plateau value will make the patient worse, for the increase in ventricular pressure will increase wall stress, distort the ventricles, and produce peripheral edema. What often is not appreciated is that the limit of the cardiac function curve occurs in most people at a right atrial pressure of less than 10 to 12 mm Hg, and in some people right ventricular function can be limited even below 5 mm Hg. Individual responses are highly variable and also affected by the measurement technique. It is thus important to determine if the patient's heart is functioning on the flat part of the cardiac function curve.

Tests of Cardiac Function Limitation and Volume Responsiveness

If measurements of cardiac output are available, the gold standard for determining the cardiac limitation is to give a volume bolus sufficient to raise right atrial pressure and then determine if there is a change in cardiac output (see Fig. 29.7). An increase in right atrial pressure of 2 mm Hg has been suggested because this magnitude of change can be determined with some confidence on most monitors, although even a change of 1 mm Hg can produce a significant change in cardiac output. A change in cardiac output in the range of 300 mL/min is a reasonable choice because it is in the range of error of repeated measurements of cardiac output by thermodilution.

There are a number of other bedside guides that can be used to determine whether right heart function is limited. Useful information can be found in the wave form of the right atrial pressure tracing. The y-descent of the atrial pressure tracing is due to the emptying of atrial volume into the ventricle at the start of diastole. If ventricular filling is restricted, as is the case on the plateau phase of the cardiac function curve, there is steep drop of the pressure wave and a rapid rise. The steep drop in pressure occurs because the ventricle is relatively compliant after the ventricle has ejected volume, but as it fills, the steep part of the pressure volume curve is again reached and there is a marked rise in pressure. In one study, a y-descent of greater than 4 mm Hg was associated with a limit to cardiac filling, but the number of subjects was small, which limits the precision of this value, although the general principle is likely valid. Similar information can be obtained from the pattern of diastolic mitral flow with the use of echocardiography.

In patients who have any spontaneous respiratory efforts, even if the effort only involves triggering a mechanical breath, the absence or presence of respiratory variations in right atrial pressure can be used to determine if the patient will be volume responsive (Fig. 29.8). The lack of an inspiratory fall in right atrial pressure as measured at the base of the "a" wave during the spontaneous effort indicates that the heart is functioning on the plateau of the cardiac function curve and volume loading will not increase cardiac output. The presence of an inspiratory fall in right atrial pressure indicates that the heart is functioning on the ascending part of the cardiac function curve and will likely but not necessarily respond to volume infusion. The reason volume loading does not always increase cardiac output in patients with an inspiratory fall in right atrial pressure is that the heart may be functioning too close to the plateau of the cardiac function curve to observe a change in cardiac output with a volume infusion, but the inspiratory fall in pleural pressure can still produce a fall in right atrial pressure because it moves to the left of the venous return curve. An important potential false positive result with this technique occurs in patients who have forced expiration, for this will produce an expiratory rise in right atrial pressure, and when the expiratory effort is released, it may appear that there was an inspiratory fall in pressure when in reality there was just a loss of the expiratory rise.

Other approaches that have been used to determine whether the heart is volume responsive and thus on the ascending portion of the cardiac function curve are the assessment of respiratory variations in systolic arterial pressure, arterial pulse pressure, or left ventricular stroke volume variation as assessed by Doppler techniques. With all these tests, the larger the fall in the pressure or stroke volume during the expiratory phase of the respiratory cycle, the more likely that the cardiac output will increase with a volume infusion. Although various values have been given in the literature to determine the likelihood of cardiac output being volume responsive, these values are highly dependent upon the ventilator settings, the pulmonary and chest wall compliance, and aortic elastance and filling. It also must be emphasized that for all tests that use a variation of arterial pressure or stroke volume to predict fluid responsiveness, the patient must have no spontaneous respiratory efforts, including inspiratory or expiratory efforts.

The tests presented in this section can be used to determine if the patient will respond to volume. However, it is important

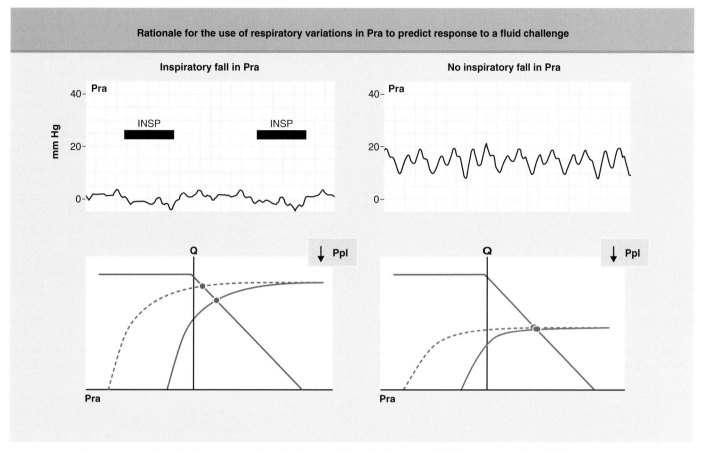

Rationale for the use of respiratory variations in Pra to predict response to a fluid challenge

Inspiratory fall in Pra

No inspiratory fall in Pra

Figure 29.8. Rationale for the use of respiratory variations in Pra to predict the response to a fluid challenge.
At left, a fall in right atrial pressure (Pra) predicts that the venous return curve intersects the ascending part of the cardiac function curve and an increase in volume (which shifts the venous return curve to the right) will likely, but not necessarily, increase cardiac output. At right, there is no inspiratory fall in Pra. This predicts that the venous return curve intersects the plateau of the cardiac function curve, and a rightward shift of the venous return curve will not change cardiac output. Ppl, Pleural pressure.

to appreciate that this does not mean that the patient needs volume. Under normal physiologic conditions, the return function intersects the cardiac function curve and thus cardiac output will increase with a volume infusion, but by definition, normal people do not need a volume infusion. Even in an unstable patient who has evidence of volume responsiveness, volume infusion is not necessarily the correct choice, and there might be advantages to increasing inotropy or increasing arterial pressure with a vasopressor rather than increasing cardiac output by giving more volume. When the arterial pressure is increased by increasing cardiac output with a volume infusion, pressure increases throughout the vasculature because the resistance profile of the vascular tree is not altered (Fig. 29.9). This means that capillary pressures will also increase, which in turn means that the force driving capillary filtration will also be increased. In contrast, when arterial pressure is increased with the use of a vasoconstrictor, the resistance profile throughout the vasculature is altered so that the pressure in vessels distal to the arterioles, including capillaries, is likely unchanged or even decreased. This will tend to decrease capillary filtration, which is especially important in patients with sepsis and increased capillary leak.

Importance of Right Ventricular Afterload
In contrast to the left ventricle, which functions as a pressure pump, the right ventricle functions more as a volume pump and does not tolerate large increases in pressure. Without any preconditioning, the right ventricle will usually fail when the pulmonary arterial systolic pressure is greater than 50 mm Hg. When the right ventricle fails, right ventricular end-systolic volume rises and consequently right ventricular end-diastolic volume rises. When the increase in end-diastolic volume is large enough so that the heart is functioning on the steep portion of the diastolic pressure-volume curve, there is no more preload reserve to allow compensation for further increases in right ventricular afterload. When that happens, further increases in pulmonary artery pressure will result in a decrease in stroke volume. Cardiac output can then only be maintained by an increase in contractility or heart rate or a decrease in pulmonary vascular resistance (Fig. 29.10).

Preload Becomes Afterload
Right ventricular preload has potential for an important paradoxical effect. An increase in right atrial pressure when the heart is functioning on the flat part of the cardiac function curve will

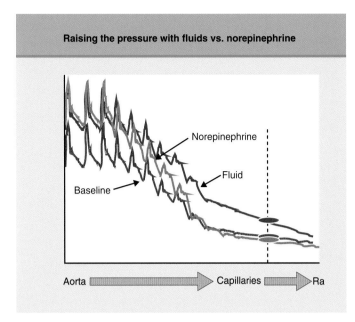

Raising the pressure with fluids vs. norepinephrine

Figure 29.9. Raising the pressure with fluids vs. norepinephrine.
Fluid infusion raises the pressure throughout the vasculature without a
change in the pressure profile. In contrast, an infusion of norepinephrine
sufficient to produce the same rise in pressure changes the pressure
profile so that at the level of the capillaries there may be no change or
even a decrease in capillary pressure. Ra, right atrium.

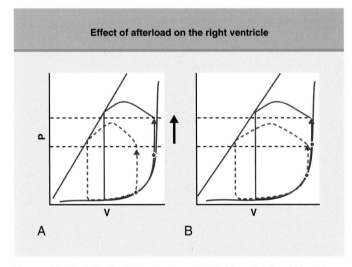

Effect of afterload on the right ventricle

Figure 29.10. Effect of afterload on the right ventricle. At left, the
rise in afterload (rise in dashed line; A) results in a small fall in stroke
volume because there are still adequate reserves in the end-diastolic
volume. At right, the EDV is on the steep portion of the diastolic pressure-
volume relationship, there are no diastolic reserves to compensate for the
increase in afterload, and there is a much larger fall in stroke volume.

be transmitted to the left heart even though the cardiac output
does not change. This occurs because of the coupling effect of
the pericardium and cardiac cytoskeleton. The consequent rise
in left atrial pressure leads to an increase in pulmonary venous
and thus pulmonary arterial pressure, which then further
increases the load on the right heart and leads to a further

decrease in right ventricular stroke volume. In this way, the pulmonary arterial pressure can remain the same even though
cardiac output falls. The expression is that "right ventricular
preload becomes right ventricular afterload."

A consequence of high right heart pressure is that coronary
venous pressure, as well as the critical closing pressure in coronary vessels, rises. This compromises perfusion to the right heart
and leads to further right heart decompensation. Furthermore,
as the right heart fails, cardiac output falls and thus arterial pressure and coronary perfusion pressure fall. On the left side of the
heart, a fall in coronary perfusion pressure due to a decrease in
arterial pressure is at least matched by a fall in left ventricular
wall tension, an important determinant of myocardial oxygen
demand. However, this is not true for the right heart, where the
load on the right ventricle and wall tension can remain elevated
even though coronary perfusion pressure decreases. For this
reason, it is critical to maintain adequate arterial pressure in
patients with right heart failure so that perfusion to the failing
right heart does not fall and to be cautious in the use of drugs
that decrease arterial pressure.

As discussed above, overdistention of the right heart can lead
to a decrease in cardiac output with increasing right atrial pressures. This may appear as if the heart is functioning on a downward part of the Starling function curve, but there is no
downward part to a Starling curve. The overdistention of the
ventricular wall actually decreases cardiac function and the heart
is operating on a new and lower cardiac function curve. This may
occur because of myocardial ischemia from the high wall pressures, because of distortion of the ventricles, or possibly from
valvular regurgitation due to ventricular dilatation and disruption of the normal function of the atrioventricular valves. The
consequence, however, is the same as if there were a downward
part to the Starling curve. Decreasing the diastolic pressure in
the heart and reducing ventricular overdistention potentially can
improve cardiac function, as demonstrated by Atherton and
coworkers.

The load on the right ventricle is more complicated than just
the pulmonary systolic pressure and is really related more to pulmonary vascular resistance. Again based on Poiseuille's law, a rise
in right heart output will lead to a rise in pulmonary arterial
pressure, but the magnitude of the change in pressure depends
upon the pulmonary resistance. The importance of this is that
pulmonary pressure can be elevated because the pulmonary vascular resistance is high or because the downstream pulmonary
artery or venous pressures are elevated and resistance is not
increased. The downstream pressure can be from the left atrium
but also can be from a critical closing pressure in the pulmonary
circuit. This in turn can be produced by air trapping and the production of West zone 2, in which case alveolar pressure is higher
than pulmonary venous pressure but less than pulmonary arterial pressure, or by disease processes that affect small pulmonary
arteries (Fig. 29.11). This is important because when pulmonary
pressure is elevated owing to a rise in the outflow pressure and
not the resistance, an increase in cardiac output will produce a
small rise in pulmonary artery pressure and be better tolerated
than when the pulmonary pressure is increased owing to high
pulmonary vascular resistance. This has particular significance
for the selection of patients for heart transplantation.

The classic clinical sign of chronic right heart dysfunction is
peripheral edema. The question arises whether the heart has a

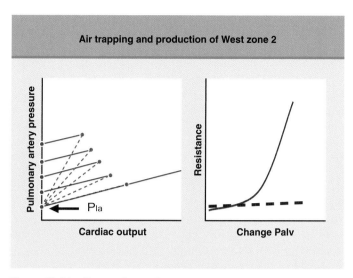

Figure 29.11. Air trapping and production of West zone 2. At left is shown the pressure-flow relationship of the pulmonary artery and cardiac output, and the figure at right shows the relationship of pulmonary vascular resistance to change in pulmonary alveolar pressure (Palv). If the "outflow" pressure is viewed as left atrial pressure, it appears that pulmonary artery resistance increases with increases in Palv. However, if the increase in pulmonary artery pressure rises because of an increase in outflow pressure due to the change in Palv, this creates a vascular waterfall phenomenon at the level of the alveoli (West zone 2) and the true resistance does not change (upward shift of parallel lines and flat dashed line in the figure at right).

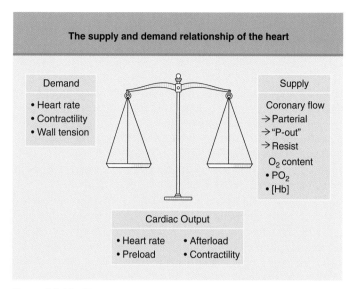

Figure 29.12. The supply and demand relationship of the heart. P-out, outflow pressure.

role in the production of this edema. This was the actual question raised by Starling (1918) when he designed his studies on cardiac function and the law of the heart. As Starling appreciated, the answer is no. Consider what happens when the cardiac output goes to zero. The right atrial pressure will rise only to the level of MCFP, which is the pressure in the small veins and venules and is normally in the range of 8 to 10 mm Hg. Even with major recruitment of unstressed volume into stressed volume, MCFP will rise only to the 12 to 15 mm Hg range, which would not cause major edema, and if edema developed this would mean a loss of vascular volume into the interstitial space. Thus, edema is caused by the retention of fluid by the kidneys or by excessive intake of fluid, which means that in critically ill patients there is often a significant iatrogenic component to edema formation. This physiologic point has important implications for patients who have initial high right atrial pressures. A high initial right atrial pressure means that the patient must have chronic right heart failure, have received a lot of intravenous fluids, or possibly has a ruptured ventricular septum so that left-sided pressures are transmitted to the right heart.

LEFT HEART DYSFUNCTION

The left heart is composed of a thick muscle that generates high pressures and has high energy demands. Thus, to understand the pathophysiology of the left heart dysfunction, it is necessary to have a good understanding of the energy supply-demand relationship of the heart (Fig. 29.12). The primary determinants of myocardial energy demand are heart rate, wall tension, and con-

tractility. Wall tension is related to the product of the pressure in the ventricle and the radius of the ventricle. The largest radius occurs during diastole, and thus diastolic volume is a major determinant of peak wall tension. The greatest pressure in the ventricle occurs during contraction, and thus the arterial pressure is the second major determinant of maximal wall tension during the cardiac cycle. The tension in the wall is decreased by an increase in wall thickness, but this in practice is not much help because when the heart hypertrophies, the microvasculature does not increase in proportion to the increase in muscle mass and the diffusion of oxygen from the blood to myocardial cells is compromised. This is especially a problem in subendocardial regions of the heart. Since contractility tends to increase with increases in heart rate, changes in the product of heart rate and arterial pressure give good estimates of the changes in energy needs of the heart, and even a change in heart rate alone gives a reasonable approximation of increases in myocardial oxygen demand. The actual need for oxygen depends upon the initial heart size and the blood pressure.

As is the case with other muscles, an increase in myocardial oxygen demand must be matched by an increase in coronary flow, and there is a linear relationship between myocardial oxygen demand and coronary flow. However, unlike other muscles, the heart works continuously at a high metabolic level. When the body functions at a basal metabolic rate and the heart is beating at the normal "resting" rate of 60 to 70 beats/min, the heart consumes 6 to 8 mL O_2/min/100 g tissue, which accounts for 10% to 12% of the resting oxygen consumption for the whole body. In contrast, the oxygen consumption of resting skeletal muscle is only 0.15 mL O_2/min/100 g. Even an asystolic heart consumes 1.5 mL O_2/min/100 g, which is 10-fold higher than resting skeletal muscle. To supply its oxygen needs, the heart requires coronary flow in the range of 70 to 80 mL O_2/min/100 g tissue (assuming a normal hemoglobin concentration), whereas resting skeletal muscle requires only a blood flow of approximately 4 to 6 mL O_2/min/100 g tissue. Because of the high energy demand and oxygen consumption of the heart, oxygen extraction in the coronary circulation is in the 70% to 80% range even at resting heart rates, whereas that of resting skeletal muscle is less than 25%. Thus, the working heart has very limited extraction reserves to compensate for inadequate coronary blood flow. Furthermore, because of the heart's high energy demands, anaerobic metabolism can provide the heart's energy needs for only very brief periods, and cardiac force generation falls very quickly when the supply of oxygen is inadequate to meet the heart's energy needs. If the oxygen supply is inadequate in a region of the heart, regional dyskinesia results and oxygen supply is inadequate for the whole heart, the result being pulseless electrical activity.

The heart tolerates volume loads (i.e., ejecting stroke volume) much more efficiently than pressure loads, which produce great demands on the heart, both in terms of energy needs and its ability to shorten. This is likely one of the reasons that the circulatory system evolved as a constant pressure system, for having a constant pressure means that one of the major determinants of the energy demands of the heart does not change. For this reason it generally is not useful to try to improve coronary flow by increasing arterial pressure above normal levels. In particular, decreasing arterial pressure often treats subendocardial myocardial ischemia, although one must be careful not to decrease arterial pressure to levels that compromise coronary flow.

Determinants of myocardial oxygen delivery are coronary arterial blood flow, hemoglobin concentration, and arterial oxygen saturation. Coronary blood flow is determined by arterial pressure, the downstream pressure in the myocardium, and the coronary vascular resistance. The downstream pressure for the coronary circulation is not actually the coronary venous pressure, although the venous pressure affects the coronary downstream pressure. The downstream pressure is produced by a critical closing pressure at the arteriolar level. A critical closing pressure occurs when the inward force on the wall of the vessel is greater than the pressure inside the vessel. The critical closing pressure in the coronary circulation has been estimated to be in the range of 20 to 25 mm Hg. It is increased when the tension in the wall of the heart is increased and also by increases in diastolic filling pressure. Coronary arterial critical closing pressure can also be increased by α-adrenergic agents, increased arterial pressure, and inhibitors of nitric oxide synthase and decreased by increased metabolic activity.

The potential flow reserves of the normal heart are very large. As noted above, the "resting" coronary flow is in the range of 70 to 80 mL/min/100 g tissue, but flow can increase to 400 to 500 mL/min/100 g tissue at peak cardiac performance; this value is almost double that obtainable in skeletal muscle. Since arterial pressure is generally regulated over a small range and the magnitude of potential variations in critical closing pressure is small, large changes in coronary flow are primarily dependent upon a decrease in coronary vascular resistance. The resistance in the large epicardial coronary vessels is small, and the main coronary vascular resistance is at the arteriolar level. Because of this, epicardial vessels need to be narrowed by at least 70% before coronary flow is significantly compromised, and the narrowing needs to be greater than 95% before resting flow is compromised. This explains why the symptoms of coronary artery disease mainly occur when myocardial oxygen demand is significantly increased. The presence of signs and symptoms of

myocardial ischemia at low heart rates indicates that there must be an almost a total occlusion of a large coronary vessel. Furthermore, if the ischemia is transient, coronary artery spasm or intermittent platelet plugs are likely playing a role.

It is worthwhile to consider the effect of changes in the magnitude of the three factors that determine oxygen delivery, which are coronary flow, hemoglobin concentration, and oxygen saturation. An increase in hemoglobin concentration from 80 to 120 g/L would increase myocardial O_2 delivery by 50%, and a change in oxygen saturation from 80% to 100% would increase O_2 delivery by 25%, but these changes are small compared to the potential increase in flow of almost 600% that is produced by a decrease in coronary arterial resistance when coronary vessels are normal. Thus, increasing hemoglobin concentration or oxygen saturation has a therapeutic benefit only when changes in coronary flow are very limited.

The heart differs from all other tissues in that during systole the high pressure in the wall of the heart impedes blood flow and coronary flow to the left heart must largely occur during diastole. Thus, the magnitude of diastolic pressure and the rate of decrease of diastolic pressure are important determinants of coronary perfusion. The magnitude of diastolic pressure is dependent upon systolic pressure, for systolic pressure determines the starting point of the diastolic run-off. However, increasing systolic pressure increases the energy demands of the heart and thus increases the need for more oxygen and flow. A useful relationship to consider when examining the energy supply-demand balance of the heart is the ratio of the area under the systolic pressure time curve, which is related to myocardial oxygen demand and the area under the diastolic pressure time curve, which is related to the supply of oxygen to the heart (Fig. 29.13). In the 1970s, attempts were made to build this into monitoring devices, but the sensitivity of specific guidelines was inadequate. However, the basic concept is still useful.

The left heart tolerates large afterloads much better than the right heart does. During daily activities, the arterial pressure can get very high for transient periods, and these rises in pressure

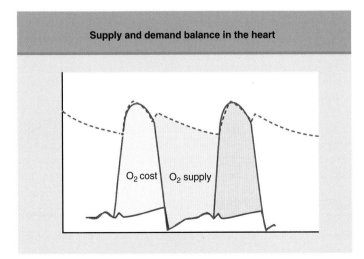

Figure 29.13. Supply and demand balance in the heart. O_2 cost is primarily determined by the area under the systolic pressure time relationship. O_2 supply is determined by the area under the diastolic pressure time curve for this determines coronary perfusion.

are well tolerated by the normal heart. High blood pressure becomes important when it is sustained because of the induction of changes in vessel walls and cardiac hypertrophy. Changes in afterload can have consequences for both forward and backward failure. The effect of afterload on both forward and backward failure depends upon the slope of the end-systolic pressure volume relationship. If the slope of this relationship is steep, there is only a small reduction in stroke volume with an increase in arterial pressure and also only a small rise in end systolic volume. Thus, when the heart is functioning normally, decreasing arterial pressure produces little gain in stroke volume. With regard to backward failure, the normal physiologic response to an increase in afterload is an increase in atrial filling pressure. The reason for this is evident from an examination of the ventricular pressure-volume relationship. When the heart ejects at a higher arterial pressure, the end-systolic volume increases. For the same return of blood per beat, the end-diastolic volume and thus end-diastolic pressure must rise unless there is a change in heart rate or contractility. As discussed above, for the effects of a change in afterload on stroke volume, the rise in magnitude of the end-diastolic volume will depend upon the slope of the end-systolic pressure volume relationship. However, the magnitude of the change in atrial pressure for a change in afterload also depends upon where the heart is functioning on the passive filling curve of the ventricle. If the left ventricular end-diastolic volume starts on the steep part of the passive filling curve, the change in atrial pressure in response to an increase in afterload will be large, even for very small changes in volume. Thus, the potential therapeutic benefit for a reduction in pulmonary capillary pressures, the driving force for pulmonary edema, will be greater. For this reason, although often not appreciated, the effect of a change in afterload is probably in many cases more important for backward failure than for forward failure.

Another factor that limits the significance of changes in left ventricular afterload on stroke volume and cardiac output is the series effect of the two ventricles. It must be remembered that the left heart can only put out what the right heart delivers. If the output from the right heart is limited, a change in left heart function will not change forward output unless the change in left-sided function results in a reduction in the load on right ventricle failure sufficient to allow the right heart to move off the plateau of the cardiac function curve. Another consequence of the series effect is that when the right heart function is limited, left heart dysfunction may not be evident until right heart function improves. The expression is that there is "no left-sided failure without right-sided success." A clinical caveat is that pulmonary edema in the presence of right heart limitation means that there is likely nonhydrostatic pulmonary edema and increased capillary leak.

As discussed above, pure left heart dysfunction can only lower cardiac output by eventually raising right atrial pressure and decreasing the gradient for venous return. For this to happen, there must be a large increase in pulmonary vascular pressures, which will greatly increase pulmonary vascular leak. Because of this, patients effectively drown before cardiac output falls. When cardiac output falls from a primary left heart problem, it is more likely because the hypoxemia and respiratory acidosis due to the respiratory failure are the cause of global cardiac failure. Failure of cardiac function leads to worsening respiratory failure because the decrease in cardiac output

limits respiratory muscle blood flow, which decreases respiratory muscle function in the face of increased respiratory demands.

An interesting consequence of ventricular interaction was studied by Scharf and coworkers as well Belenkie and coworkers. As already discussed, it is well recognized that a decrease in cardiac output induced by right ventricular dysfunction eventually leads to a decrease in arterial pressure and coronary perfusion pressure. The decrease in coronary perfusion results in progressive worsening of right ventricular function and death. To identify other potential effects of a decrease in arterial pressure on cardiac function, these investigators maintained coronary pressure constant and studied the independent effect of arterial pressure on right ventricular function. They found that an increase in arterial pressure resulted in an increase in load tolerance of the right ventricle even without a change in coronary perfusion. The explanation given is that the ventricular septum is common to both ventricles, and thus the increased force of left ventricular contraction aids right ventricular ejection by increased shortening of the septum, which is common to both chambers.

SPECIFIC CAUSES OF CARDIOVASCULAR FAILURE

Valvular Disease

A number of the effects of valvular abnormalities on cardiac dysfunction are reviewed in this section. A common problem of critically ill patients is mitral regurgitation. This can occur acutely because of ischemia or infarction of the base of the papillary muscles as well as erosion of the leaflets by bacterial endocarditis. Acute mitral insufficiency results in a marked rise in left ventricular diastolic pressures and severe acute pulmonary edema. However, the cardiac output may only be moderately depressed. The reasoning is the same as discussed for acute coronary events. For cardiac output to decrease, there ultimately must be a rise in right atrial pressure; the patient literally drowns before this happens. A more frequent problem in critically ill patients than complete disruption of the mitral valve is mitral insufficiency as a result of dilation of the ventricle and mitral ring as well as inadequate alignment of the papillary muscle–chordae apparatus. This results in another positive feedback loop. Wall stress increases as the heart dilates. Myocardial oxygen demand is increased, and the resulting supply-demand imbalance produces myocardial ischemia and decreased ventricular efficiency. These lead to further dilatation and progressive deterioration. Reduction of ventricular size thus potentially plays an important role in the management of these patients, for it reduces regurgitation and improves ventricular efficiency. Afterload reduction and increasing ventricular contractility can reduce ventricular size and thus are important components of the management strategy.

In chronic aortic insufficiency, the heart dilates in response to the increase in end-diastolic load and the end-diastolic pressures can remain normal. Peripheral dilatation due to a reflex response to the larger than normal stroke volume also occurs and helps reduce the regurgitant fraction. However, the large ventricle volume means that the wall stress is increased and so is myocardial oxygen demand. Furthermore, the decrease in peripheral resistance results in a more rapid fall in diastolic pressure and thus a decrease in coronary perfusion pressure. As discussed above in the coronary perfusion section, this means that demand is increased at a time when supply is decreased and there is potential for myocardial ischemia, especially in the subendocardial regions, where wall stress is greatest. This could especially become a problem under other conditions, such as hemorrhage or sepsis or lower arterial pressure.

Acute aortic valve insufficiency is an uncommon problem but an important one to recognize. The major causes are endocarditis and erosion of the valve and aortic dissection with disruption of the aortic valve cusps. In acute aortic insufficiency there is no cardiac or circulatory adaptation. Since arterial resistance does not fall, one of the classic signs of aortic insufficiency is absent. Importantly, when aortic insufficiency is acute, left ventricular pressure rises very quickly during diastole and produces severe pulmonary edema. The rapid rise in diastolic pressure can even close the mitral valve before the end of diastole, which produces a classic echocardiographic sign of this condition—premature closure of the mitral valve.

Patients with aortic stenosis are at increased risk when acutely ill. The high ventricular pressure required for ejection means that cardiac energy demands are high and relatively fixed, which means that decreases in coronary perfusion pressure are generally not well tolerated, although surprisingly a recent report showed that afterload reduction could improve function in patients with aortic stenosis. The gradient across the aortic valve, and thus the classic systolic ejection murmur, are related to the flow across the valve. When the ventricle fails, forward flow of aortic stenosis and the gradient across the valve decrease. Thus, the classic murmur may not be obvious in severe cases, and the physician must have a high index of suspicion and remember to consider tight aortic stenosis in patients with unexplained cardiovascular failure. A major problem for patients with aortic stenosis is that when the heart hypertrophies, the coronary microvasculature does not increase in proportion to the increase in muscle mass, and myocardial oxygen supply can easily become inadequate to the demand. These patients are particularly sensitive to hypotension. Furthermore, the heart may not be able to increase cardiac output to meet the tissue needs in distributive shock. The typical fall in peripheral resistance with sepsis will thus tend to result in more severe hypotension. Because of the decreased ventricular compliance, volume infusion in such a patient will also have a much greater likelihood of producing pulmonary edema, and the use of inotropic agents and vasoconstrictors such as norepinephrine is a preferable approach.

A less common cause of aortic outflow tract obstruction, but one that is often not recognized, is subacute aortic obstruction. In this condition, thickened myocardium, particularly in the septum, can obstruct the outflow to the left ventricle. Part of the obstruction is caused directly by myocardial muscle bulging into the outflow tract, but part is also due to the mitral valve being sucked into the narrowed outflow tract by the Bernoulli effect, which is produced by the increased ejection velocity through the aortic outflow tract. The degree of obstruction increases when the ventricle is smaller. Thus, the obstruction is increased by hypovolemia or a decrease in right heart output induced by increased intrathoracic pressure. The fall in cardiac output may tempt the clinician to use inotropic agents to improve cardiac output, but inotropes will worsen the condition. The increase in contractility will decrease ventricular size and increase obstruction. Inotropes also increase the ejection velocity and Bernoulli effect. The correct clinical solution is to give volume as well as a pure α-agonist such as phenylephrine. The α-agonist will have a minimal impact on cardiac contractility but will increase peripheral resistance and the ventricular afterload and this will increase end-systolic pressure and volume. The increase in ventricular volume will decrease the dynamic obstruction, and the improved ejection will improve coronary perfusion pressure.

Sepsis

A decrease in cardiac function in sepsis is well described. The decrease in contractility is related to expression of cytokines such as tumor necrosis factor–α and the production of nitric oxide. There are abnormalities of α-adrenergic signaling as well as the handling of intracellular calcium. Importantly, sepsis-induced cardiac dysfunction usually resolves quickly when the septic process resolves. Despite evidence of cardiac dysfunction in isolated heart preparations and cardiac myocytes in culture, most patients and volume-resuscitated animals actually have an increase in cardiac output, and cardiac function appears preserved or even increased. This apparent paradox can be partly explained by realizing that in the laboratory, maximal cardiac performance is tested, whereas in patients, the heart is likely functioning at a submaximal level, for the full capacity of the normal heart is many fold greater than that seen at rest. Thus, increases in intrinsic catecholamines can still increase contractility even with reduced reserves until the condition becomes very severe. It is likely that reflex mechanisms and other stimuli of intrinsic responses do not return the cardiac function to normal so that the increase in cardiac output is associated with higher than normal filling pressures.

It has been argued that the increase in cardiac output in sepsis is related to the decrease in systemic vascular resistance and the consequent decrease in left ventricular afterload. However, this explanation is typical of the error in reasoning that occurs when the significance of the series effect of the right and left ventricles is not considered. Although the afterload on the left ventricle is decreased in sepsis, the afterload on the right ventricle usually rises because of an increase in pulmonary artery pressure. The only way that a fall in left ventricular afterload can increase cardiac output is by decreasing pulmonary artery pressure; therefore, this clearly cannot be the explanation. It has also been noted that survivors of sepsis have dilated left ventricles, whereas nonsurvivors have less dilatation of the left ventricle. A possible explanation for this seeming paradox is that the left ventricle can only dilate if the right ventricle successfully increases flow to the left heart. Thus, patients who have more severe cardiac dysfunction and limitation of right ventricular output will not have dilatation of the left ventricle. As stated previously, there cannot be left-sided failure without right-sided success.

Cardiac Surgery

Right ventricular dysfunction is common following cardiac surgery. The cause is multifactorial. An important factor is that it is more difficult to provide myocardial protection to the right heart than to the left heart. This can especially be a problem when the patient has a major obstruction of the right coronary artery prior to surgery. In such patients there might be right ventricular dysfunction even prior to surgery, which is exacerbated by the decreased perfusion during surgery. The right heart also can easily become overdistended when the patient is put on or off the cardiac bypass circuit. The distention of the ventricle raises the pressure in the right ventricular wall, which can result in myocardial ischemia. There can also be direct injury to the right ventricle by emboli down the right coronary or problems related to the creation of a right coronary graft.

Acute Deterioration in Patients with Dyskinetic Myocardial Segments

Patients who have an area of the myocardium that bulges outward during contraction are in a potentially precarious position. If left ventricular volume is increased because of an increased load on the ventricle or decrease in contractility by a pharmacologic agent, alcohol, or a mild infection, the increase in ventricular radius will increase wall stress and myocardial oxygen demand. If coronary flow to the region is limited, there is further ischemia, which will lead to further dilatation and perpetuate the process until the patient presents in extremis. Furthermore, when ischemic segments of myocardium bulge outward, the heart becomes more inefficient because a significant amount of the work from sarcomere shortening goes into increasing the volume of the dyskinetic area rather than producing forward flow. The key to breaking this vicious cycle is to decompress the ventricle by decreasing left ventricular volume. This decreases the wall stress and reduces the wasted stroke volume and allows rebalancing of the supply-demand relationship of the heart. Decompression can be achieved acutely by pharmacologic means with drugs such as nitrates or by mechanically increasing intrathoracic pressure with positive airway pressure.

Acute Coronary Ischemia in Critically Ill Patients

It is important to consider the mechanisms of acute coronary ischemia when planning therapy for a critically ill patient. In the community, myocardial infarction is caused most often by rupture of an atherosclerotic plaque, exposure of the intravascular blood to thrombogenic factors in the vessel wall, and development of a thrombus. Thus, the main therapeutic approach is to use antiplatelet drugs to prevent platelet aggregation and antithrombotic agents to decrease thrombus formation. Attempts are also made to clear the clot by lytic agents or directly with balloon angioplasty. For these techniques to successfully open an occluded vessel and salvage ischemic myocardium, perfusion needs to be restored ideally within 4 to 6 hours and at least by around 12 hours; otherwise most of the injury is irreversible. Once the damage is irreversible, there is little advantage to the use of antithrombotic agents except to prevent clot development at the site of injury in the ventricle, for this becomes a potential source of systemic embolization in infarcted hearts. There is also little advantage at that point to urgently trying to reopen the vessel.

The increased stress of surgery and associated increase in prothrombotic factors during surgery can also lead to plaque rupture and a typical acute coronary event. However, a number of factors also increase the risk of subendocardial ischemia from a supply-demand imbalance in the perioperative and critically ill patient, even without coronary obstruction. Induction of anesthesia or pain can result in tachycardia, which will increase myocardial oxygen demand. Ischemia due to these processes is not due to a thrombotic process and generally results in more diffuse myocardial injury than that seen with plaque rupture. Thus, these patients would not be expected to respond to antithrombotic or antiplatelet therapy. Restoring the supply-demand balance is likely to be the crucial factor in management.

"Pseudocardiac" Failure

The value of right atrial pressure that determines cardiac function is the transmural right atrial pressure, which is the pressure inside the heart relative to the pressure surrounding the heart. This is accounted for in Guyton's graphic analysis by starting the cardiac function curve from a value below zero in a person who is breathing spontaneously, because at end-expiration, pleural pressure is less than atmospheric pressure. When the patient is breathing with mechanical breaths and positive pressure ventilation, the cardiac function curve is shifted to the right. An increase in pressure surrounding the heart, either due to an increase in pleural pressure or to increased compression by structures around the heart, including pericardial fluid, leads to a picture of apparent cardiac dysfunction (Fig. 29.14). Thus, the patient may have high cardiac filling pressures because of external compressive factors but actually have a low transmural pressure, which is the true determinant of preload. This can occur also when abdominal pressure is markedly increased, as in the abdominal compartment syndrome, for the high abdominal pressure can be transmitted to the pleural space. All these conditions can produce what might be called "pseudocardiac failure" because the filling pressures seem high and the cardiac output is low, but in reality the transmural pressure is not elevated and there is no abnormality of cardiac function. In such patients cardiac output may increase in response to a fluid bolus at high right atrial pressures because a high pressure relative to

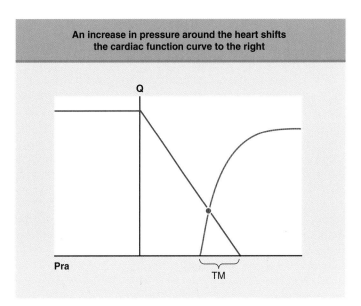

Figure 29.14. An increase in pressure around the heart shifts the cardiac function curve to the right. The single point would suggest a decrease in cardiac function; however, the shape of the cardiac function curve is not altered and the decrease in cardiac output is explained by the marked decrease in transmural pressure (TM).

atmosphere is required to overcome the external compressive forces and stretch the sarcomeres. However, there is a very important consequence of this strategy, and the therapeutic utility of this approach is limited. Although right atrial transmural pressure determines cardiac function, the downstream pressure and determinant of venous return is the right atrial pressure relative to atmospheric pressure and not the transmural pressure. For venous return to occur, the MCFP must be higher than right atrial pressure, and the capillary pressure is higher than MCFP, for the capillaries are upstream from the capacitant region of the circulation. The high venous pressure can have an important effect on renal and hepatic blood flow and greatly increase capillary filtration and edema formation. Edema formation in thoracic structures also increases with high venous pressures, and this leads to increased compression of the heart. Even higher cardiac filling pressures then are required to maintain cardiac output. Thus, a strategy of pushing central venous pressures to very high levels is ultimately doomed to fail, and instead attempts must be made to increase cardiac function by increasing either heart rate or contractility, for these will allow cardiac output to be generated at a lower transmural filling pressure. As the edema resolves in the mediastinum, the compressive forces around the heart will decrease, and gradually it should become possible to maintain normal cardiac output at lower central venous pressures.

The full magnitude of the effect of high central venous pressures on upstream venous beds, including the liver and kidney, is often not appreciated, since the standard measurement of right atrial pressure is made at the base of the "a" wave because this gives the best estimate of the cardiac preload. However, as filling pressures rise and atrial compliance decreases, the peak of the "a" and "v" waves can increase substantially and have a significant impact on the liver and kidneys.

SUMMARY AND APPROACH TO SHOCK

As discussed in the introduction, examination of the relationship of arterial pressure to cardiac output and systemic vascular resistance provides the basis for diagnosing and treating cardiovascular failure and hypotension (Fig. 29.15). The first question to ask is, what is the cardiac output? If the arterial pressure is decreased with a normal or elevated cardiac output, the problem is a decrease in SVR. The important part of the management is then to increase the SVR with an agent such as norepinephrine. One could also increase the arterial pressure by increasing cardiac output with volume if cardiac function is not limited, but as discussed above, the consequences for the microcirculation are potentially very different from what occurs with the use of a vasopressor. Furthermore, if cardiac function is limited, which is often the case, volume loading will not increase cardiac output. If the arterial pressure is decreased because of a decrease in cardiac output, the next step is to determine if the cardiac output is decreased because of a decrease in pump function or a decrease in the return function. These two are separated by examination of the right atrial pressure. If the right atrial pressure is low, or even better if cardiac output fell with a fall in right atrial pressure, the primary problem is in the return function. The most likely cause is a loss of volume, and a volume infusion is likely to be the best approach. If volume reserves are adequate, it is also possible to recruit unstressed volume

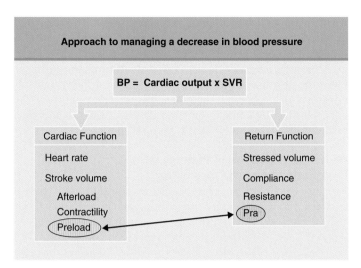

Figure 29.15. Approach to managing a decrease in blood pressure (BP). See text for details. SVR, systemic vascular resistance.

into stressed volume with norepinephrine; this can be helpful in patients with sepsis in whom there is a loss of venous tone and an increase in capacitance. If cardiac output is decreased and right atrial pressure is elevated, or even more importantly, if cardiac output falls with a rise in right atrial pressure, the primary problem is an abnormality of cardiac function. The next step is to examine the pulmonary artery and pulmonary artery occlusion pressures to determine the specific etiology. When a decrease in cardiac function is the primary problem, either use of pharmacologic agents or correction of the underlying cardiac pathology such as a coronary artery obstruction, a valve problem, or pulmonary hypertension is the best therapeutic approach.

When considering therapeutic options, the physician must be conscious of the underlying physiologic mechanisms. It is especially important to consider the limitations of the cardiovascular system, for responses can only occur within the range of limitations of cardiac function and return function. A physiologically based approach to management can allow rapid and directed management.

SUGGESTED READING

Deschamps A, Magder S: Baroreflex control of regional capacitance and blood flow distribution with or without alpha adrenergic blockade. J Appl Physiol 1992;263:H1755–H1763.

Guyton AC: Determination of cardiac output by equating venous return curves with cardiac response curves. Physiol Rev 1955;35:123–129.

Guyton AC, Jones CE, Coleman TG: Circulatory Physiology: Cardiac Output and Its Regulation. Philadelphia, WB Saunders, 1973.

Magder S: Shock physiology. In Pinsky MR, Dhainault JF (eds): Physiological Foundations of Critical Care Medicine. Philadelphia, Williams & Wilkins, 1992, pp 140–160.

Magder S: Heart-lung interactions in sepsis. In Scharf SM, Pinsky MR, Magder S (eds): Respiratory-Circulatory Interactions in Health and Disease, 2nd ed. New York, Marcel Dekker, 2001, pp 739–762.

Magder S, Scharf SM: Venous return. In Scharf SM, Pinsky MR, Magder S (eds): Respiratory-Circulatory Interactions in Health and Disease, 2nd ed. New York, Marcel Dekker, 2001, pp 93–112.

Magder SA, Georgiadis G, Cheong T: Respiratory variations in right atrial pressure predict response to fluid challenge. J Crit Care 1992;7:76–85.

Mitzner W: Resistance of pulmonary circulation. Clin Chest Med 1983; 4:127–137.

Parillo JE: Pathogenetic mechanisms of septic shock. N Engl J Med 1993; 328:1471–1477.

Permutt S, Riley RL: Hemodynamics of collapsible vessels with tone: the vascular waterfall. J Appl Physiol 1963;18:924–932.

Pierard LA, Lancellotti P: The role of ischemic mitral regurgitation in the pathogenesis of acute pulmonary edema. N Engl J Med 2004; 351:1627–1634.

Sagawa K: The ventricular pressure-volume diagram revisited. Circ Res 1978;43:677–687.

Starling EH: The Linacre Lecture of the Law of the Heart. London, Longmans, Green & Co, 1918.

Chapter 30

Acute Coronary Syndromes

Stephan Windecker

KEY POINTS

- Acute coronary syndrome signifies a clinical state characterized by acute myocardial ischemia with or without myocardial infarction, with an increased risk for cardiac death.
- Cardiogenic shock is the principal cause of in-hospital mortality from myocardial infarction and complicates approximately 7% of ST segment elevation myocardial infarction and 2% or 3% of non–ST segment elevation myocardial infarction.
- Risk factors for atherosclerotic coronary artery disease not only predispose to the development of acute coronary syndromes but also are associated with an increased risk of adverse outcome.
- Mortality and risk of reinfarction are doubled in diabetic patients with acute coronary syndromes compared with those in nondiabetic patients.
- An early invasive strategy is superior to conservative treatment in patients with acute coronary syndrome.
- Modification of lifestyle habits has an important impact on long-term prognosis.

Acute coronary syndromes encompass a wide spectrum of ischemic myocardial events, ranging from unstable angina to myocardial infarction to sudden death induced by myocardial ischemia. The common pathophysiologic substrate is coronary thrombosis following rupture or erosion of an inflamed atherosclerotic plaque, with subsequent partial or total vessel occlusion causing ischemia in the corresponding myocardial area. The extent of intracoronary thrombosis and distal embolization determines the clinical presentation, ranging from unstable angina (UA) without myocardial necrosis to non–ST segment elevation myocardial infarction (NSTEMI) to ST segment elevation myocardial infarction (STEMI) (Table 30.1). Diagnosis and risk stratification of acute coronary syndromes are based on history, electrocardiographic changes, and cardiac biomarkers. Risk stratification is useful for selection of site (outpatient vs intermediate vs intensive care unit) and type of treatment (i.e., necessity of glycoprotein IIb/IIIa antagonists) and determination of the need for revascularization procedures. The in-hospital treatment is directed at dissolution of intracoronary thrombus, reduction of inflammatory plaque activity, and improved healing of the coronary endothelium. Long-term treatment aims at modifications of the cardiac risk factor profile and lifestyle interventions to reduce morbidity and mortality.

EPIDEMIOLOGY, RISK FACTORS, AND PATHOPHYSIOLOGY

Epidemiology

With more than 2.5 million annual hospitalizations worldwide, acute coronary syndromes account for the most common cause of admission for cardiac disorders and 50% of coronary care unit admissions. Sudden death is the first manifestation of underlying heart disease in approximately 500,000 patients per year in the United States, with 80% of these deaths caused by acute coronary syndromes (Fig. 30.1). The number of hospitalizations for UA/NSTEMI continues to rise, whereas the number of STEMI is stabilizing or even declining. This change in natural history is multifactorial and has been related to more sensitive diagnostic tools (i.e., troponin) and more effective treatment strategies in recent years.

The establishment of continuous rhythm monitoring in the setting of coronary care units and improvements in pharmacologic and mechanical reperfusion therapy have dramatically lowered in-hospital mortality during the past 5 decades (Fig. 30.2). Untreated patients with acute coronary syndromes have a 5% to 10% mortality and a 10% to 20% nonfatal myocardial infarction rate within the first days to weeks of the event. However, despite modern therapy, there remains an important short-term risk for death (5%), reinfarction (5%–10%), and refractory angina (10%–20%). Furthermore, mortality is typically higher in population-based studies and registries (approximately 20%) compared to patients enrolled in controlled clinical trials, and it remains high in elderly patients (20%) and patients not eligible for reperfusion therapy (Fig. 30.3). Today, cardiogenic shock constitutes the principal cause of in-hospital mortality from myocardial infarction and complicates approximately 7% of STEMI and 2% or 3% of NSTEMI.

Risk Factors

Most of the established risk factors for atherosclerotic coronary artery disease are also indicators of risk in patients with acute coronary syndromes (Box 30.1). Thus, older age, male sex, arterial hypertension, dyslipidemia, smoking, diabetes, obesity, and physical inactivity are associated with more severe coronary artery disease. Putative markers of risk include psychosocial factors (depression, stress, and acute life events) and elevated homocysteine and lipoprotein (a) levels. These risk factors not only predispose to the development of acute coronary syndromes but also are associated with an increased risk of adverse outcome. In addition, previous manifestations of coronary artery disease—such as long-standing angina pectoris, a history of

Table 30.1 Acute Coronary Syndromes						
Type	**Symptoms**	**ECG**	**Myocardial Necrosis**	**Coronary Lesion**	**Acute Treatment**	**Prognosis**
Unstable angina	Recurrent chest pain < 20 min	No ST elevation ST depression T wave inversion	None	Severe stenosis Small thrombus	Aspirin Clopidogrel Thrombin inhibitors	Reinfarction Recurrent ischemia
Non–ST segment elevation MI	Recurrent chest pain < 20 min	No ST elevation ST depression T wave inversion	Minor	Partial thrombotic occlusion with or without distal embolization or severe stenosis	Aspirin Clopidogrel Thrombin inhibitors GP IIb/IIIa antagonists Early revascularization	Reinfarction Recurrent ischemia
ST segment elevation MI	Severe chest pain > 20 min	ST elevation Left BBB New Q wave	Large	Total and persistent thrombotic occlusion	Immediate reperfusion Primary PCI Thrombolysis	Reinfarction Heart failure Arrhythmias

BBB, bundle branch block; GP, glycoprotein; MI, myocardial infarction; PCI, percutaneous coronary intervention.

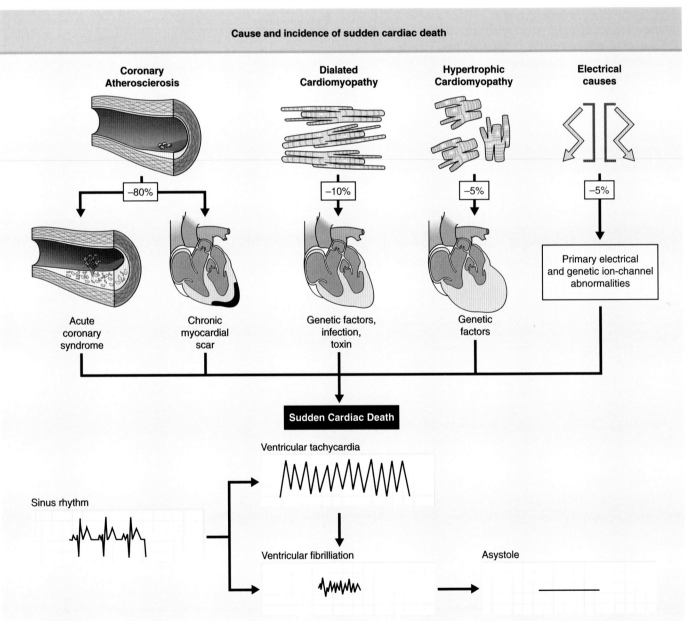

Figure 30.1. Causes and incidence of sudden cardiac death. The most prevalent mechanism of sudden death is acute myocardial infarction: More than one third of patients with evolving myocardial infarction die before reaching the hospital.

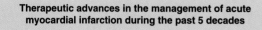

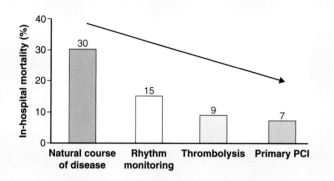

Figure 30.2. **Therapeutic advances in the management of acute myocardial infarction and their impact on short-term mortality during the past 5 decades.** PCI, percutaneous coronary intervention.

Box 30.1 Cardiovascular Risk Factors and Markers

Classical Risk Factors

Advanced age
Smoking
Arterial hypertension
Diabetes mellitus
Obesity
Increased LDL cholesterol
Decreased HDL cholesterol
Sedentary lifestyle

Emerging Serum Markers for Risk Stratification in Acute Coronary Syndromes

C-reactive protein
Interleukins
Soluble CD14 ligand
Myeloperoxidase
Plasminogen activator inhibitor
Tissue plasminogen activator
Pregnancy-associated plasma protein A
Homocysteine
Lipoprotein A
B-type natriuretic peptide

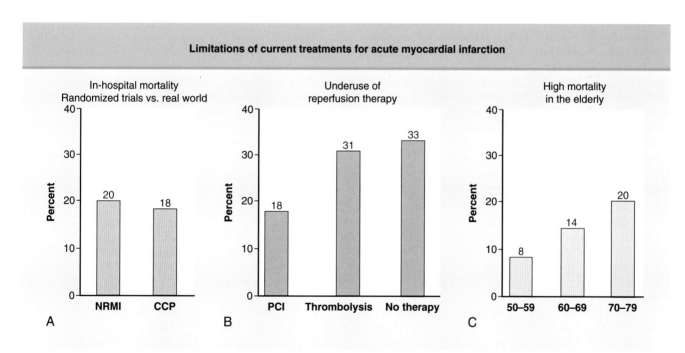

Figure 30.3. **Limitations of current treatments for acute myocardial infarction.** *A,* Mortality rates are typically higher in patients encountered in daily clinical practice than in patients included in clinical trials. Reference data from the National Registry of Myocardial Infarction (NRMI-2) and Cooperative Cardiovascular Project (CCP) registries on in-hospital mortality of patients with acute myocardial infarction. *B,* Underutilization of reperfusion therapy in patients with acute myocardial infarction. Approximately one third of patients with acute myocardial infarction do not receive any reperfusion therapy by either thrombolysis or percutaneous coronary intervention (PCI). *C,* Mortality remains high in the elderly. (*A,* Data from Every NR, Frederick PD, Robinson M, et al: A comparison of the National Registry of Myocardial Infarction 2 with the cooperative cardiovascular project. J Am Coll Cardiol 1999;33:1886–1894; *B,* Data from Eagle KA, Goodman SG, Avezum A, et al: Practice variation and missed opportunities for reperfusion in ST-segment-elevation myocardial infarction: findings from the Global Registry of Acute Coronary Events (GRACE). Lancet 2002;359:373–377; *C,* Data from Barakat K, Wilkinson P, Deaner A, et al: How should age affect management of acute myocardial infarction? A prospective cohort study. Lancet 1999;353:955–959.)

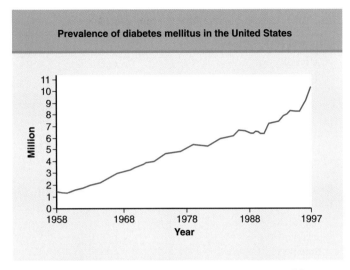

Figure 30.4. Prevalence of diabetes mellitus in the United States. Note the sixfold increase over 4 decades.

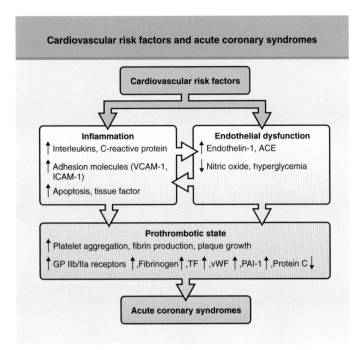

Figure 30.5. Impact of cardiovascular risk factors on the pathogenesis of acute coronary syndromes.

coronary artery bypass surgery or previous percutaneous coronary intervention, left ventricular dysfunction, and congestive heart failure—are predictive of worse prognosis.

Diabetes is a serious cardiovascular risk factor, with a prevalence that increased sixfold in the United States over the course of 4 decades (Fig. 30.4). Hematologic abnormalities in diabetic patients include increased platelet aggregation and procoagulant factors, decreased endogenous fibrinolysis, and endothelial dysfunction. More important, mortality and risk of reinfarction are doubled in diabetic patients with acute coronary syndromes compared with those in nondiabetic patients. The impaired outcome of diabetic patients has been related to a higher atherosclerotic disease burden and a higher incidence of comorbid conditions, such as renal dysfunction and obesity.

The link between risk factors and the development of acute coronary syndromes is depicted in Figure 30.5. Thus, several clinical risk factors have been recognized to induce endothelial dysfunction and promote inflammatory and thrombogenic pathways. The chronic damage to the endothelium arising from these risk factors predisposes to atherosclerotic plaque development, progression, and rupture and their thrombotic sequelae.

Risk Markers

C-reactive protein (CRP), a marker of inflammation, is a strong independent predictor of future cardiovascular risk. In patients with acute coronary syndromes, elevated CRP levels are associated with an increased risk of death, myocardial infarction, and revascularization and have incremental value beyond standard lipid screening and cardiac troponin testing.

Soluble CD-40 ligand is a biochemical marker with proinflammatory and prothrombogenic properties that is released by activated platelets. It is a marker of platelet activation and identifies an increased thrombotic activity in patients with acute coronary syndromes, independent of cardiac troponin and CRP levels. Whereas troponin levels indicate myocardial necrosis, sCD40 ligand is a marker of thrombotic activity and provides information on disease activity and cardiac risk, even in troponin-negative patients.

Myeloperoxidase levels are increased in patients with coronary artery disease and within lesions of plaques prone to rupture. Myeloperoxidase is released by activated leukocytes and thus reflects plaque vulnerability. It is used to identify patients at increased risk for myocardial infarction and adverse events independent of troponin and CRP levels.

Other emerging markers of risk include interleukins (IL-6), pregnancy-associated plasma protein A, serum amyloid A, homocysteine, lipoprotein A, tissue plasminogen activator, plasminogen activator inhibitor, and B-type natriuretic peptide (BNP) (see Box 30.1).

Pathophysiology
Atherosclerosis
Atherosclerosis involves lesions in large and medium-sized elastic and muscular arteries and is preferentially observed at sites of increased shear stress such as bifurcations. Initially, a normal or only slightly narrowed lumen will prevail due to outward remodeling in relation to plaque area, and the disease remains clinically silent for several years. With progression of atherosclerotic lesions over time, functionally important obstruction of blood flow ensues, giving rise to symptomatic coronary artery disease.

Atherosclerosis has been increasingly recognized as a chronic inflammatory disease (Fig. 30.6). The initiation of atherosclerotic lesions is preceded by endothelial dysfunction induced by mechanical and toxic stimuli and accentuated by classical clinical risk factors. Dysfunctional endothelial cells express vascular cell adhesion molecules (VCAM-1), which allow for binding and penetration of leukocytes into the intima. Monocytes, which turn into activated macrophages and T lymphocytes, secrete cytokines and growth factors, which perpetuate the inflammatory process in the subendothelium. Lipid accumulation occurs

Acute coronary syndromes are most often caused by plaque rupture (75%) and less frequently by plaque erosion (25%). Approximately two thirds of acute coronary syndromes emanate from coronary lesions without hemodynamic significance (stenosis diameter < 50%) prior to plaque rupture. Atherosclerotic plaques considered vulnerable or at high risk for rupture are characterized by a large lipid core relative to the total plaque volume (>40%) and a thin fibrous plaque (65–150 µm) depleted of smooth muscle cells and collagen. A predisposition for plaque rupture appears related to the action of physical forces such as shear stress and resistance to circumferential wall stress (cap fatigue) on the one hand, and inflammatory processes such as the release of extracellular matrix-degrading enzymes with subsequent weakening of the fibrous cap on the other hand. Rupture mostly occurs spontaneously, but external triggers such as strenuous physical exercise, severe emotional trauma, and exposure to illicit drugs have been described. Plaque rupture may be clinically silent if not accompanied by intracoronary thrombosis. Thus, in approximately 40% of cases with acute coronary syndromes, multiple plaque ruptures have been observed in arteries remote from the culprit lesion. The thrombogenicity of a ruptured atherosclerotic plaque is promoted by large tears, lipid extrusion, numerous macrophages, a high tissue factor expression, high-grade stenosis, and low blood flow.

Erosions of the endothelium overlying the atherosclerotic lesion are more prevalent in young survivors of cardiac arrest, women, and smokers. Plaques under these erosions typically have a smaller lipid core, less evidence of inflammation, and a richer extracellular matrix. Luminal narrowing in these lesions occurs by rapid proliferation and migration of smooth muscle cells in response to endothelial injury. Intracoronary thrombosis in this setting has been related to an enhanced thrombogenic state.

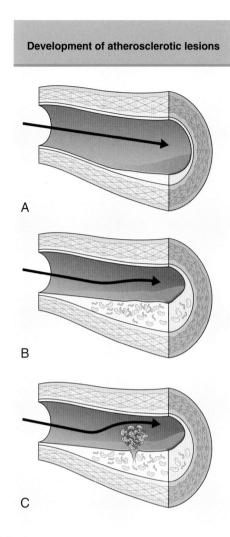

Development of atherosclerotic lesions

A

B

C

Figure 30.6. Schematic diagram of the development of atherosclerotic lesions. *A,* Endothelial dysfunction preceding the formation of atherosclerotic lesions, characterized by increased endothelial permeability, expression of vascular adhesion molecules, and migration of leukocytes into the arterial wall. *B,* Early atherosclerotic lesion with lipid-rich core, debris, leukocytes, and a fibrous cap. *C,* Ruptured fibrous cap leading to superficial thrombosis with or without distal embolization.

Thrombosis and Platelet Aggregation

The pivotal role of coronary artery thrombosis in the pathogenesis of acute coronary syndromes is supported by autopsy studies demonstrating thrombi at sites of plaque rupture/erosion, angiographic evidence of thrombus at sites of ulcerated lesions, elevated cardiac biomarkers of myocardial necrosis suggesting distal embolization of thrombotic particles, and improved clinical outcome with antithrombotic treatment. In the event of plaque rupture, the central lipid core via expression of tissue factor becomes the most potent substrate for platelet-rich thrombus formation upon exposure to plasma coagulation proteins. Tissue factor, a transmembrane glycoprotein expressed on the surface of macrophages, interacts with factor VIIa to initiate an enzymatic cascade resulting in the local generation of thrombin and deposition of fibrin.

Platelets adhere to the subendothelial matrix exposed in the case of plaque rupture by binding to collagen, von Willebrand factor, and fibronectin via their respective receptors. Platelet adhesion is followed by platelet activation, resulting in conformational changes, release of thromboxane A2 and serotonin, and expression of activated glycoprotein IIb/IIIa receptors. Platelet aggregation is mediated by binding and subsequent cross-linking between fibrinogen and glycoprotein IIb/IIIa receptors. This, and the formation of a fibrin mesh, leads to the formation of a platelet-rich thrombus.

directly by endocytosis of native and oxidized low-density lipoprotein (LDL) into macrophages and indirectly after death of lipid-rich foam cells. Subsequent smooth muscle cell migration and proliferation, extracellular matrix deposition, and further lipid accumulation give rise to complex atherosclerotic lesions composed of a lipid core, necrotic tissue, and a fibrous cap.

Plaque Rupture and Erosion

Disruption of atherosclerotic plaque may occur at any point in the chronic disease process and is central to the initiation of acute coronary syndromes. Intraluminal thrombosis at sites of atherosclerotic plaque disruption can lead to partial or total vessel occlusion, causing myocardial ischemia (Fig. 30.7). Two types of plaque damage may result in thrombosis formation in coronary arteries: rupture of the fibrous cap and superficial erosion of the endothelium overlying the atherosclerotic plaque.

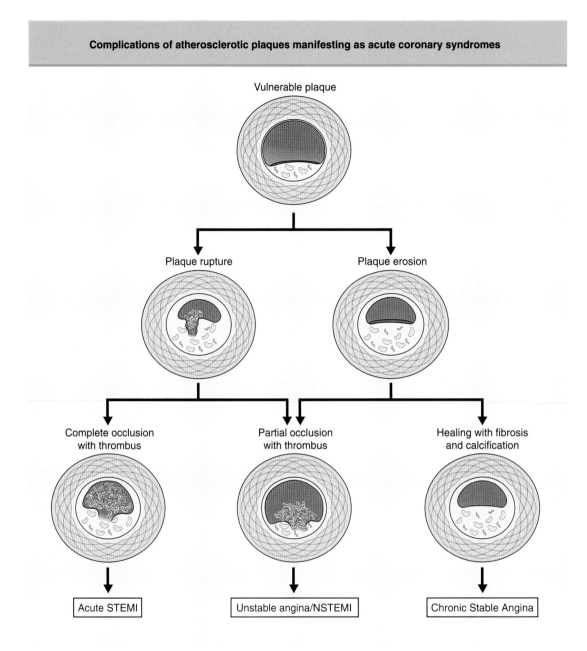

Figure 30.7. Complications of atherosclerotic plaques manifesting as acute coronary syndromes. Rupture or erosion of a vulnerable plaque results in local intracoronary inflammation and thrombus formation. Partial vessel occlusion manifests as unstable angina/NSTEMI, whereas complete vessel occlusion manifests as STEMI.

Inflammation

Acute coronary syndromes are associated with signs of increased inflammatory activity. This is supported by increased levels of cytokines such as IL-1, IL-6, and IL-8, soluble adhesion molecules, and acute phase proteins such as fibrinogen and CRP. In addition, activated platelets express P-selectin and CD40 ligand on the platelet surface, allowing for binding to leukocytes. Thus, increased amounts of platelet–granulocyte and platelet–monocyte complexes are observed in patients with acute coronary syndromes, which further promote coagulation, platelet adhesion, and inflammation by production and secretion of cytokines. Circulating inflammatory markers and cytokines may not only identify patients at increased risk for future cardiovas-

cular events but also contribute to the pathogenesis of acute coronary syndromes.

CLINICAL FEATURES AND DEFINITIONS

Acute coronary syndrome signifies a clinical state characterized by acute myocardial ischemia with or without myocardial infarction and with an increased risk for cardiac death. Myocardial infarction describes an episode of myocardial ischemia resulting in myocardial necrosis (cell death). The traditional definition of myocardial infarction drafted by the World Health Organization required the fulfillment of at least two of the following three criteria: (1) typical ischemic chest pain; (2) raised serum concentration of creatine kinase–myocardial band (CK-MB) fraction; and (3) typical electrocardiographic findings, such as pathologic Q waves. Aimed at high specificity for epidemiologic purposes, this definition omitted many patients with minor myocardial necrosis.

Cardiac troponin serum levels have been shown to be more sensitive and powerful predictors of patients' risk than CK-MB levels, and current technology is able to detect small areas of myocardial necrosis weighing less than 1.0 g. In addition, assays for troponin T and I have proved to be highly specific for myocardial necrosis. Accordingly, the Joint European Society of Cardiology/American College of Cardiology Committee has refined the contemporary definition of myocardial infarction based on cardiac troponin measurements (Box 30.2). An increased value for cardiac troponin is defined as a measurement exceeding the 99th percentile of a reference control group. The measurement of troponin has proved useful for distinguishing UA from NSTEMI (approximately 30% of patients previously classified as UA on the basis of normal CK-MB levels are now diagnosed as NSTEMI), as well as establishing prognosis and selection of therapy.

The acute coronary syndrome concept originates from a common pathophysiologic substrate (plaque rupture and its thrombotic complications) and provides a useful framework for subsequent therapeutic strategies (see Fig. 30.7). Patients with acute chest pain suggestive of coronary ischemic origin are categorized according to the presence or absence of ST segment elevation and the presence or absence of biochemical markers of myocardial necrosis (Fig. 30.8). Plaque rupture causing acute, complete thrombotic occlusion of a major epicardial coronary artery typically results in acute and persistent ST segment elevation. Most of these patients eventually develop myocardial infarction with elevated biomarkers of myocardial necrosis, and 75% of patients initially presenting with STEMI develop Q waves in the leads overlying the infarct zone, formerly referred to as Q wave MI. Rapid restoration of blood flow, preferably by mechanical (percutaneous coronary intervention) or, in case of

---

Box 30.2 ESC/ACC Definition of Myocardial Infarction

Criteria for Acute Myocardial Infarction

1. Typical increase and gradual decrease (troponin) or more rapid increase and decrease (CK-MB) of biochemical markers of myocardial necrosis, with at least one of the following:
   Ischemic symptoms
   Development of pathologic Q waves on the ECG
   ECG changes indicative of ischemia (ST segment elevation or depression)
   Coronary artery intervention
2. Pathologic findings of an acute myocardial infarction

Criteria for Established Myocardial Infarction

Either of the following criteria satisfies the diagnosis for established myocardial infarction:

1. Development of new pathologic Q waves on serial ECGs. Biochemical markers of myocardial necrosis may have normalized, depending on the length of time that has passed since the infarct developed.
2. Pathologic findings of a healed or healing myocardial infarction.

---

unavailability, pharmacological (thrombolysis) reperfusion, limits myocardial necrosis and reduces mortality.

Nonobstructive coronary thrombi overlying a ruptured plaque typically do not produce STEMI but, rather, ST segment depression and/or T wave inversion. In the case of prolonged vessel obstruction or distal embolization of thrombotic particles, biomarkers of cardiac necrosis are released, with myocardial necrosis typically being less extensive than in STEMI. Patients in this category are classified as suffering from NSTEMI, and the majority of these patients do not develop Q waves on the electrocardiogram (ECG). Previous terminology of non–Q-wave myocardial infarction (NQWMI) was based on late electrocardiographic criteria, which only poorly correlated with the

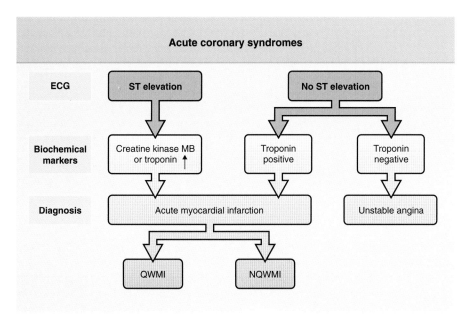

Figure 30.8. Classification of acute coronary syndromes based on electrocardiographic and biochemical markers. NQWMI, non–Q-wave myocardial infarction; QWMI, Q-wave myocardial infarction.

underlying pathology and did not assist in acute therapeutic decision making. NSTEMI patients benefit from glycoprotein IIb/IIIa receptor inhibitors and early revascularization therapy in addition to standard antiplatelet and antithrombin therapy.

Episodes of plaque rupture with spontaneous lysis and restoration of antegrade blood flow within 20 minutes usually do not result in myocardial necrosis, release of biomarkers of cardiac necrosis, or persistent electrocardiographic changes. Patients in this category are classified as suffering from UA.

DIAGNOSIS

The initial evaluation of patients with suspected acute coronary syndromes has two objectives: confirmation of the diagnosis and determination of prognosis. Approximately two thirds of patients presenting with chest pain to the emergency room will require hospitalization for treatment of an acute coronary syndrome. The early diagnosis, with repeated measurements of cardiac biological markers, 12-lead ECG, and continuous observation for symptoms and ECG monitoring for ischemia, identifies patients with ischemia within the first 6 hours.

Clinical Presentation
UA/NSTEMI
Patients with UA/NSTEMI usually present with one of three clinical patterns:
1. Rest angina (80%): Angina occurring at rest and prolonged (>20 min)
2. New-onset, severe angina: New-onset angina of at least Canadian Cardiovascular Society (CCS) class III
3. Accelerating angina: Previously diagnosed angina that has become more frequent, longer in duration, or lower in threshold

Patients with NSTEMI usually experience angina at rest. The duration and intensity of angina are graded according to the CCS classification (I–IV). The initial patient evaluation aims at determining the likelihood that signs and symptoms are related to obstructive coronary artery disease. The most important predictors of ischemia due to coronary artery disease are summarized in Box 30.3.

STEMI
Patients with acute STEMI complain of severe, nonabating chest pain with radiation to the left arm, right arm, or both arms, the mandible, the back between the scapulae, or the abdomen. The nature of the pain is oppressing, crushing, and constricting, and the usual location is midsternal. Accompanying symptoms are frequent and include anxiety, nausea, vomiting, diaphoresis, and dyspnea. The differential diagnosis of acute myocardial infarction is summarized in Table 30.2.

Physical Examination
Physical examination in a patient with suspected acute coronary syndrome is most often normal, including chest examination, auscultation, and measurement of heart rate and pulse. A high risk of adverse clinical outcome is present in patients with hemodynamic instability, the presence of pulmonary edema or an S3 heart sound, and a new or increasing mitral regurgitation murmur. Physical examination is directed to the exclusion of

---

Box 30.3 Clinical Symptoms of UA/NSTEMI Suggestive of Obstructive CAD

Characteristics of symptoms
  Chest or left arm pain, reproducing prior documented angina, relieved promptly by nitroglycerin
  Atypical chest pain does not exclude the possibility of ACS
Demographics and prior history
  Prior history of MI
Male sex
  Male patients are more likely to have obstructive coronary artery disease
Age > 65 years
  Increased risk of both underlying coronary artery disease and multivessel disease
Number of atherosclerotic risk factors present
  Diabetes mellitus
  Extracardiac manifestation of atherosclerotic disease

Table 30.2 Differential Diagnosis of Acute Myocardial Infarction

Diagnosis	Differentiating Features
Aortic dissection	Pain more severe, tearing character, radiation to back and extremities, pulse deficit, pericardial effusion, murmur of aortic regurgitation may be present
Pericarditis	Stabbing chest pain with aggravation during inspiration, cough and change in body position, slower onset, fever, pericardial rub
Pleural pain	Sharp, stabbing chest pain aggravated by inspiration; cough and change in body position
Pulmonary embolism	Pain more laterally in the chest, often pleuritic, sometimes associated with hemoptysis
Pneumothorax	Young age, unilateral impaired ventilation
Esophageal spasm	Burning sensation, epigastric origin of discomfort, related to meal intake
Costochondral pain	Superficial location, reproducible by digital pressure

---

extracardiac chest pain causes, such as pericarditis and pneumothorax, and a search for signs of hemodynamic instability and left ventricular dysfunction. Patients with inferior myocardial infarction complicated by right ventricular involvement may present with low blood pressure, distended neck veins, and right upper quadrant pain due to liver congestion. Mechanical complications, such as papillary or ventricular muscle rupture, may be detected by a harsh systolic murmur at the left sternal border or over the apex.

Electrocardiography
Electrocardiography allows for classification into STEMI and NSTEMI, with implications for the acute management strategy. Thus, patients with STEMI require immediate reperfusion therapy, preferably by percutaneous coronary intervention (PCI) or, in case of unavailability, thrombolysis. In contrast, patients with UA/NSTEMI will receive antithrombotic treatment followed by further risk stratification according to cardiac biomarker status. Of note, the sensitivity of the ECG at the time of clinical presentation does not exceed 60% with a specificity of 90%.

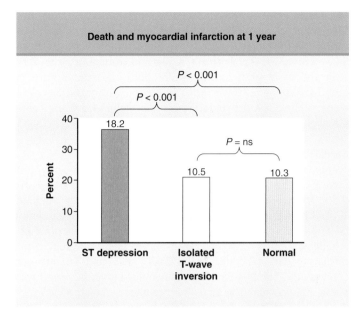

Figure 30.9. Predictive value of electrocardiographic findings in patients with NSTEMI. ST segment depression larger than 0.5 mm at the time of initial ECG recording signifies a significantly higher risk of death and myocardial infarction at 1 year compared with both the absence of ST segment changes and isolated T wave inversions. (Data as reported by the FRISC-II investigators in ST depression in ECG at entry indicates severe coronary lesions and large benefits of an early invasive treatment strategy in unstable coronary artery disease; the FRISC II ECG substudy. Eur Heart J 2002;23:41–49.)

UA/NSTEMI

A resting 12-lead ECG provides important diagnostic and prognostic information. It should be recorded in all patients presenting with suspected acute coronary syndrome and is most valuable when recorded during episodes of ongoing chest pain. Comparison with previous ECGs facilitates the diagnostic interpretation. Acute ischemic changes are primarily noted in the ST segment and T wave. ST segment depression with or without T wave changes is the most characteristic finding in UA/NSTEMI patients. Thus, ST segment depression as little as 0.05 mV is a predictor of adverse outcome, with increasing severity of ST segment depression translating into progressively increased risk (Fig. 30.9). Approximately 25% of patients with ST segment depression and elevated cardiac biomarkers develop Q wave myocardial infarction, whereas the remaining 75% of patients have a NQWMI. Widespread ST segment depression in more than 6 leads is highly specific for acute myocardial infarction, as is intermittent ST segment elevation. Furthermore, deep and symmetric T wave inversion in leads V2 through V4 usually suggests ischemia caused by a proximal lesion of the left anterior descending artery. ST segment depression in leads V1 through V3 may reveal a true posterior infarction, which should be approached like a STEMI. Of note, a normal ECG does not exclude the possibility of an acute coronary syndrome, since 1% to 6% of such patients are subsequently found to have acute myocardial infarction as evidenced by elevated biomarkers.

Nonspecific ST segment and T wave changes, defined as ST segment depression of less than 0.05 mV or T wave inversion of less than 0.2 mV, are less diagnostic for acute ischemia. In addi-

tion, alternative causes for ST segment and T wave abnormalities should be considered, such as left ventricular hypertrophy, pericarditis, myocarditis, early repolarization, electrolyte imbalances, metabolic disorders, digitalis effect, tricyclic antidepressants, phenothiazines, and central nervous system pathologies.

A resting 12-lead ECG does not reflect the dynamic nature of coronary thrombosis in patients with acute coronary syndromes. Thus, up to two thirds of ischemic episodes in acute coronary syndrome patients remain clinically silent without associated chest discomfort. Continuous 12-lead ECG monitoring studies have shown that 15% to 30% of acute coronary syndrome patients have transient episodes of ST segment depression that are associated with adverse outcome. Accordingly, continuous ST segment monitoring adds diagnostic and prognostic information in acute coronary syndrome patients.

STEMI

The electrocardiographic finding of ST segment elevation is extremely useful for the diagnosis of acute STEMI. The extent of ST segment elevation, the location of infarction, and QRS duration allow for prognostication. Even in the presence of left bundle branch block (LBBB), acute myocardial infarction may be diagnosed if excessive ST segment deviation (>5 mm) is present. ST segment depression in leads V1 through V3 may indicate true posterior myocardial infarction. Diagnostic criteria for STEMI are summarized in Box 30.4. Alternative causes of ST segment elevation are acute pericarditis, left ventricular aneurysm, early repolarization, Wolff-Parkinson-White syndrome, hyperkalemia, and Prinzmetal's angina.

Biochemical Markers of Myocardial Necrosis

Cardiac biological markers are pivotal for diagnosis, risk stratification, and management of patients with acute coronary

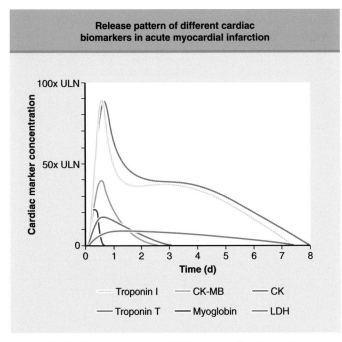

Figure 30.10. Release pattern of different cardiac biomarkers in acute myocardial infarction.

syndromes. Myocardial necrosis leads to the loss of integrity of cardiac myocyte membranes, with release of intracellular macromolecules into the interstitium and, via lymphatics and microvasculature, into the peripheral circulation. Myocardial infarction is diagnosed when blood levels of sensitive and specific markers (troponin T and I and CK-MB) are increased in the clinical setting of acute ischemia (see Box 30.2). Elevated cardiac biological markers without signs of acute ischemia should prompt the search for alternative causes of cardiac damage, such as trauma, pulmonary embolism, hypertensive crisis, and myocarditis, since these markers indicate myocardial damage without shedding light on its mechanism. Importantly, no current marker is detectable immediately upon onset of myocardial infarction, and therefore repeated measurements are required during the first 6 to 12 hours after admission. The release pattern of different cardiac biological markers is depicted in Figure 30.10.

Creatine Kinase

Creatine kinase levels increase within 4 to 8 hours after the onset of myocardial infarction and decline to near normal levels within 2 or 3 days. The peak CK level is usually observed after 24 hours, but it may occur earlier, with higher levels in patients with successful reperfusion (early washout sign). The major drawback of CK is the lack of cardiac specificity, with false-positive results being observed in patients with muscle disease and trauma, vigorous exercise, intramuscular injections, convulsions, alcohol intoxication, etc. CK-MB is the cardiac-specific isoform of CK and was the principal serum cardiac marker until the introduction of troponin. CK-MB is detected in blood of healthy people and present in minor quantities in the uterus, prostate, and small intestine; therefore, it has reduced sensitivity and specificity for cardiac myocyte necrosis.

Myoglobin

Myoglobin, a low-molecular-weight heme protein, is found in cardiac and skeletal muscle. It is more rapidly released from injured myocardial cells than CK-MB and troponin (within 2 hr after the onset of myocardial infarction), and therefore it is useful for ruling out myocardial infarction within the first 4 to 8 hours. However, the clinical value of myoglobin measurements remains limited due to its lack of specificity.

Cardiac-Specific Troponins

Troponin has become the preferred biomarker for assessment of myocardial damage due to its high cardiac specificity and sensitivity. The troponin complex consists of three subsets: troponin T (TnT), troponin I (TnI), and troponin C (TnC). Since skeletal and cardiac troponin are immunologically distinct proteins, monoclonal antibody-based tests have been developed for cardiac-specific TnT and TnI. Usually, TnT and TnI are not detectable in the blood of healthy people, and an increased troponin value is defined as a measurement exceeding the 99th percentile of a reference control group. TnT and TnI are detectable in blood within 4 to 12 hours after the onset of myocardial infarction, and peak values are observed at 12 to 48 hours. Since troponin levels may remain elevated for 7 to 10 days after myocardial necrosis, the attribution of cardiac troponin levels to other than recent clinical events proves difficult.

Small myocardial infarctions (microinfarctions) can lead to elevations of cardiac TnT and TnI in peripheral blood without detectable levels of CK-MB. The greater sensitivity of cardiac troponins as opposed to CK-MB led to an increased frequency of the diagnosis of myocardial infarction. Up to 30% of patients previously diagnosed to have UA on the basis of a normal ECG and CK-MB levels are now classified as NSTEMI due to elevated troponin levels in the clinical setting of ischemia.

For patients presenting with STEMI, the initiation of reperfusion therapy must not be withheld until the results of troponin levels become available. In this clinical condition, troponin levels may be useful for assessing prognosis, reperfusion success, and reinfarction. For patients with NSTEMI, troponin levels provide important information about prognosis, selection of therapy, and for the diagnosis of reinfarction. Thus, a positive troponin test indicates a two- to ninefold increased risk of death compared to that for troponin-negative patients (Fig. 30.11). The increased risk associated with elevated troponin levels has been related to underlying severe coronary stenoses, the presence of thrombus at the culprit lesion with distal embolization, and total vessel occlusion with large myocardial infarction. Patients with acute coronary syndromes and elevated troponin levels receive the greatest treatment benefit from an early invasive strategy with revascularization (40% reduction in recurrent cardiac events) and use of glycoprotein IIb/IIIa antagonists (50% reduction in recurrent cardiac events).

Multiple Marker Assessment

Pathophysiologic substrate of acute coronary syndromes is a vulnerable plaque complicated by intracoronary thrombosis, vascular inflammation, and myocardial damage. All three facets of this complex pathophysiologic process can be assessed by the serum markers troponin (thrombosis and distal embolization), CRP (vascular inflammation), and BNP (ventricular dysfunction) (Fig. 30.12). In retrospective and prospective analyses of

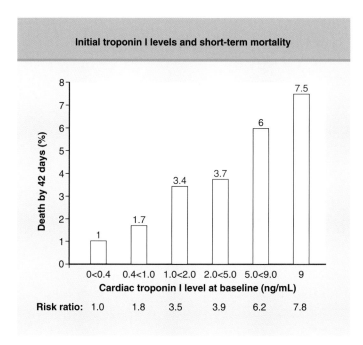

Figure 30.11. Correlation of initial troponin I levels with short-term mortality (at 42 days) in patients with acute coronary syndromes. Mortality increases significantly with each 1 ng/mL increase in troponin I level. (Data from Antman EM, Tanasijevic MJ, Thompson B, et al: Cardiac-specific troponin levels to predict the risk of mortality in patients with acute coronary syndromes. N Engl J Med 1996;335:1342–1349.)

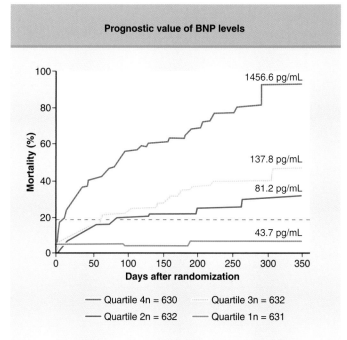

Figure 30.12. Prognostic value of B-type natriuretic peptide levels in patients with acute coronary syndromes. (Data obtained from De Lemos JA, Morrow DA, Bentley JH, et al: The prognostic value of B-type natriuretic peptide in patients with acute coronary syndromes. N Engl J Med 2001;345:1014–1021.)

patients with acute coronary syndromes, each of these markers was identified as an independent predictor of adverse outcome. Multimarker measurements may become an important future tool for risk stratification and treatment allocation.

Echocardiography

Two-dimensional transthoracic echocardiography provides valuable information in selected patients with acute coronary syndromes. Left ventricular systolic function, an important prognostic variable, and regional wall motion abnormalities are easily assessed by echocardiography. In addition, echocardiography allows for rapid exclusion of mechanical complications such as pericardial effusion, ventricular septal rupture, and acute mitral regurgitation related to papillary muscle dysfunction in hemodynamically unstable patients. Finally, other underlying conditions, such as aortic stenosis, hypertrophic cardiomyopathy, and myxoma, may be identified.

Coronary Angiography

Coronary angiography provides unique information on the presence and extent of coronary artery disease, identification of culprit lesions, and the presence of intracoronary thrombus. Patients with acute coronary syndromes have a higher incidence of complex plaque morphology, coronary artery thrombi, and multisite or multivessel involvement than patients with stable angina. In prognostic terms, patients with an increasing number of affected coronary vessels with significant stenoses have been shown to be at increased risk for adverse outcome. In addition, coronary angiography allows for selection of the most appropriate revascularization strategy—coronary artery bypass grafting versus percutaneous coronary intervention.

Risk Stratification

Early risk stratification of patients with acute coronary syndromes with the use of clinical criteria, electrocardiography, and biomarkers allows for appropriate selection of the site and intensity of therapy. Electrocardiography dichotomizes patients into those with and without ST segment elevation. Patients with STEMI require initiation of immediate reperfusion therapy (preferably PCI, but thrombolysis if PCI is not available) and are usually hospitalized in a coronary care unit. Patients with NSTEMI do not require immediate reperfusion therapy but are further stratified according to clinical, electrocardiographic, and cardiac biological markers into high- and low-risk categories (Fig. 30.13). Clinical factors indicative of increased risk for adverse outcome are resting pain, hemodynamic and rhythm instability, and diabetes mellitus. Electrocardiographic predictors of increased risk are ST segment depression and dynamic ST segment changes. Finally, troponin-positive acute coronary syndrome patients constitute a high-risk population. In contrast, patients without recurrent chest pain or ST segment depression and with negative troponin levels at two separate measurements represent a low-risk cohort.

All patients with acute coronary syndrome receive a standard antithrombotic and anti-ischemic treatment consisting of aspirin, clopidogrel, heparin (unfractionated or low molecular weight), beta blockers, and nitrates, irrespective of initial risk allocation. Patients deemed at low risk can be discharged home if, at least 12 hours after the onset of symptoms, repeat troponin measurements remain negative, ischemic symptoms have not recurred, and ECGs remain normal. A noninvasive stress test should complement the evaluation on an ambulatory basis, and

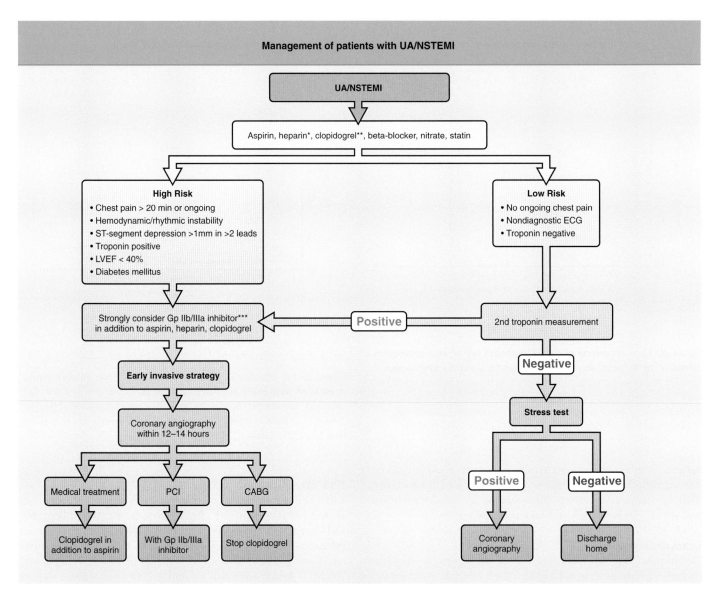

Figure 30.13. Management of patients with unstable angina/NSTEMI. *AHA/ACC class IIa recommendation: low-molecular-weight heparin (LMWH) enoxaparin preferred over unfractionated heparin. **Clopidogrel: loading dose of 300 to 600 mg followed by 75 mg daily. ***GP IIb/IIIa inhibitors: tirofiban and eptifibatide preferred over abciximab if started prior to coronary angiography; abciximab preferred over tirofiban if started at time of coronary intervention. CABG, coronary artery bypass grafting; LVEF, left ventricular ejection fraction; NSTEMI, non–ST elevation myocardial infarction; PCI, percutaneous coronary intervention; UA, unstable angina.

patients with abnormal findings should be referred for coronary angiography. In contrast, high-risk patients are hospitalized in an intermediate care unit with continuous rhythm and provisional ST segment monitoring. Early coronary angiography is advised within 12 to 24 hours to determine the need for revascularization therapy. Glycoprotein IIb/IIIa inhibitors are infused in addition to background therapy with aspirin and clopidogrel in patients likely to undergo PCI.

TREATMENT

The acute treatment strategy differs for patients with UA/NSTEMI and STEMI, with the latter requiring immediate reperfusion therapy.

UA/NSTEMI

The three pillars of acute treatment for patients with UA/NSTEMI consist of antiplatelet and anticoagulant therapy, anti-ischemic therapy, and invasive therapy.

Antiplatelet and Anticoagulant Therapy
Aspirin
Aspirin inhibits platelet cyclooxygenase-1 by irreversible acetylation, preventing the formation of thromboxane A2 and thus reducing platelet aggregation and the likelihood of arterial thrombi formation. Aspirin reduces the relative risk of death by 15%, and of nonfatal myocardial infarction by 30%, both in acute ischemic syndromes and during secondary prevention (Fig. 30.14). The benefit of aspirin has been shown to be present over

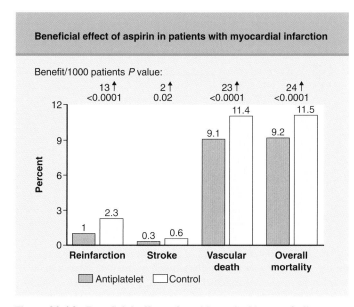

Beneficial effect of aspirin in patients with myocardial infarction

Figure 30.14. Beneficial effect of aspirin on incidence of all-cause mortality, vascular death, stroke, and reinfarction in patients with acute myocardial infarction compared to controls. (Data from 19,288 patients in 15 randomized trials as reported by the Antithrombotic Trialists Collaboration in Collaborative meta-analysis of randomised trials of antiplatelet therapy for prevention of death, myocardial infarction, and stroke in high risk patients. Br Med J 2002;324:71–86.)

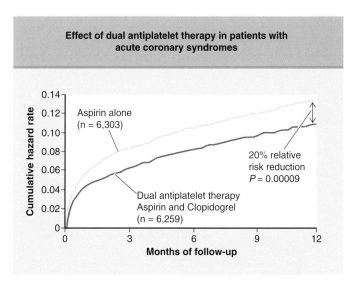

Effect of dual antiplatelet therapy in patients with acute coronary syndromes

Figure 30.15. Effect of dual antiplatelet therapy with aspirin and clopidogrel compared to aspirin treatment alone on the combined end point of vascular death, myocardial infarction, and stroke in patients with acute coronary syndromes. (Data from the CURE investigators as reported in Effects of clopidogrel in addition to aspirin in patients with acute coronary syndromes without St-segment elevation. N Engl J Med 2001;345:494–502.)

a wide range of doses, which led to the current recommendation to initiate treatment with an initial dose of at least 150 mg followed by long-term maintenance therapy with 75 to 150 mg daily. Aspirin's ability to reduce platelet aggregation is limited due to alternative pathways of platelet activation involving adenosine diphosphate, thrombin, and collagen.

Clopidogrel
Clopidogrel is a thienopyridine derivative that irreversibly binds to the $P2Y_{12}$ adenosine diphosphate (ADP) receptor and thereby inhibits ADP-dependent platelet activation. Clopidogrel has been shown to be somewhat more effective than aspirin at reducing cardiovascular events (relative risk reduction, 9%) in patients with atherosclerotic disease. More important, dual antiplatelet therapy consisting of aspirin and clopidogrel has been shown to be synergistic in preventing thrombus formation and clinical events. Thus, clopidogrel in addition to aspirin reduces the relative risk of death, nonfatal myocardial infarction, and stroke by 20% compared to aspirin alone in patients with acute coronary syndromes (Fig. 30.15). The beneficial effect of clopidogrel is present in all subgroups, including those with low- and high-risk features, emerges within hours of administration, and remains durable up to 1 year. Early administration of clopidogrel in patients undergoing PCI appears to be particularly beneficial when it precedes the intervention by more than 6 hours. The combination treatment of aspirin and clopidogrel is associated with an increased risk of bleeding, especially in patients undergoing coronary artery bypass grafting, and it is recommended to discontinue clopidogrel 5 days prior to planned coronary artery bypass grafting. In summary, it is recommended to administer clopidogrel in addition to aspirin to patients with UA/NSTEMI not deemed at increased risk of bleeding, with a

loading dose of 300 to 600 mg to achieve rapid onset of action followed by a maintenance dose of 75 mg daily for a duration of 9 to 12 months.

Glycoprotein IIb/IIIa receptor antagonists
The glycoprotein (GP) IIb/IIIa receptor is an integrin found in the platelet membrane and is conceived as the final common pathway of platelet aggregation. Platelet GP IIb/IIIa receptor antagonists are a novel class of potent antiplatelet agents interfering with this receptor, with three agents available for intravenous administration. Abciximab is a monoclonal chimeric antibody that irreversibly binds to the GP IIb/IIIa receptor, whereas tirofiban and eptifibatide are synthetic, reversible, small-molecule inhibitors of the GP IIb/IIIa receptor. Overall, these agents have shown a modest 1% absolute and 9% relative reduction of death and nonfatal myocardial infarction in patients with acute coronary syndromes, which was associated with a 1% increase in bleeding complications. Bleeding associated with GP IIb/IIIa receptor antagonists has special features beyond puncture site–related bleeding, involving mucocutaneous oozing from gums, mouth, skin, and nose. Preliminary data indicate that clopidogrel does not increase the bleeding risk of GP IIb/IIIa receptor antagonists.

Patients with high-risk features—notably troponin-positive patients (Fig. 30.16), those undergoing early revascularization by percutaneous coronary intervention (38% relative risk reduction of death and myocardial infarction) (Fig. 30.17), and diabetic patients (26% relative mortality reduction) (Fig. 30.18)—appear to derive a great benefit from the addition of GP IIb/IIIa receptor antagonists to treatment with aspirin and heparin. The two small-molecule GP IIb/IIIa receptor antagonists tirofiban and eptifibatide may be used for "upstream" therapy (i.e., 1 or 2 days prior to coronary angiography and continued for 24 hours after percutaneous coronary intervention). In contrast, abcix-

313

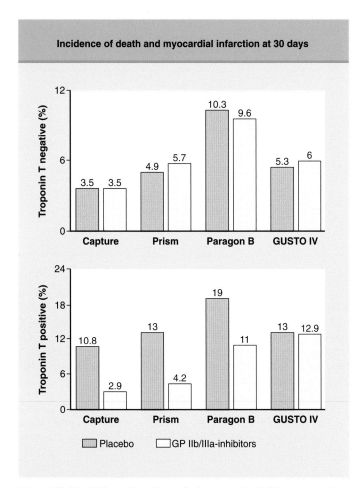

Figure 30.16. Differential effect of glycoprotein IIb/IIIa antagonists on the combined end point of death and myocardial infarction at 30 days in relation to troponin levels in four randomized clinical trials. *Top*, Lack of therapeutic effect exerted by GP IIb/IIIa antagonists in troponin-negative patients. *Bottom*, Pronounced therapeutic effect exerted by GP IIb/IIIa antagonists in troponin-positive patients.

imab is not indicated in patients treated conservatively and should be initiated at the time of coronary angiography when the decision to proceed with PCI has been made.

In summary, triple antiplatelet therapy with GP IIb/IIIa receptor antagonists in addition to aspirin and clopidogrel is indicated in patients with high-risk acute coronary syndromes undergoing PCI. In contrast, patients with low-risk acute coronary syndromes not undergoing revascularization derive no additional benefit from intravenous GP IIb/IIIa receptor blockade. Oral GP IIb/IIIa receptor antagonists have shown no evidence of benefit in patients with acute coronary syndromes.

Unfractionated heparin and low-molecular-weight heparin

Unfractionated heparin, a glycosaminoglycan made of polysaccharide chains ranging in molecular weight from 5 to 30 kDa, exerts its anticoagulant effect by binding to antithrombin and thus inactivates factor Xa and thrombin. Unfractionated heparin has to be administered intravenously and has unpredictable pharmacokinetics, requiring frequent anticoagulation monitoring. It is recommended that heparin be administered as a weight-adjusted bolus of 60 IU/kg (maximal dose, 4000 IU), followed by an infusion of 12 IU/kg/hr. Further dosing adjustments are

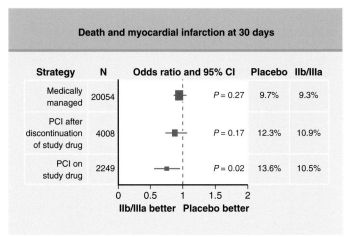

Figure 30.17. Beneficial effect of glycoprotein IIb/IIIa antagonists on the combined end point of death and myocardial infarction in relation to revascularization therapy. *Top*, Lack of therapeutic benefit exerted by GP IIb/IIIa antagonists in patients managed conservatively. *Middle*, Lack of therapeutic benefit exerted by GP IIb/IIIa antagonists in patients undergoing delayed percutaneous coronary intervention (PCI) after discontinuation of study drug. *Bottom*, Pronounced therapeutic benefit exerted by GP IIb/IIIa antagonists in patients undergoing PCI during index hospitalization while on study drug. (Data from Roffi M, Chew DP, Mukherjee D, et al: Platelet glycoprotein IIb/IIIa inhibition in acute coronary syndromes. Gradient of benefit related to the revascularization strategy. Eur Heart J 2002;23:1441–1448.)

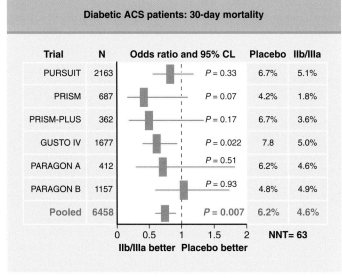

Figure 30.18. Beneficial effect of glycoprotein IIb/IIIa antagonists on 30-day mortality in diabetic patients presenting with acute coronary syndromes. Meta-analysis of six randomized trials assessing the benefit of glycoprotein IIb/IIIa antagonists in patients with acute coronary syndromes. NNT, number needed to treat. (Data from Roffi M, Chew DP, Mukherjee D, et al: Platelet glycoprotein IIb/IIIa inhibitors reduce mortality in diabetic patients with non-ST-segment-elevation acute coronary syndromes. Circulation 2001;104:2767–2771.)

based on measurements of activated partial thromboplastin time (50–70 sec). If added to aspirin, unfractionated heparin reduces the relative risk of death and myocardial infarction by 33% and has been the standard treatment for patients with acute coronary syndromes during the past 20 years.

Low-molecular-weight heparins (LMWHs) are obtained by chemical and enzymatic depolymerization of the heparin polysaccharide chains, resulting in short chain fragments with a molecular weight ranging from 4 to 6 kDa. LMWHs have a higher anti-factor Xa:anti-factor IIa activity than unfractionated heparin, which provides for more potent inhibition of thrombin generation. The pharmacokinetic profile of LMWH is predictable, with a high bioavailability and long plasma half-life without the need to monitor anticoagulation. In addition, LMWHs can be easily administered by the subcutaneous route. Clinical trials comparing LMWHs with unfractionated heparin indicate that LMWHs are at least as effective as unfractionated heparin, and that the LMWH enoxaparin may offer a modest benefit over unfractionated heparin. Furthermore, enoxaparin has been shown to be safe and effective in patients undergoing PCI and in conjunction with GP IIb/IIIa receptor antagonists. Accordingly, either LMWH or unfractionated heparin is recommended in addition to aspirin and clopidogrel during the acute treatment phase of patients with acute coronary syndromes. LMWHs should be used with caution in patients with renal insufficiency and avoided in the presence of severe renal failure (creatinine clearance < 30 mL/min).

Anti-ischemic Therapy
Nitrates
Nitrate preparations cause vasodilatation of veins, arteries, and arterioles by smooth muscle cell relaxation. They augment coronary collateral blood flow, reduce the frequency of coronary vasospasm, and potentially inhibit platelet aggregation. Both preload and afterload are reduced, improving the ratio of oxygen demand to supply and thus reducing ischemia. Intravenous nitrates are recommended for ongoing ischemic chest pain due to the ease of administration, titration, and rapid resolution of adverse effects as soon as the infusion is discontinued. Tolerance to nitrate therapy may develop as soon as 24 hours after initiation of therapy and may be overcome by increasing the dose or changing the route of administration.

Beta blockers
Beta blockade remains an important cornerstone for treatment of patients with ongoing ischemic chest pain. Intravenous beta blockade followed by oral administration is targeted to reduce the heart rate to 50 to 60 beats per minute. Beta blockers reduce the need for analgesics and relieve ischemic pain. In patients with acute myocardial infarction, beta blockade reduces mortality, the incidence of cardiac arrest, and reinfarction. Beta blockers should be used with caution in patients with heart failure, arterial hypotension, and bradyarrhythmias.

Invasive Therapy
Significant coronary artery lesions can be demonstrated in 80% to 90% of patients with acute coronary syndromes undergoing coronary angiography. The culprit lesion often reveals a stenosis with irregular borders and identifiable thrombotic material. In addition, multiple lesions in more than one epicardial vessel may be present. Accordingly, the risk of complications during revascularization procedures is higher than in stable patients, and for years there was a debate about the benefits of routine early invasive therapy compared to a noninvasive, conservative strategy.

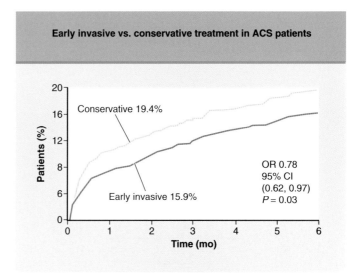

Figure 30.19. Beneficial effect of an early invasive compared to a conservative strategy on the combined end point of death, myocardial infarction, and rehospitalization in patients with acute coronary syndromes in the TACTICS-TIMI 18 trial. (Data from Cannon CP, Weintraub WS, Demopoulos LA, et al: Comparison of early invasive and conservative strategies in patients with unstable coronary syndromes treated with the glycoprotein IIb/IIIa inhibitor tirofiban. N Engl J Med 2001;344:1879–1887.)

Six randomized clinical trials have conclusively attested to the superiority of an early invasive strategy, defined as coronary angiography followed by revascularization by either PCI or coronary artery bypass grafting (CABG), with significant reductions in death, reinfarction, and rehospitalization (relative risk reduction of 20%–30%) in patients with acute coronary syndromes (Fig. 30.19). Preliminary data also indicate that an immediate (within hours) invasive strategy may be superior to a delayed (within several days) invasive strategy. The advantages of an early invasive strategy are related to the elimination of the culprit lesion, with effective restoration of blood flow and reduction of the risk for reinfarction. The greatest benefit (>50% relative risk reduction) of an early invasive strategy is observed in patients with moderate to high-risk acute coronary syndromes, notably patients with ST segment depression and/or a positive troponin test. Of note, an early invasive strategy has been shown to be very cost-effective, with a cost of $12,739 per life-year saved, even in low-risk patients.

The invasive strategy is associated with a small early hazard related to the procedure. This risk has been largely eliminated in the setting of PCIs with the advent of modern antiplatelet and antithrombotic treatment consisting of aspirin, clopidogrel, GP IIb/IIIa receptor antagonists, and heparin. In contrast, early procedure-related deaths are more common in patients undergoing CABG, and therefore only patients with a profile known to benefit from surgical revascularization should be referred for early CABG.

Current practice guidelines recommend an early invasive strategy consisting of coronary angiography followed by appropriate revascularization by either PCI or CABG as routine management in patients with intermediate to high-risk acute coronary syndromes at facilities with adequately trained staff and appropriate equipment.

Cardiovascular Problems

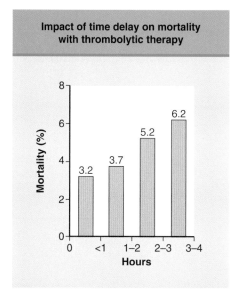

Figure 30.20. Impact of time delay until initiation of thrombolysis on early mortality in patients with acute STEMI as observed by the TIMI 2 study group.

STEMI

Since acute STEMI is caused by thrombotic occlusion of a coronary artery, therapeutic efforts have focused on effective restoration of blood flow by means of pharmacological or mechanical reperfusion therapy. Reperfusion therapy is indicated in the presence of nonabating ischemic chest pain (>20 min duration), ST segment elevation more than 0.1 mV in at least two contiguous leads (>0.2 mV in leads V1–V3) or presumably new left bundle branch block, and the onset of symptoms within 12 hours. Patients with ongoing ischemic chest pain after 12 hours of symptom onset and those in cardiogenic shock may still derive benefit from mechanical reperfusion therapy. The most important aspect of reperfusion therapy is its timely implementation. Thus, data from the Thrombolysis in Myocardial Infarction (TIMI) 2 study group and the FTT collaborators indicate that mortality increases on average by 1% per hour and that 1.6 lives per 1000 treated patients are lost per hour of treatment delay (Fig. 30.20).

Immediate treatment measures include administration of aspirin, clopidogrel, heparin, beta blockers, nitrates, and oxygen as outlined previously. In the absence of existing aspirin therapy, an intravenous bolus of 250 to 500 mg aspirin is given to completely block thromboxane A2 synthesis. Unfractionated heparin is given as a weight-adjusted bolus of 60 IU/kg (maximum dose, 4000 IU) followed by intravenous administration of 12 IU/kg/min (maximum dose, 1000 IU/hr).

Thrombolysis

Thrombolytic therapy has dramatically improved the outcome of patients with STEMI. It is readily available, may be administered during the prehospital phase, does not require specialized staff, and has been reproducibly shown to reduce mortality by more than 25%. Front-loaded alteplase was shown to be superior to streptokinase in terms of vessel patency, left ventricular function, and mortality reduction in the large-scale GUSTO I trial. Subsequent development of bolus thrombolytics, such as

tenecteplase and reteplase, allowed for easier administration than alteplase but failed to further improve survival. The combination of thrombolytic agents with GP IIb/IIIa receptor antagonists also failed to improve survival, resulted only in modest reductions of reinfarction, and was associated with considerable bleeding complications.

There are several shortcomings of thrombolytic therapy. Even the most modern thrombolytic agents achieve vessel patency in only 60% of patients. The most important adverse events related to thrombolytic therapy are bleeding complications, notably a 0.5% to 1.0% incidence of intracranial hemorrhage. Furthermore, a reocclusion rate of 20% to 30% is observed at 3 months, and the benefit of thrombolytic therapy in elderly patients remains undefined.

Invasive Therapy

Mechanical reperfusion therapy by primary PCI has emerged as the gold standard in the acute treatment of STEMI and has been shown to be superior to thrombolytic therapy at facilities with both capabilities. The advantages of primary PCI over thrombolysis are the higher vessel patency with contemporary techniques (>95% with stents and GP IIb/IIIa receptor antagonists) (Fig. 30.21) and the lower risk of intracranial hemorrhage. A meta-analysis of 23 trials comparing primary PCI with thrombolysis in approximately 8000 patients showed a significant reduction of death (27%), reinfarction (57%), stroke (50%), and

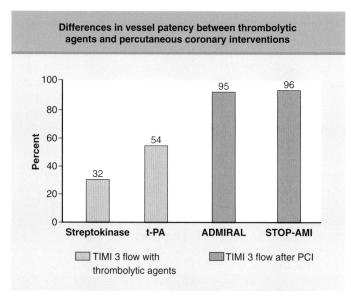

Figure 30.21. Differences in vessel patency between thrombolytic agents and percutaneous coronary interventions. Differences in vessel patency (TIMI 3 flow) achieved with different thrombolytic agents (green; data from the GUSTO I trial as reported in The effects of tissue plasminogen activator, streptokinase, or both on coronary-artery patency, ventricular function, and survival after acute myocardial infarction. N Engl J Med 1993;329:1615) compared to percutaneous coronary interventions (purple; data from the STOP-AMI trial as reported in Coronary stenting plus platelet glycoprotein IIb/IIIa blockade compared with tissue plasminogen activator in acute myocardial infarction. N Engl J Med 2000;343:385, and the ADMIRAL trial as reported in Platelet glycoprotein IIb/IIIa inhibition with coronary stenting for acute myocardial infarction. N Engl J Med 2001;344:1895) in patients with acute STEMI.

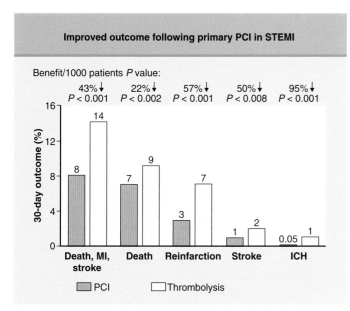

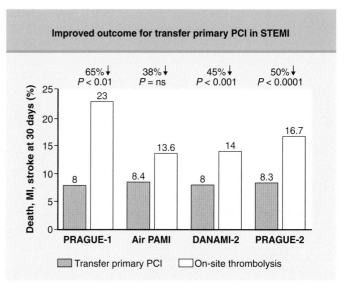

Figure 30.22. Superiority of primary percutaneous coronary intervention (PCI) compared to thrombolysis with regard to short-term outcome in patients with acute STEMI. For 1000 patients treated with primary PCI instead of thrombolysis, 23 lives are saved and 44 myocardial infarctions and 11 strokes prevented. ICH, intracranial hemorrhage. (Data from a meta-analysis of 7739 patients in 23 randomized trials as reported by Keeley EC, Boura JA, Grines CL in Primary angioplasty versus intravenous thrombolytic therapy for acute myocardial infarction: a quantitative review of 23 randomised trials. Lancet 2003;361:13.)

Figure 30.23. Benefit of percutaneous coronary intervention (PCI) in patients with acute STEMI transferred to a facility with a catheterization laboratory compared to on-site thrombolysis in four randomized trials. Data are reported for the combined end point of death, myocardial infarction (MI), and stroke at 30 days.

intracranial hemorrhage (95%) in favor of catheter-based reperfusion (Fig. 30.22). The short-term benefit appears to be maintained at long-term follow-up, with improved event-free survival, left ventricular function, and decreased rehospitalization rates. However, primary PCI is only more effective than throm-bolysis when carried out expeditiously (door-to-balloon time < 90 min) by skilled operators in experienced centers. Accordingly, current practice guidelines recommend primary PCI as first-line therapy in patients with acute STEMI when available within 90 minutes in experienced centers.

Most patients with acute STEMI present to hospitals without on-site catheterization facilities. Four randomized trials addressed the question of whether patients should be preferentially transferred on an emergency basis to a site capable of performing primary PCI compared with administering thrombolytic therapy. All trials demonstrated an unexpected benefit for catheter-based reperfusion therapy over on-site thrombolysis, with a consistent 40% to 50% reduction of the end point death, myocardial infarction, or stroke (Fig. 30.23). Accordingly, primary PCI becomes an increasingly attractive alternative to thrombolytic therapy in patients presenting to facilities without on-site catheterization if transport times of less than 60 minutes can be realized.

Catheter-based reperfusion therapy should also be considered in patients with failed thrombolysis (rescue PCI). Finally, patients presenting with acute myocardial infarction complicated by cardiogenic shock should undergo emergency revascularization. The SHOCK trial demonstrated a 39% improvement in 1-year survival (132 lives saved for 1000 treated patients) for

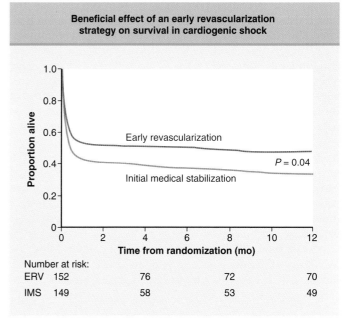

Figure 30.24. Beneficial effect on survival (39% improvement) of an early revascularization (ERV) strategy compared to conservative treatment [initial medical stabilization (IMS)] in patients with acute STEMI complicated by cardiogenic shock. For 1000 patients undergoing early revascularization instead of conservative treatment, 132 lives are saved. (Data from Hochman JS, Sleeper LA, White HD, et al: One-year survival following early revascularization for cardiogenic shock. JAMA 2001;285:190–192.)

patients assigned to emergency revascularization as opposed to conservative therapy (Fig. 30.24).

Clinical Course and Prevention

Following the acute treatment phase, patients remain hospitalized for hemodynamic and rhythm monitoring for several days.

In the hospital, approximately 5% to 15% of patients with STEMI die of heart failure (cardiogenic shock) and arrhythmic death. Another 10% to 15% of patients develop complications related to myocardial infarction, including various degrees of atrioventricular or intraventricular block, ventricular tachyarrhythmias, recurrent angina or infarction, postinfarction pericarditis, mitral regurgitation related to papillary muscle dysfunction, ventricular septal rupture, and cardiac free wall rupture. Approximately 75% of patients remain stable after myocardial infarction and can be rapidly discharged. Most recurrent cardiac events are observed during the first few months following the initial coronary event. This observation has been related to the prolonged healing process of ruptured plaques and sustained prothrombotic activity and highlights the importance of long-term antithrombotic and anti-inflammatory medical treatment.

The medical regimen at discharge should include aspirin at a dose of 75 to 150 mg daily. This is combined with clopidogrel at a dose of 75 mg per day for a duration of 9 to 12 months in patients with UA/NSTEMI and for patients with STEMI following primary PCI. Beta blockers improve prognosis following myocardial infarction by reducing mortality, reinfarction, and symptoms of angina and should be continued after acute coronary syndromes. Treatment with statins is a well-documented primary and secondary prevention strategy for reducing the future risk of cardiovascular death and myocardial infarction. Lipid-lowering therapy with statins should be initiated immediately, aiming at a cholesterol level of less than 5 mmol/liter and an LDL level of less than 1.8–2.6 mmol/dL. Statins may exert a beneficial effect beyond lipid lowering by attenuating inflammation, as reflected by decreased CRP levels after initiation of therapy. Angiotensin converting enzyme (ACE) inhibitors reduce mortality and reinfarction and improve ventricular remodeling following myocardial infarction. They are strongly recommended in patients with acute coronary syndromes. In the absence of contraindications, ACE inhibitors should be initiated early and continued long term. The efficacy appears greatest in patients at high risk, such as elderly people, patients with signs of heart failure, and asymptomatic patients with depressed left ventricular function.

Modification of lifestyle habits has an important impact on long-term prognosis. Smoking is a major cardiovascular risk factor, and the benefits of smoking cessation are well documented: The myocardial risk returns to normal at approximately 2 years. Similarly, weight control is important since increased weight interacts with lipid levels and blood pressure and has an independent effect on event-free survival. Regular physical exercise has been demonstrated in numerous studies to improve cardiovascular outcome. Current recommendations include 30 minutes of walking or jogging three to seven times per week, with the goal to increase heart rate to 70% of the predicted maximum. Finally, patients require instruction for regular blood pressure and lipid level control and, in the case of established diabetes, intensive management.

SUGGESTED READING

Alpert JS, Thygesen K, Antman E, Bassand JP: Myocardial infarction redefined—A consensus document of the Joint European Society of Cardiology/American College of Cardiology Committee for the Redefinition of Myocardial Infarction. J Am Coll Cardiol 2000;36:959–969.

Andersen HR, Nielsen TT, Rasmussen K, et al: A comparison of coronary angioplasty with fibrinolytic therapy in acute myocardial infarction. N Engl J Med 2003;349:733–742.

Boersma E, Mercado N, Poldermans D, et al: Acute myocardial infarction. Lancet 2003;361:847–858.

Braunwald E: Application of current guidelines to the management of unstable angina and non-ST-elevation myocardial infarction. Circulation 2003;108:III28–III37.

Cannon CP, Weintraub WS, Demopoulos LA, et al: Comparison of early invasive and conservative strategies in patients with unstable coronary syndromes treated with the glycoprotein IIb/IIIa inhibitor tirofiban. N Engl J Med 2001;344:1879–1887.

Corti R, Fuster V, Badimon JJ: Pathogenetic concepts of acute coronary syndromes. J Am Coll Cardiol 2003;41:7S–14S.

Hamm CW, Goldmann BU, Heeschen C, et al: Emergency room triage of patients with acute chest pain by means of rapid testing for cardiac troponin T or troponin I. N Engl J Med 1997;337:1648–1653.

Keeley EC, Boura JA, Grines CL: Primary angioplasty versus intravenous thrombolytic therapy for acute myocardial infarction: A quantitative review of 23 randomised trials. Lancet 2003;361:13–20.

Prasad A, Mathew V, Holmes DR Jr, Gersh BJ: Current management of non-ST-segment-elevation acute coronary syndrome: Reconciling the results of randomized controlled trials. Eur Heart J 2003;24:1544–1553.

Ross R: Atherosclerosis—An inflammatory disease. N Engl J Med 1999;340:115–126.

Yeghiazarians Y, Braunstein JB, Askari A, Stone PH: Unstable angina pectoris. N Engl J Med 2000;342:101–114.

KEY POINTS

- Arrhythmias occur commonly in critically ill patients, and their prompt recognition and accurate diagnosis are crucial to determining pathophysiology, treatment, and prognosis.
- Nonsustained ventricular tachycardia occurs frequently in the critical care setting and treatment is generally not necessary. Treatment with antiarrhythmic agents including amiodarone requires caution and careful patient selection.
- Sustained ventricular arrhythmias require prompt recognition of the exact type of arrhythmia and its associated "syndrome" in order to ensure correct treatment and to establish prognosis. Direct cardioversion using high-energy countershock is recommended for patients who are hemodynamically unstable. Recognition of monitoring artifact is important in the patient who is hemodynamically stable.
- Atrial tachycardia, atrial fibrillation, and atrial flutter are the most prevalent supraventricular arrhythmias in the critical care patient population. Differentiation between these and other forms of supraventricular tachycardia allows accurate diagnosis and prompt therapy.
- Although less common than tachyarrhythmias, bradyarrhythmias, both physiologic and pathologic, may occur in various settings in critical care patients. Treatment depends on the etiology, with differentiation between sinus node and atrioventricular node dysfunction being paramount.

The critical care setting is a hotbed for numerous cardiac arrhythmias. These arrhythmias frequently occur in critically ill patients because of high sympathetic tone, sepsis, cerebral injury, trauma, increased cardiac demand, cardiac ischemia, or myocardial infarction, and following out-of-hospital cardiac arrest. Accordingly, the prompt recognition of these arrhythmias, coupled with an understanding of their pathophysiologic basis, provides the backbone of understanding in order to deliver timely, effective therapy.

The types of arrhythmias that are encountered in the intensive care unit (ICU) include those that are either fast or slow and, of those that are fast, either narrow or wide, regular or irregular. All arrhythmias may be further categorized into those that are either hemodynamically stable or unstable. Slow heart rhythms can also be categorized into those that are physiologic versus pathologic, with the latter more likely requiring perma-

nent pacemaker implantation. An approach to arrhythmias is shown in Figure 31.1, which can be used to direct the reader to the appropriate arrhythmia section within this chapter. A general preamble regarding the mechanisms of action and use of common antiarrhythmic drugs is shown in Box 31.1.

SUPRAVENTRICULAR ARRHYTHMIAS

The most common supraventricular arrhythmias (SVTs) encountered in critical care patients are atrial tachycardia (AT), atrial flutter (AFL), and atrial fibrillation (AFIB). Their incidence increases with age. They have numerous cardiac and noncardiac causes (Box 31.2), although the arrhythmias can occur in the absence of secondary factors. These three arrhythmias are closely related, and often patients may cycle from one arrhythmia to the next (Fig. 31.2). Other forms of SVTs are uncommon in the critical care unit and more likely to occur in patients who have a long history of arrhythmias. These include atrioventricular nodal reentrant tachycardia (AVNRT) and atrioventricular reciprocating tachycardia (AVRT).

In general, the approach to the electrocardiographic diagnosis of SVTs, other than AFL or AFIB, rests on the relationship between the "P" and "R" waves. When speaking of SVTs with one P wave for every QRS complex, or a 1:1 atrioventricular (AV) relationship, one can differentiate between the various forms of SVTs by examining the "RP" interval, or the time from onset of QRS to onset of P wave. In general, three types of RP relationships exist: P "in" R, short RP, and long RP (Fig. 31.3). Differentiation between the various electrocardiographic features of the arrhythmias is discussed separately for each arrhythmia type.

Atrial Tachycardia
Epidemiology and Pathogenesis
Atrial tachycardias originate from a small region of abnormal electrical activity within either the left or the right atrium, brought about because of abnormal automaticity, triggered activity, or as part of a small reentrant circuit (microreentry). In general, these regions of abnormal electrical activity usually develop due to areas within the atrial musculature that have heterogeneous electrical properties. Commonly, ATs originate along the crista terminalis, the region that separates the smooth from trabeculated right atrium. Atrial tachycardias have also been shown to originate along the tricuspid annulus, in the atrioventricular nodal (AVN) region, and from within and around the pulmonary veins. The latter forms of AT may commonly precipitate atrial fibrillation. Because aging is associated with

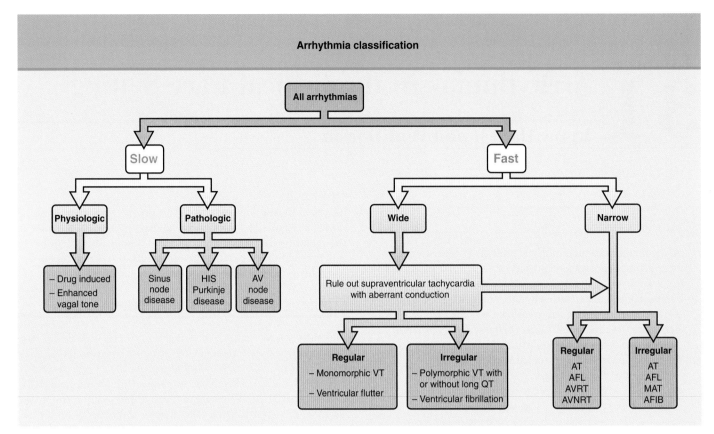

Figure 31.1. Arrhythmia classification. AFIB, atrial fibrillation; AFL, atrial flutter; AT, atrial tachycardia; AV, atrioventricular; AVNRT, atrioventricular nodal reentrant tachycardia; AVRT, atrioventricular reciprocating tachycardia; MAT, multifocal atrial tachycardia; VT, ventricular tachycardia.

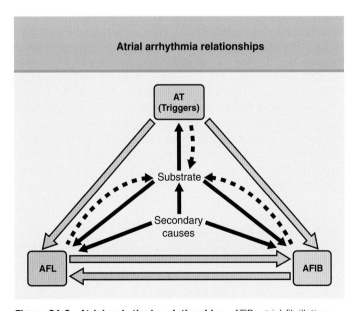

Figure 31.2. Atrial arrhythmia relationships. AFIB, atrial fibrillation; AFL, atrial flutter; AT, atrial tachycardia.

the development of atrial fibrosis, the elderly may be more prone to ATs as atrial fibrosis degrades cell-to-cell electrical communication within the atrium. Some ATs may be sensitive to catecholamine stress, making the critical care patient more prone to these arrhythmias.

Diagnosis

During AT, the relationship between atrial and ventricular activation is usually not very different from that which is present during normal sinus rhythm, and thus, in general, the RP relation is long. However, in conditions of AV node disease, very rapid ATs, or when AV node blocking medications are present, the PR may become progressively longer, making the RP interval progressively shorter. In this instance, the P wave axis becomes very useful for differentiating AT from AVNRT or AVRT since the latter two will usually have a superior axis, whereas AT commonly has an inferior axis. AT may be difficult to differentiate from AVNRT or AVRT either when the RP relation is short or when P waves are not visible because they are hidden inside the QRS complex or T wave. In this instance, administration of intravenous AV node–blocking medications, such as beta blockers, calcium channel blockers, or adenosine, may be used to increase AV block during AT. If the rapid P wave activation persists despite AV block, then the diagnosis of AT can be made since AVNRT and AVRT must maintain a 1:1 AV relationship. An example of AT initially with 1:1 AV conduction and subsequently with higher grade AV block after administration of adenosine is shown in Figure 31.4.

Treatment

Initial therapy for patients diagnosed with sustained AT should consist of control of the ventricular rate, preferably with beta blockers or calcium channels blockers (with or without digoxin) or a combination. Subsequently, treatment of the actual arrhyth-

Box 31.1 Overview of Antiarrhythmic Drugs

Antiarrhythmic drugs with class I and III action, along with amiodarone, are discussed. The most commonly used class I medications include procainamide, propafenone, lidocaine, and flecainide. These medications generally act on sodium channels to delay the upstroke of the action potential and reduce the propensity for reentrant circuits to propagate by slowing conduction. They also generally reduce automaticity to a minor degree. Although lidocaine is commonly used in patients with ventricular arrhythmias, its efficacy is poor. Sotalol is a hybrid of a class III antiarrhythmic and a nonselective beta blocker. It acts by blocking potassium channels, thereby delaying repolarization. Its main risk is that of QT prolongation and development of torsades des pointes, and thus its use should be restricted to patients with normal QT intervals and those with normal electrolytes and renal function. Amiodarone is a very unusual antiarrhythmic drug in that it has actions from virtually all classes of antiarrhythmics. It is likely the most efficacious of antiarrhythmics, beneficial for those with both atrial and ventricular arrhythmias. Orally, amiodarone has a very long half-life, and long-term accumulation is responsible for the majority of side effects. Intravenously, amiodarone has acute antiadrenergic effects, short-term antiarrhythmic effects that are useful for control of some ventricular arrhythmias, and intermediate-term antiarrhythmic effects that may take 6 to 12 hr for efficacy. Usually, loading doses of amiodarone over days to weeks are required prior to ascertaining antiarrhythmic efficacy. Rapid infusion of intravenous amiodarone may lead to hypotension, principally because of vasodilating effects of the solvent used in the intravenous preparation.

Box 31.2 Secondary Causes of Atrial Fibrillation

Cardiac

Valvular

Rheumatic heart disease
Mitral stenosis or regurgitation
Mitral valve prolapse without regurgitation
Severe tricuspid regurgitation

Nonvalvular

Arterial
    Hypertension
Myocardial
    Myocardial infarction
    Myocarditis
    Left ventricular dysfunction
    Hypertrophic cardiomyopathy
    Cardiac tumors (e.g., atrial myxoma)
Pericardial
    Pericarditis
    Postcardiac surgery
Electrical
    Wolff-Parkinson-white (WPW) syndrome with
        supraventricular tachycardia (SVT)
    Other supraventricular arrhythmias: atrial flutter, atrial
        tachycardia
    Vagal-mediated AF: AF in setting of bradycardia

Noncardiac

Pulmonary

Pulmonary embolism
Bronchopneumonia
Obstructive sleep apnea
Other nonspecified pulmonary pathology

Nonpulmonary

Hyper- or hypothyroidism
Acute alcohol intake
Catecholaminergic drugs or medications (e.g.,
    pseudoephedrine, cocaine)

mia may be accomplished by a variety of approaches. ATs may be sensitive to calcium channel blockers (e.g., those that are terminated with adenosine) or beta blockers (those triggered by sympathetic stress—catecholaminergic). Importantly, some ATs are not responsive to either of these medications, and antiarrhythmic drugs may be required. Depending on the clinical situation, one may consider medications such as sotalol, procainamide, or amiodarone. Generally, anticoagulation is not required for patients with AT because atrial contraction is preserved. However, because of the overlap between AT and AFIB, anticoagulation should be considered in at-risk individuals who have both arrhythmias.

Frequently, nonsustained episodes of AT may occur in monitored patients, especially in the setting of increased sympathetic tone. Generally, treatment is not required unless a patient becomes hemodynamically unstable or significantly symptomatic during these episodes. The prognosis of patients with AT generally depends on the underlying disease because the arrhythmia is usually benign.

Atrial Flutter

Epidemiology and Pathogenesis

Atrial flutter is a generic term for any macroreentrant circuit that is confined to the atrium. For such circuits to occur, obstacles to conduction of impulses are generally required and can be fixed or functional (physiologic). Fixed obstacles may be anatomic (e.g., the tricuspid annulus), pathologic (e.g., an atrial septal defect and extensive atrial fibrosis), or acquired (e.g., atriotomy scar from previous surgery). The usual obstacles to conduction include the superior vena cava (SVC), inferior vena cava (IVC), tricuspid annulus (TA), coronary sinus (CS), fossa ovalis (FO), crista terminalis (CT), and eustachian ridge (ER) in the right atrium and the mitral annulus (MA), fossa ovalis, and pulmonary veins (PVs) in the left atrium. Most AFLs originate in the right atrium, and this may be in part related to the greater number of obstacles to conduction compared to the left atrium. Generally, the most common kind of AFL is one that circulates around the TA in a counterclockwise or clockwise direction when the annulus is viewed from the ventricular aspect. With this type of AFL, the anterior boundary for conduction is the TA, whereas the posterior boundaries include the CT, IVC, CS, and SVC. AFL is a very stable arrhythmia, more so than AFIB, with either arrhythmia capable of degenerating or organizing into the other. During AFL, the ventricular response rate is generally

321

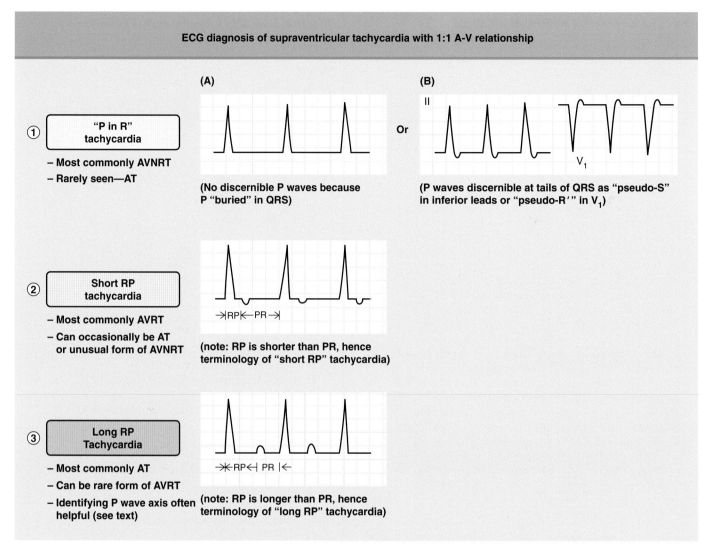

Figure 31.3. ECG diagnosis of supraventricular tachycardia with 1:1 AV relationship. AT, atrial tachycardia; AVNRT, atrioventricular nodal reentrant tachycardia; AVRT, atrioventricular reciprocating tachycardia.

faster than that of AFIB for a given patient, and it can be more difficult to control.

Diagnosis

The atrial rate during AFL usually ranges between 250 and 300 beats per minute (bpm) and, as such, is rarely able to support 1:1 AV conduction. Usually, the ventricular response is regular and is proportionally related to the atrial rate (e.g., 1:2, 1:3), although occasionally variable conduction over the AV node may occur. Because the cycle length (CL [msec] = 60,000/rate [bpm]) of AFL is equal to the time that it takes to complete one circuit around the TA, usually the atria are being depolarized throughout the entire cycle. As such, the flutter waves are seen to continually disrupt the baseline of the electrocardiogram (ECG), hence the "sawtooth" appearance of the ECG (Fig. 31.5). Of note, during AFL, one expects the flutter waves to have a consistent beat-to-beat morphology and cycle length, given the stability of the reentrant circuit. Additionally, one expects to see flutter waves in both the precordial and limb leads. During common (typical or isthmus-dependent) AFL, the flutter waves have one of two distinct morphologies, although

rare exceptions may occur: counterclockwise—predominantly negative flutter waves inferiorly, positive flutter waves in lead V1 that become progressively more negative toward V6; and clockwise—predominantly positive flutter waves inferiorly, negative flutter waves in lead V1 that become progressively more positive toward V6. Recognition of the common forms of AFL has important implications for future therapy. An example of atypical AFL is shown in Figure 31.6. If AFL occurs with 2:1 AV conduction, appreciating the flutter waves can be difficult because every second flutter wave is hidden inside the QRS complex, and in this case the administration of AV node-blocking agents (beta blockers, calcium channel blockers, and digoxin) or vagotonic maneuvers (Valsalva maneuver and carotid sinus massage) can increase the degree of AV block and make it easier to appreciate and analyze the flutter waves.

Treatment

The general approach to AFL treatment is similar to that of AFIB because both require a rate and rhythm approach to therapy. However, rate control in AFL can be significantly more difficult to achieve, mainly because the average atrial rates are

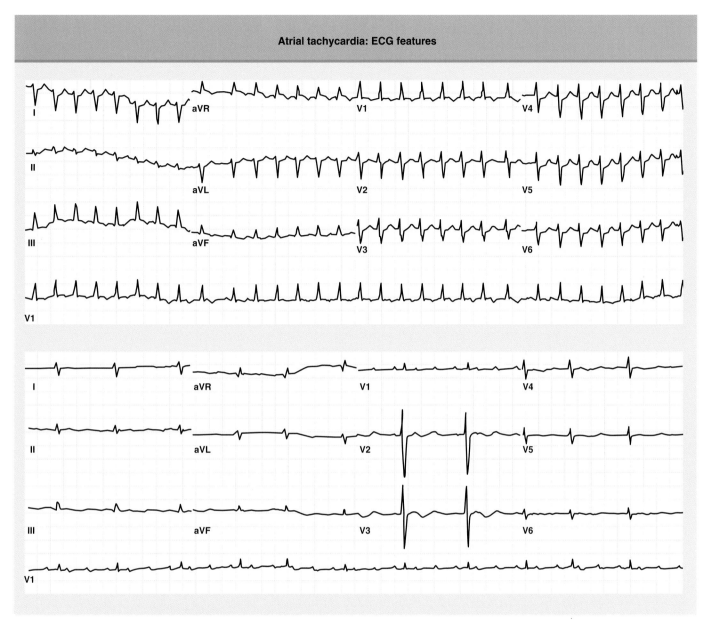

Atrial tachycardia: ECG features

Figure 31.4. Atrial tachycardia: ECG features. The top panel shows a rapid, narrow complex tachycardia at 182 bpm. P waves are difficult to discern, although there is a suggestion that the P wave is distorting the T wave, especially in leads V1 and III. The bottom panel shows the same patient after administration of an AV node-blocking agent. Clearly, the P waves are now visible, and at the same atrial rate as in the top panel. Because 3:1 AV block now exists, the arrhythmia is easily diagnosed as an atrial tachycardia. The P wave axis suggests that the atrial tachycardia originates in the inferoposterior region of the atria.

slower (250–300 bpm compared to 400–600 bpm), and thus the AV node is more reliably able to conduct a greater number of atrial activations to the ventricle. Because AFL is a very stable reentrant circuit, antiarrhythmic therapy is also often ineffective because it serves only to slow conduction, which may merely reduce the rate of tachycardia without termination. Again, like AFIB, the aggressiveness with which one desires to restore normal sinus rhythm depends on multiple factors, with the major consideration being patient symptoms. Anticoagulation should be used in a similar manner to AFIB, including around the time of cardioversion.

Chronically, once the acute illness is stabilized, one should consider electrophysiologic referral for patients with AFL

because current catheter ablation techniques are able to achieve long-term success rates of 85% to 90% in patients with typical forms of AFL. However, given the relationship between AFIB and AFL, approximately 5% to 50% of patients with successful AFL ablation may go on to develop AFIB, depending on the amount of AFIB at baseline. An algorithm for the acute treatment of AFL and AFIB is presented in Figure 31.7.

Atrial Fibrillation
Epidemiology and Pathogenesis
Atrial fibrillation can be thought of as a disease of aging. Prevalence increases with age such that more than 5% of individuals older than 80 years of age will have AFIB. This phenomenon

Typical atrial flutter: ECG features

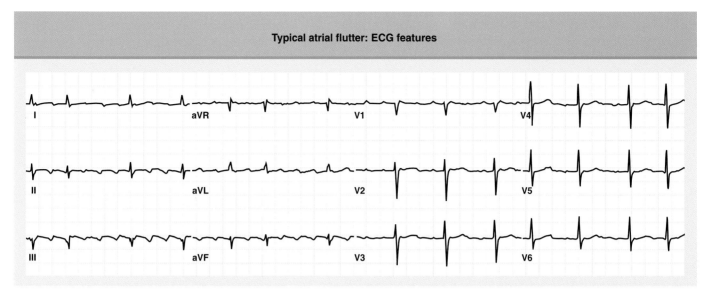

Figure 31.5. Typical atrial flutter: ECG features. This ECG demonstrates a patient with typical atrial flutter with variable AV block. The flutter rate is approximately 240 bpm, with negative flutter waves in the inferior leads, positive flutter waves in V1, and negative flutter waves in V6, suggesting a counterclockwise form of atrial flutter.

Atypical atrial flutter: ECG features

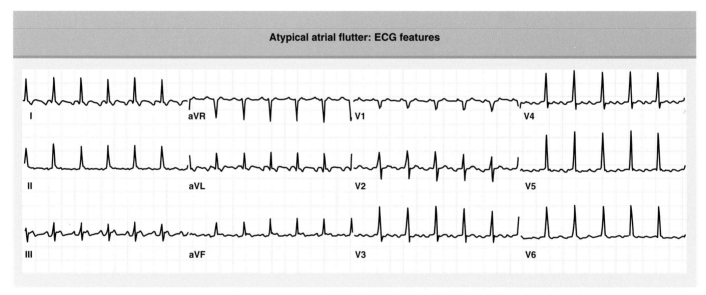

Figure 31.6. Atypical atrial flutter: ECG features. An atypical form of atrial flutter, with an atrial rate of approximately 290 bpm, positive flutter waves in the inferior leads, a positive flutter wave in V1, and a negative flutter wave in lead I. This pattern does not fit with either a clockwise or counterclockwise form, and it is likely an atypical form originating from the left atrium in a patient who is post-coronary artery bypass surgery. Compare to Figure 31.5.

may be related to development of atrial fibrosis, which may occur in the aging atrium, or increasing prevalence of risk factors for secondary causes of AFIB with age (see Box 31.2). During AFIB, multiple reentrant circuits (at least three at any one time) randomly collide, dissipate, and regenerate within both atria, leading to disorganized atrial activation and the absence of clear-cut P waves on the surface ECG. As long as the reentrant circuits continue to collide and regenerate, AFIB persists. Generally, the multiple reentrant circuits cause rapid repeated depolarization of the atrium in excess of 300 bpm, and because of the varied nature of these circuits, the ventricular response is rapid and irregular. Occasionally, these reentrant circuits can become transiently organized, especially in the region of the right atrial appendage, which can alter the appearance of AFIB of the surface ECG to look more like AFL.

Generally, patients are somewhat more hypotensive during AFIB than when in sinus rhythm (especially with rapid ventricular rates). This is likely a consequence of the combination of rapid and irregular rates as well as reduced atrial contraction, all of which lead to variable and reduced left ventricular filling, and the resultant reduction in cardiac output, with concomitant increase in left atrial pressures. Although AFIB is hemodynamically well

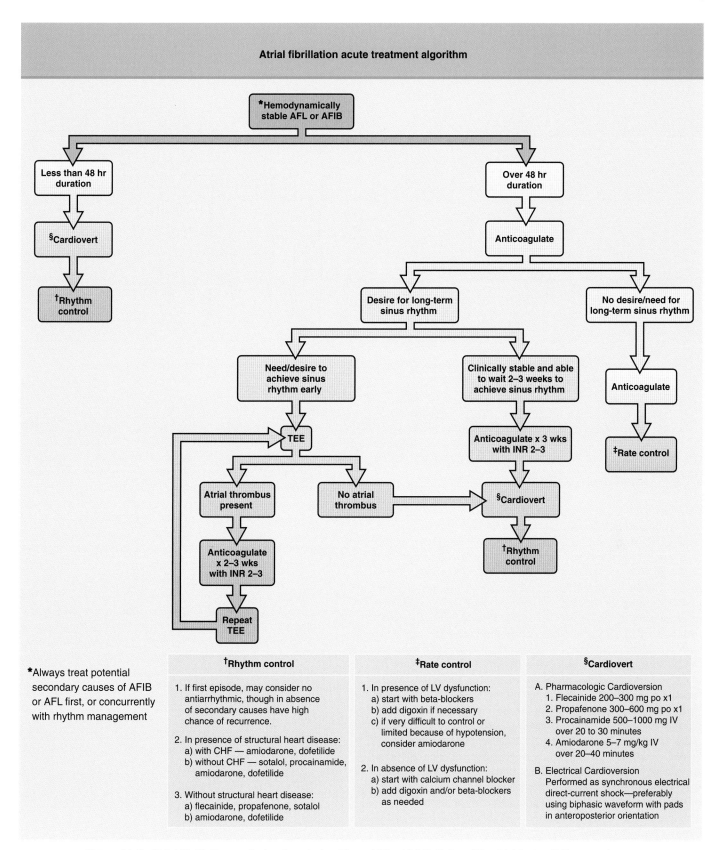

Figure 31.7. Atrial fibrillation acute treatment algorithm. AFIB, atrial fibrillation; AFL, atrial flutter; CHF, congestive heart failure; LV, left ventricular; TEE, transesophageal echocardiography.

Atrial fibrillation: ECG features I

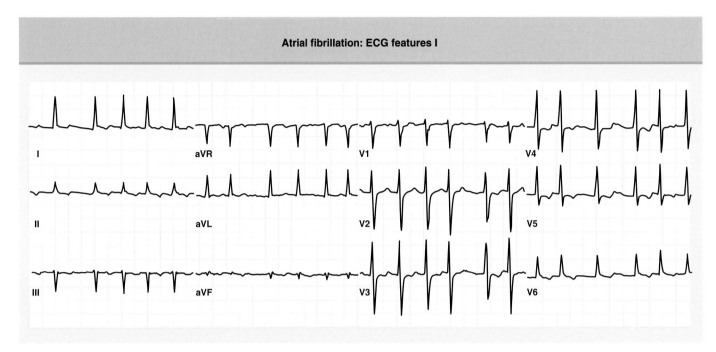

Figure 31.8. Atrial fibrillation: ECG features, I. Typical ECG of atrial fibrillation. Note the absence of discrete P waves and an irregularly irregular ventricular response.

tolerated in patients with normal left ventricular function, very rapid rates or concomitant left ventricular dysfunction can lead to significant hypotension and/or pulmonary venous congestion.

Diagnosis

The hallmark of AFIB on the surface ECG is the lack of discernible P waves, or undulating baseline, with an irregularly irregular ventricular response rate (Fig. 31.8). Importantly, at very high ventricular response rates, the degree of irregularity may not easily be appreciable, and the use of calipers or faster ECG recording speeds (e.g., 50 mm/sec) may be required. One must be wary of a baseline that appears like AFIB with a completely regular QRS response because this may represent AFIB with complete heart block and a junctional escape rhythm, as can be seen in the case of digoxin toxicity (typically causes AV block and increased junctional automaticity). Occasionally, the reentrant circuits of AFIB can lead to organized depolarization within the atria, especially along the trabeculated muscle of the right atrial appendage. This organized conduction over the right atrial appendage may lead to the transient appearance of "P waves"—especially in lead V1 because it overlies the right atrial appendage—and must be differentiated from AFL. Distinct from AFL, these P waves have variable morphologies, variable P-P intervals, and may not be appreciable in the limb leads. An example is shown in Figure 31.9. AFIB must also be distinguished from multifocal AT, shown in Figure 31.10.

Treatment

In the critical care setting, increased right and left atrial pressures, AV increased cardiac output secondary to sepsis, ventilation, pericarditis, and other conditions that increase sympathetic tone often lead to AFIB that requires acute treatment but often

do not require long-term treatment once the underlying cause improves. Although treatment of AFIB first includes the removal and treatment of any secondary causes, this may prove difficult in critically ill patients. Certainly, an attempt should be made at withdrawing central lines from the right atrium to avoid direct irritation, removal of pulmonary artery catheters when no longer necessary, and normalization of left ventricular (and left atrial) pressures whenever possible. Subsequently, amelioration of symptoms of AFIB is achieved by control of the ventricular rate, with or without restoration of sinus rhythm. Acutely, if the patient is hemodynamically compromised, then synchronous direct-current electrical cardioversion is indicated. This is best accomplished by placing defibrillation pads in the anteroposterior orientation (Fig. 31.11) and using the maximum energy from the defibrillator to avoid the need for repeat shocks. Sedation of the patient with a short-acting anesthetic such as propofol is ideal. If available, a defibrillator capable of delivering biphasic energy should be used because this type of defibrillator has been shown to be successful with reduced energy requirements.

Occasionally, patients with AFIB cannot be cardioverted, and one of several "tricks" may be used. One option is to apply manual pressure to the anterior defibrillator pad, and defibrillate the patient at end expiration. This technique will lessen the impedance to defibrillation and may make defibrillation more successful. Second, in a patient who is very difficult to convert, one may consider using two sets of pads and two defibrillators to effectively deliver twice the energy (with two simultaneous shocks) of only one defibrillator. However, this technique is imperfect because of potentially inadequate synchronization between the devices, and it should only be performed with the correct equipment (including cables and connections) and usually with cardiology or cardiac electrophysiology consultation.

Atrial fibrillation: ECG features II

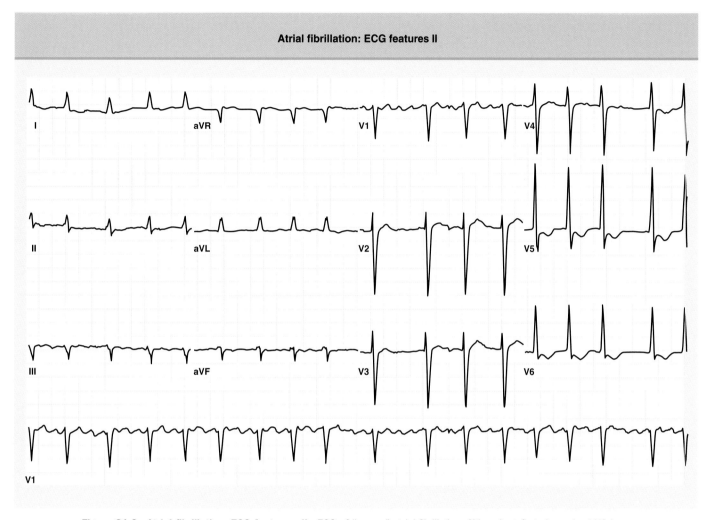

Figure 31.9. Atrial fibrillation: ECG features, II. ECG of "coarse" atrial fibrillation. Although at first glance lead V1 is suggestive of atrial flutter, clearly the P wave morphology is variable and irregular, even in lead V1, with the absence of discernible P waves in any other lead and an irregularly irregular ventricular response.

When cardioversion of AFIB is successful but AFIB recurs within 60 seconds, this phenomenon is termed immediate recurrence of AFIB (IRAF). IRAF tends to be more common when AFIB duration is less than 1 hour, in comparison to patients who have AFIB that lasts more than 24 hours. IRAF may be reduced by the administration of antiarrhythmic medications at steady state prior to cardioversion. In the critical care setting, ibutilide (a class III potassium channel blocker) may be used to aid in cardioversion of AFIB because it has a direct effect on AFIB termination, effectively reduces defibrillation thresholds, thereby reducing the energy required to defibrillate with electrical cardioversion, and can help prevent IRAF. Ibutilide can be administered as a 1 mg bolus in normal saline or 5% dextrose in water over 10 minutes, and this dose can be repeated once 10 minutes after the end of the first infusion. It is important to note that ibutilide should be avoided when the patient is bradycardic, has QT prolongation, is taking other antiarrhythmic medication (although it appears safe in the setting of chronic amiodarone intake), or has significant left ventricular dysfunction because of the 1% to 4% risk of torsades des pointes (TdP). Pretreatment with magnesium may improve the efficacy of ibutilide at converting AFIB but has no effect in reducing

proarrhythmia. The main QT-prolonging effect of ibutilide resolves after approximately 1 hour, but patients should be monitored for the development of TdP for up to 4 hours.

If the patient is not hemodynamically compromised, the need to achieve "rhythm control" (conversion of AFIB to sinus rhythm) is less clear and depends on the long-term goals for patient management. An algorithm for the approach to acute AFIB without the need for immediate therapy, including agents for chemical cardioversion, is shown in Figure 31.7.

Several studies have suggested that long-term rhythm control may not be superior to rate control alone (in association with anticoagulation) for chronic management of patients with paroxysmal or persistent AFIB. Importantly, these studies do suggest that anticoagulation is equally important for those at-risk patients who have AFIB, regardless of the ability to achieve sinus rhythm. All patients in whom AFIB has persisted for longer than 48 hours should be anticoagulated if electrical or chemical cardioversion is contemplated. In patients who have had more than 48 hours of AFIB, cardioversion should generally be attempted only after 3 weeks of therapeutic anticoagulation. However, if cardioversion is desired prior to this time point, then transesophageal echocardiography (TEE) may expedite car-

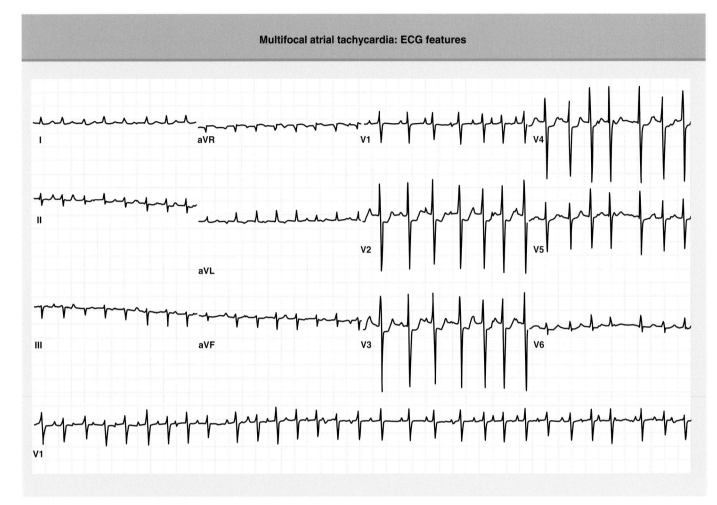

Figure 31.10. Multifocal atrial tachycardia: ECG features. ECG of multifocal atrial tachycardia. Note that in lead V1, P waves are easily discernible, and there appears to be one P wave for each QRS complex. This ECG is a good example of the criteria for multifocal atrial tachycardia, including at least three different P wave morphologies, with variable PR and PP intervals. This type of ECG must be differentiated from atrial fibrillation because pharmacologic management is difficult and cardioversion generally not successful.

dioversion if atrial thrombus can be excluded. It is important to note that even this population of patients must be anticoagulated prior to and for at least 4 weeks after cardioversion. Importantly, the risk of stroke during cardioversion, whether therapeutically anticoagulated or TEE guided, ranges between 0.5% and 1%. If AFIB has lasted less than 48 hours, it may be reasonable to perform cardioversion without anticoagulation.

In patients who have recurrent AFIB despite cardioversion, pretreatment with an antiarrhythmic medication to maintain sinus rhythm may be helpful if rate control alone cannot provide adequate hemodynamic management. In the critical care patient, this is best achieved with intravenous amiodarone, with 900 to 1200 mg loaded over 24 hours. Importantly, intravenous amiodarone has multiple effects, including some antiadrenergic effects acutely; thus, it is potentially also useful for rate control. One must be careful in the hypotensive patient, however, because the solvent used for the intravenous form of amiodarone is a potent vasodilator and may cause significant hypotension. The use of intravenous amiodarone is also limited by its propensity to cause thrombophlebitis, and thus it should be administered via central line access whenever possible.

Patients with AFIB have a significantly higher long-term mortality compared to age-matched controls. However, it is likely that the majority of this excess mortality is related to the thromboembolic complications associated with AFIB, emphasizing the importance of anticoagulation in appropriate individuals. Certainly, in the acute setting, prognosis is directly related to the underlying illness and less to the arrhythmia.

Other Paroxysmal Supraventricular Tachycardias
Generally, the term paroxysmal supraventricular tachycardia (PSVT) refers to a sudden-onset, sudden-offset reentrant arrhythmia during which the ventricles are activated via the atria (hence the term supraventricular). Although somewhat of a misnomer, the term PSVT is usually reserved to describe reentrant circuits caused by abnormal electrical connections, typically located between the atria and ventricles, either within the AV node (as in AVNRT) or on the tricuspid or mitral annulus (atrioventricular connection or accessory pathway), as in AVRT.

These forms of tachycardia are rare in the ICU setting, and thus a detailed discussion is beyond the scope of this chapter. Suffice to say they are typically benign arrhythmias that are

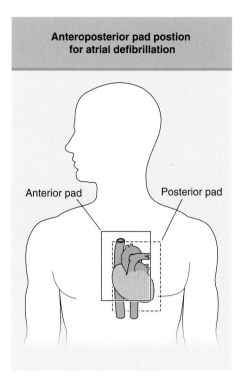

Figure 31.11. Anteroposterior pad position for atrial defibrillation.
This diagram indicates the preferred defibrillation pad setup for atrial defibrillation. The solid square indicates the position of the anterior defibrillation pad, whereas the dotted square indicates the position of the posterior pad. Note that the right and left atria in their entirety are within the defibrillation zone between the two pads.

readily treatable with the administration of medications that slow or block conduction in the AV node, such as adenosine, beta blockers, and some calcium channel blockers (diltiazem and verapamil). Rarely, if ever, are class I or III antiarrhythmics

required to control these arrhythmias. Each arrhythmia has a distinct RP relation, as noted in Figure 31.3. Examples of AVNRT and AVRT are shown in Figures 31.12 and 31.13.

Wolff-Parkinson-White Syndrome

Wolff-Parkinson-White syndrome involves an atrioventricular connection or accessory pathway that has the added ability to conduct in the anterograde direction (atrium to ventricle) and is associated with symptoms of PSVT. Although AVRT is the most common arrhythmia in these patients, they are also prone to AFIB and other atrial arrhythmias. During AFIB, if the accessory pathway is able to conduct rapidly, the QRS morphology may become very wide as the relative contribution of the AV node to ventricular activation diminishes, and thus the arrhythmia may be very difficult to distinguish from a ventricular arrhythmia. Patients who are able to conduct very rapidly over the accessory pathway in an anterograde manner (over 240 bpm) may be at risk for such atrial arrhythmias to degenerate to ventricular arrhythmias, and they should be referred for further evaluation. Medications that block or slow AV node conduction should not be used during preexcited tachycardia because they may lead to development of ventricular arrhythmias. In this situation, treatment should consist of true antiarrhythmic drugs, such as intravenous procainamide or amiodarone, or direct current cardioversion.

VENTRICULAR (WIDE COMPLEX) ARRHYTHMIAS

Wide complex arrhythmias can be classified as those that truly originate from the ventricle(s) and those that are supraventricular in origin but conducted aberrantly. Several different methods exist to distinguish SVT with aberrancy from ventricular tachycardia; these are presented in Table 31.1. Once aberrantly conducted SVTs have been excluded, wide complex

	Table 31.1 Differentiating Ventricular Tachycardia (VT) from Supraventricular Tachycardia (SVT) with Aberrancy	
	VT	**SVT**

AV dissociation	Usually present but may be difficult to identify
	 Presence of AV dissociation 100% specific for VT
	 Manifests in three ways
	   P waves marching through QRS complexes
	   Presence of capture beats
	   Presence of fusion beats
		Never present

Rate	120–250	110–250
Axis	Can be anywhere Predictive of VT if between −45 and 180	Usually normal (−30 to 90)
QRS width	Usually > 130 msec Can be < 130 msec if fascicular in origin Predictive value increases as QRS width > 140–150 msec	Usually < 120 msec If structural heart disease, QRS may be > 130 msec

QRS Morphology: Evaluate the QRS morphology during the wide complex tachycardia. If ***any*** of the following three characteristics are present, then the most likely diagnosis is VT, whereas if ***all*** of the features are absent, then the most likely diagnosis is SVT with aberrancy. The sensitivity and specificity of this evaluation are 98.7% and 96.5%, respectively.

1. Absence of rS pattern of QRS complex in all precordial leads (i.e., either monophasic R wave or QS or QR pattern in all precordial leads).
2. Onset of QRS complex to the nadir of the S wave in any precordial lead is greater than 100 msec.
3. Morphology criteria as stated below are fulfilled for both V1 or V2 and V6 for either right bundle branch or left bundle branch pattern of QRS complex:
   Left bundle pattern (predominantly negative in V1)
      V1 or V2: R wave is over 30 msec wide ***or*** onset of QRS complex to nadir of S wave is over 60 msec ***or*** S wave is notched; ***and***
      V6: QR or QS pattern ***or*** monophasic R wave
   Right bundle pattern (predominantly positive in V1)
      V1 or V2: monophasic R wave ***or*** triphasic R wave ***or*** QR or QS complex; ***and***
      V6: R:S ratio is less than 1 ***or*** QR or QS complex ***or*** monophasic or triphasic R wave

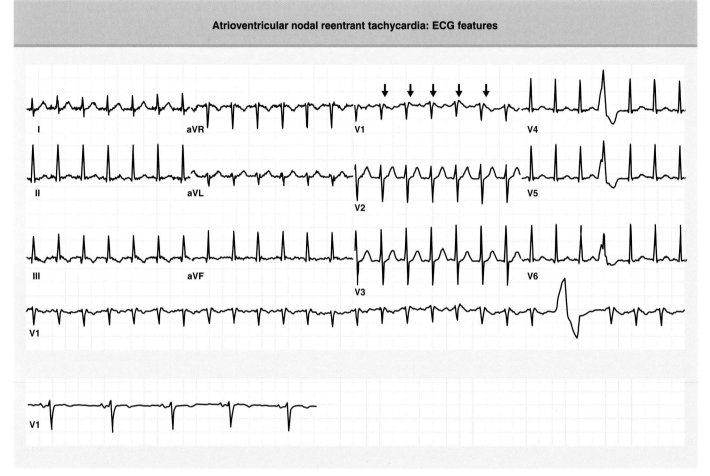

Atrioventricular nodal reentrant tachycardia: ECG features

Figure 31.12. Atrioventricular nodal reentrant tachycardia (AVNRT): ECG features. The ECG in the top panel shows a regular, narrow complex supraventricular tachycardia at a rate of 160 bpm. Careful examination suggests that there may be a P wave (arrows) at the terminal part of the QRS; this is manifested as a "pseudo-R'" pattern in lead V1. Note that when the patient has been converted to sinus rhythm (bottom), the QRS morphology in lead V1 is different, and the pseudo-R' pattern no longer exists. Thus, it is likely that the pseudo-R' was created by a P wave during this typical ECG of AVNRT.

arrhythmias can be evaluated on a syndromal basis by assessing the clinical scenario in which they arise and combining this with the ECG features of the arrhythmia. Several of the syndromes relevant to the care of critically ill patients are presented next, categorized first by the ECG manifestation.

Nonsustained Ventricular Arrhythmias

Nonsustained ventricular arrhythmias are the most common form of wide complex arrhythmias and are defined as those that occur for at least three beats and last for less than 30 seconds. As a rule, treatment is not required for nonsustained ventricular tachycardia (NSVT) unless hemodynamically unstable or polymorphic (see Box 31.3 for a description of monomorphic and polymorphic ventricular arrhythmias). Polymorphic forms of nonsustained ventricular arrhythmias are discussed in the section on sustained polymorphic ventricular arrhythmias. Nonsustained monomorphic ventricular tachycardia can occur in various scenarios, including cardiac ischemia, underlying myocardial disease, congestive heart failure exacerbation, excessive catecholamine tone secondary to stress (e.g., infection and trauma), and in response to adrenergic stimulating medications.

> **Box 31.3 Monomorphic versus Polymorphic Ventricular Arrhythmias**
>
> *Monomorphic* ventricular arrhythmias have a single QRS morphology that does not vary from beat to beat, with stable beat-to-beat intervals (cycle length). Occasionally, especially at onset, offset, or when short-lived, monomorphic ventricular arrhythmias may display some irregularity. Monomorphic ventricular arrhythmias can be further differentiated into monomorphic ventricular tachycardia (MVT) and ventricular flutter (VFL). By definition, MVT occurs at rates of between 120 and 260 beats per minute (bpm), whereas VFL occurs at rates in excess of 260 bpm.
>
> *Polymorphic* ventricular arrhythmias can be divided into two groups: polymorphic ventricular tachycardia (PVT) and ventricular fibrillation (VF). Generally, PVT is a rapid, irregular rhythm originating from the ventricles with beat-to-beat variability in QRS morphology and cycle length, although discrete ventricular depolarization is always noted, ranging in rate from 180 to 280 bpm. VF is generally faster than 280 bpm, with difficult-to-discern QRS complexes that are highly irregular in rate and morphology.

Atrioventricular reciprocating tachycardia: ECG features

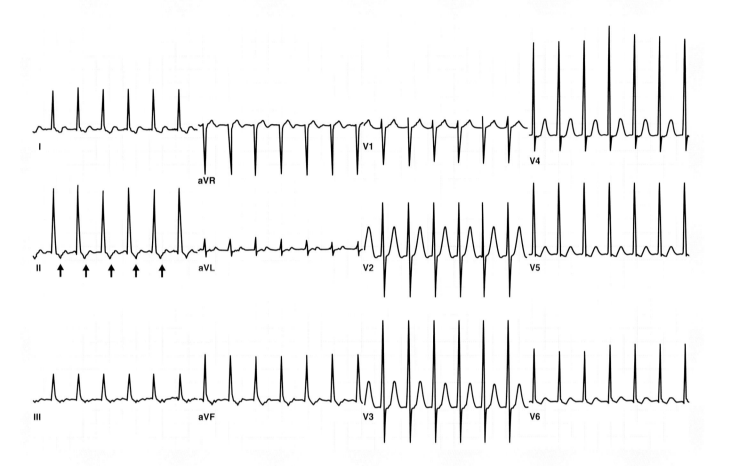

Figure 31.13. Atrioventricular reciprocating tachycardia: ECG features. This ECG demonstrates a regular, narrow complex supraventricular tachycardia at a rate of 155 bpm. A P wave is clearly seen approximately 80 msec after the end of the QRS complex (arrows). It is easily visible in the inferior leads as a negative deflection, and it causes a very "pointy" T wave in lead V1. The short RP relation is highly suggestive of AVRT as the mechanism of this tachycardia.

A relatively slow nonsustained ventricular arrhythmia that occurs at a rate of 80 to 120 bpm is termed accelerated idioventricular rhythm and may occur after ischemia and reperfusion, especially after thrombolysis or percutaneous intervention at the time of acute myocardial infarction. No treatment is required for this type of arrhythmia because it rarely causes hemodynamic instability and is not associated with an unfavorable prognosis. More rapid forms of NSVT may occur in some of the other scenarios previously mentioned and are most common in patients with structural heart disease, especially ischemic heart disease with previous myocardial infarction. Although in these patients the presence of frequent ventricular ectopy is associated with reduced long-term survival, treatment with antiarrhythmic drugs such as flecainide or moricizine has been shown to cause excess mortality. Although treatment with amiodarone does not have this adverse effect, there does not seem to be a direct benefit of amiodarone therapy in these patients, and thus its use is not warranted for NSVT. In patients who do not have structural heart disease, the prognosis of NSVT is benign and does not warrant further management or antiarrhythmic treatment.

Sustained Ventricular Arrhythmias

Sustained ventricular arrhythmias are best discussed by first distinguishing the arrhythmia as either monomorphic or polymorphic (see Box 31.3) and then approaching the arrhythmia based on the clinical scenario in which it arises. The following sections are to be used in conjunction with Figure 31.1 so that the reader can identify the type of arrhythmia and understand the pathophysiology, which then guides the treatment.

Monomorphic Ventricular Tachycardia (Wide and Regular)

Monomorphic ventricular tachycardia (MVT) can occur in various settings, most importantly in the setting of structural heart disease. In these patients, MVT occurs as a result of a reentrant mechanism, usually because of areas of scar interspersed with areas of slow conduction, which are the prerequisite substrates for reentry to occur. More than 50% of MVT occurs in

331

the setting of coronary artery disease with a fixed scar, usually secondary to a previous myocardial infarction, with or without intervening ischemia. Ischemia may rarely be a precipitant for this arrhythmia, although it cannot by itself usually be responsible for reentrant forms of MVT. Other forms of structural heart disease that increase the risk of MVT are shown in Box 31.4.

Box 31.4 Forms of Structural Heart Disease Predisposing to Monomorphic Ventricular Tachycardia

Ischemic cardiomyopathy
Myocardial disorders
   Hypertrophic cardiomyopathy
   Dilated cardiomyopathy
   Infiltrative disorders (e.g., sarcoid, amyloid, hemochromatosis)
   Right ventricular dysplasia/cardiomyopathy
Valvular disorders
   Mitral valve prolapse
   Aortic stenosis
   Prosthetic valves
Congenital heart disease, especially with ventricular dysfunction

The most common forms of structural heart disease that may lead to the development of monomorphic ventricular tachycardia are shown in bold text.

MVT is characterized as a wide complex tachycardia with a stable cycle length and consistent beat-to-beat QRS morphology. Differentiation of MVT from SVT with aberrancy is best done by the demonstration of AV dissociation, either by evident P waves that are dissociated from the QRS complexes or by the presence of capture or fusion beats (Fig. 31.14). Unfortunately, AV dissociation is noted in a minority of wide complex tachycardias, and thus other features, including axis, QRS width, and QRS morphology, may help differentiate VT from SVT with aberrancy (see Table 31.1).

Any patient with a hemodynamically unstable ventricular arrhythmia should promptly be electrically cardioverted. Cardioversion should be synchronous, unless the arrhythmia is disorganized [polymorphic ventricular tachycardia (PVT) or ventricular fibrillation (VF)], and it is ideal to use the maximum output of the device. Failure to use maximum output may lead to subsequent failure with further deterioration of the arrhythmia and persistent cerebral hypoperfusion, potentially worsening anoxic brain injury. Once the baseline rhythm has been restored by either chemical or electrical methods, further evaluation of the patient will guide ongoing management. Generally, the prognosis of patients with ventricular arrhythmias is related to the degree of structural heart disease and left ventricular function and also the presence or absence of coronary artery disease. An algorithm for the approach to therapy of the patient with MVT is shown in Figure 31.15.

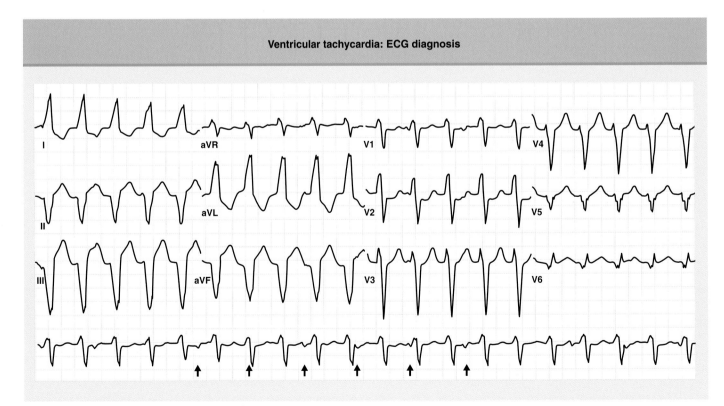

Ventricular tachycardia: ECG diagnosis

Figure 31.14. Ventricular tachycardia: ECG diagnosis. This ECG demonstrates a wide complex tachycardia at approximately 120 bpm, with clear-cut AV dissociation visible in lead V1. The arrows point to the P waves, which march through the QRS complexes and are unrelated to ventricular activation. Additionally, the left bundle pattern of this wide complex rhythm meets morphology criteria for VT because the R wave in lead V1 is approximately 80 msec wide, and a QR complex is present in lead V6 (see Table 31.1 for a summary of morphology criteria for VT).

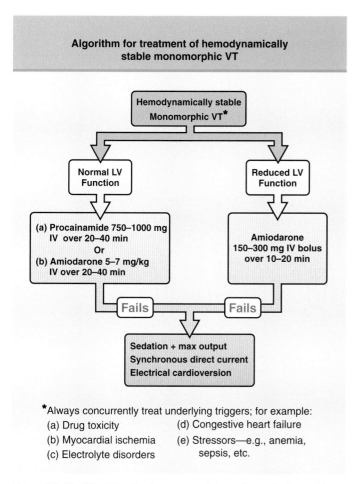

Algorithm for treatment of hemodynamically
stable monomorphic VT

Hemodynamically stable
Monomorphic VT*

Normal LV
Function

Reduced LV
Function

(a) Procainamide 750–1000 mg
IV over 20–40 min
Or
(b) Amiodarone 5–7 mg/kg
IV over 20–40 min

Amiodarone
150–300 mg IV bolus
over 10–20 min

Fails   Fails

Sedation + max output
Synchronous direct current
Electrical cardioversion

*Always concurrently treat underlying triggers; for example:
(a) Drug toxicity   (d) Congestive heart failure
(b) Myocardial ischemia   (e) Stressors—e.g., anemia,
(c) Electrolyte disorders   sepsis, etc.

Figure 31.15. Algorithm for treatment of hemodynamically stable monomorphic VT. IV, intravenous; LV, left ventricular.

Box 31.5 Major Causes of Acquired Long QT Syndrome

Drugs (Abbreviated List of Common Drugs)
Cardiac
　　Class I: disopyramide, procainamide, quinidine, bretylium
　　Class II: dofetilide, ibutilide, azimilide, sotalol, amiodarone
Anti-infective
　　Antibiotics: clarithromycin, cotrimoxazole, erythromycin, doxorubicin
　　Antifungals: ketoconazole, fluconazole, itraconazole
　　Antimalarials: chloroquine
Antihistamines: terfenadine, astemizole, diphenhydramine, hydroxyzine
Psychiatric
　　Antidepressants: amitriptyline, imipramine, fluoxetine, doxepin
　　Antipsychotics: chlorpromazine, haloperidol, droperidol, lithium, pimozide, prochlorperazine, thioridazine, sertindole, trifluoperazine
Other: cisapride, fenoxidil, prednisone, probucol, salbutamol, amantadine, aminophylline

Marked Bradycardia

Electrolyte Disorders
Hypokalemia
Hypomagnesemia
Hypocalcemia

Left Ventricular Hypertrophy

Miscellaneous
Anorexia
Hypothyroidism
Cerebrovascular injury

For a complete updated listing of drugs that may cause long QT syndrome or drugs that should be avoided in patients with long QT syndrome, see www.qtdrugs.org.

Rarely, forms of VT can occur in patients without structural heart disease. Two common forms are those that originate from the region of the right ventricular outflow tract and those that involve the His–Purkinje network in the left ventricle. Generally, these forms of VT are benign and do not require inpatient management, although occasionally a patient may present in the critical care setting because these arrhythmias can be sensitive to excess catecholamine tone.

Polymorphic Ventricular Tachycardia and Ventricular Fibrillation (Wide and Irregular)

PVT is likely the most common form of VT in the critical care setting and is classified into two groups based on the length of the baseline QT interval.

Torsades des pointes is a specific syndrome of PVT occurring in the setting of a prolonged QT interval. Translated, TdP refers to "twisting of the points." As the name suggests, this refers to the varying morphology of the QRS complexes during PVT, which look as though they are twisting around the horizontal axis. It is important to note, however, that this type of ECG signature can occur with any form of PVT, and thus the term TdP should be used only to describe the specific syndrome of PVT that occurs when the baseline QT interval is prolonged. Although it can be inherited, the prolonged QT is usually acquired and is caused by a reduction in potassium channel repolarizing current, resulting in delayed repolarization. When repo-

larization is altered in this manner, early afterdepolarizations within the ventricular myocardium that occur at a critical time of repolarization—the so-called vulnerable period—trigger the initiation of PVT.

Generally, the duration of repolarization is directly linked to the length of the preceding RR interval. Initiation of PVT usually occurs when a pause following a premature beat leads to an excessive QT interval of the beat after the pause. During this markedly prolonged repolarization time, an early afterdepolarization may occur and thus trigger PVT. Thus, TdP is usually initiated with a "short–long–short" sequence of events and can frequently be nonsustained. An example of this arrhythmia is shown in Figure 31.16.

Causes of acquired long QT syndrome, as well as the various medications that prolong the QT interval, are noted in Box 31.5. Since this syndrome is easily treated if promptly recognized, a careful examination of the initiating sequence of all PVTs and the 12-lead ECG recorded at the time of the arrhythmia is crucial to effective management. A review of all medications being administered to the patient is essential. Usually, removal of the cause of prolonged QT (if acquired), correction of electrolytes (especially to maintain optimal potassium and

Polymorphic ventricular tachycardia with long QT: ECG features

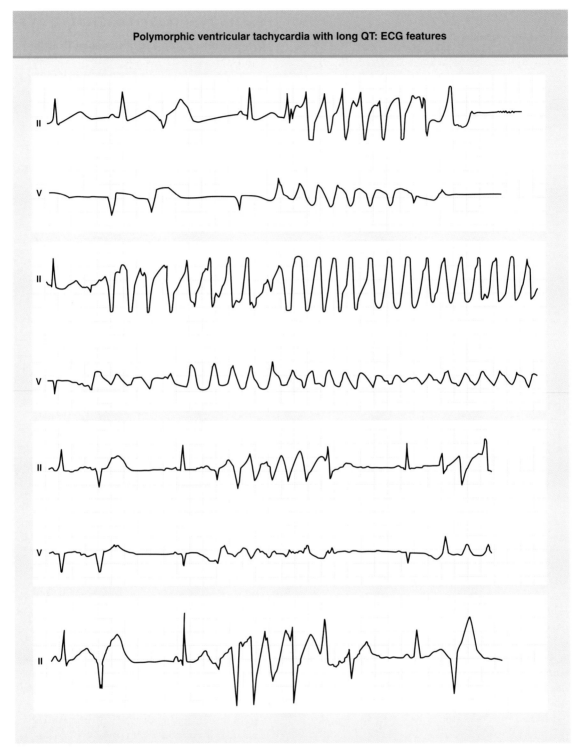

Figure 31.16. Polymorphic ventricular tachycardia with long QT: ECG features. Two-lead ECG telemetry strips, with upper two strips continuous and lower two strips continuous but at a different period in time. Notice the salvos of nonsustained polymorphic ventricular tachycardia, with one episode that appears more sustained. Each episode starts with a late coupled ventricular beat that occurs on top of an exceedingly prolonged QT interval (over 600 msec). Note that the initiating sequence is always short (PVC)–long (pause)–short (PVC on very long QT interval starts tachycardia).

magnesium concentrations), and administration of intravenous magnesium will allow stabilization and control of the arrhythmia. However, in some cases, overdrive pacing (preferably in the atrium if AV node conduction is preserved) to prevent bradycardia and promote shortening of the QT interval may be required. Of course, if at any time the patient is hemodynamically unstable, direct current cardioversion should be performed to revert the patient back to baseline rhythm.

The prognosis of PVT in the setting of a prolonged QT interval is generally good, especially when the QT interval can be corrected by removal of offending agents. Rarely, some patients with congenital forms of long QT syndrome require further management or risk stratification because of increased risk of recurrent ventricular arrhythmias.

The most common cause of PVT without baseline prolongation of the QT interval is cardiac ischemia. Although ischemia can occasionally prolong the QT interval (frequently in association with marked abnormalities in the ST-T complex), ischemia-induced PVT generally does not occur with prolongation of the QT. PVT can be a common arrhythmia in the critical care environment, and ischemia should always be considered as a cause when PVT occurs in the absence of a baseline prolonged QT interval. Usually, with forms of polymorphic VT that occur during ischemia, the coupling interval of the last normal beat to the first beat of tachycardia is "short," less than 400 msec. This is different from that of TdP, which usually has a coupling interval that is longer than 450 msec. In addition, these forms of PVT will occur during sinus tachycardia, at a time when cardiac demand is high and supply may be compromised, whereas TdP usually occurs during relative bradycardia. An example of the initiation of PVT without prolongation of the baseline QT interval is shown in Figure 31.17.

Treatment of this form of PVT requires treatment of the underlying cause, usually cardiac ischemia. Thus, intravenous beta blocker therapy, with or without intravenous nitrates, in combination with intravenous magnesium and correction of electrolytes should be first-line therapy to control the arrhythmia. Subsequently, specific ischemia evaluation and treatment is also essential. Isoproterenol is generally contraindicated for this form of PVT, and overdrive pacing is rarely, if ever, required. Again, however, if the patient is hemodynamically unstable at any time, direct current cardioversion will be required to restore baseline rhythm.

Ventricular fibrillation is an extreme form of PVT that usually occurs at rates in excess of 250 bpm, with QRS complexes that may be very difficult to distinguish from one another. This arrhythmia occurs most frequently in the setting of profound myocardial ischemia, although it may occur in the setting of significant sympathetic stimulation, as with large doses of epinephrine or cocaine overdose, especially when associated with coronary artery vasoconstriction. VF may also result from PVT, either monomorphic or polymorphic, as an end-stage arrhythmia related to progressive breakdown of reentrant wavelets and fibrillatory conduction or because of significant ischemia associated with the previously hemodynamically unstable rhythm. Generally, any condition that significantly reduces myocardial oxygen supply will lead to VF. Rarely, unusual myocardial disorders, or disorders of sodium or potassium channel function, may lead to primary VF without left ventricular dysfunction.

Treatment for VF universally requires direct current cardioversion, with treatment of the underlying cause being paramount in order to prevent recurrent episodes. Prognosis of VF and PVT without long QT depends entirely on the underlying condition and is generally very good if the arrhythmia triggers

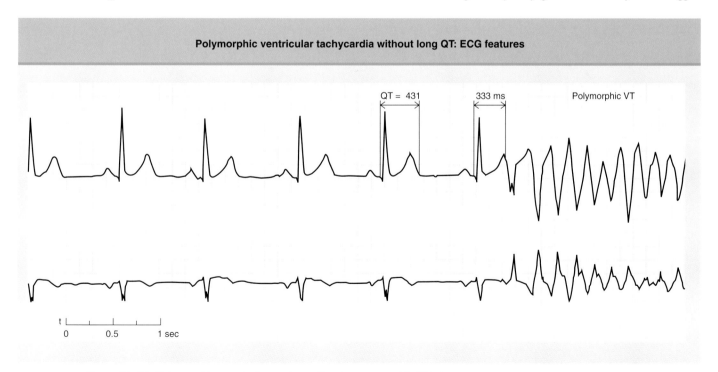

Polymorphic ventricular tachycardia without long QT: ECG features

QT = 431   333 ms   Polymorphic VT

t
0   0.5   1 sec

Figure 31.17. Polymorphic ventricular tachycardia without long QT: ECG features. Two-lead ECG telemetry strip of an initiation of polymorphic ventricular tachycardia in a patient with a resting rate of 60 to 70 bpm and a normal baseline QT (431 msec). Note that the initiating sequence occurs with an "early" coupled PVC (<400 msec). Ischemia is the most common cause of polymorphic VT in the patient with a normal baseline QT interval.

can be treated, prevented, or reversed. Patients with significant underlying heart disease may require further evaluation for risk stratification by cardiac catheterization and coronary angiography, echocardiographic assessment of cardiac function, invasive electrophysiologic studies, or a combination of these.

Ventricular Arrhythmias: Special Scenarios

A small fraction of ventricular arrhythmias may be drug induced. These can obviously occur with or without the presence of structural heart disease, which eventually determines the prognosis. The patient who does not have structural heart disease is more likely to recover spontaneously and have a more benign course. Frequently, adrenergic agents that are administered in the ICU (e.g., inotropic agents) can cause automatic ventricular arrhythmias—usually slow monomorphic VT at variable rates that disappear when the medication is stopped. In this scenario, it is prudent to rule out the possibility of underlying myocardial ischemia or left ventricular dysfunction. Other β agonists, such as salbutamol, may also predispose to ventricular arrhythmias but usually only when used in excess. Numerous illicit and over-the-counter stimulant medications, such as pseudoephedrine, cocaine, crack cocaine, and methamphetamines, have also been implicated in the setting of ventricular arrhythmias, not only as a direct result of catecholamine surge but also because of coronary vasoconstriction and subsequent cardiac ischemia, which

may lead to PVT or VF. In extreme circumstances, such as overdose, these arrhythmias may be fatal. After control of the ventricular arrhythmia and removal of the offending substance, the future risk of arrhythmias depends on the presence of underlying structural heart disease.

Many patients treated in the critical care setting have suffered out-of-hospital cardiac arrest or resuscitated sudden cardiac death (SCD). The majority of patients with SCD do not survive to hospitalization, and of those who do, a minority survive to hospital discharge. Increasing evidence suggests that the majority of these patients likely have primary VF or PVT as their index arrhythmia. However, as time to resuscitation elapses, PVT degenerates to VF, which further deteriorates to asystole or pulseless electrical activity. Thus, time to treatment is paramount because rapid diagnosis and treatment of VF or PVT can have a major effect on patient survival. Once such patients have been stabilized and have recovered neurologically, further cardiac evaluation is required to evaluate prognosis, which is dependent on the underlying cardiac condition.

Monitoring Artifacts

In the monitored setting of the critical care unit, sources of interference may lead to disruptions of the ECG baseline, potentially leading to the misdiagnosis of arrhythmias (Fig. 31.18). These types of disruptions may appear as asystole or as

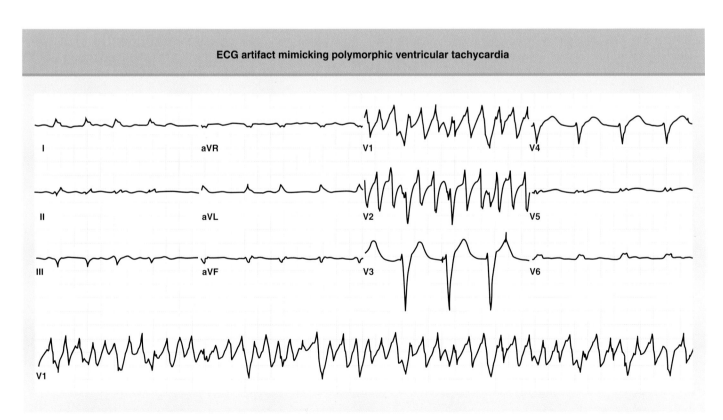

ECG artifact mimicking polymorphic ventricular tachycardia

Figure 31.18. ECG artifact mimicking polymorphic ventricular tachycardia. Twelve-lead ECG shows significant wide complex fluctuations secondary to artifacts in lead V1 and, to a lesser extent, lead V2. If V1 was the only lead being monitored, this could easily be mistaken for a ventricular arrhythmia. The cause in this situation is likely poor skin-to-electrode contact with leads V1 and V2 because the artifact is not visible on the other leads. Analysis of lead V1 shows that several of the "complexes" have coupling intervals that are nonphysiologic (i.e., <150 msec), and this is a clue indicating artifact. Additionally, the true QRS complex can be noted to march through the artifact, although because of the baseline atrial fibrillation in this patient, this may be difficult to identify without help from the nonartifactual leads.

supraventricular or ventricular tachycardia. Frequently, the cause of these artifacts is related to the limited number of leads, usually visible on telemetered patients, coupled with poor skin–lead contact and body movement. Occasionally, these artifacts may lead to inappropriate investigations or therapy, and thus careful analysis of arrhythmias to ensure against incorrect interpretation of artifact is necessary. In the critical care setting, simultaneous monitoring of multiple ECG leads and arterial blood pressure or pulse oximetry may be a useful tool to aid in correctly diagnosing electrocardiographic monitoring artifacts.

Electrical Storm

Electrical storm refers to ventricular arrhythmias (usually MVT) that continue to recur despite initial medical therapy. Usually, such ventricular arrhythmias occur in the setting of ischemic heart disease, with prior myocardial scar tissue that acts as the "arrhythmogenic substrate." It is unclear why electrical storm occurs in patients who may have had previous stable arrhythmias, but precipitants such as myocardial ischemia, electrolyte disturbances, worsening congestive heart failure, medication toxicity, and other underlying conditions including sepsis or thyrotoxicosis must be ruled out and concomitantly treated. Such arrhythmias can usually be controlled by administration of one or more antiarrhythmic agents, with the most popular and effective drug being amiodarone. Even if the patient is already taking amiodarone, additional intravenous amiodarone may be effective at terminating and controlling the arrhythmias. Subsequently, various other antiarrhythmics, including intravenous or oral procainamide or quinidine or oral mexiletine, may be used either alone or, more commonly, in conjunction with amiodarone to treat the "storm." Intravenous beta blockers should be used universally, except where contraindicated, to reduce both the effect of the sympathetic nervous system on the heart and myocardial ischemia. Sedatives and, rarely, general anesthesia may be required to "quiet the storm" if the preceding measures have not been effective. Difficult-to-manage patients may be candidates for percutaneous catheter ablation therapy. There is evidence that the prognosis of patients who suffer from electrical storm is worse than that of matched patients with stable ventricular arrhythmias, although in general, aggressive antiarrhythmic management usually leads to effective control of the patient's arrhythmia burden.

BRADYCARDIA AND PACING

In general, pacing—both temporary and permanent—is appropriate in the setting of symptomatic bradycardia. Although this is a simplified approach, several types of bradycardia present as potential "gray zones," and thus we hope to shed light on this area with a brief summary of bradycardia epidemiology, diagnosis, and management.

Terminology

Bradycardia is a very vague term, and thus to be more exact, one must try to examine the site of bradycardia, the degree of bradycardia, and hemodynamic consequences in order to better communicate its importance or severity. A classification scheme of bradycardia location and degree is shown in Figure 31.19. Essentially, the classification scheme requires that the site of bradycardia be localized to the level of either the sinus node or the

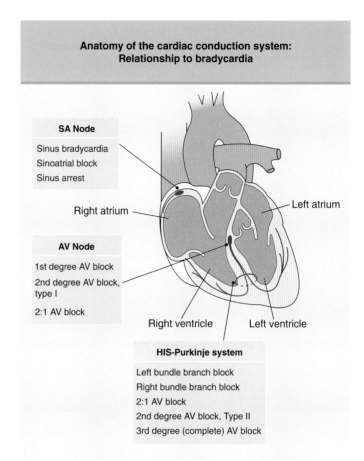

Figure 31.19. Anatomy of the cardiac conduction system: Relationship to bradycardia. This diagram shows the representative "electrical centers" of the heart: the SA node, AV node, and His–Purkinje system, which are the target sites for various forms of bradycardia. Higher levels of AV block, including second-degree Mobitz type II and complete or third-degree AV block, generally require pacing. When 2:1 AV block occurs in the His–Purkinje system, pacing is likely also required. Any level of conduction slowing, with the exception of first-degree AV block, is an indication for permanent pacing in the symptomatic patient.

AV junction (including the AV node and His–Purkinje system). Once location and degree of bradycardia have been identified, it is important to determine whether the bradycardia has resulted in any hemodynamic compromise. Generally, if bradycardia has caused hemodynamic compromise in the absence of reversible causes, then pacemaker implantation is indicated.

Sinus node (SA) dysfunction manifests as sinus bradycardia, sinus pauses, or prolonged periods of asystole and is usually transient, readily treatable, and rarely causes serious compromise. Examples of SA dysfunction are shown in Figure 31.20. Conversely, the diagnosis of AV block requires differentiation of physiologic block from pathologic block; the latter usually occurs in the presence of severe AV node or His–Purkinje disease and almost universally requires pacing. Examples of AV block are shown in Figure 31.21.

In the following sections, several important scenarios of bradycardia that may be encountered in the critically ill patient are discussed.

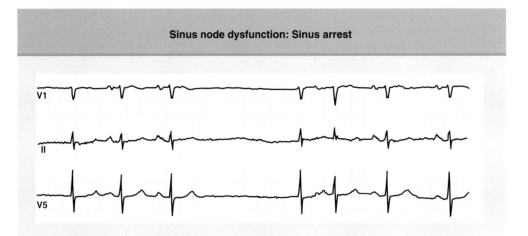

Figure 31.20. Sinus node dysfunction: Sinus arrest. Note that in this three-lead rhythm strip the first beat is a junctional beat, followed by two sinus beats at a rate of approximately 80 bpm, followed by a pause with no discernible P wave that ends with a junctional beat after 2 seconds. This is an example of sinus arrest, and it does not usually require pacing unless it is frequent, recurrent, and prolonged (usually more than 4 sec) and associated with hemodynamic compromise. Occasionally, such patients also have episodes of tachycardia, and thus the intermittent pauses may make antiarrhythmic treatment difficult, leading to the need for permanent pacing to allow medication adjustment.

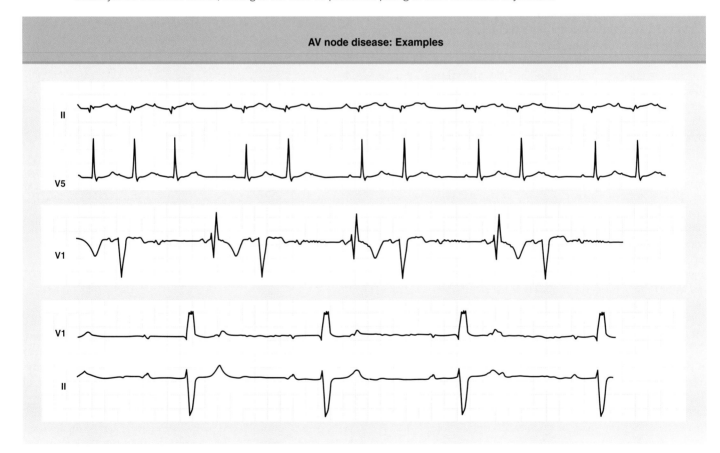

Figure 31.21. AV node disease: Examples. The top panel shows a patient with 3:2 AV Wenckebach (three P waves for every two QRS complexes, with progressive lengthening of the PR interval until P wave with AV block occurs, and then the cycle repeats) with a narrow QRS, suggesting that the conduction delay resides within the AV node. Pacemaker implantation is generally not required for this type of conduction delay. The middle panel shows 3:2 AV block but without PR lengthening, suggesting second-degree Mobitz type II block. This type of block generally occurs in the His–Purkinje system. Additionally, this patient has an alternating right bundle and left bundle branch block pattern, also suggesting significant His–Purkinje system disease. Thus, this patient is more likely to progress to complete AV block and likely requires permanent pacing. The bottom panel shows complete AV block with no relation between atrial and ventricular rates. In addition, the escape rhythm is wide and slow, suggesting a ventricular (not junctional) origin. This is an indication for temporary pacing as a bridge to permanent pacemaker implantation, given the high risk of worsening bradycardia.

Medication-Induced Bradycardia

When bradycardia occurs in conjunction with drug toxicity or drugs that affect conduction, it is generally reasonable to wait until five half-lives of the drug have passed before deciding whether the drug alone was responsible for the bradycardia. If bradycardia-causing drugs are necessary to prevent tachy-arrhythmias (so-called tachy-brady syndrome), then permanent pacing may be used to prevent the bradycardic effect of the required medications.

Bradycardia during Cardiac Ischemia

Myocardial ischemia may cause bradycardia through a variety of mechanisms: direct effect on the AV node or SA node by affecting vascular supply, direct effect on the His–Purkinje system by affecting vascular supply, or indirect effect on the SA node or AV node by triggering nocireceptors in the myocardium that stimulate vagal tone (i.e., Bezold–Jarisch reflex). Often, when hemodynamic stability is compromised, temporary pacing may be required in these scenarios. However, permanent pacing is only required if the condition persists despite the correction of ischemia or if ischemia cannot be corrected.

Bradycardia after Cardiac Surgery

Cardiac surgery may cause direct trauma, usually to the AV node or His–Purkinje system, and subsequently cause heart block. Most commonly, this occurs with valvular surgery, usually on the mitral or aortic valve, and may be related to edema. As such, it is prudent to wait at least 5 to 7 days after cardiac surgery before declaring that damage is permanent and proceeding with permanent pacemaker implantation. In addition, sinus node dysfunction may occur in patients in the early postoperative period after cardiac surgery, likely as a result of the effects of cardioplegia on the sinus node, usually on a background of mild, previously asymptomatic sinus node disease. Generally, these patients do not require temporary or permanent pacing. Because AFIB is common in patients after cardiac surgery, and many of these patients may already have mild sinus node dysfunction, a period of sinus arrest may occur during transitions from AFIB to sinus rhythm. In this case, if the pauses are less than 4 seconds or if they are completely asymptomatic, pacemaker implantation can usually be avoided. It may be prudent to treat such patients with antiarrhythmic drugs to prevent AFIB and, as such, prevent the pauses (during AFIB, the sinus node is suppressed, and when AFIB terminates, sinus node recovery may be delayed). Usually, a treatment period of up to 3 months suffices because the AFIB post-cardiac surgery is usually related to pericardial inflammation and should resolve after that period of time.

Physiologic AV Block

One of the most common forms of bradycardia is that which is induced by excess vagal tone. Usually, vagal tone is increased in young, healthy individuals and declines with age, accounting for resting bradycardia and occasional sinus pauses in athletic individuals. In the ICU setting, various maneuvers can frequently increase vagal tone, including suctioning through the endotracheal tube, coughing or "bucking the ventilator" while intubated, or severe pain without adequate analgesia. In these situations, if the vagal stimulus is powerful enough, then sinus node slowing and prolongation of the PR interval may occur. In severe cases,

---

Box 31.6 Secondary Causes of Bradycardia

Sinus Node

Acute myocardial infarction, myocarditis
Drugs: beta blockers, digoxin, class I and III antiarrhythmics
Increased intracranial pressure
Sick sinus syndrome: idiopathic fibrosis
Increased vagal tone (e.g., athletes)
Hypothyroidism
Hyperkalemia
Hypothermia
Postcardiac surgery, secondary to cardioplegia or mechanical trauma

AV Node

Acute myocardial infarction or ischemia (especially inferior)
Increased vagal tone
Idiopathic degeneration
Drugs: beta blockers, calcium channel blockers (e.g., diltiazem, verapamil), digoxin, amiodarone
Infection: Lyme disease, diphtheria, endocarditis (especially aortic valve)
Immunological: systemic lupus erythematosus
Hyperkalemia

His–Purkinje System

Acute myocardial infarction—usually extensive, involving septum
Idiopathic degeneration of conduction system
Cardiomyopathy: dilated, hypertrophic, other
Infiltrative myocardial disease: sarcoid, amyloid
Trauma (e.g., post-cardiac surgery, especially with mitral or aortic valve surgery)
Congenital heart disease (e.g., atrial septal defect)
Rheumatic heart disease

This is a partial list of the secondary causes of bradycardia most commonly encountered in clinical practice.

---

sinus arrest or transient complete AV block may occur. An example of this phenomenon is shown in Figure 31.22. Rarely, for extremely prolonged episodes, temporary pacing may be required, although removal of the vagal stimulus is usually all that is needed and no further rhythm-specific therapy is required.

Other secondary causes of bradycardia, some of which are reversible, are shown in Box 31.6. Ideally, if the secondary cause can be removed, then pacemaker implantation is not warranted. In some cases, the secondary cause cannot be treated effectively, such as cardiac sarcoidosis or other infiltrative diseases that affect the conduction system, and as such permanent pacing may be warranted.

Acute Treatment of Bradycardia

In the acute situation, temporary relief of bradycardia may be essential, either as a bridge to permanent pacemaker implantation or to allow the removal of secondary causes of bradycardia. Specific antidotes for certain types of drug toxicity are available, including isoproterenol for beta blocker toxicity and Digibind (a monoclonal antibody against digoxin) for digoxin toxicity.

Vagal mediated AV block (physiologic): ECG features

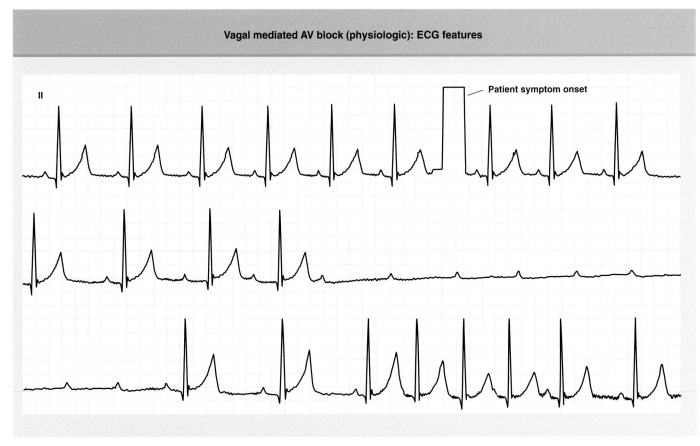

Figure 31.22. Vagal-mediated AV block (physiologic): ECG features. This continuous ECG tracing shows the hallmarks of bradycardia caused by excess vagal tone. Note that immediately prior to the onset of complete AV block (no QRS complexes), an increase in the PP and PR intervals is noted. These features point to the level of block being within the AV node and not within the His–Purkinje system. Also, during asystole, the sinus node response is blunted (faster sinus rates would be expected given that complete asystole is present). Usually, permanent pacing is not warranted in this syndrome but, rather, conservative measures are taken to prevent situations in which excess vagal tone may prevail. This includes maintaining euvolemia, use of compression stockings to prevent venous blood pooling, and avoidance of aggressive suctioning maneuvers that may increase vagal tone.

Additionally, agents that increase adrenergic tone, including dopamine, dobutamine, phenylephrine, isoproterenol, and other stimulants, including caffeine or theophylline, may be useful for temporarily increasing automaticity in the case of sinus bradycardia.

Temporary transvenous pacing is often necessary to support hemodynamics until permanent pacing can be performed or secondary causes of bradycardia can be treated or removed. This is likely best accomplished by fluoroscopic guidance of a 5- or 6-Fr temporary pacing catheter positioned at the right ventricular apex via a catheter and sheath assembly inserted into the right or left internal jugular vein. The right or left femoral vein may also be used, although the risk of catheter-related infection is somewhat higher at this site. Thresholds should be tested daily and the catheter repositioned if thresholds increase substantially. Ideally, the catheter should be positioned in an area where the threshold to capture the ventricle is below 1 to 1.5 mA. When fluoroscopy is not available, a balloon-tipped transvenous pacing catheter may be used to help guide the catheter safely, with lower risk of perforation. However, in this instance it is useful to use ECG guidance to determine whether the pacing wire has reached the appropriate location. If temporary transvenous pacing may be required for a prolonged period, there is evidence that active fixation leads (screw-in, as opposed to passive fixation, which are simply "placed" against the endocardium) have lower dislodgment rates and a lower incidence of pacing-related adverse events.

Troubleshooting Temporary Pacemakers
When adjusting temporary pacemakers, it is important to program the rate as low as possible (e.g., 40–50 ppm) to avoid overdrive suppression of the patient's own sinus node or escape rhythm. Frequently, when temporary pacemakers are set to high rates, patients can be declared "pacemaker dependent" simply because of overdrive suppression. Also, when trying to ascertain whether the patient is pacemaker dependent, it is important not to simply inhibit pacing but to gradually lower the paced rate to 30 bpm and then, as long as the patient is hemodynamically stable, to leave it at a low rate for 1 or 2 minutes to allow the patient's native rhythm to emerge.

In the ICU, temporary pacemakers may be subject to external electromagnetic interference (EMI), which may inappropriately be sensed as cardiac activity and thus suppress pacemaker output when in the demand mode. Thus, in the patient who is truly pacemaker dependent, programming the pacemaker to an asynchronous mode such as "VOO" may help to prevent unexpected bradycardia secondary to EMI.

There is a false perception that patients should be paced at faster rates when hypotensive. Although it is true that faster rates will improve cardiac output, stroke volume during right ventricular pacing may actually decrease, especially in the patient who has impaired left ventricular filling or significant left ventricular systolic dysfunction. Thus, in the pacemaker-dependent patient, it is rarely necessary to pace faster than 75 bpm, especially in the presence of left ventricular dysfunction. If faster rates are required, it is advantageous to pace in the atrium when AV node conduction is preserved, although temporary atrial pacing is technically challenging because of instability of pacemaker leads in the atrial position.

SUGGESTED READING

Brugada P, Brugada J, Mont L, et al: A new approach to the differential diagnosis of a regular tachycardia with a wide QRS complex. Circulation 1991;83(5):1649–1659.

Da Costa D, Brady WJ, Edhouse J: Bradycardias and atrioventricular conduction block. Br Med J 2002;324:535–538.

Fuster V, Ryden LE, Asinger RW, et al: ACC/AHA/ESC guidelines for the management of patients with atrial fibrillation: Executive summary. J Am Coll Cardiol 2001;38:1231–1266.

Jafri SM, Kruse JA: Temporary transvenous cardiac pacing. Crit Care Clin 1992;8:713–725.

Lip GY, Hart RG, Conway DS: Antithrombotic therapy for atrial fibrillation. Br Med J 2002;325:1022–1025.

Mittal S, Ayati S, Stein KM, et al: Transthoracic cardioversion of atrial fibrillation: Comparison of rectilinear biphasic versus damped sine wave monophasic shocks. Circulation 2000;101:1282–1287.

Sarkozy A, Dorian P: Advances in the acute pharmacologic management of cardiac arrhythmias. Curr Cardiol Rep 2003;5:387–394.

Chapter 32

Hypertensive Emergencies

Catherine L. Kelleher and Stuart L. Linas

KEY POINTS

- The clinical presentation of hypertensive crisis is variable and related to any end-organ damage.
- The preferred treatment for hypertensive crisis includes parenteral hypotensive therapy with intensive care monitoring by arterial cannulation or automated blood pressure (BP) cuff measurement.
- The primary objective is to lower BP to alleviate ischemia of vital organs; however, the desired rate of BP lowering is also determined by the clinical setting.

Nearly 28.7% of the adult population in the United States was hypertensive in 1999–2000 (age-adjusted hypertension prevalence), and only 59% of these affected individuals were being treated. Furthermore, of those individuals being treated for hypertension, only 34% had blood pressure (BP) controlled to less than 140/90 mm Hg. The risk of hypertensive crisis is estimated to be less than 1%.

Hypertensive crisis is defined as an elevated BP with evidence of acute arteriolar damage. With acute ischemic damage to vital organs such as the kidney, heart, central nervous system (CNS), and gastrointestinal (GI) tract, the risk of morbidity in hours without therapeutic intervention is significant. The development of hypertensive crisis is determined by both the absolute level of BP and the rate of rise of BP elevation. The diastolic BP is usually greater than 130 mm Hg with hypertensive crisis. However, hypertensive crisis may also occur with minor increases in BP in children, gravid females, and previously normotensive individuals. *Malignant hypertension* is a specific syndrome in which markedly elevated BP is associated with hypertensive neuroretinopathy.

PATHOPHYSIOLOGY

Hypertension from any cause may enter a malignant phase. Although the precise pathophysiology is not known, one of the initiating events in the transition from simple hypertension or normotension to hypertensive crisis is an acute increase in BP (Fig. 32.1). BP is determined by the product of cardiac output and peripheral vascular resistance. An increase in peripheral vascular resistance is likely the first event to occur. This causes mechanical stress in the arteriolar endothelium and disruption of endothelial integrity in a number of vascular beds including the kidney, retina, brain, and GI tract. Diffuse microvascular lesions develop with fibrinoid necrosis, which is considered the histologic hallmark of hypertensive crisis.

Other factors likely contribute to the development of hypertensive crisis but their exact role is unclear. Activation of the renin-angiotensin-aldosterone system increases peripheral vascular resistance. Angiotensin II activates the genes for both proinflammatory cytokines (interleukin 6) and nuclear factor κB, causing direct injury to the vascular wall. Hyperviscosity, immunologic factors, and other hormones including catecholamines, vasopressin, and endothelin also likely increase peripheral vascular resistance.

The impact of BP on cerebrovascular physiology influences treatment decisions in hypertensive crisis. Autoregulation of cerebral blood flow refers to the ability of the brain to maintain a constant cerebral blood flow as the cerebral perfusion pressure varies between 60 and 150 mm Hg by dilation or constriction of the blood vessels (Fig. 32.2). It is a function of cerebral perfusion pressure (CPP) (mean arterial pressure minus the venous pressure) divided by cerebral vascular resistance. This range of cerebral autoregulation is increased from 60 to 150 mm Hg to 80 to 160 mm Hg in the setting of chronic hypertension. Autoregulation is generally impaired when the mean arterial pressure is greater than 140 mm Hg.

The backflow in the cerebral venous system, or venous pressure, is near zero so that arterial pressure normally determines the CPP. It is when the systemic pressure exceeds the ability of the brain to autoregulate cerebral blood flow that ischemic brain injury may develop, as for example, in the setting of hypertensive encephalopathy.

MEDICAL HISTORY, PHYSICAL EXAMINATION, AND LABORATORY EVALUATION

Hypertensive crisis is a syndrome that usually develops in the setting of essential hypertension but is also seen in the setting of secondary hypertension. Hypertensive crisis may also develop in previously normotensive individuals who acquire preeclampsia, a pheochromocytoma, or acute glomerulonephritis or who experience drug withdrawal. The medication history detailing use of over-the-counter medications and illicit drugs is important to discuss with every patient. Risk factors associated with the development of malignant hypertension include age between 30 and 50 years, male gender, African-American ethnicity, and smoking (increases the risk by 2.5- to 5-fold).

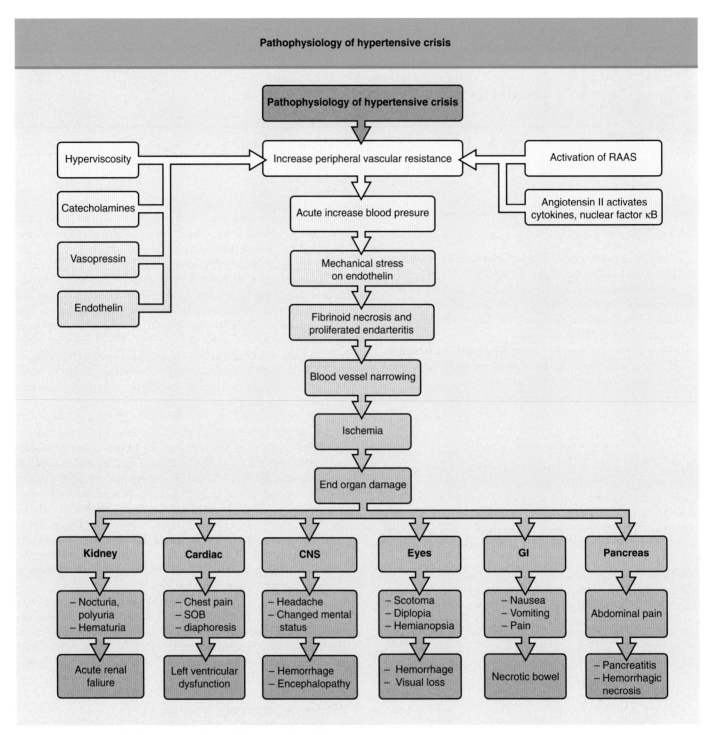

Figure 32.1. Pathophysiology of hypertensive crisis.

The clinical presentation of hypertensive crisis is variable and related to end-organ damage (see Fig. 32.1). One of the most common complaints is headache, often increased in the morning, sudden in onset, and usually different in character from the patient's usual headache. Symptoms of hypertensive encephalopathy include headache, visual changes, and seizures. Individuals with hypertensive crisis may also complain of ischemic chest pain, renal symptoms, and GI problems (see Fig. 32.1). Early on, many patients experience spontaneous diuresis and often have intravascular volume depletion.

To exclude coarctation, the BP is measured in both arms. It is also important to exclude "pseudohypertension." Pseudohypertension (caused by stiffening of the vascular wall that prevents vessel compression by a BP cuff) refers to an artificial increase (at times extreme) in the systolic and diastolic BP. Pseudohypertension can occur in atherosclerosis, Monckeberg's medial calcification, and metastatic calcification as experienced in end-stage renal disease. Pseudohypertension should be suspected when severe hypertension is noted in an individual without evidence of end-organ damage. The diagnosis is sug-

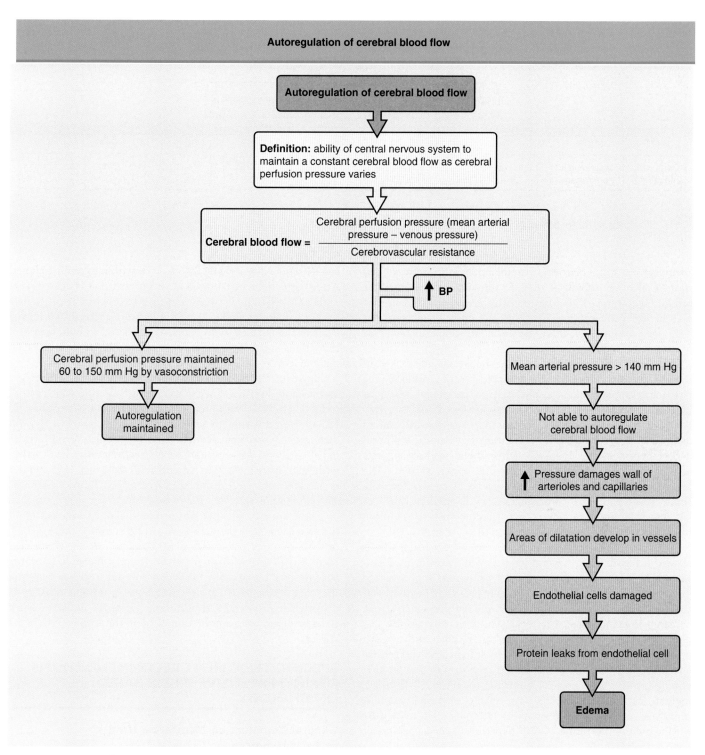

Autoregulation of cerebral blood flow

Autoregulation of cerebral blood flow

Definition: ability of central nervous system to maintain a constant cerebral blood flow as cerebral perfusion pressure varies

$$\text{Cerebral blood flow} = \frac{\text{Cerebral perfusion pressure (mean arterial pressure} - \text{venous pressure)}}{\text{Cerebrovascular resistance}}$$

↑ BP

Cerebral perfusion pressure maintained 60 to 150 mm Hg by vasoconstriction

Autoregulation maintained

Mean arterial pressure > 140 mm Hg

Not able to autoregulate cerebral blood flow

↑ Pressure damages wall of arterioles and capillaries

Areas of dilatation develop in vessels

Endothelial cells damaged

Protein leaks from endothelial cell

Edema

Figure 32.2. Autoregulation of cerebral blood flow.

gested by a palpable radial artery after proximal compression (Osler's maneuver).

There are distinct funduscopic changes in hypertension. Funduscopic changes in chronic hypertension include arteriolar thickening (manifested by increased light reflex), vascular tortuosity, and arteriovenous nicking (grades I and II). Increased arteriole damage results in decreased blood flow manifested by a silver wire pattern to the vessels. These funduscopic changes seen with chronic hypertension do not impact prognosis or treat-

ment with regard to hypertensive crisis. On the other hand, with loss of cerebral autoregulation in malignant hypertension, evidence of vasculitis occurs in the retinal arteriolar and venous circulation. Acute changes including flame-shaped hemorrhages, white cotton-wool spots, yellow-white exudates, and eventually papilledema may be seen.

Other important physical examination findings include evidence of left ventricular hypertrophy (suggesting chronic hypertension), and the abdomen should be examined to exclude aortic

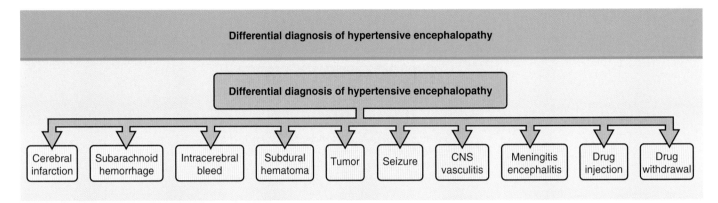

Figure 32.3. Differential diagnosis of hypertensive encephalopathy.

aneurysm. A careful neurologic examination, including a mental status evaluation, should be done to rule out a cerebrovascular insult. Hypertensive neuroretinopathy is usually present but may be absent in patients in whom the pressure increase has been very abrupt, such as in cases of acute glomerulonephritis or catecholamine excess states.

The initial laboratory evaluation should include a serum sodium, chloride, potassium, bicarbonate, creatinine, blood urea nitrogen, complete blood count (with a peripheral smear to identify schistocytes), electrocardiogram, and urinalysis. Evidence of microangiopathic hemolysis may make it difficult to distinguish hypertensive crisis from primary vasculitis with secondary hypertension. Hypokalemic metabolic alkalosis suggests activation of the renin-angiotensin-aldosterone system. The blood urea nitrogen and creatinine levels are often elevated. The acute development of proteinuria and hematuria (20% of patients have gross hematuria, 50% microhematuria) is often found on urinalysis with occasional erythrocyte casts.

The differential diagnosis of hypertensive encephalopathy is shown in Figure 32.3. Several important diagnostic considerations help narrow the diagnosis: (1) symptoms of generalized brain dysfunction usually develop slowly (12–24 hr) with hypertensive encephalopathy and more acutely with ischemic stroke or cerebral hemorrhage; (2) focal neurologic findings are less common with hypertensive encephalopathy than with a CNS bleed; (3) papilledema is almost always noted with hypertensive encephalopathy and, if absent, should raise suspicion of another etiology; and (4) in comparison with an acute CNS bleed, mental status with hypertensive encephalopathy generally improves within 24 to 48 hours of treatment. Ultimately, an MRI should be performed. With hypertensive encephalopathy, edema may occur in the posterior regions of the cerebral hemispheres, particularly in the parieto-occipital regions, a finding called posterior leukoencephalopathy on MRI. However, brainstem involvement on MRI has also been reported.

GENERAL TREATMENT OF HYPERTENSIVE CRISIS

The preferred treatment of hypertensive crisis includes parenteral hypotensive therapy with intensive care monitoring by arterial cannulation or automated BP cuff measurement (Fig. 32.4). The primary objective is to lower the BP at a rate that arrests or alleviates ischemia of vital organs. In most settings, BP can be reduced acutely by 20% to 25% within minutes to hours. After the patient is stabilized at this pressure, it is decreased to 160/100–110 mm Hg over the next 2 to 6 hours. If the patient remains clinically stable, the BP may be decreased to a normal BP over the next 24 to 48 hours. With these carefully measured reductions in BP, autoregulation of cerebral blood flow is usually maintained.

However, the desired rate of BP lowering is also determined by the clinical setting. Specific clinical situations in which a rapid reduction in BP is warranted include acute aortic dissection. The BP is lowered within 15 to 30 minutes in an effort to stop the dissection. More rapid reductions in BP are also recommended in patients with active unstable angina or congestive heart failure with pulmonary edema. In patients with malignant hypertension or hypertensive encephalopathy, a more controlled titration of BP reduction over 1 to 3 hours is satisfactory.

There are clinical situations in which caution in lowering BP is advised. In older patients with carotid stenosis, there is a risk of CNS hypoperfusion with rapid reduction in BP. BP management in patients with stroke or intracranial bleeding is controversial, since the loss of CNS blood flow autoregulation and the presence of brain edema require high systemic pressures to provide adequate cerebral perfusion. There are no large clinical trials to support rapid reduction of BP in the setting of ischemic stroke.

SPECIFIC TREATMENT RECOMMENDATIONS FOR HYPERTENSIVE CRISIS BASED ON ETIOLOGY

General Comment on Medication Used to Treat Hypertensive Crisis

The classes of parental antihypertensive agents available to treat hypertensive crisis include direct vasodilators (sodium nitroprusside, nitroglycerin), α- and β-adrenergic blockers (labetalol), α-adrenergic blockade (phentolamine), angiotensin-converting enzyme inhibitors (enalaprilat), calcium channel blockers, and dopamine agonist (fenoldopam). More information on these medications is given in Table 32.1. The most widely used agent is the vasodilator sodium nitroprusside because of its rapid onset of action (1–2 min) and short half-life (2–5 min). It is effective in most hypertensive emergencies but should be used with caution in the setting of renal disease and liver dysfunction. There is no consensus on the most effective antihypertensive

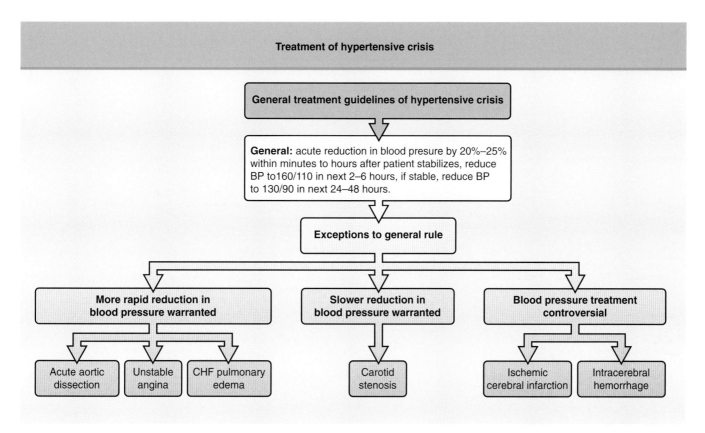

Treatment of hypertensive crisis

General treatment guidelines of hypertensive crisis

General: acute reduction in blood presure by 20%–25% within minutes to hours after patient stabilizes, reduce BP to160/110 in next 2–6 hours, if stable, reduce BP to 130/90 in next 24–48 hours.

Exceptions to general rule

More rapid reduction in blood pressure warranted

Slower reduction in blood pressure warranted

Blood pressure treatment controversial

Acute aortic dissection

Unstable angina

CHF pulmonary edema

Carotid stenosis

Ischemic cerebral infarction

Intracerebral hemorrhage

Figure 32.4. General treatment guidelines for hypertensive crisis.

medications in the setting of a CNS insult, and there are no randomized trials comparing different agents in the setting of hypertensive crisis and CNS insult. However, the use of nitroprusside in the setting of increased intracranial pressure (ICP) is cautioned. Animal and human studies show no effect of nitroprusside on ICP in the setting of a normal ICP. Studies on animals and humans with preexisting increased ICP suggest that nitroprusside increases the ICP. This is likely secondary to systemic vasodilatation in the setting of decreased cranial compliance. Other treatment options include labetalol, nicardipine, and fenoldopam. Fenoldopam shares with nitroprusside a rapid onset and short duration of action. In addition, fenoldopam, in contrast to nitroprusside, possibly increases renal blood flow, induces natriuresis, and produces no toxic metabolites.

Malignant Hypertension

Malignant hypertension is characterized by markedly elevated pressures with hypertensive neuroretinopathy. Funduscopic examination reveals acute vasculitis manifested by flame-shaped hemorrhages, cotton-wool spots, or papilledema. Other findings include nephropathy, encephalopathy, microangiopathic hemolytic anemia, and cardiac ischemia. Without treatment, malignant hypertension results in a greater than 90% 1-year mortality rate. In the classic series by Kincaid-Smith (1980), deaths from untreated malignant hypertension resulted from renal failure (19%), congestive heart failure (13%), renal failure plus congestive heart failure (48%), stroke (20%), and myocardial infarction (1%).

The primary goal is to reduce BP while preserving target organs at risk. The autoregulatory range of cerebral blood flow

is increased in chronic hypertension, but the lower limit remains approximately 25% below the resting mean arterial pressure (MAP) in patients with both normotension and chronic hypertension. Symptoms of low cerebral blood flow include nausea, yawning, hyperventilation, clamminess, and syncope. After initial reduction of BP by 20% within the first hour, BP is further reduced over the next 2 to 6 hours to the 160/110 mm Hg range as long as there is no evidence of alterations in cerebral perfusion. Nitroprusside is the most useful intravenous agent for hypertensive crises. Since malignant hypertension is associated with intravascular volume depletion, nitroprusside should be started at low doses and titrated slowly (0.25 µg/kg/min or less with titration every 3 to 5 minutes). Alternatives to nitroprusside include labetalol, fenoldopam, and nicardipine. Rebound hypertension can occur if parental therapy is terminated early. Oral therapy is started after the pressure has been stabilized on parenteral therapy. Parenteral therapy is then slowly removed and oral therapy titrated to maintain BP control.

Renal failure is common with malignant hypertension and may exacerbate the hypertension (Fig. 32.5). Fibrinoid necrosis develops in afferent arterioles, and proliferative endarteritis develops in interlobular arteries. As a result, the vessel lumen becomes narrowed, resulting in decreased renal blood flow. The arteriolopathy of malignant hypertension results in fixed anatomic lesions so that when the BP is initially lowered the creatinine may increase. Renal function begins to improve after several weeks of therapy in most patients and may continue to improve for up to 26 months. Of the patients who require dialysis, 50% regain sufficient function to discontinue dialysis. Recovery of renal function is more likely when the combined

Table 32.1 Treatment of Hypertensive Crisis: Intravenous Medication*

Medication Mechanism/Use	Disadvantages/Adverse Effects/Metabolism/Cautions
Direct Vasodilators	
Sodium Nitroprusside **Mechanism:** Nitric oxide compound, vasodilates arteriolar resistant vessels and venous capacitance vessels, decreases systemic vascular resistance (SVR) **Use:** Most hypertensive crises	Contraindicated in high-output cardiac failure, congenital optic atrophy. Liver disease—at risk for cyanide toxicity. Symptoms—acidosis, tachycardia, and change in mental status; almond smell on breath. Renal disease—at risk for thiocyanate toxicity. Symptoms—psychosis, hyperreflexia, seizure, tinnitus. Cautious use with increased intracranial pressure. Do not use maximum dose for more than 10 min. Crosses the placenta.
Hydralazine **Mechanism:** Primarily dilates arteriolar vasculature **Use:** Primarily in pregnancy/eclampsia	Reflex tachycardia, give β-blocker concurrently, may exacerbate angina. Half-life 3 hr. Depends on hepatic acetylation for inactivation.
Nitroglycerin **Mechanism:** Directly interacts with nitrate receptors on vascular smooth muscle, primarily dilates venous bed, decreases SVR **Use:** Cardiac ischemia, perioperative hypertension in cardiac surgery	Contraindicated in angle-closure glaucoma, increased intracranial, pressure, aortic dissection, myocardial ischemia. Blood pressure decreased secondary to decreased preload, cardiac output—avoid when cerebral or renal perfusion is compromised. Use caution with right ventricular infarct.
α- and β-Adrenergic Blockade	
Labetalol **Mechanism:** α/β Blocking ratio is 1:7, decreases SVR **Use:** Malignant hypertension, hypertensive encephalopathy, aortic dissection, alternative to nitroprusside	Avoid in bronchospasm, bradycardia, congestive heart failure, greater than first-degree heart block, avoid after cardiac surgery, oral only in pregnancy, IV in pregnancy associated with fetal bradycardia, hypoglycemia, hyperkalemia with renal failure. Use caution with hepatic dysfunction, inhalational anesthetics (myocardial depression). Enters breast milk.
Selective β₁-Blockade	
Esmolol **Mechanism:** Selective beta 1 beta blocker **Use:** Aortic dissection. Used during intubation, intraoperative and postoperative hypertension.	See labetalol. Not dependent on renal or hepatic function for metabolism (metabolized by hydrolysis in red blood cells)
Dopamine Agonists	
Fenoldopam **Mechanism:** Postsynaptic dopamine-1 agonist, decreases peripheral vascular resistance. Ten times more potent than dopamine as vasodilator. **Use:** May be advantageous in kidney disease, increases renal blood flow, increases sodium excretion, no toxic metabolites, decreases SVR	Contraindicated in glaucoma (may increase intraocular pressure) or allergy to sulfites, hypotension especially with concurrent β-blocker. Check serum potassium every 6 hr. No CNS effects. Concurrent acetaminophen may significantly increase blood levels. Dose-related tachycardia.
α-Adrenergic Blockade	
Phentolamine **Mechanism:** Nonselective α-adrenergic blocking agent, dilatation of arteriolar resistance vessels and venous capacitance vessels, decreases SVR **Use:** Excessive catecholamine, e.g., pheochromocytoma	β-Blockade is generally added to control tachycardia or arrhythmias. As in all catecholamine excess states, β-blockers should never be given first, as the loss of β-adrenergically mediated vasodilatation will leave β-adrenergically mediated vasoconstriction unopposed and result in increased pressure.
Dihydropyridine Calcium Channel Blockers	
Nicardipine **Mechanism:** Inhibits transmembrane influx of calcium ions into cardiac and smooth muscle **Use:** Postoperative hypertension	Avoid with congestive heart failure, cardiac ischemia, cardiac surgery. Adverse effects include tachycardia, flushing, headache.
Angiotensin-Converting Enzyme (ACE) Inhibitors	
Enalaprilat **Use:** Scleroderma kidney	Response not predictable, with high renin states may see acute hypotension. Hyperkalemia in setting of reduced glomerular filtration rate. Avoid in pregnancy.
Nondepolarizing Ganglionic Blockade	
Trimethaphan **Mechanism:** Competes with acetylcholine for postsynaptic receptors **Use:** Aortic dissection, autonomic hyperreflexia with spinal cord injury	Does not increase cardiac output. No inotropic cardiac effect. Disadvantages include parasympathetic blockade resulting in paralytic ileus and bladder atony, and development of tachyphylaxis after 24–96 hr of use.

*Data from Up to Date Inc.; Varon J, Marik PE: The diagnosis and management of hypertensive crisis. Chest 2000;118:214–227; and Abdelwahab W, Frishman W, Landau A: Management of hypertensive urgencies and emergencies. J Clin Pharmacol 1995;35:747–762.

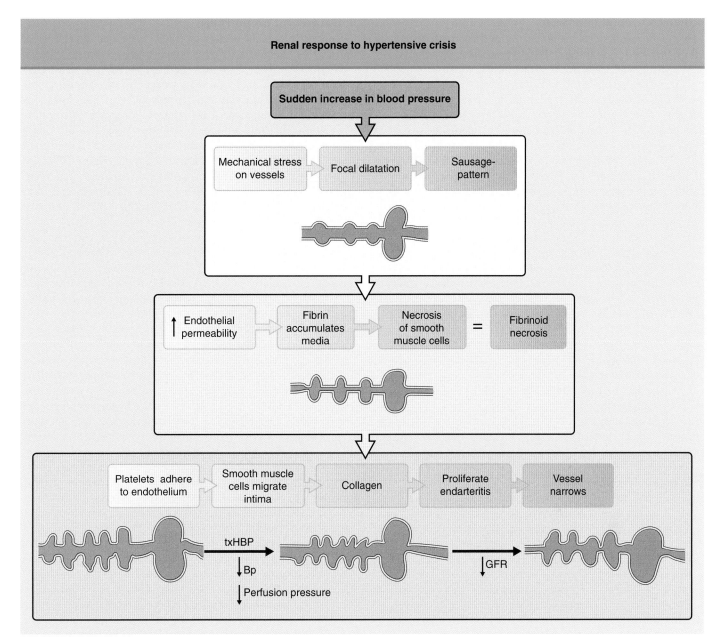

Figure 32.5. Renal response to hypertensive crisis.

length of both kidneys is 20.2 cm or more and less likely when the kidney length is 14.2 cm or less. If renal failure is secondary to malignant hypertension, adequate BP control may reverse renal failure. However, when malignant hypertension is secondary to underlying kidney disease (e.g., glomerulonephritis), the primary renal disease may cause progress to end-stage renal disease (ESRD) regardless of BP control. In the past, nitroprusside has been the preferred agent to treat hypertension and renal failure. The metabolism of nitroprusside results in the production of cyanide, which is taken up by red blood cells and conjugated to thiocyanate in the liver. Cyanide toxicity occurs in patients with anemia or liver disease, whereas thiocyanate toxicity is seen in the setting of renal disease. Thiocyanate levels should be monitored and the duration of therapy kept to less than 72 hours whenever possible. Alternatively, both fenoldopam and labetalol have no toxic metabolites and may protect renal function.

Hypertensive Encephalopathy

Hypertensive encephalopathy may occur with or without malignant hypertension. In hypertensive encephalopathy, the mean arterial pressure exceeds the limits of autoregulation and brain edema develops from extravasation of plasma proteins (see Fig. 32.2). Left untreated, coma and death may follow. The challenge of hypertensive encephalopathy is appropriate lowering of BP in the setting of CNS ischemia and edema. The hallmark of hypertensive encephalopathy is clinical improvement within 12 to 24 hours of adequate BP reduction. The mean arterial pressure should be reduced by no more than 15% over 2 to 3 hours. Neurologic complications have been reported from reductions in MAP of 40% or more. If an acute decline in mental status occurs with treatment, the BP should be allowed to increase until neurologic symptoms resolve. It should then be reduced over several days to allow restoration of autoregulation.

Ischemic Cerebral Infarction

Cerebral ischemia develops when the perfusion pressure falls below the level of autoregulation. On occasion, hypoperfusion results in marked increases in systemic BP, which often spontaneously resolve in 24 to 48 hours. The treatment of BP in the setting of cerebral infarction is controversial. In animals, in the area surrounding the infarct there are "neurons at risk" that depend on collateral circulation to maintain perfusion. These neurons are nonfunctional, not dead, with the potential to be "rescued" by reperfusion, a phenomenon referred to as "ischemic penumbra." The impact of the "ischemic penumbra" in humans is not known. Moreover, in acute ischemic stroke, autoregulation is generally impaired. The net effect is that cerebral blood flow is unpredictable. As a result of these changes, there is concern that acute reductions in BP may actually increase the area of infarct and severely compromise clinical outcome. Recommendations for treatment from the American Stroke Association include the recommendation that in individuals with a recent ischemic infarct and a BP greater than 220/120–140 mm Hg, the BP may be decreased by 10% to 15%. During this period of reduction, the patient must be closely monitored for evidence of neurologic deterioration. In conclusion, most clinicians do not treat hypertension in the setting of ischemic stroke unless the BP elevation is extreme (systolic BP > 220 mm Hg, diastolic BP > 120 mm Hg) or there is acute ischemic damage to vital organs (cardiac ischemia, aortic dissection). Hypotensive agents used in this setting include nitroprusside and labetalol. Intravenous labetalol may not elevate intracranial pressure as much as nitroprusside.

Subarachnoid Hemorrhage

Subarachnoid hemorrhage accounts for approximately 10% of cerebrovascular accidents and carries an estimated mortality rate of 40% to 50%. The most common cause of subarachnoid hemorrhage is ruptured congenital berry aneurysm, and the treatment of choice is surgical clipping. Subarachnoid hemorrhage increases intracranial pressure and decreases cerebral perfusion, resulting in global ischemia. Intracerebral hemorrhage and hydrocephalus are potential complications. The risk of a repeat bleed in the first 24 hours is significant. In contrast to cerebral ischemia, intracranial bleed induces intense vasospasm in neighboring vessels 4 to 12 days after the initial bleed, increasing the risk for significant cerebral ischemia during this period. As a result, treatment of hypertension with subarachnoid hemorrhage differs significantly from that with ischemic cerebral infarction.

Markedly elevated pressures increase the risk of rebleeding. The goal is 20% to 25% reduction in MAP over 6 to 12 hours, but not to less than 160–180/100 mm Hg. An intact mental status is evidence of adequate cerebral perfusion and may be used to guide therapy.

Labetalol is the preferred agent because it does not elevate ICP or CPP. Given the potential increase in cerebral blood volume and intracranial pressure associated with vasodilators, sodium nitroprusside and nitroglycerin are not usually first-line treatments. Nimodipine may be the preferred medication in the setting of neurologic insult given clinical evidence suggesting that it decreases vasospasm and cerebral ischemia. Nimodipine may also directly protect ischemic damage to nerve cells by blocking calcium uptake into cells.

Intracerebral Hemorrhage

Seventy-five percent of affected individuals who experience an intracerebral hemorrhage have preexisting hypertension. Intracerebral hemorrhage accounts for 10% to 20% of all strokes. Symptoms of intracerebral hemorrhage include nausea, vomiting, change in mental status, hypertension, headache, and a focal neurologic examination. The definitive diagnosis is made by neuroimaging. With intracerebral hemorrhage, the BP rapidly declines in the first 24 hours but may not return to normal for 7 to 10 days (as opposed to ischemic stroke, where BP generally returns to normal in 24 to 48 hours). Hematoma compresses normal tissue, causing ischemia, ICP increases, and CPP decreases. Autoregulation is altered, making cerebral perfusion critically dependent on systemic BP.

There is no consensus or randomized trial on the treatment of hypertension in intracerebral hemorrhage. One argument is that lowering BP decreases risk of hemorrhage extension and edema, particularly when systolic BP exceeds 200 mm Hg, a level shown to be associated with hematoma growth. Others argue that not treating hypertension allows continued perfusion of neurons at risk. Rebleeding in the first 24 hours is more common than thought, occurring in up to one third of affected individuals. The greatest risk is in the first few hours after the initial insult. Risk factors for a rebleed include an initial large irregular bleed, coagulopathy, liver disease, and a low platelet count. A clear relationship between acute hypertension after an intracerebral bleed and the risk of rebleeding has not been demonstrated. Extreme elevations of pressure (mean arterial pressure ≥ 130 mm Hg) should probably be treated with reduction of BP limited to 20%. With regard to the antihypertensive agent of choice, the major concern is the impact on intracranial pressure. Common to all agents is a decrease in mean arterial pressure and a decrease in cerebral perfusion pressure. As discussed above, vasodilating agents may increase cerebral blood flow and, in the setting of decreased cranial compliance, increase intracranial pressure, further decreasing cerebral perfusion pressure. The combination of decreased cerebral compliance, decreased cerebral blood flow, and altered autoregulation as occurs in chronic hypertension makes the administration of any antihypertensive agent potentially dangerous. Combination α- and β-blockers are recommended when antihypertensive treatment is indicated in intracerebral hemorrhage. The primary risk is bradycardia associated with the Cushing response. In the setting of normal cranial compliance and an increased intracranial pressure, vasodilators are probably safe. With intracerebral bleed, catecholamine levels are elevated and β-blockade should be added to vasodilators when indicated. In one study, barbiturates were found to modestly reduce MAP while markedly reducing the intracranial pressure, and should be considered in cases of severe hemorrhage.

Head Trauma

Skull fractures, epidural hematomas, subdural hematomas, intracerebral hematomas, and diffuse axonal damage are all potential complications of head trauma. Acute increases in ICP are initially prevented by flow of blood and cerebrospinal fluid (CSF) from the cranial vault. However, with increasing edema, ICP eventually increases. Defective autoregulation has been noted in 31% to 61% of patients with a closed head injury. With intact autoregulation, increasing the MAP results in vasoconstriction and no change in ICP. However, if autoregulation is not intact, increases in MAP are not compensated and may increase blood volume, leading to edema and increased ICP. The goal is to maintain a minimum CPP of 70 mm Hg and a mean arterial pressure greater than 90 mm Hg. If an antihypertensive agent is indicated, an important consideration is its impact on ICP. With decreased intracranial compliance and increased intracranial pressure, a combination α- and β-blocker is preferred. In the absence of increased intracranial compliance, vasodilators may be preferred.

Aortic Dissection

Aortic dissection begins with a tear in the intima of the aorta. The aortic pulse wave (dP/dt), determined by myocardial contractility, heart rate, and BP, contributes to propagation of dissections. Two types of aortic dissection are described: A and B. Type A dissections often begin with a tear in the intima of the proximal aorta next to a coronary artery that may extend to the aortic arch. Type B dissections begin in the descending aortic arch with an intimal tear next to the subclavian artery. Risk factors for dissection include advanced atherosclerosis, Marfan syndrome, Ehlers-Danlos syndrome, and coarctation of the aorta. As the expanding hematoma causes pressure on the vasculature, signs and symptoms occur including myocardial infarction, stroke spinal cord/bowel infarction, and acute renal failure. Renal ischemia may develop, leading to refractory hypertension. Dissection to the aortic root can precipitate acute aortic insufficiency. Rupture of the ascending aorta leads to hemopericardium and tamponade.

The clinical presentation of both types of dissection may include severe, often tearing pain in the chest, back, or abdomen with diaphoresis, nausea, or vomiting. Physical examination is usually remarkable for hypertension, a discrepancy in peripheral pulses, and sometimes an expanding pulsatile aortic mass. A recent analysis showed that a widened mediastinum on the chest radiograph was present in only one half of individuals with type B dissection. The diagnosis is confirmed by computed tomography (CT) or magnetic resonance imaging (MRI). Multiplanar transesophageal echocardiography is also used.

Treatment for type A dissection usually includes surgery to prevent the catastrophic consequences of great vessel occlusion, aortic insufficiency, or tamponade. Type B dissections are usually treated medically.

Given the very high mortality associated with aortic dissection, treatment decisions are made rapidly on the basis of clinical suspicion and later confirmed by radiologic examination. β-Blockers are given initially to decrease myocardial contractility and heart rate. Propranolol is often used. Labetalol is also a good choice but given the potential for emergency surgery, its longer duration of action may be problematic. The treatment goal is the lowest tolerable BP until pain is relieved. Absence of pain suggests arrest of active aortic dissection. The most widely used agent is nitroprusside. Nitroprusside is titrated to systolic pressure of 100 to 120 mm Hg or to as low as 70 to 80 mm Hg. Prior treatment with β-blockers prevents reflex cardiac stimulation and a potential increase in the aortic pulse wave seen with nitroprusside.

An alternative treatment is the ganglionic blocking agent trimethaphan. It is used to treat hypertension with aortic dissection because of its potent reduction in the steepness of the pulse wave contour. This agent prevents increases in cardiac output and left ventricular ejection rate. The rapid onset (1 to 2 minutes) and short duration of action (10 minutes) allow precise pressure control. Any mild reflex increase in heart rate may be treated with subsequent β-blockade. Hydralazine is avoided because it causes reflex cardiac stimulation. Even normotensive individuals should be treated with antihypertensive medications to keep the heart rate and shear forces low.

Pulmonary Edema

In the setting of chronic hypertension, patients often develop concentric left ventricular hypertrophy and well-preserved systolic contraction. When the BP acutely increases, as with hypertensive crisis, acute diastolic dysfunction occurs in response to abrupt increases in cardiac afterload. With impairment of diastolic relaxation, the left ventricle requires markedly elevated filling pressures, leading to pulmonary venous hypertension and edema. The treatment goal is to decrease afterload, improve diastolic relaxation, and decrease pulmonary pressure, making vasodilators the agent of choice. β-Blockers are also used. Nitroprusside is sometimes used because it reduces preload and afterload, improving left ventricular function and decreasing myocardial oxygen demand. Modest decreases in pressure improve symptoms markedly. In less emergent settings, angiotensin-converting enzyme (ACE) inhibitors or calcium channel antagonists have been shown to improve diastolic function and cause regression of concentric ventricular hypertrophy.

When left ventricular failure is secondary to poor systolic function, vasodilators are preferred. Nitroglycerin is preferred for cardiac ischemia. Nitroglycerin dilates intercoronary collateral vessels more than small resistance arterioles and improves perfusion of ischemic myocardium. In patients refractory to nitrites, nitroprusside may be used. However, nitroprusside dilates resistance arterioles predominantly, which may cause potential steal of blood flow from ischemic areas. Diuretics are used to reduce left ventricular end-diastolic volume.

In the setting of acute myocardial infarction, acute catecholamine release and sympathetic outflow contribute to hypertension. The initial treatment is sedation and pain control. This is often followed by lowering of BP within a few hours. However, most clinicians would treat a diastolic blood pressures greater than 100 mm Hg with nitroglycerin. The goal is to lower BP to near normotensive levels and avoid overshoot hypotension, which can decrease coronary perfusion. Therapy can usually be terminated within 24 hours. There is considerable evidence that the early use of β-blocking agents may reduce ultimate infarct size independently of BP control.

Perioperative Hypertension

Perioperative hypertension is a major risk factor for the development of postoperative hypertension. Elective surgery should be deferred until the diastolic pressure is below 110 mm Hg. A diastolic BP below 110 mm Hg is not associated with increased surgical risk unless there are coexisting conditions such as ischemic heart disease, cerebrovascular disease, or congestive heart failure. In the presence of additional risk, surgery should be canceled until the BP has been adequately controlled for several weeks. In patients with chronic hypertension on ade-

351

quate treatment, oral medications should be taken on the morning of surgery.

The impact of anesthesia on BP is an important consideration. In patients with hypertension who receive anesthesia, rapid and wide fluctuations in BP are common. For example, induction of anesthesia is associated with increased sympathetic activity and increased BP. This response may be exaggerated in the setting of chronic hypertension. After continued anesthesia, a decline in BP generally occurs.

Hypertensive therapy should continue after surgery, with a change to an equivalent intravenous medication when indicated. Patients previously on a β-blocker or clonidine should have these medications continued postoperatively to prevent "rebound" hypertension. If intravenous medication is necessary, propranolol or methyldopa may be used. The high incidence of post-surgical hypertension is in part related to the decreased use of "deep" anesthesia and the absence of prolonged sedation following surgery. As a result, there is increased sympathetic response to surgical stimuli such as pain, hypoxia, and the anesthetic agents themselves. Effective pain control and avoidance of hypoxia is often sufficient to treat the hypertension. Adequate BP control reduces the risk of bleeding from suture lines, premature graft closure, and ischemic damage to organs at risk. Nitroprusside is widely used. Nitroglycerin is preferred for the post–coronary bypass patient. Fenoldopam is also recommended, especially in clinical settings where renal ischemia is a risk.

Catecholamine-Associated Hypertension

Hypertensive crisis related to excess catecholamine secretion occurs with ingestion of sympathomimetic agents such as cocaine, amphetamines, phencyclidine, phenylpropanolamine (diet pills), decongestants such as ephedrine and pseudoephedrine, and other agents including atropine, ergot alkaloids, and tricyclic antidepressants. It may also be caused by tyramine ingestion in conjunction with monoamine oxidase (MAO) inhibitor therapy (Fig. 32.6), autonomic dysfunction, withdrawal from certain antihypertensive medications, and pheochromocytoma. Critically elevated pressures can cause myocardial infarction, aortic dissection, and stroke.

Pheochromocytoma is a very rare cause of hypertension. The tumor produces excess catecholamines, causing a sustained elevation of BP in most patients. Paroxysmal symptoms occur when catecholamines are released in response to stimuli. Symptoms of pheochromocytoma include headache, palpitations, anxiety, abdominal pain, and diaphoresis. On physical examination, hypertension, often with orthostatic changes, may be appreciated. With hypertensive crisis secondary to pheochromocytoma, the preferred agent is the short-acting parenteral β-antagonist phentolamine. As in all catecholamine excess states, β-blockers should not be used as initial therapy. This is because loss of β-adrenergic-mediated vasodilatation leaves β-adrenergically mediated vasoconstriction unopposed, increasing BP. However, after the BP is initially lowered, a β-blocker may be added to control tachycardia and arrhythmias. An oral regimen of the nonselective β-antagonist phenoxybenzamine can be used in nonemergent situations. Labetalol has been effective in treating hypotension related to pheochromocytoma in selected patients. However, since its β-blockade exceeds its β-blocking effect, severe hypertension has been reported.

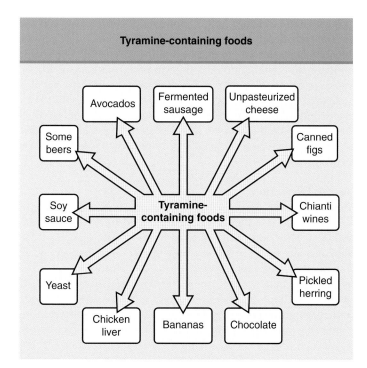

Figure 32.6. Tyramine-containing foods that may cause hypertension in patients taking MAO inhibitor therapy.

Significant rebound hypertension may develop 12 to 72 hours after abrupt discontinuation of high-dose centrally acting β-agonist antihypertensives such as clonidine or methyldopa. In cases of moderate hypertension, restarting the antihypertensive agent may control the BP. With more severe BP elevations, intravenous therapy should be used.

In patients taking MAO inhibitor therapy, ingestion of foods containing tyramine or sympathomimetic amines can result in hypertension (see Fig. 32.6). Tyramine is metabolized by an alternative pathway to octopamine, which releases catecholamines from peripheral sites by acting as a false neurotransmitter. Nitroprusside or phentolamine is used, with the addition of β-blockade as needed for tachycardia. The episodes are self-limited and last 6 hours or less.

Gestational Hypertension/Preeclampsia/Eclampsia

During the course of a normal pregnancy, BP initially declines and then slowly increases toward the normal range during the third trimester. Gestational hypertension is defined as a systolic BP of at least 140 mm Hg and a diastolic BP of at least 90 mm Hg on two separate BP measurements done 6 hours apart. Gestational hypertension develops after 20 weeks of pregnancy in patients with no prior history of hypertension. Up to 50% of women who develop gestational hypertension before 30 weeks of pregnancy will go on to develop preeclampsia. Preeclampsia is defined as gestational hypertension with 300 mg of protein on a 24-hour urine (urine dipstick 1+). A 24-hour urine is necessary because urine protein on dipstick correlates poorly with 24-hour urine protein in gestational hypertension. Preeclampsia should also be suspected in patients with hypertension developing after 20 weeks of gestation and associated with nausea, vomiting, cerebral symptoms, abnormal liver function tests, or thrombocytopenia, even in the absence of proteinuria.

Preeclampsia develops in 7% of all pregnancies: 70% in nulligravidas and 30% in multigravidas. Up to 70% of individuals with molar pregnancies develop preeclampsia. In preeclampsia, intravascular volume is low despite peripheral edema, and the renin-angiotensin system is activated. Progression to seizures indicates eclampsia and may occur with diastolic pressures of as low as 100 mm Hg. Clinical treatment includes bed rest and parenteral magnesium. The goal is to keep the systolic BP between 140 and 150 mm Hg and diastolic BP between 90 and 105 to assure adequate placental blood flow. Hydralazine is the preferred agent. Labetalol may also be used. Nitroprusside should be avoided owing to the risk of cyanide toxicity in the fetus. ACE inhibitors should also be avoided.

Other Hypertensive Situations

The renal crisis of scleroderma is an aggressive form of malignant hypertension occurring in 8% to 13% of patients with scleroderma and is more common in blacks. The first event, which proceeds the hypertension, is proliferative endarteritis. Hypertension occurs because of ischemic-induced activation of the renin-angiotensin system. Progression to ESRD occurs in 1 to 2 months without treatment. Aggressive pressure control with ACE inhibitors leads to a long-term survival of about 50% to 70%.

Hypertension is a feature of both primary and secondary antiphospholipid antibody syndromes occurring in up to 93% of patients. Both microvasculopathy and emboli to the renal artery contribute to the malignant hypertension. Antihypertensive treatment is similar to that for malignant hypertension. Successful treatment outcomes have been reported with anticoagulation.

One fourth of patients with extensive second- or third-degree burns develop severe hypertension in the first few days probably secondary to elevated levels of circulating catecholamines and renin.

Patients with transverse spinal cord lesions at the T6 level or higher, including patients with Guillain-Barré syndrome, have autonomic hyperreflexia. In this setting, noxious stimuli in dermatomes below the level of the lesion trigger a massive sympathetic discharge with severe hypertension, bradycardia, diaphoresis, and headache. Autonomic hyperreflexia may occur 4 to 6 months after the acute injury and may recur throughout life. In 90% of patients, distention of the bladder or bowel causes the dysreflexia, and prompt decompression leads to resolution of hypertension. Drugs that have been used successfully in treating this condition include nitroprusside, phentolamine, and labetalol.

Hypertension in the renal transplant recipient may be caused by acute rejection, vascular anastomotic stenosis, obstructive uropathy, corticosteroid use, cyclosporine, and native-kidney renin release. Oral calcium channel antagonists are effective and well tolerated in these patients. Other rare causes of hypertension include erythropoietin-associated hypertension. This is treated with phlebotomy and dose reduction in conjunction with antihypertensive drugs. Diabetic patients taking β-blockers can experience severe hypertension with hypoglycemic episodes, presumably as a result of catecholamine release.

SUGGESTED READING

Abdelwahab W, Frishman W, Landau A: Management of hypertensive urgencies and emergencies. J Clin Pharmacol 1995;35:747–762.

Adams RE, Powers WJ: Management of hypertension in acute intracerebral hemorrhage. Crit Care Clin 1997;13:131–161.

Adams HP Jr, Adams RJ, Brott T, et al: Guidelines for the early management of patients with ischemic stroke: a scientific statement for the Stroke Council for the American Stroke Association. Stroke 2003;34:1056–1083.

Chobanian AV, Bakris GL, Black HR, et al: The Seventh Report of the Joint National Committee on Prevention, Detection, Evaluation, and Treatment of High Blood Pressure. JAMA 2003; 289:2560–2572.

DeSanctis RE, Doroghazi RM, Austen WG, Buckley MJ: Aortic dissection. N Engl J Med 1987;317:1060.

Kincaid-Smith P: Malignant hypertension: mechanisms and management. Pharmacol Ther 1980;9:245.

Kincaid-Smith P, McMichael J, Murphy EA: The clinical course and pathology of hypertension with papilledema (malignant hypertension). Q J Med 1958;27:117.

Marsh ML, Shapiro HM, Smith RW, et al: Changes in neurologic status and intracranial pressure associated with sodium nitroprusside administration. Anesthesiology 1979;51:336.

Murphy MB, Murray C, Shorten GD: Fenoldopam: a selective peripheral dopamine-receptor agonist for the treatment of severe hypertension. N Engl J Med 2001;345:1548–1557.

Whelton PK, Klag MJ: Hypertension as a risk factor for renal disease: review of clinical and epidemiological evidence. Hypertension 1989;13:119.

Acute Cardiovascular Emergencies

Vanessa Cobb, Greg McAnulty, and Andrew Rhodes

KEY POINTS

- The Frank-Starling law of the heart states that, under normal circumstances, the heart is able to increase its stroke volume appropriately according to venous return. Understanding the factors that influence preload and afterload may suggest therapeutic strategies in cardiogenic shock.
- Trauma is the leading cause of death of children and adults under 45 years of age. Advanced Trauma Life Support (ATLS) training has been introduced by the American College of Surgeons Committee on Trauma to optimize management using a systematic approach to the injured patient and includes guidelines on the management of cardiac and great vessel trauma.
- Management of clinical cardiac tamponade is pericardiocentesis. Serious complications of pericardiocentesis include myocardial perforation, coronary artery laceration, pneumothorax, and puncture of upper abdominal organs.
- The majority of patients with acute aortic dissection complain of pain that is typically sudden and maximal at the time of onset. Pain may be limited to the anterior chest, may radiate to the posterior chest, or involve only the interscapular region, back, or abdomen. The site of pain can change with extension of the dissection. The return of pain after subsidence may indicate impending rupture.

Regardless of the primary physiologic insult resulting in patients being admitted to an intensive care unit (ICU), restoration and maintenance of optimal hemodynamic status are crucial determinants of eventual outcome.

This chapter discusses cardiogenic shock, describing the final common pathway of a process of deterioration following cardiac or great vessel injury. Cardiovascular emergencies resulting from myocardial disease, trauma, and valvular abnormalities are considered, together with cardiac tamponade and aortic dissection. Acute coronary syndromes, arrhythmias, congestive cardiac failure, and hypertensive emergencies are addressed in detail elsewhere, but there is necessarily some overlap with other chapters.

CARDIOGENIC SHOCK

Cardiogenic shock is defined by failure of the heart to pump an adequate amount of blood for the body's metabolic requirements, leading to general tissue hypoxia. The physiologic concept of "preload" refers to the precontraction length of a myocyte and is taken to be equivalent to left ventricular end diastolic volume. The observation that the precontraction length of a cardiac muscle fiber is proportional to the energy of contraction has been extrapolated to describe the relationship between left ventricular end-diastolic volume and stroke volume. The Frank-Starling law of the heart states that, under normal circumstances, the heart is able to increase its stroke volume appropriately according to venous return. "Afterload" is the resistance against which the ventricle contracts and describes the tension generated in the ventricular wall in systole. Understanding the factors that influence preload and afterload may suggest therapeutic strategies in cardiogenic shock.

Preload is determined largely by venous return but is also affected by factors such as heart rate (tachycardia reduces filling time), valvular disease (atrioventricular valve stenosis may reduce ventricular filling, aortic or pulmonary valve incompetence may increase preload), atrial fibrillation (which may reduce filling time as well as removing the normal active atrial contribution to filling at high heart rates), and ventricular ejection (reduced ejection increases end diastolic volume).

Cardiogenic shock is most commonly precipitated by the conditions listed in Box 33.1.

Myocardial infarction associated with cardiogenic shock is fatal in approximately 60% of cases. Patients may have symptoms of myocardial ischemia together with signs of tissue hypoperfusion, sympathetic activation, hypotension, and frequently altered level of consciousness. Patients are generally oliguric and cool and clammy to the touch and may be cyanotic.

Neurohumoral compensatory mechanisms activated to maintain perfusion of vital organs can further compromise the ratio between myocardial oxygen demand and supply by increasing afterload. Since the heart's blood supply is dependent on its own function, a vicious cycle is created wherein the heart struggles to perform with a dwindling supply of energy.

It is important to exclude other causes of shock (hemorrhage, other fluid loss, sepsis, pulmonary embolism) and to recognize and treat reversible, immediately life-threatening problems such as tamponade or tension pneumothorax and to correct any compounding problems such as arrhythmia.

Treatment of cardiogenic shock should follow standard resuscitation procedure, paying attention to maintaining the patient's

Box 33.1 Causes of Cardiogenic Shock

Ischemia- or infarction-induced ventricular wall hypokinesia
Arrhythmias
Valvular pathology
Tamponade
Ventricular septal or free wall rupture
Myocardial trauma
Drug toxicity
Metabolic derangements
Hypoxemia
Hypertension
Sepsis

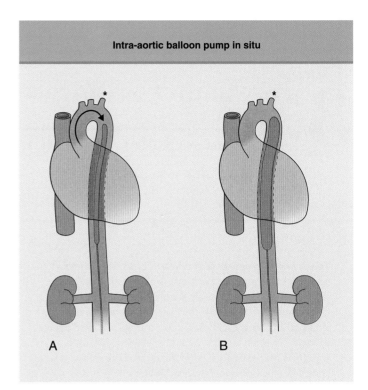

Intra-aortic balloon pump in situ

A   B

Figure 33.1. Schematic diagram of intra-aortic balloon pump in situ within the descending aorta. The balloon tip is distal to the left subclavian artery (*). *A,* Balloon deflation occurs prior to ventricular contraction and remains deflated throughout systole. *B,* The balloon inflates at the onset of diastole.

airway breathing and circulation. Oxygen should be given by mask, but if oxygenation is still inadequate, continuous positive airway pressure by mask or intubation and positive pressure ventilation may improve ventilation-perfusion matching in the lung as well as reduce left ventricular filling pressure.

By definition, a patient in cardiogenic shock has inadequate organ perfusion and treatment with vasoactive and inotropic drugs normally is required. Invasive monitoring of right and, frequently, left (via a pulmonary artery catheter) atrial pressures may assist management of fluids and vasodilators. Hypovolemia is poorly tolerated by a failing ventricle and is frequently present. It should be corrected with careful monitoring of filling pressures. Echocardiography is an alternative or an additional tool in the assessment of right and left ventricular preload and may allow diagnosis of cardiac tamponade, valvular disease, and myocardial infarction or ischemia. Vasoconstrictors may be required to preserve adequate perfusion pressure for organ perfusion. Inotropic agents may increase myocardial oxygen consumption but, if improved myocardial contractility results in improved ejection and a reduction in end-diastolic volume, the overall effect may be to reduce myocardial wall tension.

Inotropes exploit mechanisms such as stimulation of β-adrenergic receptors, inhibition of intracellular phosphodiesterase, and recently increasing intracellular calcium sensitivity. All but the last mechanism increase myocardial oxygen consumption.

Mechanical devices that improve myocardial oxygen supply while decreasing myocardial work are an attractive therapeutic strategy in cardiogenic shock. The most commonly deployed such device is the intra-aortic counter-pulsation balloon pump.

INTRA-AORTIC BALLOON PUMP

The intra-aortic balloon pump (IABP) is a cardiac mechanical assist device consisting of a balloon mounted on a catheter attached to a console. The balloon is placed just distal to the left subclavian artery (Fig. 33.1). The balloon is rapidly inflated and deflated with a gas (generally helium because of its low density and, therefore, low resistance to flow) timed according to the events of the cardiac cycle.

The balloon is inflated during diastole, increasing diastolic aortic pressure and improving coronary perfusion. Just before ventricular ejection the balloon deflates, reducing the proximal aortic pressure and reducing left ventricular afterload. The

overall effect is to increase myocardial oxygen delivery while at the same time reducing myocardial oxygen consumption (Fig. 33.2).

The observed secondary effects of intra-aortic balloon counter-pulsation include increase in mean arterial pressure, decrease in pulmonary artery wedge pressure, increase in cardiac output, and reduction in heart rate.

Indications for Use

Although the IABP has been used since the 1960s as a treatment for cardiogenic shock following myocardial infarction, evidence for benefit in this circumstance is limited. However, data from registries and post hoc analyses of clinical trials suggest that the use of IABP in patients who have suffered myocardial infarction and who receive emergency revascularization therapy is associated with a reduction in mortality.

Use of the IABP

The IABP can be inserted percutaneously (usually via a femoral artery) or during cardiac surgery. Percutaneous insertion is best performed under fluoroscopic control by an experienced operator. If fluoroscopy is not used to confirm correct placement, a chest radiograph is required following insertion. The ideal position is 2 to 3 cm distal to the left subclavian artery and proximal to the renal arteries. The device may be inserted without a sheath if the arteries are of small caliber, but this method should not be used if there is significant fatty or scar tissue at the site of insertion.

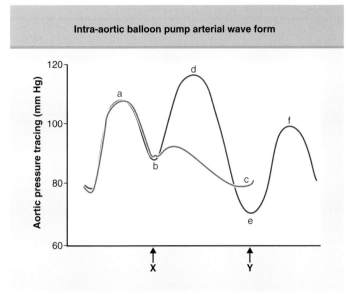

Figure 33.2. The intra-aortic balloon pump arterial waveform. The red line represents the normal arterial waveform with dicrotic notch. The blue line shows unassisted systole followed by a pump-generated assisted diastole with subsequent reduced end-diastolic and systolic aortic pressure. *a*, Unassisted systole. *b*, Dicrotic notch (inflation point). *c*, Unassisted aortic end-diastolic pressure. *d*, Assisted diastole. *e*, Assisted aortic end-diastolic pressure. *f*, Assisted systole. X, Aortic valve closes. Y, Aortic valve opens.

IABP function is timed to coincide with use of electrocardiography (ECG) or arterial waveform as a guide. In most cases it is preferable to set the console to follow the ECG trace. When ECG is used, balloon inflation is set to occur at the peak of the T wave, corresponding to aortic valve closure, and deflates just before or on the R wave, corresponding with ventricular systole.

When the arterial waveform is used, balloon inflation is timed to occur at the dicrotic notch on the arterial trace to coincide with the closure of the aortic valve. Deflation is just before the aortic upstroke. An adequate pulse pressure and gradient of upstroke is necessary for sensing to occur. In addition, it is important to be aware of the time delays involved in the transmission of waveforms when using peripheral arteries to generate signals for the console.

The console has the facility to generate its own rhythm in the absence of signals generated by the heart such as during cardiopulmonary bypass. The use of pacing spikes as a method of generating signals for the console is recommended only in selected circumstances.

IABP weaning can be achieved by reducing the ratio of augmented to nonaugmented beats. In addition, the amount of volume assist provided can be altered. It is important to check coagulation and platelet count before removal.

Contraindications for IABP Use

IABP use is contraindicated in aortic valve insufficiency, aortic dissection, and severe calcific disease of the aorta or iliac vessels (due to potential for balloon membrane damage). Further considerations include need for anticoagulation and existing comorbidities.

Box 33.2 Complications of Intra-aortic Balloon Pump

Limb ischemia
Infection
Gas embolism
Thrombotic embolism
Thrombocytopenia
Aortic dissection
Renal artery occlusion

Complications of IABP Use

The most common complication associated with percutaneous devices is limb ischemia (Box 33.2). This has been reduced by the development of smaller catheters. Sheathless insertion can also be used to reduce this complication. Limb ischemia is more likely to occur in females and in patients with peripheral vascular disease or diabetes. It is important in all cases to monitor foot perfusion.

In the Benchmark Counterpulsation Outcomes Registry, major limb ischemia (defined as ischemia requiring surgical arterial repair or amputation) occurred in 1.2% of cases using the IABP. Infection is uncommon and is an indication for device removal.

Balloon rupture with gas embolism is rare. It may be indicated by blood tracking into the lumen. If gas embolism is suspected, the patient should be placed in the Trendelenburg position and the IABP removed. The console is designed to alarm if it detects a gas leak. However, small defects in the membrane may be difficult to detect. If blood and helium come into contact, a solid mass may form that may impede catheter removal.

Other complications include embolic events and compartment syndrome. Thrombocytopenia can occur and is thought to result from mechanical platelet damage. Aortic dissection and subintimal placement of the catheter have been described.

VENTRICULAR SEPTAL RUPTURE

Ventricular septal rupture (VSR) is an uncommon complication of myocardial infarction. It is associated with advanced age and female sex and is more common following anterior myocardial infarction (MI). Patients with VSR are more likely to have complete occlusion of the involved coronary artery without evidence of a collateral circulation.

VSR can occur following both anterior and inferior MI. Typically, the defect in anterior MI is apical. VSR complicating inferior MI tends to be a more complex lesion with greater tissue destruction. It occurs in the basal region of the septum and has a higher associated operative mortality.

The incidence of VSR has decreased since the introduction of thrombolysis as a treatment for MI, although it appears to occur earlier after thrombolysis than in patients who do not receive this therapy for MI. VSR complicates 0.2% of acute MIs (compared with 1% to 2% before thrombolysis was introduced [GUSTO-1 trial]). Primary percutaneous intervention may also reduce the incidence of this complication in acute MI.

The septal defect causes a left-to-right shunt, and this leads to right ventricular volume overload. Pulmonary blood flow increases, leading to pulmonary congestion. Compensatory peripheral vasoconstriction as a result of reduced cardiac output predictably worsens left-to-right shunt.

Patients may experience chest pain and develop clinical signs of congestive heart failure. A harsh systolic murmur at the left sternal edge with palpable thrill may become apparent. Acute mitral regurgitation (MR) and acute VSR present with similar features and may be clinically indistinguishable. They may also occur together.

The defect may be detected using two-dimensional echocardiography with color flow mapping. It is also useful to make an assessment of right ventricular function, which has some prognostic significance in VSR following MI. Right heart catheterization demonstrates an oxygen step up between the right atrium and right ventricle/pulmonary artery and helps quantify the shunt. Left ventricular catheterization is also used to visualize coronary arteries where there is a view to concomitant bypass grafting.

The current trend is toward early surgical intervention. No clear patient subgroup has been identified as suitable for deferred surgery. Preoperative use of an IABP will reduce left ventricular afterload and reduce the shunt size. Operative mortality is high but significantly lower than mortality without surgery. Successful percutaneous repair of VSR with a prohibitively high surgical risk has been reported, but this is not an established treatment.

LEFT VENTRICULAR FREE WALL RUPTURE

Left ventricular free wall rupture (LVFWR) is responsible for 10% to 15% of in-hospital deaths after acute MI. It occurs more frequently than either papillary muscle rupture or ventricular septal rupture. Risk factors include first MI, advanced age, and transmural infarct.

The lateral wall is the most common site of rupture, which usually occurs up to 7 days after MI but earlier in cases treated with thrombolytic therapy. However, there is evidence that early thrombolysis reduces the risk of LVFWR. The converse is true with later thrombolysis. Primary percutaneous intervention is associated with a lower risk of cardiac rupture.

Clinical presentation in many cases is catastrophic with electromechanical dissociation (pulseless electrical activity) or asystole. Signs include hypotension and poor peripheral perfusion, jugular venous distention, pulsus paradoxus, and muffled heart sounds. The diagnosis is often made clinically and corroborated using echocardiography or pericardiocentesis. Prompt resuscitation, pericardiocentesis as a temporizing measure, and emergency surgery to repair the defect may save the patient.

Approximately one third of patients with LVFWR follow a subacute course. This may present with episodic or prolonged chest pain, hypotension, and arrhythmia. Symptoms suggestive of impending rupture include nausea and vomiting, restlessness, and agitation. Surgical repair is the definitive treatment.

Rarely, there may be a slow or episodic leak into the pericardial space to produce a pseudoaneurysm. A murmur may be heard as a result of blood flow through the neck connecting it to the left ventricle. This requires surgical repair because it is at risk of rupture.

MYOCARDITIS

Myocarditis is an inflammatory, nonischemic condition of the myocardium. The etiology in most cases is infective, but it can also occur with autoimmune disease or exposure to certain agents such as anthracyclines and α-interferon. The most likely infective agent in the developed world is viral, in particular, coxsackie B enterovirus. Myocardial damage probably results from a combination of direct viral cytotoxicity and immune-mediated pathology. Giant cell myocarditis is thought to be autoimmune mediated.

Clinical features of acute myocarditis may range from subclinical to cardiac failure and shock (fulminant myocarditis) and may include conduction disturbances and malignant arrhythmias. There is often a history of preceding flu-like symptoms, chest pain, and dyspnea. The erythrocyte sedimentation rate, CKMB fraction, cardiac troponin, and white blood cell count may be raised. A fourfold rise in IgG antienterovirus titer over 4 weeks is supportive of acute infection.

On 12-lead ECG, diffuse T-wave abnormalities, sinus tachycardia, and conduction abnormalities are nonspecific findings. Echocardiography may demonstrate left ventricular systolic dysfunction and regional wall motion abnormalities, mimicking an ischemic etiology. Endomyocardial biopsy can support the diagnosis, but normal histologic findings do not exclude it.

Treatment is supportive. Some also advocate use of antiviral agents in selected cases. Immunosuppression is indicated in specific cases such as giant cell myocarditis and in some autoimmune disorders.

Fulminant myocarditis is characterized by rapid development of profound hemodynamic compromise but has a good prognosis if the patient survives the acute phase. Therefore, in cases of severe acute cardiac compromise secondary to myocarditis, it is worthwhile to provide bridging mechanical support in the form of an intra-aortic balloon pump or even a ventricular assist device, since the patient may predictably recover. The natural history of acute myocarditis can range from restoration of normal cardiac function to progression to dilated cardiomyopathy and heart transplantation or death.

PRIMARY CARDIOMYOPATHY

Hypertrophic Cardiomyopathy

Hypertrophic cardiomyopathy (HCM) describes the presence of myocardial hypertrophy. The majority of cases result from mutations in genes encoding cardiac sarcomere proteins and are inherited in an autosomal dominant fashion. The prevalence is approximately 1 in 500 adults. Sporadic cases also occur. HCM can present at any age and may be asymptomatic.

In addition to myocardial hypertrophy, there is abnormal myocyte structure and organization. The condition is also associated with abnormal myocardial calcium handling and small vessel disease. In a subtype of HCM known as hypertrophic obstructive cardiomyopathy (HOCM), there is thickening of the interventricular septum, which may cause left ventricular outflow tract obstruction.

In HCM the left ventricle is stiff, causing high diastolic pressures and impaired filling. This can lead to diastolic heart failure. Anginal symptoms result from an oxygen demand-supply mismatch due to the bulk of myocardial tissue, even if there is not coronary artery disease. Outflow tract obstruction can lead to syncopal episodes as in severe aortic stenosis. HCM is also associated with sudden death, probably due to arrhythmia.

Twelve-lead ECG demonstrates left ventricular hypertrophy. The chest radiograph may be normal or show pulmonary congestion. Echocardiography may demonstrate hypertrophy of the left ventricle. In most cases this will be asymmetric and involve the interventricular septum more than the free wall. Abnormal systolic anterior motion (SAM) of the mitral valve leaflet is another feature of HCM detectable on an echocardiogram.

Management aims to improve ventricular relaxation and diastolic filling and reduce heart rate, usually with β-blockers or calcium antagonists. Verapamil is a rational choice, since it is thought that excess calcium contributes to impaired myocardial relaxation. Dihydropyridines have greater vasodilatory properties than verapamil and can have a deleterious hemodynamic effect. Inotropes such as epinephrine (adrenaline) produce tachycardia and reduced diastolic relaxation and are avoided. Dual ventricular pacing and septal ablation may be effective.

Dilated Cardiomyopathy

Dilated cardiomyopathy (DCM) describes dilatation and impaired systolic function of the left ventricle or both ventricles. It may be idiopathic or result from myocarditis, excess alcohol intake, thiamine deficiency, thyrotoxicosis, or hemochromatosis and also may occur in association with some neuromuscular disorders. Anthracycline treatment can result in DCM, and the incidence is increased at higher cumulative doses. Peripartum cardiomyopathy is a form of DCM. It has a higher incidence in older mothers, hypertension, and twin pregnancies. Diagnosis requires cardiac failure (LVEF < 40%) to develop during pregnancy or within 6 months of delivery without an alternative explicable etiology. It is estimated to lead to death or heart transplantation in 20% of cases and to significant improvement in 50%. Poorer prognosis is related to the age of the mother and the degree of cardiac impairment. It should be treated as for cardiac failure but with attention given to potential contraindications in pregnancy, such as ACE inhibitors.

CARDIAC TRAUMA

Trauma is the leading cause of death of children and adults under 45 years of age. Advanced Trauma Life Support (ATLS) training has been introduced by the American College of Surgeons Committee on Trauma to optimize management using a systematic approach to the injured patient and includes guidelines on the management of cardiac and great vessel trauma. Cardiac trauma can be the result of blunt or penetrating injury.

Blunt Trauma

Myocardial Contusion

Myocardial contusion should be considered following blunt chest trauma and may be indicated by angina-like chest pain that is unrelieved by nitrates. Significant complications of contusion include cardiac failure and life-threatening arrhythmias.

The right ventricle is most commonly injured. The left ventricle may be indirectly affected, as a result of reduced left ventricular preload and septal shift.

Patients with suspected blunt cardiac injury should have an ECG. Various nonspecific abnormalities are possible in contusion: The most common is sinus tachycardia. Continuous ECG monitoring for 24 to 48 hours is recommended when abnormalities are found. Malignant arrhythmias may occur although in a minority of cases. Acid-base/electrolyte abnormalities and hypoxia should be treated. Inotropes, if required, should be used with caution.

Echocardiography may demonstrate wall motion abnormalities and can give an indication of left ventricular function and the presence of other cardiac injuries. Most authorities agree that troponin measurement has some value in the assessment of blunt cardiac injury. Conclusive diagnosis of contusion is only possible with direct inspection or histologic examination, which is not warranted in the majority of cases. The incidence of myocardial contusion in blunt chest trauma is not known, since standardized diagnostic criteria do not exist.

Valve Damage

A murmur or features of congestive heart failure following severe blunt trauma to the chest may suggest valve damage. Injury to the aortic valve is most commonly reported. Repair may be possible, but replacement is the usual surgical treatment. Traumatic mitral regurgitation is usually due to papillary muscle or chordae tendineae damage rather than to direct injury to valvular cusps. Valve replacement can be avoided in some cases. Aortic, mitral, or tricuspid valvular insufficiency may not always be apparent immediately following injury, and all can present subacutely.

Coronary Artery Damage

Coronary artery damage from blunt trauma usually affects the left anterior descending or right coronary arteries and may result in dissection and subsequent ischemia or pericardial effusion. Repair by stent deployment has been described.

Chamber or Vessel Rupture

Rupture of a cardiac chamber or great vessel usually rapidly leads to death. It is likely that chamber rupture results from impact during a vulnerable time in the cardiac cycle. It is suggested that the ventricles are most susceptible at the end of diastole, when the atrioventricular and outflow valves are closed. The presentation is one of cardiac tamponade (which may be slower to develop in cases of atrial chamber rupture) hemorrhagic shock, or traumatic VSR. Other significant injuries are often present.

Aortic Rupture

Traumatic aortic rupture is usually rapidly fatal. Survival is possible if the bleed is contained. Survivors of traumatic aortic rupture are likely to have an incomplete laceration near the ligamentum arteriosum. The chest radiograph may be normal, but clues include widened mediastinum, loss of normal aortic outline, deviation of trachea to the right, loss of space between pulmonary artery and aorta, depression of the left main-stem bronchus, and presence of left hemothorax. Imaging options include angiography, contrast-enhanced CT scan, and transesophageal echocardiography (TOE). Esophageal, cervical spine, or maxillofacial trauma may preclude the use of the latter.

Surgical management is by repair or resection and grafting of the aorta.

Penetrating Trauma

Penetrating wounds to the thorax, neck, or upper abdomen should raise suspicion for cardiac injury. The patient may have shock due to hemorrhage or cardiac tamponade. Pericardiocentesis or a subxiphoid pericardial window can provide a temporizing measure for cardiac tamponade prior to definitive surgery. Resuscitative thoracotomy can be performed in the emergency room if greater access to cardiac structures is necessary. It allows evacuation of hematoma, digital pressure on bleeding points, cardiac massage, and aortic cross-clamping. Management, as with blunt trauma, should follow ATLS guidelines.

INFECTIVE ENDOCARDITIS

Infective endocarditis describes the invasion by microorganisms of either native or prosthetic heart valves with the formation of vegetations and valvular destruction. Vegetations typically contain a mixture of fibrin and platelets together with the culprit microorganism. The usual infecting organisms are gram-positive cocci: the viridans and enteric streptococci and staphylococci.

The annual incidence in developed countries is roughly 2 to 4 per 100,000 and is greater in men than women. The incidence has not appreciably decreased over recent decades, perhaps related in part to increased detection and an increased life span in individuals with predisposing conditions. Mortality remains high related to hemodynamic or central nervous system complications.

The typical presentation is subacute with nonspecific features such as fever, malaise, arthralgia, and anorexia. There are likely to be additional clues in the history (Box 33.3). Occasionally, the course of infection is acute with rapid onset of fever and sepsis.

Fever and new or changed murmurs are the most common clinical findings. Extracardiac manifestations include cutaneous and retinal lesions, splenomegaly, hematuria, renal impairment, and neurologic abnormalities. These are thought to reflect embolism, stimulation of the immune system, and/or immunocomplex deposition.

Complications

Complications requiring ICU admission include congestive cardiac failure, renal failure, septic shock, and neurologic deterioration.

Box 33.3 Risk Factors for Bacterial Endocarditis

Intravenous drug abuse
Prosthetic valve
Congenital heart disease (especially cyanotic conditions)
History of previous endocarditis
Native valvular heart disease
Hypertrophic obstructive cardiomyopathy
Catheters or shunts in dialysis patients

Congestive Cardiac Failure

Congestive cardiac failure in infective endocarditis can result from damage to native or bioprosthetic valves and valvular apparatus, leading to valvular incompetence, and also from dehiscence of prosthetic valves. These phenomena are described elsewhere in this chapter. Additional causes of cardiac failure include large vegetations causing valvular obstruction and intracardiac shunts resulting from perivalvular extension of infection.

Perivalvular Infection and Abscess

Perivalvular infection and abscesses are particularly associated with prosthetic valve and native aortic valve endocarditis. In native aortic valve disease, spread of infection can lead to conduction disturbances, which may require pacing.

Fistula

In the presence of perivalvular infection, fistulas may form, leading to structural disruption and intracardiac shunting. Pericardial effusion and aortocardiac fistulas are rare complications of infective endocarditis.

Extracardiac Complications

Extracardiac complications include emboli and metastatic infection. Embolization of vegetations and thrombi leads to tissue infarction. Virtually any organ can be affected. Seeding of infection can lead to extracardiac abscesses and persistence of fever. Neurologic complications are common and may result from emboli, abscesses, rupture of mycotic aneurysms, and vasculitic processes.

Diagnosis and Management

Multiple blood cultures should be taken. Special microbiology laboratory techniques can be employed to detect the slower growing and more fastidious organisms. Serologic tests and analysis of surgically removed valve tissue or embolized material can also be performed to identify the organism. Inflammatory markers are often raised. Serial measurements are useful to assess response to infection. Normocytic anemia and microscopic hematuria are commonly present.

ECG can detect conduction disturbances, indicating septal involvement, and ischemia secondary to coronary artery embolism. The chest radiograph may show pulmonary congestion or lung abscesses.

Echocardiographic assessment is an important part of the diagnostic workup and can demonstrate vegetations, pericardial effusion, periannular abscess, and shunts. Transthoracic echocardiography (TTE) has the advantage of accessibility and is useful for detection of right-side lesions. However, it cannot easily detect small vegetations, and image quality can be affected by factors such as obesity and chest wall deformities. Transesophageal imaging is more sensitive (Fig. 33.3) and should be used if there is suspicion of perivalvular involvement and in the assessment of prosthetic valves. Echocardiography should not be used alone to rule out infective endocarditis. Repeat echo studies can be performed when the index of suspicion remains high following a "negative" test.

Management of infective endocarditis requires collaboration among the disciplines of infectious disease, microbiology, cardiology, and cardiac surgery. In bacterial endocarditis, high-dose bacteriocidal antibiotics are recommended and long treatment

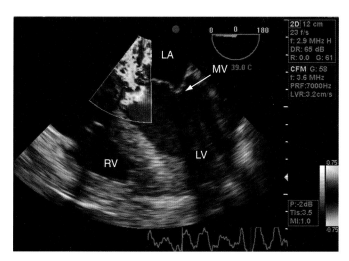

Figure 33.3. Transesophageal echocardiogram of mitral regurgitation. This two-dimensional view demonstrates coaptation of mitral valve leaflets, but color flow mapping shows a significant regurgitant jet via leaflet perforation. LA, left atrium; LV, left ventricle; MV, mitral valve leaflet; RV, right ventricle.

There is substantial evidence that surgical intervention in congestive cardiac failure (CCF) due to endocarditis reduces mortality. It is the most common indication for proceeding to early surgery. CCF also predicts poor outcome following surgery. In some cases, it is possible to delay surgery in well-controlled CCF secondary to native mitral valve involvement. Native aortic valve involvement is less well tolerated and can often be accompanied by extension of infection. Tricuspid involvement rarely leads to surgery.

Early surgery is indicated in the presence of valvular obstruction or prosthetic dehiscence, because they are likely to result in rapid hemodynamic compromise. Surgery is indicated if there is evidence of recurrent septic emboli, but in some cases the decision to go ahead with early surgery must be balanced by the increased risk of further neurologic deterioration or death, particularly in the presence of large or hemorrhagic cerebral lesions.

Decisions for surgery based on the characteristics of the vegetation are not clear cut but should take into account whether embolic events have already occurred, particularly in the presence of very large or mobile vegetations, and the site of the vegetation. (There is some evidence that vegetations on the anterior mitral valve leaflet are associated with a greater risk of embolization.) Fungal infection is often complicated by large vegetations and embolic phenomena and often requires early surgery.

Failure to respond to medical therapy (persistence of fever or positive blood cultures) without evidence of an extracardiac nidus of infection is an indication for cardiac surgery. Assessment of response should be made after a week of targeted antibiotic therapy.

Figure 33.4 shows surgical repair of a perforated mitral valve leaflet following endocarditis.

duration is standard. The intravenous route increases bioavailability and is therefore used, at least initially. Most drug regimens require blood level monitoring. Description of specific antimicrobial regimens is beyond the scope of this chapter but takes into account the drug susceptibility of the organisms, whether the valve is native or prosthetic, and any drug idiosyncrasies of the patient.

Indications for Surgery

In previous years, it was usual to delay surgery until completion of antibiotic treatment. It is now common practice to perform surgery during active infection (Box 33.4).

Box 33.4 Indications for Surgery in Infective Endocarditis

Refractory congestive cardiac failure (most common indication, often secondary to acute AR or MR)

Failure to respond to medical therapy (persistent fever/bacteremia without evidence of extracardiac infection)

Recurrent emboli despite adequate antibiotic therapy

Valvular obstruction

Prosthetic dehiscence

Extension beyond valve annulus (abscess/fistula/ruptured sinus of Valsalva/perforation of septum)

Evidence of new atrioventricular block on ECG indicating septal involvement (pacemaker implantation may be required)

Surgery is usually indicated for

　Fungal infection

　Very large or mobile vegetations (particularly if evidence of embolic event)

　Prosthetic valve endocarditis involving *Staphylococcus aureus*

　Infective endocarditis due to gram-negative organisms

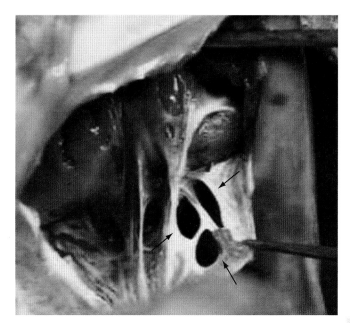

Figure 33.4. Intraoperative image of perforated mitral valve leaflets. Arrows indicate perforations resulting from endocarditis.

Prognosis

The overall estimated mortality with infective endocarditis is 20%. In particular the presence of congestive cardiac failure (CCF) is a predictor of poor outcome. Mortality is 56% to 86% with moderate to severe CCF with nonsurgical therapy. The presence of CCF also predicts poor perioperative outcome as do renal impairment, advanced age, and delay to surgery. In the long term following surgery, reoperation rate is 2% to 3% per year due to recurrence of infective endocarditis or prosthetic valve dysfunction. Prognosis also depends on the culprit organism, speed of initiation and adequacy of therapy, and the affected site.

ACUTE NATIVE AORTIC REGURGITATION

Aortic dissection, infective endocarditis leading to leaflet perforation, ruptured sinus of Valsalva, and trauma may all give rise to acute native valve aortic regurgitation (AR), which can also be iatrogenic.

Diastolic backflow of blood into the left ventricle leads to left ventricular volume overload. In chronic disease, the left ventricle compensates by dilating. In acute AR, left ventricular end-diastolic pressure rapidly increases, leading to pulmonary edema. Acute volume overload reduces left ventricular stroke volume so that cardiac output decreases. Cardiogenic shock may ensue.

Patients may have features of pulmonary edema or cardiogenic shock. Typical features of chronic AR are often absent.

In true acute cases, the chest radiograph shows a normal heart size with pulmonary congestion. Echocardiography can provide information on both the etiology and severity. Doppler studies are employed to measure the regurgitant jet and detect diastolic reversal of aortic flow. An additional feature of detectable AR using echocardiography is early diastolic closure of the mitral valve resulting from a rapid rise in LVEDP from the regurgitant jet, and this is a marker of severity, particularly if it occurs before the Q wave.

Acute AR is a surgical emergency. Medical management is directed at hemodynamic optimization. Vasodilators such as sodium nitroprusside or dobutamine may improve forward flow, but their use may be limited by hypotension. IABP is contraindicated. Multiple blood cultures should be taken before antibiotics are administered.

It may be possible to delay emergency surgery so that coronary angiography can be performed when coronary artery disease is likely or so that antibiotics have time to reduce the septic load.

AORTIC STENOSIS

Aortic stenosis may present acutely after decompensation precipitated by ischemia, arrhythmia, dehydration, or sepsis.

A normal valve may undergo degenerative calcification, but stenosis is more likely in a congenitally bicuspid valve. Rheumatic heart disease rarely leads to aortic stenosis in isolation.

Aortic stenosis creates an increase in afterload to which the ventricle responds over time by hypertrophy to maintain stroke volume. The increase in muscle mass results in an oxygen demand and supply mismatch and ischemia. Diastolic compliance is reduced, making the heart dependent on adequate preload to maintain stroke volume, and as pressures rise, pulmonary congestion can occur.

Box 33.5 Causes of Acute Native Mitral Regurgitation
Complication of Myocardial Infarction
Papillary muscle ischemia/rupture
Rupture of chordae tendineae
Dilatation of mitral annulus
Geometrical changes in left ventricle
Infective Endocarditis
Vegetations inhibiting normal leaflet coaptation
Leaflet obstruction
Chordal rupture
Connective Tissue Disease Affecting Mitral Valve Apparatus
Marfan syndrome
Myxomatous degeneration
Systemic lupus erythematosus
Left Atrial Myxoma (poor leaflet closure)
Infiltrative Disease Affecting Papillary Muscle
Amyloid/sarcoid/infiltrative cardiomyopathies
Trauma
Iatrogenic
Valvuloplasty/surgery

The most common symptom is angina. Effort-related lightheadedness, dizziness, syncope, and dyspnea also occur. Typically a crescendo-decrescendo murmur is heard at the base of the heart. If systolic function is compromised, the murmur is less prominent. Twelve-lead ECG usually demonstrates left ventricular hypertrophy. Left bundle branch block is common.

On a chest radiograph, the cardiac silhouette size is usually normal. Echocardiography can be used to estimate valve surface area and transvalvular pressure gradients. Cardiac catheterization provides direct pressure measurements and detailed information on coronary arteries. This is, in many cases, useful prior to valve replacement surgery because bypass grafting can be performed within the same operation.

Percutaneous balloon valvotomy is associated with a high incidence of early restenosis and is not usually recommended. It can be performed in specific circumstances such as in patients with severe comorbidity not expected to survive a graft procedure or as a bridge procedure before valve replacement in very unstable patients. Medical management is generally directed toward reversal of the cause of decompensation.

ACUTE NATIVE MITRAL REGURGITATION

Failure of both functional and anatomic relationships between the valve leaflets and their supporting structures can result in mitral regurgitation. Etiologies include trauma and iatrogenic causes, infiltrative conditions such as amyloid and sarcoid, connective tissue diseases, and infective endocarditis. Wall motion abnormalities and altered geometry affecting the structural relationships between the different elements of the mitral valve apparatus following acute myocardial infarction can lead to acute mitral regurgitation as can papillary muscle ischemia or necrosis and chordae tendineae rupture. Box 33.5 summarizes the different etiologies of acute native mitral valve regurgitation.

Papillary muscle tissue has a vulnerable blood supply, since it is far from the origin of the coronary arteries. As a result it is at risk of ischemia or infarction. There are two papillary muscles in the left ventricle. The anterolateral muscle is supplied by the left anterior descending artery, often with an additional contribution from the left circumflex. The posteromedial muscle is supplied by the posterior descending artery. The anterolateral muscle benefits from the dual blood supply and is less prone to ischemic injury than the posteromedial muscle.

Acute MR can rapidly lead to pulmonary edema and cardiogenic shock. The underlying pathophysiology involves loading of a nondilated, noncompliant left atrium with regurgitant blood. This is transmitted to the pulmonary vasculature, resulting in pulmonary congestion and edema. With a portion of the intended stroke volume regurgitating into the left atrium, forward flow is also compromised. This can lead to cardiogenic shock, particularly if left ventricular function is otherwise compromised, such as in acute myocardial infarct.

Many cases do not have an easily detectable murmur. This is in part related to high pressure within the noncompliant left atrium, reducing the pressure differential between the two chambers. Furthermore, the regurgitant jet may be passing through a large hole. If a murmur is present, it tends to die away before S_2, since the noncompliant left atrium limits regurgitation.

Echocardiography is the diagnostic method of choice (Fig. 33.5). Transesophageal echo may provide more useful information on the severity and mechanism of mitral insufficiency than transthoracic views. The chest radiograph may show a normal heart size with pulmonary edema. Pulmonary artery catheterization may reveal a high PCWP with prominent v waves (the v wave represents an increase in left atrial pressure in systole), although this is not specific to MR.

The aim of management is prompt hemodynamic stabilization with timely corrective surgery where appropriate. Inotropic support, mechanical ventilation, and an intra-aortic balloon pump may be required. Afterload reduction with vasodilators can be useful if tolerated.

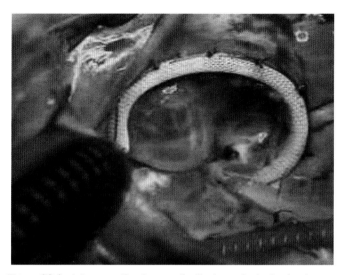

Figure 33.6. Intraoperative image of mitral annuloplasty ring in position. The mitral valve leaflets are preserved.

Surgical options depend on the underlying mechanism and the extent of damage. Options include chordal transfer, Goretex chordal insertion, mitral annuloplasty (Fig. 33.6), and mitral valve replacement. In some cases, a ruptured papillary muscle may be sutured if there is not extensive tissue damage. Intermittent acute MR as a result of ischemia may be simply resolved by a percutaneous or surgical revascularization procedure.

MITRAL STENOSIS

Rheumatic heart disease is the most common cause of mitral stenosis. Progression to mitral stenosis following childhood rheumatic carditis tends to be more rapid in developing countries. It is important to be aware that it can be accompanied by abnormalities in other valves, which may affect clinical presentation.

The most common presenting symptoms are dyspnea and fatigue. Chest discomfort for which the cause is not entirely clear may also occur. The hemodynamic effects of mitral stenosis include increased left atrial pressure and reduced cardiac output. The increase in left atrial pressure leads to pulmonary congestion and reactive pulmonary hypertension with eventual right heart failure. Left atrial dilatation predisposes to atrial fibrillation and systemic embolism.

Acute decompensation may result from an insult such as arrhythmia or sepsis, which compromises diastolic filling of the left ventricle. Hemodynamic deterioration is also a well-recognized phenomenon in pregnancy.

Twelve-lead ECG may demonstrate atrial fibrillation and right ventricular hypertrophy. A chest radiograph may reveal left atrial enlargement and pulmonary congestion. Echocardiography can confirm the diagnosis and demonstrate severity (Fig. 33.7). TOE is superior to TTE in detection of left atrial thrombus. Measured PCWP often overestimates the true transmitral pressure gradient.

β-Blockers are the staple treatment because they improve diastolic filling. If the condition is refractory to medical treatment, options for direct intervention should be considered.

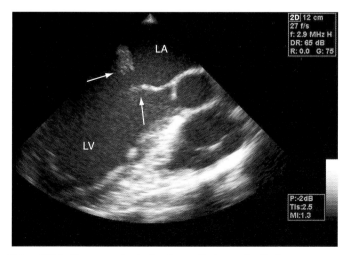

Figure 33.5. Transesophageal echocardiogram of mitral regurgitation. Failure of coaptation of the mitral valve leaflet tips is shown (arrows). LA, left atrium; LV, left ventricle.

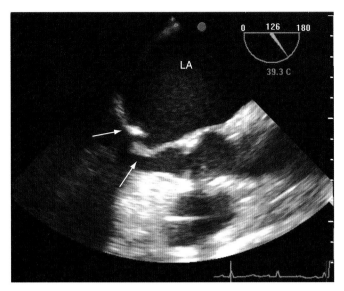

Figure 33.7. Two-dimensional transesophageal image of the mitral valve leaflet in mitral stenosis. The leaflets are thickened and have a characteristic "hockey stick" appearance in diastole. This results from wider separation of the basal portions of the leaflets with increased left atrial pressure and relative immobility of the leaflet tips. The arrows show the leaflet tips. LA, left atrium.

Many acutely decompensated patients will not tolerate surgical commissurotomy. However, there are reports emerging of successful balloon mitral valvotomy in patients with cardiogenic shock and resistant pulmonary edema or following cardiac arrest. Balloon valvotomy can be used as a bridging procedure or as the sole therapy. In pregnancy, balloon valvotomy involves less risk for the fetus than does a surgical procedure.

PROSTHETIC VALVE COMPLICATIONS

Valve Obstruction

A valve obstruction can lead to restricted movement or sticking of the valve in the open or closed position. The restriction of movement may be intermittent. The material causing the obstruction can be thrombus but can also be pannus (fibrous tissue growth). Very rapid development is more suggestive of predominantly thrombotic rather than tissue composition.

Many thrombogenic surfaces are associated with a prosthetic valve. These include the materials inserted and the exposed perivalvular tissue. Additionally, associated abnormalities of blood flow increase the predisposition to thrombus formation.

Bioprosthetic valves are less thrombogenic than mechanical valves. The likelihood of this complication depends on type and from greatest to least is as follows: first-generation ball and cage valves, tilting disc types, and bileaflet valves. Thrombotic complications are more likely when the valve is in the mitral position, when more than one valve is replaced, in the setting of low cardiac output or atrial fibrillation, and in hypercoagulable states such as pregnancy. Identification of a period of inadequate anticoagulation may suggest thrombosis as a cause for valve failure. Normal clicking of the valve may be lost or a new murmur may be auscultated.

Presentation can range from mild heart failure to shock. Choices for treatment in cases of hemodynamic compromise

include thrombectomy and prosthetic valve replacement. Thrombolysis can be used in selected cases but is not without its own risks—in particular, embolic and hemorrhagic complications. It is often reserved for high-risk surgical candidates.

Disc Escape

Fracture or fatigue of the strut supporting the disc may lead to valve failure (often with dramatic hemodynamic sequelae) and disc embolism. Björk-Shiley 60 convexo-concave valve and models welded between January 1981 and July 1982, especially larger sizes in the mitral position, were prone to this complication. It is rarely reported in other valve models.

Prosthetic Valve Endocarditis

Infective endocarditis involving a prosthetic valve carries a higher risk than that involving a native valve. The infective agent in early endocarditis post surgery is often *Staphylococcus epidermidis*, which colonizes the graft perioperatively. Gram-negative bacilli and fungi can also be responsible. Streptococci are more likely in late endocarditis. Vegetations may obstruct the valve or embolize to the systemic circulation. Periannular infection may lead to a paravalvular leak, abscesses, and fistulas.

Valve Dehiscence

This is usually an early event following surgery and often is a reflection of suture failure, but it may also result from prosthetic valve endocarditis or from Marfan syndrome due to underlying tissue friability. Valve dehiscence requires surgical correction. Medical supportive therapy and the intra-aortic balloon pump can be used as interim measures.

Bioprosthetic Valve Failure

Likelihood of structural damage to the bioprosthetic valve increases over the time since operation and is greater in patients who were young at the time of implantation. It is also greater in patients with renal failure and hypercalcemia. The mitral position is the most likely site of complications. Deterioration can be rapid, especially if the cusp is torn. Echocardiography is the investigation of choice.

CARDIAC TAMPONADE

Acute cardiac tamponade results from rapid external compression of the heart, usually by fluid contained within an intact pericardium (Box 33.6).

Box 33.6 Causes of Cardiac Tamponade
Post–cardiac surgery
Tumors (primarily lung cancer)
Pericarditis (viral or bacterial)
Uremia
Hypothyroidism
Connective tissue diseases
Ventricular free wall rupture following acute myocardial infarction
Tuberculosis

The reserve volume of the pericardial space can be filled without an appreciable increase in intrapericardial pressure. With continued filling the tissue can stretch. If the rate of accumulation exceeds the compliance of the pericardium, the filling of the heart chambers is reduced. At first, the right side chamber diastolic pressures are exceeded, leading to a compensatory increase in systemic venous pressure to fill the right side chambers. Eventually, diastolic pressure in all four chambers equalizes and the space occupied by the heart cannot increase to allow for diastole. Filling of all four chambers is then compromised. Neurohormonal compensatory mechanisms initially maintain cardiac output in tamponade by increasing heart rate and contractility, and shock ensues.

Typically the patient has tachypnea, tachycardia, hypotension, or shock. The classical sign of jugular venous distention may be absent in hypovolemia.

Pulsus paradoxus (a decrease in systolic arterial pressure of more than 10 mm Hg during inspiration) may be evident. A negative intrathoracic pressure is created during inspiration that reduces pulmonary venous pressure and, secondarily, reduces left ventricular diastolic filling on which cardiac output is dependent. At the same time, an increase in venous return to the right ventricle during inspiration can impair left ventricular filling, since it will do so at the expense of the left side owing to ventricular interdependence. Note that, in particular, this sign may not be reliably elicited in the ventilated patient nor in the patient with acute aortic insufficiency complicating dissection.

An enlarged cardiac silhouette and a notable absence of evidence of pulmonary congestion may be seen on a chest radiograph. Low-voltage QRS complexes and electrical alternans are associated findings on 12-lead ECG. Electrical alternans is uncommon and occurs in effusions large enough to cause swinging motion of the heart. Pulseless electrical activity or electromechanical dissociation precedes death.

Echocardiography is the investigation of choice, although it may miss localized effusions and compression. Localized posterior effusions may not be visible on transthoracic echo and may require transesophageal views. Supportive evidence of cardiac tamponade includes right ventricular early diastolic collapse, straightening of the interventricular septum, early closure of the aortic valve, and respiratory variation in flow across atrioventricular valves.

Management of clinical cardiac tamponade is pericardiocentesis. Interim hemodynamic support in the form of inotropes and intravenous fluid can be offered but is controversial. It is preferable to use imaging such as echocardiography or fluoroscopy to guide needle insertion. Blind percutaneous pericardiocentesis should be avoided except in a dire emergency such as imminent cardiac arrest. Serious complications of pericardiocentesis include myocardial perforation, coronary artery laceration, pneumothorax, and puncture of upper abdominal organs.

When an acute tamponade is not amenable to pericardiocentesis, urgent surgical drainage via a subcostal approach is an option. When managing tamponade it is important to note that anesthesia and positive pressure ventilation can further compromise cardiac function. Recurrent episodes of tamponade can be treated by the creation of a surgical pericardial window or via closed balloon pericardotomy.

A special problem is tamponade following cardiothoracic surgery and is an indication for urgent mediastinal reexploration. On occasion emergency sternotomy is indicated in the ICU.

AORTIC DISSECTION

Aortic dissection is demonstrated in less than 1% of autopsy cases and accounts for fewer than 1 in 10,000 admissions to hospital. However, it has a high associated untreated mortality.

Predisposing Factors
Chronic systemic hypertension is a major predisposing factor (Box 33.7). Aortic dissection is more common in men and rare in the young. Mechanisms that predispose to aortic wall weakening and stress can lead to aortic dissection. These include inherited, congenital, and acquired inflammatory conditions. Cocaine use is thought to cause dissection by causing rapid elevation of blood pressure. Aortic dissection can also occur following clinical procedures involving the aorta. There is a possible association with pregnancy.

Pathogenesis
It is thought that in nontraumatic cases of aortic dissection a common underlying theme is damage to or degeneration of the medial layer of the aortic wall, predisposing to separation of wall layers. Classically aortic dissections are described as having an intimal flap through which blood enters the media of the aortic wall, creating a false lumen. The false lumen can propagate in both a retrograde and anterograde direction. As it spreads, it may compromise branch vessels, cause aortic insufficiency, or rupture.

The tear occurs at sites of greatest mechanical stress and pressure fluctuation. These include the proximal ascending aorta and the proximal descending aorta just beyond the origin of the left subclavian artery. Studies have shown that dP/dt (rate of pressure change) is of importance in the propagation of dissection. Aortic atherosclerosis is not a risk factor for classic aortic

---

Box 33.7 Aortic Dissection: Predisposing Factors

Age
Male sex
Chronic systemic hypertension
Hereditary connective tissue disorder
    Marfan syndrome, Ehlers-Danlos syndrome, annuloaortic ectasia
Congenital abnormalities of the aorta
    Bicuspid aortic valve, coarctation of the aorta, aortic arch hypoplasia
Syndromic
    Turner's syndrome, Noonan's syndrome
Inflammatory conditions
    Syphilis/giant cell arteritis, Takayasu arteritis, Behçet's disease
Trauma (deceleration injuries)
Iatrogenic
    Cardiac surgery, cardiac catheterization, IABP use
Cocaine use

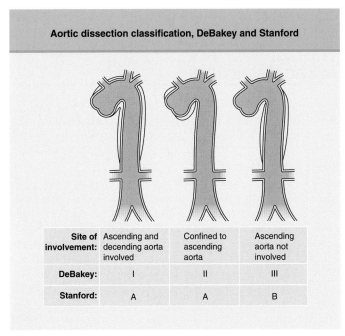

Aortic dissection classification, DeBakey and Stanford

Site of involvement:	Ascending and decending aorta involved	Confined to ascending aorta	Ascending aorta not involved
DeBakey:	I	II	III
Stanford:	A	A	B

Figure 33.8. Schematic drawing of aortic dissection classification according to DeBakey and Stanford. The Stanford system grades all dissections involving the ascending aorta as type A regardless of entry site location.

dissection, and the typical distribution of atherosclerotic plaques does not correspond to the most common sites of intimal flaps.

Alternative mechanisms have been proposed to explain the existence of aortic dissections without intimal flaps. Intramural hemorrhages are believed to result from bleeding into the media from the vasa vasorum. The hemorrhage can then rupture into the aortic lumen. An alternative mechanism is the development of penetrating atherosclerotic ulcers. These occur predominantly in the descending thoracic and abdominal aortas and rarely extend or lead to complications of branch vessel involvement.

Classification
Classification of aortic dissections is based on the site and extent of involvement, which has therapeutic implications. There are two established classification systems. The DeBakey classification describes three types of dissection, and the Stanford classification recognizes two. Both systems differentiate ascending from nonascending aortic involvement (Fig. 33.8). A further classification system was proposed by the European Society of Cardiology Task Force on Aortic Dissection in 2001. This system encompasses five classes of dissection describing the different proposed underlying mechanisms.

Aortic dissection is also classified as acute or chronic. Chronic dissection is defined if the presentation is two or more weeks following the acute event. It is an important milestone, since mortality associated with untreated aortic dissection begins to plateau around this time.

Clinical Features
The majority of patients with acute aortic dissection complain of pain, which is typically sudden and maximal at the time of

onset. The patient may describe it as sharp or tearing in nature. Pain may be limited to the anterior chest, may radiate to the posterior chest, or may involve only the interscapular region, back, or abdomen. The site of pain can change with extension of the dissection. The return of pain after subsidence may indicate impending rupture.

Functional aortic regurgitation (AR) can result from dilatation of the annulus or root, dissection involvement of the annulus or valves, cusp displacement due to pressure from the false lumen, or the presence of an intimal flap at this site interfering with normal opening and closing. A pericardial effusion may result from transudation of fluid or from rupture of blood into the pleural cavity. Tamponade may be rapidly fatal. Coronary arteries, frequently the right, may be involved in the dissection and lead to myocardial ischemia and infarction.

The function of other organ systems may be compromised by ischemia or direct compression from blood either contained within the dilated aortic serosa or after leakage into a confined space.

Neurologic complications include cerebral ischemia and stroke, altered mental status, and syncope. Spinal cord infarction can occur, and peripheral nerve involvement may manifest as paresthesias, Horner syndrome (if there is involvement of the superior cervical sympathetic ganglion), or hoarse voice (from compression of the left recurrent laryngeal nerve).

The dissection may involve the renal arteries and can result in oligoanuria. Similarly, mesenteric ischemia may be due to involvement of mesenteric vessels. Syncope may be due to pain, cardiac tamponade, aortic baroreceptor involvement, or cerebral vessel involvement.

Physical Findings
In cases of aortic dissection, blood pressure is typically high unless complicated by severe AR, tamponade, aortic rupture, or myocardial ischemia. Blood pressure may be asymmetric in the upper limbs. These findings can be transient. A pleural effusion (usually left sided) may be detectable clinically. It may be reactive or be due to a hemothorax. Other physical findings depend on organ system involvement.

Diagnosis
ECG may be normal or demonstrate nonspecific ST segment or T-wave abnormalities. ECG criteria for LVH are common. If the coronary ostium is involved, changes due to ischemia or infarction may be apparent. Acute coronary syndrome and MI are important differential diagnoses and can coexist with aortic dissection. Thrombolytic therapy is withheld in cases in which this is suspected.

No features on a plain chest radiograph are diagnostic, and it may be normal, especially when only the proximal ascending aorta is involved. The most common abnormality is widening of the superior mediastinum, which is nonspecific. Other abnormalities include haziness of the aortic knob, irregular aortic shadow, and right side shift of trachea. Intimal calcium may be separated from the outer contour of the descending aorta by more than 5 mm. Evidence of pericardial and pleural effusions may also be visible on plain film.

The choice of imaging depends on availability, local expertise, the information the test can provide, and urgency. More than

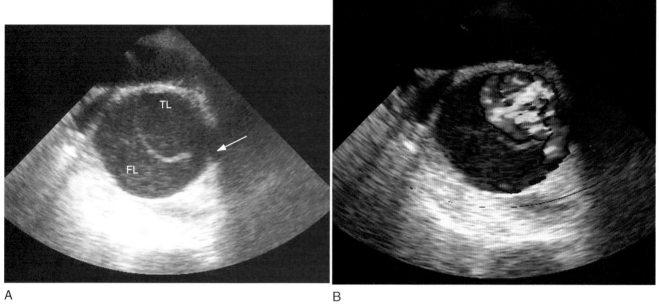

A B

Figure 33.9. Cross-sectional transesophageal echo view of aortic dissection in descending aorta. *A,* The intimal flap is clearly visible separating the false and true lumina. The arrow marks the site of communication. *B,* Color Doppler demonstrates flow into the false lumen. FL, false lumen; TL, true lumen.

one imaging modality may be required to gain the necessary information.

Diagnostic Imaging Modalities

Adequate transthoracic echocardiographic visualization can be impeded by chest wall deformities, obesity, emphysema, and mechanical ventilation. Transesophageal echocardiography (Fig. 33.9) is limited by operator experience and cannot visualize the entire descending aorta. In severely compromised patients, TOE may be the only diagnostic imaging procedure, performed in the operating theater immediately before surgery.

Computerized axial tomography (CT) is a rapid test in comparison with MRI and aortography and has a sensitivity of greater than 90% and specificity of greater than 85%. However, detailed views of the aortic valve are not possible, and tears may not be detected. Furthermore, radiocontrast material is required, which may worsen renal function.

Magnetic resonance imaging (MRI) provides high-quality images and has very high sensitivity and specificity. Scanning time is prolonged, making it less attractive in the context of hemodynamic instability. Its availability is limited. Its value as a follow-up test is greater than for diagnosis.

Angiography is invasive and requires the use of contrast media. It may fail to demonstrate noncommunicating dissections and where flow is slow in the false lumen. Entry and reentry sites may not be identified.

Management

The aim of medical therapy is to lower systemic blood pressure, reducing shear stress in the aortic wall. A target systolic blood pressure of 100 can be set but titrated to avoid compromise of perfusion of vital organs such as brain and heart (and kidneys). Adequate opiate analgesia is important.

β-Blockers are suitable first-line antihypertensives. They can be used in combination with vasodilators such as sodium nitroprusside. Labetalol is an alternative to this combination. If β-blockers are contraindicated, verapamil or diltiazem can be administered. Arterial pressure should be monitored invasively, particularly during transfer to a cardiothoracic center.

Surgery is indicated in Stanford type A dissection (DeBakey I and II). The aim of surgery is to prevent aortic rupture and tamponade and treat aortic insufficiency. A limited portion of the ascending aorta is resected, preferably including the intimal tear. In selected cases, the aortic arch is included in the repair. When possible the aortic valve leaflets are spared and resuspended, but this can be technically difficult in an emergency. In a previously ectatic aorta, such as in Marfan syndrome, a composite graft is usually used, incorporating tube graft and prosthetic valve.

Dissection limited to the descending aorta (type B or III) is usually treated medically. Indications for surgery include dissection extension during medical treatment, suspicion of impending rupture, intractable pain, and major branch artery occlusion. The latter complication may be amenable to percutaneous intervention.

Endovascular therapies are increasingly employed and include stent placement and balloon fenestration procedures. Their role continues to be investigated and is not fully defined. Balloon fenestration is the creation of a tear between the false and true lumina. It can be used to connect the true lumen with a dead-end false lumen with the aim of preventing thrombosis where the false lumen is supplying blood to an important branch artery. It can be used in combination with aortic stents in the treatment of dynamic obstruction to major side branches. Aortic stents can also be deployed to cover entry tears and enlarge the compressed true aortic lumen and may reduce propagation of

367

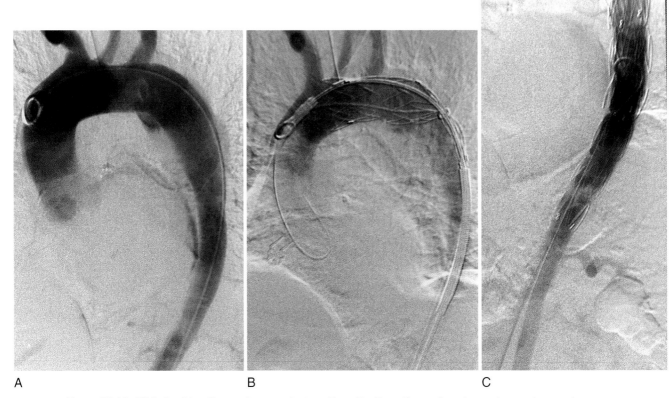

A   B   C

Figure 33.10. Digital subtraction angiogram of a type B aortic dissection undergoing endovascular repair.
A, Dissection present in descending aorta. *B*, Deployment of stent. *C*, Stent positioned over tear.

dissection (Fig. 33.10). Static obstruction from propagation of the dissection into a branch artery is treated by branch vessel stenting.

Prognosis

The International Registry of Aortic Dissection found in-hospital mortality of surgically treated type A dissection to be 26% (and 58% in those not treated surgically). High mortality (31%) also occurred in surgically treated type B dissection, which is likely to be a reflection of the complications leading to surgery. Lowest mortality was found in medically treated type B dissection (10.7%). Common causes of death for both dissection types included aortic rupture and visceral ischemia. Cardiac tamponade also contributed to mortality in type A dissection.

Survivors of aortic dissection require close long-term follow-up, since the risk of dissection, aneurysmal dilatation, and rupture persist.

SUGGESTED READING

Bonow RO, Carobello D, de Leon AC, et al: ACC/AHA guidelines for the management of patients with valvular heart disease. J Am Coll Cardiol 1998;32:1486–1488.

Crenshaw BS, Granger CB, Birnbaum Y, et al: Risk factors, angiographic patterns and outcomes in patients with ventricular septal defect compli-cating acute myocardial infarction. GUSTO-I (global utilisation of streptokinase and T-PA for occluded coronary arteries). Circulation 2000;101:27–32.

Erbel R, Alfonso F, Boileau C, et al: Diagnosis and management of aortic dissection. Recommendations of the Task Force on Aortic Dissection, European Society of Cardiology. Eur Heart J 2001;22:1642–1681.

Ferguson JJ III, Cohen M, Freedman RJ Jr, et al: The current practice of intra-aortic balloon counterpulsation: results from the Benchmark Registry. J Am Coll Cardiol 2001;38:1456–1462.

Hagan PG, Nienaber CA, Isselbacher EM, et al: The International Registry of Aortic Dissection (IRAD): new insights into an old disease. JAMA 2000;283:897–903.

Hasdai D, Berger PB, Battler A, et al (eds): Cardiogenic Shock: Diagnosis and Treatment. Contemporary Cardiology series. Totowa, NJ: Humana Press; 2002.

Leprince P, Combes A, Bonnet N, et al: Circulatory support for fulminant myocarditis: consideration for implantation, weaning and explantation. Eur J Cardiothorac Surg 2003;24:399–403.

Menon V, Webb JG, Hilis LD, et al: Outcome and profile of ventricular septal rupture with cardiogenic shock after myocardial infarction: a report from the SHOCK trial registry. J Am Coll Cardiol 2000;36:11110–11116.

Sanborn TA, Sleeper LA, Jacobs AK, et al: Impact of thrombolysis, intra-aortic balloon counterpulsation and their combination in cardiogenic shock complicating acute myocardial infarction: a report form the SHOCK Trial Registry. Should we emergently revascularise occluded coronaries in cardiogenic shock? J Am Coll Cardiol 2000;36 (3 suppl A):1123–1129.

Spodick DH: Acute cardiac tamponade. N Engl J Med 2003;349:684–690.

KEY POINTS

- Intubation and mechanical ventilation, when adjusted to the metabolic demands of the patient, will decrease the work of breathing, resulting in increased O_2 delivery to vital organs and decreased serum lactic acid levels.
- An important factor central to understanding heart–lung interactions is the relation between airway pressure (Paw) and intrathoracic pressure (ITP), the transpulmonary pressure.
- Assuming some constant fraction of Paw transmission to the pleural surface as a means of calculating the effect of increasing Paw on ITP is inaccurate and potentially dangerous if used to assess transmural intrathoracic vascular pressures.
- Changing lung volume changes pulmonary vascular resistance, but the reasons for these changes are complex, often conflicting, and reflect both humoral and mechanical interactions.
- Increases in lung volume progressively increase alveolar vessel resistance, becoming measurable above normal functional residual capacity.
- Hyperinflation can create significant pulmonary hypertension and may precipitate acute right ventricular failure (acute cor pulmonale) and right ventricular ischemia.

Heart–lung interactions include the effect of the circulation on ventilation and the effect of ventilation on circulation. However, most references to heart–lung interactions usually refer to the effect of ventilation on the circulation. Still, cardiovascular dysfunction alters ventilation.

EFFECTS OF CARDIOVASCULAR DYSFUNCTION ON VENTILATION

Cardiogenic shock can induce secondary, or hydrostatic, pulmonary edema, impairing gas exchange by reducing the number of aerated alveolar units available for gas exchange. Also, circulatory shock by limiting blood flow to the respiratory muscles can induce respiratory muscle failure and respiratory arrest independent of any effect of the circulation on pulmonary edema formation. These interactions are usually discussed within the framework of traditional determinants of cardiovascular performance: contractility, preload, afterload, vasomotor tone, circulating blood volume, and perfusion pressure. However, a fundamental aspect of ventilation is that it is exercise, and like any form of exercise, it must place a certain metabolic demand on the cardiovascular system. If cardiovascular reserve is limited or compromised, it may not be able to increase O_2 delivery needed to meet the increased metabolic activity associated with spontaneous ventilation. Accordingly, subjects with cardiovascular insufficiency may not be able to breathe spontaneously because the metabolic demand is too great. Importantly, failure to wean from mechanical ventilation often reflects cardiovascular insufficiency and may not be identifiable beforehand by measures of the work cost of breathing, such as airway resistance, airflow obstruction, thoracic system compliance, or Vaseline cardiovascular status on mechanical ventilatory support because at those times the increased workload of breathing is not present.

Spontaneous ventilation requires respiratory muscle contraction. Blood flow to the respiratory muscles comes from several arterial circuits whose absolute flow is believed to exceed the highest metabolic demand of maximally exercising skeletal muscle. Thus, under conditions of normal cardiovascular conditions, blood flow is not the limiting factor determining maximal ventilatory effort. Although ventilation normally requires less than 5% of total O_2 delivery to meet its demand, in lung disease states in which the work of breathing is increased, such as pulmonary edema or bronchospasm, the work cost of breathing can increase O_2 demand to 25% of total O_2 consumption. If cardiac output is limited, blood flow to all organs, and specifically to the respiratory muscles, may be compromised, inducing both tissue hypoperfusion and lactic acidosis. Finally, if cardiac output is severely limited, respiratory muscle failure develops despite high central neuronal drive, such that many heart failure patients die a respiratory death prior to cardiovascular standstill. Supporting ventilation externally by the use of mechanical ventilation will reduce metabolic demand, increasing SvO_2 for a constant cardiac output and CaO_2. Intubation and mechanical ventilation, when adjusted to the metabolic demands of the patient, will decrease the work of breathing, resulting in increased O_2 delivery to other vital organs and decreased serum lactic acid levels. These cardiovascular benefits can also be realized with the effective use of noninvasive ventilation mask continuous positive airway pressure (CPAP). If O_2 demand decreases, then SvO_2 will increase, resulting in an increase in PaO_2 if fixed right-to-left shunts exist, even if mechanical ventilation does not alter the ratio of shunt blood flow to cardiac output.

Ventilator-dependent patients who fail to wean may have impaired baseline cardiovascular performance that is readily apparent, but routinely patients develop overt signs of heart

Effect of a spontaneous breathing trial on pulmonary artery occlusion pressure and esophageal pressure in a patient failing to wean

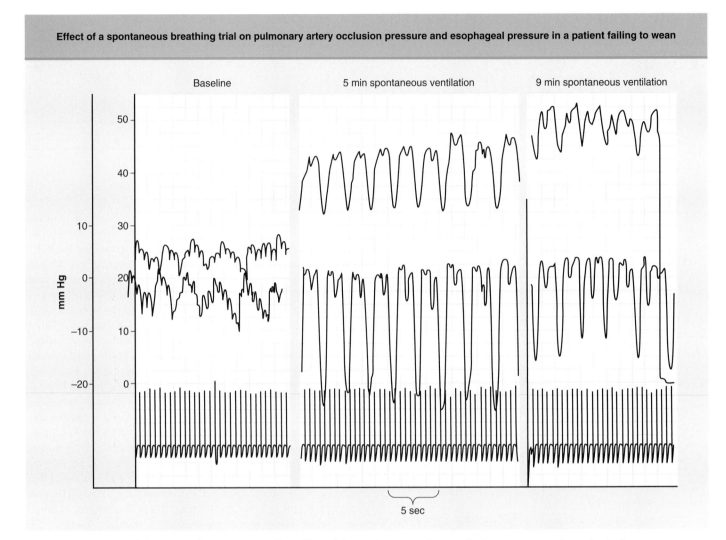

Figure 34.1. Effect of a spontaneous breathing trial on pulmonary artery occlusion pressure and esophageal pressure in a patient failing to wean. Effect of spontaneous ventilation (SV) on esophageal pressure (Peso), as a marker of intrathoracic pressure (ITP), and pulmonary artery occlusion pressure (Ppao) in a patient who rapidly deteriorates during a spontaneous breathing trial. (Reproduced with permission from LeMaire F, Teboul JK, Cinotti L, et al: Acute left ventricle dysfunction during unsuccessful weaning from mechanical ventilation. Anesthesiology 1988;69:171–179.)

failure during weaning, such as pulmonary edema, myocardial ischemia tachycardia, and gut ischemia. Figure 34.1 describes one subject who rapidly deteriorated during a spontaneous breathing trial. Note that pulmonary artery occlusion pressure rose to nonphysiological levels within 5 minutes of instituting weaning. Although all subjects increase their cardiac outputs in response to a weaning trial, those who subsequently fail to wean demonstrate a reduction in mixed venous O_2 saturation, consistent with a failing cardiovascular response to an increased metabolic demand (Jabran and colleagues, 1998). Weaning from mechanical ventilatory support can be considered a cardiovascular stress test. Again, investigators have documented weaning-associated ECG and thallium cardiac blood flow scan-related signs of ischemia in both subjects with known coronary artery disease and in otherwise normal patients. Using this same logic, placing patients with severe heart failure and/or ischemia on ventilatory support by either intubation and ventilation

(Rasanen and associates, 1984) or noninvasive CPAP can reverse myocardial ischemia. Importantly, the increased work of breathing may come from the endotracheal tube flow resistance. Thus, some subjects who fail a spontaneous breathing trial may actually be able to breathe on their own if extubated.

HEMODYNAMIC EFFECTS OF VENTILATION AND VENTILATORY MANEUVERS

Ventilation can profoundly stress cardiovascular function dependent on myocardial reserve, circulating blood volume, blood flow distribution, autonomic tone, endocrinological responses, lung volume, intrathoracic pressure (ITP), and the surrounding pressures for the remainder of the circulation. This understanding has been described since mechanical ventilation was introduced in the 1940s and still results in new perspectives today. An important factor central to understanding heart–lung interactions is the relation between airway pressure (Paw) and ITP, the transpulmonary pressure. Airway pressure, as an estimate of alveolar pressure, is relatively easy to measure, whereas ITP is not.

Increases in Paw do not necessarily equate to proportional increases in ITP. The primary determinants of the hemodynamic responses to ventilation are due to changes in ITP and lung volume, not Paw. The relation between Paw, ITP, pericardial pressure (Ppc), and lung volume varies with spontaneous ventilatory effort and lung and chest wall compliance. Only lung and thoracic compliance determine the relation between end-expiratory Paw and lung volume in the sedated and paralyzed patient. However, if a ventilated patient actively resists lung inflation or sustains expiratory muscle activity at end inspiration, then end-inspiratory Paw will exceed resting Paw for that lung volume. Similarly, if the patient activity prevents full exhalation by expiratory breaking, then for the same end-expiratory Paw, lung volume may be much higher than predicted from end-expiratory Paw values alone. The difference between measured Paw and alveolar pressure is called intrinsic positive end-expiratory pressure (PEEP). Finally, even if inspiration is passive and no increased airway resistance is present, Paw may rapidly increase over minutes as chest wall compliance decreases. During inspiration, positive pressure Paw increases as a function of both total thoracic compliance and airway resistance. Subjects with marked bronchospasm will display a peak Paw greater than end-inspiratory (plateau) Paw.

Lung expansion during positive pressure inspiration pushes on the surrounding structures, distorting them and causing their surface pressures to increase, thus increasing lateral wall, diaphragmatic, and juxtacardiac pleural pressure (Ppl), as well as Ppc. The degree of increase in each of these surface pressures will be a function of the compliance and inertance of their opposing structures. Changes in Ppl induced by positive pressure inflation are different among lung regions (Fig. 34.2). Pleural pressure on the diaphragm increases least during inspiration and juxtacardiac P_{pl} increases most, presumably because the diaphragm is very compliant, whereas mediastinal contents are not. However, if abdominal distention develops, then the diaphragm will become relatively noncompliance and ITP will increase similarly across the entire thorax. Increasing Paw to overcome chest wall stiffness (abdominal distention) in secondary acute respiratory distress syndrome (ARDS) should increase ITP more, giving greater hemodynamic consequences, but should not improve gas exchange since the alveoli are not damaged. If lung compliance is reduced, as in primary ARDS, then for a similar increase in Paw ITP will increase less, creating less hemodynamic effects but also recruiting more collapsed and injured alveolar units, improving gas exchange.

A hydrostatic pressure gradient exists in the pleural space. Dependent regions have a higher baseline pressure than nondependent regions in proportion to their height above or below the heart in centimeters and equate to an equal cm H_2O pressure difference. In the supine subject, steady-state apneic Ppl along the horizontal plane from apex to diaphragm are similar, whereas anterior Ppl is less and posterior gutter Ppl is greater (Fig. 34.3).

Since the heart is fixed within a cardiac fossa, juxtacardiac Ppl increases more than lateral chest wall or diaphragmatic P_{pl}. Ppc and ITP may not be similar nor increase by similar amounts with the application of positive Paw, if the pericardium acts as a limiting membrane. With pericardial restraint, Ppc will exceed juxtacardiac Ppl. Pinsky and Guimond demonstrated in a canine model that the induction of heart failure was associated with a greater increase in Ppc than juxtacardiac Ppl, presumably because of pericardial restraint (Fig. 34.4). With progressive increases in PEEP, juxtacardiac Ppl increased toward Ppc levels, whereas Ppc initially remained constant. Once these two surface pressures became equal, further increases in PEEP increased both juxtacardiac Ppl and Ppc in parallel. Thus, if pericardial volume restraint exists, then juxtacardiac Ppl will underestimate Ppc. However, with sustained lung compression of the heart, the increase in juxtacardiac Ppl will override tamponade, such that juxtacardiac Ppl and Ppc will become similar as cardiac volumes decrease.

The interaction of Paw, lung volume, and ITP in the setting of lung disease is complex and can be different for the same pathologic setting depending on the tidal volume, inspiratory flow rate, ventilatory frequency, and body position. The presence of parenchymal disease, airflow obstruction, and extrapulmonary processes that directly alter chest wall–diaphragmatic contraction also profoundly alter these interactions. Static lung expansion occurs as Paw increases because the transpulmonary pressure (Paw relative to ITP) increases. If lung injury induces alveolar flooding or increased pulmonary parenchymal stiffness, then greater increases in Paw will be required to distend the lungs to a constant end-inspiratory volume. Romand and coworkers demonstrated that although Paw increased more during acute lung injury (ALI) than in control conditions for a constant tidal volume, both lateral chest wall Ppl and Ppc increased similarly between both conditions if tidal volume was held constant (Fig. 34.5). The primary determinant of the increase in Ppl and Ppc during positive pressure ventilation is lung volume change, not Paw change.

Since the distribution of alveolar collapse and lung compliance in ALI is nonhomogeneous, lung distention during positive pressure ventilation must reflect overdistention of some regions of the lung at the expense of noncompliant or poorly compliant regions. Accordingly, Paw will reflect lung distention of lung units that were aerated prior to inspiration but may not reflect the degree of lung inflation of nonaerated lung units. Pressure-limited ventilation assumes that this is the case and aims to limit Paw in ALI states so as to prevent overdistention of aerated lung units, with the understanding that tidal volume, and thus minute ventilation, must decrease. Thus, pressure-limited ventilation will hypoventilate the lungs, leading to "permissive" hypercapnia. It is not surprising, therefore, that in an animal model of ALI, in which tidal volume was reduced to match preinjury plateau Paw (pressure-limited ventilation), both Ppl and Ppc increased less compared to both prelung injury states or in ALI when tidal volume remained at preinjury levels. These points underlie the fundamental hemodynamic differences seen when different modes of mechanical ventilatory support are compared to each other.

As stated previously, because ALI is often nonhomogeneous, with aerated areas of the lung displaying normal specific compliance, increases in Paw above approximately 30 cm H_2O will overdistend these aerated lung units. Vascular structures that are distended will have a greater increase in their surrounding pressure than collapsible structures that do not distend. However, Romand and colleagues and Scharf and Ingram demonstrated

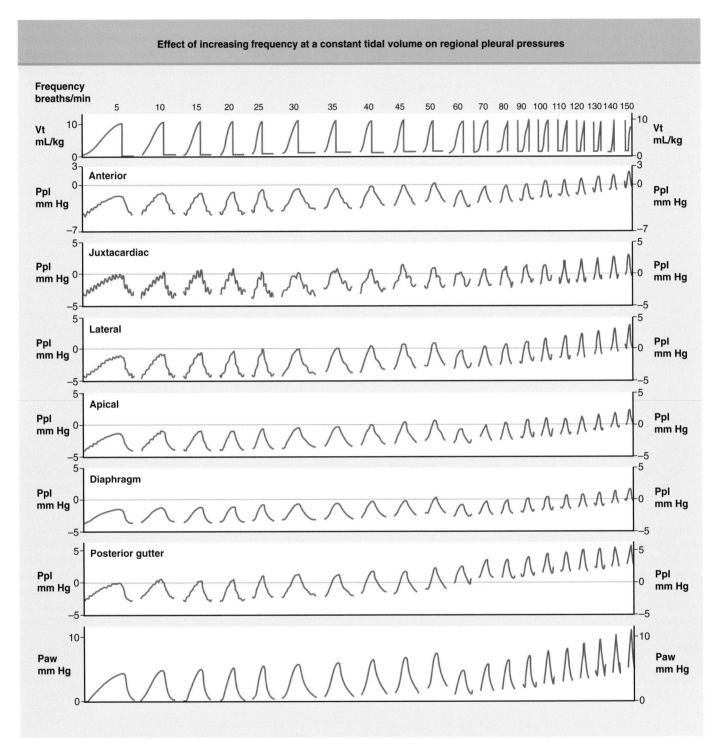

Figure 34.2. Effect of increasing frequency at a constant tidal volume on regional pleural pressures. Effect of increasing ventilatory frequency on regional pleural pressure (Ppl) changes in the lung of an intact dog. Ppl (mean ± SE) in Torr for six pleural regions of the right hemithorax of an intact supine canine model. (Reproduced with permission from Novak R, Matuschak GM, Pinsky MR: Effect of positive-pressure ventilatory frequency on regional pleural pressure. J Appl Physiol 1995;65:1314–1323.)

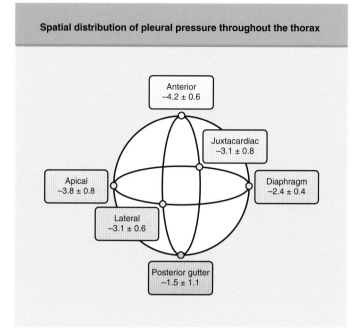

Figure 34.3. Spatial distribution of pleural pressure throughout the thorax. Apneic pleural pressure (Ppl) (mean ± SE) in Torr for six pleural regions of the right hemithorax of an intact supine canine model. (Reproduced with permission from Novak R, Matuschak GM, Pinsky MR: Effect of positive-pressure ventilatory frequency on regional pleural pressure. J Appl Physiol. 1995;65:1314–1323.)

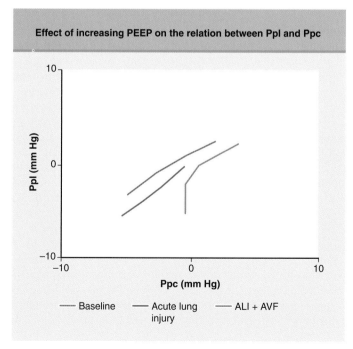

Figure 34.4. Effect of increasing PEEP on the relation between Ppl and Ppc. Relation between pericardial pressure (Ppc) and juxtacardiac pleural pressure (Ppl) as PEEP is progressively increased under conditions of normal cardiac function, oleic acid-induced acute lung injury (ALI), and ALI plus propranolol-induced acute ventricular failure (ALI + AVF) in an intact canine model. Data represent the mean of six animals. (After Pinsky MR, Guimond JG: Effects of positive-pressure on heart–lung interactions. J Crit Care. 1991;6:1–11.)

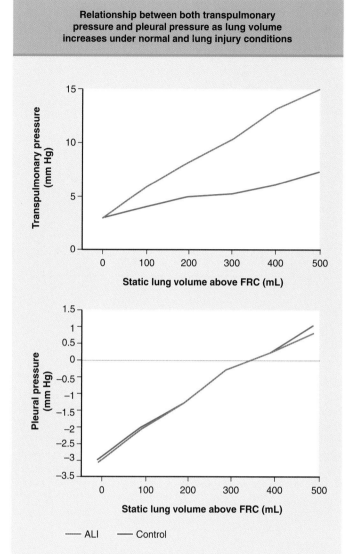

Figure 34.5. Relationship between both transpulmonary pressure and pleural pressure as lung volume increases under normal and lung injury conditions. Relation between airway pressure (Paw) and tidal volume (V_T) and between pleural pressure (Ppl) and V_T in control and oleic acid-induced acute lung injury (ALI) conditions in a canine model. Note that despite greater increases in Paw for the same V_T during ALI compared to control conditions, Ppl and Ppc increase similarly during both control and ALI conditions for the same increase in V_T. (Reproduced with permission from Romand JA, Shi W, Pinsky MR: Cardiopulmonary effects of positive pressure ventilation during acute lung injury. Chest 1995;108:1041–1048.)

that despite this nonhomogeneous alveolar distention, if tidal volume is kept constant, then Ppl will increase equally, independent of the mechanical properties of the lung. Thus, under constant tidal volume conditions, changes in peak and mean Paw will reflect changes in the mechanical properties of the lungs and patient coordination but may not reflect changes in ITP. Similarly, these changes in Paw may not alter global cardiovascular dynamics. Underscoring this limitation of Paw to reflect either ITP or Ppc, Pinsky and colleagues (1983) demonstrated in postoperative patients that the percentage of Paw increase that will

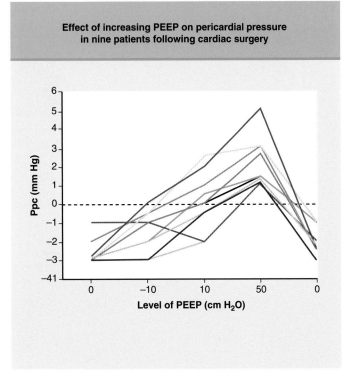

Figure 34.6. Effect of increasing PEEP on pericardial pressure in nine patients following cardiac surgery. Relation between pericardial pressure (Ppc) and airway pressure as apneic levels of PEEP were progressively increased from zero to 15 cm H₂O and then back to zero in 5 cm H₂O increments in patients immediately following open heart surgery. (Reproduced with permission from Pinsky MR, Vincent JL, DeSinet JM: Estimating left ventricular filling pressure during positive end-expiratory pressure in humans. Am Rev Respir Dis 1991;143:25–31.)

intrathoracic vascular pressures by calculating the airway pressure transmission index to the pleural space or by briefly removing PEEP while these pressures are directly measured is reviewed elsewhere.

HEMODYNAMIC EFFECTS OF VENTILATION

Heart–lung interactions can be grouped into interactions that involve three basic concepts that usually coexist. First, as described previously, spontaneous ventilatory efforts are exercise: They require O_2 and blood flow, thus placing demands on cardiac output and producing CO_2, adding additional ventilatory stress on CO_2 excretion. Second, inspiration increases lung volume above resting end-expiratory volume. Thus, some of the hemodynamic effects of ventilation are due to changes in lung volume and chest wall expansion. Third, spontaneous inspiration decreases ITP, whereas positive pressure ventilation increases ITP; thus, the differences between spontaneous ventilation and positive pressure ventilation primarily reflect the differences in ITP swings and the energy necessary to produce them.

Hemodynamic Effects of Changes in Lung Volume
Changing lung volume, whether induced passively by positive pressure ventilation or volitionally during spontaneous ventilation, alters autonomic tone and pulmonary vascular resistance, and at high lung volumes the enlarged lungs compress the heart in the cardiac fossa, limiting absolute cardiac volumes analogous to cardiac tamponade. However, unlike cardiac tamponade, in which Ppc selectively increases in excess of Ppl, with hyperinflation both juxtacardiac Ppl and Ppc increase together.

Autonomic Tone
The lungs are richly enervated with integrated somatic and autonomic fibers that originate, traverse through, and end in the thorax. These neuronal networks mediate multiple homeostatic processes through the autonomic nervous system that alter both instantaneous cardiovascular function and steady-state cardiovascular status. Inflation induces immediate changes in autonomic output. Inflation chronotropic responses act through vagal-mediated reflex arcs. Lung inflation to normal tidal volumes (<10 mL/kg) induces withdrawal of basal parasympathetic tone and increases heart rate. This inspiration-induced cardioacceleration, referred to as respiratory sinus arrhythmia, is used to document normal autonomic control, especially in diabetics with peripheral neuropathy. However, inflation to larger tidal volumes (>15 mL/kg) decreases heart rate by a combination of both increased vagal tone and sympathetic withdrawal. The sympathetic withdrawal also creates arterial vasodilation (Shepherd, 1981). This inflation–vasodilatation response has been shown to induce expiration-associated reductions in left ventricular (LV) contractility in healthy volunteers and ventilator-dependent patients with the initiation of high-frequency ventilation or hyperinflation (Shepherd, 1981). Humeral factors, including compounds blocked by cyclooxygenase inhibition, released from pulmonary endothelial cells during lung inflation may also induce this depressor response. However, these interactions do not appear to grossly alter cardiovascular status. Although overdistention of aerated lung units in patients with ALI may induce such cardiovascular depression, unilateral lung hyperinflation (unilateral PEEP) does not appear

be transmitted to the pericardial surface is not constant from one subject to the next as PEEP is increased (Fig. 34.6). Thus, one cannot predict the amount of change in ITP or Ppc that will occur in patients as PEEP is varied. Accordingly, assuming some constant fraction of Paw transmission to the pleural surface as a means of calculating the effect of increasing Paw on ITP is inaccurate and potentially dangerous if used to assess transmural intrathoracic vascular pressures.

Although it may be difficult to determine the actual Ppl, it is possible to determine the ventilation-induced change in Ppl. Since if lung volume does not change, transpulmonary pressure is constant, during airway occlusion strain maneuvers the change in ITP is equal to the change in Paw (Buda and associates, 1979). Furthermore, esophageal pressure is often used to estimate swings in both Ppl and Ppc during ventilation. Although esophageal pressure is accurate at reflecting negative swings in Ppl during spontaneous inspiration in upright seated individuals and in recumbent dogs in the left lateral position, esophageal pressure changes underestimate both the positive swings in Ppl and the mean increase in Ppl seen with increases in lung volume during positive pressure ventilation and in the supine position. During Müller and Valsalva maneuvers, however, because lung volume does not change, swings in esophageal pressure will accurately reflect swings in ITP. The ability to measure on-PEEP

to influence systemic hemodynamics. Thus, these cardio-vascular effects are of uncertain clinical significance.

Ventilation also alters control of intravascular fluid balance via hormonal release. The right atrium functions as the body's effective circulating blood volume sensor. Both positive pressure ventilation and sustained hyperinflation decrease right atrial stretch, stimulating endocrinological responses that induce fluid retention. Plasma norepinephrine, plasma rennin activity, and atrial natriuretic peptide increase during positive pressure ventilation because of right atrial collapse. Interestingly, when subjects with congestive heart failure (CHF) are given nasal CPAP, plasma atrial natriuretic peptide activity decreases in parallel with improvements in blood flow, suggesting that some of the observed benefit of CPAP therapy in heart failure patients is mediated, in part, through humoral mechanisms.

Right Ventricular Afterload and Pulmonary Vascular Resistance

Right ventricular (RV) ejection is very sensitive to changes in ejection pressure, and sudden increases in pulmonary vascular resistance can induce cardiovascular collapse. Changing lung volume changes pulmonary vascular resistance. The reasons for these changes are often complex, often conflicting, and reflect both humoral and mechanical interactions. Increasing lung volume occurs due to increasing transpulmonary pressure. Transpulmonary pressure is the pressure difference between alveolar pressure and ITP. Thus, occlusion respiratory strain maneuvers, such as a Valsalva maneuver (positive ITP) or obstructive inspiratory efforts (Müller maneuver), do not alter pulmonary vascular resistance. Although obstructive inspiratory efforts, such as occur during obstructive sleep apnea, are usually associated with increased RV afterload, the increased afterload is due primarily to either increased vasomotor tone (hypoxic pulmonary vasoconstriction) or backward LV failure.

RV afterload can be defined as the maximal RV systolic wall stress during contraction, which is determined by the maximal product of the RV free wall radius of curvature (a function of end-diastolic volume) and transmural pressure (a function of systolic RV pressure) during ejection. Systolic RV pressure equals transmural pulmonary artery pressure. Increases in transmural Ppa impede RV ejection, decreasing RV stroke volume (Pinksy, 1984) and inducing RV dilation and passive impedance to venous return. If not relieved quickly, acute cor pulmonale rapidly develops. Furthermore, if RV dilation and RV pressure overload persist, RV free wall ischemia and infarction can develop. Importantly, rapid fluid challenges in the setting of acute cor pulmonale can precipitate profound cardiovascular collapse due to excessive RV dilation, RV ischemia, and compromised LV filling.

During normoxic conditions ($Pao_2 > 65$ mm Hg) and with the application of low levels of PEEP (<7.5 cm H_2O), transmural pulmonary artery pressure increases minimally at end inspiration of a mechanical breath. If these slight increases in transmural Ppa are sustained, however, fluid retention occurs either by intrinsic humeral mechanisms (increased atrial natriuretic peptide secretion) or by iatrogenic intravascular volume infusion necessary to sustain cardiac output. Transmural pulmonary artery pressure can increase without an increase in pulmonary vasomotor tonc if blood flow increases, as during exercise, or if left atrial pressure increases due to LV failure. Although both of these conditions are often present during spontaneous ventilation, usually during instantaneous positive pressure ventilation neither cardiac output nor LV filling increase (Buda and colleagues, 1979). Thus, any increase in transmural pulmonary artery pressure seen during positive pressure ventilation is usually due to an increase in pulmonary vascular resistance.

Hypoxic Pulmonary Vasoconstriction

Unlike systemic vascular beds that dilate in the setting of tissue hypoxia, pulmonary vasculature constricts. If alveolar PO_2 (PAo_2) decreases below 60 mm Hg, local pulmonary vasomotor tone increases, reducing blood flow to those alveoli. This process of hypoxic pulmonary vasoconstriction is mediated, in part, by variations in the synthesis and release of nitric oxide by endothelial nitric oxide synthase localized on pulmonary vascular endothelial cells. The pulmonary endothelium normally synthesizes a low basal amount of nitric oxide, keeping the pulmonary vasculature actively vasodilated. Loss of nitric oxide allows the smooth muscle to return to its normal resting vasomotor tone. Nitric oxide synthesis is dependent on adequate amounts of O_2 and is inhibited by both hypoxia and acidosis. Hypoxic pulmonary vasoconstriction, by reducing pulmonary blood flow to hypoxic lung regions, minimizes shunt blood flow. However, if generalized alveolar hypoxia occurs, then pulmonary vasomotor tone increases, increasing pulmonary vascular resistance and impeding RV ejection. Importantly, at low lung volumes, alveoli spontaneously collapse as a result of loss of interstitial traction and closure of the terminal airways. This collapse causes both absorption atelectasis and alveolar hypoxia. Patients with acute hypoxemic respiratory failure have small lung volumes and are prone to spontaneous alveolar collapse (Hakim and associates, 1982). Therefore, pulmonary vascular resistance is often increased in patients with acute hypoxemic respiratory failure (e.g., ALI).

Mechanical ventilation may reduce pulmonary vasomotor tone and pulmonary artery pressure by many related processes. First, hypoxic pulmonary vasoconstriction can be inhibited if O_2-enriched inspired gas increases PAo_2 or if the mechanical breaths and PEEP, by recruiting collapsed alveolar units, increase PAo_2 in those local alveoli. Second, mechanical ventilation often reverses respiratory acidosis by increasing alveolar ventilation. Finally, decreasing central sympathetic output by sedation during mechanical ventilation will also reduce vasomotor tone. These effects do not require endotracheal intubation to occur because they merely reexpand collapsed alveoli. Thus, PEEP, CPAP, recruitment maneuvers, and noninvasive ventilation may all reverse hypoxic pulmonary vasoconstriction.

Volume-Dependent Changes in Pulmonary Vascular Resistance

Changes in lung volume directly alter pulmonary vasomotor tone by compressing the alveolar vessels (Hakim and associates, 1982). The actual mechanisms by which this occurs have not been completely resolved but appear to reflect differential extraluminal pressure gradient-induced vascular compression. Pulmonary circulation occurs in two environments, which are separated from each other by the pressure that surrounds them. The small pulmonary arterioles, venules, and alveolar capillaries sense alveolar pressure as their surrounding pressure and are called alveolar vessels. The large pulmonary arteries and veins,

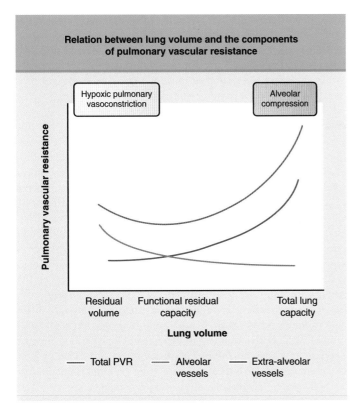

Figure 34.7. Relation between lung volume and the components of pulmonary vascular resistance. Schematic diagram of the relation between changes in lung volume and pulmonary vascular resistance, where the extraalveolar and alveolar vascular components are separated.

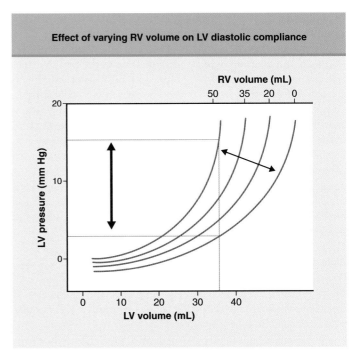

Figure 34.8. Effect of varying right ventricular volume on left ventricular diastolic compliance. Schematic diagram of the effect of changing right ventricular (RV) volumes on the left ventricular (LV) diastolic pressure–volume relationship. (After Taylor RR, Corell JW, Sonnenblick EH, Ross J Jr: Dependence of ventricular distensibility on filling the opposite ventricle. Am J Physiol 1967;213:711–718.)

as well as the heart and intrathoracic great vessels of the systemic circulation, sense ITP as their surrounding pressure and are called extraalveolar vessels. Alveolar pressure minus ITP is the transpulmonary pressure, and increasing lung volume requires increased transpulmonary pressure. Thus, the extravascular pressure gradient between alveolar and extraalveolar vessels varies proportionally with changes in lung volume. Increases in lung volume progressively increase alveolar vessel resistance, becoming clinically relevant above normal functional residual capacity (FRC) (Fig. 34.7). As lung volume increases, this extraluminal pressure difference increases as well. Since the intraluminal pressure in the pulmonary arteries is generated by RV ejection relative to ITP but the outside pressure of the alveolar vessels is alveolar pressure, if transpulmonary pressure increases enough to exceed intraluminal vascular pressure, the pulmonary vasculature will collapse where extraalveolar vessels pass into alveolar loci, reducing the vasculature cross-sectional area and thus increasing pulmonary vascular resistance. Similarly, increasing lung volume by stretching and distending the alveolar septa may also compress alveolar capillaries, although this mechanism is less well substantiated. Hyperinflation can create significant pulmonary hypertension and may precipitate acute RV failure (acute cor pulmonale) and RV ischemia. Thus, PEEP may increase pulmonary vascular resistance if it induces overdistention of the lung above its normal FRC. The effect of inflation on RV input impedance has been validated in humans using echocardiographic techniques. Similarly, if lung volumes are reduced, increasing lung volume to baseline levels by the use

of PEEP decreases pulmonary vascular resistance by reversing hypoxic pulmonary vasoconstriction.

Also important are the radial interstitial forces of the lung that keep the airways patent. These radial forces also act on the extraalveolar vessels, causing them to remain dilated. Thus, as lung volume increases, the radial interstitial forces increase, resulting in an increase in the diameters of both extraalveolar vessels and airways. This results in a reduction in airway resistance and extra-alveolar vessel vascular resistance, as well as an increase in extra-alveolar vessel capacitance. This interstitial tethering effect is reversed with lung deflation, thereby increasing pulmonary vascular resistance. The collapse of small airways also induces alveolar hypoxia. Thus, at small lung volumes, pulmonary vascular resistance is increased due to the combined effect of hypoxic pulmonary vasoconstriction and extraalveolar vessel collapse.

Ventricular Interdependence

Although LV preload can be directly altered by changes in RV output because the two ventricles are serially linked through the pulmonary vasculature, changes in RV end-diastolic volume can also alter LV preload by altering LV diastolic compliance. Changes in RV volume reciprocally alter LV diastolic compliance by the mechanism of ventricular interdependence. Ventricular interdependence functions through two separate processes. First, increasing RV end-diastolic volume will induce an intraventricular septal shift into the LV, thereby decreasing LV diastolic compliance (Fig. 34.8). Thus, for the same LV filling pressure, RV dilation will decrease LV end-diastolic volume and,

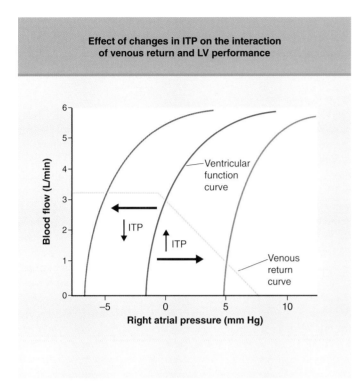

Figure 34.9. Effect of changes in intrathoracic pressure on the interaction of venous return and left ventricular performance. Schematic representation of the effects of increasing intrathoracic pressure (ITP), as would occur during positive pressure inspiration, or decreasing ITP, as would occur during spontaneous inspiratory efforts, on steady-state venous return as defined by the left ventricular (LV) function curve at that level of ITP. Note that decreases in ITP, which decrease right atrial pressure to below zero relative to atmospheric pressure, will only increase venous return by a limited amount, whereas increases in ITP will progressively decrease venous return to a complete circulatory standstill.

therefore, cardiac output. Second, if pericardial restraint limits absolute biventricular filling, then RV dilation will increase Ppc without septal shift. This ventricular interaction is believed to be the major determinant of the phasic changes in arterial pulse pressure and stroke volume seen in tamponade, referred to as pulsus paradoxus, which can be easily demonstrated during loaded spontaneous inspiration in normal subjects. Spontaneous inspiration increases venous return, causing RV dilation and decreasing LV end-diastolic compliance. Since RV volumes usually do not increase during positive pressure inspiration, ventricular interdependence is usually less. These differences in LV outflow between spontaneous and positive pressure ventilation are illustrated in Figure 34.9. Maintaining a relatively constant rate of venous return, either by volume resuscitation or by vasopressor infusion, will minimize this effect. Thus, the presence of pulsus paradoxus can be used as a marker of functional hypovolemia, even if actual intravascular volume status is not reduced.

Mechanical Heart–Lung Interactions
As absolute lung volume increases, the heart is compressed between the two expanding lungs, increasing juxtacardiac ITP. Because the chest wall and diaphragm can move away from the expanding lungs, whereas the heart is trapped within its cardiac

fossa, juxtacardiac ITP may increase more than lateral chest wall or diaphragmatic ITP. This compressive effect of the inflated lung can be seen with either spontaneous or positive pressure-induced hyperinflation. In this scenario, both Ppc and ITP are increased and no pericardial restraint exists. This decrease in apparent LV diastolic compliance was previously misinterpreted as impaired LV contractility because LV stroke work for a given LV end-diastolic pressure or pulmonary artery occlusion pressure is decreased. However, when such patients are fluid resuscitated to return LV end-diastolic volume to its original level, both LV stroke work and cardiac output also return to their original levels (Jardin and colleagues, 1981), despite the continued application of PEEP. In postoperative cardiac surgery patients, PEEP and, by extension, lung expansion compress the heart within the cardiac fossa in a manner analogous to pericardial tamponade.

Hemodynamic Effects of Changes in Intrathoracic Pressure
The heart within the thorax is a pressure chamber within a pressure chamber. Therefore, changes in ITP will affect the pressure gradients for both systemic venous return to the RV and systemic outflow from the LV, independent of the heart. Increases in ITP, by increasing right atrial pressure and decreasing transmural LV systolic pressure, will reduce the pressure gradients for venous return and LV ejection, decreasing intrathoracic blood volume. Using the same argument, decreases in ITP will augment venous return and impede LV ejection and increase intrathoracic blood volume.

Systemic Venous Return
Blood flows back from the systemic venous reservoirs into the right atrium through low-pressure, low-resistance venous conduits. Right atrial pressure is the backpressure or downstream pressure for venous return. Ventilation alters both right atrial pressure and venous reservoir pressure. These changes in right atrial and venous capacitance vessel pressure induce most of the observed cardiovascular effects of ventilation. Pressure in the upstream venous reservoirs is called mean systemic pressure, and it is a function of blood volume, peripheral vasomotor tone, and the distribution of blood within the vasculature. Mean systemic pressure does not change rapidly during positive pressure ventilation, whereas right atrial pressure does so due to concomitant changes in ITP. Accordingly, variations in right atrial pressure represent the major factor determining the fluctuation in pressure gradient for systemic venous return during ventilation. Positive pressure inspiration increases ITP and right atrial pressure, decreasing the pressure gradient for venous return, venous blood flow (Pinsky, 1984), RV filling, and, consequently, RV stroke volume (Pinsky, 1984; Jardin and Viellard-Baron, 2003) (see Fig. 34.9). During normal spontaneous inspiration, the converse occurs: With decreases in ITP, right atrial pressure decreases, accelerating venous blood flow and increasing RV filling and RV stroke volume (Pinsky, 1984) (see Fig. 34.9).

Importantly, the decrease in venous return during positive pressure ventilation is often lower than might be expected based on the increase in right atrial pressure, whereas the increase in venous return during spontaneous inspiration is often higher than predicted by a decrease in right atrial pressure. The reason for these apparent paradoxes is the effect of diaphragmatic

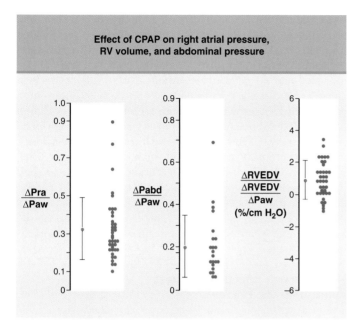

Figure 34.10. Effect of CPAP on right atrial pressure, right ventricular volume, and abdominal pressure. Effect of increasing levels of CPAP on the relations between increasing airway pressure and right atrial pressure (*left*), airway pressure and intraabdominal pressure (*middle*), and airway pressure and changes in right ventricular end diastolic volume (RVEDV) (*right*) in 43 postoperative fluid-resuscitated cardiac surgery patients. (Derived from data in Van den Berg P, Jansen JRC, Pinsky MR: The effect of positive-pressure inspiration on venous return in volume loaded post-operative cardiac surgical patients. J Appl Physiol 2002;92:1223–1231.)

descent and abdominal muscle contraction of intra-abdominal vascular capacitance. PEEP increases intra-abdominal pressure by causing the diaphragm to descend, increasing the pressure surrounding the intra-abdominal vasculature. Because a large proportion of venous blood is in the abdomen, the net effect of PEEP is to increase mean systemic pressure and right atrial pressure in a parallel manner. Accordingly, the pressure gradient for venous return may not be reduced by PEEP, especially in patients with hypervolemia. In fact, abdominal pressurization by diaphragmatic descent may be the major mechanism by which the decrease in venous return is minimized during positive pressure ventilation. Thus, ventilation may have less of an effect on venous return than originally postulated. Sustained increases in airway pressure may have even less detrimental effects than positive pressure swings during breathing. Van den Berg and corworkers (2002) documented that up to 20 cm H_2O CPAP did not significantly decrease cardiac output, as measured 30 seconds into an inspiratory hold maneuver, in postoperative cardiac surgery patients. They demonstrated that although CPAP induced an increase in right atrial pressure, intraabdominal pressure also increased, preventing a significant change in RV volumes (Fig. 34.10). Finally, with exaggerated swings in ITP, as occur with obstructed inspiratory efforts, venous return behaves as if abdominal pressure is additive to mean systemic pressure in defining total venous blood flow. Interest in inverse ratio ventilation has raised questions regarding its hemodynamic effect because its application includes a large component of hyperinflation. However, Mang and coworkers demonstrated in

an animal model of ALI that when total PEEP (intrinsic PEEP plus extrinsic PEEP) was similar, no hemodynamic difference between conventional ventilation and inverse ratio ventilation was seen.

Right Ventricular Filling
Under normal conditions, it is difficult to document any relation between RV filling pressure and volume. In fact, when measured carefully in cardiac surgery patients, volume loading-induced increases in RV volumes do not alter the pressure gradient between the RV intraluminal pressure and Ppc, although both increase in a parallel manner. Similar parallel change in volume pressures and Ppc are seen when RV volumes are reduced by the application (Rankin and associates, 1982). Thus, RV diastolic compliance is normally very high, and most of the increase in right atrial pressure seen during volume loading reflects pericardial compliance and cardiac fossa stiffness more than changes in RV distending pressure. Presumably, conformational changes in the RV more than wall stretch are responsible for RV enlargement. Accordingly, changes in right atrial pressure do not necessarily follow changes in RV end-diastolic volume. RV filling pressure does not increase until RV volume exceeds a certain threshold value. When cardiac contractility is reduced and intravascular volume is expanded, RV filling pressure increases as a result of decreased RV diastolic compliance, increased pericardial compliance, increased end-diastolic volume, or a combination of these three.

Venous return is the primary determinant of cardiac output. Since right atrial pressure is the backpressure to venous return, venous return is maintained near maximal levels at rest (Shepherd 1981; Jardin and Viellard-Baron, 2003) because RV filling occurs with minimal changes in filling pressure (Fig. 34.11). The closer right atrial pressure remains to zero relative to atmospheric pressure, the maximal is the pressure gradient for systemic venous blood flow. For this mechanism to operate efficiently, RV output must equal venous return; otherwise, sustained increases in venous blood flow would overdistend the RV, increasing right atrial pressure. Under normal conditions of spontaneous ventilation, the increase in venous return is in phase with inspiration, decreasing again during expiration as ITP increases. Likewise, the pulmonary arterial inflow circuit is highly compliant and can accept large increases in RV stroke volume without changing pressure (Pinsky, 1984). Thus, any increase in venous return is proportionally delivered to the pulmonary circuit without forcing the RV to increase its force of contraction or myocardial O_2 demand. This compensatory system rapidly becomes dysfunctional if RV diastolic compliance decreases or if right atrial pressure increases independent of changes in RV end-diastolic volume. RV diastolic compliance decreases in acute RV dilation or cor pulmonale (pulmonary embolism, hyperinflation, and RV infarction). These conditions are characterized by profound decreases in cardiac output not responsive to fluid resuscitation. Dissociation between right atrial pressure and RV end-diastolic volume occurs during either tamponade or positive pressure ventilation because right atrial pressure is artificially increased by increasing ITP or Ppc. Accordingly, positive pressure ventilation impairs normal circulatory adaptive processes. Restoration of normal right atrial pressure to RV volume coupling by using partial ventilatory support modes of ventilation will increase cardiac output only if the RV

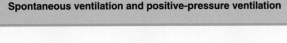

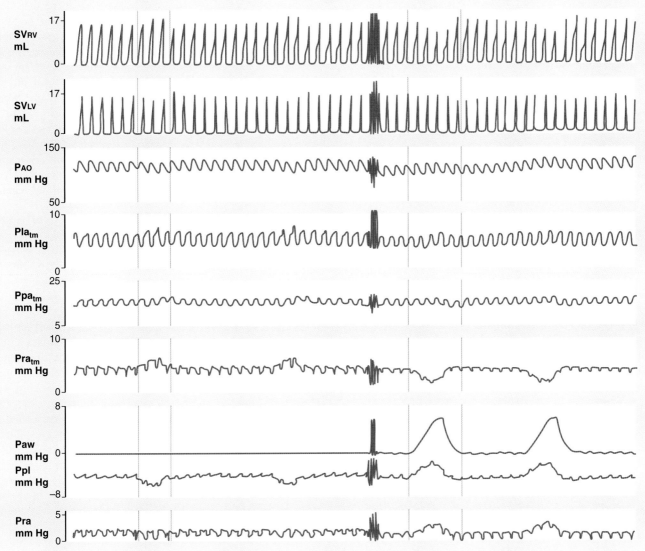

Figure 34.11. Spontaneous ventilation and positive-pressure ventilation. Strip chart recoding of right and left ventricular stroke volumes (SVrv and SVlv, respectively), aortic pressure (Pao), left atrial, pulmonary arterial, and right atrial transmural pressures (Pla$_{tm}$, Ppa$_{tm}$, and Pra$_{tm}$, respectively), airway pressure (Paw), pleural pressure (Ppl), and right atrial pressure (Pra) during spontaneous ventilation (*left*) and similar tidal volume positive pressure ventilation (*right*) in an anesthetized, intake canine model. (Reproduced with permission from Pinsky MR, Matuschak GM, Klain M: Determinants of cardiac augmentation by increases in intrathoracic pressure. J Appl Physiol 1985;58:1189–1198.)

can transduce the associated increase in venous return to forward blood flow. Thus, during weaning from mechanical ventilation, occult RV failure may be exposed in a previously stable ventilator-dependent patient. Clinically, indications suggesting acute RV failure are a rapid increase in right atrial pressure and a decrease in cardiac output, coupled with inspiration-associated tricuspid regurgitation. The detrimental effect of positive pressure ventilation on cardiac output can be

minimized by either fluid resuscitation to increase mean systemic pressure (Van den Berg and associates, 2002) or by keeping both mean ITP and swings in lung volume as low as possible. Accordingly, prolonging expiratory time, decreasing tidal volume, and avoiding PEEP all minimize the decrease in systemic venous return to the RV.

Spontaneous inspiratory efforts usually increase venous return because of the combined decrease in right atrial pressure and increase in intra-abdominal pressure. Interestingly, negative pressure ventilation, by augmenting venous return, was shown to increase cardiac output by 39% in 23 intubated children following repair of tetralogy of Fallot. In this condition, impaired RV filling secondary to RV hypertrophy and reduced RV chamber size are the primary factors limiting cardiac output. However, this augmentation of venous return is limited because as ITP decreases below atmospheric pressure, venous return becomes flow limited because the large systemic veins collapse as they enter the thorax. This vascular flow limitation is a safety valve for the heart because ITP can decrease greatly with obstructive inspiratory efforts and if not flow limited, the RV could become overdistended and fail.

LV Preload and Ventricular Interdependence

Changes in systemic venous return to the right ventricle must eventually result in directionally similar changes in LV preload because the two ventricles are linked in series. During a Valsalva maneuver, initially RV filling is reduced by the increase in ITP and right atrial pressure, but LV filling is unaltered (Buda and coworkers, 1979). However, as the strain is sustained, LV filling and cardiac output both begin to decrease (Sharpey-Schaffer, 1955). This phase delay in changes in output from the RV to the LV is exaggerated if tidal volume or respiratory rate is increased and in the setting of hypovolemia (Rankin and coworkers, 1982). Direct ventricular interdependence can also occur. As described previously, increasing RV volume decreases LV diastolic compliance. During positive pressure ventilation, RV volumes are usually decreased, minimizing ventricular interdependence (Rankin and coworkers, 1982) (see Figs. 34.9 and 34.11). Although PEEP results in some degree of right-to-left intraventricular septal shift, echocardiographic studies demonstrate that the shift is small (Jardin and colleagues, 1981). In fact, increases in lung volume during positive pressure ventilation primarily compress the two ventricles into each other, decreasing biventricular volumes. The decrease in cardiac output commonly seen during PEEP is due to a decrease in LV end-diastolic volume, since both LV end-diastolic volume and cardiac output are restored by fluid resuscitation without any measurable change in LV diastolic compliance. Positive pressure ventilation decreases intrathoracic blood volume, and PEEP decreases it even more without altering LV diastolic or contractile function (Dhainaut and associates, 1986).

However, during spontaneous inspiration RV volumes increase transiently, shifting the intraventricular septum into the LV, thus decreasing LV diastolic compliance and LV end-diastolic volume. This transient RV dilation-induced septal shift is the primary cause of inspiration-associated decreases in arterial pulse pressure that, if greater than 10 mm Hg or 10% of the mean pulse pressure, are referred to as pulsus paradoxus (see Fig. 34.9). Spontaneous inspiratory efforts can occur during positive pressure ventilation and especially during partial ventilatory assist. Thus, pulsus paradoxus can also be seen in mechanically ventilated patients.

LV Afterload

LV afterload, like RV afterload, can be defined as the maximal LV systolic wall tension, which, by the Laplace equation, is proportional to both transmural LV pressure and LV volume. Maximal LV wall tension normally occurs at the end of isometric contraction with the opening of the aortic value. Normally, LV ejection decreases LV afterload by rapidly decreasing LV volume. Importantly, when LV dilation exists, as in CHF, maximal LV wall stress occurs during LV ejection since the maximal product of pressure and volume occurs at that time. LV ejection pressure is the transmural LV systolic pressure, which can be estimated as transmural arterial pressure. Since normal baroreceptor mechanisms located in the extrathoracic carotid body function to maintain arterial pressure constant with respect to atmosphere, if arterial pressure were to remain constant as ITP increased, then transmural LV pressure would decrease. Similarly, if transmural arterial pressure were to remain constant as ITP increased, then LV wall tension would decrease. Thus, increases in ITP decrease LV afterload, and decreases in ITP increase LV afterload (Buda and associates, 1979; Pinsky and colleagues, 1983). These two opposing effects of changes in ITP on LV afterload have important clinical implications.

Processes associated with decreases in ITP must also be associated with increased LV afterload and myocardial O_2 consumption (MVO_2). Thus, spontaneous ventilation not only increases global O_2 demand by its exercise component but also increases MVO_2. Profound decreases in ITP commonly occur during spontaneous inspiratory efforts with bronchospasm and obstructive breathing. These conditions rapidly deteriorate into acute heart failure and pulmonary edema. Since weaning from positive pressure ventilation to spontaneous ventilation may reflect dramatic changes in ITP swings from positive to negative, independent of the energy requirements of the respiratory muscles, weaning from mechanical ventilation is a selective LV stress test. Similarly, improved LV systolic function is observed in patients with severe LV failure placed on mechanical ventilation. Very negative swings in ITP, as seen in vigorous inspiratory efforts in the setting of airway obstruction (asthma, upper airway obstruction, and vocal cord paralysis) or stiff lungs (interstitial lung disease, pulmonary edema, and ALI), selectively increase LV afterload and may be the cause of LV failure and pulmonary edema, especially if LV systolic function is already compromised.

Although the pulsus paradoxus seen during spontaneous inspiration under conditions of marked pericardial restraint reflects primarily ventricular interdependence, the negative swings in ITP also increase LV ejection pressure, thus increasing LV end-systolic volume (Buda and associates, 1979). Other systemic factors may influence LV systolic function during loaded inspiratory efforts, including an increase in aortic input impedance, altered synchrony of contraction of the global LV myocardium, and hypoxemia-induced decreased global myocardial contractility. Hypoxia also directly reduces LV diastolic compliance. Experimental repetitive periodic airway obstructions induce pulmonary edema in normal animals. Furthermore, removing the negative swings in ITP by applying nasal CPAP results in improved global LV performance in patients with combined obstructive sleep apnea and CHF.

If ITP were to increase rapidly, such as during a cough, then arterial pressure would also increase by a similar amount, such that both arterial pressure relative to ITP (transmural arterial pressure or LV ejection pressure; Buda and associates, 1979; Denault and coworkers, 2001) and aortic blood flow would remain constant. However, sustained increases in ITP must eventually decrease aortic blood flow and arterial pressure due to the associated decrease in venous return (Buda and associates, 1979). If ITP increased arterial pressure without changing transmural arterial pressure, then baroreceptor-mediated vasodilation would occur to maintain a constant extrathoracic arterial pressure–flow relation. Since coronary perfusion pressure reflects the intrathoracic pressure gradient for blood flow, it is not increased by ITP-induced increases in arterial pressure. However, compression of the coronaries by the expanding lungs may obstruct coronary blood flow. Thus, the combined decrease in coronary blood flow may induce myocardial ischemia.

One cannot readily apply increasing ITP to augment LV performance because the effect rapidly becomes self-limited as venous return declines. However, removing large negative levels of ITP does not have the same effect on venous return as does increasing ITP. Since venous return is flow limited below an ITP of zero, removing large negative swings in ITP will not alter venous return. However, the effect of removing negative ITP swings on LV afterload will be identical to adding positive ITP. Thus, any relative increase in ITP from very negative values to zero, relative to atmosphere, will minimally alter venous return but markedly reduce LV afterload. Removing large negative swings in ITP by either bypassing upper airway obstruction (endotracheal intubation) or by the institution of mechanical ventilation or PEEP-induced loss of spontaneous inspiratory efforts should selectively reduce LV afterload without significantly decreasing either venous return or cardiac output (Sharpey-Shaffer, 1955). The cardiovascular benefits of positive airway pressure on nonintubated patients can be seen by withdrawing negative swings in ITP, as created by using increasing levels of CPAP. Even CPAP levels as low as 5 cm H_2O can increase cardiac output in CHF patients, whereas cardiac output decreases with similar levels of CPAP in both normal subjects and heart failure patients without volume overload. Patients with CHF but in whom forced diuresis has induced a relative hypovolemic state, as manifest by a pulmonary artery occlusion pressure of 12 mm Hg or less, will decrease their cardiac outputs equally whether they receive CPAP or BiPAP at the same mean airway pressure. Nasal CPAP can also achieve the same results in patients with obstructive sleep apnea and heart failure, although the benefits do not appear to be related to changes in obstructive breathing pattern. Prolonged nighttime nasal CPAP can selectively improve respiratory muscle strength, as well as LV contractile function, if patients have preexisting heart failure (Kaneko and colleagues, 2003). These benefits are associated with reductions of serum catecholamine levels.

Using Changes in ITP to Define Cardiovascular Performance

Since the cardiovascular response to positive pressure breathing is determined by the baseline cardiovascular state, this response can be used to define such cardiovascular states. Sustained increases in airway pressure will reduce venous return, allowing one to assess LV ejection over a range of end-diastolic volumes. If echocardiographic measures of LV volumes are made simultaneously, then one can use an inspiratory hold maneuver to measure cardiac contractility, as defined by the end-systolic pressure–volume relation, which is similar to that created by transient inferior vena caval occlusion. Furthermore, these measures can be made during the ventilatory cycle to define dynamic

interactions. If positive airway pressure augments LV ejection in heart failure states, then systolic arterial pressure should not decrease but actually increase during inspiration, which is the so-called reverse pulsus paradoxus. This was what Abel and colleagues found in 10 postcardiac surgery patients. Perel and colleagues suggested that the relation between ventilatory efforts and systolic arterial pressure may be used to identify which patients may benefit from cardiac assist maneuvers. Patients who increase their systolic arterial pressure during ventilation relative to an apneic baseline tend to have a greater degree of volume overload and heart failure, whereas those in whom systolic arterial pressure decreases tend to be volume responsive. In a series of ventilator-dependent septic patients, Michard and associates found that the greater the degree of arterial pulse pressure variation during positive pressure ventilation, the greater the subsequent increase in cardiac output in response to volume expansion therapy.

Any hemodynamic differences between different modes of total mechanical ventilation at a constant airway pressure and PEEP are due to differential effects on lung volume and ITP. Importantly, when two different modes of total or partial ventilatory support have similar changes in ITP and ventilatory effort, their hemodynamic effects are also similar despite markedly different airway waveforms. Partial ventilatory support with either intermittent mandatory ventilation or pressure support ventilation gives similar hemodynamic responses when matched for similar tidal volumes. Similar tissue oxygenation occurred in ventilator-dependent patients when they were switched from assist-control, intermittent mandatory ventilation, and pressure support ventilation with matched tidal volumes. Numerous studies have documented cardiovascular equivancy when different modes of ventilatory support were matched for tidal volume and level of PEEP. Different modes of mechanical ventilation will affect cardiac output to a similar extent for similar increases in lung volume. However, when pressure control with a smaller tidal volume was compared to volume control, pressure control was associated with a higher cardiac output. Davis and associates studied the hemodynamic effects of volume control versus pressure-controlled ventilation in 25 patients with ALI. When matched for the same mean Paw, both methods gave the same cardiac outputs. However, when Paw was increased during volume-controlled ventilation by sign wave to square wave flow pattern, cardiac output declined. Furthermore, Kiehl and associates found cardiac output to be better with biphasic positive airway pressure than volume-controlled ventilation, leading to an increased Svo_2 and indirectly increasing PaO_2. Singer and colleagues showed that in 18 ventilator-dependent but hemodynamically stable patients, the degree of hyperinflation, not Paw, determined the decrease in cardiac output.

Increases in cardiac output with Paw increases suggest the presence of CHF. Grace and Greenbaum noted that giving PEEP to patients with heart failure did not decrease cardiac output, and it actually increased cardiac output if pulmonary artery occlusion pressure exceeded 18 mm Hg. Similarly, Calvin and colleagues noted that patients with cardiogenic pulmonary edema had no decrease in cardiac output when given PEEP. Rasanen and coworkers (1984) documented that decreasing levels of ventilatory support in patients with myocardial ischemia and acute LV failure worsened ischemia and could be

Cardiovascular Problems

minimized by preventing spontaneous inspiratory effort-induced negative swings in ITP.

Acknowledgment

This work was supported in part by NIH grants NHLBI K-24 HL67181 and NRSA 2-T32 HL07820.

REFERENCES

Buda AJ, Pinsky MR, Ingels NB, et al: Effect of intrathoracic pressure on left ventricular performance. N Engl J Med 1979;301:453–459.

Denault AY, Gorcsan J 3rd, Pinsky MR: Dynamic effects of positive-pressure ventilation on canine left ventricular pressure–volume relations. J Appl Physiol 2001;91:298–308.

Dhainaut JF, Devaux JY, Monsallier JF, et al: Mechanisms of decreased left ventricular preload during continuous positive pressure ventilation in ARDS. Chest 1986;90:74–80.

Hakim TS, Michel RP, Chang HK: Effect of lung inflation on pulmonary vascular resistance by arterial and venous occlusion. J Appl Physiol 1982;53:1110–1115.

Jabran A, Mathru M, Dries D, Tobin MJ: Continuous recordings of mixed venous oxygen saturation during weaning from mechanical ventilation and the ramifications thereof. Am J Respir Crit Care Med 1998; 158:1763–1769.

Jardin F, Farcot JC, Boisante L: Influence of positive end-expiratory pressure on left ventricular performance. N Engl J Med 1981;304:387–392.

Jardin F, Viellard-Baron A: Right ventricular function and positive-pressure ventilation in clinical practice: From hemodynamic subsets to respirator settings. Intensive Care Med 2003;29:1426–1434.

Kaneko Y, Floras JS, Usui K, et al: Cardiovascular effects of continuous positive airway pressure in patients with heart failure and obstructive sleep apnea. N Engl J Med 2003;348:1233–1241.

Pinsky MR: Determinants of pulmonary arterial flow variation during respiration. J Appl Physiol 1984;56:1237–1245.

Pinsky MR, Summer WR, Wise RA, Permutt S, Bromberger-Barnea B: Augmentation of cardiac function by elevation of intrathoracic pressure. J Appl Physiol 1983;54:950–955.

Rankin JS, Olsen CO, Arentzen CE, et al: The effects of airway pressure on cardiac function in intact dogs and man. Circulation 1982;66:108–120.

Rasanen J, Nikki P, Heikkila J: Acute myocardial infarction complicated by respiratory failure. The effects of mechanical ventilation. Chest 1984;85:21–28.

Romand JA, Shi W, Pinsky MR: Cardiopulmonary effects of positive pressure ventilation during acute lung injury. Chest 1995;108:1041–1048.

Sharpey-Schaffer EP: Effects of Valsalva maneuver on the normal and failing circulation. Br Med J 1955;1:693–699.

Shepherd JT: The lungs as receptor sites for cardiovascular regulation. Circulation 1981;63:1–10.

Van den Berg P, Jansen JRC, Pinsky MR: The effect of positive-pressure inspiration on venous return in volume loaded post-operative cardiac surgical patients. J Appl Physiol 2002;92:1223–1231.

Chapter 35

Intracranial Pressure and Cerebral Blood Flow Autoregulation

Marco Fontanella and Luciana Mascia

KEY POINTS

- Cerebral blood flow (CBF) is mainly guaranteed by an adequate cerebral perfusion pressure (CPP), which is the difference between mean arterial pressure and intracranial pressure (ICP).
- Uncontrollable ICP is a frequent cause of death in severely brain-injured patients. Consequently, ICP management is mainly oriented to maintain CPP above a minimum threshold in order to guarantee oxygen delivery to neural tissue.
- The assessment of intracranial compliance has the advantage of detecting pending herniation and characterizing parameters leading to raised ICP.
- The balance between cerebral oxygen supply and demand is reflected by changes of jugular oxygen saturation ($SjVO_2$). If $CMRO_2$ remains constant, changes in $SjVO_2$ can be interpreted as changes in CBF.
- Pressure autoregulation is defined as the ability of cerebral circulation to maintain total and regional CBF nearly constant despite major changes in CPP. Static measurements evaluate the overall effect (efficiency) of the autoregulatory action (i.e., the change in cerebrovascular resistance in response to the manipulation of arterial blood pressure), whereas measurement of the dynamic response yields information about the latency, which may be relevant in certain clinical conditions, including head injury.

In the 1960s, the introduction of mechanical ventilation and the strain gauge transducer to produce a continuous record of arterial pressure represented fundamental tools for the development of general intensive care. Similarly, the introduction of continuous monitoring of intracranial pressure (ICP) in the 1970s led to the definition of neurologic critical care as a specific branch of critical care medicine. Current research on applied computer technology, molecular biology, and their "translation" to the bedside characterizes the profile of the actual approach to neurocritical care medicine.

PRINCIPAL OF USE OF INTRACRANIAL PRESSURE MONITORING

Pathophysiology of the Intracranial Space

Intracranial pressure, represented by cerebrospinal fluid (CSF) pressure, is defined as the pressure that must be exerted against a needle introduced into the CSF space to prevent escape of fluid. The physiological basis of ICP is best explained by the Monroe–Kellie theory, which describes the adult skull as a rigid closed box system containing four compartments in a state of volume equilibrium: cells (neurons, glia, etc.) occupying a volume of approximately 1500 mL, CSF occupying 100 to 150 mL, and interstitial fluid and blood occupying a volume of 50 to 100 mL. An increase in the volume of any of these components must lead to a decrease in the space available to the others according to the following formula:

$$V_{tot} = V \text{ blood} + V \text{ tissue} + V \text{ CSF}$$

For example, when an intracerebral mass lesion is present, CSF is forced out of the intracranial compartment. This compensatory mechanism will be evident on cerebral computer tomography (CT) scan, where the basal cisterns and cortical sulci will be hardly visible and the cerebral ventricles will be reduced in volume.

The fundamental components of the intracranial pressure equilibrium are represented by the volume homeostasis of the CSF system and the vascular compartment.

CSF System

The CSF space consists of two communicating compartments: the interstitial space that surrounds cellular elements and the larger one consisting of ventricles, cisterns, and subarachnoid space. CSF is produced by the choroid plexus and the ventricular ependyma; the rate of formation is estimated to be 0.35 mL/min. The driving force propelling fluid along the CSF pathways is referred to arterial pulsations; absorption takes place at the arachnoid villi. Under normal conditions, the rate of formation is balanced by an equal rate of absorption. This condition of equilibrium results in the storage component equal to zero so that resting pressure and resting CSF volume remain unchanged. When CSF volume is altered, CSF pressure changes depending on three factors: rate of volume change, amount of volume change, and intracranial compliance. The change in CSF volume per unit change in CSF pressure defines the intracranial compliance, which can be expressed mathematically as follows:

Neurologic Problems

Compliance = change in volume/change in pressure
$$= \Delta V/\Delta P$$

Ideally, change in pressure should correspond linearly to change in volume, but the intracranial system shows an exponential variation of pressure with volume (Fig. 35.1). The relationship between intracranial volume and pressure was described in 1964 by Langfitt and colleagues. The authors observed that when ICP was low, an increase in volume produced a small change in pressure, but when intracranial compensatory mechanisms were exhausted, the same change in volume produced much larger increases in pressure. The Langfitt curve is best applied to rapid increases in ICP due to the presence of an intracranial acute hematoma, whereas a slow-growing mass lesion, such as a meningioma, may cause no increase in ICP until it becomes extremely large. In this case, different compensatory mechanisms may play a role, such as a decrease in extracellular fluid and eventually loss of neurons and glia. In addition, elderly patients may more easily tolerate the presence of a cerebral mass compared to younger patients because of cerebral atrophy. Intracranial compliance can be measured by injecting small quantities of fluid into the CSF space and recording the instantaneous rise in ICP. A new method has been proposed based on the use of multiple time-averaged small-volume pulses with the advantage of providing less perturbation in pressure. The assessment of intracranial compliance has the advantage of detecting pending herniation and characterizing parameters leading to raised ICP. The other approach used to derive more information from ICP monitoring is a system analysis in which the craniospinal axis is considered as a closed box in which the input is the arterial blood pressure waveform and the output is the ICP waveform. Both waveforms are subjected to spectral analysis to resolve them in the fundamental and higher harmonic waves to analyze changes in amplitude and phase that may occur when the waves pass through the cerebrovascular bed.

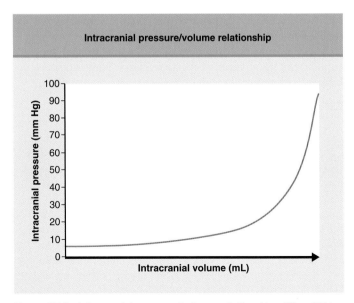

Figure 35.1. Intracranial pressure/volume relationship. When ICP is low, an increase in volume (ΔV) produces a small change in pressure (ΔP). If intracranial compensatory mechanisms are exhausted, a small change in volume produces much larger increases in pressure.

Vascular Compartment

The second fundamental component of ICP equilibrium is the vascular compartment. In the past, the terms *water content* and *vascular engorgement* were used interchangeably to define brain edema. Recently, Marmarou and coworkers distinguished the two components in an MRI study and concluded that brain edema is primarily responsible for brain swelling. The increase in tissue water (brain edema) can be classified as neurotoxic and ischemic edema of cellular origin and edema of extracellular origin due to blood–brain barrier disruption. The increase in blood volume is discussed later together with cerebral blood flow (CBF) regulation.

Uncontrollable ICP remains a frequent cause of death in severely brain-injured patients. Mortality and morbidity of severe brain-injured patients are related to the time spent above the critical threshold of 20 mm Hg. CBF is indeed mainly guaranteed by an adequate cerebral perfusion pressure (CPP), which is the difference between mean arterial pressure (MAP) and ICP. Consequently, ICP management is mainly oriented to maintain CPP above a minimum threshold in order to guarantee oxygen delivery to neural tissue, particularly in boundary regions, which are more sensitive to perfusion changes.

The cranium is partially divided into three compartments by the falx and tentorium. Mass lesions may induce different brain shifts due to compression against the falx or tentorium. If the lesion causes tentorial (uncal, transtentorial) herniation, compression of the third cranial nerve will cause ipsilateral fixed dilated pupils and the shift of the midbrain and brainstem will cause loss of consciousness due to ischemia of the reticular activating system. If the temporal lobe is pushed down onto the midbrain through the tentorium incisura with the cerebellar peduncles being forced down through the foramen magnum, the front-to-back shift will cause severe brainstem ischemia with loss of consciousness and failure of brainstem reflexes. If the lesion is located in the posterior fossa, obstruction of CSF outflow causes an increase in supratentorial ICP; clinical signs include neck stiffness and respiratory arrest, and lumbar puncture may worsen the symptoms. In the absence of significant mass lesions, herniation usually does not occur until ICP reaches extremely high levels.

Indications and Contraindications of ICP Monitoring

No general guidelines for ICP monitoring can be applied to the different intracranial pathologies (Table 35.1).

Traumatic Brain Injury

For severe traumatic brain-injured patients, defined as those with a Glasgow Coma Scale between 3 and 8 after cardiopulmonary resuscitation, the Brain Trauma Foundation suggests monitoring ICP if brain CT scan shows hematomas, contusions, and edema indirectly indicated by compressed basal cisterns and in patients with normal CT scan if two or more of the following features are present on admission: age older than 40 years, unilateral or bilateral motor posturing, and systolic blood pressure lower than 90 mm Hg. ICP monitoring is not routinely indicated in patients with mild or moderate head injury. However, a physician may choose to monitor ICP in conscious patients with traumatic mass lesions or in patients with concomitant extracranial lesions that require sedation and eventually muscle

Table 35.1 Indications for ICP Monitoring				
Pathology	CT Findings	Cause of Intracranial Hypertension	First-Choice ICP Monitoring System	Duration
TBI	Brain edema Basal cisterns and cortical sulci hardly visible. Cerebral ventricles reduced in volume	Brain swelling	Intraventricular catheter	3 days 7–10 days in select cases
TBI	Cerebral mass lesions or hematomas with midline shift	Mass lesion	Intraparenchymal catheter	3 days 7–10 days in select cases
SAH	Diffuse subarachnoid hemorrhage with/without intraventricular hemorrhage in patients with severe neurologic conditions	Brain edema Hydrocephalus	Intraventricular catheter	3 days 7–10 days in select cases
Postoperative	Brain edema after brain hematoma or tumor removal in select cases	Mass lesion	Intraparenchymal or subdural catheter	24 hr to 3 days
Hydrocephalus	Ventricular enlargement	Hydrocephalus	Lumbar catheter Epidural catheter	24 hr
Liver failure	Brain edema Basal cisterns and cortical sulci hardly visible. Cerebral ventricles reduced in volume	Brain edema	Intraventricular catheter	3–4 days

CT, computed tomography; ICP, intracranial pressure; SAH, subarachnoid hemorrhage; TBI, traumatic brain injury.

paralysis for mechanical ventilation and hemodynamic instability precluding neurological assessment.

Subarachnoid Hemorrhage

After *subarachnoid hemorrhage*, ICP monitoring is useful in patients with severe neurological conditions, hydrocephalus, and risk for cerebral vasospasm to measure and titrate CPP. After surgery for intracerebral hematoma, tumors, or vascular malformations, intraparenchymal or subdural ICP sensors may be positioned in select unconscious patients.

Liver Failure

Intracranial hypertension secondary to cerebral edema is the cause of death in 50% to 80% of patients with fulminant hepatic failure. Ventricular ICP monitoring should be implemented according to the coagulation status. The main indications for ICP monitoring are patients with grade III or IV encephalopathy and patients undergoing liver transplantation. Generally, ICP higher than 40 mm Hg with CPP lower than 50 mm Hg for more than 2 hours represents a contraindication for liver transplant.

Normotensive Hydrocephalus

ICP monitoring can be performed in select cases. A good correlation was found between the number, peak, and pulse pressures of B waves and the mean ICP. However, the presence of B waves is not a good predictor of the degree of clinical improvement postshunting. A lumbar catheter may be used to measure intracranial compliance during lumbar saline infusion.

Contraindications

Relative contraindications include severe infection, severe hemodynamic instability, immunosuppression, severe coagulopathy, or other conditions associated with an unacceptably high risk of intracranial hemorrhage related to the insertion procedure. Patients' complete blood count, bleeding indices (PT, PTT, and bleeding time), and infectious status should be investigated before starting the procedure. Coagulation parameters that represent a contraindications are platelet count lower than

75,000, PT higher than 16, and INR higher than 1.2. The decision regarding the duration of ICP monitoring in each patient should be based on the balance between the risk of infection and the benefits obtained by continuing the measurement. In general, infection rates become significant after 3 days; therefore, if ICP is below the threshold value for active treatment for more than 24 hours, monitoring should be discontinued. However, ICP monitoring can be required for 1 week to 15 days to orient specific therapy, such as osmotics, hyperventilation, or barbiturates administration.

Techniques and Equipment

Two methods are commonly used for ICP monitoring: fluid-filled catheters and catheter tip transducer systems. ICP can be detected from five different sites: intraventricular, intraparenchymal, subdural, extradural, and lumbar. To compare pressure sensors, static and dynamic characteristics should be considered. Static characteristics include zero drift, linearity, sensitivity, and accuracy, whereas dynamic characteristics include frequency response and damping (Table 35.2).

Fluid-Filled Catheter System

This was the first method used to drain CSF from the ventricles and to measure ICP. The catheter is inserted under sterile conditions via a twist-drill hole, usually in a lateral ventricle with the zero level at the external ear meatus. Stiff-walled catheters are preferable to the soft Silastic catheters to reduce damping errors. The catheter should be connected to a Luer-Lok three-way tap and then to the transducer (Fig. 35.2). Subdural pressure catheters are inaccurate more than 40% of the time, usually underestimating high ICP. Lumbar ICP monitoring is indicated only for diagnostic monitoring of patients with communicating hydrocephalus. A Tuohy needle is inserted into the lumbar subarachnoid space and the catheter is placed. This method is not indicated in the presence of an intracranial mass due to the risk of a cerebellar herniation into the spinal canal.

The Spiegelberg ICP monitoring system is a special type of fluid-filled catheter transducer system with an air pouch balloon

Table 35.2 Standard Devices for ICP Measurement					
Type	**Invasiveness/Risk**	**Cost**	**Accuracy**	**Calibration**	**Drainage**
Fluid-filled					
Ventricular catheter	Low	Low	High	In vivo zeroing required	Possible
Spiegelberg	Medium	High	High	In vivo zeroing possible	Possible with double-lumen intraventricular catheter
Fiberoptic					
Camino	Low	High	High	In vivo zeroing not possible	Possible with intraventricular catheter
InnerSpace	Medium–high	High	High	In vivo zeroing not possible	Possible with intraventricular catheter
Strain gauge					
Codman	Low	High	High	In vivo zeroing not possible	Possible with intraventricular catheter
Gaeltec	Medium	High	Low	In vivo zeroing possible	Drainage not possible
Rehau	Low	High	High	In vivo zeroing not possible	Possible with intraventricular catheter

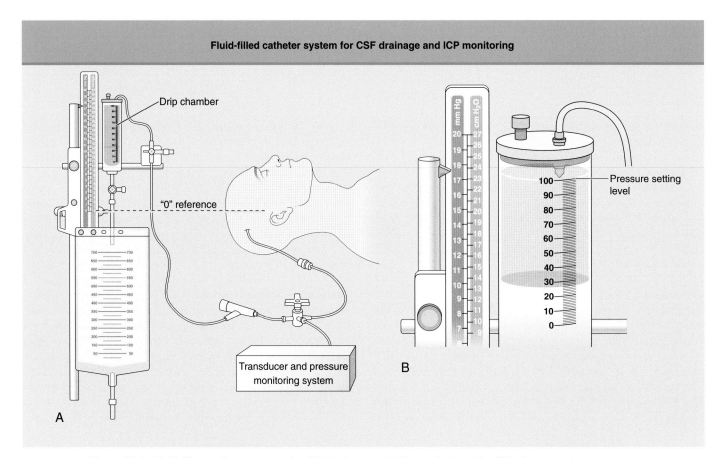

Figure 35.2. Fluid-filled catheter system for CSF drainage and ICP monitoring. The "0" reference point the outer ear canal corresponds to the outer ear canal (A). B, The drip chamber is then adjusted up or down until it is at a level equal to the maximum desired ICP (pressure setting level). If the system is open to drainage, CSF will drain as soon as the intracranial pressure exceeds the pressure determined by the height of the drip chamber. This system may be utilized for continuous pressure monitoring, continuous drainage, or both. To obtain an accurate pressure measurement, the stopcock should be turned "off" to drainage and "open" to the patient catheter and pressure monitoring system. If pressure is measured when the drainage unit is open in all three directions, the pressure measured will be a reflection of the patient and drainage bag.

situated at the tip. By maintaining a constant known volume of fluid within the air pouch, the pressure within the air pouch balloon is equivalent to the surrounding pressure (i.e., ICP). The internal air pouch balloon is transduced by an external strain gauge transducer, and because the fluid used for pressure transduction is air, the error in the pressure reading caused by an air column is low. It consists of a 2-mm probe with a 16-mm catheter tip. The placement of the catheter requires at least an 11-mm bur hole. The accuracy is high (±2 mm Hg) in more than 90% of cases. The device allows automatic in vivo zeroing, CSF drainage through a double-lumen catheter, and, with a dedicated software, continuous compliance measurement. Epidural, subdural, intraparenchymal, and intraventricular systems are available.

Catheter Tip Transducer Systems

These systems can be categorized as fiberoptic [(Camino and InnerSpace InnerSpace Medical, Inc., Irvine, CA) and strain gauge [(Codman (Codman & Shurtleff, Inc., Raynham, MA) and Gaeltec (Gaeltec, Ltd., Dunvegan, Isle of Skye, Scotland)].

The InnerSpace OPX 100 system has good zero drift and high sensitivity but requires large probes that may cause hematoma formation. Therefore, its use is indicated for postoperative patients because its positioning can be done at the end of surgery.

The Camino system consists of a fiberoptic sensor approximately 1.5 mm in diameter that can be placed in the ventricle, the subdural space, or the brain parenchyma. The manufacturer's specification for zero drift of the catheter is ±2 mm Hg for the first day and ±1 mm Hg/day thereafter, but some authors have reported a daily drift rate of 3.2 mm Hg. The temperature drift of the device is significant (0.3 mm Hg/1°C). Technical complications with failure rates ranging from 10% to 25% are also reported.

The Codman system consists of a 1.1-mm probe that has in its distal part a microprocessor inserted inside a silicon-coated titanium capsule mounted at the top of a nylon-coated copper wire, with an electronic connector on the proximal end; it can be inserted into a dedicated ventricular catheter. Accuracy is high (±1 mm Hg). The probe is the same for intraparenchymal, intraventricular, and subdural measurement. Clinical evaluations have revealed inter- and intrapatient variability compared with an intraventricular catheter transducer system.

The Gaeltec ICP/B system has a solid-state miniature strain gauge ICP transducer (6–7 mm) with a coaxial rubber diaphragm near the tip, which is used for in situ calibration and can be reused after ethylenoxide sterilization. The epidural catheter is made of a flat silicone rubber membrane, or balloon, covering the pressure-sensing diaphragm. Measurement artifacts and poor quality associated with repeated use are reported.

The Rehau system uses a pressure-sensitive semiconductor chip placed on the distal tip of the probe. It has different probes for the detection of intraparenchymal, ventricular, and epidural ICP. The parenchymal catheter has a diameter of 1.45 mm, and the epidural probe has a circular tip of 6×2.1 mm. The system can be connected to any monitor.

Complications and Controversies

The fluid-filled catheter system placed into the ventricle is considered the "gold standard" method of measuring ICP in the absence of mass lesions because ICP should be equally distributed and transmitted to the ventricles. In the presence of mass lesions, particularly in the posterior fossa, the main advantage of the catheter tip transducer systems placed in the parenchyma is the possibility of detecting an increase in ICP early and directly in the site of the cerebral lesion. The fluid-filled catheter system allows checking for zero drift after placement and to drain CSF if required, although CSF drainage should be done carefully in cases of midline shift or posterior fossa lesion because it can increase the shift and produce cerebral herniation. The Brain Trauma Foundation recommended intraventricular ICP measurement as the first-line approach to monitoring ICP. This is a low-cost system in comparison to the transducer-tipped system, but a higher risk of infection (approximately 1%) and higher risk of blockage are reported in comparison with the transducer-

tipped systems. Positioning of the catheter tip system with the intraparenchymal probe is a bedside procedure that avoids the transport of the patient to the operating theater. With these systems, the calibration cannot be performed in vivo. They are zeroed during a preinsertion calibration, and then the pressure output will be dependent on zero drift of the sensor. A catheter transducer system can be described as a second-order mechanical system that, if underdamped, oscillates at its own natural frequency that is close to the frequency of the recorded signal, producing significant amplitude and phase distortion of the pressure signal. The degree of distortion depends on the damping factor of the system. Catheter tip transducers have high resonant frequencies; therefore, amplitude and phase distortion usually do not occur.

No prospective randomized controlled trials have been conducted to demonstrate that ICP monitoring improves outcome of patients with suspected intracranial hypertension, but there is sufficient evidence that mortality and morbidity of severe brain-injured patients are related to the time spent above the critical ICP threshold of 20 mm Hg. Therefore, indications for ICP monitoring remain controversial in many centers. Factors contributing to this controversy are its invasiveness, a paucity of specific therapies to lower ICP, and the fact that intracranial hypertension represents the consequence of many different pathological conditions.

PRINCIPLE OF USE OF CEREBRAL BLOOD FLOW MEASUREMENTS

Cerebral Circulation

In humans, the cerebrovascular bed is supplied by blood flowing through the two internal carotid arteries and the two vertebral arteries that join to form the basilar artery. These major arteries communicate with each other through arterial anastomoses that form the circle of Willis. Blood is then distributed distally via the paired anterior, middle, and posterior cerebral arteries and by branches that penetrate the parenchyma. Regions of cerebral cortex bordering the areas supplied by the anterior, middle, and posterior cerebral arteries represent boundary zones. These areas are particularly vulnerable to reductions in CBF; indeed, during episodes of prolonged hypotension, ischemia is most pronounced in these areas. Experimental studies indicate that in physiological conditions blood from the internal carotid artery supplies the ipsilateral cerebral hemisphere and blood from the vertebrobasilar system supplies structures in the posterior fossa with little mixing through the circle of Willis. When a proximal vessel is occluded, the circle of Willis provides important collateral circulation. The actual pattern of collateral blood flow depends on the site of stenosis and on available collateral channels; in general, the recruitment of collateral channels is more effective if the major vessel occlusion occurs over weeks or months rather than suddenly. The cerebral veins are thin walled and distensible and have no valves. They are influenced by the surrounding presssure (ICP); therefore, intravascular pressure of superficial veins must be greater than ICP to guarantee venous drainage. Venous blood flows via superficial and deep cerebral veins into thick-walled, nonelastic collecting ducts, the venous sinuses that reach the internal jugular and vertebral veins. Several venous connections are present between cerebral veins, dural sinuses, and the venous system of meninges, skull, scalp, and nasal sinuses that may facilitate propagation of thrombus or infection.

Although the normal weight of the human adult brain is only 2% of body weight, it utilizes 25% of the glucose and approximately 20% of the oxygen required by the whole body at rest (3.3 mL O_2/min/100 g). There is a tight coupling between oxygen supply (CBF) and demand ($CMRO_2$) and the utilization of glucose by the brain. CBF measurement improved our knowledge of the pathophysiology of severe brain injury, although this measure has never been considered part of clinical monitoring because of its complexity.

Techniques and Equipment

Many techniques have been proposed to measure CBF in humans and can be classified as direct measurements based on the Fick principle, which first used nitrous oxide and later radioactive inert gases (xenon[133] and krypton[85]); tomographic methods, such as Xe CT scan, single-photon emission computed tomography (SPECT), and photon emission tomography (PET); and indirect measurements, such as jugular bulb venous oxygen content and transcranial Doppler flow velocity (Table 35.3). In this context, we consider only those of clinical relevance; therefore, other techniques, such as hydrogen clearance, autoradiography, and microspheres, used only in the experimental setting are not discussed in this chapter.

Kety–Schmidt Technique

The first quantitative method to measure CBF in humans was used by Kety and Schmidt in 1945. The method is based on the Fick principle, which states that "the quantity of a substance taken up by an organ per unit time is equal to the product of the blood flow through that organ and the arteriovenous concentration difference of the substance." That is:

$$Q_t = F_t(C_a - C_v)$$

where Q_t is the quantity of substance taken up per unit time; F_t is blood flow per unit time, and C_a and C_v are the arterial and venous concentrations of the substance.

The method consists of the inhalation of a tracer (N_2O, Xe^{133}, or krypton[85]) that is absorbed by the brain via the lungs and the circulation and, because it is inert, does not alter the metabolic rate of the brain. The numerator of the Fick equation (Q_t) is the product of concentration of the tracer in the brain, the weight of the brain, and the blood–brain coefficient (λ) for the tracer. The denominator has to be integrated with respect to time until equilibration is achieved between arterial blood, venous blood, and brain tissue. CBF can be determined (per unit weight of brain tissue) by the sequential sampling of arterial blood and cerebral venous blood (obtained from the jugular bulb) and by measurement of the N_2O concentrations throughout the equilibration process (usually 10 min for the saturation technique) or during the desaturation phase, which occurs when inhalation of N_2O is stopped (the desaturation technique). Limitations of the Kety–Schmidt technique include the following: It is invasive, requiring cannulation of an artery and the jugular bulb; it is time-consuming because it requires analysis of multiple arterial and venous samples; and it assesses global CBF. To reduce the invasiveness, the use of radioactive inert gases such as krypton[85] or xenon[133] has been proposed. Removal of these gases from the brain depends only on physical properties such as diffusion and solubility. The use of external detectors determines the decay in radioactivity; the rate of this "washout" depends on the blood flow. Originally, the tracer was administered through carotid infusion, without recirculation problems. Currently, the isotope is administered by inhalation or intravenous injection, and therefore the isotope is distributed not only to the brain but also throughout the body. Consequently, during the desaturation phase, CBF measurement must be corrected for the recirculation of the isotope. This method allows investigation of regional blood flow.

Xenon-Enhanced Computed Tomography

Stable (nonradioactive) xenon can absorb x-rays and is used to enhance the images that can be obtained with standard CT scan. A subanesthetic mixture of xenon and oxygen is inhaled. The resultant changes in the absorption coefficients of the x-rays depend on the solubility of the xenon and the perfusion of the tissue. These differences, together with the measurement of the end-tidal xenon concentration, can be used to calculate absolute values of regional CBF with excellent anatomical specificity. It is noninvasive, but the inhalation of high concentrations of xenon

---

Table 35.3 Techniques for CBF Measurement					
Technique	**Tracer**	**Invasiveness**	**Bedside**	**Intermittent Continuous**	**Global/Regional**
Kety–Schmidt	Nitrous oxide	Yes	Yes	Intermittent	Global
	Xe^{133}	No	Yes	Intermittent	Regional
SPECT	^{99m}Tc-HMPAO	No	No	Intermittent	Regional
PET	^{15}O or $^{15}CO_2$	No	No	Intermittent	Regional
Sjo$_2$	Oxygen	Yes	Yes	Continuous	Global
TCD	—	No	Yes	Continuous	Regional
NIRS	Oxygen	No	Yes	Continuous	Regional
Perfusion MRI	Gadolinium	No	No	Intermittent	Regional
Perfusion CT	Iodine contrast	No	No	Intermittent	Regional

NIRS, near-infrared spectroscopy; perfusion CT, cerebral perfusion computed tomography; perfusion MRI, cerebral perfusion weighted magnetic resonance imaging; PET, dual-photon emission tomography; Sjo$_2$, jugular bulb venous oxygen saturation; SPECT, single-photon emission computed tomography; TCD, transcranial Doppler.

may increase ICP, inducing vasodilation, and requires the use of low levels of inspired fraction of oxygen.

Single-Photon Emission Computed Tomography

Xenon[133] or technetium-[99]m-hexamethylene-propyleneamine oxime ([99]mTc-HMPAO) produce particles that can be detected by conventional gamma cameras. [99]mTc-HMPAO is lipophilic, diffuses passively across the blood–brain barrier, and is retained by the brain in the "first pass" for at least the acquisition time of the gamma camera. Once it diffuses through the blood–brain barrier, it is converted to a hydrophilic form that is unable to pass the barrier and remains stable over the subsequent 24 hours. The tracer is distributed in proportion to the regional CBF; therefore, this technique assesses relative values of CBF, but the high background activity prevents subsequent measurements.

Dual-Photon Emission Tomography

The cyclotron can be used to generate short-lived positron-emitting radionuclides, such as ^{15}O (half-life, 2.1 min), ^{13}N (half-life, 10 min), ^{11}C (half-life, 20.3 min), and ^{18}F (half-life, 1.83 hr). These can be used to measure regional CBF (intravenous ^{15}O or inhalation of $^{15}CO_2$), cerebral blood volume (inhalation of ^{11}C-labeled CO_2), $CMRO_2$ (inhalation of ^{15}O-labeled oxygen), and cerebral metabolic rate for glucose [^{18}F-labeled 2-fluoro-2-deoxy-D-glucose (FDG) or ^{11}C-labeled glucose]. The technique is based on the detection of the dual high-energy ray photons, which result from the collision between the positrons (released as the isotope decay) and the electrons. After the inhalation of gas labeled with ^{15}O, the tracer is distributed to all regions of the brain in proportion to the blood flow. The oxygen extraction ratio (OER) can be calculated; using CBF and arterial oxygen content (CaO_2), regional cerebral metabolic rate for oxygen ($CMRO_2$) can be derived: $OER \times CaO_2 = CMRO_2/CBF$.

Regional cerebral metabolism can be quantified using FDG or ^{11}C-labeled glucose. Neurons absorb glucose in relation to their metabolic activity. FDG is taken up by active cells and then stored in the cells in the phosphorylated form. The amount of accumulated radioactivity is a measure of glucose utilization and neuronal functional activity.

Jugular Bulb Venous Oxygen Saturation

Oxygen supply (CBF) and demand ($CMRO_2$) are linked as follows:

$$AjVDO_2 = CMRO_2/CBF$$

where $AjVDO_2$ is the difference in oxygen content measured in the arterial blood and jugular blood and indicates the coupling between metabolism and flow. If the ratio between supply and demand does not change (i.e., if the coupling flow/metabolism is preserved), $AjVDO_2$ remains constant (normal value, 7 mL O_2/100 mL blood in adults). Values of $AjVDO_2$ higher than 9 mL O_2/100 mL usually indicate an increased extraction of oxygen due to impending cerebral ischemia. Conversely, values lower than 4 mL O_2/100 mL indicate global hyperemia. If arterial oxygen saturation is 100%, we may approximate $AjVDO_2$ to jugular bulb venous oxygen saturation ($SjVO_2$). The balance supply/demand is then reflected by changes of $SjVO_2$:

$$SjVO_2 = CBF/CMRO_2$$

If $CMRO_2$ remains constant, changes in $SjVO_2$ can be interpreted as changes in CBF. The venous blood is drained by the jugular bulb with the tip of the catheter above the lower border of C1 to avoid extracranial contaminations. Continuous monitoring of $SjVO_2$ can be obtained using fiberoptic catheters. The value obtained will be the average of cerebral venous oxygen saturation without a regional resolution. In the absence of focal lesion, the catheter should be placed on the dominant side, which can be defined with the jugular compression test or by defining the larger jugular foramen on CT scan. In the presence of a focal lesion, the catheter should be placed on the ipsilateral side of the lesion. After brain injury, CBF and metabolism may be uncoupled. Because of reduced synaptic activity, $CMRO_2$ consistently falls in proportion to coma depth, whereas CBF varies independently. Hence, CBF may exceed metabolic requirements, resulting in hyperemia.

Transcranial Doppler

Transcranial Doppler (TCD) sonography is a bedside, noninvasive technique that continuously measures blood flow velocity in the major intracranial vessels using extracranial probes. The method was introduced by Aaslid to assess vasospasm after subarachnoid hemorrhage (Fig. 35.3) and then used for the diagnosis of cerebral artery stenosis, to test cerebrovascular reactivity, and to detect emboli. The technique is based on the principle that velocity is inversely related to flow if the vessel diameter is constant. Blood velocity is determined by calculating the shift in frequency between the transmitted and the reflected ultrasound. Systolic, diastolic, and mean velocity can be obtained and the direction of flow can be determined. A pulsed-range gated probe is used to select the depth of recording in order to insonate the cerebral arteries of the circle of Willis. The use of 2 MHz probes allows penetration in the skull bone. The internal carotid artery and the middle, anterior, and posterior cerebral arteries are insonated through the temporal bone, whereas the transoccipital approach is used to insonate vertebral and basilar arteries. Data can be recorded continuously but absolute values of CBF cannot be obtained. A daily TCD examination in patients with subarachnoid hemorrhage may give accurate information about the onset and presence of vasospasm, whereas during intracranial hypertension there is a decrease in the diastolic value of the TCD waveform that suggests high peripheral resistances. In brain-dead patients, the arrest of the cerebral circulation is associated with a biphasic waveform of low amplitude, an anterograde flow during systole, and a reversal flow during diastole. TCD can also be useful for assessing pressure autoregulation and cerebrovascular reactivity to carbon dioxide.

During neurosurgical procedures such as after aneurysm clipping to detect a stenosis of a vessel near the clip or to exclude arteriovenous malformations, 16 or 20 MHz Doppler probes can be used to record velocities from small arteries. Alternatively, perivascular probes (Transonic) consisting of a probe body that houses ultrasonic transducers and a fixed acoustic reflector can be positioned on one side of the vessel and the reflector positioned at a fixed position between the two transducers on the opposite side. An electrical excitation causes the downstream transducer to emit a plane wave of ultrasound. This ultrasonic

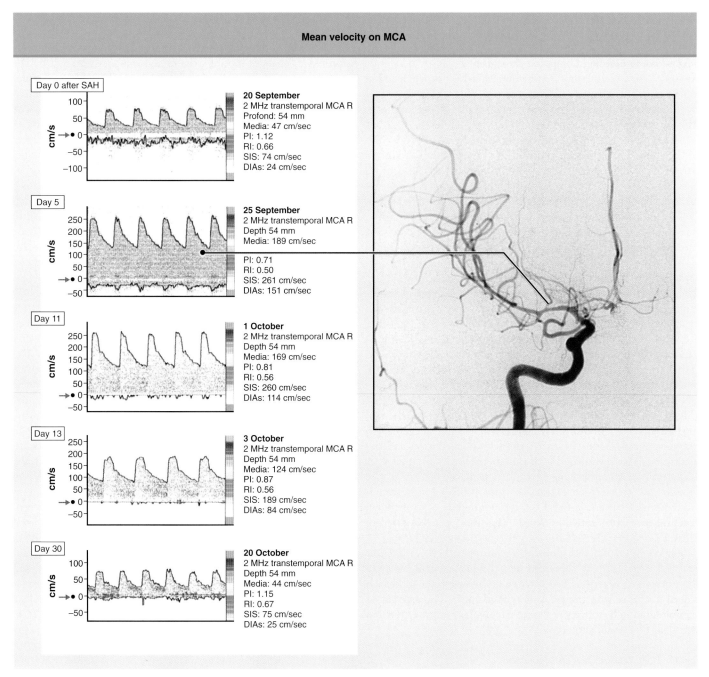

Mean velocity on MCA

Figure 35.3. Transcranial Doppler and cerebral angiography. TCD shows an increase in mean flow velocity of the middle cerebral artery, whereas the angiography shows a reduction in the caliber of the vessel.

wave intersects the vessel in the upstream direction and then bounces off the fixed "acoustic reflector." It again intersects the vessel and is received by the upstream transducer, where it is converted into electrical signals. From these signals, the flowmeter derives an accurate measure of the "transit time."

Near-Infrared Spectroscopy

In 1977, Jöbsis first demonstrated that transmittance measurements of near-infrared (NIR) radiation could be used to monitor the degree of oxygenation of certain metabolites. A compound that absorbs light in the spectral region of interest is known as a chromophore. Each chromophore has its own particular absorption spectrum that describes the level of absorption at each wavelength. The concentration of some absorbers, such as water, melanin, and bilirubin, remains virtually constant with time, whereas oxygenated hemoglobin (HbO_2), deoxyhemoglobin (Hb), and oxidized cytochrome oxidase (CtOx) have concentrations in tissue that are strongly linked to tissue oxygenation and metabolism. Specific extinction coefficients of HbO_2 and Hb are in the 450- to 1000-nm wavelength range. The difference in the absorption spectra explains the well-recognized phenomenon of arterial blood (containing approximately 98% HbO_2) having a bright red appearance, whereas venous or deoxygenated blood appears more blue. Within the 650- to 1000-nm window, it is possible with sensitive instrumentation to detect light that has traversed up to 8 cm of tissue. Measurement of regional CBF can be obtained using oxyhemoglobin as the intravascular tracer. If a sudden increase in the arterial saturation of hemoglobin (approximately 5%) is produced by an acute increase in the inspired fraction of oxygen, the resultant increase in the cerebral oxyhemoglobin concentration can be detected and measured. The rate of cerebral hemoglobin delivery can be calculated in millimoles per liter per minute, and this can be converted to CBF in mL/100 g/min. The technique is noninvasive and can be performed without risk.

Cerebral Perfusion Weighted MRI

Perfusion MRI (pMRI) is an imaging technique used for measuring blood flow through the brain. Two types of PWI techniques are widely used: bolus tracking with exogenous contrast agents (BT-PWI), extensively used in the clinical setting, and arterial spin labeling techniques (ASL-PWI). With BT-PWI, serial multislice T2-weighted images are obtained every 1 or 2 seconds over 1.5 to 2 minutes to monitor the signal decrease associated with the passage of the contrast bolus. From the time curve of the signal change, various hemodynamic parameters, such as the time to peak (TTP), relative mean transit time (MTT), and relative cerebral blood flow (rCBF) and volume (rCBV), can be calculated. Information on any areas in the brain can be obtained if the blood flow is delayed relative to the rest of the brain (Fig. 35.4). BT-PWI should be regarded as a semiquantitative technique when applied to patients with cerebrovascular disease. However, new multislice ASL-PWI methods are becoming available, and future technical improvements should further reduce the acquisition times while increasing the slice coverage, resolution, and stability of the images.

Cerebral Perfusion Computed Tomography

This technique allows rapid qualitative and quantitative evaluation of cerebral perfusion by generating maps of CBF, CBV, and MTT. The technique is based on the central volume principle (CBF = CBV/MTT) and requires the use of commercially available software employing complex deconvolution algorithms to produce the perfusion maps. Some controversy regarding which artery should be used as input vessel and the accuracy of quantitative results and their reproducibility exists. However, perfusion CT is a useful tool for noninvasive diagnosis of cerebral ischemia and infarction and for evaluation of vasospasm after subarachnoid hemorrhage. Perfusion CT has also been used for assessment of cerebrovascular reserve by using acetazolamide in patients with intracranial vascular stenoses who are potential candidates for bypass surgery or endovascular treatment, for the evaluation of patients undergoing temporary balloon occlusion to assess collateral flow and cerebrovascular reserve, and for the assessment of microvascular permeability in patients with intracranial neoplasms. Perfusion studies are obtained by monitoring the first pass of an iodine contrast agent bolus through the cerebral vasculature. There is a linear relationship between contrast agent concentration and attenuation, with the contrast agent causing a transient increase in attenuation proportional to the amount of contrast agent in a given region. Contrast agent time–concentration curves are generated in an arterial region of interest (ROI), a venous ROI, and in each pixel. Deconvolution of arterial and tissue enhancement curves, a complex mathe-

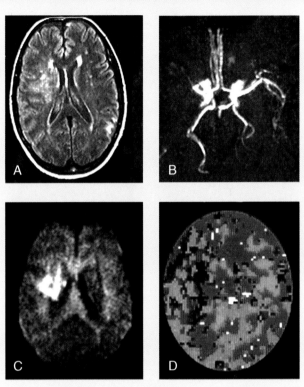

Cerebral blood-flow regulation

Figure 35.4. Cerebral blood-flow regulation. Right middle cerebral artery occlusion. *A*, MRI flair image showing only slight signal differences in the right hemisphere. *B*, Angio-MRI showing right middle cerebral artery occlusion. *C*, Diffusion MRI showing only the core of the ischemic lesion. *D*, Perfusion MRI showing a hypoperfusion in whole middle cerebral artery territory.

matic process, gives the MTT. CBV is calculated as the area under the curve in a parenchymal pixel divided by the area under the curve in an arterial pixel. The central volume equation can then be solved for CBF. Good quality perfusion maps have been obtained with injection rates as low as 1.5 mL/sec.

Cerebral Blood Flow Autoregulation

The cerebral circulation is regulated by perfusion pressure, metabolic stimuli, chemical stimuli, and neural stimuli. Pressure autoregulation is defined as the ability of cerebral circulation to maintain total CBF nearly constant despite large changes in CPP (Fig. 35.5B). This mechanism can be defined by the relationship between CBF and CPP where CPP is calculated as the difference between MAP and cerebral outflow pressure. Because the cerebral venous system is compressible and behaves as a "Starling resistor," outflow pressure is whichever pressure is higher—ICP or venous outflow pressure. CBF can be expressed as

$$CBF = CPP/CVR$$

where CVR is defined by

$$(8/\pi) \times (hl/r^4)$$

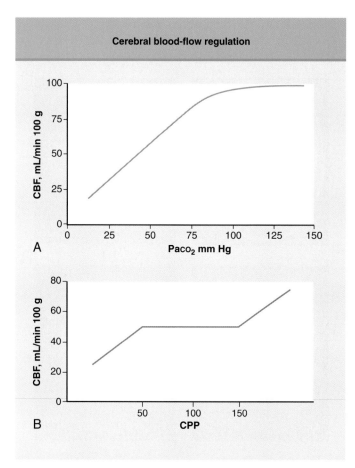

Figure 35.5. CBF regulation. *A,* The relationship between CBF and Paco$_2$: CBF increases linearly with Paco$_2$ increases in the range of 20 to 80 mm Hg. *B,* The pressure autoregulation curve: CBF is nearly constant despite changes in CPP in the range of 60 to 150 mm Hg, whereas below and above these limits CBF follows passively CPP changes

where $(8/\pi)$ is a constant, h the blood viscosity, and l is the length and r the radius of the vessel. The radius is expressed as the fourth power in the equation, making it the most efficient means of controlling vascular resistance. Under physiological conditions, autoregulation is obtained by active alteration of the caliber of the resistance vessels in the brain. This process typically operates between MAP on the order of 60 and 150 assuming normal ICP, whereas in hypertensive patients the autoregulation curve is shifted to the right. Many authors have proposed myogenic and/or metabolic mechanisms to explain this response of the vasculature. The involvement of vasodilators (nitric oxide) and vasoconstrictors (endothelin) has been proposed in the regulation of the cerebrovascular tone. At the lower limit of autoregulation, cerebral vasodilation is maximal, and below this level CBF falls passively with CPP. Beyond the upper limit where vasoconstriction is maximal, the elevated intraluminal pressure may force the vessels to dilate, leading to an increase in CBF and damage to the blood–brain-barrier. To assess "static" autoregulation, CBF has to be measured at baseline and after manipulation of CPP until higher or lower CPP values are reached. However, CBF measurement techniques are not easily available in the clinical settings; therefore, a "dynamic"

approach has been proposed. Aaslid and colleagues introduced a noninvasive method using TCD. This dynamic approach uses the rapid decreases in MAP caused by the release of high blood pressure cuffs as an autoregulatory stimulus and compares MAP and CBF velocity during the autoregulatory process. The transfer function analysis between the arterial and ICP or TCD signals has been proposed to assess dynamic autoregulation. Static measurements evaluate the overall effect (efficiency) of the autoregulatory action (i.e., the change in CVR in response to the manipulation of ABP), but they do not address the time in which this change in CVR is achieved (its latency). Measurement of the dynamic response yields information about the latency as well, which may be relevant in certain clinical conditions including head injury. Many reports suggest that progressive impairment in autoregulation first affects the latency and then the efficiency of the autoregulatory response, indicating the relevance of continuous monitoring of autoregulation following head trauma and other neurological diseases.

Metabolic regulation is an adaptative mechanism of CBF to the cerebral metabolic demand. CBF is linked to brain function and varies in parallel with CMRO$_2$. This coupling of flow to metabolism implies that local increases in metabolic demand can be rapidly met by a local increase in CBF and substrate delivery.

Chemical stimuli include arterial blood gases, circulating vasoactive substances, and neurotransmitters.

Arterial CO$_2$

Because of its powerful vasodilator effect on the cerebral vasculature, arterial CO$_2$ (PaCO$_2$) is a major determinant of CBF (Fig. 35.5*A*). At normotension, CBF increases 2% to 4% for each mm Hg increase in PaCO$_2$ in the range of 20 to 80 mm Hg. Arteriolar tone has an important influence on how PaCO$_2$ affects CBF; indeed, hypotension impairs the response of the cerebral circulation to changes in PaCO$_2$. The response of the cerebral vessels to CO$_2$ is used by anesthesiologists and intensivists to decrease CBF, cerebral blood volume, and then ICP. CO$_2$ reactivity has also been used to assess adequacy of brain perfusion in patients with internal carotid artery stenosis or cerebrovascular disease. In severe head injury, intact CO$_2$ vasoreactivity is a good predictor of the effectiveness of hyperventilation or barbiturate therapy, and impaired cerebral CO$_2$ vasoreactivity is associated with a poor outcome.

Arterial PO$_2$ (hypoxic vasodilation)

In the normoxemic range, moderate changes in arterial PO$_2$ (PaO$_2$) do not significantly alter CBF, whereas CBF increases if PaO$_2$ decreases below 50 mm Hg to maintain constant cerebral oxygen delivery.

Neurogenic regulation

Intracranial arteries are innervated by sympathetic fibers. The adrenergic innervation originates from the upper cervical ganglion, whereas the cholinergic innervation is limited to the extracranial arteries. There is a relative lack of humoral and autonomic control on normal cerebrovascular tone and a maximal stimulation of the sympathetic or parasympathetic nerves alters CBF only by approximately 5% to 15%. Stimulation of some intracerebral sites, such as locus coeruleus, and upper cervical stimulation can increase CBF. Sympathetic nerves protect the cerebral circulation from hyperemia associated with even modest elevations in arterial blood pressure.

SUGGESTED READING

Brain Trauma Foundation, American Association of Neurological Surgeons, Joint Section on Neurotrauma and Critical Care: Guidelines for the management of severe head injury. J Neurotrauma 1996;13:641–734.

Chan KH, Miller JD, Dearden NM, et al: The effect of changes in cerebral perfusion pressure upon middle cerebral artery blood flow velocity and jugular bulb venous oxygen saturation after severe brain injury. J Neurosurg 1992;77(1):55–61.

Czosnyka M, Smielewski P, Kirkpatrick P, et al: Monitoring of cerebral autoregulation in head injured patients. Stroke 1996;27:1829–1834.

Foulkes MA, Eisenberg HM, Jane JA, et al: The traumatic Come Data Bank: Design, methods and baseline characteristics. J Neurosurg 1991;75: S1–S13.

Kety SS, Schmidt CF: The nitrous oxide method for the quantitative determination of cerebral blood flow in man: Theory, procedure and normal values. J Clin Invest 1948;29:476–483.

Luce JM, Huseby JS, Kirk W, et al: Starling resistor regulates cerebral venous outflow in dogs. J Appl Physiol. 1982;53(6):1496–1503.

Marmarou A, Fatouros P, Barzó P, et al: Contribution of edema and cerebral blood volume to traumatic brain swelling in injured patients. J Neurosurg 2000;93:183–193.

Muizelaar JP, Ward JD, Marmarou A, et al. Cerebral blood flow and metabolism in severely head-injured children part 2: Autoregulation. J Neurosurg 1989;71:72–76.

Piper I, Spiegelberg A, Whittle I, et al: A comparative study of the Spiegelberg compliance device with a manual volume-injection method: A clinical evaluation in patients with hydrocephalus. Br J Neurosurg 1999;13:581–586.

Robertson CS, Gopinath S, Goodman G, et al: SjvO₂ monitoring in head injured patients. J Neurotrauma 1995;12:891–896.

Tiecks FP, Lam AM, Aaslid R, et al: Comparison of static and dynamic cerebral autoregulation measurements. Stroke 1995;26(6):1014–1019.

KEY POINTS

- Resuscitation, triage and transportation, identification and evacuation of hematomas, and good supportive critical care are responsible for improved outcome.
- Pathophysiology and empirical epidemiologic data suggest severe traumatic brain injury is particularly vulnerable to a second injury of hypotension or hypoxia.
- Intracranial pressure monitoring and cerebral perfusion pressure management are central to modern critical care of severe traumatic brain injury.
- Be vigilant and avoid fever and hypotonic fluid, and monitor the injured patient with a contusion for sudden delayed deterioration.
- Multimodal monitoring provides a physiological basis for interventions.

Traumatic brain injury (TBI) is the leading cause of death for young people in industrialized countries and is rapidly becoming so in developing countries. Furthermore, because it commonly affects the young, not only is it the leading cause of potential years of life lost but also it is responsible for among the greatest number of years lost to disability from any cause. There have been substantial improvements in the clinical outcome from TBI during the past 25 years that many attribute in part to the improved critical care of these patients. Nevertheless, there remains variation in the critical care approaches to TBI and wide variation in outcome. These facts taken together present the critical care clinician with the compelling challenge to become expert in this area of practice.

EPIDEMIOLOGY

By any measure, TBI is a significant medical problem. In North America, there are approximately 50,000 deaths annually and 80,000 neurologically impaired survivors from TBI. The incidence of severe brain injury [Glasgow Coma Scale (GCS) of 8 or less] is approximately 32 per 100,000 annually, with a mortality of approximately 17 per 100,000. However, approximately 2 million people suffer some degree of TBI annually in North America. Whereas the rates are similar in all industrialized countries, there has been a dramatic increase in the incidence in developing countries, attributed to the "advances" in the use of motor vehicles without necessarily the benefit of preventive qualities in the infrastructure.

RISK FACTORS

TBI occurs more commonly in males and in individuals 15 to 45 years of age. There are also lesser peaks in young children and the elderly older than 75 years of age, largely based on falls. Other mechanisms account for many of the risk factors. For example, 50% of severe brain injuries are related to motor vehicle accidents. Substance abuse and previous head injuries increase relative risks. Work-related injuries figure prominently, and there is also a surprisingly significant sports-related incidence. Firearm-related head injuries also constitute a definite portion of many etiologic surveys; head injuries, including closed head injuries, have become a significant and leading cause of death in combat situations. The risks of repeated concussions are increasingly documented.

PATHOGENESIS

The pathogenesis of TBI is commonly described as primary and secondary injury mechanisms. The primary injury constitutes the immediate sequelae of the impact, including the absorption of energy, changes in momentum (especially angular momentum) (Fig. 36.1), compression, tears, and hemorrhages. The adult brain weighs 1.5 kg, is made largely of lipids and water, and can be easily deformed at body temperature. With impact to the skull, the brain's change in momentum will lag behind that of the skull, and as the brain compresses and rebounds, a contusion occurs that often referred to as the coup injury (Fig. 36.2A). With greater changes in momentum, brain regions at the opposite side of impact will experience negative pressure injury as the change in momentum lags behind that of the skull, and this is called contrecoup (Fig. 36.2B). These manifest as contusions, affecting all layers of the brain, eventually leaving tissue necrosis and a fibroglial scar.

Subdural hematoma formation is common in TBI, especially with axial forces to the brain, arising from injuries to the cortical veins or pial arteries (Fig. 36.3A). Epidural hematoma formation is generally secondary to transverse forces and temporal bone fracture, and it arises from laceration to the dural arteries or veins and the fractured bone surface or commonly the middle meningeal artery (Fig. 36.3B). This arterial bleeding accumulates quickly, leading to rapid neurological impairment. Intraparenchymal hematomas occur with laceration of the superficial or deep cerebral vessels or arise from contusions.

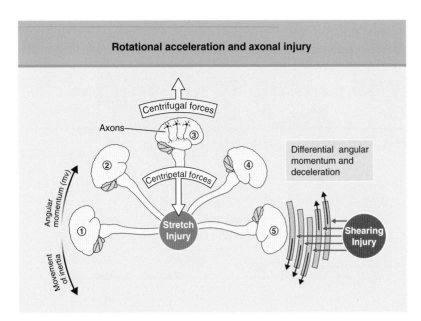

Rotational acceleration and axonal injury

Figure 36.1. Mechanism of injury with rotational acceleration and deceleration. Angular momentum is generated with rotational movement, but the magnitude varies with distance from the center of rotation and with different tissue densities. Shearing occurs between layers with differing momentum. Stretch injury occurs with centrifugal and centripetal forces.

Intraventricular hemorrhage and subarachnoid hemorrhage associated with trauma reflect severe injury and are associated with a poor prognosis.

Diffuse axonal injury is a devastating clinical syndrome reflecting generalized white matter damage. The injury to white matter includes deep punctuate hemorrhages ("Strich hemorrhages") that are concentrated in areas where there is a cleavage plane. This occurs where there is variation in angular momentum because of the different density (and velocity)

between these surfaces. Common areas of injury in diffuse axonal injury are the parasagittal regions of the cerebral hemispheres, the corpus callosum, and the focal lesions in the cerebral peduncle (classified by Gennarelli as grades I, II, and III, respectively) (Fig. 36.4; see Fig. 36.1). Shear forces of the tentorium and falx from high deceleration motion and especially axial momentum deceleration result in these injuries. Axonal stretch of 20% or more leads to primary axotomy in less than 1 hour. Lesser stretch leads to membrane dysfunction, with loss

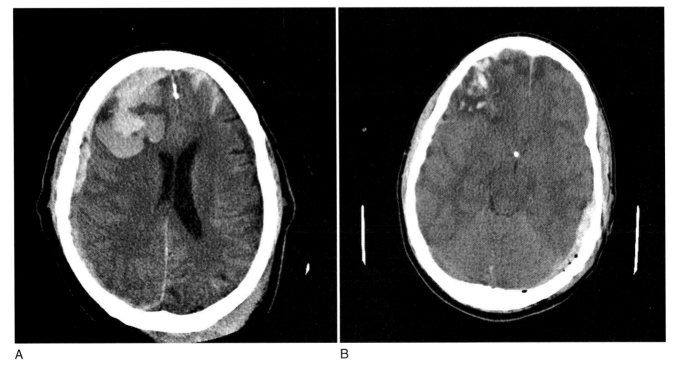

A   B

Figure 36.2. Coup and contrecoup injury. *A,* Bifrontal contusions representing coup injury occurring after a motor vehicle accident. Diabetes insipidus occurred in this case. *B,* Following an assault, this person suffered frontal contusions and a contrecoup phenomenon.

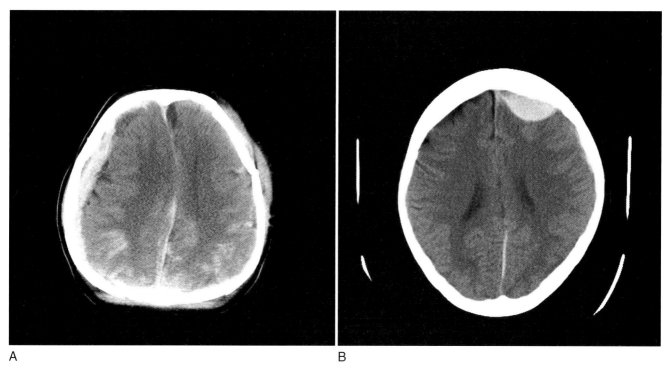

A   B

Figure 36.3. Traumatic intracranial hemorrhages. *A,* A pedestrian was hit by a car and developed a subdural hematoma with traumatic subarachnoid hemorrhage and midline shift. *B,* Following a fall, this patient exhibits an epidural hematoma, with typical elliptical shape.

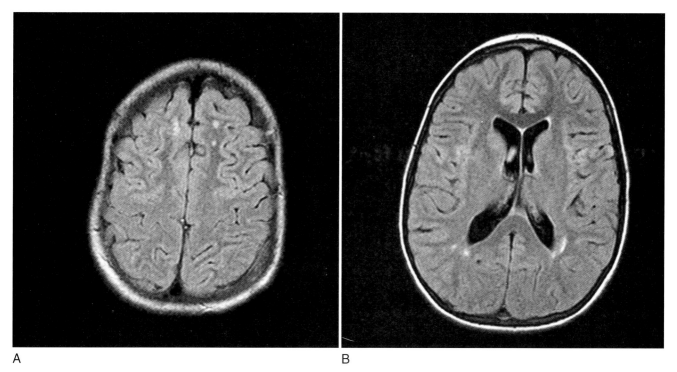

A   B

Figure 36.4. Diffuse axonal injury. A 12-year-old boy suffered diffuse injuries following a motor vehicle accident. This magnetic resonance image shows features typical of diffuse axonal injury. *A,* Magnetic resonance imaging in acute phases of injury shows hyperintense focal lesions in T2 sequences, which correspond to the Strich bleed. *B,* In chronic phases, these lesions become hypointense in T2 magnetic resonance imaging. The presence of lesions in chronic phases has been correlated with worse prognosis.

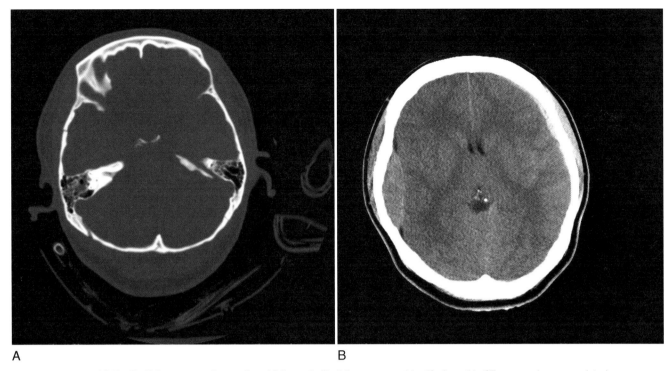

A   B

Figure 36.5. Skull fracture and associated injury. *A,* Skull fractures are identified on this CT scan and are associated with an epidural hematoma. *B,* This patient also suffered a contralateral subdural hematoma and presented with obvious signs of rising intracranial pressure. The isodensity of the epidural hemorrhage suggests ongoing active bleeding.

of ion homeostasis and subsequent focal loss of axonal transport within minutes, axonal swelling, neurofilament compaction, and proteolysis culminating in secondary axotomy. This process of secondary axotomy can be found in patients from hours to weeks and months following concussion.

Open head injuries include penetrating foreign bodies piercing dura, with the attendant injuries arising from tears and energy absorption. Skull fractures include basilar or vault fractures, and when depressed these can injure underlying brain tissue (Fig. 36.5). Vault fractures can also extend into the venous sinuses. Complications include infection, cerebrospinal fluid leak, and coagulopathies.

The concept of secondary injury is central to the understanding of the pathogenesis of TBI and to the subsequent rationale behind treatment approaches. Secondary injuries are understood to be the events that follow primary injury leading to further brain damage and a further source of critical pathophysiology. However, the distinction between primary and secondary is much more difficult to make as one looks closer at the biology of the evolution of primary injuries. Key features of the secondary injury include changes in cerebral blood flow and its autoregulation, edema formation and intracranial hypertension, and a series of metabolic cascades beginning with immediate early gene expression and including inflammation, excess excitatory neurotransmitter release, and the initiation of other biochemical pathways. In addition, abnormal systemic physiology plays a key role, both exacerbating and as a consequence of these brain events.

Immediately following trauma, at least one third of patients will exhibit cerebral ischemia as evidenced by the cerebral blood flow reduction to less than 20 mL/100 g/min (normal, 33–55)

and a decrease in the oxygen content of jugular venous blood compared with arterial (>9 vol% difference). This leads to the risk of further ischemia in the brain tissue surrounding hematomas and contusion regions. These are thought to be the reasons why episodes of hypotension and hypoxia, otherwise tolerable, confer a significantly worse prognosis and are the most relevant systemic clinical factors.

Cerebral perfusion pressure is the difference between mean arterial pressure and intracranial pressure and is a determinant (along with cerebrovascular resistance) of cerebral blood flow. Elevations in intracranial pressure or decreases in mean arterial blood pressure result in lower cerebral perfusion pressure and cerebral blood flow. Therefore, blood pressure, oxygen content, and intracranial pressure are all central determinants of brain oxygen supply.

In addition to hematoma formation, the rapid development of cerebral edema following trauma is responsible for intracranial hypertension. Membrane failure, excitotoxic depolarization, and ion channel dysfunction lead to early intracellular sodium accumulation, followed by calcium accumulation. Cellular edema, especially of astrocytic foot processes, not only worsens intracranial hypertension but also impairs microcirculation. Inflammation is initiated, which includes impaired white cell capillary travel resulting in further microcirculatory impairment. Excessive intracellular calcium triggers the activation of proteases, lipases, free oxygen radicals, and membrane lipid peroxidation. There is release of endogenous opioid peptides that in turn cause further release of neurotransmitters and activate muscarinic receptors in the rostral pons that mediate behavioral responses. An endogenous catecholamine release occurs, stimulating the sympathicoadrenomedullary axis as well as augmenting serotoninergic system activity. This highly imbalanced metabolic state is thought to lead to, among many other processes, sudden excessive glucose utilization followed by severe extracellular hypoglycemia and subsequent hypoglycemic injury. All these processes continue the cycle of secondary injury begetting further injury.

Injury to blood vessel structures and the blood–brain barrier leads to a nonpreserved blood flow/pressure autoregulation. A vasogenic response ensues, which includes early hypoperfusion followed by a phase of hyperemia (days 2–4) and a third phase of possible vasospasm (days 4–15). Vasogenic edema develops from the disrupted blood–brain barrier and the loss of autoregulation, adding further to the cycle of secondary injury.

CLINICAL FEATURES

The main clinical features of TBI include amnesia, decreased level of consciousness, and focal neurological deficits. These can be followed by signs of raised intracranial pressure (see Chapter 35), including signs of herniation. The GCS (Table 36.1) has become the standard means of rapidly communicating the depth of coma and presumed degree of injury. With the use of the GCS, in combination with specific signs of focal deficits and basic systemic vital signs, patients can be quickly triaged. The

postresuscitation GCS correlates well with clinical outcome, which is often described by the Glasgow Outcome Score (see Table 36.1). Despite good interrater reliability, it is frequently not possible to fully assess all aspects of the score. The motor component is a useful substitute.

Focal signs suggest the existence and location of focal central lesions. Expanding focal hemispheric lesions can lead to contralateral weakness and temporal lobe tentorial herniation resulting in third nerve palsy and an ipsilateral dilated pupil. Infrequently, an expanding lesion (e.g., an epidural hematoma) can shift the brain stem away from the mass compressing the opposite cerebral peduncle on the tentorial notch, resulting in ipsilateral weakness; this is described as Kernohan's notch and is a false localizing sign. Focal findings in the absence of an explanatory finding on computed tomography (CT) should trigger the clinician to consider traumatic injury to major arteries because signs of regional ischemia may be clinically manifest prior to ischemic CT findings. Severe TBI occurs with forces that are often sufficient to cause significant neck and spinal cord injuries as well as significant intrathoracic and intraabdominal injuries, and so the presence of TBI mandates a complete trauma assessment.

Following clinical examination, neurosurgical consultation and CT scanning are central to diagnosis. Figures 36.2 through 36.6 demonstrate examples of possible diagnoses. Although surgical triage is the first step in the diagnosis of potential surgically remedial lesions, the intensivist should always be alert to the diagnosis of rising intracranial pressure, especially in the absence of direct invasive intracranial pressure monitoring. In addition to clinical features (see Chapter 35), transcranial Doppler and evidence on CT scans can be helpful (see Fig. 36.6). The patient with contusions, especially bifrontal contusions, who has a GCS of 9 or 10 and does not have invasive intracranial pressure monitoring represents a special challenge of vigilance. Suddenly fatal surges of intracranial pressure can occur with minor expansions of contusions because many of these patients are on the cusp of the pressure–volume curve.

TREATMENT

It is widely believed that the improvement observed during the past 25 years in the outcome of patients with TBI is largely attributable to the advances in trauma resuscitation, early imaging and diagnosis, integrated health care systems that allow early transportation to neurosurgical centers for definitive surgical intervention, and improved supportive critical care. As such, some believe that the combination of good early resuscitation, surgical intervention, and critical care is sufficient in the overall approach to the patient with a head injury. However, many care algorithms relate directly to the various pathophysiologic mechanisms. Patient care should be individualized and respond to the temporal phases of secondary mechanisms. To do this requires multimodal monitoring—the cornerstone of modern care of the TBI patient.

Resuscitation, Triage, and Transport

There is increasing evidence that early hypoventilation and low cerebral blood flow occur immediately following TBI. Furthermore, there is good evidence that hypoxia, hypotension, and low cerebral blood flow multiply the risk of poor outcome. Thus, the

Table 36.1 Glasgow Coma Scale and Glasgow Outcome Scale[a]		
Glasgow Coma Scale		
Eye opening		
Spontaneous		4
To voice		3
To pain		2
None		1
Verbal response		
Oriented		5
Confused		4
Inappropriate		3
Incomprehensible sounds		2
None		1
Motor response		
Obeys commands		6
Localizes pain		5
Withdraws to pain		4
Abnormal flexor response		3
Extension response to pain		2
None		1
Clinical classification		
Mild		14–15
Moderate		9–13
Severe		3–8
Glasgow Outcome Scale and distribution after severe injury		
1	Dead	45%
2	Vegetative	5%
3	Severely dependent	15%
4	Moderately dependent	15%
5	Good	20%

[a]The Glasgow Coma Scale (summed from 3 to 15) is a widely used score to rapidly convey depth of traumatic coma. The outcome scale is broadly defined. Typical outcomes from severe injury are presented; however, outcomes vary between centers and have improved during the past 25 years.

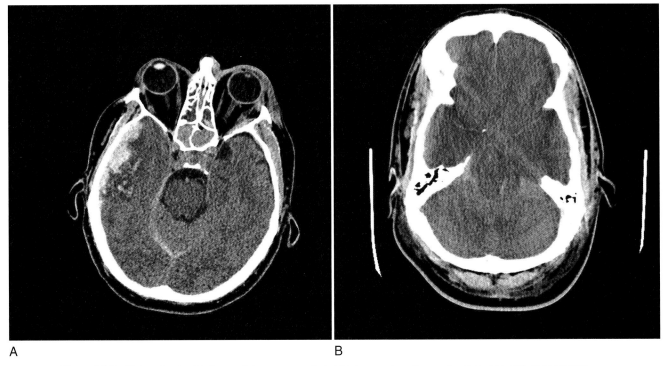

A   B

Figure 36.6. Signs of raised intracranial pressure. *A,* A right temporal posttraumatic contusion with open cisterns.
B, Generalized swelling after diffuse, prolonged decrease in cerebral blood flow demonstrating closed basal cisterns.

priorities in the approach to the patient with severe TBI are airway and ventilation management, adequate hemodynamic resuscitation, neurologic assessment including CT scanning, followed by surgical triage including transport to a neurosurgical center.

Supportive Critical Care

Patients with severe TBI should have a secured protected airway with mechanical ventilation. Prophylactic and unguided hyperventilation should not be employed, especially in the first 24 hours. The avoidance of positive end-expiratory pressure is not necessary and should be used and titrated as usual to achieve optimal oxygenation. The avoidance of a systolic blood pressure below 90 mm Hg is a minimum starting point; more specific targets for blood pressure are discussed later. Intravascular volume correction is a priority followed by vasopressors as required. Avoidance of "free water" or hypotonic solutions is important to avoid the exacerbation of brain edema. The avoidance of fever, even low grade, has been widely recommended. This is partly based on some human data that indicate that following TBI, parenchymal brain temperatures can exceed core temperatures by 1 to 1.5°C, and partly based on both experimental and clinical data that suggest hyperthermia worsens secondary injury. Elevated blood glucose levels are associated with worse neurological outcome, and tight control is generally advocated. Early enteral nutrition has been shown to improve outcomes. Some severe injuries are associated with difficult to treat coagulopathies, and these must be aggressively treated to avoid fatal delayed intracranial hemorrhage. Seizure prophylaxis is helpful for the first 7 days and thereafter should be discontinued in the absence of seizures. It does not decrease the

incidence of late-onset seizures. Some advocate its use only when traumatic intracranial hemorrhage is present.

Intracranial Hypertension Focus

Intracranial pressure measurement can serve as a surrogate patient end point, as a physiologic variable important in the management and avoidance of secondary injury, and as a statistical index of severity of injury and outcome. Persistently elevated intracranial pressure is associated with poor outcomes. Uncontrolled intracranial hypertension is the final common pathway of death by neurologic criteria following TBI, and it is undoubtedly involved in the mechanisms of secondary injury. Finally, a threshold of 20 mm Hg of intracranial pressure is often employed to determine whether more involved approaches to the injured brain are necessary. Given these aspects of intracranial pressure monitoring, it is not surprising that beyond the surgical, resuscitative, and general critical care measures already mentioned, the control of intracranial pressure is the major focus in many intensive care units.

In order to treat raised intracranial pressure, patients should be maintained in the 30-degree head up position if possible. Intermittent drainage of cerebrospinal fluid through an external ventricular drain that is also used for intracranial pressure monitoring is a simple and effective maneuver. Hypertonic solutions, such as mannitol (0.25–1 g/kg) or hypertonic saline (3 mL/kg of 3%), are effective, but total serum osmolarity must be monitored to avoid injury to renal function. Sedation and paralysis are also extremely effective, followed by guided hyperventilation and, in resistant cases, induced barbiturate coma. Removal of hematomas should always be considered at the outset, but subsequent lobectomies may be an option. The role of decompressive craniectomy remains controversial and is still actively studied.

Cerebral Perfusion Pressure Focus

Cerebral perfusion pressure is the difference between the mean arterial pressure and intracranial pressure. Until recently, many advocated directly manipulating the cerebral perfusion pressure, based on observed associations between patients with cerebral perfusion pressures higher than 70 mm Hg and better outcomes. The Rosner concept of vasodilatory cascade occurs only in patients with preserved autoregulation. A vasodilatory cascade occurs with low cerebral perfusion pressure when compensatory vasodilation increases cerebral blood volume, which in turn increases intracranial pressure leading to an even lower cerebral perfusion pressure. Maintaining an adequate cerebral perfusion pressure is achieved by lowering the intracranial pressure and supporting the mean arterial blood pressure through fluid resuscitation and direct-acting vasoconstrictors. Caution has been advised as a result of a study that found an increased incidence of acute respiratory distress syndrome when this strategy was employed, and North American guidelines suggest the lower minimum goal of 60 mm Hg unless there is evidence of brain ischemia. Therefore, optimal cerebral perfusion pressure management should be individualized, with confirmation that it is improving a desired end point. For patients with an intracranial pressure higher than 20 mm Hg, one practical recommendation is to target a cerebral perfusion pressure that minimizes the amount of time this pressure falls below 60 mm Hg.

Blood and Oxygen Flow

The importance of cerebral perfusion pressure is demonstrated by its effect on cerebral blood flow and oxygen delivery. Therefore, a more advanced approach to managing patients with severe TBI is to guide the treatments of both intracranial pressure and cerebral perfusion pressure with indices of blood flow and tissue oxygenation. This includes the recommendation of guided hyperventilation. Jugular venous saturation by intermittent sampling or continuous oximetry can be used to determine the balance between cerebral oxygen extraction and delivery. Transcranial Doppler is a daily noninvasive monitor used to evaluate the circulation for low perfusion, hyperemia, or trends suggesting vasospasm. The transcranial Doppler pulsatility index has a linear correlation with the trends of intracranial pressure beyond the critical pressure point of the volume–pressure curve, and this allows the progression of these patients to be followed, even until the onset of brain death. Tissue oxygen tension probes have been employed in either pericontusion tissue or "normal" tissue in cases of diffuse injury. Microdialysis probes sampling the parenchymal extracellular fluid can demonstrate metabolic activity that suggests energy imbalance. Each of these monitors is used to provide feedback for decisions regarding cerebral perfusion pressure target, treatments of intracranial hypertension, transfusion, whether CT scanning should be performed, etc. (Fig. 36.7).

Lund Approach

There are reports from Lund, Sweden, with recommendations that are in contrast to many guidelines on managing TBI. A central theme of this approach is the avoidance of brain tissue edema. Treatment principles are partly based on the Starling equation, which relates edema to both hydrostatic and osmotic pressure differences. This approach advocates maintaining a lower minimum cerebral perfusion pressure of 50 mm Hg and maintaining good osmotic pressures with either albumin or plasma. It involves strategies to reduce capillary pressures through the use of agents such as clonidine and metoprolol and a precapillary vasoconstrictor dihydroergotamine. The published results are impressive but have not been reproduced in a randomized trial. Although this approach has not been adopted in some areas of the world, in other areas it has become part of an armamentarium for use in a guided and reevaluated individualized manner.

Tissue Preservation

In general terms, the goal of critical care for the severely brain injured patient is the prevention of secondary neuronal injury and the preservation of tissue. Initially, this involves the surgical removal of expanding or compressive hematomas and is followed by manipulating the intracranial physiology. In addition, directly preserving brain tissue has been a long-pursued clinical goal. Although many modalities based on the cellular pathophysiology of TBI have been tested, there is little evidence of success. Meta-analysis of the use of corticosteroids in TBI did not support their use. Free radical scavengers and excitotoxic neurotransmitter blockers have been tried without clear benefit. Calcium channel blockers have also been evaluated, and there was some improved outcome in a group identified with significant traumatic subarachnoid blood. Nevertheless, they are not routinely employed in TBI. Barbiturates remain as the single therapeutic agent recommended for tissue preservation. They were found to confer survival benefits in resistant uncontrolled intracranial hypertension.

Therapeutic hypothermia is also an important consideration for brain tissue preservation. Recent trials have not resulted in a clear set of recommendations regarding its safe and effective use in TBI. Nevertheless, some mildly hypothermic patients, who remained so as part of a trial, had better outcomes. This suggests potential benefits of early hypothermia and/or the dangers of the metabolically fragile condition of rewarming. The benefits of hypothermia for brain tissue preservation continue to be demonstrated in other conditions and will no doubt be the subject of further trials of TBI.

CLINICAL COURSE AND PREVENTION

The clinical course of patients with severe TBI depends on the degree of injury, underlying pathology, and the development of complications. The clinical course reflects the evolution of the underlying pathophysiology as described previously. Ninety percent of the mortality of patients with TBI who make it to the hospital occurs by 48 hours. Later deaths occur due to the combination of other injuries, complications of head injury, uncontrolled intracranial hypertension, and clinical utility decisions. The long-term outcome of severe head injury can be measured by various scoring systems; a simplified method is the Glasgow Outcome Score (see Table 36.1).

Long-term features of people recovering from TBI include not only neurologic disabilities but also an important range of neuropsychological dysfunction. There are a growing number of studies that aim to identify anatomic and physiologic imaging

401

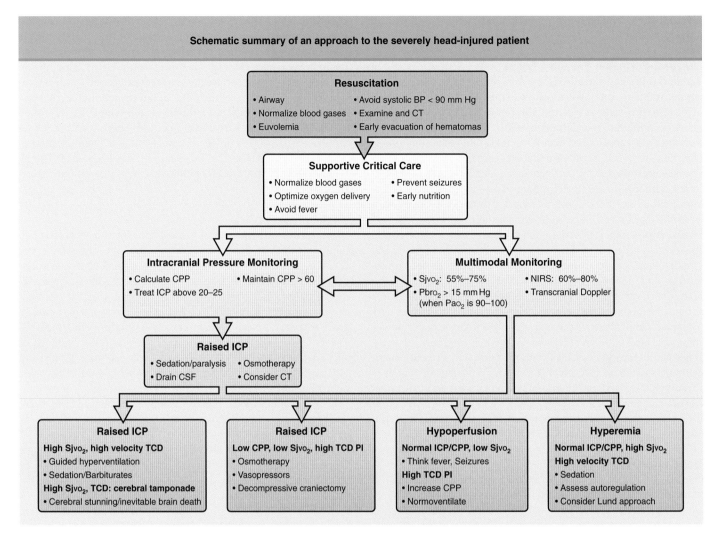

Figure 36.7. Schematic summary of an approach to the severely head-injured patient. Early effective resuscitation with appropriate triage and removal of hematoma is central to management. Careful supportive care can minimize secondary injury and improve outcomes. Intracranial pressure monitoring is important in order to direct treatment and to calculate the cerebral perfusion pressure. Concurrent multimodal monitoring provides a more detailed physiologic picture and can guide the choice of different therapies. CPP, cerebral perfusion pressure; ICP, intracranial pressure; NIRS, near infrared spectroscopy measuring brain tissue oxygen saturation; Pbro$_2$, oxygen saturation of brain tissue; Sjvo$_2$, oxygen saturation of the jugular venous blood; TCD PI, transcranial Doppler pulsatility index.

correlates of these problems. Cognitive impairment involves the loss of focus and the retention and speed of processing of new knowledge. Diminished judgment as well as chronic pain disorders and migraine are common. Depression arises from several neurotransmitter imbalances. Long-term problems also include sleep disorders, dizziness, and substance abuse disorders. Post-traumatic epilepsy is a common complication in survivors of severe TBI.

Prevention of TBI is divided into primary, secondary, and tertiary prevention. Advocacy for primary prevention measures and identification of new risks (related to newer sources of high momentum experiences) should be a part of the larger professional role of the intensivist, especially given the high public health impact of head injury and our clinical responsibility for this patient population. Secondary prevention is aimed at reducing the total neurologic injury and includes all the measures aimed at reducing secondary injury and reducing the occurrence

of complications. Neurorehabilitation and tertiary preventive measures are central in the continuum of care and allow patients and their families to maximize function given their injury. All patients warrant consideration for appropriate rehabilitation programs.

COMPLICATIONS

The pathophysiology of TBI includes the generation of circulating inflammatory mediators, neurohumoral factors, and endocrine changes that result in systemic morbidity. In addition, central regulatory functions may be disrupted, leading, for example, to diabetes insipidus or temperature dysregulation. A net production of inflammatory mediators measurable in the jugular veins is likely responsible for many features that are characteristic in patients with the systemic inflammatory response syndrome. Most notably, in addition to associated direct lung injuries and aspiration or ventilator-associated pneumonia, the severely head-injured patient frequently displays acute respiratory distress syndrome arising from TBI. *Staphylococcus aureus* is the most common pathogen in infectious pneumonia in this population. This group of patients frequently displays a disrupted breathing pattern and spontaneous hyperventilation.

Cardiac function can be impaired as a consequence of either humoral depressant factors or subendocardial ischemia associated with high sympathetic states. An elevated metabolic rate combined with catabolism occurs. Gastric paresis is common and can lead to delayed enteral nutrition unless a postpyloric feeding tube is used early. Gastric stress ulcer prophylaxis should be routine. Deep venous thrombosis risk is elevated in patients with TBI, and prophylaxis, especially in the sedated, paralyzed, or immobile patient, should be introduced as soon as feasible. Seizure prophylaxis is employed in the first 7 days, especially when there is traumatic intracranial hemorrhage.

Patients with TBI are commonly young and active, and the injury is sudden with devastating long-term personal and family implications. A proactive approach to family crisis intervention and family-centered care is a central aspect of the modern critical care of this disorder. Early comprehensive assessment of the needs of the family is critical in order to help them cope with the crisis and to improve their understanding of the implications of prognosis and of death by neurological criteria, for example. Dysfunctional relationships and family dynamics are common following TBI.

CONTROVERSIES

Wide variation exists across industrialized countries in the use of intracranial pressure monitoring and in the application of guidelines. This may reflect problems of knowledge transfer also seen in other areas of critical care. Although there are many examples of good evidence of the association between physiologic variables and outcome, examples of strong evidence that interventions actually affect outcome are few. Centers agree that good resuscitation, surgical triage, and good supportive critical care are advisable, but some controversy exists regarding the impact of each of the subsequent strategic approaches listed previously. North American guidelines, however, certainly support the importance of intracranial pressure monitoring and treatments and indicate that a minimum cerebral perfusion pressure may also be important. The use of mild hypothermia remains actively investigated with some promising results. Corticosteroids are used in some centers internationally but are not advocated by guidelines and are the focus of a large international study. The use of free radical scavengers and anti-inflammatory mediators such as tetracannabinoid is under investigation. New transcranial Doppler techniques are emerging, such as laser Doppler, which is used to define interhemispheric perfusion asymmetries, or the harmonic Doppler, which is used to identify brain tissue penumbra and vessel vasoreactivity in perilesional areas. Principles of the Lund protocols have intuitive appeal, but their uniform application has not been widely accepted. Translating basic science into clinical application has been a challenge. New ideas regarding resuscitation of white matter in diffuse axonal injury, prehospital use of hypertonic saline, and the emerging evidence of the clinical significance of delayed cerebellar dysfunction may have future relevance. The application of the various principles and approaches to each patient and over the different phases of secondary injury has become the focus of discussion in the modern approach to the patient with TBI.

SUGGESTED READING

Alvarez del Castillo M: Monitoring neurologic patients in intensive care. Curr Opin Crit Care 2001;7(2):49–60.

Andrews PJD: Potential end points of treatment after acute brain injury: Should we be using monitors of metabolism? Curr Opin Crit Care 2003; 9(2):83–85.

Bouma GJ, Muizelaar JP: Cerebral blood flow, cerebral blood volume, and cerebrovascular reactivity after severe head injury. J Neurotrauma 1992; 9(Suppl 1):S333–S348.

Chan KH, Dearden NM, Miller JD: The significance of posttraumatic increase in cerebral blood flow velocity: A transcranial Doppler ultrasound study. Neurosurgery. 1992;30:697–700.

Clifton GL, Miller ER, Choi SC, Levin HS. Fluid thresholds and outcome from severe brain injury. Crit Care Med 2002;30(4):739–745.

Cruz J: The first decade of continuous monitoring of jugular bulb oxyhemoglobin saturation: Management strategies and clinical outcome. Crit Care Med 1998;26(2):344–351.

Cruz J, Jaggi JL, Hoffstad OJ: Cerebral blood flow and oxygen consumption in acute brain injury with acute anemia: An alternative for the cerebral metabolic rate of oxygen consumption? Crit Care Med 1993;21: 1218–1224.

Gopinath SP, Valadka AB, Uzura M, et al: Comparison of jugular venous oxygen saturation and brain tissue PO_2 as monitors of cerebral ischemia after head injury. Crit Care Med 1999;27:2337–2345.

Leker RR, Shohami E: Cerebral ischemia and trauma—Different etiologies yet similar mechanisms: Neuroprotective opportunities. Brain Res Brain Res Rev 2002;39:55–73.

Martin NA, Patwardhan RV, Alexander MJ, et al: Characterization of cerebral hemodynamic phases following severe head trauma: Hypoperfusion, hyperemia, and vasospasm. J Neurosurg 1997;87:9–19.

Obrist WD, Langfitt TW, Jaggi JL, et al: Cerebral blood flow and metabolism in comatose patients with acute head injury. Relationship to intracranial hypertension. J Neurosurg 1984;61:241–253.

Robertson CS, Valadka AB, Hannay HJ, et al: Prevention of secondary ischemic insults after severe head injury. Crit Care Med 1999; 27(10):2086–2095.

Rosner MJ, Rosner SD, Johnson AH: Cerebral perfusion pressure: Management protocol and clinical results. J Neurosurg 1995;83:949–962.

Chapter 37

Management of Subarachnoid Hemorrhage

Thorsteinn Gunnarsson and Christopher Wallace

KEY POINTS

- Spontaneous subarachnoid hemorrhage (SAH) is a devastating condition that often occurs in young individuals.
- Intensive care management of SAH has a central role in the avoidance, detection, and management of brain injury.
- Many of the most serious consequences of SAH are predictable, easily identified, and treatable.
- Among the most important factors for preventing vasospasm is maintenance of relatively normal physiology and aggressive treatment of changes toward hypovolemia and hyponatremia.
- Despite best efforts, many patients with aneurysmal SAH still die or suffer from severe disability; the optimal treatment for SAH remains elusive.

Spontaneous subarachnoid hemorrhage (SAH) is a devastating condition that often occurs in young individuals. After the primary neuronal injury caused by the SAH, multiple pathophysiological mechanisms are initiated that can lead to further brain damage referred to as secondary brain injury. Intensive care management of SAH has a central role in the avoidance, detection, and management of secondary brain injury. Thorough understanding of the pathophysiology and management of SAH is thus essential to the intensive care physician because many of the most serious consequences of SAH are predictable, easily identified, and, most important, treatable. This chapter focuses on the clinical aspect of the management of aneurysmal SAH, but the principles outlined apply to any patient with significant SAH.

EPIDEMIOLOGY, RISK FACTORS, AND PATHOGENESIS

Epidemiology

Spontaneous SAH occurs in approximately 1 in 10,000 individuals per year. The incidence increases with age (mean age, approximately 50 years), it is more common in females, and the incidence is probably higher in African Americans compared with white Americans. Rupture of an intracranial aneurysm is the cause of 75% to 80% of spontaneous SAHs. Approximately 90% of ruptured aneurysms are found in the anterior circulation in the following locations in order of decreasing frequency: anterior communicating artery/anterior cerebral artery, internal carotid artery, and middle cerebral artery. Although SAH only accounts for 3% of all strokes and 5% of all stroke deaths, it is responsible for more than one fourth of lives lost through stroke and affects younger people than most other forms of stroke.

Approximately 10% to 15% of patients with spontaneous SAH have no aneurysm demonstrated on angiography. Many of these patients have a minor SAH with a typical perimesencephalic distribution. Perimesencephalic SAH has a very favorable natural history compared to aneurysmal SAH. The majority of these patients make an excellent recovery, and the risk of rebleeding is extremely low. Other causes of SAH include head injury, bleeding from an arteriovenous malformation, and pituitary apoplexy.

Risk Factors for Aneurysmal SAH and Factors Affecting Outcome

Risk factors associated with aneurysmal SAH include smoking and high blood pressure. Patients with heritable disorders such as polycystic kidney disease, Marfan syndrome, and Ehlers–Danlos syndrome are also thought to be at a higher risk for aneurysm formation and subsequent SAH. There are also well-documented families with multiple individuals with intracranial aneurysms and SAH who tend to suffer from SAH at a younger age than those without a positive family history. The risk of rupture of incidentally discovered aneurysms is not well established but appears to be low.

In patients with SAH, there are several known risk factors that lead to an unfavorable outcome and a "rough" clinical course. The patient's clinical grade after resuscitation and treatment of hydrocephalus, if present, is a very important prognostic factor. The worse the neurological condition, the poorer the prognosis. The amount of subarachnoid blood seen on computed tomography (CT) scan affects outcome and is discussed later in detail. Intraventricular blood and intracerebral blood also have a negative impact on outcome. One of the most significant negative prognostic factors in patients with aneurysmal SAH is age. In the Cooperative Aneurysm Study, 86% of the patients between 18 and 29 years old made a good recovery, with a 7% mortality rate, whereas only 26% of patients between the ages of 70 and 87 years had a similar outcome, with a mortality rate of 49%. Any associated comorbidities also inversely affect prognosis in patients with SAH. In summary, young, otherwise healthy, patients in good clinical grade with minimal SAH and small aneurysms are most likely to make a good recovery.

Pathogenesis

During rupture of an intracranial aneurysm, intracranial pressure (ICP) rises to diastolic blood pressure levels and cerebral blood flow (CBF) only occurs during systole. The aneurysm then seals off, but in some cases the bleeding is extensive or does not stop, causing immediate death, and approximately 12% of patients die before they can obtain medical attention. Many patients lose consciousness for a brief period of time and in some cases they also have seizures. The immediate loss of consciousness with or without seizures can cause respiratory arrest. This period is also often associated with cardiac arrhythmias. The direct mechanical destructive effects of the bleeding on brain tissue, poor oxygenation, and the low cerebral perfusion pressure lead to global ischemic neuronal injury and, in combination, cause the primary neuronal injury. The presence of subarachnoid blood then activates mechanisms that can lead to secondary brain injury, which are responsible for the greater part of the resulting morbidity and mortality in this patient group.

CLINICAL FEATURES AND CLASSIFICATION

Patients who complain of sudden-onset severe headache or those who suffer from a sudden decrease in the level or loss of consciousness, seizures, or new neurological deficits should have a high-resolution CT scan of the head. In cases in which the CT scan is negative and the diagnosis of SAH is still suspected, a lumbar puncture is mandatory to rule out SAH. In confirmed cases of SAH, further diagnostic tests are warranted to rule out an intracranial aneurysm or other vascular malformations as the cause of the bleeding. These are most commonly in the form of conventional cerebral angiogram, but some centers use CT angiography as the first study of choice. SAH is usually classified according to the patient's clinical condition and the amount and location of the intracranial hemorrhage. The most commonly used classifications for clinical grading are those of Hunt and Hess (modified from Botterell's initial classification from 1956) and the World Federation of Neurological Surgeons (WFNS) (Tables 37.1 and 37.2). The WFNS classification is

Table 37.2 World Federation of Neurological Surgeons Grading Scale[a]

Grade	GCS Score	Motor Deficit
I	15	Absent
II	14–13	Absent
III	14–13	Present
IV	12–7	Present or absent
V	6–3	Present or absent

GCS, Glascow Coma Scale.
[a]Adapted from Drake CG: Report of World Federation of Neurological Surgeons Committee on a Universal SAH Grading Scale. J Neurosurg 1988;68:985.

more objective and is based on the Glasgow Coma Scale. The amount and location of the bleeding seen on the initial CT scan are classified by the Fisher grading scale (Fig. 37.1). The Fisher grade as well as the clinical grading scales are highly predictive of the clinical course and outcome and therefore serve as useful clinical tools.

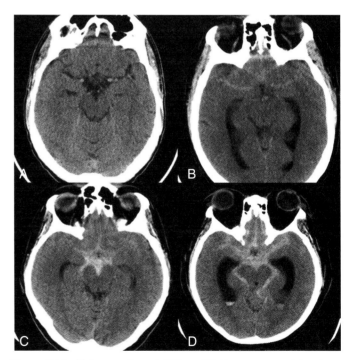

Figure 37.1. Fisher grading of SAH on CT. The amount and location of blood on a CT scan in patients with ruptured intracranial aneurysms are used to assess the severity of the bleeding and for prognostic purposes. The classification described by Fisher has four grades (Fisher CM, Kistler JP, Davis JM: Relation of cerebral vasospasm to subarachnoid hemorrhage visualized by computerized tomographic scanning. Neurosurgery 1980;6:1–9). *A*, Grade 1, no subarachnoid blood is seen. *B*, Grade 2, diffuse or vertical layers of blood less than 1 mm in thickness. *C*, Grade 3, localized clot and/or vertical layers more than 1 mm. *D*, Grade 4, intracerebral or intraventricular blood with or without diffuse SAH. Patients with grade 3 and 4 SAH are most likely to develop clinically significant vasospasm.

Table 37.1 Modified Hunt and Hess Classification of Patients with SAH[a]

Grade	Condition
0	Unruptured aneurysm
1	Asymptomatic or minimal headache and slight nuchal rigidity
2	Moderate to severe headache, nuchal rigidity, no neurologic deficit other than cranial nerve palsy
3	Drowsiness, confusion, or mild focal deficit
4	Stupor, moderate to severe hemiparesis, possible early decerebrate rigidity, vegetative disturbances
5	Deep coma, decerebrate rigidity, moribund appearance

[a]Serious systemic illnesses (hypertension, atherosclerotic heart disease, diabetes, chronic pulmonary disease, and severe vasospasm seen on angiography) place the patient in the next less favorable category. Adapted from Hunt WE, Hess EM: Surgical risk as related to time of intervention in the repair of intracranial aneurysms. J Neurosurg 1968;28:14.

TREATMENT

Initial Management and Level of Monitoring

The initial management including resuscitation of unstable patients with SAH follows the same steps as for any unstable patients in the intensive care unit (ICU), where breathing and circulation are the first priority. All patients with confirmed SAH should be kept in a monitored unit until proper imaging studies have ruled out an aneurysm, an arteriovenous malformation (AVM), or any pathological condition that needs emergency surgical or endovascular treatment to prevent further bleeding. The level of monitoring should be based on the clinical condition of the patients. Patients who are neurologically well and physiologically stable can be monitored in a step-down unit and in most cases do not need arterial line monitoring for blood pressure or central lines. Patients who are either neurologically or physiologically unstable should have more aggressive clinical and physiological monitoring, including arterial and central venous lines, because they can deteriorate quickly. Patients with SAH commonly have severe headache and nausea, which should be treated aggressively. Agitated patients and intubated patients are sedated with short-acting drugs such as propofol or midazolam. This allows for "waking up" the patients for repeated neurological assessments. Gastric stress ulcer prophylaxis with sucralfate is routinely administered because neurosurgical patients are particularly prone to developing stress ulcers.

All patients are treated with nimodipine (Nimotop), a calcium channel blocker used for the prevention and treatment of vasospasm. It has been shown to be beneficial in several clinical trials in patients with SAH, and a meta-analysis of the literature indicated that nimodipine improves outcome. The standard regimen for patients with SAH is 60 mg per os or in the nasogastric tube every 4 hours initiated within the first 96 hours of the bleeding. The treatment should be continued for 21 days or until the patient is discharged home in a good condition, whichever occurs first. An intravenous form of nimodipine is also available.

Pulmonary Management

Medical complications account for approximately one fourth of deaths in patients with SAH. Of these, the majority are caused by pulmonary and cardiovascular complications. These conditions may by themselves be life threatening and cause hypoxemia and hypotension; in addition, they can aggravate the neurological injury already caused by the SAH. Risk factors for cardiopulmonary complications include poor clinical grade, amount of hemorrhage, hypertension, age, and ventricular repolarization abnormalities.

Unconscious patients or patients who cannot protect the airways because of a neurological deficit need to have the airways secured. Hypoventilation causes cerebral vasodilation and an increase in ICP. Hyperventilation, on the other hand, can cause vasoconstriction, which may lead to aggravation of cerebral ischemia and should not be routinely used. Patients on ventilators should therefore be kept normocapnic; hyperventilation should only be used temporarily, for example, in an emergency situation such as during sudden neurological deterioration due to elevation in ICP or in special situations in which all other steps have been taken to lower high ICP.

Cardiac dysfunction and pulmonary edema may occur together or independently. Clinical and experimental evidence suggests that the main underlying mechanism is "catecholamine storm" that occurs as a result of ischemia or infarction in the posterior hypothalamus. This mechanism is different from the inflammatory response that creates acute lung injury and acute respiratory distress syndrome, although SAH can also trigger a systemic inflammatory response. This neurogenic pulmonary edema, defined as bilateral pulmonary infiltrates on chest x-ray and reduced PaO_2 not attributable to another cause, is a serious complication after SAH. Although positive pressure ventilation and diuretics have been used to treat this condition, systemic circulating volume overload is not considered to be the cause of neurogenic pulmonary edema. The pulmonary circulation may be severely overloaded due to redistribution of blood volume as a result of catecholamine release so that the systemic circulation is rendered acutely hypovolemic. Therefore, volume resuscitation may be more appropriate than diuretic therapy to restore circulating volume acutely and optimize right ventricular preload. Figure 37.2 shows a management protocol for cardiorespiratory compromise in SAH.

Cardiovascular Management

Patients with SAH commonly have increased ICP and high blood pressure; actively lowering blood pressure can cause cerebral ischemia by lowering cerebral perfusion pressure (CPP) (CPP = mean arterial pressure − ICP). Therefore, lowering blood pressure aggressively in patients with SAH is usually not indicated, even in patients with ruptured unsecured aneurysms. Systolic blood pressure less than 180 mm Hg should therefore not be actively lowered in patients with SAH. After the aneurysm has been repaired, systolic blood pressure up to 220 mm Hg or even higher can be accepted. Approximately 20% of patients with ruptured intracranial aneurysms have more than one aneurysm. If the aneurysm that ruptured has been treated, the presence of other unruptured intracranial aneurysms should not affect the blood pressure management during the stay in the ICU.

Rhythm and conduction disturbances seen on electrocardiogram (ECG) are extremely common in SAH, but their clinical relevance is often questionable. Common findings include QRS, ST segment, and T wave abnormalities and prolongation of the QT interval. These changes may mimic myocardial infarction or ischemia but are usually reversible in survivors of SAH. The ECG abnormalities have no consistent association with mechanical hypokinesis found on echocardiography, histological cardiac lesions, or serum markers of cardiac injury. Arrhythmias causing hemodynamic changes have been found in approximately 40% of patients. Life-threatening arrhythmias are uncommon, however, occurring in approximately 5% of patients. Given the relatively benign nature of most ECG changes and arrhythmias seen in aneurysmal SAH, these should not generally be used as a contraindication for delaying endovascular or surgical treatment of a ruptured aneurysm.

An increase in plasma creatine phosphokinase–myocardial fraction and troponin I is commonly seen, more so in patients with echocardiographic evidence of wall motion abnormalities and in patients with neurogenic pulmonary edema. Such ventricular dysfunction is commonly seen in patients with SAH and

407

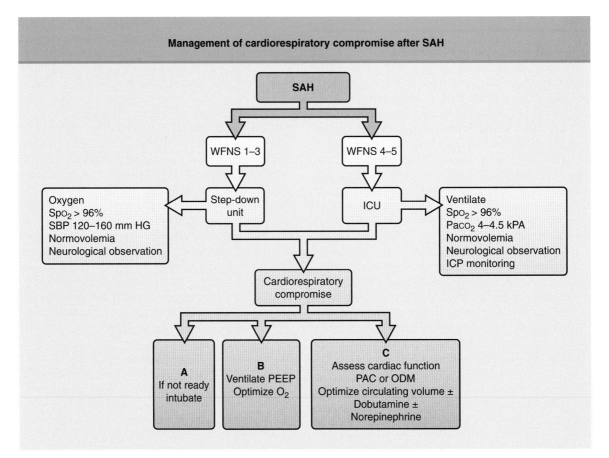

Figure 37.2. Management of cardiorespiratory compromise after SAH. Neurogenic pulmonary edema and cardiac dysfunction can manifest clinically as separate entities or together. They should be considered together as a part of a clinical syndrome that requires assessment of cardiac function for optimal treatment. OMD, esophageal Doppler monitor; PAC, pulmonary artery catheter; WFNS, World Federation of Neurosurgeons grading for SAH; SBP, systolic blood pressure. (Modified from Macmillan CS, Grant IS, Andrews PJ: Pulmonary and cardiac sequelae of subarachnoid haemorrhage: Time for active management? Intensive Care Med 2002;28:1012–1023.)

can be fatal. The term "myocardial stunning" has been applied to such sudden and sometimes unexpected ventricular hypokinesis. The most commonly seen wall motion abnormality is left ventricular dysfunction and is usually not due to coronary artery disease. Inotropic support may cause improvement, despite catecholamines causing ventricular injury and neurogenic pulmonary edema. In patients with reduced left ventricular work, dobutamine has proved effective. In one series, SAH patients with pulmonary edema, increased pulmonary artery occlusion pressure, and variable cardiac index (all with low ejection fractions on echocardiography) were treated successfully with dobutamine and a combination of epinephrine and/or norepinephrine. Patients with any clinical evidence of neurogenic pulmonary edema and/or cardiac impairment should have a pulmonary artery catheter or esophageal Doppler assessment of cardiac function to guide therapy (see Fig. 37.2).

Seizures

Patients with SAH and seizures should be treated with antiseizure medications. Our first drug of choice is phenytoin (Dilantin). Seizures should be treated aggressively because they cause secondary brain injury by aggravating cerebral ischemia.

Antiseizure treatment before the aneurysm is excluded from the circulation can be considered as a treatment option, although there is no evidence supporting this practice. Prophylactic seizure treatment after the aneurysm has been excluded from the circulation has no role in the management of SAH.

Prevention of Rebleeding

If untreated, ruptured intracranial aneurysms are at a high risk of rupture, with a case fatality rate of approximately 70% for people who rebleed. In the prospective cooperative aneurysm study, rebleeding was 4% on the first day and then 1% or 2% per day during the next 4 weeks. After 6 months, approximately 50% of untreated ruptured intracranial aneurysms have reruptured.

Despite the fact that antifibrinolytic therapy has been found to effectively reduce the incidence of rebleeding after aneurysmal SAH, its efficacy is dampened by the increased number of cerebral infarcts and hydrocephalus with long-term treatment. However, a randomized multicenter trial showed a reduction in the ultra-early rebleeding rate from 10.8% to 2.4% and an 80% reduction in the mortality rate from early rebleeding with short-term (maximum of 72 hr) treatment with tranexamic acid

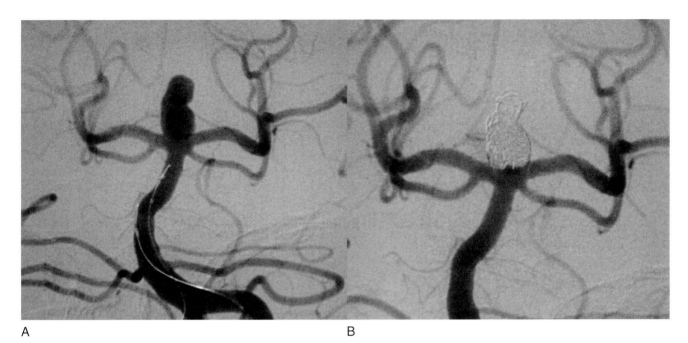

A   B

Figure 37.3. Endovascular treatment of an intracranial aneurysm. Endovascular treatment is now generally the favored treatment modality for ruptured and unruptured aneurysms. Endovascular treatment has technical limitations, and currently 20% to 50% of aneurysms are treated with surgical clipping. *A*, Ruptured basilar tip aneurysm prior to coiling. *B*, After the procedure, the aneurysm is no longer filling and only a small neck remnant is seen on the final angiogram. This prevents the aneurysm from rebleeding.

without any increase in the number of vasospasm or cerebral infarcts in patents who had an early operation for their aneurysms. The percentage of patients with favorable outcomes increased from 70.5% to 74.8%. Whether this applies to patients who will subsequently undergo endovascular treatment, where thromboembolic complications are one of the main concerns, is not known.

The aneurysm that caused the SAH should be excluded from the circulation as soon as practically possible. Aneurysms can be closed using microsurgical techniques by placing a clip around the neck of the aneurysm or by endovascular techniques most often by filling the aneurysm from the inside with coils (Fig. 37.3). A randomized international multicenter trial (ISAT) showed that patients with aneurysmal SAH who underwent coiling had a 6.9% absolute risk reduction for death or dependency compared to the surgical group. The main concern with endovascular treatment is the unknown long-term efficacy because many of the aneurysms treated are left with a small remnant that may increase in size and potentially cause a future rupture, although this risk seems to be small according to our current understanding. Current practice favors endovascular treatment of ruptured aneurysms with endovascular techniques if it is believed that these are safe and going to produce good immediate results. If not, they are treated with surgical clipping. Detailed descriptions of these treatment modalities are beyond the scope of this chapter. With endovascular treatments, especially when aneurysms have been treated with microstents, all patients are currently treated with antiplatelet agents. This approach requires special consideration if subsequent surgical treatment is necessary, with increased risk of hemorrhagic com-

plications. If it is anticipated that the patient will need an external ventricular drain, it is preferable to place it before the antiplatelet treatment is started.

Hydrocephalus

Approximately 500 mL of cerebrospinal fluid (CSF) is produced in the ventricles every 24 hours. SAH can block the pathways and the drainage of CSF leading to the development of hydrocephalus, seen as dilated ventricles on a CT scan (Fig. 37.4). This increases ICP and consequently causes reduction in cerebral perfusion pressure and a decreased level of consciousness. The presence of large amounts of thick subarachnoid or intraventricular blood increases the risk of acute hydrocephalus and is sometimes seen on the initial CT scan but can develop at any stage after SAH or even after discharge from the hospital.

In patients with symptomatic hydrocephalus, the first treatment choice is insertion of an external ventricular drain (EVD) to reduce ICP and to clear any blood from the ventricles (see Fig. 37.4). Standard treatment is to keep the drain open initially at a 10- to 15-cm height. Once the blood has cleared, the drain is then elevated and finally closed, and ICP and the patient's neurological status are monitored carefully. In case of elevated ICP or neurological deterioration, the drain is reopened and a decision has to be made whether the patient needs a permanent ventriculoperitoneal shunt or whether the patient should keep draining for a few more days before a new trial of closing. Once the intraventricular blood has cleared, another temporary solution for CSF diversion is to insert a lumbar drain. CSF should be routinely sent for analysis. A controversial issue is whether EVDs need to be changed after a certain period of time to

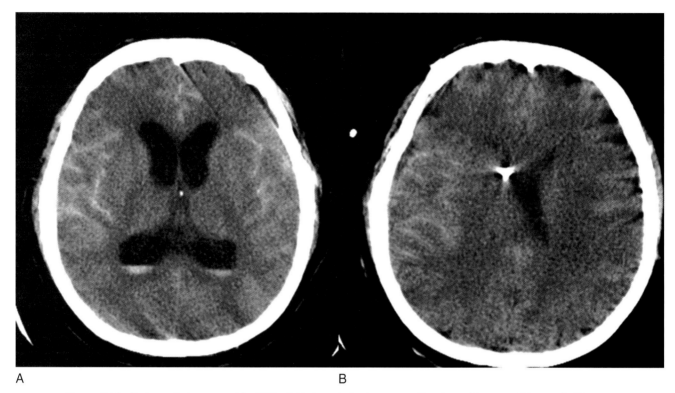

A   B

Figure 37.4. Hydrocephalus caused by SAH. *A,* Hydrocephalus is seen as dilated ventricles on a CT scan. *B,* After placement of an external ventricular drain, the ventricles are reduced in size. This also allows for recording of intracranial pressure.

reduce the risk of infection. Some surgeons routinely change the drain every 7 days, whereas others do not; there are no data available on the best approach.

Diagnosis and Treatment of Clinical Vasospasm

After an aneurysm has been excluded from the circulation, and rebleeding thus prevented, the major cause of morbidity and mortality in SAH is clinically significant vasospasm, also referred to as delayed ischemic deficit (Fig. 37.5). The risk of developing clinical vasospasm is directly related to the amount of blood seen on CT and the patients with greatest risk are those with thick subarachnoid blood and a poor clinical grade (see Tables 37.1 and 37.2 and Fig. 37.1). Other risk factors implicated but not as well confirmed are smoking, preexisting hypertension, older age, female gender, and hydrocephalus. Clinically significant vasospasm occurs in approximately 30% of patients with aneurysmal SAH and typically starts between days 3 and 14. It is associated with severe arterial narrowing seen on conventional angiogram. Since blood flow in a vessel varies directly and resistance inversely with the fourth power of the radius, blood flow and resistance are obviously affected by small changes in vessel caliber. Clinically significant vasospasm should not be confused with angiographic vasospasm, which is seen in up to two thirds of all patients with aneurysmal SAH and in many cases is entirely asymptomatic because it does not reduce CBF sufficiently to decrease neurological function. The cause of vasospasm is under intense investigation but clearly is related to the presence and breakdown of blood in the subarachnoid space.

Patients with SAH commonly deteriorate during their stay in the ICU. Neurological deterioration after SAH is a medical emergency and needs rapid evaluation and treatment. Because there are many causes of neurological deterioration, several diagnostic tests should be ordered simultaneously. Blood work should include electrolytes, blood gases, and levels of drugs that may alter level of consciousness such as phenytoin. A CT scan should be done acutely to rule out bleeding, new infarcts, brain swelling, and hydrocephalus. If the patient has an external ventricular drain or has had a neurosurgical procedure, CSF should be sent for biochemistry, cell count, and culture to rule out central nervous system infection such as postoperative meningitis. If the drain is closed and the ICP is high, it can be opened to release a few milliliters of CSF to reduce ICP while the CT scan is being arranged. In rare cases, the cause of the deterioration is a seizure without muscle twitching, and this can only be diagnosed with an electroencephalogram. If no cause is found for the deterioration, the most common reason is clinically significant vasospasm. The first symptom of vasospasm is most commonly increasing headache followed by signs such as increasing confusion and drowsiness and focal neurological deficits caused by decreasing blood flow to the vascular territory involved. The most common vasospasm syndromes are listed in Box 37.1.

The gold standard test for the diagnosis of vasospasm is conventional cerebral angiography, which by itself carries an approximately 0.5% risk of permanent neurological complications. It can show concentric narrowing of the intracranial vessels that can be focal, segmental, or diffuse. Vasospasm is classified as mild narrowing (<25%), moderate (25–50%), or severe (>50%).

Transcranial Doppler ultrasonography (TCD) is a noninvasive bedside monitoring technique that is routinely used to follow patients with SAH. TCD detects blood flow direction and veloc-

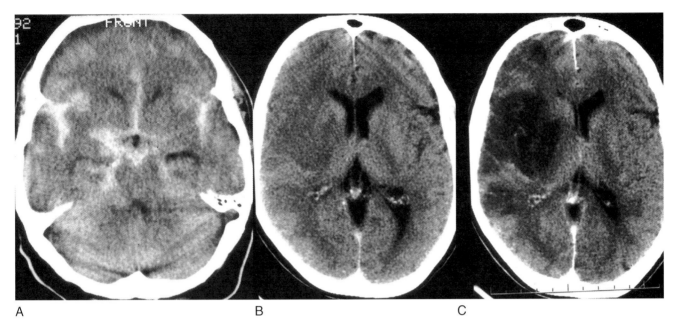

Figure 37.5. Evolution of a cerebral infarct caused by vasospasm. This patient had an initial CT scan showing a Fisher grade 3 SAH from a ruptured intracranial aneurysm (*A*). *B*, Seven days later, increased swelling and low density are seen in the right hemisphere. *C*, On day 11, an area of low density (infarct) is seen in the right middle cerebral artery territory.

ity in the middle cerebral artery, and there is a close correlation between flow velocity and the degree of arterial narrowing seen on angiograms. It should be done daily and during neurological deterioration. Mean velocity of more than 120 cm/sec and/or an increase of 50 cm/sec/day are highly suggestive of vasospasm. The sensitivity and specificity of the TCD findings are a subject of intense debate. There are studies demonstrating that commonly used TCD indices used to diagnose vasospasm do not always reflect cerebral perfusion values. Nevertheless, TCD has been found to be useful as a early warning tool for the detection of an impending clinical vasospasm, but the results from cerebral angiography and TCD studies have to be put into clinical context since neither measures CBF and positive findings do not necessarily indicate a reduction in cerebral ischemia. The importance of repeated neurological examinations cannot be overemphasized in this patient group. There are ways to quantitatively measure CBF, such as Xe CT scan and positron emission tomography. If available, these may further guide in the treatment and especially in the assessment of the efficacy of the treatment instituted to reverse the cerebral ischemia.

"Triple H" Therapy

The goal of treatment for clinically significant vasospasm is to increase CBF to reverse the neurological deficit that has occurred. In 1990, Origitano introduced the concept of hypertensive hypervolemic hemodilution, or triple H therapy. It is now considered first-line treatment for vasospasm, although there is no evidence from large randomized controlled clinical trials to support this type of treatment. Every neurosurgeon or intensive care physician who has been involved in the management of patients with SAH has anecdotal experience of patients who markedly improve neurologically with this treatment and deteriorate when it is discontinued. There are also small

prospective clinical series showing that triple H can improve CBF and reverse neurological deficits. In light of the severe nature of this condition, and the suggestive evidence in its favor, this treatment is justified in most patients with vasospasm. The three H's are now discussed in greater detail according to a treatment protocol for the management of vasospasm (Fig. 37.6).

Hypervolemia

Patients with SAH routinely become hypovolemic, and this must be aggressively corrected because blood volume status is a key factor in predicting patients who will develop vasospasm. One should aim at a central venous pressure of 8 to 12 mm Hg or pulmonary wedge pressure of 18 to 20 mm Hg. The primary fluids used are usually isotonic crystalloids such as normal saline or Ringer's lactate. For further volume expansion, 5% albumin is probably the most commonly used colloid solution. Other alternatives are fresh frozen plasma or red blood cells. Many centers use hydroxyethyl starch (HES) instead of albumin. The use of HES in the management of SAH is controversial. The advantages are twofold: HES is not made from human blood products, and it costs much less than albumin. There is very limited information in the literature on the differences between different colloids in the treatment of SAH, but the main concern with the use of HES is that it may cause coagulopathy. A Cochrane review of the current literature found no evidence that one colloid solution was more effective or safe than any other.

Electrolytes

Counteracting hyponatremia and hypovolemia in patients with vasospasm deserves special attention. The most common electrolyte disturbance seen in patients treated for SAH is hyponatremia (Na$^+$ < 135 mmol/liter), seen in up to 43% of patients.

Box 37.1 Differential Diagnosis of Affected Vascular Territories in Intracranial Vasospasm

Anterior Circulation

Middle cerebral artery (MCA)

Complete MCA occlusion
Contalateral hemiplegia with face and upper and lower extremities equally affected; head and eye deviation toward the side of the lesion; hemianopia; global aphasia if dominant hemisphere; contralateral neglect if nondominant

Upper trunk of MCA
Hemiparesis with face and arm more than leg; if dominant hemisphere, expressive aphasia; nondominant hemisphere, neglect.

Inferior trunk of MCA
Weakness or sensory changes less marked; hemianopia or upper quadrant anopia; nondominant hemisphere, constructional apraxia, and delirium

Anterior cerebral artery

Sensory motor disturbances of the leg and foot, loss of control of the urinary bladder; abulia in bifrontal dysfunction; lack of responsiveness to verbal stimuli; if Heubner's artery is involved, dysarthria as well as behavioral and cognitive disturbances

Anterior choroidal artery

Contralateral hemiparesis; hemisensory loss; and homonymous hemianopia

Posterior cerebral artery

Obtundation; contralateral visual defects

Posterior Circulation

Highly variable symptoms; altered conciousness, confusion, delirium, dizziness, vertigo, ocular and pupillary abnormalities, hemifacial paresis, bilateral motor weakness, ataxia, dysarthria, dysphagia, crossed sensory loss, visual field defects

---

It tends to occur between days 2 and 10, paralleling the period of vasospasm. Severe hyponatremia (Na^+ < 120 mmol/liter) is rarely seen and hyponatremia is seldom the sole cause of neurological deterioration. Studies have shown that most of these patients are volume depleted and have a negative sodium balance and therefore do not have syndrome of inappropriate secretion of ADH but, rather, a condition called cerebral salt wasting syndrome (CSWS) (Table 37.3).

CSWS and iatrogenic-induced hyponatremia are both caused by excessive natriuresis associated with hypovolemia and should be treated with volume and sodium replacement. Sodium replacement conversely provokes further natriuresis and osmotic diuresis. Avoiding hypovolemia can therefore be challenging in this setting. Hydrocortisone (1200 mg/day) or fludrocortisone (maximal dose, 0.4 mg/day) cause sodium retention and have been found to be helpful, causing positive sodium balance and hypervolemia in this patient group.

Hemodilution

Hemodilution and hypervolemia are related because hypervolemia induces hemodilution. The rationale for inducing hemodilution is to decrease blood viscosity and improve CBF. This comes at a cost of decreased oxygen-carrying capacity and therefore might decrease oxygen delivery to the brain. The optimal hematocrit (Hct) for providing optimal O_2 delivery to ischemic brain tissue is not known. For normal tissues, it is approximately 30% to 33%, but for the brain it may be higher. We do not actively phlebotomize our patients but try to keep the Hct at approximately 35% and transfuse patients who have hemoglobin values under 10 g/dL.

Hypertension

Raising blood pressure is reserved for patients who have already been optimally treated with fluids to reach a state of hypervolemia and who have not responded with improvement in neurological status. The blood pressure is raised to a level at which the neurological deficit resolves, but it should not be more than 240 mm Hg systolic (or MAP < 150 mm Hg). In patients who have not had their ruptured aneurysm repaired, we do not recommend raising the systolic blood pressure above 180 mm Hg. This should be done while the patient is carefully monitored because some studies have shown that patients can paradoxically deteriorate with a decrease in CBF with this treatment. If the neurological deficit does not resolve and CT scan does not show an already established infarct, one should consider other treatment options such as angioplasty. However, if the CT scan or perfusion scans (PET, CT, or MRI-based perfusion scans) do reveal an already established infarct, aggressive blood pressure treatment should be discontinued. What inotropes and vasopressors to use is usually a matter of personal or institutional preference. Most units start either with dopamine or dobutamine and then add phenylephrine or norepinephrine if needed. Others immediately start with phenylephrine.

Increasing Cardiac Output Alone vs. Blood Pressure

Triple H therapy is associated with numerous complications, which are mostly pulmonary, cardiac, and intracranial in nature. It is estimated that 25% of patients suffer from complications associated with triple H therapy. Pulmonary complications such as pulmonary edema and cardiac arrhythmias along with cardiac ischemia are the most common. CBF studies have shown that triple H in some patients may exacerbate brain ischemia by reducing CBF (seen on Xe CT) and cause reduction in O_2 delivery (seen on PET). Hemorrhagic complications also occur. It can also cause or exacerbate cerebral edema in the presence of blood–brain barrier disruption and even cause iatrogenic hypertensive encephalopathy.

One study showed that increasing cardiac output with dobutamine in patients with delayed ischemic deficit (DID) reversed CBF deficits as much as elevating blood pressure with phenylephrine. This may prove to be a step one could consider before elevating blood pressure in patients with DID because it is probably safer than elevating the blood pressure with phenylephrine.

When Triple H Fails

If the patient has a persistent neurological deficit after maximal triple H treatment, percutaneous balloon dilatation of the

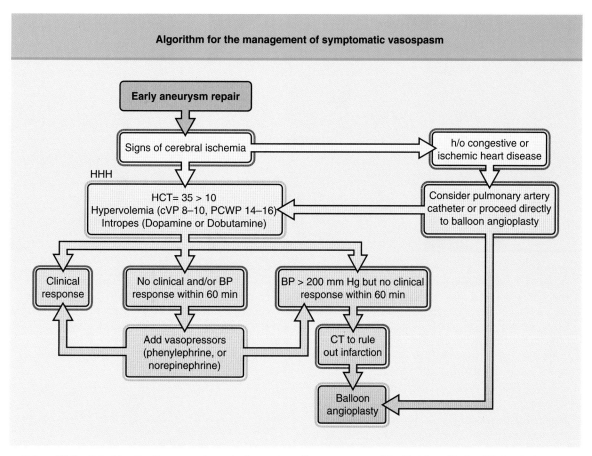

Figure 37.6. Algorithm for the management of symptomatic vasospasm. (Modified from Findlay JM: Cerebral Vasospasm. In Winn HR (ed): Youmans Neurological Surgery, 5th ed. Philadelphia, Elsevier, 2004.)

Table 37.3 Differential Diagnosis of Cerebral Salt Wasting Syndrome (CWS) and Inappropriate Secretion of ADH (SIADH)[a]		
	CSW	**SIADH**
Extracellular fluid volume	↓	↑
Body weight	↓	↑
Fluid balance	Negative	Negative
Urine volume	↔ or ↑	↔ or ↓
Tachycardia	+	−
Hematocrit	↑	↔
Albumin	↑	↔
Serum bicarbonate	↑	↔ or ↓
Blood urea nitrogen	↑	↔ or ↓
Serum uric acid	↔ or ↓	↓
Urinary sodium	↑	↑
Sodium balance	Negative	Negative or +
Central venous pressure	↓	↔ or slightly ↑
	(<6 cm H2O)	(6–10 cm H2O)
Wedge pressure	↓	↔ or slightly ↑

[a]Modified from Rabinstein AA, Wijdicks EFM: Hyponatremia in critically ill neurological patients. Neurologist 2003;9:290–300.

spastic intracranial vessels should be considered. A CT scan or a perfusion study showing an established infarct is a contraindication to this treatment. This treatment modality can be used to dilate the larger proximal intracranial arteries (Fig. 37.7) and has been shown in several small clinical series to be effective in reversing otherwise persisting neurological deficits in 30%

to 70% of patients and improves CBF (studied with Xe CT). It is clearly effective in reversing angiographic vasospasm. This approach, however, is not without risk. The procedure is technically difficult and carries up to a 5% risk of mortality mainly caused by intraprocedural rupture of the vessel's being dilated. The key to a successful angioplasty is careful patient selection and timing because this should not be done in a delayed fashion. In summary, the management of vasospasm should focus on prompt recognition of the condition, prompt triple H therapy, and angioplasty if triple H therapy fails.

CLINICAL COURSE AND PREVENTION

The clinical course for many cases of SAH is a challenging one, both for the patient and for the treating physician. The first 2 weeks usually give a good indication about the prognosis. One of the most important factors for preventing vasospasm is maintenance of relatively normal physiology and aggressive treatment of any changes toward hypovolemia and hyponatremia, even to the point of modest hypervolemia and increased cardiac output. Hct should also be normalized. It is important to reduce ICP, treat hypotension, and not treat hypertension, especially when the patient is at maximal risk of vasospasm. Fever and infections should also be actively treated. All of these measures are necessary to optimize CBF to prevent secondary brain injury. In our view, there is no indication for prophylactic triple H therapy other than inducing modest hypervolemia. Close monitoring in

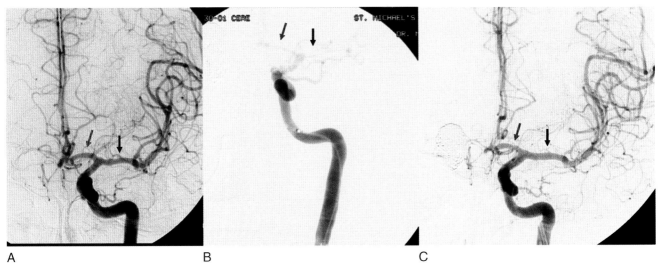

A   B   C

Figure 37.7. Vasospasm on angiography treated with balloon angioplasty. This 50-year-old woman suffered from a Fisher grade 3 SAH. A large right-sided posterior communicating artery aneurysm was treated with coils. Clinically, she was doing well until day 7, when she rapidly became comatose. *A,* Initial angiogram at the time of the aneurysm treatment. *B,* Angiogram of the left internal carotid artery on day 7 showing severe narrowing of the anterior cerebral artery (red arrow) and the middle cerebral artery (blue arrow). The patient was treated with balloon angioplasty, which has a long-lasting effect on vessel diameter. *C,* Three days later, an angiogram shows that the diameter of the previously narrowed vessels is now almost back to normal.

a neuro-ICU or a neuro-step-down unit is also essential to detect quickly any subtle deterioration in neurology that may indicate the beginning of DID.

Despite our best effort, many patients with aneurysmal SAH still die or suffer from severe disability. An international population-based study found that only 56% of patients with SAH were alive at 1-year follow-up. Of those who survived, 46% reported incomplete recovery. The optimal treatment for SAH remains elusive.

SUGGESTED READING

Hillman J, Fridriksson S, Nilsson O, et al: Immediate administration of tranexamic acid and reduced incidence of early rebleeding after aneurysmal subarachnoid hemorrhage: A prospective randomized study. J Neurosurg 2002;97:771–778.

Joseph M, Ziadi S, Nates J, et al: Increases in cardiac output can reverse flow deficits from vasospasm independent of blood pressure: A study using xenon computed tomographic measurement of cerebral blood flow. Neurosurgery 2003;53:1044–1051.

Kassell NF, Torner JC, Haley EC Jr, et al: The International Cooperative Study on the Timing of Aneurysm Surgery. Part 1: Overall management results. J Neurosurg 1990;73:18–36.

Macdonald RL, Weir B. Cerebral Vasospasm. London, Academic Press, 2001.

Macmillan CS, Grant IS, Andrews PJ: Pulmonary and cardiac sequelae of subarachnoid haemorrhage: Time for active management? Intensive Care Med 2002;28:1012–1023.

Molyneux A, Kerr R, Stratton I, et al: International Subarachnoid Aneurysm Trial (ISAT) Collaborative Group. International Subarachnoid Aneurysm Trial (ISAT) of neurosurgical clipping versus endovascular coiling in 2143 patients with ruptured intracranial aneurysms: a randomised trial. Lancet 2002;360:1267–1274.

Rabinstein AA, Wijdicks EF: Hyponatremia in critically ill neurological patients. Neurologist 2003;9:290–300.

Treggiari MM, Walder B, Suter PM, Romand JA: Systematic review of the prevention of delayed ischemic neurological deficits with hypertension, hypervolemia, and hemodilution therapy following subarachnoid hemorrhage. J Neurosurg 2003;98:978–984.

van Gijn J, Rinkel GJ: Subarachnoid haemorrhage: Diagnosis, causes and management. Brain 2001;124:249–278.

Wiebers DO, Whisnant JP, Huston J 3rd, et al: International Study of Unruptured Intracranial Aneurysms Investigators: Unruptured intracranial aneurysms: Natural history, clinical outcome, and risks of surgical and endovascular treatment. Lancet 2003;362:103–110.

- Seizures in the critical care setting are a symptom that should be treated promptly, before most diagnostic testing is even ordered.
- Seizure can be mimicked by other movements, including tremors, shivering, reflexes, tics, and volitional motor events.
- Given sufficient metabolic or neurological derangement, anyone can have a seizure.
- It is not unusual for the comatose patient to be in an unrecognized, subtle status epilepticus (as many as 40% by continuous electroencephalogram).
- Because morbidity and mortality increase after the first 30 minutes, convulsive and subtle status epilepticus must be treated aggressively with target phenytoin levels of 20 to 30 mg/mL.

Organized, synchronous electrical activity has long been feared in intensive care unit (ICU) settings, usually in the form of ventricular tachycardia. When this occurs, personnel and algorithms are immediately mobilized to prevent a lethal outcome. Warning alarms and systems designed for the early detection of arrhythmias have led to increased survival of patients in the critical care setting. Organized, synchronous electrical activity in the brain (i.e., seizures) may have a similarly devastating outcome if unrecognized and untreated. Just as with arrhythmias, it is important to look beyond the obvious presentation and to establish a heightened level of awareness for all types of seizures (Fig. 38.1). The goal of this chapter is to help establish a consistent and aggressive protocol for addressing seizures in the ICU.

EPIDEMIOLOGY, RISK FACTORS, AND PATHOGENESIS

Epidemiology

A seizure is the clinical manifestation of abnormal, synchronous neuronal firing. This term is not specific with regard to etiology and may be genetic or provoked. The term epilepsy describes a condition in which a patient develops a propensity for unprovoked seizures that are ultimately genetic or acquired.

Any stress able to create sufficient neuronal hyperexcitability may lead to a seizure. It is not surprising, therefore, that

"normal" individuals have a 9% cumulative risk of having a single seizure in a lifetime. Also, the prevalence of epilepsy in the general population is approximately 1%. The risk of developing status epilepticus (SE) is 0.4% by age 75 years. One percent of patients with epilepsy will experience at least one episode of SE annually, and they likewise have a 20% chance of experiencing SE within the first 5 years of their epilepsy diagnosis. Overall, this translates to 152,000 patients with at least one episode of SE in the United States per year, or an incidence of 61 in 100,000. There appears to be no sex or geographic predilection. As might be expected, the highest incidences of seizures and SE occur at the extremes of age. Comprehensive data regarding seizures and SE stratified along socioeconomic lines are not available.

Risk Factors

Of people who have seizures, approximately one third are children with febrile convulsions, one third are patients with epilepsy, and one third are symptomatic from medical issues. As more is learned about the neurogenetics of epilepsy, all these patients may be related by a reduced, multifactorial "seizure threshold." Currently, however, one should consider disturbances in any of the systems listed in Table 38.1 and Box 38.1 as placing a patient at risk for a provoked seizures or SE. It can be argued that any disturbance sufficient to require an ICU bed is sufficient to place that patient at risk for seizure.

Trauma and stroke are the most common causes of new-onset symptomatic seizures in adults, followed by drug withdrawal, central nervous system infection, drug intoxication, metabolic derangements, central nervous system (CNS) neoplasms, and hypoxic–ischemia. In the ICU, however, drug effects and toxic-metabolic disturbances are most common.

Pathogenesis

Seizures are presumed to be generated by cerebral gray matter and therefore often have signs and symptoms based on the location in the cortex where they occur. For instance, seizures with symptomatology from the occipital lobe may involve flashing lights or lines, those from the temporal lobes may have gustatory or emotional sensations, and those from the posterior frontal lobe may have a progressive spread of motor activity following the homunculus (Fig. 38.2).

Seizure pathogenesis can be thought of as an abnormal pattern of normal neuronal firing. This short circuit creates an aberrant loop, which results in a brain region with synchronous depolarization. Clinically, this is a focal seizure. When this region is located in an area with widespread interconnection with other

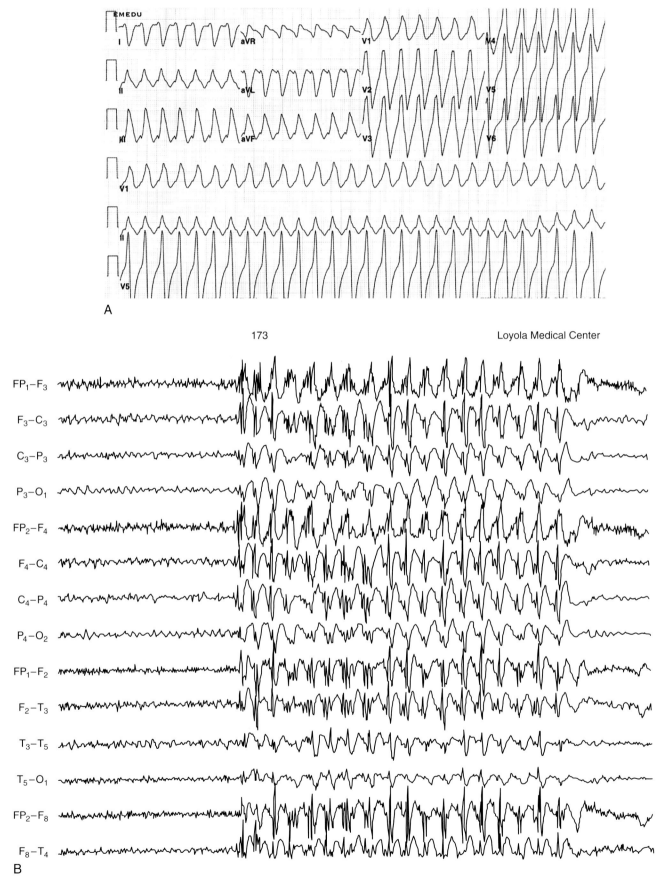

Figure 38.1. Ventricular tachycardia and generalized spike-and-wave seizure. This figure illustrates the similarities in appearance of (*A*) ventricular tachycardia and (*B*) generalized spike-and-wave seizure.

Table 38.1 Triggers for Symptomatic Seizures	
Organ System	**Conditions**
General	Medication and drug intoxication or withdrawal
	Fever
	Electrolytes ($\downarrow$ Na, Ca, Mg; $\uparrow$ Na)
	Glucose abnormalities
Cardiovascular	Global ischemia
	Embolic disease
	Acute hypertension
Pulmonary	Hypoxemia
	SIADH ($\downarrow$ Na)
Renal	Uremia
	Dialysis
	Electrolyte imbalance
	Coagulopathy
Gastrointestinal	Diarrhea/vomiting (electrolyte imbalance)
	Hepatic failure, coagulopathy
Heme/Onc	Coagulopathy
	Hypercoagulable state
	Metastatic disease
	Chemo/XRT
	Paraneoplastic
Endocrine	Glucose abnormalities
	Thyrotoxicosis/myxedema
	Adrenal electrolyte disturbance
	Pheochromocytoma
	Ca metabolism alteration
	Porphyria
Rheumatologic	Collagen vascular disease (CVD) vasculitis
Obstetric	Toxemia
	Embolic disease
	Coagulopathy
	Hypercoagulable state
Neurologic	
Vascular	Hemorrhage
	Ischemic
	Hypertensive
Inflammatory/infection	Parenchymal
	Meningeal
	Parameningeal
Traumatic	Hematoma
	Contusion
Neoplastic	Primary
	Metastatic
	Chemo/surgical/XRT
Congenital	Focal or generalized

Box 38.1 Drugs Associated with Lowering Seizure Threshold

Antiasthmatics
Theophylline

Antibiotics
INH (without B_6 supplementation)
Lindane
Metronidazole
PCN
Acyclovir
Quinolones

Antidepressants
TCA (rare)
SSRI (rare)
Buproprion

Hormones
Insulin ($\downarrow$ glucose)
Prednisone ($\downarrow$ Ca)
Estrogen

Immunosuppressants
Cyclosporine A
Tacrolimus

Anesthetics
Lidocaine ($\uparrow$ dose)
Enflurane
Ketamine

Narcotics
Meperidine
Pentazocine

Stimulants
Amphetamines
Cocaine
Methylphenidate
Phenylpropanolamine
Phencyclidine

Neuroleptics
Clozapine
Phenothiazines
Butyrophenones

Other
Anticholinergics
Anticholinesterases
Antihistamines
Baclofen
Lithium
Oral hypoglycemics
Heavy metals
Mexiletine

CLINICAL FEATURES

Classification

Clinical features of seizures are dependent on the anatomic origin of symptomatology. For this reason, a system of classification was established to both codify and provide a common language when discussing seizures.

The first delineation is that of a partial-onset and that of a generalized-onset seizure. Partial seizures begin in a specific unilateral focus, clinically associated with stereotypical functions of that specific brain region. Generalized seizures occur bilaterally and synchronously, and when used to describe a primary disorder, the seizure usually has a genetic origin. More commonly, however, generalized seizures evolve from partial seizures that spread from a localized area of cortex to the whole brain.

The next delineation involves impairment (complex) or preservation (simple) of consciousness. When electrical activity spreads bilaterally, consciousness becomes impaired so that generalized seizures are "complex" by definition, but the "complex" label is redundant and not used. Simple partial seizures may become complex when they spread to bilateral limbic circuits.

Last, seizures are classified by their clinical symptoms, having motor, sensory, or limbic flavors. Motor seizures are subdivided into tonic (stiffening), clonic or convulsive (alternating flexion and extension), myoclonic (rapid and large-amplitude contrac-

cortical regions, rapid spread of synchronous discharges can evolve into a secondarily generalized seizure. As with all kinds of neurochemical learning, the circuit becomes reinforced and may represent the mechanism of the clinical observation that "seizures beget seizures."

Creation of these aberrant connections can occur with any stress that can cause instability in cellular membrane function, leading to hyperexcitability and unpredictable firing. Conversely, any stress that impairs the brain's inhibitory mechanisms may also create aberrant circuitry. For example, GABA, an inhibitory neurotransmitter, has suppressed activity in EtOH withdrawal, a condition that creates provoked focal and generalized seizures in the nonepileptic patient.

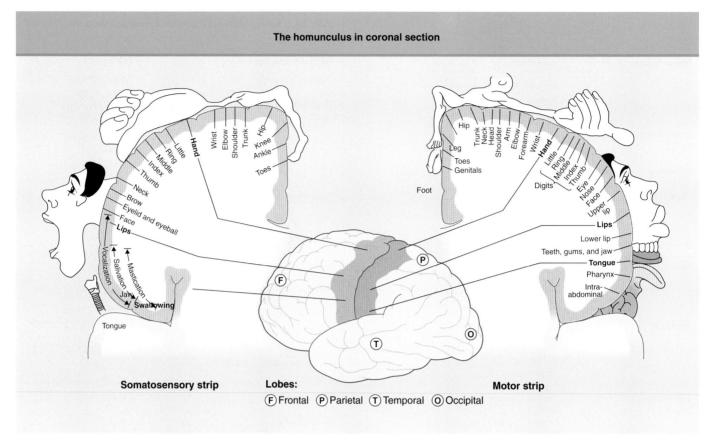

The homunculus in coronal section

Somatosensory strip

Lobes:
(F) Frontal (P) Parietal (T) Temporal (O) Occipital

Motor strip

Figure 38.2. The homunculus in coronal section.

tions), and so on. Sensory seizures may include visual disturbances or parasthesias. Limbic seizures can have gustatory sensations, déjà vu, jamais vu, fear, autonomic disturbances or bizarre and complex motor movements.

Due to the rich interconnections of the limbic circuits, seizures can develop there and rapidly spread to other areas or develop elsewhere and spread into this region. Sensory areas, which may be more evolutionarily stable, seem to be less epileptogenic. Motor areas, which are the primary output of the brain, have widespread connections from motivational (limbic) and sensory centers and therefore readily exhibit activity during many seizure types.

Clinical presentations of SE are similarly described by the previously discussed nomenclature. The definition, however, has evolved in recent times. Observations from antiquity recognized the potentially lethal outcome of continuous seizure activity. In the mid-20th century, Gastaut believed that seizures lasting longer than 1 hour constituted SE. Not until Meldrum's primate studies in the 1970s did the current definition of SE become fully accepted. Based on his pathologic studies, irreversible neuronal injury begins approximately 30 minutes after the onset of continuous seizure. Any seizure lasting longer than 30 minutes or, alternatively, having any two seizures without return of consciousness between the two seizures for more than 30 minutes has been defined as SE. Since typical generalized tonic–clonic seizures stop on their own after 2 minutes, there is a new push for redefining SE as any tonic–clonic seizure lasting longer than 5 minutes.

For the typical patient in the ICU, sedated, ventilated, and critically ill, there may actually be little practical difference between an isolated seizure and SE. For convenience, it is appropriate to categorize any seizure in the ICU as convulsive, subtle, or nonconvulsive.

Generalized Convulsive Status Epilepticus

Due to the tremendous electrical activity coursing across the cerebral cortex and the resultant major motor output (rapid alternating rhythmic flexion and extension), significant physiologic changes are also observed. Catecholamine-driven hypertension, tachycardia, hyperglycemia, and cardiac arrhythmias are seen in the first phase of generalized convulsive status epilepticus (GCSE) (<30 min). Hyperthermia, pulmonary edema, and lactic acidosis soon follow. Serum and cerebrospinal fluid leukocytosis may occur secondary to demargination. Cerebral blood flow increases by 200% to 600%. In the second phase (approximately 30–60 min later), hypotension and neuronal death from cytotoxic glutamate release are seen because the body is no longer able to compensate. With continuation of major motor activity, the amplitude and synchronicity of the convulsions begin to diminish. This may evolve into subtle SE, a condition that the critical care setting of dressings, lines, and endotracheal tubes can mask (Box 38.2).

Subtle Status Epilepticus

Subtle SE should be assumed if consciousness is not regained 20 to 30 minutes following a generalized seizure. Obviously, trying

Box 38.2 Physiologic Changes in Status Epilepticus

<30 Min of SE	>30 Min of SE
Hypertension	Hypotension
Tachycardia	Neuronal injury
Hyperglycemia	
Cardiac arrhythmias	
Hyperthermia (>42°C)	
Pulmonary edema	
Lactic acidosis (pH < 7)	
Serum leukocytosis (12.7–28.8 with normal differential)	
CSF pleocytosis (<30 with normal differential)	
CSF blood flow increases 200%–600%	

to distinguish between a single seizure and SE is a daunting task in the ICU. Subtle status is easily missed in the hustle and bustle of a typical ICU because the motor manifestations are minute. They can vary from unilateral to bilateral eyelid twitching to rhythmic vertical or horizontal nystagmoid eye movements beneath closed eyelids, platysmal or lip twitching, toe, thumb, or finger rhythmic movements, or nothing at all. Unexplained vital sign changes, pupillary dilation, and poor pupillary reactivity to light may be other clues. Although no movements may be witnessed, for prognostic value, subtle status (associated with a recent history of a tonic–clonic seizure) should be distinguished from nonconvulsive SE.

Nonconvulsive Status Epilepticus

Nonconvulsive SE (NCSE) consists of absence SE (ASE) or complex partial SE (CPSE). Both present with a clear change in consciousness. Most patients are not comatose but, rather, confused and lethargic with decreased spontaneity of speech. Stereotyped automatisms and eye fluttering are seen with both conditions, although the automatisms may be more complex with CPSE. ASE may occur in 10% of adults with a history of absence seizures as a child. Seventy-five percent of ASE occurs before the age of 20 years, and the remainder occurs in the elderly. It is believed that 15% of patients with complex partial epilepsy have a history of CPSE. The distinction between these two entities is important because there has been no morbidity or mortality associated with ASE, whereas CPSE is occasionally associated with morbid outcomes. Combined, however, these entities are clearly distinct prognostically from GCSE and subtle status.

Myoclonus

As seen in the ICU, this movement is associated with an almost uniformly dismal prognosis. The rapid and irregular, sometimes high-velocity startle-like movements typically accompany hypoxic–ischemic coma. These movements may have the appearance of GCSE, but despite treatment they only really resolve on their own. Over the course of several hours, the movements seem to diminish, leaving the false sense of the "seizure" getting better. Unfortunately, the clinical presentation can appear much like the transition of GCSE to subtle status.

Only continuous electroencephalogram (EEG) monitoring will differentiate these conditions.

Decorticate and Decerebrate Posturing

Both conditions portend serious brain injury. The arched back and extended legs seen in these conditions have the appearance of a tonic seizure or the tonic phase of a generalized convulsive seizure. The difference is seen in the upper extremities, with flexion (decorticate) and extension (decerebrate) postures. These are not usually rhythmical conditions, and they are often stimulus induced.

Nonepileptic Seizures

Surprisingly, psychogenic nonepileptic seizures (NES) occasionally enter the differential in the ICU patient. Unfortunately, unresponsiveness and lack of movement are the major presentations in this situation. More telling signs include asynchronous extremity movement, forward pelvic thrusting, and "geotropism" or downward eye deviation despite the head being manually turned from side to side. Short of these nonphysiologic behaviors, continuous EEG may be the only way to distinguish NES from subtle status or coma.

Other Findings in the ICU

Tables 38.2 and 38.3 present other findings in the ICU.

DIAGNOSIS

The suspicion of an ongoing seizure or SE should initiate treatment with actual diagnosis concurrent to or following seizure stoppage (Fig. 38.3). Otherwise, diagnosis proceeds along the typical history, physical, and laboratory study methodology with specific features outlined next.

History

The patient is rarely able to provide verbal information in this situation, but chart review often elicits a history of epilepsy. Systemic or CNS infections, head trauma, CNS neoplasms, metabolic disorders, toxic ingestions, alcohol abuse, and recent cessation are also common features. For patients with epilepsy, noncompliance with medications is the most common cause of increased seizure activity and SE. Witnessed accounts of sudden changes of mental state, tonic or clonic activity, any rhythmic movements, or unexplained vital sign changes may also provide historical clues of the presence of a seizure.

Physical

Most lay persons can easily describe the clonic phase of a generalized convulsive seizure. Additional findings include the Bell's phenomenon (eyes rolling back with eyelid closure), tongue biting, and urinary or fecal incontinence. In addition to a change in mental state, subtle physical findings may include pupillary dilation or poor reactivity of enlarged pupils, rhythmic or deviated eye movements often beneath closed eyelids, or rhythmic twitches of a variety of small muscle groups (including facial and digital muscles). Asymmetric tone in the extremities can be increased in a subtle focal motor seizure, decreased in a postictal Todd's paralysis. Signs of trauma to the face, head, or limbs may also be noted. Signs of healed injection tracks may be important in drug-induced seizures, and rashes or sores may

Table 38.2 A Differential of Common Movements in the ICU

	Focal Seizure	Generalized Seizure	Nonconvulsive Seizure	Postanoxic Myoclonus	Posturing, Spasticity	Parkinsonism	Shivers, Rigors, Shakes
Distribution	Typically hemibody, can start in face, arm, or leg	Involves both sides, can start unilaterally and spread	May have loss or change in consciousness. May see flicker in eyes, mouth	Affect multiple areas in random patterns at the same time	Hemibody, or bilateral	Hands and face most obvious spontaneously, increased tone throughout, obvious with movements	Bilateral and more trunk than extremities
Rhythm	Rhythmic, synchronous	Rhythmic, synchronous	Rhythmic or none	Irregular in rhythm and asynchronous	Rhythmic, can get single jerks that can appear to be withdrawal or volitional	Tremor is rhythmic. Tone increases reflect rhythm of task or passive movement and can "catch" from "clasp-knife" phenomena	Rhythmic
Amplitude	Crescendo-decrescendo pattern	Crescendo-decrescendo pattern	Very subtle movements, if any. Automatism. May have postictal period of confusion, headache, fatigue	Typically small movements, but can have trunk movements that appear more violent	Typically large, whole limb and whole body/hemibody. Partial cases can pervert a volitional movement	Mild tremors can become exaggerated times. Tone is not obvious until a passive or active movement is attempted	Shivers are mild, with rigors being the larger trunk jerks that can lift the patient off of the bed
Duration	Motor lasts seconds	Motor lasts around a minute or two, then fades away	30–60 seconds, can be sustained	Sustained. Begins soon after resuscitation and spontaneously burns out over hours to a few days	Sustained	Sustained	Typically crescendos to increase temperature, then decrescendos with deeffervescence
Response to external stimulation	No changes	No changes	May alter patient's interaction with environment	Often stimulus sensitive in direct manner (increases to motion) or less direct (more during nursing interventions, less when left alone for a while)	Can induce with classic maneuvers	Tone not obvious without passive range of motion exam	Unaffected
Consciousness	Preserved. If lost/changed it is really a generalized event	Unconscious	Reduced or lost	Coma is generally required for this type of myoclonus	No changes per se, but most often these movements are a result of profound hemispheric injury	No effect in Parkinson's disease, but when drug or hepatic induced, the consciousness will reflect that underlying cause	Consciousness often reduced, but may be alert or nearly alert
Sustained	Focal motor status is also called epilepsia partialis continua. If unresponsive, this is usually a generalized event with PLEDS on the EEG	The classic "status epilepticus" with increased morbidity/mortality with longer duration	Nonconvulsive status epilepticus is dangerous more from iatrogenic injury than from attempts to treat alternative causes of unconsciousness	This is typically sustained and stops before death or discharge from the ICU	Typically sustained, can be episodic in unusual cases	Typically sustained after acquired	Sustained during the fever-generating cycle
Comment	Indicates a focal brain lesion is new or active. May be very refractory to treat, especially PLEDS	Most respond quickly to the algorithm, but refractoriness can be brain or metabolic	Responds easily to small benzodiazepine IV doses	Unless this is misdiagnosed or in part drug induced (sympathomimetic, lithium, etc.) there is little hope for an outcome beyond chronic coma or death	Decorticate, from the midbrain, has flexed arm posture. Decerebrate (pontine) extends the legs are extended in both types	Can be confused with mild tremulousness from sympathomimetic over-modulation in the frightened or recovering patient	Can mimic the last part of a generalized seizure

Table 38.3 Transient Neurologic Phenomena

	Seizure	TIA	Migraine	Psychiatric	Cardiovascular
Onset	Immediate	Immediate	Builds over minutes	Varies, often fluctuates	Immediate
Duration	Minutes	Seconds to minutes; longer than an hour or two typically results in some cellular death	Complicated portion lasts 10–20 minutes, sometimes longer	Time duration fits with the underlying need or goal	Depends on underlying cause: Syncope is seconds, arrythmias may be sustained
Residual Deficits	Postictal headache, confusion, fatigue, incontinence, and trauma	None, by definition	Headache, neausea, fatigue	Normal. Often a bit euphoric or proud, rarely concerned unless an obvious manipulation	Normal
Clinical Presentation	Very stereotypical	Duration, severity, and/or distribution typically vary significantly	Very stereotypical	Quite variable	Stereotypical
Notes	Large anion gap that closes spontaneously. Prolactin rise that resolves	Baseline blood pressure or pulse may remain elevated for a while after event is over	Autonomic phenomena	Unexpected emotional response to the event	Low baseline blood pressure for syncope, ECG abnormalities

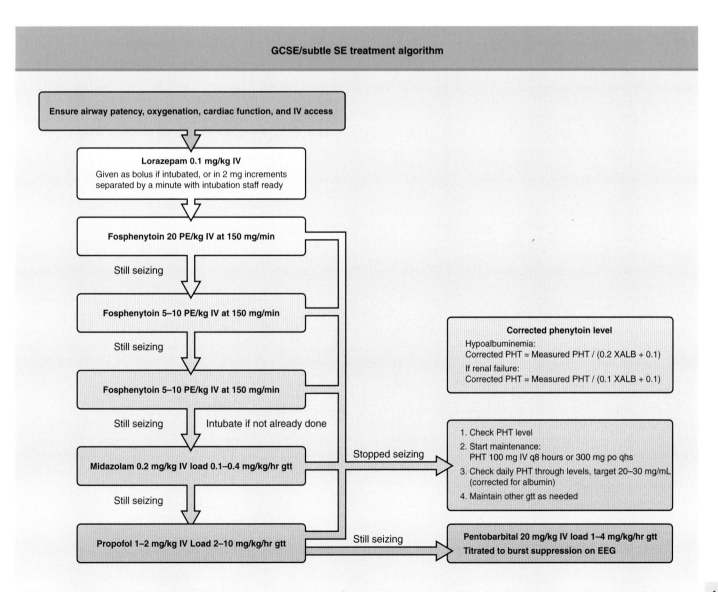

Figure 38.3. GCSE/subtle SE treatment algorithm.

indicate systemic or CNS infection. Additional physical findings were described previously.

Labs

Fortunately, chemistries are easily drawn during the process of seizure management and rarely inhibit infusion of appropriate medications. A rapid chemistry panel, including Na, Mg, Ca, glucose, and renal indices, should identify any easily reversible electrolyte disturbance. Toxicology panels for drugs of abuse, and antiepileptic medications, will also provide important management information.

Other labs are dictated by the clinical situation and are not necessarily ordered in all cases. An arterial blood gas (ABG) will often reveal a profound metabolic acidosis that easily reverses with seizure cessation as the lactic acid buildup from major motor activity is metabolized. Any residual anion gap acidosis should be investigated further (isoniazid poisoning is an example because the seizures are easily reversible with pyridoxine). Urinalysis and complete blood count (CBC) with blood cultures are indicated with a history of infection, liver function tests and an ammonia level may be considered with a history of liver injury, PT/PTT are indicated for patients with known coagulopathies or on anticoagulation, and so on.

Additional Studies

Assuming seizure stoppage, imaging should be performed unless the seizure or SE is typical for the patient with epilepsy. Computed tomography without contrast is the image of choice due to its speed and widespread availability. It is most useful in the diagnosis of trauma and intracranial hemorrhage. Large space-occupying tumors or ischemic strokes older than 12 hours are also usually identified. With time, patient stability, and availability permitting, magnetic resonance imaging offers better resolution of the cranial vault. Gadolinium enhancement may be used to elucidate infectious, inflammatory, or neoplastic etiologies. Diffusion weighted imaging may be used to age and identify injury from stroke.

If CNS infection is suspected, lumbar puncture should be performed. Again, after seizure stoppage and imaging rules out a space-occupying lesion, lumbar puncture may safely be performed. Bacterial and viral infections as well as subarachnoid hemorrhage (very irritating to the cerebral cortex) may be responsible for seizures. In addition to bacterial cultures, a variety of viral polymerase chain reaction (PCR) studies are available for diagnosis of meningitis/encephalitis. Most common offenders include the enteroviruses and herpes simplex virus encephalitis, which has a propensity for localizing in the epileptogenic temporal lobes. Many other possibilities exist, and their diagnosis should be guided by the appearance of their clinical presentation and spinal fluid analysis.

Electroencephalogram

EEGs are useful for distinguishing epileptic from nonepileptic activity and are usually obtained through a neurologic consultation. Rarely needed to diagnose generalized tonic–clonic SE, the EEG's main utility is the ability to differentiate subtle or nonconvulsive SE from other causes of obtundation, to establish partial versus complete antiepileptic therapy, to categorize the various movements seen in the ICU, and to provide general neurologic prognostication.

A study utilizing continuous EEG monitoring in a neuro-ICU demonstrated that 29% of patients had nonconvulsive seizures and 65% were in NCSE. Another study showed that 74 of 198 patients who developed alteration of mental status, but had no clinical evidence of convulsion, had EEG evidence of SE. Even more disconcerting is a prospective study of 64 patients who were treated for SE. These patients remained comatose without evidence of overt clinical seizure; however, electrographically 48% showed persistent NCSE. A study using continuous EEG documented NCSEs in 101 of 570 consecutive patients in a neuro-ICU; 88% of these seizures occurred in the first 24 hours, an additional 5% in the next 24 hours, and the remaining 7% were seen more than 48 hours after onset of monitoring.

EEG Patterns

Spike and Wave

Rhythmic wave forms are the hallmark of ongoing electrographic seizure activity. The classic morphology is an upward deflecting spike followed by an upward deflecting slow wave seen in a continuous run. This activity may be seen in specific and related leads or they may be generalized. With clinical convulsions, the motor artifact typically obscures this trace, and often this pattern is seen in the obtunded patient in subtle or NCSE (Fig. 38.4).

Interictal Spikes

Sharply contoured waves that seem to localize to a specific cortical region overlie suspicious hyperirritable neurons. This activity indicates a strong propensity for seizure genesis rather than ongoing seizure activity. These wave forms are seen in both primary and symptomatic seizures and correlate with focal or generalized onset, depending on the anatomic distribution (Fig. 38.5).

Periodic Lateralized Epileptiform Discharges

Periodic lateralized epileptiform discharges (PLEDs) occur in acute unilateral disorders such as infarcts, tumors, or infections. They may also be seen in chronic seizure disorders, alcohol withdrawal, or toxic–metabolic states. The complexes consist of sharp waves or spikes followed by a slow wave and then relative flattening, and they occur every 1 or 2 seconds. Many believe that PLEDs are actually an interictal pattern because seizures are often seen associated with a faster and continuous rhythmic activity. There may be a synchronous reflection of PLED activity to the contralateral side (Fig. 38.6).

Bilateral Independent PLEDs

These PLEDs are bilateral but independent. They often have different morphologies and are not synchronous. They are typically caused by hypoxic–ischemic injury, meningitis/encephalitis, or chronic seizure disorders. The presence of bilateral PLEDs is associated with a higher likelihood of coma and morbidity compared with PLEDs. PLEDs are believed to be an interictal phenomenon (Fig. 38.7).

Periodic Epileptiform Discharges

Bisynchronous sharp complexes, often at a frequency near 1 Hz, are seen in a variety of toxic–metabolic conditions, following anoxic brain injury, associated along the continuum of convulsive SE, or occasionally in Creutzfeld–Jakob disease. These

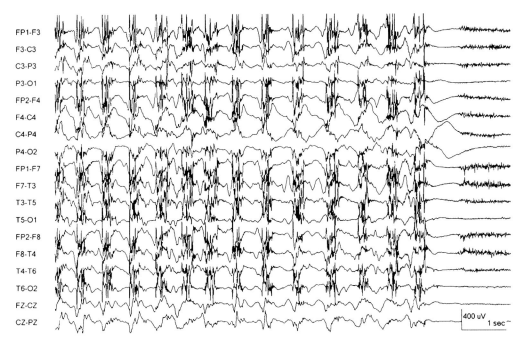

Figure 38.4. Generalized spike and wave. Generalized spike and wave, best seen in the midline electrodes, with prominent superimposed repetitive muscle artifact during the clonic phase, followed by postictal suppression in a 22-year-old woman with a primary generalized tonic–clonic seizure. (From Brenner RP: EEG in status epilepticus. J Clin Neurophysiol 2004;21(5):320.)

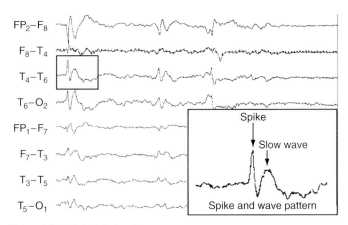

Figure 38.5. Interictal spikes.

waves often have a triphasic configuration, and their candidacy as treatable ictal activity is debated (Fig. 38.8).

Triphasic Waves

Because of the confusion and inconsistency surrounding the true three phases of this wave, it may best be thought of as a blunted spike followed by a slow wave. Triphasic waves (TWs) typically imply the presence of a toxic–metabolic encephalopathy, usually due to severe hepatic or renal dysfunction. TWs may be stimulus driven, and the EEG technician may utilize loud noises or painful stimuli to elicit an increase in activity. Unfortunately, this pattern is often difficult to distinguish from epileptic sharp and slow wave activity, and it is even believed by some to straddle the border between seizure and encephalopathy (Fig. 38.9).

Diagnostic Flow Chart

Figure 38.10 presents a diagnostic flow chart.

Differential Diagnosis

Clinical diagnosis of seizure is based on the appropriate event, confirmed by personally witnessing the event or an acceptable description from another witness. Due to the long list of seizure mimics (Table 38.4) that can fool even an experienced observer, the critical care event presents a difficult differential diagnosis. Helpful adjuncts include an assessment of the individual's risk of seizures from epilepsy, medical factors, and treatment risks. Laboratory testing can yield an anion gap after a generalized motor seizure that goes away without intervention. Such an observation is unusual in other medical diseases. There can be a transient prolactin increase that may be helpful in some cases. This is not specific, however, and can be seen in nonepileptic seizures, syncope, or other events that trigger a brief hormonal change.

The gold standard of diagnosis is to record the seizure with EEG, preferably with video recording. This is done routinely in epilepsy monitoring units that are designed for localization of seizures in ablative surgery candidates and characterization of nonepileptic events. In the critical care unit, portable monitoring can record brief periods of time, but if no seizure occurs, the EEG can only detect interictal discharges that correlate with seizure propensity but are not diagnostic. Newer computerized EEG units can continuously record events with or without time-synchronized video recording.

TREATMENT

Typical convulsive seizures stop on their own after approximately 2 minutes. Seizures that are prolonged or followed by more than 20 minutes of unresponsiveness should be assumed to be SE and treated as a medical and neurological emergency.

Various treatment regimens exist, but there are no double-blind, randomized, controlled studies to compare them. The advantage of lorazepam in the initial treatment of SE has been

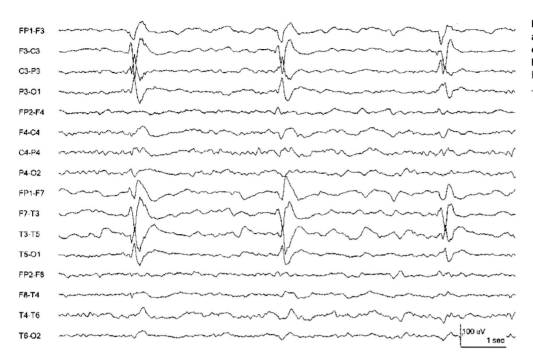

Figure 38.6. Left-sided PLEDs in a 74-year-old woman after evacuation of a left subdural hematoma 4 days earlier. (From Brenner RP: EEG in status epilepticus. J Clin Neurophysiol 2004;21(5):325.)

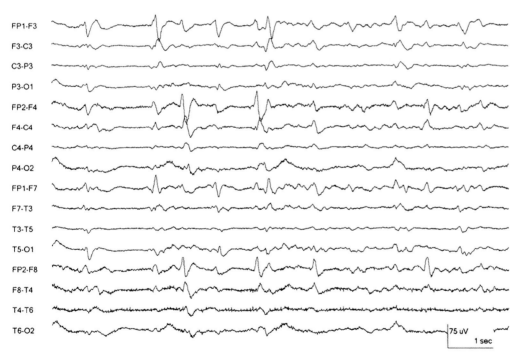

Figure 38.7. Bilateral independent PLEDs in a 72-year-old woman after anoxia. (From Brenner RP: EEG in status epilepticus. J Clin Neurophysiol 2004;21(5):326.)

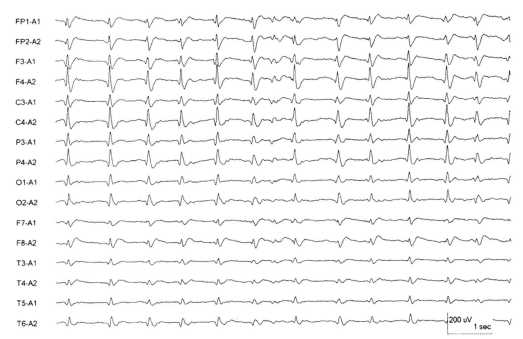

Figure 38.8. Generalized PLEDs (maximal right) in a 33-year-old man after anoxia secondary to a motor vehicle accident. Initially he had eyelid twitching. This EEG pattern was present after the administration of lorazepam and phenytoin and was unassociated with clinical changes. (From Brenner RP: EEG in status epilepticus. J Clin Neurophysiol 2004;21(5):326.)

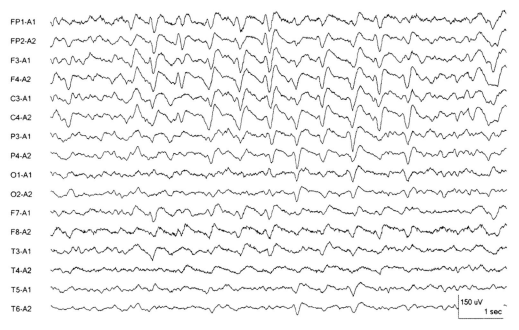

Figure 38.9. Triphasic waves in a 74-year-old man in renal failure. (From Brenner RP: EEG in status epilepticus. J Clin Neurophysiol 2004;21(5):326.)

Figure 38.10. Diagnostic flow chart.

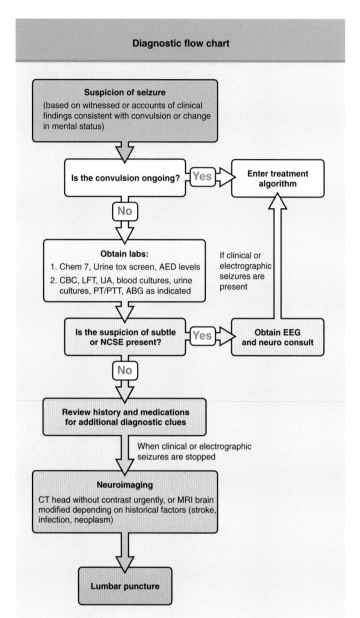

Diagnostic flow chart

Suspicion of seizure
(based on witnessed or accounts of clinical findings consistent with convulsion or change in mental status)

Is the convulsion ongoing? → Yes → **Enter treatment algorithm**

No

Obtain labs:
1. Chem 7, Urine tox screen, AED levels
2. CBC, LFT, UA, blood cultures, urine cultures, PT/PTT, ABG as indicated

If clinical or electrographic seizures are present

Is the suspicion of subtle or NCSE present? → Yes → **Obtain EEG and neuro consult**

No

Review history and medications for additional diagnostic clues

When clinical or electrographic seizures are stopped

Neuroimaging
CT head without contrast urgently, or MRI brain modified depending on historical factors (stroke, infection, neoplasm)

Lumbar puncture

demonstrated. A response rate of 64.9% for lorazepam was superior to the other combinations, including phenobarbital alone (58.2%), diazepam plus phenytoin (55.8%), and phenytoin monotherapy (43.6%). Unfortunately, this study was done before fosphenytoin became available. Clearly what is needed in the critical care setting, in which rapid treatment is required, is a standardized algorithm of medications, listed sequentially and in good therapeutic doses (which for SE exceeds the normal outpatient expectation of appropriate serum levels). This avoids treatment delays and identifies agents that offer the best safety and efficacy.

For GCSE and subtle SE, the consensus includes a combination of lorazepam 0.1 mg/kg given rapidly in 2-mg boluses, followed, when available, by fosphenytoin at 20 PE/kg at 150 mg/min. Fosphenytoin is preferable to phenytoin because of its increased water solubility. This characteristic allows quicker loading (150 vs. 50 mg/mL) and fewer complications (fewer cases of compartment syndrome from infiltrated lines

and less severe hypotension). Seizures are expected to stop with the infusion of benzodiazepines, and cessation is maintained with antiepileptic medications. For seizures that persist through the initial regimen, studies indicate that true therapeutic levels of fosphenytoin, particularly in the critically ill, may be higher than the established 20 mg/mL. Target levels of 20 to 30 mg/mL should be sought. Correction for hypoalbuminemia is important, and if free phenytoin levels are not available the same day, the following calculation can be used:

$$\text{Corrected PHT} = \text{measured PHT}/(0.2 \times \text{ALB} + 0.1)$$

In renal failure,

$$\text{Corrected PHT} = \text{measured PHT}/(0.1 \times \text{ALB} + 0.1)$$

If seizures become refractory to these supratherapeutic doses, use of general anesthesia is reasonable. Protocols including phe-

Table 38.4 Seizure Classification

| | Epilepsies | | | |
	Primary Generalized Epilepsies: Unprovoked Recurrent Seizures of These Types	Partial Epilepsies: Unprovoked Recurrent Seizures of These Types	Provoked Seizures	Seizure Mimics
Pathogenesis	An inborn defect causes seizures of different types to be expressed in a bilateral, synchronous 3 Hz pattern	An acquired lesion causes focal electrical instability that can spread to generate a partial seizure (typically an aura) and can further spread to the entire brain causing a generalized tonic-clonic seizure with focal features	Typically a generalized tonic-clonic seizure. May have a focal start	These are not seizure or electrical events
Common types	Seizure types include absence, myoclonic, and generalized tonic-clonic without aura	Seizure types include simple partial (motor, sensation, etc., without a change in consciousness) and complex partial (consciousness change required). Either can quickly generalize into a generalized tonic-clonic seizure. The partial seizure is the aura in these cases	Metabolic disruption: any acute organ failure (chronic failure unlikely to cause). Laboratory: sodium, calcium, magnesium, and glucose. Drug toxicity and withdrawl. CNS lesions of any type, especially new. Fluid shift from resuscitation, hypertension (eclampsia, hypertensive encephalopathy), dialysis. Hypertension sufficient to break down the blood-brain barrier. Sympathomimetic use essential or secondary hypertension, especially with new worsening	Psychiatric causes: anxiety, psychosis, and mania can mimic partial seizures. Outright malingering or somatiform disorders will perform a voluntary "pseudoseizure" for secondary gain. Movement disorders: tremor, hemiballism, myoclonus with syncope, spasticity, dystonia. Sleep phenomena: nightmares, somnombulism, narcolepsy, dreams. TIA, syncope, arrhythmia. Reflex movements, withdrawal, spasticity normal
Imaging	Often normal, can have congenital malformation, some of which are subtle and require special imaging protocols	Can be normal, but epilepsy protocols often demonstrate mesial temporal sclerosis. Any significant brain lesion also will be evident, if perinatal or recently acquired	Normal in most metabolic, toxic, drug seizures. May reveal some transient and permanent brain abnormalities	
EEG	Bilateral 3 spike-and-wave discharges/sec	Focal slowing or spike-and-wave over the seizure focus. Can be normal	Typically reflects underlying neurologic or metabolic condition without chronic signs of an epilepsy	Reflects underlying illness. Video EEG often clarifies confusing movements as nonseizure
Treatment	IV depakote, then select best long-term medication	IV phenytoin load, then select best long-term medication	IV phenytoin load, short term use until provoking mechanism is treated and resolved	Treat primary condition

nobarbital, valproic acid, midazolam or propofol drips, and pentobarbital coma have all been proposed, with pros and cons associated with each. With the exception of valproic acid, central respiratory drive is impaired with all of these medications and intubation is necessary prior to proceeding to these other medications. Midazolam is rapidly reversible and has no effect on intracranial pressure, but it frequently causes hypotension. Propofol is also quickly reversible, decreases intracranial pressure, and causes hypotension. Pentobarbital coma, on the other hand, requires days to clear secondary to its half-life, but it is also protective by lowering intracranial pressure and is neutral with regard to systemic blood pressure. Choice of second- and third-line medications typically depends on concurrent medical factors.

For NCSE, due to the relatively benign prognosis of ASE and CPSE, the level of aggression as well as medications may differ. Valproic acid at 25 to 50 mg/kg following careful infusion of lorazepam is the therapy of choice for ASE. Intubation is typically avoided because morbidity and mortality from ASE are not

expected, and cases of ASE stopped with valproic acid alone have been documented. CPSE should be treated similarly to GCSE, except that measures that fall short of intubation are typically favored. Practically speaking, however, the distinction between subtle SE, ASE, and CPSE in the ICU is rarely possible without EEG, and the delay in treating would not be justified to identify these rare cases of SE (Table 38.5).

CLINICAL COURSE AND PREVENTION

Clinical Course

The awareness of SE as a medical and neurological emergency is lagging behind the awareness of other notorious medical events. In one study of SE patients, the reported mean duration from seizure onset to paramedic arrival was 30 minutes (range, 15–140 min). Time from seizure onset to ED arrival was 50 minutes, and treatment initiation averaged an unimpressive 85 minutes after seizure onset. This delay in treatment is important to recognize because many studies have shown that increas-

Table 38.5 Medications Used in the Treatment of Status Epilepticus

Class	Dose/Route/Level	Contraindications/ Precautions	Adverse Effects	Other
Benzodiazepines				
Lorazepam	0.1 mg/kg IV at 2 mg/min	Hypersensitivity to class, acute narrow angle glaucoma, sleep apnea syndrome	Transient memory impairment, dizziness, drowsiness, GI upset, respiratory depression, propylene glycol toxicity	Antiseizure effect is prolonged (12 hr) compared with diazepam
Diazepam	0.2 mg/kg IV or IM in 5 to 10-mg increments every 10 min Diastat Rectal Gel also available	Hypersensitivity to class, acute narrow angle glaucoma, sleep apnea syndrome	Ataxia, drowsiness, hypotension, respiratory depression, fatigue	Antiseizure effect is short-lived (15 min) with rapid redistribution into fat stores
Midazolam	200 µg/kg IV load, then 0.75–10 µg/kg/min IV gtt	Hypersensitivity to class, acute narrow angle glaucoma	Respiratory depression, apnea, involuntary movements, cardiac and respiratory arrest, hypotension, cough, hiccups/ nausea/vomiting	Intubation and continuous EEG are needed
Antiepileptic drugs				
Phenytoin (PHT)	20 mg/kg IV load, then 100 mg IV q8hr maintenance Rate 50 mg/min with PHT or 150–200 mg/min with fosphenytoin. Therapeutic level 10–20 mg/mL as outpatient, 20–30 mg/mL in ICU	Hypersensitivity to hydantoins, sinus bradycardia, SA block, second- and third-degree AV block	Ataxia, slurred speech, choreathetosis, encephalopathy, insomnia, osteomalacia, nephro/ hepatotoxcity, Stevens–Johnson syndrome, toxic hepatitis, pancytopenia	Hypoalbuminemia causes increased free PHT levels. Zero-order kinetics creates a narrow therapeutic window. Inadvertent or intended abrupt cessation carries a high risk of SE
Valproic acid (VPA)	25–50 mg/kg IV load at 20 mg/min with 10–15 mg/kg/day IV divided q6hr maintenance Therapeutic level 50–100 µg/mL as outpatient, 100–150 µg/mL in ICU	Hypersensitivity to VPA, urea cycle disorders, pregnancy, hepatic disease, pancreatitis, use in conjunction with meds that affect platelet fixation	GI upset, anorexia, alopecia, rash, tremor, ataxia, diplopia, nystagmus, weight gain, somnolence, hepatic failure, hemorrhagic pancreatitis, dose-related thrombocytopenia	Anecdotal usage in first-line SE therapy with easier transition to outpatient regimen reported. Success rate vs. PHT is unknown
Barbiturates				
Phenobarbital (PB)	20 mg/kg IV load at 75 mg/min with 10–60 mg IV daily maintenance Therapeutic level 10–40 µg/mL	Hypersensitivity to barbiturates, porphyria, marked liver failure, severe pulmonary disease	Profound CNS sedation, GI complaints, dizziness, anxiety, Stevens–Johnson syndrome, hepatic damage, osteopenia, agranulocytosis, thrombocytopenia	Complete withdrawal of PB is difficult with h/o prolonged exposure. SE commonly occurs in the setting of cessation
Pentobarbital	5–20 mg/kg IV load followed by 1–4 mg/kg/hr	Hypersensitivity to barbiturates, h/o porphyria	Bradycardia, hypotension, apnea, hepatic injury, Stevens–Johnson syndrome, agranulocytosis	Requires continuous EEG to titrate until burst suppression. This coma is induced in the most refractory SE
Novel anesthetic				
Propofol	1–2 mg/kg IV load followed by 2–10 mg/kg/hr	Hypersensitivity to propofol or when general anesthesia is contraindicated	Risk of seizure during recovery phase, apnea, bradycardia, hypotension, anaphylaxis, GI complaints, involuntary movements (peds), arrhythmia, metabolic acidosis, rhabdomyolosis	Intubation and continuous EEG are needed

ing delay leads to increasing refractoriness to therapy. First-line therapy was successful in 80% of patients when initiated within 30 minutes of onset, 75% within 60 minutes, 63% within 90 minutes, 44% within 120 minutes, and 37% more than 120 minutes after seizure onset.

First-month mortality estimates following SE range from 3% to 50%. In the modern critical care era, estimates are probably more accurately in the 3% to 20% range. Interestingly, the mortality from SE itself is less than 1% because mortality is usually attributed to the underlying etiology. This may help explain the relatively low mortality in children (3%) compared to adults (30%–40%). Morbidity following an episode of SE is commonly reported, but these effects are as broad reaching as they may be

subtle, and it is not clear if they are due to the inciting injury or due to the prolonged seizure.

Prevention

In the ICU, prevention of SE and its complications centers around awareness. For patients with known epilepsy that are NPO for surgery or other reasons, it is important that a parenteral antiepileptic medication is utilized. To reiterate, the major cause of SE in this population is noncompliance or sudden cessation of the antiepileptic drug. There should be a heightened level of suspicion for SE for patients with sudden changes in mental status or failure to arouse after a witnessed, reported, or even treated convulsive seizure. Maintenance of maximal

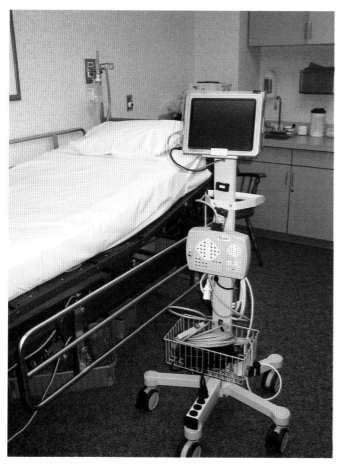

Figure 38.11. A mobile continuous EEG machine, approximately 4 feet tall, makes constant patient monitoring possible in the ICU.

Box 38.3 Pitfalls and Complications

Recognizing physical findings of subtle status (SS) is essential.

Patients with SS under sheets and cooling blankets may have their minor motor clues hidden.

Lack of EEG services is common in ICU settings.

Undertreatment of seizures and SE should be avoided (a typical mistake is ordering "one gram of dilantin," which is only good for a 50-kg person).

Recognize that the true therapeutic level of PHT in a critically ill patient is >20 mg/ml.

Treating lactic acidosis with HCO_3 is not necessary because, even with the low pH's seen in SE, it resolves on its own very quickly.

Using an incorrect AED or a correct AED incorrectly:

    Carbamazepine has a tendency to exacerbate primary generalized seizure disorders.

    Starting only the home regimen medications for an ongoing seizure without additional medications to stop the seizure.

    Giving a patient with known epilepsy a smaller loading dose on the assumption that the patient already has some on board.

Epilepsy patients admitted to the hospital and made NPO still need seizure coverage.

Hypotension and suppressed respiratory drive are associated with most therapies in acute seizure control.

Mistakenly using a paralytic instead of an antiepileptic anesthetic to stop convulsions, only to allow the electrographic seizure to continue unnoticed and untreated.

Taking time to obtain studies before the seizure or SE is stopped (CT/MRI/LP).

---

medical therapy should be practiced because even minor metabolic disturbances when taken in combination in the critically ill may predispose to seizure and SE. Frequent neuro checks, as utilized in a neuro-ICU, often provide the first warning that a neurological disturbance is present. Despite the studies of subtle and NCSE in comatose patients discussed previously, most ICUs are not equipped for continuous EEG monitoring. Fortunately, technology is rapidly advancing, creating smaller and less obtrusive mobile EEG monitoring devices. Some even have the capability of remote and Internet viewing. As these devices become smaller and more automated, continuous EEG may become as common as cardiac telemetry monitoring, which seems reasonable given the frequency and similarities of cardiac and cerebral dysfunction in the ICU (Fig. 38.11).

PITFALLS/COMPLICATIONS AND CONTROVERSIES

Boxes 38.3 and 38.4 present pitfalls/complications and controversies.

Box 38.4 Controversies

Treatment of PEDs/PLEDs/BiPLEDs may not be warranted if these are interictal patterns.

Use of phenobarbital coma is sometimes avoided when premorbid prognosis is dismal because the prolonged half-life requires days to weeks to clear from the system, before which brain function determination is impossible.

Treatment of myoclonic seizures in hypoxic ischemic coma is ineffectual and these typically burn out without treatment. These are disturbing for the family to view, however, and antiepileptic anesthetics, valproic acid, and paralytics with cEEG have been used.

Use of paralytics to remove motor artifact from convulsive or pseudoconvulsive movements (while intubated) during EEG monitoring may reveal ictal vs nonictal rhythms, but it makes the neurological exam more difficult.

SUGGESTED READING

Brenner R: EEG in convulsive and nonconvulsive status epilepticus. J Clin Neurophysiol 2004:21:319–331.

Bromfield E: Seizures. In Samuels M (ed): Hospitalist Neurology. Boston, Butterworth-Heinemann, 1999, pp 79–105.

Chin F, Neville B, Scott R: A systematic review of the epidemiology of status epilepticus. Eur J Neurol 2004;11:800–810.

Claassen J, Mayer S, Kowalski R, et al: Detection of electrographic seizures with continuous EEG monitoring in critically ill patients. Neurology 2004;62:1743–1748.

Holtkamp M, Othman J, Buckkeim K: Predictors and prognosis of refractory status epilepticus treated in a neurological intensive care unit. J Neurol Neurosurg Psychiatr 2005;76:534–539.

Huff J: Status epilepticus. Emedicine. March 2005. Retrieved June 18, 2005, from www.emedicine.com/emerg/topic554.htm.

Nowack W: EEG in status epilepticus. Emedicine. January 2005. Retrieved June 18, 2005, from www.emedicine.com/neuro/topic114.htm.

Wong M. Evidence-based epilepsy: An epilepsy reference source. Retrieved June 18, 2005, from Washington University, Pediatric Epilepsy Center: www.neuro/wustl.edu/epilepsy/pediatric/EvidenceBasedEpilepsy-VII.html.

KEY POINTS

- The diagnosis of spinal cord injury can be missed because of an inadequate or incomplete history or physical examination. However, there are many other factors that may obscure the diagnosis. "Spinal clues" can help raise the suspicion of spinal cord injury.
- Imaging modalities available today can provide further information about the degree of instability and risk of worsening injury, but one must assume instability until proven otherwise; a complete and meticulous neurological examination cannot be replaced by imaging technologies.
- Tracheostomy should be coordinated with the surgical team in advance, because the procedure may interfere with possible surgical management of some cervical spine fractures.
- The intensive care setting provides the optimal environment to monitor and treat fluctuations in blood pressure. We strongly recommend mandatory admission of all spinal cord injury patients to the intensive care unit.
- Pressure sores and decubitus ulcers in dependent areas can become a major concern with prolonged immobilization. The risks of infection and systemic complications cannot be trivialized.
- Prevention of secondary injury to the spinal cord involves specific measures to minimize the damage already inflicted. Prevention of secondary injury can also be viewed as creating the optimal environment for recovery.

Effective management of acute spinal cord injury (SCI) requires an understanding of the epidemiology and clinical features of these injuries. Knowledge of the epidemiology will alert the physician or surgeon to the possible occurrence of such an injury. Detection of an SCI can be difficult in the acute phase, particularly in the context of multiple traumas or in the setting of preexisting disease such as metastatic disease of the vertebral column, congenital anomalies, or spinal arthropathy (ankylosing spondylitis).

Acute SCI is relatively uncommon, affecting approximately 1 in 40 patients presenting to a major trauma center. The annual incidence in developed countries varies from approximately 10 to 50 cases per 1 million population. Despite their relatively low incidence, these injuries have profound consequences for patients, their families, and society in general. For example, the mortality rates, both immediate and delayed, are high: The immediate fatality rate approaches 50%, and approximately 80% of the fatalities occur at the scene of the trauma or on arrival at the hospital. For immediate survivors, mortality ranges up to 15% at hospital admission. Morbidity rates for SCI are also very high, and survivors may require prolonged and/or multiple hospitalizations in acute treatment units and rehabilitation centers.

There are additional significant effects on the social and psychological well-being of the patients and their families. Furthermore, the financial burden to the individual patient and to the health care system is very high. For example, a major SCI in the cervical region will cost several million dollars for acute care, rehabilitation, and in lost earnings.

EPIDEMIOLOGY

The epidemiology of SCI varies considerably between countries, and even within a given country there are variations in causation depending on location. Also, the causes differ among different age groups, with younger victims showing a greater preponderance of injuries due to high-velocity, high-impact activities, such as motor vehicle crashes and diving. Younger victims may be subject to different physiological factors that affect the spine, such as undeveloped paraspinal musculature and increased elasticity of ligaments. In contrast, older victims tend to have lower velocity injuries, such as from falls down stairs, and have more rigid spines and additional pathological features, such as osteoarthritis or spondylosis, that tend to make the spinal cord more vulnerable to space-occupying lesions such as herniated disks.

The most common cause of SCI in developed countries is associated with motorized vehicles, whereas in less developed countries falls are the most common cause. Worldwide, traffic mishaps—including motor vehicle crashes and injuries to bicyclists and pedestrians—account for the largest number of SCIs; in most countries, these represent approximately half of all cases (Table 39.1). In some locations, violence is a major cause of SCI. For example, in some cities in the United States, gunshot wounds are the most frequent causes of SCI. In developed countries, sports and recreational activities have become much more frequent causes as leisure time has increased, whereas work-related SCIs appear to be on the decline, possibly due to prevention efforts from organized labor and/or employer associations.

In almost all countries, the vast majority of victims (up to 80%–85%) are males, and younger patients account for more than half. Indeed, the usual mean and median ages range from the late 20s to the early 30s in most countries.

Table 39.1 Clinical Features of Spinal Cord Injuries	
Feature	**%**
Cause	
Traffic (motor vehicle, bicycle, pedestrian)	40–50
Work	10–25
Sports and recreation	10–25
Falls (home, elsewhere)	20
Violence	10–25
Level of injury	
Cervical (C1 to C7–T1)	55
Thoracic (T1–T11)	15
Thoracolumbar (T11–T12 to L1–L2)	15
Lumbosacral (L2–S5)	15
Severity of neurological injury—ASIA grades	
Complete injury—grade A	45
Incomplete injuries	
Grade B	15
Grade C	10
Grade D	30
Types of bony injuries	
Minor fracture (including compression)	10
Fracture–dislocation	40
Dislocation only	5
Burst fracture	30
SCIWORA	5
SCIWORET (including osteoarthritis and cervical spondylosis)	10

LEVEL AND SEVERITY OF INJURY

Approximately 50% of injuries to the spinal cord occur in the cervical region from C1 to C7–T1. Of the remaining injuries, approximately 15% occur in each of three regions: from T1 to T11, in the thoracolumbar region from T11–T12 to L1–L2, and in the lumbosacral region from L2 to S5 (see Table 39.1). Some causes produce injuries in specific locations of the spinal column. For example, diving produces almost exclusively cervical SCIs, whereas injuries in mining and logging tend to crush the thoracic and thoracolumbar regions.

There are many types of fractures and dislocations of the vertebral column in patients with SCI. The diagnosis of both vertebral column and spinal cord injuries has been greatly facilitated by computed tomography (CT) and magnetic resonance imaging (MRI). The most common type of bony injury is the fracture–dislocation, which occurs in approximately 40% of patients, followed by burst fractures in 30%, minor fractures in 10%, and dislocations in approximately 5% (see Table 39.1). In the remaining 15%, there is an SCI but without definite evidence of radiological abnormality [spinal cord injury without radiological abnormality (SCIWORA)] or an SCI with a radiological abnormality but not one associated with trauma. These latter cases are termed spinal cord injury without radiological evidences of trauma (SCIWORET), and the radiological abnormality in most of these cases is osteoarthritis or cervical spondylosis.

The current method of grading the severity of the neurological injury is based on the International Classification of Spinal Cord Injury (ICSCI). In North America, this system of grading is known as the American Spinal Injury Association (ASIA) system (Fig. 39.1). ASIA grade A implies a complete SCI without any voluntary motor function below the level of the injury and with no retained sensation, including anesthesia in the sacral segments. It occurs in approximately 45% of cases. ASIA grade B describes a patient with absent voluntary motor function below the level of injury but with some sensory preservation. Grade B comprises approximately 15% of cases. ASIA grade C implies a patient with some retained motor and sensory function below the lesion, but the majority of the weakened muscles have grade strength of 2 or less on average. ASIA grade D, comprising approximately 30% of cases, indicates preserved motor and sensory function below the level of the lesion but average retained motor function of grade 3 or more. The reader should be reminded that the motor grading is primarily based on the muscle groups being tested to overcome gravity (= 3). Normal is 5 out of 5, whereas just visible contractions are graded 1 out of 5 (see Fig. 39.1).

These percentages of cases of ASIA grades A through D represent a marked improvement compared with previous eras. The change began in the 1970s, when there appeared to be a change in the relative incidence of complete and incomplete SCIs. Previously, approximately two thirds of SCIs were complete, whereas currently approximately 45% are complete. The reasons for this improvement are multifactorial and include the use of seat belts, air bags, and child restraint systems. Also, there has been improved first aid and ambulance retrieval. These latter factors include better management of spinal shock, with its accompanying systemic hypotension, and better management of hypoxia. There has also been greater awareness among the general public about the possibility of causing increased damage to the injured spinal cord by injudicious movement of the injured and unstable spine.

THE PRESENCE OF OTHER INJURIES

Management of patients with SCI in the presence of multiple trauma is a major challenge. For example, establishment of an adequate airway may be extremely difficult and hazardous in the presence of a cervical SCI. Hypoxia due to respiratory failure is common in these patients because of diaphragmatic and/or intercostal muscle paralysis. Abdominal distention, ileus, or vomiting and aspiration may add to the hypoxia. Hypotension is often present in SCI with multiple trauma due to spinal neurogenic shock and/or systemic shock. Patients with SCI, especially those with cervical injuries, have a sympathectomy effect with unopposed vagotonia that may cause cardiac arrhythmia or even reflex cardiac arrest. Intra-abdominal hemorrhage or visceral rupture in patients with SCI may be overlooked because of the absence of the typical findings associated with these conditions. Approximately 20% to 50% of patients with SCI will have multiple trauma, and the common additional injuries are brain injuries and chest injuries. Indeed, some studies have reported that 25% to 50% of spinal cord-injured patients have an associated head injury.

The most common mechanism of injury in patients with SCI and additional injuries is motor vehicle crashes. Some series have

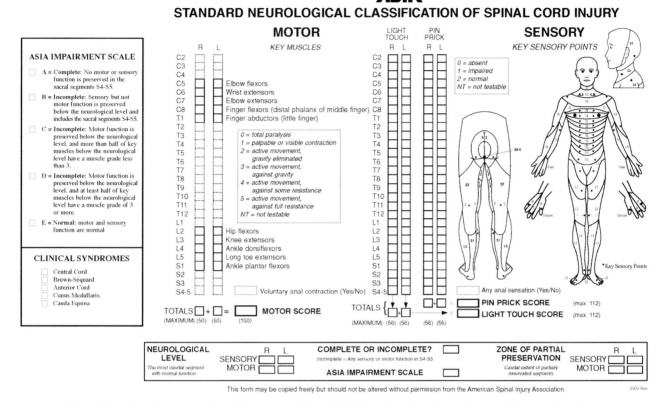

Figure 39.1. American Spinal Cord Injury Association (ASIA) impairment scale and neurological classification of spinal cord injury. (Reproduced with permission from ASIA.)

found that the chance of neurological recovery is decreased and the chance of death is increased in patients with SCI in the presence of multiple trauma. Reasons for the reduced neurological recovery include hypoxia and hypotension, which are especially frequent in patients with multiple trauma. In addition, the SCIs in patients with multiple trauma tend to be more severe than in those with isolated SCI.

Alcohol is a significant factor in the etiology of SCI. Indeed, alcohol consumption appears to be a factor for approximately 25% of patients with SCI. Drugs play a much smaller role.

CLINICAL EXAMINATION

There are a number of "safe assumptions" that examiners should make when examining a trauma victim in order to avoid a missed diagnosis of SCI. Box 39.1 highlights some of the physical signs often associated with SCI, and the following list focuses on historical information that should make the treating physician suspicious. The importance of early diagnosis of an SCI lies in prevention of secondary insult.

- Mechanism of injury: The level of energy or forces involved. Examples of high energy transfer include motor vehicle accidents, whereas a fall from the standing position is low energy transfer in conscious individuals.
- Serial assessment, with particular attention to deterioration in function.
- Unconscious patient, not possible to make accurate neurological assessment.

- Distracting injuries, which would mask spinal pain or neurological deficits.

The diagnosis of SCI may also be missed because of an inadequate or incomplete history or physical examination. There are many other factors that may obscure the diagnosis. The combination of a head injury and inebriation will make it very difficult to examine the patient. Also, the presence of multiple trauma may divert the examiner's attention toward more obvious but often less important injuries, such as limb fractures.

Box 39.1 Physical Signs Associated with Spinal Cord Injury

Hypotension and bradycardia (spinal shock)
Paradoxical respiration
Low body temperature and high skin temperature
Priapism
Bilateral paralysis of arms and legs, especially flaccid
Bilateral paralysis of arms only, or arms weaker than legs
Bilateral paralysis of legs, especially flaccid
Lack of response to painful stimuli
An anatomic level in response to painful stimuli
Only head movement or facial grimacing in response to painful stimulation
Anatomic level for sweating
Horner's syndrome
Brown–Séquard syndrome

Other situations leading to difficulty in diagnosis include patients who are psychologically upset by the injury or those who are hypoxic, restless, uncooperative, or agitated. In all these instances, the practitioner's diagnostic acumen is severely taxed. Indeed, the patient's reactions may be so bizarre that the diagnosis of hysteria may be mistakenly made. A diagnosis of hysteria is extremely dangerous in situations involving trauma. In the presence of alcohol, multiple trauma, head injury, or bizarre behavior, it is wise to make the assumption that there is an accompanying SCI.

The history provided by the trauma victim, witnesses, or ambulance personnel may provide important clues for diagnosing the presence and severity of an SCI. At the scene of the mishap, the first aid personnel may report that there was leg movement and that this function disappeared later. Conversely, the legs may have been motionless at the scene of the trauma, with subsequent improvement. The former situation would indicate an unstable spine with severe pressure on the cord from progressive dislocation, whereas the latter may indicate a period of spinal shock that is now passing. Symptoms such as the inability to move one or more limbs or the relative lack of movement of one or more limbs are highly suspicious. Complaints of weakness, tingling, and loss of sensation are extremely important. Similarly, posttraumatic urinary retention and incontinence are danger signs.

The physical examination can yield specific indications of the presence of SCI (see Box 39.1). These "spinal clues" are obtained from a detailed testing of the vital signs as well as testing of strength, sensation, and reflexes in all four limbs. The spine must be palpated in its entirety, with the examiner paying special attention to tenderness, step deformity (disruption in the alignment of the bony spinous processes), or crepitus. It is important to realize that the examiner's hand can be safely passed between the patient and the mattress or stretcher and the spine palpated from the foramen magnum to the sacrum. This must be done in every case.

Hypotension, bradycardia, and warm extremities are due to a cervical SCI and not systemic shock, which usually causes hypotension, tachycardia, and cold extremities. A cervical injury causes paradoxical respiration in which inspiration causes the chest cage to be drawn in while the abdomen expands due to intercostal muscle paralysis and preserved diaphragmatic contraction. Also, the examiner should not misinterpret reflex withdrawal of the limbs in response to painful stimulation of the extremities as being due to voluntary movement.

Spinal clues also include low body temperature, priapism, and the unusual instance of bilateral paralysis of either the arms only or greater paralysis of the arms than the legs (see Box 39.1). These features indicate a central cord syndrome or an injury at the foramen magnum. A lack of response to painful stimulation should alert the examiner to the possible presence of an SCI. Detection of an anatomical level in response to painful stimulation or painful stimulation that produces only head movement or facial grimacing should also be regarded as a spinal clue. The presence of a unilateral or bilateral Horner's syndrome and the presence of Brown–Séquard syndrome are strong spinal clues.

IMAGING STUDIES

The basis of diagnosis is the ability of the treating physician to assess the patient accurately. As noted previously, spinal clues

can help raise the suspicion of SCI. A complete and meticulous neurological examination cannot be replaced by imaging technologies. Diagnosis of an SCI can be suspected based on the mechanism of injury and confirmed by the neurological examination. Further information about the degree of instability and risk of worsening injury can be provided by the imaging modalities available today, but one must assume instability until proven otherwise.

Imaging studies provide a wide range of information but require the judicious application of indications. Basic investigations in the form of plain x-rays can be divided into static and dynamic studies. Multiple views of the bony anatomy of the spine can be provided by this simple and quick technique. Limitations are encountered in certain levels of the spine that are more difficult to image. For example, the occipitocervical junction, cervicothoracic junction, and lateral views of the midthoracic spine may hide fractures because of the overlying structures. Dynamic views allow assessment of the integrity and structural stability of the spine. The more common views include flexion and extension lateral x-rays of the cervical and lumbar spine. In our opinion, dynamic views are contraindicated in the acute phase in the presence of a neurological deficit. Conclusions regarding the ligamentous integrity are made when the alignment of the bony elements of the spine is within certain acceptable parameters. The next level of sophistication with imaging is CT scan. We recommend axial images and subsequent reconstructions in sagittal and coronal planes (Fig. 39.2). The level of precision and detail, without relying on overlapping images such as in the conventional x-ray, provides more accu-

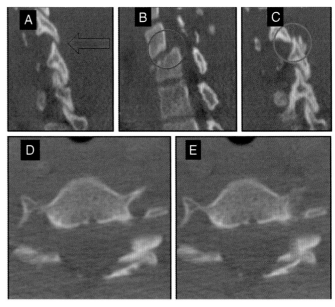

Figure 39.2. CT images of a patient with a traumatic spinal fracture dislocation and spinal cord injury. *A,* The sagittal reconstruction right of the midline showing the normal orientation of the facet joint *(arrow).* *B,* Midline sagittal reconstruction from the axial images showing the subluxation of C6 on C7 *(red circle).* *C,* Sagittal reconstruction left of midline showing the dislocated facet joint *(green circle).* *D,* Axial image at the level of C6, with the black line showing the level of the reconstruction for A. *E,* Axial image at the same level (C6), with the black line showing the level of the reconstruction for C.

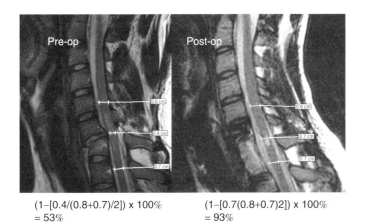

(1–[0.4/(0.8+0.7)/2]) x 100%
= 53%

(1–[0.7(0.8+0.7)2]) x 100%
= 93%

Figure 39.3. MRI with spinal cord measurements. T2-weighted MRIs show a patient with a spinal cord injury both pre- *(left)* and postoperatively *(right)*. The measurements of the actual cervical spinal cord are taken above and below the greatest area of compression. The surgical decompression can be analyzed quantitatively.

rate information about the anatomy being studied. Due to their density, the bony elements can be imaged with great detail, and fractures are seldom overlooked. The speed of image acquisition makes this technique more conducive to dealing with trauma patients. MRI provides greater anatomical detail with respect to the soft tissues, such as the nervous tissues, disks, and ligaments, but requires more time for acquisition of information. The ability to measure the thickness of the spinal cord is demonstrated in Figure 39.3. This has certain implications in the trauma setting for a hemodynamically unstable patient. The management algorithm provided in Figure 39.4 guides the treating physician through the various imaging studies necessary for early identification of injury.

TREATMENT

The management of the patient with SCI can be divided into diagnosis and treatment. In the trauma setting, time can be limited, and the need to provide treatment and assessment simultaneously is essential. The initial treatment is the provision of supportive measures, which can be grouped into three broad categories: oxygenation, circulatory support, and prevention of secondary injury.

Oxygenation includes airway management and ventilatory support, the end point of which is the delivery of oxygen to the blood. Indications for immediate emergency intubation are clear in some situations, whereas sometimes intubation may be delayed until optimal intubation conditions are present. In the setting of an apneic patient with a SCI, the indications are obvious. Other scenarios may also be encountered, and the situation can change quickly. An example is the patient who can protect his or her airway but due to hemodynamic instability may require intubation. The patient with a midcervical injury can in some cases present initially with the ability to breathe, but due to the loss of the accessory breathing muscles, the patient may gradually lose endurance. This will be observed by serial monitoring of tidal volume. Intubation in the setting of cervical fractures requires immobilization to prevent further injury to the spinal cord. In-line traction and awake fiberoptic

intubation provide the means to achieve oral or nasal intubation by minimizing the risk of moving the cervical spine. Using minimal sedation and/or short-acting agents allows the treating physicians to assess the patient following intubation to ensure that no further insult to the spinal cord has occurred. Securing an airway will in some circumstances require tracheostomy. This technique is used not only in the acute setting but also after prolonged intubation. This procedure should be coordinated with the surgical team in advance, since the tracheostomy may interfere with possible surgical management of some cervical spine fractures. Once the airway is secured, ventilation should also be instituted in accordance with the aim of optimal oxygen delivery. Ventilatory settings are based on FIO_2, tidal volumes, positive end-expiratory pressure, and respiratory rate. Optimization of ventilatory settings is beyond the scope of this chapter. Adjuncts to ventilatory support include phrenic nerve pacers for the chronic ventilator-dependent SCI patient, although the indications for this type of pacer are limited.

Circulatory management or blood pressure support is fundamental in the delivery of oxygenated blood to the tissues. Studies have demonstrated the deleterious effect of hypotension. For example, neurological deterioration may occur with an episode of 15 minutes with a systolic blood pressure below 85 mm Hg. The intensive care setting provides the optimal environment to monitor and treat fluctuations in blood pressure. We strongly recommend mandatory admission of all SCI patients to the intensive care unit (ICU). The etiology for the variations in blood pressure can be neurogenic and/or hypovolemic. Treatment of both will require aggressive administration of intravenous fluid in the form of normal saline, volume expanders, or blood product. In some circumstances, inotropic support is required to achieve adequate blood pressure. A variety of agents can be used. However, pure alpha agonists can cause severe constriction of spinal cord vasculature, which is counterproductive to the ultimate goal. Dopamine is the agent preferred by most centers for SCI patients, despite the potential systemic complication profile.

Prevention of secondary injury to the spinal cord involves specific measures to minimize the damage already inflicted. Immobilizing the patient with a collar and/or a spinal board reduces the risk of further damage. Routinely, after motor vehicle accidents patients are placed in a collar and treated as having an unstable spine until proven otherwise. In the situation of a comatose or sedated patient, ensuring that the cervical spine is stable can be challenging. The algorithm for clearing the cervical spine provides general guidelines (see Fig. 39.4). One of the imaging studies recommended in our algorithm is the CT scan with fine cuts of 3 mm or less from the occiput to the T1 level. The time required to image this area of the spine, the low dose of radiation, and the potential need to place the patient in the CT scan unit to image other areas, such as the head, thorax, or abdomen, provide a strong argument for a more liberal use of this technique in difficult or comatose patients. The strongest arguments for using the CT scan lie in the ability to maintain immobilization and the quality of the images, which justifies our departure in part from the guidelines established by the Eastern Association for the Surgery of Trauma. Once the CT scan has ruled out fractures, the possibility of ligamentous instability still exists. The incidence of SCI without fracture is low (0.7%) but still warrants attention. To assess stability, dynamic x-rays can

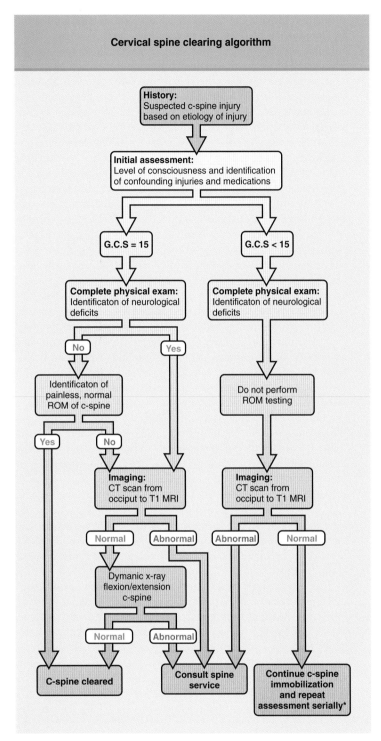

Cervical spine clearing algorithm

History:
Suspected c-spine injury based on etiology of injury

Initial assessment:
Level of consciousness and identification of confounding injuries and medications

G.C.S = 15

G.C.S < 15

Complete physical exam:
Identificaton of neurological deficits

Complete physical exam:
Identificaton of neurological deficits

No

Yes

Identificaton of painless, normal ROM of c-spine

Do not perform ROM testing

Yes

No

Imaging:
CT scan from occiput to T1 MRI

Imaging:
CT scan from occiput to T1 MRI

Normal

Abnormal

Abnormal

Normal

Dymanic x-ray flexion/extension c-spine

Normal

Abnormal

C-spine cleared

Consult spine service

Continue c-spine immobilization and repeat assessment serially*

Figure 39.4. Cervical spine clearing algorithm. A number of logical steps are required to address the issue of cervical spine stability, and numerous factors need to be considered. The algorithm provides guidance to the treating physician; navigating from top to bottom allows the reader to systematically address each factor. Initial steps involve gathering information, including the etiology of the injury; complete neurological assessment; and identification of pain. In the cooperative patient, assessment of the range of motion (ROM) is essential. CT scan and MRI will assist the spinal surgeon in making a determination of the stability. Proper interpretation of these studies is essential since these must be normal prior to proceeding with dynamic x-rays of the cervical spine. *"Clearing the cervical spine" refers to identification of patients who no longer need the cervical spine immobilized. A cleared cervical spine does not mean the complete absence of injury to the cervical spine but simply that the injury has a low probability of resulting in neurological compromise. Emphasis is on serial and frequent assessments, since a patient with a spinal cord injury can deteriorate quickly. The primary goal of this management tree is to expedite treatment and minimize complications with cervical spine trauma.

provide more information. The ability of the spine to maintain normal alignment of its bony elements in flexion and extension infers normal ligamentous integrity. The risk of obtaining dynamic x-rays and causing further injury must be weighed against the disadvantages of leaving the patient supine and in a collar. Pressure sores and decubitus ulcers in dependent areas can become a major concern with prolonged immobilization. The risks of infection and systemic complications cannot be trivialized.

Prevention of secondary injury can also be viewed as creating the optimal environment for recovery. This goal can be achieved by optimal perfusion to the spinal cord. In theory, the use of steroids in the setting of SCI targets the deleterious effect of the inflammatory cascade. In practice, the therapeutic benefits of steroids have been the subject of randomized studies, such as the National Acute Spinal Cord Injury Study by Bracken and colleagues (1998). Treatment with methylprednisolone for 24 or 48 hours has not been universally accepted, and methylprednisolone is considered a treatment option. This area of controversy has been fueled in part by the initial acceptance of this treatment option as a standard of care, with significant medicolegal implications. There is no unanimity about the use of steroids.

Surgical intervention is designed to achieve decompression and stabilization. There are controversies regarding timing and technique, but the ultimate goal of relieving pressure on the neural elements to create an environment best suited for recovery and preservation of neurological function is generally accepted. The timing of surgical decompression is the principal focus of attention for the Surgical Treatment of Acute Spinal Cord Injury Study group. Animal studies support early intervention; however, human studies have been less convincing. Our ability to perform early decompression of the neural elements and spinal stabilization has been demonstrated to be safe when vigilance over the oxygenation and vascular support is exercised.

A stable spine protects the neural elements in the setting of physiological loads. Advances in technology and surgical techniques have provided the spine surgeon with the ability to accurately reconstruct the injured spinal column in most instances. Anatomical levels previously left untouched are now being approached with more confidence, such as the craniocervical junction. Older techniques of immobilization, such as the halo vest, play a more limited role. The principle of early decompression and stabilization allows a faster transition to rehabilitation for the injured patient. Early implementation of physiotherapy has many benefits for the SCI patient. Respiratory complications can be minimized and functional recovery maximized.

PHASES OF CARE AND PREVENTION OF COMPLICATIONS

The clinical course of SCI patients can be subdivided into acute, subacute, and chronic, or rehabilitative, phases. At each period, the treatment team focuses on specific obstacles faced by the SCI patient. The objective in the acute phase is to save the patient's life and prevent worsening of the injury due to secondary injury processes such as ischemia. Transition into the subacute phase places more emphasis on prevention of complications. Complications in SCI patients can affect multiple systems. The cardiovascular system is faced with a significant increase in volume to compensate for the loss in sympathetic tone. The sympathectomy effects can be seen to varying degrees, based on the level of the SCI. Denervation of the muscles of respiration will affect the mechanics of breathing and can lead to atelectasis, which will predispose the lung to infection. Pneumonia can also result from aspiration or difficulty with managing secretions. Chest physiotherapy plays a critical role in minimizing these risks. Surgery, with early decompression and stabilization, allows the patient to be nursed in the sitting position and mobilized more aggressively. Early mobilization will also help prevent skin breakdown. Pressure sores can lead to life-threatening infections and interfere with rehabilitation. Ideally, patients should be nursed on special beds with pneumatic pumps for a smooth and controlled rotation allowing frequent repositioning.

Box 39.2 Pitfalls in the Management of Spinal Cord Injury Patients

Missed or delayed diagnosis of spinal fracture and/or spinal cord injury
Steroid use for prolonged period or use in penetrating trauma, resulting in complications such as infection
Performing surgical decompression without adequate blood pressure support, resulting in hypotension and further insult to the injured spinal cord
Cervical manipulation of unstable spine during intubation
Aspiration pneumonia
Inadequate feeding
Respiratory insufficiency
Fluid imbalance and overload leading to pulmonary edema
Prolonged immobilization and pressure sores
Severe bradycardia and/or cardiac arrest
Severe hypotension

Box 39.3 Areas of Controversy in Management of Spinal Cord Injury Patients

Diagnosis

Confirmation of cervical spine stability in comatose or sedated patients
Timing and use of MRI in suspected spinal cord injury patients

Treatment

Mandatory admission to the ICU for all spinal cord injury patients
Benefit of steroids in spinal cord injury
Timing of surgical decompression in spinal cord injury
Centralized admission of all spinal cord injury patients to specialized centers only

---

CONCLUSION

The pitfalls are numerous and present at every stage in the management of SCI patients. Box 39.2 provides a comprehensive list. Vigilance and serial examinations are essential when treating patients with SCIs. Controversies in the management of SCIs are listed in Box 39.3 and represent areas of research. This list emphasizes the important ones; however, the need for attention to details is critical.

SUGGESTED READING

Ball PA, Chicoine RE, Gettinger A: Anesthesia and critical care management of spinal cord injury. In Tator CH, Benzel E (eds): Contemporary Management of Spinal Cord Injury: From Impact to Rehabilitation. Park Ridge, IL, American Association of Neurological Surgeons, 2000, pp 99–108.
Bracken MB, Shepard MJ, Holford TR, et al: Methylprednisolone or tirilazad mesylate administration after acute spinal cord injury: 1-year follow-up. Results of the third National Acute Spinal Cord Injury randomized controlled trial. J Neurosurg 1998;89:699–706.

Chiu WC, Haan JM, Cushing BM, et al: Ligamentous injuries of the cervical spine in unreliable blunt trauma patients: Incidence, evaluation, and outcome. J Trauma 2001;50:457–463.

Fehlings MG, Sekhon LHS: Cellular, ionic, and biomolecular mechanisms of the injury process. In Tator CH, Benzel E (eds): Contemporary Management of Spinal Cord Injury: From Impact to Rehabilitation. Park Ridge, IL, American Association of Neurological Surgeons, 2000, pp 33–50.

Fehlings MG, Tator CH: An evidence-based review of decompressive surgery in acute spinal cord injury: Rationale, indications, and timing based on experimental and clinical studies. J Neurosurg Spine 1999;91:1–11.

Kiss Z, Tator C. Neurogenic shock: In Geller ER (ed): Shock and Resuscitation. New York, McGraw-Hill, 1993, pp 421–440.

Neurosurgery (Suppl.) 2002;50(3):s1–s199.

Singh RVP, Suys S, Villanueva PA: Prevention and treatment of medical complications. In Tator CH, Benzel E (eds): Contemporary Management of Spinal Cord Injury: From Impact to Rehabilitation. Park Ridge, IL, American Association of Neurological Surgeons, 2000, pp 253–272.

Tator C: Clinical manifestations of acute spinal cord injury. In Tator CH, Benzel E (eds): Contemporary Management of Spinal Cord Injury: From Impact to Rehabilitation. Park Ridge, IL, American Association of Neurological Surgeons, 2000, pp 21–32.

Tator C, Fehlings M: Clinical trials in spinal cord injury. In Biller J, Bogousslavsky J (eds): Clinical Trials in Neurologic Practice, Blue Books of Practical Neurology. Boston, Butterworth-Heinemann, 2001, pp 99–120.

KEY POINTS

- The term *brain stem death* should be used rather than *brain death*. A vegetative state implies a working brain stem. Patients may breathe spontaneously, open eyes, swallow, grimace, and have intact corneal reflexes; such patients may live for months or years. Patients with brain stem death are in deep coma and have irreversibly lost the ability to breathe; they will inevitably die within hours or days.
- It is important to establish as quickly as possible whether or not the donor has organs that are suitable for donation. Fewer exclusions occur today because organs can be accepted from HIV-positive and hepatitis C-positive patients when transplanting them into recipients who are infected with the same virus.
- Much of the care of the organ donor is a continuation of good intensive care practice. Thus, strict asepsis, chest physiotherapy, maintenance of normovolemia, treatment of hypo- or hyperthermia, and maintenance of normoglycemia are all extremely important.

The advent of mechanical ventilation and cardiovascular support has led to confusion in the diagnosis of death. Previously, irreversible failure of heart and lungs was easily observable and sufficient to make a diagnosis of death, irrespective of which organ system failed, because irreversible failure of the heart and lungs or brain precluded the continued function of the other. Today, however, despite irreversible failure of the brain, the heart and lungs can be artificially supported for considerable time. In these circumstances, death is recognized as the irreversible and complete loss of brain function.

In an attempt to standardize statutes and the judicial process throughout the United States, the American Bar Association, the American Medical Association, the National Conference of Commissioners on Uniform State Laws, and the President's Commission for the Study of Ethical Problems in Medicine and Biomedical and Behavioural Research proposed the following model statute, which has also been endorsed by the American Academy of Neurology and the American Electroencephalographic Society (Anonymous, 1979):

Uniform Determination of Death Act

An individual who has sustained either (1) irreversible cessation of circulatory and respiratory functions or (2) irreversible cessation of all functions of the entire brain, including the brain stem, is dead. A determination of death must be made in accordance with accepted medical standards.

The statute relies on the existence of accepted medical standards and that death can be determined by either cardiopulmonary or neurological criteria.

The tests used to determine cessation of brain function will continue to evolve as new research and technologies appear. The Harvard criteria (Pallis, 1996) are widely accepted, but advances have led to the demand for other criteria to be adopted. The time of death is a matter of local practice and not covered in this document (Department of Health, 1998; Kennedy, 1994):

THE CRITERIA FOR DETERMINATION OF DEATH

A. Cardiopulmonary: An individual with irreversible cessation of circulatory and respiratory function is dead.
   i. Cessation is recognized by an appropriate clinical examination of responsiveness, heart beat, and respiratory effort, with or without confirmatory tests such as ECG.
   ii. Irreversibility is recognized by persistent cessation of functions during an appropriate period of observation and/or trial of therapy.
B. An individual with irreversible cessation of all functions of the entire brain, including the brain stem, is dead.
   i. Cessation is recognized when both
      a. Cerebral function is absent, including unresponsivity, unreceptivity, and may require the use of EEG or cerebral blood flow studies, and
      b. Brain stem functions are absent. Testing requires an experienced physician, testing pupillary light, corneal, oculocephalic, oculovestibular, oropharyngeal, and respiratory [apnea when $PaCO_2 \geq 60$ mm Hg (Ad Hoc Committee of Harvard Medical School, 1968)] reflexes. When these reflexes cannot be adequately assessed, confirmatory tests are required.
   ii. Irreversibility is recognized when evaluation ascertains a, b, and c.

439

a. The cause of coma is known and is sufficient to account for the loss of brain functions. Etiology of the coma is a prerequisite and may require brain CT scan, drug toxicology screen, EEG, angiography, or other appropriate investigation.

b. The possibility of recovery of any brain functions is excluded—consider drugs, hypothermia, and shock—and can be confirmed by determination of cerebral blood flow.

c. The cessation of all brain functions persists for an appropriate period of trial observation and/or trial of therapy. Even where coma is known to have commenced before the period of observation, an experienced physician must establish cessation of all brain function at the beginning of the period of observation. Where drug intoxication, hypothermia, young age, or shock have been excluded, a period of 6 hours' observation with confirmatory EEG is recommended and 12 hours where no confirmatory test is available. In the case of cerebral hypoxia (cardiac arrest), a longer period of up to 72 hours is recommended.

Established Confirmatory Tests

i. Electrocerebral silence in the absence of brain stem functions confirms the diagnosis of brain death.

ii. Four-vessel intracranial angiography is definitive for diagnosing cessation of circulation to the entire brain. Complete cessation of circulation to the normothermic adult brain for more than 10 minutes is incompatible with survival of brain tissue.

iii. Absent cerebral blood flow in the hemispheres only, in conjunction with the determination of the cessation of all brain functions for 6 hours, is diagnostic of death.

Caution Required

Drug and metabolic intoxication: In cases where there is any likelihood of sedative presence, toxicology screening for all likely drugs is required. Death cannot be declared until the intoxicant is metabolized or intracranial circulation is tested and found to have ceased.

Hypothermia: Criteria for reliable recognition of death are not available at core temperatures below 32.2°C.

Children: Physicians should be particularly cautious in applying neurological criteria to determine death in children younger than 5 years.

Shock: Clinical and laboratory tests are unreliable in determining neurological criteria for death because of the associated reduction in cerebral circulation.

DIAGNOSIS OF BRAIN STEM DEATH

We can define death as the irreversible loss of the capacity for consciousness combined with irreversible loss of the capacity to breathe. We should use the term "brain stem death" rather than brain death. A vegetative state, which may occur because of cortical damage, implies a working brain stem, and patients may breathe spontaneously, open eyes, swallow, grimace, and have intact corneal reflexes. Such patients may live for months or years. Patients with brain stem death are in deep coma and have irreversibly lost the ability to breathe. They will inevitably die within hours or days. Studies that have examined brain stem death patients, whose ventilation is continued, confirm this.

Functions of the brain stem include the following:

a. The brain stem is essential for respiration and for mechanisms responsible for maintenance of blood pressure.

b. Projection from the upper part is responsible for alerting mechanisms, generating the capacity for consciousness.

c. All motor outputs from the cerebrum pass through, as do all sensory inputs other than sight/smell.

A diagnosis of brain stem death is based on satisfying certain preconditions and exclusions and then testing brain stem function. The preconditions and exclusions consider any reversible cause of brain stem failure. If the brain stem tests show no function and the preconditions and exclusions have been met, then a diagnosis of brain stem death can be made.

Preconditions

a. The patient is deeply unconscious.

b. There is no doubt that this is due to irremediable structural brain damage of known etiology.

c. The patient is on a ventilator and is not breathing.

Exclusions

a. Drug intoxication—alcohol, sedatives, muscle relaxants, and analgesics

b. Hypothermia

c. Circulatory, metabolic, and endocrine disturbances (electrolytes, acid–base, and BSL)

Tests of Brain Stem Function

a. Pupils unresponsive to light

b. No corneal reflex

c. No vestibuloocular reflex on caloric testing

d. No motor responses in cranial nerve distribution; no limb responses to supraorbital pressure

e. No gag response or response to tracheal suction

f. No spontaneous respiration when patient disconnected from ventilator long enough for $PaCO_2$ to reach 6.7 kPa (hypoxia should be prevented by giving O_2 via a catheter into the trachea)

Pitfalls and Safeguards

a. Inadequate consideration of preconditions and exclusions. There must be no doubt.

b. When eliciting signs of brain stem function:

Pupils: Use a bright light, and remember the actions of drugs (e.g., atropine may cause papillary dilation) and the possibility of local damage to eye/nerves.

Corneal reflexes: Use firm pressure (but avoid damaging cornea).

Caloric testing: Ensure by direct vision a wax-free external auditory meatus; remember gentamicin damage.

Apnea: Sufficient time must be allowed for CO_2 to rise (rate of rise is approximately 0.27 kPa/min). If possible, measure blood gases before and after disconnection to ensure no hypoxia and sufficiently high $PaCO_2$.

c. Remember that spinal reflexes can be present even though brain stem is dead.

Who Tests and When

The diagnosis of brain stem death should be made by at least two medical practitioners who have been registered or licensed for more than 5 years, are competent in the field, and are not members of the transplant team. At least one of the doctors should be a consultant or the equivalent. Testing is not normally considered until at least 6 hours after the onset of coma. If the causative problem was a cardiac arrest, hypoxia, or severe circulatory insufficiency with an indefinite period of cerebral hypoxia, it may take much longer to establish the diagnosis and be confident of the prognosis. In such cases, it may be necessary to wait 72 hours or longer after the circulation has been restored before testing.

Declaration of Death

Testing should be repeated to remove the risk of observer error. The timing of the interval between tests is a matter of clinical judgment but should be adequate for the reassurance of all concerned. If the second testing confirms brain stem death, the relatives can be informed that death can be declared and a certificate issued. The time of death is stated as the time that the first test indicated brain stem death. If organ donation is not planned, the patient need not be reconnected to the ventilator. If organ donation is planned, then ventilation should be reestablished until the organs are removed from the beating heart cadaver. Pressor agents and antibiotics may still be given, and anesthesia and muscle relaxants may be required to prevent spinal reflexes during surgery.

CARE OF THE ORGAN DONOR

This section deals with the care of the brain stem dead organ donor, although organs for donation are also provided by living donors or those without beating hearts. The objective of managing the brain stem dead donor is to preserve the organs to be donated by preventing damage from the changes that occur following brain stem death (Box 40.1). It perhaps seems logical that the management would also reduce the incidence of late rejection by increasing the quality of transplanted organs; however, this has not proven to be the case. A pilot study examining the use of a management protocol for organ donors found that use of such a protocol increased the number of organs available for donation but did not improve the rejection rate of transplanted organs. This is presumably because the protocol-managed and non–protocol-managed pathways converge at the point of selection of organs for donation, and at this

point evaluation allows selection of suitable organs and avoidance of those that are unsuitable and likely to be rejected.

The range of organs and tissues transplanted from brain stem dead donors includes the cornea, skin, small intestine, bones, liver, pancreas, heart, and lungs. Not all of these require critical management, but the heart, liver, and pancreas are vulnerable to hypoxia, and the changes following brain stem death may result in pulmonary damage that is preventable with active treatment. Optimal management aimed at preserving one organ may conflict with preservation of another. For example, using inotropes to maintain blood pressure and perfusion of the kidneys may render the heart less suitable for donation. Where such conflicts occur, they should be resolved based on which organs are the highest priority for donation.

It is important to establish as quickly as possible whether or not the donor has organs that are suitable for donation. There are fewer exclusions today because organs can be accepted from HIV-positive and hepatitis C-positive patients when transplanting them into recipients who are infected with the same virus. Organs will not be accepted from donors with the following conditions:

- Age > 75 years
- Malignant disease outside the central nervous system
- Systemic sepsis

HIV- and hepatitis C–positive potential donors should be reviewed with the organ transplant coordinator as soon as possible to determine if a potential recipient is on the waiting list with the same infection. Knowing this information early on will minimize the distress to the family and friends of the donor should no appropriate recipient be available. The following parameters and treatment details represent an amalgamation from the references listed at the end of this chapter. Although they give a guide to safe and appropriate management of the organ donor, there is increasing use of protocols in this field, and the majority of transplant centers likely have a donor management protocol. The specifications of the specific donor organs center should take precedence over the information given here.

Pathophysiological Changes Associated with Brain Stem Death

A transient period of parasympathetic activity occurs when brain stem death occurs, followed by intense sympathetic activity with release of large quantities of catecholamines lasting from 15 to 30 minutes (Box 40.2). These catecholes, in conjunction with changes in endocrine function that occur after brain stem death, may cause defective myocardial oxidative metabolism, myocardial ischemia, and consequent neurogenic pulmonary

---

Box 40.1 General Care of the Organ Donor

- Confirm suitability for donor status ASAP
- Discuss with family/next of kin
- Good ICU practice
- Optimal management will increase number of viable organs available for donation

---

Box 40.2 Physiological Management

- Tailor care to which organs will be donated
- Invasive monitoring including CVP/PA catheter
- Hormone replacement regime
- Treat hypovolemia and hypotension
- Chest physiotherapy and tracheal toilet
- Maintain normoglycemia
- Treat hypo-/hyperthermia

Table 40.1 Pathophysiological Changes Following Brain Death

Condition	Percent
Hypotension	81
Diabetes insipidus	65
DIC	28
Arrhythmias	27
Pulmonary edema	18
Metabolic acidosis	11

edema (Table 40.1). Blood pressure, heart rate, cardiac output, and systemic vascular resistance rise markedly with the increased autonomic activity, but these are followed by loss of sympathetic tone and consequent profound vasodilation secondary to death of the vasomotor centers. Combined with myocardial depression, this causes hypotension in approximately 80% of cases. Both atrial and ventricular dysrrhythmias are common, as are ECG changes that may include ST segment and T wave abnormalities and conduction problems. ECG changes suggestive of ischemia should not be taken to preclude organ donation because they may be reversible consequences of the hormonal failure that follows brain stem death. If the brain stem dead patient is ventilated but otherwise unsupported, the clinical course is usually short, with asystolic cardiac arrest generally occurring within 72 hours.

Anterior and posterior pituitary failure occur. Failure of ADH production results in diabetes insipidus in 65% of patients. If untreated, the consequent diuresis can cause hypovolemia, further contributing to the hypotension observed and causing plasma hyperosmolality and hypernatremia. There is also loss of the ADH contribution to maintaining vasomotor tone. Failure of TSH production results in reduced circulating levels of triiodothyronine and thyroxine, and loss of ACTH production leads to reduced circulating cortisol. Insulin levels are also decreased. The lower levels of tri-iodothyronine, insulin, and cortisol cause a change from aerobic to anaerobic metabolism that contributes to myocardial and plasma lactic acidosis. The reduced stress response, with its associated reduction in insulin levels, commonly leads to hyperglycemia. Brain stem death is also associated with increased immunogenicity of solid organs. The mechanism for this is unclear.

Pulmonary pathology may be present even before brain stem death occurs as a result of pulmonary trauma, aspiration of gastric contents, pneumonia, or neurogenic pulmonary edema. The intense sympathetic activity associated with brain stem death may cause acute left ventricular failure with functional mitral reflux. Pulmonary venous hypertension may briefly reach the level at which left atrial pressure exceeds pulmonary artery pressure with consequent pressure damage to the pulmonary vascular bed, disruption of the pulmonary capillary membranes, and the formation of protein-rich exudate in the alveoli. This is the probable mechanism of neurogenic pulmonary edema.

Disseminated intravascular coagulation occurs in 28% of brain stem dead organ donors, presumably due to the release of tissue thromboplastin from the ischemic or necrotic brain. Hypothalamic failure impairs temperature regulation, generally resulting in hypothermia because the reduction in metabolic rate and the loss of muscular activity both reduce heat production while vasodilation increases heat loss.

Monitoring
Invasive monitoring is essential for active management of the donor's circulation and pulmonary function. Because of the order in which the great vessels are ligated during the donor harvest, it is preferable to place the arterial cannula in the left brachial or radial artery and the central venous pressure (CVP) catheter or pulmonary artery catheter in the right internal jugular vein. Although a CVP may be used for hemodynamic monitoring, evidence supports using a pulmonary artery catheter.

General Management and Nursing Care
Much of the care of the organ donor is a continuation of good intensive care practice. Thus, strict asepsis, chest physiotherapy, maintenance of normovolemia, treatment of hypo- or hyperthermia, and maintenance of normoglycemia are all extremely important.

Hormone Replacement Therapy
Hormonal replacement facilitates the management of the cardiovascular changes associated with brain stem death (e.g., vasopressin can reverse the changes resulting from lack of ADH, and triiodothyronine can improve the function of the donor heart).

The "Papworth" regime includes
- Triiodothyronine: 4 µg bolus followed by an infusion of 3 µg per hour.
- ADH bolus of 1 unit followed by 1 to 4 units per hour
- Insulin: minimum of 1 unit per hour, adjusted to maintain normal blood glucose

With this regime, there is often stabilization or improvement in the hemodynamic state of the donor, and weaning of inotropic support is often possible.

Cardiovascular Support
The following are targets for hemodynamic values:
- Mean arterial pressure: >60 mm Hg
- Systolic blood pressure: <130 mm Hg
- Cardiac index: >2.5 liters/min/m^2
- Heart rate: 70 to 120 bpm in sinus rhythm
- Pulmonary capillary wedge pressure (or CVP if PCWP not available): <13 cm H$_2$O
- Systemic vascular resistance: 800 to 1200 dyn/sec/cm^5
- Left ventricular stroke work: >15 g

Hemodynamic support should begin by treating hypovolemia using colloids and/or blood guided by the CVP or PAOP readings. Where this is insufficient to achieve the previously discussed targets, inotropes may be used within the following limits:
- Dopamine: <5 pg/kg/min
- Dobutamine: <15 µg/kg/min
- Epinephrine: <0.2 µg/kg/min

When it is necessary to increase the systemic vascular resistance, vasopressin should be used rather than norepinephrine because it is less detrimental to the heart. Arrhythmias should be treated. Hypertension should be treated by reducing inotrope dosage whenever the cardiac index allows. If this is insufficient, an infusion of glyceryl trinitrate up to 30 mg/hr or sodium nitro-prusside up to 10 μg/kg/min may be used. If the patient is in the operating room, isoflurane up to an inspired concentration of 5% may be used.

Respiratory Support

Frequent chest physiotherapy and regular tracheal suctioning should be used to prevent or reduce retention of pulmonary secretions, mucous plugging, and subsequent segmental collapse. Differing ventilation regimens are recommended: The "Papworth" recommendations are to use a high tidal volume (12–15 mL/kg) and positive end-expiratory pressure (PEEP) of 5 cm H_2O, whereas the Scottish Cardiopulmonary Transplant Unit recommends a tidal volume of 6 mL/kg body weight and PEEP of up to 15 cm H_2O. The inspired oxygen level should be kept as low as possible, consistent with maintaining PaO_2 above 12 kPa. The $PaCO_2$ should be kept between 3.5 and 6.0 kPa.

Renal Support

Urine output should be maintained between 1 and 2 mL/kg/hr using fluid replacement and maintenance of cardiovascular parameters as previously described. The Scottish Cardiopulmonary Transplant Unit recommends the use of furosemide or mannitol if necessary. With urine output above 2 mL/kg/hr, the output should be matched with 0.9% saline and a bolus of vasopressin plus an increase in the vasopressin infusion rate. Serum electrolyte levels should be maintained as follows:

- Potassium: 3.5 to 6.0 mmol/liter
- Calcium: >0.7 mmol/liter
- PO_4: >0.8 mmol/liter

Careful attention to electrolyte levels may reduce the incidence of dysrrhythmias.

Hematological Support

Blood, fresh frozen plasma, and platelets should be used when necessary to achieve the following targets:

- Hemoglobin: >9.0 g/dL
- INR: <1.5
- Platelet count: >50 × 10^9/liter

Temperature

Hypothermia (i.e., core temperature below 35°C) should be prevented by using air-fed warming blankets, humidification of inspired gases, a warming mattress while in the operating room, and/or control of the ambient temperature. Occasionally, it may be necessary to cool the patient. When pyrexia occurs, the temperature should be kept below 39°C.

Communication

Communication with relatives is particularly important in such distressing circumstances. By providing information in an easily understood and reassuring manner, medical and nursing staff can help relatives understand the reasons for, and components of, brain stem testing. Regardless of the timing of the request for organ donation, relatives need time to consider and discuss these matters.

SUGGESTED READING

Ad Hoc Committee of the Harvard Medical School; A definition of irreversible coma. JAMA 1968;205:87–88.

Alvarez LA: Controversies in the diagnosis of brain death in children. Int Pediatr 1990;5:197–202.

Anonymous: Conference of Medical Royal Colleges and their faculties (UK). Br Med J 1979:1;332.

Anonymous: Multi-organ retrieval. A guide for the retrieval team. Papworth Hospital NHS Trust 2001 Conference of Medical Royal Colleges and their Faculties (UK). Br Med J 1976;2:1187.

Anonymous: Report of the medical consultants on the diagnosis of death to the President's Commission for the Study of Ethical Problems in Medicine and Biomedical and Behavioural Research. Guidelines for the determination of death. JAMA 1981;246:2184–2187.

Bates D: Coma and brain death. Curr Opin Neurol Neurosurg 1991;4:17–20.

Department of Health: A Code of Practice for the Diagnosis of Brain Stem Death (Including Guidelines for the Identification and Management of Potential Organ and Tissue Donors). London: Department of Health, 1998.

Kennedy S. Declaration of brain death. Anesthesiol Clin North Am 1994;12:643–654.

Morgan G, Smith M: Donation of Organs for Transplantation. The Management of the Potential Organ Donor. A Manual for the Establishment of Local Guidelines. London: Intensive Care Society, 1999.

Pallis C: ABC of Brain Stem Death, 2nd ed. Anapolis Junction MD: BMJ, 1996.

Walker AE: Brain death. An American viewpoint. Neurosurg Rev 1989;12:259–264.

<table>
<tr><td>

Chapter

41

</td><td>

Acid-Base Disorders

Thomas John Morgan

</td></tr>
</table>

Interpretation of acid-base data and management of acid-base disorders are fundamental to critical care practice. Cellular enzyme structure and kinetics depend on a tightly controlled intracellular pH. However, this aspect of cell physiology is difficult to monitor. To add complexity, there is no single intracellular pH, but rather a range of values in the cytosol and various organelles. Consequently, most tests are conducted on extracellular fluid, usually by sampling arterial blood. Plasma pH is on average about 0.6 pH units above intracellular values.

EPIDEMIOLOGY AND PATHOPHYSIOLOGY

Epidemiology

Data on the prevalence of acid-base disorders in specific populations are scarce. In intensive care, case mix has an important effect. Much also depends on how these disturbances are defined. Table 41.1, based on unpublished Australian data and using definitions set out in this chapter, gives an idea of the distribution of acid-base disorders in a surgical/medical intensive care unit (ICU).

Pathophysiology

The diagnostic algorithm normally commences with an examination of arterial PCO_2 ($PaCO_2$) and pH. The $PaCO_2$/pH relationship is thus a fundamental acid-base property.

CO_2 interacts with plasma water as follows:

$$CO_2 + H_2O \leftrightarrow H_2CO_3 \leftrightarrow H^+ + HCO_3^-$$

By applying the law of mass action and substituting [dissolved CO_2] for $[H_2CO_3]$, the following expression can be derived:

$$pH = pK_1 + \log_{10}([HCO_3^-]/\alpha\, PCO_2)$$

This is the Henderson-Hasselbalch equation, where α is the plasma CO_2 solubility coefficient, and pK_1 the negative logarithm of the dissociation constant. With it we can calculate the plasma $[HCO_3^-]$ from measured $PaCO_2$ and pH values.

However, the Henderson-Hasselbalch equation is an incomplete description of the $PaCO_2$/pH relationship (Fig. 41.1). To illustrate, consider a patient undergoing mechanical ventilation. If the $PaCO_2$ is 40 mm Hg and the arterial plasma pH is 7.4, we can show with the Henderson-Hasselbalch equation that the arterial $[HCO_3^-]$ is 24 mEq/L. If hyperventilation reduces the $PaCO_2$ to 20 mm Hg, this equation on its own cannot predict either the new pH or the new $[HCO_3^-]$. At the new acid-base equilibrium there are at least five other equations that must be satisfied simultaneously; they deal with water dissociation and the physical chemistry of proteins and electrolytes in plasma, red cells, and the interstitial space. They are discussed later in this chapter.

By convention, acid-base disorders are divided into respiratory ($PaCO_2$) and metabolic (non-$PaCO_2$) disturbances. Most practitioners use $PaCO_2$ as the sole index of respiratory acid-base status. However two "schools" (Boston and Copenhagen) have formed around the identification and quantification of metabolic acid-base disturbances. The advent of the physical chemical approach of the late Peter Stewart has added confusion for some. This is quite unnecessary. The Stewart approach is a help rather than a hindrance.

Table 41.1 Sample Distribution of ICU Acid-Base Abnormalities

Abnormality	Percentage (%)
No abnormality	35
Respiratory alkalosis	15
Respiratory acidosis	10
Metabolic acidosis	10
Metabolic alkalosis	5
Mixed disorders	25

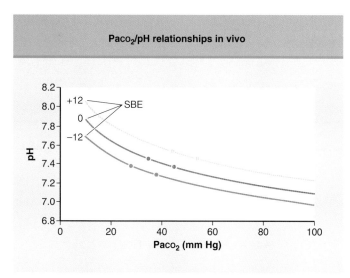

Figure 41.1. Paco₂/pH relationships in vivo. The middle curve (red, SBE = 0 mEq/L) shows the normal relationship. The left-shifted curve (green, SBE = −12 mEq/L) illustrates metabolic acidosis. The right-shifted curve (yellow, SBE = +12 mEq/L) shows metabolic alkalosis. Curve shifts arise either as primary metabolic acid-base disturbances, or as compensation for respiratory acid-base disturbances. The normal Paco₂ range is illustrated *(filled circles)* on the middle curve, along with the alterations expected as respiratory compensation for metabolic acidosis and alkalosis *(filled circles,* left- and right-shifted curves, respectively; see Table 41.2).

The important thing to realize is that the Boston and Copenhagen schools describe the same processes from different vantage points. Stewart's concepts do not invalidate either approach but rather help us understand their physiologic basis.

The Physical Chemistry of Acid-Base

More than 20 years ago, Peter Stewart pointed out that, from the perspective of physical chemistry, $[HCO_3^-]$ and pH in body fluids are controlled by just three independent variables: PCO_2, the total concentration of nonvolatile weak acid (A_{TOT}), and the strong ion difference (SID) (Fig. 41.2). $PaCO_2$ represents the respiratory acid-base status, as in the traditional classification scheme. SID and A_{TOT} acting together constitute the metabolic acid-base status.

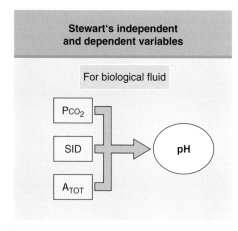

Figure 41.2. Stewart's independent and dependent variables. SID is strong ion difference, whereas A_{TOT} is the total concentration of weak acid (see text).

PaCO₂

$PaCO_2$ is an equilibrium value determined by the balance between CO_2 production (15,000 mmol/day) and its rate of elimination via the lungs.

A_TOT

Body fluid compartments have varying concentrations of nonvolatile (i.e., non-CO_2) weak acids. In plasma, they consist mainly of albumin and inorganic phosphate. These same weak acids are present in interstitial fluid, although concentrations are smaller. In red cells the predominant nonvolatile weak acid is hemoglobin. For convenience Stewart lumped together all nonvolatile weak acids in each compartment and modeled them as having a single anionic form (A^-) and a single conjugate base form (HA), with a single pKa (in plasma around 6.8).

$$HA \leftrightarrow H^+ + A^-$$

Stewart termed the total concentration of nonvolatile weak acid in any compartment "A_{TOT}," where $A_{TOT} = [HA] + [A^-]$

SID

The SID concept arose because certain elements such as Na^+, K^+, Ca^{2+}, Mg^{2+}, and Cl^- exist in body fluids as completely ionized entities. At physiologic pH this is also effectively true of anions with pKa values of 4 or less, e.g., sulfate, lactate, and β-hydroxybutyrate. Stewart described all such compounds as "strong ions." In body fluids there is a surfeit of strong cations, the excess quantified by SID. In other words, SID = [strong cations] − [strong anions]. Being a "charge" space, SID is expressed in mEq/L. SID calculated from measured strong ions in normal plasma is 42 mEq/L.

SID is under constant attack by the metabolic production of approximately 1 mEq/kg/day of sulfate. Without renal elimination of these anions, SID would be steadily reduced.

Weak ions and buffer base

The SID space is filled by weak ions. They include H^+, OH^-, HCO_3^-, CO_3^{2-}, and the A^- component of A_{TOT}. To preserve electrical neutrality, their total net charge must always equal SID. However, unlike strong ions, their individual concentrations vary with pH by dissociation/association of their respective parent molecules. Stewart set out six equations to describe their acid-base behavior. They are applications of the law of mass action to the dissociation of water, H_2CO_3, HCO_3^-, and nonvolatile weak acids, coupled with the expression for A_{TOT} and a statement of electrical neutrality.

However, HCO_3^- and A^-, together known as the "buffer base" anions, occupy virtually all of the SID "space" (Figs. 41.3 and 41.4), since the other ions in the space are measured in either micromoles per liter or nanomoles per liter. This means that SID not only dictates the buffer base concentration but is also virtually identical to it, so that SID = $[HCO_3^-] + [A^-]$. In fact the quantitative insignificance of all but the buffer base anions allows us to reduce Stewart's equations from six to three, without loss of accuracy. The three simplified plasma equations are set out in Box 41.1.

We can use these equations in a number of ways. For example, we can substitute measured values of pH, [Alb], [Pi], and $PaCO_2$, and solve for $[A^-]$ and $[HCO_3^-]$ (note that

Gamblegram of plasma strong and weak ions

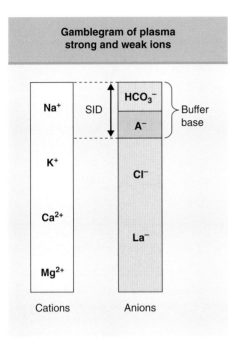

Figure 41.3. **Gamblegram of plasma strong and weak ions.** The strong ion difference (SID) is an electrical space, filled primarily by the weak buffer base anions HCO₃⁻ and A⁻.

Influence of Stewart's independent variables on buffer base components

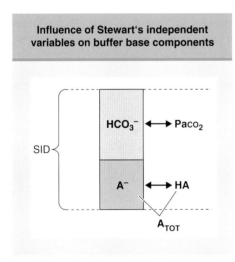

Figure 41.4. **Influence of Stewart's independent variables on buffer base components.** The relative values of [HCO₃⁻] and [A⁻] (nonvolatile weak acid anion) within the SID space are strongly influenced by Paco₂ and A_TOT, respectively.

Box 41.1 Physical-Chemical Equations Simplified for Plasma

$$[A^-] = [Alb] \times (0.123 \times pH - 0.631) + [Pi] \times (0.309 \times pH - 0.469)$$

$$[HCO_3^-] = 0.0301 \times PCO_2 \times 10^{(pH-6.1)}$$

$$SID = [HCO_3^-] + [A^-]$$

[Alb] is albumin concentration expressed in g/L, [Pi] is phosphate concentration in mmol/L, and PCO₂ is in mm Hg.

Effect of isolated SID changes on plasma pH

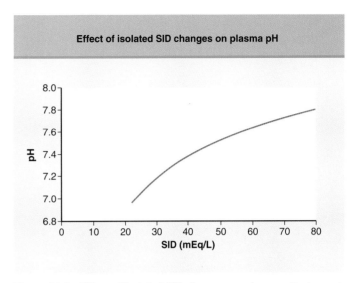

Figure 41.5. **Effect of isolated SID changes on plasma pH.** A_TOT and Paco₂ are held constant at 20 mEq/L and 40 mm Hg, respectively. A rising SID increases pH.

[HCO₃⁻] is the "actual" bicarbonate concentration, not "standard" bicarbonate, which is discussed below). SID can then be calculated as [HCO₃⁻] + [A⁻]. This is the most convenient method for determining SID, when it is termed the "effective" SID, or SIDe. If SID is calculated more laboriously from measured plasma strong ion concentrations, it is termed the "apparent" SID, or SIDa. Discrepancies between SIDe and SIDa imply the presence of unmeasured ions, as will be discussed.

Isolated changes in SID and A_TOT

Another use of the equations in Box 41.1 is to test the effect of isolated variations in SID or A_TOT on plasma pH. These are shown in Figs. 41.5 and 41.6. They illustrate important Stewart concepts. At any given Paco₂, a falling SID or a rising A_TOT reduces pH (and [HCO₃⁻]) and moves the equilibrium towards a metabolic acidosis. Conversely, a rising SID or a falling A_TOT creates a metabolic alkalosis. Interestingly, despite these physical chemical "truths," which are easy to demonstrate in vitro, variations in A_TOT in vivo seem to reset the normal value for SID rather than cause primary acid-base disturbances. Presumably this adjustment is via altered renal chloride handling.

Determinants of the Paco₂/pH Relationship

Since plasma pH at any given Paco₂ is defined solely by A_TOT and SID, Stewart's six equations (or the three simplified equations in Box 41.1) go a long way toward defining the Paco₂/pH relationship (see Fig. 41.1). However, if Paco₂ is suddenly altered, the equations described so far still cannot make an accurate prediction of the new plasma pH. The reason is that as Paco₂ changes, plasma SID also changes.

The dependence of plasma SID on Paco₂ stems from the interaction via Donnan equilibria of the plasma compartment (volume 3 L) with the adjacent erythrocyte compartment (volume 2 L) and with the interstitial space (volume 13.5 L). Each compartment has different concentrations of nondiffusible protein anions, mainly albumin or hemoglobin. Their negative

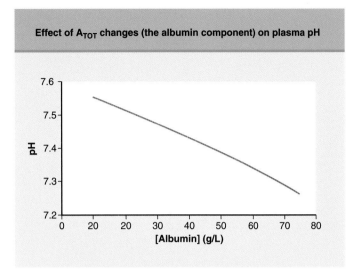

Figure 41.6. Effect of isolated A_{TOT} changes (the albumin component) on plasma pH. SID and $PaCO_2$ are held constant at 40 mEq/L and 40 mm Hg, respectively. A rising A_{TOT} decreases pH.

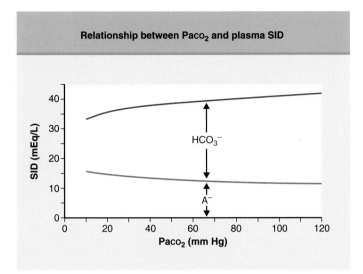

Figure 41.7. Relationship between $PaCO_2$ and plasma SID (here calculated as SIDe [see text]) when metabolic acid-base status is held constant. Plasma SID increases with $PaCO_2$, primarily because of chloride shifts (see text). The progressive $[HCO_3^-]$ increase with $PaCO_2$ is accompanied by a progressive decrease in A^- (nonvolatile weak acid anion).

charges vary with pH (Box 41.1, first equation). As a result, whenever pH changes there is a redistribution of diffusible ions (mainly Cl^-) between compartments. These pH-driven Cl^- shifts cause plasma SID to go up and down in synchrony with $PaCO_2$ (Fig. 41.7). When added to Stewart's equations, they complete the definition of the $PaCO_2$/pH relationship.

Importantly, extracellular SID remains unaffected by Donnan phenomena, since the ionic shifts are contained within the extracellular space. Thus extracellular SID taken as a whole is independent of sudden changes in $PaCO_2$. (We can regard red cells as part of the extracellular space for this exercise.) The immunity of extracellular SID from sudden $PaCO_2$ changes is fundamental to the notion of standard base excess (see below).

How Acid-Base Disturbances are Reflected in the PaCO₂/pH Relationship

Acute respiratory disturbances move data points up (respiratory alkalosis) and down (respiratory acidosis) the prevailing $PaCO_2$/pH curve (see Fig. 41.1). In contrast, metabolic disturbances (altered SID and/or A_{TOT}) shift the curve to the left or right (see Fig. 41.1). A left-shifted curve means the pH at any given $PaCO_2$ is lower than normal, which depending on the $PaCO_2$ represents either a primary metabolic acidosis or else metabolic compensation for a respiratory alkalosis. With a right-shifted curve, the pH at any given $PaCO_2$ is higher than normal, signifying a primary metabolic alkalosis or else compensation for a respiratory acidosis.

Quantifying Metabolic Acid-Base Disturbances

It is important to realize that SID on its own does not give us the current metabolic acid-base status in any patient. This can be determined only by the interplay between SID and A_{TOT}. For example, a plasma SID of 42 mEq/L is normal in a healthy individual, but in the presence of hypoalbuminemia (reduced A_{TOT}) it represents a right-shifted curve and a metabolic alkalosis. For

this reason, clinicians prefer to use metabolic indices that integrate the effects of SID and A_{TOT} on the $PaCO_2$/pH relationship. The best of these is standard base excess. However, it is also possible (with some caveats) to use bicarbonate-based indices such as the "rules of thumb" of the Boston school, or else "standard bicarbonate." We will touch on each of these in turn.

Standard base excess

An ideal metabolic acid-base index is independent of $PaCO_2$ and identifies and quantifies shifts in the $PaCO_2$/pH curve. By these criteria, standard base excess (SBE), developed by the Copenhagen "school," is the best single index. In reality it expresses the deviation from normal of the buffer base concentration ($[HCO_3^-]$ + $[A^-]$) in the total extracellular space. It is thus identical to the abnormality in extracellular SID, since buffer base and SID are interchangeable terms. SBE is calculated from a single set of arterial blood gases by assuming a mean extracellular hemoglobin concentration of 50 g/L. A useful formula is

$$SBE = 0.93 \times ([HCO_3^-] + 14.84 \times (pH - 7.4) - 24.4)$$

(SBE and $[HCO_3^-]$ values in mEq/L)

A typical reference range is −3.0 to +3.0 mEq/L. If SBE is less than −3.0 mEq/L, there is a left-shifted curve. As already stated, this shift could represent either a primary metabolic acidosis or else compensation for a primary respiratory alkalosis, depending on the $PaCO_2$ and the pH. The SBE abnormality quantifies the increase in extracellular SID needed to shift the curve back to the normal position without changing A_{TOT}. SBE is thus really "extracellular SID excess," or SIDex.

To illustrate, if the SBE is −9 mEq/L, extracellular SID must be increased by 9 mEq/L to bring SBE back to zero. This value should be close to the number of mmol of $NaHCO_3$ solution

Table 41.2 Primary Acid-Base Disturbances and Expected Compensation			
Primary Disorder	**Initiating Factor**	**Compensation Mechanism**	**Compensation Rules of Thumb**
Acute respiratory acidosis	Pa_{CO_2} increase	Nil (extracellular SID unchanged, $[HCO_3^-]$ increased and $[A^-]$ decreased)	(1) $\Delta SBE = 0$ (2) $\Delta HCO_3^- = 0.1 \times (Pa_{CO_2}-40)$
Chronic respiratory acidosis	Prolonged Pa_{CO_2} increase	Extracellular SID increased due to increased renal Cl^- excretion	(1) $\Delta SBE = 0.4 \times \Delta Pa_{CO_2}$ (2) $\Delta HCO_3^- = 0.35 \times (Pa_{CO_2}-40)$
Acute respiratory alkalosis	Pa_{CO_2} decrease	Nil (extracellular SID unchanged, $[HCO_3^-]$ decreased and $[A^-]$ increased)	(1) $\Delta SBE = 0$ (2) $\Delta HCO_3^- = 0.2 \times (Pa_{CO_2}-40)$
Chronic respiratory alkalosis	Prolonged Pa_{CO_2} decrease	Extracellular SID decreased due to decreased renal Cl^- excretion	(1) $\Delta SBE = 0.4 \times \Delta Pa_{CO_2}$ (2) $\Delta HCO_3^- = 0.5 \times (Pa_{CO_2}-40)$
Metabolic acidosis	SID decrease and/or A_{TOT} increase	Pa_{CO_2} reduction	(1) $\Delta Pa_{CO_2} = \Delta SBE$ (2) $Pa_{CO_2} = 1.5 \times (HCO_3^-) + 8$ (3) $Pa_{CO_2} = $ last 2 digits of pH.
Metabolic alkalosis	SID increase and/or A_{TOT} decrease	Pa_{CO_2} increase	(1) $\Delta Pa_{CO_2} = 0.6 \times \Delta SBE$ (2) $Pa_{CO_2} = 0.6 \times (HCO_3^--24)$ (3) $Pa_{CO_2} = $ last 2 digits of pH

required per liter of extracellular fluid to achieve this correction. ($NaHCO_3$ increases extracellular SID because it contains the strong cation Na^+ but no strong anion.) In fact, slightly more is needed—an amount corresponding to an extracellular volume of 30% body weight rather than 20%, the reason being that hypertonic fluid such as 1 M $NaHCO_3$ expands the extracellular space by transmembrane shifts.

Similarly, if SBE is greater than 3.0 mEq/L, the curve is right-shifted (either a primary metabolic alkalosis or else compensation for a chronic respiratory acidosis). SBE then quantifies the reduction in extracellular SID necessary to normalize the curve position and bring SBE back to zero.

Bicarbonate-Based Approaches to Metabolic Acid-Base—the Boston "Rules of Thumb" and Standard Bicarbonate

These methods ignore the A^- component of the buffer base concentration. By focusing on plasma bicarbonate they take on more qualitative characteristics. In other words, they can tell us that the Pa_{CO_2}/pH curve is shifted, but unlike SBE they cannot tell us exactly how much. As a dosage guide for interventions such as $NaHCO_3$ administration, they are therefore less reliable.

Boston-school devotees calculate the $[HCO_3^-]$ from the measured pH and Pa_{CO_2} and compare that with the $[HCO_3^-]$ deemed appropriate for the measured Pa_{CO_2}, using "rules of thumb" based on data from patients and volunteers with acid-base derangements (Table 41.2). An offset denotes a metabolic acid-base disturbance. "Standard bicarbonate" was developed by the Copenhagen school prior to SBE. It is the $[HCO_3^-]$ after in vitro P_{CO_2} correction to 40 mm Hg. Any difference from 24 mmol/L is regarded as a metabolic acid-base abnormality.

Within its qualitative limitations, the Boston method works quite well. However, because standard bicarbonate is an in vitro parameter, the more abnormal the Pa_{CO_2}, the less qualitatively reliable it becomes. As an illustration, consider the following arterial blood gas result:

Hb 150 g/L, pH 7.086, Pa_{CO_2} 100 mm Hg, $[HCO_3^-]$ 29.1 mEq/L, SBE 0 mEq/L

This patient has a severe respiratory acidosis. The SBE of 0 mEq/L indicates that there is no metabolic acid-base disturbance, compensatory or otherwise. Using the Boston approach, the expected $[HCO_3^-]$ for a Pa_{CO_2} of 100 mm Hg is 30 mEq/L (see Table 41.2). The actual $[HCO_3^-]$ of 29.1 mEq/L is slightly lower, suggesting at most a slight metabolic acidosis, but largely in agreement with the SBE findings. However, the standard bicarbonate is 21.4 mEq/L, which by comparison with 24 mEq/L gives the (false) impression that there is a significant metabolic acidosis.

Primary Acid-Base Disorders

Primary acid-base disorders are those that dictate the direction of the pH disturbance. They can be either respiratory (Pa_{CO_2}) or metabolic. With opposing primary disorders, the pH can be normal.

Compensation

Compensation is a response to a primary acid-base disorder, reducing the severity of the pH disturbance. The pH is rarely brought back to the normal range, apart from in chronic respiratory alkalosis, so that a normal pH combined with an abnormal Pa_{CO_2} usually means there are two primary acid-base disorders, one respiratory and one metabolic.

Respiratory compensation

Metabolic acid-base disturbances normally activate feedback loops that alter alveolar ventilation and thus Pa_{CO_2} in a way that reduces the impact on pH. The loops are via CSF pH and plasma pH, acting on the central and peripheral chemoreceptors, respectively. In metabolic acidosis, minute ventilation can increase by more than 8-fold, the resultant hypocapnia reducing the severity of the acidemia. In contrast, metabolic alkalosis suppresses minute ventilation, the hypercapnia blunting the pH rise.

In both cases the full response evolves over 12 to 24 hours. The delay comes about because the signal from the central chemoreceptors takes time to develop, since SID equilibration between plasma and CSF is gradual. Initial respiratory compensation is thus driven entirely by the peripheral chemoreceptors. In fact, because P_{CO_2} equilibration between plasma and CSF is immediate, the early peripheral chemoreceptor response overcorrects the CSF pH. As a result, the action of the central chemoreceptors is more like that of a slow-release brake.

449

Metabolic compensation

Metabolic compensation for respiratory acid-base disturbances is achieved by renal adjustment of plasma SID. Prolonged hypocapnia causes renal retention of Cl^- and a fall in SID, whereas in sustained hypercapnia, the kidneys increase SID by eliminating Cl^- accompanied by NH_4^+. Metabolic compensation is much slower than respiratory, taking up to 5 days to develop fully (see Table 41.2).

Role of Kidneys in Acid-Base Balance

The role of the kidneys in acid-base homeostasis is to

1. Regulate plasma and extracellular SID by
   a. maintaining the separation between $[Na^+]$ and $[Cl^-]$, mainly by regulation of Cl^- excretion.
   b. eliminating other strong anions (in company with NH_4^+) that reduce SID, especially sulfate.
2. Participate in plasma phosphate regulation (an A_{TOT} component).

The kidneys can affect acid-base only by altering SID or A_{TOT}. From the Stewart perspective, talk of H^+ or HCO_3^- "balances" is misleading, since H^+ and HCO_3^- are dependent variables and not directly exchangeable commodities.

DIAGNOSIS

Over the past 50 years, definitions of primary and compensatory acid-base processes have been the subject of dispute, despite attempts at consensus. Tables 41.2 and 41.3 set out the definitions adopted in this chapter. They are based on widespread current usage.

It is usual to classify deviation from the expected level of respiratory compensation (see Table 41.2) as a primary respiratory acid-base disturbance. For example, consider a patient with diabetic ketoacidosis. If the arterial pH is 7.20 and the $PaCO_2$ is 20 mm Hg, the patient has a metabolic acidosis with normal respiratory compensation (see Table 41.2). [Some still argue that this compensation should be called "partial," since the pH has not been corrected, but normal compensation for metabolic acidosis *never* fully corrects the plasma pH (see Table 41.2)]. If, however, we find that the pH is 7.20 with a $PaCO_2$ of

Table 41.4 Gaps Used in Acid-Base Diagnosis

Gap	Calculation	Common Reference Range
AG[a]	$([Na^+] + [K^+]) - ([Cl^-] + [HCO_3^-])$	7–17 mEq/L (subtract 4 if K^+ not used)
AGc[b]	$AG + 0.25 \times (40 - [Alb])$	7–17 mEq/L (subtract 4 if K^+ not used)
SIG[c] (SIDa – SIDe)	$[Na^+] + [K^+] + [Ca^{++}] + [Mg^{++}] - [Cl^-] - [lactate] - [A^-] - [HCO_3^-]$	Not established
Osmolal gap	Measured osmolality – $(1.86 \times ([Na^+] + [K^+]) + [urea] + [glucose])$	<10 mOsm/kg

[a] $[K^+]$ omitted in many laboratories.
[b] Assumes normal $[Alb] = 40$ g/L.
[c] $[A^-]$ calculated as in Box 41.1.

32 mm Hg, modern usage classifies this as a metabolic acidosis with an accompanying respiratory acidosis (despite the hypocapnia). Such a patient should raise more concern, since the impaired respiratory response may herald impending respiratory failure. Conversely, if the $PaCO_2$ is 12 mm Hg at the same pH, there is a metabolic acidosis with an accompanying respiratory alkalosis.

Gaps

Certain calculated gaps can assist in acid-base diagnosis (Table 41.4). They are either electrical or osmolal.

Electrical gaps such as the anion gap (AG), corrected AG (AGc), and strong ion gap (SIG) are primarily scanning tools for abnormal concentrations of unmeasured strong anions, e.g., lactate and β-hydroxybutyrate. In health, the AG represents $[A^-]$ plus small contributions from lactate, keto acid, and urate anions. Unmeasured strong anions increase the AG.

However, the AG is influenced by many other factors, especially albumin fluctuations, reducing its specificity for unmeasured strong anions (Table 41.5). The AGc corrects for albumin fluctuations, whereas the SIG adjusts for several other factors as well (see Table 41.5). A third parameter known as the BE gap is really an alternative version of SIG, the main difference being that it does not incorporate lactate. Both SIG and the BE gap have not yet achieved widespread clinical use.

The osmolal gap can help when there is a metabolic acidosis with an unexplained high anion gap. If the osmolal gap is also raised, it suggests poisoning by methanol or ethylene glycol. However, a number of other conditions elevate the osmolal gap (Table 41.6).

Temperature Correction of Blood Gas Data— Alpha-Stat versus pH-Stat Approach

Blood gas analyzers perform all measurements at 37°C, despite the fact that many ICU patients are febrile and some are hypothermic. Analyzer software algorithms can convert measured values mathematically to the patient's core temperature for interpretation and action. This is the "pH-stat" approach. However, most practitioners prefer to act on values as originally measured at 37°C, irrespective of the patient's temperature. This practice is known as the "alpha-stat" approach. The logic is as follows:

Table 41.3 Definitions of Acid-Base Processes

Term	Definition
Normal arterial pH	7.35 to 7.45
Acidemia	Arterial pH < 7.35
Alkalemia	Arterial pH > 7.45
Normal $PaCO_2$	35–45 mm Hg
Hypercapnia	$PaCO_2$ > 45 mm Hg
Hypocapnia	$PaCO_2$ < 35 mm Hg
Respiratory acidosis	$PaCO_2$ > 45 mm Hg if SBE normal, or >5 mm Hg above expected compensation for metabolic acid-base disturbance (see Table 41.2).
Respiratory alkalosis	$PaCO_2$ < 35 mm Hg if SBE normal, or >5 mm Hg below expected compensation for metabolic acid-base disturbance (see Table 41.2).
Metabolic acidosis (primary or compensatory)	SBE < −3 mEq/L
Metabolic alkalosis (primary or compensatory)	SBE > +3 mEq/L

Table 41.5 Factors Affecting Electrical Gaps

Factor	Anion Gap (AG)	Corrected AG (AGc)	Strong Ion Gap (SIG)
Lactate	Increased	Increased	No effect
Other unmeasured strong anions (e.g., keto acids, salicylate)	Increased	Increased	Increased
Unmeasured weak anions (e.g., polygelinate, myeloma IgA band)	Increased	Increased	Increased
Unmeasured strong cations (e.g., lithium)	Decreased	Decreased	Decreased
Unmeasured weak cations (e.g., THAMH$^+$, myeloma IgG band)	Decreased	Decreased	Decreased
Chloride overestimation (bromism, hyperlipidemia)	Decreased	Decreased	Decreased
Sodium underestimation (severe hypernatremia)	Decreased	Decreased	Decreased
[Pi] ⇑	Increased	Increased	No effect
[Pi] ⇓	Decreased	Decreased	No effect
pH ⇑	Increased	Increased	No effect
pH ⇓	Decreased	Decreased	No effect
[Ca^{2+}] and [Mg^{2+}] ⇑	Decreased	Decreased	No effect
[Ca^{2+}] and [Mg^{2+}] ⇓	Increased	Increased	No effect
[Alb] ⇑	Increased	No effect	No effect
[Alb] ⇓	Decreased	No effect	No effect

Table 41.6 Causes of a Raised Osmolal Gap

Condition	Causes
Drugs and ingestions (poisoning)	Ethylene glycol
	Methanol
	Isopropanol
	Ethanol
	Diethyl ether
	Paraldehyde
	Formaldehyde
	Mannitol
	Glycine
	Sorbitol
Metabolic disturbances	Ketoacidosis (acetone, glycerol)
	Lactic acidosis (unknown solutes)
	Renal failure (unknown solutes)
Factitious	Pseudohyponatremia (hyperlipidemia and hyperproteinemia)

reality, there will be in vivo hypocapnia at the lower temperature, while the actual pH will be high (about 7.55 at 30°C). This technique mimics the way ectothermic (cold-blooded) animals respond to hypothermia.

For all variations in core temperature (high or low), it is now usual to monitor pH and PaCO$_2$ values as measured at 37°C and maintain them in the normal reference ranges for 37°C. This approach should ensure that alpha remains at 0.55 (hence the term "alpha-stat" approach).

Steps in the Laboratory Assessment of Acid-Base Status

The clinician should follow a methodical sequence, such as that set out in Tables 41.7 and 41.8. Of note, increases in AGc and reductions in SBE, although similar, are not truly stoichiometric (in other words, not "one for one"). The AGc is a plasma value, whereas SBE is an extracellular concentration. Boston-

In protein molecules, the ratio of protonated imidazole to total imidazole on histidine moieties is called alpha. At 37°C, under normal acid-base conditions, the mean intracellular pH is 6.8 (which is the neutral pH at this temperature). Alpha is then approximately 0.55.

Maintaining an alpha value close to 0.55 is important for enzyme structure and function.

Arterial blood awaiting analysis is often placed on ice. Although with cooling the blood pH will rise and the PCO$_2$ fall progressively, measurement at 37°C remains unchanged until lactate accumulates, especially if the syringe is glass. Importantly, inside the syringe the alpha value of the cooled blood proteins stays at 0.55. This is because the change in the imidazole dissociation constant with temperature is about half the change in the water dissociation constant and in the same direction. As the blood cools, CO$_2$ content does not alter, whereas PCO$_2$ falls owing to the increasing solubility coefficient.

An effective way to keep alpha optimal during induced hypothermia is to maintain the PaCO$_2$ and pH measured at 37°C in their normal reference ranges for 37°C. In

Table 41.7 The Acid-Base Diagnostic Sequence

Step	Explanation
1. Scan the pH and PaCO$_2$	Identifies overt (but not all) primary acid-base disturbances (see Table 41.8).
2. Check the SBE	Quantifies overt metabolic disturbances, either primary or compensatory.
3. Apply "rules of thumb" (see Table 41.2) where appropriate	Evaluates compensation for primary acid-base disturbances.
4. Calculate the AGc (see Table 41.4)	If elevated, unmeasured anions are likely. If low or negative, suspect laboratory error, but consider lithium intoxication, IgG myeloma, and others (see Table 41.5).
5. Compare any AGc elevation with the degree of SBE or [HCO$_3^-$] reduction	An elevated AGc should be accompanied by a similar reduction in SBE or [HCO$_3^-$]. If not, there are dual disorders.
6. Perform specific assays as indicated	If no obvious cause for an elevated AGc, specific assays may be necessary (e.g., lactate, β-hydroxybutyrate, salicylate). A raised osmolal gap suggests methanol or ethylene glycol toxicity. Urinary organic anions may reveal pyroglutamate.

Renal and Metabolic Problems

Table 41.8 Initial Scan Results of pH and Paco₂		
pH	Paco₂	Overt Primary Process
Normal	Normal	None
Normal	Hypercapnia	Respiratory acidosis, metabolic alkalosis
Normal	Hypocapnia	(1) Respiratory alkalosis, metabolic acidosis, or
		(2) Chronic respiratory alkalosis
Low	Hypocapnia	Metabolic acidosis
Low	Hypercapnia	Respiratory acidosis
Low	Normal	Respiratory acidosis, metabolic acidosis
High	Hypercapnia	Metabolic alkalosis
High	Hypocapnia	Respiratory alkalosis
High	Normal	Respiratory alkalosis, metabolic alkalosis

school followers track the $\Delta AG/\Delta HCO_3^-$ inverse relationship. Again, these are similar in a pure anion gap metabolic acidosis but not exactly "mirror image." Using either method, an obvious discrepancy points to a dual metabolic disorder (e.g., a combined normal and raised anion gap metabolic acidosis).

METABOLIC ACIDOSIS

Risk Factors

In metabolic acidosis, the fall in SID can be due to a simple narrowing of the difference between [Na⁺] and [Cl⁻] (normal AGc; Table 41.9) or due to the accumulation of unmeasured anions (elevated AGc; Table 41.10). Although a normal AGc acidosis is usually hyperchloremic, if there is hyponatremia, the [Cl⁻] can be normal or even low.

Clinical Features

Clinical features are those of acidemia itself, combined in some cases of raised AGc acidosis with the toxicities of individual anions. Specific anion toxicities include blindness and cerebral edema (formate); crystalluria, renal failure and hypocalcemia (oxalate); and tinnitus, hyperventilation and uncoupling of oxidative phosphorylation (salicylate).

Acidemia has a number of important adverse effects, mainly when pH is below 7.2 (Fig. 41.8). However, the case is less clear cut with milder acidemia, which might even be beneficial,

Table 41.9 Risk Factors for Normal AGc Metabolic Acidosis	
Condition	Mechanism
Large volume saline infusions	Admixture and equilibration with zero SID crystalloid
Diabetic ketoacidosis post-resuscitation	(1) High effective SID urine (urinary keto-anions)
	(2) Large volume saline infusion
Small intestinal, pancreatic, and biliary losses	Loss of high SID fluid
Ureteral/enteric diversion (especially ureterosigmoidostomy)	High SID urine (enteric reservoir resorption of Cl⁻ accompanied by NH₄⁺)
Renal tubular acidosis	Urine SID high (see Table 41.11)
Post-hypocapnia	Urine SID high during hypocapnia (by renal tubular Cl⁻ resorption)
Total parenteral nutrition and NH₄Cl administration	Metabolic release of Cl⁻

Table 41.10 Causes of a Raised AGc Acidosis	
Condition	Unmeasured Anions
L-Lactic acidosis	L-Lactate
Ketoacidosis	β-Hydroxybutyrate, acetoacetate
Renal failure	Sulfate, urate, hippurate, other organic acids (plus phosphate accumulation, which raises A_TOT)
Salicylic acid	Salicylate, L-lactate, keto-anions
Methanol	Formate
Ethylene glycol	Glycolate, oxalate
Ingestion of paracetamol, flucloxacillin, or vigabatrin in patient with liver and renal dysfunction	Pyroglutamate
Toluene (glue sniffing)	Hippurate (if seen early)
Short bowel syndrome	D-Lactate
Paraldehyde	L-Lactate, acetate, formate

at least in theory. The Bohr effect increases tissue oxygen availability, although this is rapidly counteracted by reduced 2,3-diphosphoglycerate concentrations. There is also experimental evidence that lowering pH can protect against hypoxic stress.

Infusion-Related Acidosis

Large volumes of intravenous saline often cause a normal AGc metabolic acidosis. The SBE rarely falls below −10 mEq/L. There is debate about whether this is severe enough to be harmful. The mechanism relates to the "effective" SID of the crystalloid, which is either its [HCO₃⁻] or, in fluids that contain a bicarbonate surrogate (such as lactate), that part that is metabolized on infusion. For example, effective SID values are 0 mEq/L for saline, 27 mEq/L for Ringer's lactate, and 1000 mEq/L for 1 M NaHCO₃.

Rapid infusion alters plasma SID toward the effective SID of the crystalloid but also causes a metabolic alkalosis by diluting A_TOT. Balanced crystalloids need an effective SID higher than that of saline (zero), but lower than plasma SID (normally 42 mEq/L), so that the fall in plasma SID precisely counteracts the A_TOT dilutional alkalosis. Experimentally this value is 24 mEq/L.

Renal Tubular Acidosis

Renal tubular acidosis (RTA) is due to inadequate renal tubular Cl⁻ excretion, which increases urinary SID (Fig. 41.9 and Table 41.11). The high urinary SID causes plasma SID to fall.

Lactic Acidosis

About 1500 mmol of L-lactate is added to the blood every day as an end product of cytoplasmic glycolysis. L-lactate-exporting tissues include the red blood cells, renal medulla, skin, and muscle. Exported L-lactate is converted back to pyruvate (its glycolytic precursor) in the liver (70%); the renal cortex (20%); and resting muscle, heart, and brain (10%).

The normal [L-lactate]:[pyruvate] ratio (L/P ratio) in plasma is 10:1. It is increased during low redox states. High L-lactate concentrations occur when
- The mitochondrial NADH/NAD ratio is high (oxygen lack, low redox state, L/P ratio increased).

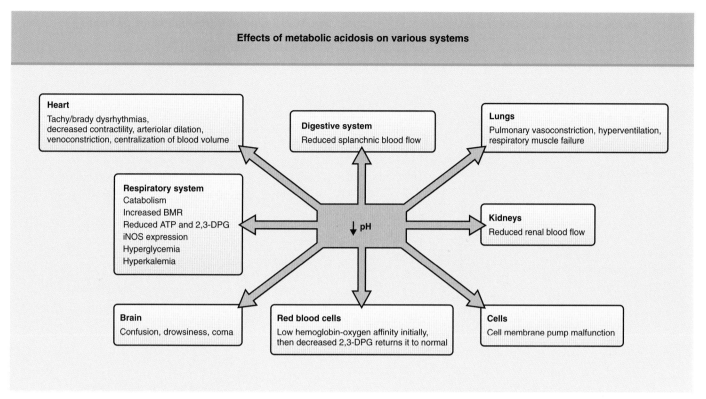

Figure 41.8. Effects of metabolic acidosis on various systems. BMR, basal metabolic rate; DPG, diphosphoglycerate.

Table 41.11 Causes of Renal Tubular Acidosis (RTA)	
RTA Type	**Cause**
1 (distal)	Idiopathic, hypercalciuric
	Amphotericin B, lithium carbonate
	Rheumatoid arthritis, Sjögren's syndrome, systemic lupus erythematosus, cirrhosis, renal transplantation, hyperglobulinemia
2 (proximal)	With other proximal tubular defects, e.g., aminoaciduria (Fanconi syndrome): genetic diseases, myeloma light chain nephropathy, heavy metals, aminoglycosides, renal transplantation, amyloidosis, paroxysmal nocturnal hemoglobinuria.
	Isolated defect: genetic, carbonic anhydrase inhibitors
4	Hyporeninemia, adrenal insufficiency
	ACE inhibitors, NSAIDs, cyclosporine, heparin, amiloride, spironolactone, triamterene, pentamidine
	Diabetes, obstructive uropathy, interstitial nephritis

- Concentrations of pyruvate are high (glycolytic stress, normal redox state, L/P ratio normal).
- There are large (>100 mmol/hr) exogenous L-lactate loads (normal redox state, L/P ratio high).

Because pyruvate concentrations are difficult to measure accurately, the L/P ratio is rarely used in clinical practice. High plasma L-lactate concentrations, whether endogenous or exogenous, and whether aerobic or anaerobic in origin have identical tendencies to reduce plasma SID, raise the AGc, and cause a metabolic acidosis. Apart from exogenous loads, elevated plasma

levels always mean increased lactate production, which may or may not be accompanied by reduced clearance. Causes of hyperlactatemia are listed in Box 41.2.

Hyperlactatemia not due to exogenous sources predicts a high mortality, especially if above 5 mmol/L and not trending downward. Treatment should be directed at the underlying cause (see Box 41.2). In particular, regional and global reductions in oxygen delivery should be searched for and corrected. Many novel therapies, such as intravenous dichloroacetate and methylene blue, have been tried without benefit.

Treatment
Sodium Bicarbonate (NaHCO₃) Administration
NaHCO$_3$ administration is either strongly indicated or should be considered for a number of conditions (Table 41.12). SBE increases by 3 mEq/L per mmol NaHCO$_3$ administered per kilogram of body weight. Adverse effects include transient venous and myocardial hypercapnia, increased hemoglobin-oxygen affinity, hyperosmolar states, reduced $[Ca^{2+}]$ and $[Mg^{2+}]$, and rebound alkalosis if given for organic acidoses.

Alternatives to NaHCO₃
Carbicarb
Carbicarb is an equimolar mixture of Na_2CO_3 and NaHCO$_3$. Side effects are similar to those of NaHCO$_3$ but with less venous and intracellular hypercapnia. Its use is still under evaluation.

THAM
THAM is tromethamine or tris buffer, a weak base with a pKa of 7.7 at 37°C. At pH 7.4, it exists as a 1:2 mixture of THAM

453

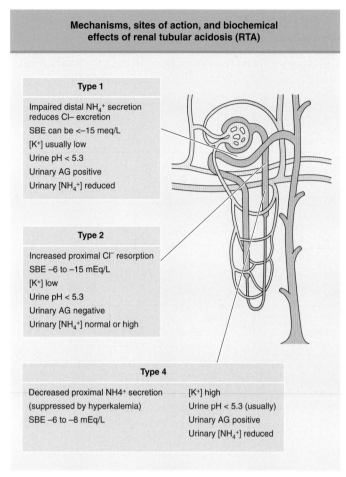

Mechanisms, sites of action, and biochemical effects of renal tubular acidosis (RTA)

Type 1

Impaired distal NH_4^+ secretion reduces Cl^- excretion

SBE can be <-15 meq/L

$[K^+]$ usually low

Urine pH < 5.3

Urinary AG positive

Urinary $[NH_4^+]$ reduced

Type 2

Increased proximal Cl^- resorption

SBE -6 to -15 mEq/L

$[K^+]$ low

Urine pH < 5.3

Urinary AG negative

Urinary $[NH_4^+]$ normal or high

Type 4

Decreased proximal NH4$^+$ secretion (suppressed by hyperkalemia)

SBE -6 to -8 mEq/L

$[K^+]$ high

Urine pH < 5.3 (usually)

Urinary AG positive

Urinary $[NH_4^+]$ reduced

Figure 41.9. Mechanisms, sites of action, and biochemical effects of renal tubular acidosis (RTA).

Box 41.2 Causes of Increased Plasma L-Lactate

Oxygen Lack Likely

Global or regional reductions in oxygen delivery

> Shock
> Cardiac arrest
> Severe anemia
> Severe hypoxemia
> Limb or splanchnic ischemia

Excessive muscle activity

> Severe exercise
> Grand mal epilepsy

Oxygen Lack Absent or Unlikely

Hereditary

> Glucose-6-phosphatase deficiency
> Fructose-1,6-diphosphatase deficiency
> Pyruvate carboxylase and pyruvate dehydrogenase deficiencies
> Mitochondrial myopathies

Acquired

> Sepsis
> Thiamine deficiency
> Alkalemia
> Leukemia, lymphoma, other malignancies
> Hepatic failure
> Excessive L-lactate administration, e.g., L-lactate-based renal replacement fluids

Drugs and toxins

> β_2-agonists
> Phenformin, metformin
> Salicylates
> Acetaminophen
> Fructose, sorbitol, xylitol
> Isoniazid, streptozocin, nalidixic acid
> Antiretroviral drugs
> Ethanol, methanol
> Cyanide
> Carbon monoxide

and THAMH$^+$. After addition of THAM, the equation for electrical neutrality shown in Box 41.1 changes to SID = $[A^-]$ + $[HCO_3^-]$ − $[THAMH^+]$. In other words, [buffer base] = SID + $[THAMH^+]$. Hence, addition of THAM increases buffer base concentrations and thus SBE without changing SID or A_{TOT}. Unlike adding $NaHCO_3$ or carbicarb, there is no generation of CO_2 with venous and intracellular hypercapnia. More than 75% is excreted in the urine in 3 hours, and accumulation occurs in renal failure. Problems include hyperosmolality, coagulation and potassium disturbances, hypoglycemia, and occasional apnea. Like carbicarb, the use of THAM in metabolic acidosis requires further evaluation.

METABOLIC ALKALOSIS

Metabolic alkalosis has been described as the most common acid-base disturbance. With modern definitions it is perhaps more often seen as part of a "mixed" disorder (see Table 41.1).

Risk Factors

Risk factors (Fig. 41.10) can be broadly grouped into those that cause low urinary SID, loss of low (or even negative) SID enteric fluid, or gain of strong cation without strong anion.

Table 41.12 Indications for NaHCO₃ Administration		
Condition	**Strongly Indicated**	**Consider**
Severe hyperkalemia	Yes	
RTA (types 1 and 2)	Yes (normally given enterally)	
Methanol and ethylene glycol poisoning	Yes	
Severe tricyclic overdose	Yes	
Normal AGc metabolic acidosis		Yes
Salicylate overdose		Yes
Severe acidemia (pH < 7.0) with circulatory compromise		Yes
Cardiac arrest with prolonged or preexisting severe metabolic acidosis		Yes

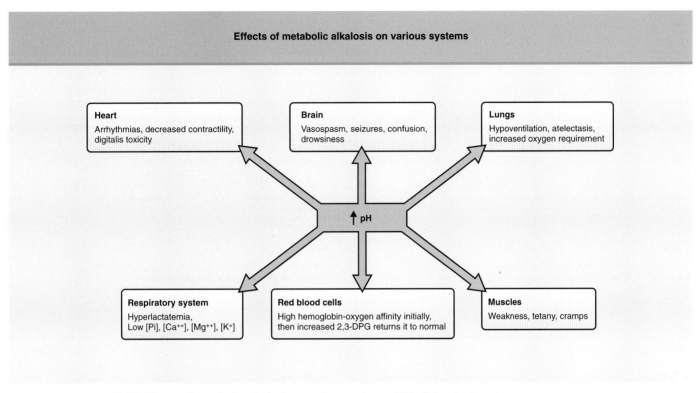

Figure 41.10 Effects of metabolic alkalosis on various systems. DPG, diphosphoglycerate.

Clinical Features

A high plasma pH (>7.55) has a number of adverse effects (Fig. 41.11).

Treatment

The first step is to remove the cause (see Fig. 41.10). However, other factors will facilitate reversal of the alkalotic state when corrected. These include effective volume depletion with secondary aldosteronism, potassium depletion, and renal failure.

Diagnosis of effective volume depletion is based on clinical and biochemical evaluation of volume status (skin turgor, postural hypotension, systolic pressure variability, high urea-to-creatinine ratio). Urinary [Cl⁻] is normally less than 20 mmol/L. Patients with effective volume depletion have been termed "saline responsive." In fact, all metabolic alkaloses are saline responsive if sufficient saline can be administered (see section on infusion-related acidosis). This is safe and practical only if there is extracellular fluid depletion.

Other measures to increase speed of correction include

- Acetazolamide administration (causes hypokalemia, requires adequate renal function)
- Infusion of NH_4Cl, arginine hydrochloride, or lysine hydrochloride (all require hepatic deamination)
- Infusion of HCl. The dose in mmol ($0.3 \times SBE \times$ weight in kg) can be infused over 24 hours as a 0.2M solution in dextrose through a central venous catheter. Regular checks of SBE are advisable.
- Renal replacement therapy

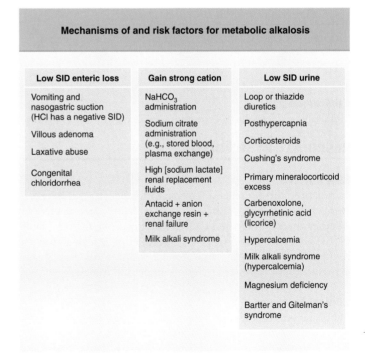

Mechanisms of and risk factors for metabolic alkalosis		
Low SID enteric loss	**Gain strong cation**	**Low SID urine**
Vomiting and nasogastric suction (HCl has a negative SID)	NaHCO₃ administration	Loop or thiazide diuretics
Villous adenoma	Sodium citrate administration (e.g., stored blood, plasma exchange)	Posthypercapnia
Laxative abuse		Corticosteroids
	High [sodium lactate] renal replacement fluids	Cushing's syndrome
Congenital chloridorrhea		Primary mineralocorticoid excess
	Antacid + anion exchange resin + renal failure	Carbenoxolone, glycyrrhetinic acid (licorice)
	Milk alkali syndrome	Hypercalcemia
		Milk alkali syndrome (hypercalcemia)
		Magnesium deficiency
		Bartter and Gitelman's syndrome

Figure 41.11 Mechanisms of and risk factors for metabolic alkalosis.

Renal and Metabolic Problems

Table 41.13 Causes of Respiratory Acidosis		
Mechanism	Acute Respiratory Acidosis (Examples)	Chronic Respiratory Acidosis (Examples)
Respiratory center suppression	Sedative and narcotic drugs, CNS injury, CNS infection, brainstem vasculitis or infarction	Obesity hypoventilation syndrome
Upper airway obstruction	Inhalational injury, postextubation stridor, Ludwig's angina, laryngeal trauma	Obstructive sleep apnea, vocal cord paresis
Mechanical ventilation	Permissive hypercapnia, inadvertent hypoventilation	
Neural and neuromuscular	Guillain-Barré syndrome, myasthenia gravis, nondepolarizing and depolarizing relaxants, envenomation, acute poliomyelitis, critical illness polyneuropathy	Phrenic nerve injury, paraneoplastic syndromes, postpolio syndrome
Muscular	Acute myopathy, low $[K^+]$, high $[Mg^+]$, ruptured diaphragm, shock states	Muscular dystrophy, motor neuron disease
Decreased chest wall compliance	Abdominal distention, burns, pneumothorax, large pleural effusions	Kyphoscoliosis, ankylosing spondylitis
Loss of chest wall integrity	Flail segment	Thoracoplasty
Increased airway resistance	Asthma, bronchiolitis	Chronic obstructive pulmonary disease
Decreased lung compliance	Acute lung injury, pneumonia, pulmonary vasculitis, pulmonary hemorrhage	Restrictive lung disease

---

Box 41.3 Risk Factors for Respiratory Alkalosis

Acute Conditions	Chronic Conditions
Hypoxemia	Pregnancy
Acute hepatic failure	High altitude
Pain	Chronic lung disease
Sepsis	CNS trauma
Asthma	Chronic hepatic failure
Pulmonary embolism	

Pneumonia, acute lung injury
CNS disorders: stroke, infection, trauma
Drugs: salicylate, SSRI
Drug withdrawal states
Mechanical hyperventilation: intentional or inadvertent
Anxiety, acute psychosis

CNS, central nervous system; SSRI, selective serotonin reuptake inhibitor.

Box 41.4 Acid-Base Controversies

Controversy	Comment
Applicability of Stewart approach	Enhances understanding of acid-base physiology in general. Enhances understanding of acid-base effects of fluids for resuscitation and dialysis. Casts doubt on conventional explanations of renal acid-base handling and proton and HCO_3^- pumps and their inhibitors.
Boston versus Copenhagen schools of acid-base analysis	Peaceful cohabitation is possible. Both schools describe the same processes from different standpoints. SBE is the most meaningful single metabolic acid-base index.
Normal SIG value	Conceptually should be close to zero, but actually 3 to 4 mEq/L in most centers.
Superiority of SIG over AG and AGc	SIG likely to have wide reference range due to summed variability of analytes.
Management of hypothermic cardiopulmonary bypass: pH-stat versus alpha-stat	Main debate is over effects on cerebral perfusion.

AG, anion gap; AGc, corrected anion gap; SBE, standard base excess; SIG, strong ion gap.

Clinical Course

Metabolic alkalosis has a reported associated mortality of 40%.

RESPIRATORY ACIDOSIS

Risk Factors

In practice, the presence of respiratory acidosis always indicates some degree of respiratory "pump" failure, irrespective of whether there is increased CO_2 production. Risk factors (Table 41.13) are exacerbated when CO_2 production is high and when ventilation is inefficient (large alveolar or apparatus dead space, hyperinflation causing respiratory muscle disadvantage).

Clinical Features

These include the generic effects of acidemia (see Fig. 41.8). However, acute hypercapnia is especially likely to cause

1. Confusion and drowsiness with asterixis, and occasionally seizures.
2. Reductions in renal blood flow, glomerular filtration rate and urine output (via the sympatho-adrenal and renin-angiotensin systems).
3. Raised intracranial pressure.

Treatment

Management is directed at the underlying cause (see Table 41.13). Mechanical ventilation may be required.

RESPIRATORY ALKALOSIS

Risk Factors

Respiratory alkalosis arises in a number of clinical scenarios (Box 41.3).

Clinical Features

Figure 41.11 illustrates the adverse effects of alkalemia. They all apply in respiratory alkalosis, except complications of hypoventilation.

Treatment

Management should be directed toward the underlying cause (see Box 41.3).

CONTROVERSIES

From the beginning, the field of acid-base disorders has been beset by controversies in definitions, terminology, and explanations of underlying mechanisms. Some current issues are set out in Box 41.4.

SUGGESTED READING

Fencl V, Jabor A, Kazda A, Figge J: Diagnosis of metabolic acid-base disturbances in critically ill patients. Am J Respir Crit Care Med 2000;162:2246–2251.

Forrest DM, Walley KR, Russell JA: Impact of acid-base disorders on individual organ systems In: Ronco C, Bellomo R, eds. Critical Care Nephrology. Dordrecht, Kluwer Academic Publishers, 1998, pp 313–326.

Gluck SJ: Acid-base. Lancet 1998;352:474–479.

Koch SM, Taylor RW: Chloride ion in intensive care medicine. Crit Care Med 1992;20:227–240.

LeBlanc M, Kellum J: Biochemical and biophysical principles of hydrogen ion regulation. In: Ronco C, Bellomo R (eds): Critical Care Nephrology. Dordrecht, Kluwer Academic Publishers, 1998, pp 261–277.

Rose BD, Post TW: Clinical Physiology of Acid-Base and Electrolyte Disorders, 5th ed. New York, McGraw-Hill, 2001.

Schlichtig R, Grogono AW, Severinghaus JW: Current status of acid-base quantitation in physiology and medicine. Anesthesiol Clin North Am 1998;16:211–233.

Schlichtig R, Grogono AW, Severinghaus JW: Human $PaCO_2$ and standard base excess compensation for acid-base imbalance. Crit Care Med 1998;26:1173–1179.

Siggaard-Andersen O, Fogh-Andersen N: Base excess or buffer base (strong ion difference) as measure of a nonrespiratory acid-base disturbance. Acta Anesth Scand 1995;39(suppl 107):123–128.

Stewart PA: How to understand acid-base. In Stewart PA (ed); A quantitative acid-base primer for biology and medicine. New York, Elsevier,1981, pp 1–286.

Disorders of Water, Sodium, and Potassium Homeostasis

Kamel S. Kamel, Andre F. Charest, Shih-Hua Lin, and Mitchell L. Halperin

KEY POINTS

- Urgent therapy with hypertonic saline (raise P_{Na} by ~5 mmol/liter) is needed for the patient with acute hyponatremia that is not due to retained lavage solutions.
- To design therapy for an acute change in the P_{Na}, calculate a tonicity balance if data are available because this reveals the basis for the change in P_{Na} and the goals for its therapy.
- Identify patients with chronic hyponatremia (P_{Na} < 125 mmol/liter) in whom vasopressin action may disappear and/or distal delivery of filtrate may increase because they are at risk of a rapid rise in P_{Na} during therapy. Give vasopressin very early in therapy to avoid a sudden water diuresis.
- In therapy for chronic hyponatremia, the values for the rise in P_{Na} are not targets; rather, they are maximum levels that must not be exceeded. Set much lower maximum levels in patients who might be malnourished or those who are K^+ depleted.
- To make a diagnosis of polyuria, the urine volume should be interpreted in conjunction with the physiological stimulus for the excretion of water. Calculate the osmole excretion rate. If high, identify whether their concentration in plasma was high enough, and identify their source.
- A high or low P_K can lead to a life-threatening cardiac arrhythmia. If the electrocardiogram (ECG) has significant changes, therapy must be given prior to the full diagnostic workup.
- In the patient with acute hypokalemia due to thyrotoxic hypokalemic periodic paralysis or an adrenergic surge, there is an effective therapy—high-dose propranolol. In patients with acute hypokalemia in whom beta-blockers should not be used, enough K^+ must be infused to reverse cardiac electrical disturbances. In the treatment of acute hypokalemia with a serious cardiac arrhythmia, infuse KCl via a central vein to achieve a target for the P_K of 3.0 mmol/ liter very quickly. Be cautious; K^+ will shift out of cells later when the stimulus for K^+ entry abates.
- In the treatment of hyperkalemia with a cardiac arrhythmia or significant ECG findings, intravenous calcium and insulin are the main therapeutic agents to be used.

- In patients with a chronic dyskalemia, evaluate both the flow rate and the luminal $[K^+]$ after back-correcting to reflect values in the terminal cortical collecting dust (CCD). This helps to determine leverage for therapy.

This chapter is divided into two sections; one deals with disorders of water and sodium (Na^+) balance and the other with disorders involving potassium (K^+) homeostasis. Each section begins with a succinct description of pertinent physiology to help the reader understand the pathophysiology of the disorder and to develop our clinical approach.

DISORDERS OF WATER AND Na^+ PHYSIOLOGY

Polyuria

Definition

The definition of polyuria should be based on physiological principles rather than a volume that is larger than "usual" or "normal" values.

Synopsis of Pertinent Physiology

Body composition

Water represents 50% to 70% of body mass. Nevertheless, it is not possible to relate total body water strictly to weight because of variations in the relative proportions of fat (which contains little water) and skeletal mass (which contains the bulk of water).

To move water and/or ions across membranes, there must be a driving force and a pathway for that substance to move across a lipid-containing membrane. The force that drives water movement is very large (~20 mm Hg/mOsmol = ~6000 mm Hg per liter of body fluids). Thus, the effective osmolality is always equal on both sides of the cell membrane. Effective osmoles have an identical concentration in the extracellular fluid (ECF) and intracellular fluid (ICF) compartments. Hence, their abundance in each compartment determines that compartment volume. The major "effective" osmoles in the ECF compartment are Na^+ and its attendant anions, chloride (Cl^-) and bicarbonate (HCO_3^-). The major effective osmoles that determine the

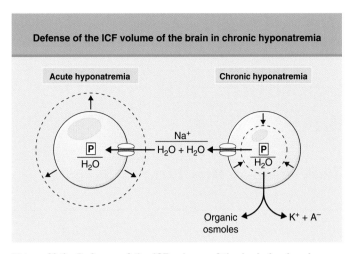

Defense of the ICF volume of the brain in chronic hyponatremia

Figure 42.1. Defense of the ICF volume of the brain in chronic hyponatremia. The solid circle represents the normal size of brain cells. Water crosses cell membranes and achieves osmotic equilibrium because of the presence of water channels. The effective osmoles in the ECF compartment are Na^+ and its attendant anions Cl^- and HCO_3^-, whereas K^+ and organic osmoles are the particles (P) that are effective osmoles in cells. In acute hyponatremia (*left*), brain cells swell, as shown by the shaded area and the dashed line. In chronic hyponatremia (*right*), brain cells have decreased in size by exporting some of their effective osmoles, K^+ salts, and small organic compounds.

volume of the ICF compartment are potassium ions (K^+) and small organic molecules such as carnosine, ATP, phosphocreatine, and amino acids. Macromolecular organic phosphate anions (DNA, RNA, and phospholipids) constitute the bulk of the anions that cause K^+ to be retained in cells. These compounds, however, are essential for cell function and hence only small net changes in their content occur in most cells. The Na^+ concentration in plasma (P_{Na}) is the best indicator of a change in the ICF volume, but with an inverse relationship (Fig. 42.1).

Water control system
To achieve water homeostasis, the body must detect a positive or negative balance for water (change in the P_{Na}) and send a message to the kidney (vasopressin) that modifies the permeability of the distal nephron to water. This system is largely independent of control mechanisms for the excretion of electrolytes.

Excretion of dilute urine
Two factors influence the volume of hypoosmolar urine: (1) the delivery of water to distal diluting sites and (2) the absence of vasopressin, which ensures that only a minimal amount of water is absorbed in the distal nephron.

Excretion of concentrated urine
Vasopressin makes the distal nephron permeable to water. This, together with the presence of a hypertonic medullary interstitial compartment, leads to the excretion of concentrated urine and the conservation of water. Quantitatively, however, most of the water delivered to the distal nephron is reabsorbed in the renal cortex when vasopressin acts. The urine flow rate when

vasopressin acts is determined by the rate of excretion of effective urine osmoles:

$$\text{Urine flow rate} = \text{No. of effective urine osmoles/concentration of effective urine osmoles} \qquad \text{(Equation 1)}$$

Urea accounts for approximately half of the osmoles in the urine in subjects who consume a typical Western diet. Nevertheless, because urea is permeable across cell membranes of the inner medullary collecting duct (MCD) when vasopressin acts, urea is not usually an effective osmole and hence will not obligate the excretion of water. Urea may become an effective urine osmole if the urine is electrolyte poor or if the rate of excretion of urea is high enough to exceed the Vmax of these urea transporters.

Tools to Assess the Renal Handling of Water
Three parameters should be examined: the urine flow rate, the number of effective osmoles in the urine, and the concentration of these osmoles in the urine (see Equation 1).

Urine flow rate
Typically, the urine volume in an adult is 1 to 1.5 liters/day. This is an average flow rate of ~1 mL/min, but with large variations throughout the day.

Expected values
When there is a deficit of water, the daily osmole load should be excreted in the smallest possible urine volume. If the maximum U_{osm} is 1200 mOsmol/kg H_2O and 800 mOsmol are excreted per day, the urine flow rate should be about 0.67 liters/day or 0.5 mL/min. Conversely, when there is a surplus of water, the urine flow rate can increase to more than 10 mL/min (extrapolated to 15 liters/day) with maximal suppression of vasopressin.

Urine osmolality and osmole excretion rate
The usual osmole excretion rate is 600 to 900 mOsmol per day. When polyuria is due to an osmotic diuresis, the U_{osm} is higher than the plasma osmolality (P_{osm}) and the osmole excretion rate is greater than 900 mOsmol/day.

Clinical Approach to the Patient with Polyuria
The differential diagnosis of polyuria is provided in Table 42.1. The steps to take are outlined here and in Figure 42.2.

What is the U_{osm}?
Water diuresis (low U_{osm})
If the U_{osm} is sufficiently lower than the P_{osm}, polyuria is due to a water diuresis. The absolute value of the U_{osm} in this setting depends on the rate of excretion of osmoles. For example, if a person excretes 800 mOsmol/day, the U_{osm} will be 80 mOsm/kg H_2O with a 10 liter/day urine volume. In contrast, if the person excretes 400 mOsmol/day, the U_{osm} will be 40 mOsmol/kg H_2O with the same 10 liters/day urine output. In other words, the rate of excretion of osmoles influences the U_{osm} but it does not influence the urine flow rate when vasopressin does not act. The major factor that influences the urine flow rate in this setting is the volume of hypotonic fluid delivered to the distal nephron.

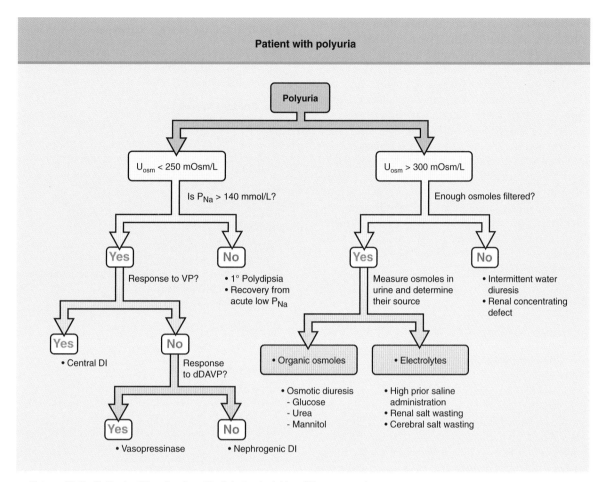

Figure 42.2. Patient with polyuria. DI, diabetes insipidus; VP, vasopressin.

Is the P_{Na} high enough to stimulate the release of vasopressin?
A water diuresis with a P_{Na} less than 138 mmol/liter indicates that at least a component of the polyuria is due to primary polydipsia. On the other hand, if the P_{Na} is more than 140 mmol/liter, diabetes insipidus (DI) is present.

What is the renal response to exogenous vasopressin? This is used to differentiate central versus nephrogenic DI. Vasopressin should only be given to a patient with polyuria who has an elevated P_{Na}. Patients with circulating vasopressinase (released from necrotic tissue) respond to dDAVP but not to the usual administered low dose of vasopressin. A lack of response to dDAVP indicates that nephrogenic DI is present. On the other hand, if the urine volume declines and the U_{osm} rises to be equal to or greater than the P_{osm}, central DI is present. Be careful when interpreting the response to vasopressin: Occasionally, the blood pressure may fall and, as a result, the urine flow rate may decrease.

Osmotic diuresis (high U_{osm})

If the U_{osm} is greater than 300 mOsmol/kg H_2O and the osmole excretion rate significantly exceeds 900 mOsmol/day, an osmotic diuresis is present.

Estimate the rate of filtration of the major urine osmoles: One can make a reasonable estimate of a solute's likelihood of causing polyuria if its concentration in plasma is measured, the GFR is estimated, and the renal handling of that solute is known. For example, a patient with a glucose concentration in plasma (P_{Glu}) of 360 mg/dL (20 mmol/liter) and a GFR of about 100 liters/day will filter 2000 mmol of glucose. The maximum amount of glucose that

Table 42.1 Differential Diagnosis of Polyuria		
Basis	**Key Features**	**Tools**
Water diuresis		
Primary polydipsia	Lack of stimulus for VP	P_{Na} < 138 mmol/L
Central DI	CNS pathology	Responds to exogenous VP
Vasopressinase	Necrotic tissue	Responds to dDAVP, not VP
Nephrogenic DI	Frequent lithium intake, inherited disorders	Does not respond to dDAVP
Osmotic diuresis		
Organic agents (glucose, urea, mannitol)	U_{osm} > 300 mOsm/L and osmole excretions > 900 mOsm/L/day	Osmole excretion rate Seek nature of the urine osmoles
Electrolytes ($Na^+ + Cl^-$)		
Renal concentrating defect	U_{osm} max 300–600 mOsm/L	Search for diseases or drugs affecting the renal medulla

CNS, central nervous system; DI, diabetes insipidus; VP, vasopressin.

461

can be reabsorbed is close to 10 mmol/liter GFR, or 1000 mmol/day in that patient. With a urine glucose concentration (U_{Glu}) of 300 mmol/liter, the expected urine volume is 3.3 liters/day (1000 mOsmol/300 mOsmol/liter). A greater degree of polyuria indicates a lower U_{osm} (low medullary interstitial osmolality) and/or that other solutes are being excreted at a high rate.

Measure urine osmoles and determine the source of extra osmoles: In a patient with a urea-induced osmotic diuresis, determine if the source of urea is from exogenous protein or tissue catabolism. In a patient with a saline-induced osmotic diuresis, one needs to determine why so much saline is being excreted. Some potential causes are prior excessive saline administration [a common situation in the intensive care unit (ICU) patient receiving volume replacement for circulatory instability], cerebral salt wasting, and renal salt wasting.

Hypernatremia

Definition
Hypernatremia is present when the P_{Na} exceeds 144 mmol/liter.

Synopsis of the Pertinent Physiology
The plasma Na+ concentration
This is the ratio of Na+ to water in the ECF compartment. Hypernatremia can be caused by a positive balance for Na+ and/or a negative balance for water, although often both are responsible (Box 42.1). Hypernatremia is associated with a low ICF volume unless its basis is a shift of water into cells due to a gain of osmoles in the ICF compartment (seizure and rhabdomyolysis). The ECF volume, on the other hand, may be increased (positive Na+ balance) or decreased (negative water balance). The plasma Na+ concentration should therefore be evaluated in context with the clinical assessment of the volume status and the history.

Physiological response to hypernatremia
Thirst
It is virtually impossible to increase the P_{Na} by more than a few millimoles per liter if water is available and the thirst mechanism is intact. Therefore, patients will only develop hypernatremia if they cannot appreciate thirst (e.g., patients who are unconscious), if they are unable to communicate their desire for water (e.g., infants, elderly suffering from a stroke, and intubation), or if they do not have access to water (e.g., iatrogenic hypernatremia in critically ill patients). Occasionally, the basis for the reduced intake of water is due to vomiting or mechanical obstruction of the upper gastrointestinal (GI) tract (e.g., due to an esophageal tumor). Rarely, hypernatremia occurs in patients with a central defect in the osmostat or the thirst center (e.g., primary hypodipsia following a subarachnoid hemorrhage).

Release of vasopressin
The second "expected" central response in a patient with hypernatremia is the release of vasopressin. Vasopressin increases the permeability of the late distal nephron to water. Hence, the urine volume should be as low as possible and the U_{osm} should be as high as possible (equal to the osmolality in the renal medullary interstitial compartment). On a typical Western diet, one expects a urine flow rate of close to 0.5 mL/min and a U_{osm}

Box 42.1 Causes of Hypernatremia

The most important aspect is that hypernatremia is always accompanied by a water intake problem. The danger is from brain cell shrinkage.

Net Primary Water Loss

Reduced water intake

Defective thirst due to altered mental state, psychological disorder, disease involving the osmoreceptor, or disease involving the thirst center

Inability to drink water

Lack of water

Increased water loss

Renal loss: central DI, nephrogenic DI (usually due to lithium), osmotic diuresis, circulating vasopressinase

Gastrointestinal loss: vomiting and osmotic diarrhea

Cutaneous loss: sweating and fever

Respiratory loss: hyperventilation and fever

Water shift into the ICF due to gain of osmoles in ICF

Convulsion, rhabdomyolysis

Net Primary Na+ Gain

Hypertonic NaCl or $NaHCO_3$ infusion

Ingestion of seawater or NaCl replacing sugar in the feeding formula

Isotonic NaCl input during osmotic diuresis or in patients with a renal concentrating defect

---

exceeding 800 mOsmol/kg H_2O. Nevertheless, patients in the ICU often have other factors that modify this response, such as a higher rate of excretion of osmoles and/or drugs that might compromise the function of the loop of Henle [e.g., loop diuretics, ligands that bind to the calcium-sensing receptor (CaSR) such as in hypercalcemia, or the use of cationic drugs such as gentamicin]. Alternatively, the osmolality of the medullary interstitial compartment may be lower if it was "washed out" by prior water or osmotic diuresis.

Assess the Basis for a High P_{Na} in the ICU
Assess the ECF volume to determine the basis of hypernatremia
There are two ways to raise the P_{Na}: a positive Na+ balance and a negative water balance. To distinguish between these two possibilities, one must have a reliable estimate of the volume of the ECF compartment. Clinical assessment of the ECF volume, although imprecise, is basic for this evaluation. Hemodynamic measurements occasionally provide useful information, but they lack the quantitative data that are needed. Although urine electrolytes are useful in many patients (Table 42.2), the caveats of using drugs that inhibit the renal reabsorption of Na+—such as loop diuretics, agents that bind to the CaSR in the loop of Henle—and disorders that lead to renal or cerebral salt wasting make them less reliable indicators of the effective circulating volume in these patients. A high hematocrit or total protein level can provide quantitative information concerning a low ECF volume.

Changes in weight do not accurately reflect changes in the ECF volume because there are often large changes in the ICF

Table 42.2 Urine Electrolytes in the Differential Diagnosis of ECF Volume Contraction

Condition	Urine Electrolyte[a]	
	Na+	Cl−
Vomiting		
Recent	High	Low
Remote	Low	Low
Diuretics		
Recent	High	High
Remote	Low	Low
Diarrhea or laxative abuse	Low	High
Bartter's or Gitelman's syndrome	High	High

[a]You must adjust values for the urine electrolyte concentration in polyuric states: high urine concentration > 15 mmol/liter; low urine concentration < 15 mmol/liter.

volume due to a change in the P_{Na} or catabolism. Moreover, there would be no change in weight if there was a shift of water into cells (e.g., due to mild rhabdomyolysis or a seizure) that causes hypernatremia. On the other hand, weight gain suggests that Na+ (+ water) gain is the basis for hypernatremia.

Calculate tonicity balance to determine the quantitative contributions of Na+ and water balances

To calculate a tonicity balance, one needs to measure the water and electrolyte contents of all inputs and outputs. Mass balance for Na+ plus K+ rather than just Na+ must be included because Na+ may enter cells in conjunction with the exit of K+.

When considering Na+ + K+ in isolation, for every millimole retained per liter of total body water, the rise in P_{Na} will be 1 mmol/liter. Similarly, a deficit of 1 liter of water, when considered in isolation, should raise the P_{Na} by the following formula: $P_{Na} \times (TBW/TBW -1 \text{ liter})$. A tonicity balance provides reliable information to guide the goals for therapy, not only to correct the hypernatremia but also to return the ICF and ECF compartment volumes and composition to normal.

Clinical Approach to the Patient with Hypernatremia

Determine the relative importance of a gain of Na+ and a deficit of water

A tonicity balance is especially useful in an ICU setting. If you have balance data for just water from recorded volumes of input and output, you can deduce the balance data for Na using the change in P_{Na} and an estimate of total body water.

Possible causes of Na+ gain

A positive balance of Na+ typically occurs during volume resuscitation in injury, sepsis, and surgical patients. It can also occur when there is an infusion of a large volume of fluid with a concentration of Na+ that is higher than the $U_{Na} + U_K$ in a patient with polyuria due to diabetes mellitus ($U_{Na} + U_K \sim$ 70 mmol/liter) or DI (often a much lower $U_{Na} + U_K$). Another example in the ICU is the administration of a large amount of hypertonic $NaHCO_3$ during cardiopulmonary resuscitation.

Possible causes of a deficit of water

A large loss of electrolyte-poor urine usually occurs through the kidney in patients with DI or during an osmotic diuresis, espe-

cially if there is a defect in the renal concentrating mechanism (see Table 42.1). Other sites of a large loss of hypotonic fluid are the GI tract (e.g., gastric suction or osmotic diarrhea) and the skin (sweat). Loss of water via the lungs can occur with hyperventilation, but this volume closely approximates metabolic water production.

There is a rare form of water loss from the ECF compartment in which water shifts into the ICF compartment. The driving force is a gain of intracellular osmoles, usually due to a seizure or rhabdomyolysis.

Assess the water control system in the central nervous system

The objective here is to define whether there is a lesion involving the central osmostat, the thirst control center, and/or the site of synthesis of vasopressin in the hypothalamus or the pathway to the posterior pituitary.

Is the urinary flow rate very low? In response to hypernatremia, vasopressin should be released and the urine output should be about 0.5 mL/min in an adult.

Does the patient complain of thirst? The expected response to hypernatremia is thirst, but thirst may be absent because of a generalized disturbance of central nervous system (CNS) function (e.g., sedation and coma) or because of a localized lesion involving the central osmostat and/or the thirst center. Thirst may be present, but water intake might be inadequate if water is not available or the patient cannot communicate adequately—a typical situation in the ICU.

Assess renal response in a patient with high P_{Na}

For a patient who has hypernatremia and a large urine output, the steps to follow to distinguish between a water or an osmotic diuresis are outlined in Figure 42.2.

Treatment of the Patient with Hypernatremia

A tonicity balance is essential to design therapy because one knows whether a positive balance for Na+ or a negative balance for water is the basis for the hypernatremia. Avoid a rapid correction of hypernatremia because there is a risk of brain cell swelling, even if the hypernatremia was not very prolonged.

ICF analysis

Hypernatremia indicates that there is a water deficit in the ICF compartment, with rare exceptions (see Fig. 42.1). The amount of water needed to restore the ICF tonicity and volume can be estimated as in Equation 2. To perform this calculation, an estimate of normal ICF volume (two thirds of body water) is required. Another assumption is that the number of particles in the ICF does not change appreciably:

$$\text{ICF water deficit} = \text{normal ICF volume} \times (\text{current } P_{Na} - 140 \text{ mmol/liter})/140 \text{ mmol/liter} \quad \text{(Equation 2)}$$

ECF analysis

The goals for therapy are based on an assessment of the ECF volume. Nevertheless, clinical estimates of ECF volume provide only rough guidelines.

Sample calculation

Let us assume that two 50-kg females each has a P_{Na} of 154 mmol/liter.

Patient 1 has a normal ECF volume (10 liters): Correction of hypernatremia in this patient will require the loss of 140 mmol of Na^+ from her ECF (154 – 140 mmol/liter × 10 liters).

Patient 2 has an estimated ECF volume of 8 liters instead of 10 liters: Because the Na^+ content in her ECF is 1232 mmol (154 mmol/liter × 8 liters), she will require a positive balance of 168 mmol of Na^+ (1400 – 1232 mmol) plus a positive balance of 2 liters of water to restore the tonicity and the volume of the ECF compartment to normal.

ICF Analysis: Because the P_{Na} increased by 10%, both patients will need a positive balance of approximately 10% of their ICF volume of 20 liters: They must retain 2 ls of electrolyte-free water.

Hyponatremia

Definition

Hyponatremia is present when the P_{Na} is less than 136 mmol/liter.

Synopsis of the Pertinent Physiology

Basis for hyponatremia

A low P_{Na} can be due to a negative balance for Na^+ or a positive balance for water, although both are almost always present. To reveal the basis for hyponatremia and to identify the goals for its therapy, the ECF volume must be assessed or a tonicity balance must be calculated. The major cause of acute hyponatremia is an excessive water input (~3–5 liters in an adult) together with a cause to diminish its excretion, the release of vasopressin. The basis for the release of vasopressin is usually obvious (Box 42.2).

Maintaining a low P_{Na}

A large intake of water is not enough to cause chronic hyponatremia; there must also be a decreased capacity to excrete water. The cause of release of vasopressin is an important issue for the treatment of patients with chronic hyponatremia (see Box 42.2). In the short term, one is primarily concerned that vasopressin might disappear, which will lead to a water diuresis, a too rapid increase in P_{Na}, and the development of the osmotic demyelination syndrome. In the long term, one is concerned about the reason why vasopressin was present because this may suggest the presence of a serious underlying lesion.

Changes in ICF and ECF volumes

In general, hyponatremia implies that the volume of cells in the body has increased; this applies to brain cells if the duration of hyponatremia is short (<48 hr) (see Fig. 42.1). Nevertheless, brain cells have a unique response to chronic hyponatremia. They extrude effective ICF osmoles; approximately half of them are K^+ salts and the other half comprises a family of small organic solutes. The most important issue now is that, once the P_{Na} rises, it will take time to reaccumulate these effective osmoles. Therefore, the major danger in the patient with chronic hyponatremia is a rise in P_{Na} that is too rapid because this may cause the osmotic demyelination syndrome.

> **Box 42.2 Causes of High Vasopressin Levels in Patients with Hyponatremia**
>
> **Vasopressin Release in Response to Physiologic Stimuli**
>
> Low "effective" circulating volume
>   ECF volume depletion
>   Blood loss
>   Hypoalbuminemia
>   Low cardiac output
> Excessive pain, nausea, vomiting, or anxiety
>
> **Vasopressin Release without a Physiologic Stimulus**
>
> CNS or lung lesions
> Neoplasms and granulomas such as tuberculosis
> Metabolic disorders such as acute intermittent porphyria
> Administration of agents that have an antidiuretic effect
>   dDAVP (e.g., treatment for diabetes insipidus or urinary incontinence)
> Drugs that augment or stimulate the release of vasopressin
>   Examples include nicotine, clofibrate, tricyclic antidepressants, antineoplastic agents (probably via nausea and emesis), anticonvulsants such as tegretol, morphine
> Drugs that promote the actions of vasopressin on the kidney by increasing cyclic AMP levels or augmenting its bioactivity
>   Examples include oral hypoglycemics (e.g., chlorpropamide), methylxanthines (e.g., caffeine, aminophylline), analgesics that inhibit prostaglandin synthesis (e.g., aspirin, nonsteroidal anti-inflammatory drugs)

The ECF volume may be high, normal, or low in the patient with hyponatremia, depending on the balances of Na^+ and water and whether other effective osmoles are present in the ECF compartment.

Assess the Basis of Hyponatremia

Use P_{osm} to decide if hyponatremia is associated with cell swelling

There are three possible scenarios to consider:

1. Gain of effective osmoles in a solution that is isotonic to plasma (iso-osmolar mannitol): The result will be a decrease in P_{Na}, but the ICF volume will not change. We recognize this picture by finding no change in P_{osm}.

2. Gain of effective osmoles in a solution that has an effective osmolality which is lower than that of the ECF (e.g., half iso-osmolar mannitol): In this setting, the decrease in P_{Na} is associated with a rise in ICF volume. The rise in ICF volume, however, is much less than anticipated simply from the decrease in P_{Na}. The change in ICF volume can be deduced from the measured P_{osm}.

3. Gain of effective osmoles in a solution that has an osmolality greater than that of the ECF: An example is the administration of hyperosmolar mannitol. In this example, the ICF volume will decrease despite the presence of hyponatremia.

   Another clinical example is the hyponatremia in patients with hyperglycemia. To minimize the risk of cerebral edema in children with diabetic ketoacidosis, one should prevent a decrease in the effective plasma osmolality ($2 P_{Na} + P_{glucose}$ in millimoles per liter) when the blood sugar level declines. The calculation that adjusts the P_{Na} for the $P_{glucose}$ should not be performed because it only reflects glucose addition while ignoring the influences of water and Na balance.

Look for laboratory clues for a low effective circulating volume

The results from the following laboratory tests might suggest that the effective circulating volume is contracted (vasopressin effect). Nevertheless, one does not obtain quantitative information from these data:

1. Urine electrolytes: Although one would expect a low rate of excretion of Na^+ and Cl^- when the ECF volume is low, there are notable exceptions to this rule. Na^+ may be excreted if there is a high rate of excretion of another anion such as HCO_3^- in the patient with recent vomiting. In this case, the excretion of Cl^- should be low. In contrast, if the loss of $NaHCO_3$ was due to diarrhea, the associated metabolic acidosis will cause a high rate of excretion of NH_4^+, and because this NH_4^+ is excreted with Cl^-, the urine may be Cl^- rich but Na^+ poor (Table 42.2). On the other hand, if the ECF volume is contracted and the urine contains both Na^+ and Cl^-, one should suspect the use of diuretics, agents that might occupy the Ca-SR, adrenal insufficiency, other causes of renal salt wasting, or cerebral salt wasting (see Table 42.2).

2. Plasma K^+ concentration (P_K): Either hypokalemia or hyperkalemia can suggest the reason for a contracted ECF volume that could cause the release of vasopressin. When hyponatremia is associated with the use of diuretics or vomiting, hypokalemia and renal K^+ wasting are often present. On the other hand, patients who have hyponatremia and hypokalemia due to diarrhea may have a low rate of excretion of K^+ if their loss of K^+ occurred via the GI tract. One should take extra care to avoid rapid correction of hyponatremia in a patient with a deficit of K^+. Therefore, the maximum allowable rise in P_{Na} in these patients should not exceed 4 mmol/liters/day. Hyperkalemia is usually present in patients with Addison's disease.

3. Plasma HCO_3^- concentration: The P_{HCO3} may be high in patients who have vomiting or who have diuretic-induced hyponatremia. In contrast, hyponatremia of hypoaldosteronism is generally accompanied by a mild fall in P_{HCO3} to close to 20 mmol/liter because of a low rate of excretion of NH_4^+ consequent to renal effects of hyperkalemia.

4. P_{Urea} or blood urea nitrogen (BUN): In patients with the syndrome of inappropriate antidiuretic hormone secretion (SIADH), the clearance of urea increases, probably as a result of ECF volume expansion. This, together with a low protein intake, results in a fall in P_{urea} or BUN. In hyponatremia associated with a low effective circulating volume, there is a higher plasma urea level (BUN) because the stimulus to vasopressin release (ECF volume contraction) leads to a fall in GFR and an enhanced rate of reabsorption of filtered urea in the PCT and in the inner MCD.

5. Plasma urate level: The plasma urate level may be quite low in patients with hyponatremia caused by SIADH; the

mechanism is thought to be the expanded ECF volume in these patients.

Initial Approach to the Patient with Hyponatremia

The initial approach is outlined in Figure 42.3.

Is the duration of hyponatremia known to be less than 48 hours? If the answer is yes, the situation can be potentially catastrophic, even if symptoms are mild (e.g., headache, drowsiness, and mild confusion).

Is it likely that lavage fluid was retained? To answer this question, measure the P_{osm} to determine the likelihood that the acute fall in P_{Na} is associated with brain swelling. If P_{osm} is appropriately low, hyponatremia is acute, and one must act quickly before the rise in intracranial pressure causes irreversible brain damage. Urgent therapy with hypertonic saline is needed to raise P_{Na} by 5 mmol/liter quickly to shrink the size of brain cells before seizures and/or respiratory arrest develop. We would give 5 mmol NaCl per liter of body water.

Can there be a component of acute hyponatremia? This may be difficult to determine. If the patient has significant symptoms, one may need to give hypertonic saline as described previously. On the other hand, if the answer is no, the main danger will appear after therapy begins—too rapid or an excessive rise in P_{Na} that may result in the osmotic demyelination syndrome. One must identify conditions in which vasopressin levels may decline rapidly (see Box 42.2) and/or distal volume delivery will increase, which leads to a large excretion of water and predisposes the patient to the danger of developing osmotic demyelination syndrome.

The level of vasopressin will decline suddenly: The level of this hormone might decline abruptly when the ECF volume is reexpanded, nonosmotic stimuli for vasopressin release disappear (chronic nausea, vomiting, anxiety, and/or stress), or because dDAVP is discontinued (e.g., to a patient in a nursing home to minimize the effects of urinary incontinence).

Low distal delivery of filtrate: Even if the effective circulating volume is not appreciably low, the distal delivery of filtrate can be low enough to reduce the excretion of water to a major extent. Because the inner medullary collecting duct has intrinsic permeability to water even in the absence of vasopressin, water can be reabsorbed from it if the interstitial fluid compartment has a high osmolality; this is called "trickle-down hyponatremia." A water diuresis will ensue if distal delivery rises appreciably.

Diagnostic Approach in the Patient with Hyponatremia

Before applying the approach summarized in Figure 42.4, one should calculate the magnitude of the deficit of Na^+ and the gain in water to understand why P_{Na} was so low.

Is the ECF volume obviously contracted? To answer this question, search for major changes on physical examination and the laboratory tests described previously. If the answer is no, this implies that an important basis of the hyponatremia is a positive balance of water. To have a positive balance one needs an intake and a reduced output.

Is the excretion of osmoles low? There are two groups of causes for a low excretion of water: the presence of vasopressin

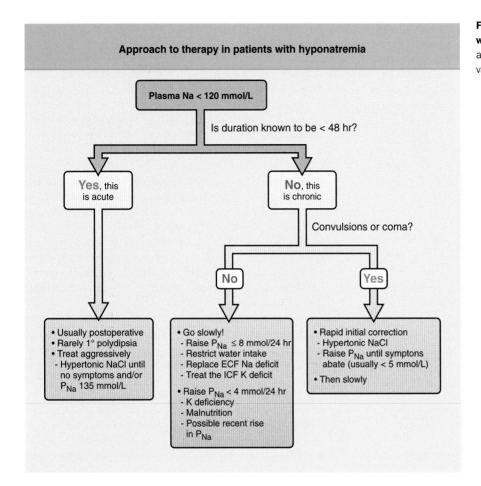

Approach to therapy in patients with hyponatremia

Plasma Na < 120 mmol/L

Is duration known to be < 48 hr?

Yes, this is acute

No, this is chronic

Convulsions or coma?

No

Yes

- Usually postoperative
- Rarely 1° polydipsia
- Treat aggressively
  - Hypertonic NaCl until no symptoms and/or P_{Na} 135 mmol/L

- Go slowly!
  - Raise P_{Na} ≤ 8 mmol/24 hr
  - Restrict water intake
  - Replace ECF Na deficit
  - Treat the ICF K deficit
- Raise P_{Na} < 4 mmol/24 hr
  - K deficiency
  - Malnutrition
  - Possible recent rise in P_{Na}

- Rapid initial correction
  - Hypertonic NaCl
  - Raise P_{Na} until symptons abate (usually < 5 mmol/L)
- Then slowly

Figure 42.3. Approach to therapy in patients with hyponatremia. Hyponatremia due to the addition of organic solutes should be ruled out. VP, vasopressin.

and/or a low distal delivery of filtrate. The latter usually implies a mildly contracted ECF volume and suspicion rises if there is a low osmole excretion rate. If this is not the case, hypothyroidism and hypoadrenalism should be ruled out, and then one is concerned with disorders causing SIADH.

Contracted ECFV: What is the U_{Na} *and the* U_{Cl}*?* Because the ECF volume is contracted, the urine electrolytes are very helpful to understanding its basis. If both U_{Na} and U_{Cl} are low, loss of NaCl by nonrenal routes such as the GI tract or in sweat is likely. It is also possible that the loss of NaCl occurred during a prior use of diuretics. On the other hand, if the urine contains appreciable Na$^+$ and Cl$^-$, proceed to the next question.

Might the patient have adrenal insufficiency? Although we recognize that diuretic use or occupancy of the Ca-SR is more common in this setting, we emphasize this question because of the danger of not recognizing this potentially important condition. Patients with adrenal insufficiency might have hyperkalemia and a low rate of excretion of K$^+$. Nevertheless, one should be aware of the fact that hyperkalemia is not present in as many as one third of patients with adrenal insufficiency.

Clinical Settings with Acute Hyponatremia
Hyponatremia associated with intense exercise
Acute hyponatremia may develop in healthy young people who run long distances in a hot environment, sweat profusely, and drink large quantities of fluid with a Na$^+$ concentration that is lower than that in sweat. Occasionally, this type of acute hyponatremia has devastating results.

Hyponatremia associated with the use of ecstasy
It is not uncommon for acute hyponatremia to develop in young females who take the drug Ecstasy at rave parties. Two well-known actions of this drug can predispose these patients to acute hyponatremia. First, it causes the release of vasopressin. Second, the mood-altering effects of this drug may permit normal subjects to overcome the strong aversion to drink water once P_{Na} falls below 136 mmol/liter.

In addition to these well-known effects, there is also a diminished rate of loss of hypotonic fluid via sweat, perhaps secondary to a contracted ECF volume. A lower ECF volume could be due to diffusion of Na$^+$ into the luminal fluid of the GI tract. Another problem to consider in this setting is that water with a lower Na$^+$ concentration than P_{Na} may be absorbed later, leading to a further decrease in P_{Na} with potentially devastating results. Furthermore, when there is a rapid absorption of water from the intestinal tract, P_{Na} in arterial blood (to which the brain is exposed) may be significantly lower than venous P_{Na} (sampled by the clinician). There may be an additional important factor in this pathophysiology that permits the noted higher incidence in women—their much smaller muscle mass (especially if they suffer from anorexia). In this setting, less water can be "stored" in muscle cells. Hence, the risk of brain cell swelling is significantly higher with a given positive water balance.

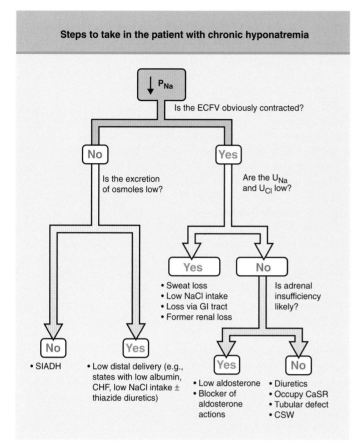

Steps to take in the patient with chronic hyponatremia

↓ P_{Na}

Is the ECFV obviously contracted?

No — **Yes**

Is the excretion of osmoles low?

Are the U_{Na} and U_{Cl} low?

Yes — **No**

- Sweat loss
- Low NaCl intake
- Loss via GI tract
- Former renal loss

Is adrenal insufficiency likely?

No — **Yes**

- SIADH

- Low distal delivery (e.g., states with low albumin, CHF, low NaCl intake ± thiazide diuretics)

Yes — **No**

- Low aldosterone
- Blocker of aldosterone actions

- Diuretics
- Occupy CaSR
- Tubular defect
- CSW

Figure 42.4. Steps to take in the patient with chronic hyponatremia. The focus in chronic hyponatremia is to determine why vasopressin is present. If the reason for the release of vasopressin is reversible, patients might be at risk of having a water diuresis if the release of vasopressin is suppressed (e.g., when their ECF volume is reexpanded). CaSR, calcium-sensing receptor; CSW, cerebral salt wasting.

Postoperative acute hyponatremia

The most common in-hospital setting for acute and potentially life-threatening hyponatremia is the acute perioperative period. There are three sources of water in this setting: the intravenous administration of glucose in water (D_5W) or hypotonic saline, an intake of water in the form of ice chips or "sips" of water, and the generation of electrolyte-free water, which occurs when the kidney excretes urine that is hypertonic to the administered fluids (or to body fluid in the absence of intravenous infusions).

The best way to prevent acute perioperative hyponatremia in hospitalized patients is to avoid giving solutions that are hypotonic to the urine if there is appreciable urine output or giving solutions that are hypotonic to body fluids in the oliguric patient. Isotonic fluids should be given only to maintain systemic hemodynamics during surgery and to replace losses if they occur. In this regard, P_{Na} should be monitored, particularly in patients who excrete more than 1 or 2 liters of urine per day.

Hyponatremia after transurethral resection of the prostate

The main reason for hyponatremia in this setting is that many liters (often as much as 20–30 liters) of half-iso-osmotic solutions of organic compounds are used under pressure as nonconductive solutions to lavage the prostatic bed. When a vein in the prostatic bed is cut, some of this lavage fluid may be absorbed.

There are two components to explain the development of hyponatremia; they become obvious after dividing the absorbed fluid into its two constituent parts:

1. Gain of osmole-free (and electrolyte-free) water: This simple water gain causes cells to swell, but it is not the major cause for the hyponatremia with lavage solutions.
2. Gain of isosmolar fluid: Solutes such as glycerol or glycine will eventually distribute in the ICF compartment. Initially, however, when they remain in the ECF compartment, they cause hyponatremia because these solutions are Na$^+$-free. This early hyponatremia is not associated with a major change in brain cell volume and does not pose an early threat of brain herniation. If P_{osm} is close to normal, one should not be alarmed by the severity of the hyponatremia. A low P_{osm}, however, indicates that the acute hyponatremia following transurethral resection of the prostate poses a threat of brain cell swelling and one must cause the P_{Na} to rise acutely.

Therapy for Acute Hyponatremia
Emergency setting

A note of caution is needed. If blood was drawn immediately after a seizure, P_{Na} might have increased by 10 to 15 mmol/liter because of a shift of water into muscle cells. This may give the false impression that hyponatremia was not the cause of the seizure.

The immediate goal of therapy is to shrink the expanded ICF volume of the brain sufficiently to prevent serious CNS damage. If acute hyponatremia is severe ($P_{Na} < 120$ mmol/liter) or if even mild symptoms are present, one should administer hypertonic saline until P_{Na} rises acutely by approximately 5 mmol/liter. When calculating the amount of Na$^+$ required, one must assume that its volume of distribution "behaves" as if the Na$^+$ will be dissolved in total body water because cell membranes are permeable to water but not to Na$^+$. Do not forget that water might be present in the lumen of the GI tract and cause a decrease in P_{Na} later when it is absorbed.

Sample calculation

Consider a 50-kg person who had a seizure 24 hours after surgery; the P_{Na} was 120 mmol/liter. The initial aim of therapy is to shrink the size of brain cells over 1 or 2 hours to the level before this seizure occurred. A reasonable target is to raise P_{Na} by 5 mmol/liter in 1 or 2 hours. In order to achieve this, 150 mmol of Na$^+$ should be administered as hypertonic saline if the total body water is 30 liters (60% of body weight). After this emergency therapy, slow the rate of infusion, raising P_{Na} toward 140 mmol/liter over the next 24 hours. Again, consider water that may exist in the lumen of the GI tract.

Having dealt with the acute emergency, there are two general strategies to prevent a further decline in P_{Na} in a patient who is excreting a large volume of hypertonic urine:

Input: If the input is equal to the output with respect to Na$^+$, K$^+$, and water, there will be no change in P_{Na}. If hypertonic saline is being excreted, the same volume and the same tonicity of hypertonic saline should be administered.

Output: When U_{Na+K} is very high, one can lower its concentration in the urine so that it becomes isotonic to plasma by administering a loop diuretic (e.g., furosemide) or an osmotic diuretic (e.g., urea). Isotonic intravenous fluids

467

should be given at the same rate as the urine output to preserve water balance. Once the cause of the release of vasopressin is no longer present, this therapy will not be required; the patient will begin to excrete dilute urine and hence P_{Na} will rise.

There are two considerations for therapy if there is a chronic component to the hyponatremia. First, if the contracted ECF volume needs to be reexpanded rapidly, infuse "isotonic to the patient" saline. Second, a large water diuresis due to the disappearance of vasopressin and/or an enhanced distal delivery of filtrate must be avoided by administering dDAVP very early in therapy.

Chronic Hyponatremia

To minimize the risk of too rapid a rise in P_{Na}, one should set limits on the maximum permissible rise in P_{Na} in a patient with chronic hyponatremia. In an uncomplicated patient, the upper limit should be 8 mmol/liter/day. In a patient who is malnourished and/or K depleted, the upper limit should be 4 mmol/liter/day. We emphasize that these are upper limits and not targets to be achieved. One final point merits mention. If one can anticipate that distal delivery of filtrate might increase and ADH levels decrease during initial therapy, administer dDAVP at the outset of therapy to prevent the development of an unwanted, large water diuresis.

POTASSIUM

Dyskalemias are common electrolyte disorders in the critical care setting, and they may have serious sequelae, notably cardiac arrhythmias. Regulation of K^+ homeostasis has two important aspects. First is the control of the transcellular distribution of K^+, which is vital for survival because it acts to limit acute changes in the P_K. Second, there is longer term regulation of K^+ excretion by the kidney, which maintains overall K^+ balance.

Shift of K^+ across Cell Membranes

Approximately 98% of total body K^+ resides in the ICF compartment. K^+ are kept inside the cell by an electrical force (a negative voltage in cells). To shift K^+ into cells, a more negative voltage is required in cells. This can be achieved by increasing the flux of cations through Na-K-ATPase. This is an active and electrogenic pump: It exports 3 Na^+ from cells while importing 2 K^+ into cells. The activity of this cation pump is enhanced by an increase in the concentration of one of its substrates (intracellular Na^+) or by covalent modification (phosphorylation via a kinase). Entry of Na^+ into cells needs to occur in an electroneutral manner via the Na^+/H^+ exchanger (NHE).

Hormones that Affect Na-K-ATPase

Insulin leads to activation of the NHE, whereas β_2-adrenergic agonists activate Na-K-ATPase by phosphorylation. Hence, insulin and β_2-adrenergic agonists can be used to cause an acute shift of K^+ into cells in the emergency treatment of patients with hyperkalemia. Similarly, a fall in P_K can be seen in patients with an insulinoma or in conditions associated with a surge of catecholamines (e.g., patients with a subarachnoid hemorrhage, traumatic brain injury, myocardial infarct, and/or an extreme degree of anxiety).

Acid–Base Influences

When an acid is added to the body, most of the H^+ is buffered in the ICF compartment. Monocarboxylic acids (e.g., L-lactic acid or β-hydroxybutyric acid) enter cells via a specific transporter; this is an electroneutral event and hence there is no change in cell voltage to cause a shift of K^+. To shift K^+ out of cells, the mechanism of entry of H^+ into cells (HCO_3^- exit) should become electrogenic (i.e., cause a less negative voltage in cells). This seems to be the case with inorganic acids and organic acids that have more than one carboxyl group (e.g., citric acid). When Cl^- ions enter cells in exchange for HCO_3^-, these Cl^- ions exit cells via Cl^- channels, creating a negative voltage in cells.

Tissue Anabolism/Catabolism

Hypokalemia may be seen in conjunction with rapid cell growth if insufficient K^+ is given. Examples include the use of total parenteral nutrition, rapidly growing malignancies, and during treatment of DKA or pernicious anemia. On the other hand, hyperkalemia may be seen with crush injury and the tumor lysis syndrome. In these patients, factors that compromise the kidney's ability to excrete K^+ are usually present as well.

Excretion of K^+ in the Urine

Control of renal excretion of K^+ maintains overall daily K^+ balance. Although the usual rate of excretion of K^+ in adults eating a typical Western diet is approximately 1 mmol/kg body weight, K^+ excretion can decline to a nadir of 10 to 15 mmol/day when there is virtually no K^+ intake, whereas the rate of excretion of K^+ can match an intake of more than 200 mmol/day with only a minor increase in P_K. Control of K^+ secretion occurs primarily in the late distal convoluted tubule (DCT) and the cortical collecting duct (CCD). Two factors influence the rate of excretion of K^+: the flow rate in the terminal CCD (Equation 3) and the net secretion of K^+ by principal cells in the CCD, which raises its luminal concentration of K^+ ($[K^+]_{CCD}$).

$$K^+ \text{ excretion} = \text{flow rate}_{CCD} \times [K^+]_{CCD} \qquad \text{(Equation 3)}$$

Flow Rate in the CCD

When vasopressin acts, the flow rate in the CCD is reflected by the rate of excretion of osmoles because the osmolality of fluid in the terminal CCD is fixed and is equal to P_{osm} (Equation 4) and most of the osmoles delivered to the terminal CCD are excreted (see Fig. 42.2). The two major urinary osmoles are urea and Na^+ (+ Cl^-):

$$(\text{Flow rate})_{CCD} = (U_{osm} \times \text{urine volume})/P_{osm}$$
$$\text{(Equation 4)}$$

$[K^+]$ in the Lumen of the Terminal CCD

The secretory process for K^+ in principal cells has two elements. First, a lumen negative voltage must be generated via electrogenic reabsorption of Na^+ via the epithelial Na^+ channel. Second, open K^+ channels must be present in the luminal membranes of principal cells. The reabsorption of Na^+ in the CCD can be electroneutral or electrogenic, depending on whether Cl^- is reabsorbed as fast as Na^+ (electroneutral) or slower than Na^+ (electrogenic). A faster reabsorption of Na^+ than Cl^- in the CCD can occur for three reasons. First, Na^+ is delivered to the CCD with little Cl^-. A key finding in these patients is a Cl^--poor urine.

Second, reabsorption of Cl^- in the CCD may be inhibited; this mechanism is suspected when the urine is not Cl^- poor. It appears that HCO_3^- and/or an alkaline luminal pH in the CCD could inhibit Cl^- reabsorption. Third, a higher lumen-negative voltage in the CCD could develop when the delivery of Na^+ and Cl^- is very high and if the capacity for Cl^- reabsorption is less than that for Na^+. This requires a stimulated reabsorption of Na^+ via the epithelial Na^+ channel in the CCD (high aldosterone level due to low effective circulating volume). Aldosterone increases the activity of the epithelial Na^+ channel.

Glucocorticoids do not usually stimulate the secretion of K^+ in the CCD because principal cells have the enzyme 11β-hydroxysteroid dehydrogenase (11β-HSDH). This enzyme converts cortisol to a metabolite (cortisone) that does not bind the mineralocorticoid receptor. Cortisol, however, can exert a mineralocorticoid effect if the activity of 11β-HSDH is decreased (e.g., apparent mineralocorticoids excess syndrome), if it is overwhelmed by an extreme abundance of cortisol (e.g., patients with an ACTH-producing tumor), or if it is inhibited (e.g., by glycyrrhizic acid in licorice). In Liddle's syndrome, there is electrogenic reabsorption of Na^+ in the CCD because of a constitutively active epithelial Na^+ channel.

If Na^+ is reabsorbed at the same rate as Cl^- in the CCD, a lumen-negative voltage cannot develop. The hyperkalemia in patients with type II pseudohypoaldosteronism (Gordon's syndrome) may be an example of this pathophysiology. Two factors are important to achieve this near equal rate of ion transport in the CCD. First, low delivery of Na^+ and Cl^- to the CCD occurs because the reabsorption of Na^+ and Cl^- was augmented in the distal convoluted tubule due to increased activity of the Na^+–Cl^- cotransporter. Second, ECF volume expansion suppresses the release of aldosterone, which leads to a diminished rate of excretion of K^+.

Assess the Control of the Renal Excretion of K^+

There are four steps in assessing the renal response in a patient with an abnormal P_K:

1. Examine the rate of excretion of K^+. To assess the renal response in a patient with hypokalemia or hyperkalemia, we use the expected rate of K^+ excretion when these electrolyte abnormalities are due to nonrenal causes. With a K^+ deficit, the expected response is to excrete less than 15 mmol/day. With a surfeit of K^+, the expected response is to excrete more than 200 mmol/day. To assess the rate of excretion of K^+, a 24-hour urine collection is not necessary. One can use $U_K/U_{creatinine}$ (despite the diurnal variation in K^+ excretion) because creatinine is excreted at a near constant rate throughout the day. Moreover, a $U_K/U_{creatinine}$ in a spot urine provides information that is more relevant because the stimulus to drive K^+ excretion (e.g., P_K) should be known at that time. The expected value in a patient with hypokalemia is approximately 1 mmol K^+/mmol creatinine (~10 mmol K^+/g creatinine), whereas in a patient with hyperkalemia the expected $U_K/U_{creatinine}$ ratio is more than 15 mmol K^+/mmol creatinine (>150 mmol K^+/g creatinine).

2. Estimate the flow rate in the terminal CCD. The critical factor in urine with a U_{osm} greater than the P_{osm} is the rate of excretion of osmoles (see Fig. 42.2 and Equation 4), typically about 0.5 mOsmol/min or 720 mOsmol/day. A minimum estimate of the flow rate in the terminal CCD is obtained by dividing the rate of excretion of osmoles by the osmolality of luminal fluid in the terminal CCD (which equals P_{osm} when vasopressin acts).

3. Estimate $[K^+]_{CCD}$. A reasonable approximation of $[K^+]_{CCD}$ can be obtained by adjusting U_K for water reabsorbed in the MCD (see Fig. 42.2). This is done by dividing U_K by $(U/P)_{osm}$ (Equation 5). Another way to evaluate the driving force for the net secretion of K^+ in the CCD is to calculate the transtubular $[K^+]$ gradient (TTKG). In this calculation, $[K^+]_{CCD}$ is divided by P_K (Equation 6). The expected value for the TTKG in a patient with hypokalemia due to a nonrenal cause is less than 2, whereas the appropriate renal response in a normal subject given a K^+ load is greater than 7:

$$[K^+]_{CCD} = [K^+]_{urine}/(U/P)_{osm} \qquad \text{(Equation 5)}$$

$$TTKG = [K^+]_{CCD}/P_K \qquad \text{(Equation 6)}$$

4. Establish the basis for the abnormal $[K^+]_{CCD}$. In a patient with hyperkalemia, a lower than expected $[K^+]_{CCD}$ implies that the lumen-negative voltage is abnormally low due to less electrogenic reabsorption of Na^+. The converse is true in a patient with hypokalemia. The basis for the change in the rate of electrogenic reabsorption of Na^+ can be deduced from an assessment of the ECF volume, the ability to conserve Na^+ and Cl^- in response to a contracted effective ECF volume, and measurement of the activity of renin and the level of aldosterone in plasma. Alternatively, one can focus on this differential diagnosis based on the presence or absence of hypertension.

Hyperkalemia

Clinical Approach to the Patient with Hyperkalemia

It is imperative to recognize when hyperkalemia (or hypokalemia) represents a medical emergency because therapy must take precedence over diagnosis.

Are there laboratory or technical problems? Hemolysis, megakaryocytosis, fragile tumor cells, a K^+ channel disorder in red blood cells, and excessive fist clenching during blood sampling should be excluded. Pseudohyperkalemia can be present in cachectic patients because the normal T-tubule architecture in skeletal muscle may be disturbed. This permits more K^+ to be released into venous blood, even without excessive fist clenching.

Is hyperkalemia due to a shift of K^+? This is suspected if hyperkalemia developed acutely or if the intake of K^+ was known to be very low.

What is the rate of K^+ excretion? If the rate is considerably less than 200 mmol/day or less than 15 mmol K^+/mmol creatinine, it is inappropriately low in the presence of hyperkalemia.

Is the flow rate in the CCD low? The answer will be yes if the rate of excretion of osmoles is low. The information can be used to design treatment; usually this entails increasing the urine flow rate by giving a loop diuretic to obtain a larger excretion of electrolytes while ensuring that the ECF volume does not become contracted.

Box 42.3 Causes of Hyperkalemia
High Intake of K⁺
Only if combined with low excretion of K⁺
Shift of K⁺ out of Cells
Cell necrosis or diminished magnitude of the resting membrane potential
Lack of insulin, β-adrenergic blockers
Metabolic acidosis where the anion does not distribute in the ICF compartment
Rare causes (e.g., hyperkalemic periodic paralysis)
Diminished K⁺ Loss in the Urine
Low flow rate in terminal CCD [low osmole excretion rate (e.g., a low-protein low-salt diet)]
Low $[K^+]_{CCD}$
Slow Na⁺ type of defect in the CCD
Very low delivery of Na⁺ to the CCD
Low levels of aldosterone (e.g., Addison's disease)
Blockade of the aldosterone receptor (e.g., spironolactone)
Low ENaC activity (hereditary disease)
Blockade of ENaC (e.g., amiloride, triamterene, trimethoprim-like drugs)
Cl⁻ reabsorbed at a similar rate as Na⁺
Gordon's syndrome (e.g., WNK kinase-4 and/or −1 mutations)
Drugs (e.g., cyclosporine)
Cl⁻ shunt disorder in the CCD

ENaC, epithelial Na⁺ channel in the CCD.

Why is $[K^+]_{CCD}$ low? There are two major groups of causes: a defect that leads to slow reabsorption of Na⁺ via the epithelial Na⁺ channel or a defect in which Cl⁻ is reabsorbed at a similar rate to Na⁺ in the CCD (Box 42.3).

Specific Causes of Hyperkalemia

A list of the causes of hyperkalemia based on their possible underlying pathophysiology is provided in Box 42.3.

Therapy for Hyperkalemia

Medical emergency

The major danger of a severe degree of hyperkalemia is a cardiac arrhythmia. Because mild electrocardiogram (ECG) changes may progress rapidly to a dangerous arrhythmia, any patient with an ECG abnormality related to hyperkalemia should be considered as a potential medical emergency. In certain circumstances, we would treat patients with a P_K higher than 7.0 mmol/liter aggressively, even in the absence of ECG changes; the exceptions include patients with hyperkalemia due to extremes in exercise (the supermarathon), most patients on chronic hemodialysis, and possibly infants.

Antagonize the cardiac effects of hyperkalemia

Ca²⁺ is the best agent, and its effects are usually evident within minutes. It is usually given as 20 to 30 mL of a 10% calcium gluconate solution (2 or 3 ampoules) or 10 mL of 10% CaCl₂ (1 ampoule). This dose can be repeated after 5 minutes if ECG changes persist. The effect usually lasts 30 to 60 minutes.

Extreme caution should be exercised for patients on digitalis because hypercalcemia may aggravate digitalis toxicity.

Induce a shift of K⁺ into the ICF

There are three modes of therapy to consider:

Insulin: A number of studies support the use of insulin to treat acute hyperkalemia. Large doses of insulin (20 units of regular insulin) are needed to obtain the supraphysiological levels of insulin in plasma that are required for a maximal shift of K⁺ into cells. Administration of intravenous glucose and monitoring P_{Glu} should avoid the development of hypoglycemia.

β₂-Adrenergic agonists: β₂-Adrenergic stimulation lowers P_K. However, 20% to 40% of patients with renal failure are resistant to this therapy, and it is not possible to predict nonresponders; hence, we do not recommend its use as a sole emergency therapy. Moreover, we are concerned about the safety of these drugs in the doses used for the treatment of hyperkalemia (20 mg of nebulized albuterol), which are four to eight times that prescribed for the treatment of acute asthma.

NaHCO₃: A number of studies have found NaHCO₃ therapy to be ineffective as the sole treatment of hyperkalemia. It is noteworthy that these studies were performed in stable hemodialysis patients who did not have significant acidosis (hence, NHE was presumably inactive). Studies that examined the combined use of NaHCO₃ with insulin also have obtained conflicting results. Thus, the question remains: Would NaHCO₃ be effective in patients with a more significant degree of acidosis? There are no data in the literature to answer this question definitively. Given this uncertainty, we only use NaHCO₃ in addition to other therapies to treat emergency acute hyperkalemia in patients with a significant degree of acidosis. Caution is warranted because excessive administration of NaHCO₃ has the risk of inducing hypernatremia, ECF volume expansion, carbon dioxide retention, and hypocalcemia.

No medical emergency

Remove K⁺ from the body

It is important to appreciate that much less K⁺ loss is needed to lower P_K from 7.0 to 6.0 mmol/liter than to lower it from 6.0 to 5.0 mmol/liter. Hence, creating a small K⁺ loss can be very important when there is a severe degree of hyperkalemia.

Enhance the excretion of K⁺ in the urine

If K⁺ excretion is low because of a low urine volume, but with a high U_K, a loop diuretic may induce kaliuresis by increasing the flow rate in the CCD. One can avoid unwanted ECF volume contraction by replacing the NaCl lost in the urine. This NaCl should be given at the same tonicity as the urine to avoid creating a dysnatremia. If U_K is unduly low, giving an exogenous mineralocorticoid (100 μg florinef) and possibly inducing bicarbonaturia with a carbonic anhydrase inhibitor may cause a substantial kaliuresis. If HCO₃⁻ is lost in the urine, it might need to be replaced.

Cation exchange resins to promote the loss of K⁺

A cation exchange resin can exchange bound Na⁺ (Kayexalate) or Ca²⁺ (calcium resonium) for K⁺. Kayexalate contains 4 mEq of Na^+ per gram, but only 1 mEq of Na^+ appears to exchange for K^+ in the GI tract. The only favorable location for the exchange of Na^+ for K^+ is in the lumen of the colon, but a number of factors limit the magnitude of this process. For example, other cations, such as NH_4^+, Ca^{2+}, and Mg^{2+}, may exchange for resin-bound Na^+ apart from K^+. Even if K^+ were secreted in the colon, the low stool volume would limit the total K^+ loss. Hence, we believe that there is virtually no benefit of resins in the treatment of acute hyperkalemia and little benefit of adding resins to cathartics to treat chronic hyperkalemia.

Dialysis

Hemodialysis is more effective than peritoneal dialysis for removing K^+. Removal rates of K^+ can approximate 35 mmol/hr with a dialysate bath K^+ concentration of 1 or 2 mmol/liter. A glucose-free dialysate is preferable to avoid the glucose-induced release of insulin and the subsequent shift of K^+ into cells, lessening the removal of K^+.

Hypokalemia

Clinical Approach to the Patient with Hypokalemia

Shift of K^+ into cells

The initial goal is to decide if a shift of K^+ into cells is playing an important role in the clinical picture. The following point to a shift of K^+ into cells.

Is hypokalemia known to be acute?

Both the time frame and the clinical setting are important elements to consider. An acute shift of K^+ into cells may occur where there is a large surge of catecholamines (e.g., post-myocardial infarction and head trauma) or in patients with hypokalemic periodic paralysis.

Is there an acid–base disorder and a high rate of excretion of K^+?

If the answer is no: Hypokalemia is due to an acute shift of K^+ into cells. One of the disorders that can cause an acute shift of K^+ into cells is hypokalemic periodic paralysis. This can be familial or associated with thyrotoxicosis. The major clues to suggest that you are dealing with thyrotoxic hypokalemic periodic paralysis are the ethnic origin (most common in Asians), gender (males most often), signs associated with hyperthyroidism (e.g., tachycardia), and a low plasma phosphate level in conjunction with a high urine calcium-to-phosphate ratio. Drugs that result in prolonged adrenergic action, such as amphetamine, cocaine, and caffeine, should also be considered.

If the answer is yes: One must seek an explanation for both the chronic hypokalemia and the acute component of the shift of K^+ into cells. For the former, the list of causes with either metabolic alkalosis or metabolic acidosis can be found in Box 42.4. The reason for the acute shift of K^+ will most likely be a surge of adrenaline and/or high levels of insulin.

Chronic hypokalemia

In this setting, the first step is to define whether there is an important renal abnormality.

If the rate of K^+ excretion is considerably higher than 1 mmol/mmol of creatinine, we examine the two components of K^+ excretion formula once they are back-calculated to reflect events in the CCD (Fig. 42.5).

Box 42.4 Causes of Hypokalemia

Decreased Intake of K^+

Rarely a primary cause unless K^+ intake is very low and duration is prolonged

Can augment the degree of hypokalemia if there is ongoing K^+ loss

Shift of K^+ into Cells

Hormones (insulin and β-adrenergics are most important)

Metabolic alkalosis

Anabolic state (e.g., recovery from diabetic ketoacidosis)

Rare (e.g., hypokalemic periodic paralysis)

Excessive Renal K^+ Loss

Faster reabsorption of Na^+ in the CCD
  High aldosterone levels (a number of causes)
  Cortisol acts as a mineralocorticoid
    Low 11-βHSDH activity (AME)
    Inhibitors of 11-βHSDH (e.g., licorice)
    Very high cortisol level (e.g., ACTH-producing tumor)
  Constitutively active ENaC (e.g., Liddle's syndrome)
  Artificial ENaC (e.g., amphotericin B)
Slower reabsorption of Cl^- in the CCD
  Delivery of Na^+ without Cl^- to the CCD and a low ECF volume
  Inhibition of Cl^- reabsorption in the CCD (e.g., bicarbonaturia)
  High delivery of Na^+ and Cl^- to the CCD and a V_{max} for Na^+ reabsorption that exceeds that for Cl^- (inhibition of NaCl reabsorption in an upstream nephron segment plus ECF volume contraction)

Loss of K^+ Via the Gastrointestinal Tract or Skin

ENaC, epithelial Na^+ channel in the CCD; V_{max}, maximum velocity.

Is there a high flow rate in the CCD?

If the osmole excretion rate is much greater than 0.5 mOsmol/min, there is a high distal flow rate. We should then analyze the urine to determine which osmoles are responsible for the high flow rate in the CCD: organic compounds (glucose, urea, or mannitol if it was administered), or electrolytes.

What is the $[K^+]_{CCD}$?

A high $[K^+]_{CCD}$ in the presence of hypokalemia indicates a higher lumen-negative voltage in the CCD (see Fig. 42.2). If the ECF volume is not low, there is a "fast" Na^+-type lesion. Confirm this impression by finding a low plasma renin activity and possibly hypertension (note that patients with renal artery stenosis or renin-producing tumors have high plasma renin activity). The differential diagnosis is summarized in Box 42.4. In contrast, if the ECF volume is low, suspect a lesion in which Cl^- is not reabsorbed as fast as Na^+ in the CCD. The clinical scenario is one of a markedly enhanced delivery of Na^+ and Cl^- to the CCD together with a maximum velocity of Na^+ reabsorption that exceeds that for Cl^- in the CCD (a more open epithelial Na^+ channel induced by aldosterone, which was released in response to a contracted ECF volume) (see Box 42.4). Confirm this impression by finding a high plasma renin activity. Clues to the

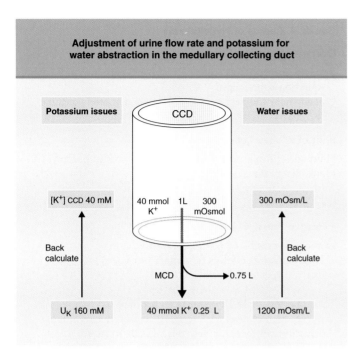

Adjustment of urine flow rate and potassium for water abstraction in the medullary collecting duct

Figure 42.5. Adjustment of urine flow rate and potassium [K⁺] for water abstraction in the medullary collecting duct. The barrel-shaped structure represents the CCD and the arrow below the CCD is the medullary collecting duct (MCD). When vasopressin acts, the osmolality in the lumen of the terminal CCD is equal to that of plasma. As shown on the left, the luminal K⁺ concentration is 40 mM. Consider what happens when 1 liter of fluid traverses the MCD, where 75% of the water is reabsorbed and no K⁺ is reabsorbed or secreted in the MCD. Therefore, the U_K is fourfold higher (160 mM), as is the U_{osm} (1200 mOsmol/kg H_2O). This should be taken into account when assessing the U_K. As shown on the right, multiplying the urine flow rate by the urine osmolality (1200 mOsmol/liter × 0.25 liter) yields the osmole excretion rate. When this value is divided by the plasma osmolality of 300 mOsmol/liter, one can deduce that the volume that exited from the terminal CCD was 1 liter in this time interval.

cause of the contracted ECF volume can be obtained from the urine electrolytes (see Table 42.2).

Specific Causes of Hypokalemia
Hypokalemia may be caused by diuretics, diarrhea, laxative abuse, vomiting, and osmotic diuresis. A summary of the causes of hypokalemia based on their pathophysiology is provided in Box 42.4.

Therapy for Hypokalemia
Our approach is to first recognize when hypokalemia may be life threatening.

Medical emergency
The major emergencies include cardiac arrhythmias and extreme weakness causing respiratory failure. When either is present, enough K⁺ must be given to raise P_K quickly to a safe range (~3.0 mmol/liter). The total body K⁺ deficit should be replaced much more slowly. Because large doses and high concentrations of K⁺ might be needed, K⁺ must be administered via a central vein and the patient should be on a cardiac monitor. In general,

the infusion should not contain glucose or HCO_3^- because this might aggravate the degree of hypokalemia.

Hypokalemic periodic paralysis
In the absence of a cardiac or respiratory emergency, small doses of KCl should be given to patients with hypokalemic periodic paralysis to minimize the risk of severe rebound hyperkalemia because they do not have a deficit of K⁺. If associated with hyperthyroidism or drugs with sustained adrenergic actions, a nonselective β-blocker (propranolol 3 mg/kg) can provide effective therapy. Clues to suggest the presence of an "occult" hyper-adrenergic state were listed previously.

No medical emergency
Magnitude of the K⁺ deficit
There is no useful quantitative relationship between P_K and total body K⁺ deficit because there may also be a shift of K⁺ into cells. Hence, careful monitoring of P_K during replacement of the K⁺ deficit is mandatory.

Route of K⁺ administration
The oral route is preferred if bowel sounds are present. When a peripheral intravenous route is used, the K⁺ concentration should not be more than 40 mmol/liter. The rate of K⁺ administration should not be more than 60 mmol/hr in all but emergency settings.

K⁺ preparations
Oral KCl (e.g., salt substitutes such as cosalt, which provides 14 mmol of K⁺ per gram) is generally well tolerated and is inexpensive. Liquid K⁺ supplements have an unpleasant taste and are often poorly tolerated. Most preparations used are "slow-release," either microencapsulated or in a wax matrix. Although usually well tolerated, they may cause ulcerative or stenotic lesions in the GI tract.

In patients with a deficit of KCl (e.g., chronic vomiting or diuretics), KCl is needed, whereas in patients with a $KHCO_3$ deficit (e.g., diarrhea), $KHCO_3$ may be needed in addition to KCl. Because the administration of HCO_3^- may lead to a shift of K⁺ into cells, KCl should be given initially and alkali should be withheld until P_K approaches a safe level (~3 mmol/liter) unless there are ongoing and large losses of HCO_3^-. K⁺ phosphate may be needed when there is rapid anabolism and little oral intake. We give K⁺ as KCl in treatment of DKA and rely on the patient's diet to supply the phosphate needed to restore a normal ICF composition later. If given, limit phosphate infusion to less than 50 mmol/8 hr to minimize the risk of hypocalcemia and metastatic calcification.

Adjuncts to therapy
Using K⁺-sparing diuretics may reduce renal loss of K⁺. This is only useful on a chronic basis. Amiloride and triamterene are better tolerated than spironolactone because they lack the gastrointestinal and hormonal (amenorrhea, gynecomastia, and decreased libido) complications of spironolactone. Nevertheless, hyperkalemia may develop, especially when K⁺ is given with K⁺-sparing diuretics and if other conditions that compromise K⁺ excretion are present; note that these drugs have a long half-life. On the other hand, there is a problem when blockers of the luminal epithelial Na⁺ channel are combined with diuretics that

cause a high distal flow rate because the luminal concentration of these epithelial Na^+ channel blockers declines due to the higher volume delivered to the CCD. As a result, the epithelial Na^+ channel might not be inhibited sufficiently to reduce the excretion of K^+.

Risks of therapy

With prolonged hypokalemia, the CCD may become temporarily hyporesponsive to the kaliuretic effect of aldosterone. Hence, it is important to monitor P_K frequently during the treatment of hypokalemia. Hyperkalemia has been observed in approximately 4% of patients taking K^+ supplements. The risk is highest in patients with renal failure and diabetes mellitus. The simultaneous use of ACE inhibitors or angiotensin II receptor blockers, β-blockers, or nonsteroidal anti-inflammatory drugs and K^+-sparing diuretics (e.g., spironolactone) may also predispose to the development of hyperkalemia.

SUGGESTED READING

Carlotti APCP, Bohn D, Mallie J-P, et al: Tonicity balance and not electrolyte-free water calculations more accurately guide therapy for acute changes in natremia. Intensive Care Med 2001;27:921–924.

Carlotti APCP, Bohn D, Halperin ML: Importance of timing of risk factors for cerebral oedema during therapy for diabetic ketoacidosis. Arch Dis Child 2003;88:170–173.

Cherney DZI, Davids MR, Halperin ML: Acute hyponatraemia and MDMA ("Ecstasy"): Insights from a quantitative and integrative analysis. Q J Med 2002;95:475–483.

Halperin ML, Kamel KS: Potassium. Lancet 1998;352:135–142.

Halperin ML, Kamel KS: Dynamic interactions between integrative physiology and molecular medicine: The key to understand the mechanism of action of aldosterone in the kidney. Can J Physiol Pharmacol 2000; 78:587–594.

Halperin ML, Davids MR, Kamel KS: Interpretation of urinary electrolyte and acid–base parameters. In Brenner BM (ed): Brenner and Rector's The Kidney, 7th ed. Philadelphia, Saunders, 2003, pp 1151–1181.

Kamel KS, Wei C: Controversial issues in treatment of hyperkalemia. Nephrol Dialysis Transpl 2003;18:2215–2218.

Lin S-H, Lin Y-F, Halperin ML: Hypokalemia and paralysis: Clues on admission to help in the differential diagnosis. Q J Med 2001;94:133–139.

Ponce S, Jennings A, Madias N, et al: Drug-induced hyperkalemia. Medicine 1985;64:357–370.

Soupart A, Decaux G: Therapeutic recommendations for management of severe hyponatremia: Current concepts on pathogenesis and prevention of neurologic complications. Clin Nephrol 1996;46:149–169.

Chapter 43

Acute Renal Failure

Rinaldo Bellomo and Claudio Ronco

KEY POINTS

- Acute renal failure (ARF) is not simply an expression of overall illness severity, but in and of itself, it significantly and independently increases mortality inside and outside of the intensive care unit (ICU).
- In order to confirm "renal dysfunction" or "renal failure," one must be able to measure renal function and detect that it has been altered.
- The tests commonly used to diagnose ARF can produce inaccurate values but are still worthwhile because absolute values are less important than monitoring change and direction of change.
- The most practically useful approach to the etiological diagnosis of ARF is to divide its causes according to the probable source of renal injury: prerenal, renal (parenchymal), and postrenal.
- The principles of management of established ARF are the treatment or removal of its cause and the maintenance of physiological homeostasis while recovery takes place.
- In the critically ill patient, renal replacement therapy should be initiated early, prior to the development of complications.

Acute renal failure (ARF) remains one of the major therapeutic challenges for the critical care physician. The term describes a syndrome characterized by a rapid (hours to days) decrease in the kidney's ability to eliminate waste products through glomerular filtration. Such loss of excretory function is biochemically and clinically manifested by the accumulation of end products of nitrogen metabolism (urea and creatinine), which are routinely measured in intensive care unit (ICU) patients and serve as markers of glomerular filtration rate (GFR). Other typical clinical manifestations include decreased urine output (not always present), the development of metabolic acidosis, and the tendency for hyperkalemia and hyperphosphatemia to occur.

ARF is one of the major critical care syndromes. In its frequency, implications, morbidity, and mortality, it rivals acute lung injury and acute respiratory distress syndrome.

DEFINITION

Depending on the criteria used to define its presence, ARF has been reported to occur in 15% to 20% of ICU patients. ARF severe enough to require the initiation of dialysis occurs in approximately 5% of ICU patients. However, its epidemiology in the ICU and elsewhere has been beset by the extreme variability in the choice of definition. In fact, approximately 30 different definitions of ARF have been used in the literature. This lack of agreement on the operative definition of ARF has significantly hindered research in this field of intensive care medicine, especially with regard to the design and execution of randomized controlled trials. Through the work of the Acute Dialysis Quality Initiative (www.ADQI.net), a consensus definition has been developed and published. It is hoped that this definition (Fig. 43.1) will lead to the development of consistency, reproducibility, and generalizability in future epidemiological and interventional studies of ARF.

EPIDEMIOLOGY

Despite the previously discussed problems, several observations can be made about the epidemiology of ARF. First, a degree of acute renal injury (manifested by albuminuria, loss of small tubular proteins, inability to excrete a water load, sodium load, or amino acid load, or any combination of these) can be demonstrated in most critically ill patients. This can be seen in patients undergoing simple and successful cardiac surgery with cardiopulmonary bypass or in those patients with severe sepsis but a normal serum creatinine.

The significance of such markers of renal dysfunction is unclear beyond the observation that some of them, such as albuminuria, have been associated with increased mortality and represent almost as good a marker of illness severity as do general illness severity scores when applied to ARF. Similarly, increased acute loss of GFR is also associated with increased mortality, as demonstrated by studies of several illness severity scores, such as APACHE I, II, and III, SAPS I and II, and the SOFA approach. There is also evidence that when dialysis becomes necessary, mortality is further increased. The population incidence of such severe acute renal failure (ARF treated by renal replacement therapy) has been reported to be between approximately 80 and 130 cases/million people/year in epidemiological studies performed first in the state of Victoria, Australia, and then throughout the country. It is also important to realize that the ARF seen in critically ill patients represents only a fraction of the total burden of ARF seen in the hospital setting, with up

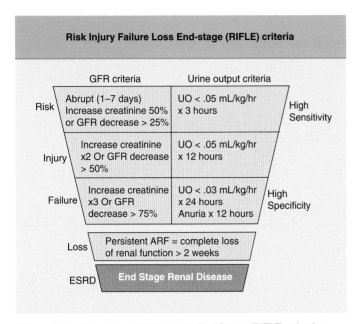

Figure 43.1. Risk Injury Failure Loss End-Stage (RIFLE) criteria: Classification scheme for acute renal failure (ARF). The classification system includes separate criteria for creatinine and urine output. The criteria that lead to the worst possible classification should be used. Note that RIFLE-F (F, failure) is present even if the increase in serum creatinine concentration (S_{Crt}) is more than threefold, as long as the new S_{Crt} is more than 4.0 mg/dL (350 μmol/L) in the setting of an acute increase of at least 0.5 mg/dL (44 μmol/L). The designation RIFLE-F_C should be used in this case to denote "acute-on-chronic" disease. Similarly, when RIFLE-F classification is reached by urine output criteria only, a designation of RIFLE-F_O should be used to denote oliguria. The shape of the figure denotes the fact that more patients (high sensitivity) will be included in the mild category, including some without actually having "renal failure" (less specificity). In contrast, at the bottom, the criteria are strict and therefore specific, but some patients with renal dysfunction may be missed. GFR, glomerular filtration rate.

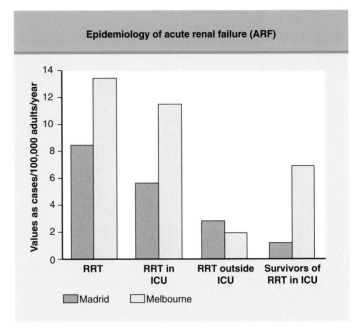

Figure 43.2. Epidemiology of acute renal failure (ARF). Diagram illustrating the differences in the epidemiology and outcomes of severe ARF in two different cities. RRT, renal replacement therapy.

ASSESSMENT OF RENAL FUNCTION

As highlighted previously, in order to confirm "renal dysfunction" or "renal failure," one needs to be able to measure renal function and detect that it has been altered. Renal function, however, is extremely complex. The kidneys control calcium and phosphate balance, acid–base balance, water balance, erythropoiesis, excretion of waste products, blood pressure, electrolyte balance, and probably, to a degree, immune function by their excretion or degradation of immunologically active peptides. However, almost all of these functions are shared with other organs and do not specifically or sensitively detect acute loss of renal function.

In the clinical context, monitoring of renal function is therefore reduced to the indirect assessment of GFR by the measurement of urea and creatinine in blood. These waste products are relatively inaccurate markers of GFR and are heavily modified by nutrition, the use of steroids, the presence of gastrointestinal blood, or the presence of muscle injury. Furthermore, they become abnormal only when more than 50% of GFR is lost; they do not reflect real-time dynamic changes in GFR and are grossly modified by aggressive fluid resuscitation. The use of creatinine clearance (2- or 4-hr collections) or of calculated clearance by means of formulae adjusted for body weight, gender, or age might increase accuracy but rarely, if ever, changes clinical management. The use of more sophisticated radionuclide-based tests is cumbersome in the ICU and only useful for research purposes. The urine output is also of limited sensitivity and specificity with patients capable of developing severe renal failure, as detected by a markedly elevated serum creatinine while maintaining normal urine output (so-called polyuric ARF).

The use of cystatin C has been proposed as a more accurate diagnostic test for renal failure. Cystatin C is a polypeptide that has many ideal features for use as a diagnostic tool, especially

to 8% of hospitalized patients showing evidence of an acute increase in nitrogen waste products. As such, the overall burden of ARF in the overall population may be up to 250 to 300 cases/million people/year. Consistent with these calculations, the Madrid ARF Study Group found an overall incidence of 209 cases/million people/year when using a definition of either a sudden increase to a serum creatinine greater than 177 μmol/L in patients with normal premorbid renal function or a 50% or greater increase in patients with chronic renal dysfunction (Fig. 43.2). If these observations apply across the developed world, which has a population of approximately 1 billion people, then the yearly incidence of ARF is more than 200,000 cases/year worldwide in economically developed countries. Little information is available from less developed countries. Several studies also show that ARF is not simply an expression of overall illness severity but that, in and of itself, it significantly and independently increases mortality inside and outside of the ICU. This effect on mortality is also independent of the use of renal replacement therapy (RRT).

its constant rate of production, exclusive renal excretion, and the good inverse correlation of its blood levels with radionuclide-derived measurements of GFR. However, this test has been developed only recently, and no large multicenter studies have been conducted to assess its role in the diagnosis and management of ARF. Therefore, clinicians continue to rely on the measurement of serum creatinine, plasma urea, and urine output as the three clinical pillars to help them diagnose ARF. They accept and understand the inaccuracy of these tests because absolute values are less important than change and direction of change.

ETIOLOGY AND CLINICAL CLASSIFICATION

The most practically useful approach to the etiological diagnosis of ARF is to classify its causes according to the probable source of renal injury: prerenal, renal (parenchymal) and postrenal (Fig. 43.3).

Prerenal ARF
So-called prerenal ARF is by far the most common cause of ARF in the ICU. The term typically indicates that the kidney malfunctions predominantly because of systemic factors that, through variable mechanisms, decrease the GFR. The most common systemic factors causing ARF in ICUs of developed countries are sepsis and septic shock. They account for approximately 50% of all cases. Other common systemic causes of ARF include a low cardiac output state (myocardial infarction,

tamponade, and valvular disease), cardiac surgery, major vascular surgery, trauma with hypovolemia, any cause of shock (anaphylactic, hemorrhagic, and hypovolemic), hemodynamic instability in association with surgery, liver failure, increased intraabdominal pressure, and rhabdomyolysis. The mechanisms by which these events induce ARF are variable according to the causative trigger and are poorly understood. Experimental studies also suggest that such mechanisms are likely to be complex and to involve multiple pathways of renal injury.

If the systemic cause of prerenal ARF is rapidly removed or corrected, renal function usually improves and, over a period of time (days), returns to near normal levels. However, if intervention is delayed or unsuccessful, renal injury becomes established, dialytic therapy may become necessary, and, if the patient survives, several days or weeks are then required for recovery. However, clinicians also loosely use terms such as prerenal azotemia or prerenal ARF to indicate not only that the cause or trigger of ARF is outside the renal parenchyma but also that a given patient has "functional" loss of GFR (no structural cell injury) as opposed to "structural" loss of GFR. Such suspected structural injury to the kidney is typically labeled acute tubular necrosis (ATN).

It is likely that this clinical subdivision does not reflect a true separation of pathophysiological states, which are much more likely to lead to a continuum of renal injury. Furthermore, no biopsy studies of ARF in patients treated in the ICU have been conducted to demonstrate that so-called ATN is the histopathological substrate of prolonged renal dysfunction.

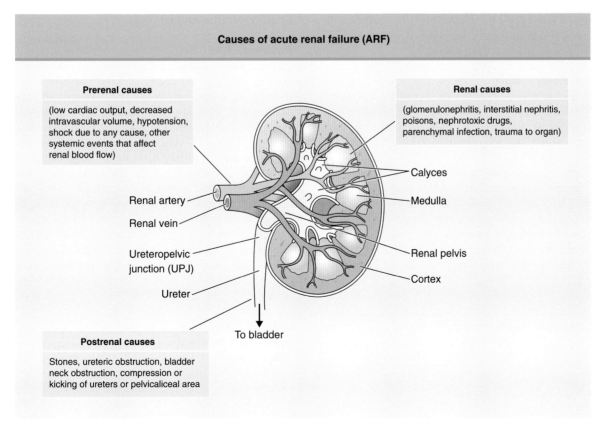

Causes of acute renal failure (ARF)

Prerenal causes

(low cardiac output, decreased intravascular volume, hypotension, shock due to any cause, other systemic events that affect renal blood flow)

Renal causes

(glomerulonephritis, interstitial nephritis, poisons, nephrotoxic drugs, parenchymal infection, trauma to organ)

Calyces

Medulla

Renal artery

Renal vein

Ureteropelvic junction (UPJ)

Ureter

Renal pelvis

Cortex

To bladder

Postrenal causes

Stones, ureteric obstruction, bladder neck obstruction, compression or kicking of ureters or pelvicaliceal area

Figure 43.3. Causes of acute renal failure (ARF). Pictorial summary of possible major categories of causes of renal dysfunction in the ICU.

Table 43.1 Laboratory Tests Used to Help Diagnose "Established" ARF

Test	Prerenal ARF	Acute Tubular Necrosis
Urine microscopy	Normal	Epithelial casts
Specific gravity	High (>1.020)	Low (<1.020)
Urine sodium	Low	High
U:P creatinine ratio	High (>40)	Low (<10)
P urea:creatinine ratio	High	Normal

P, plasma; U, urine.

Box 43.2 Drugs That May Cause ARF in the ICU

Radiocontrast agents
Aminoglycosides
Amphotericin
Nonsteroidal anti-inflammatory drugs
β-Lactam antibiotics (interstitial nephropathy)
Methotrexate
Cisplatin
Cyclosporin A
FK-506 (tacrolimus)

Nonetheless, several tests have been used to help clinicians identify the development of such ATN. These tests are included in this chapter for the sake of completeness (Table 43.1) and are often discussed in textbooks. However, these tests and their accuracy were tested in the 1970s in non-ICU patients and small cohorts from a single center. Even in these patients, the tests demonstrated variable levels of specificity and sensitivity for recovery of function within 72 hours, not histopathological confirmation of ATN. The accuracy and clinical utility of these tests in ICU patients who receive vasopressor infusions, massive fluid resuscitation, and, increasingly, loop diuretic infusions remain completely untested and, therefore, unknown. Furthermore, it is important to observe that the separation of "prerenal" ARF and ATN has limited clinical implications. The treatment is the same: treatment of the cause while promptly resuscitating the patient using invasive hemodynamic monitoring to guide therapy. Finally, rapid postmortem data in a cohort of ICU patients with ARF showed no evidence of ATN, raising further doubts about ATN as an entity in some, if not many, ICU patients with persistent renal dysfunction.

Parenchymal Renal Failure

The term *parenchymal renal failure* is used to define a syndrome in which the principal source of damage is within the kidney and in which typical structural changes can be seen on microscopy. Disorders that affect the glomerulus or the tubule may be responsible (Box 43.1).

Among these, nephrotoxins are particularly important, especially in hospitalized patients. The most common nephrotoxic drugs affecting ICU patients are listed in Box 43.2. Many cases of drug-induced ARF rapidly improve upon removal of the offending agent. Accordingly, a careful history of drug administration is mandatory in all patients with ARF. In some cases of parenchymal ARF, a correct working diagnosis can be obtained

Box 43.1 Causes of Parenchymal ARF

Glomerulonephritis
Vasculitis
Interstitial nephropathy
Malignant hypertension
Pelvicaliceal infection
Bilateral cortical necrosis
Amyloidosis

from history, physical examination, and radiological and laboratory investigations. In such patients, one can proceed to a therapeutic trial without the need to resort to renal biopsy. However, prior to aggressive immunosuppressive therapy, renal biopsy is recommended to allow histological confirmation of the etiology of ARF. Renal biopsy in ventilated patients under ultrasound guidance does not carry additional risks compared to standard conditions.

In this context, it is useful to note that more than one third of patients who develop ARF have chronic renal dysfunction with chronic parenchymal changes due to factors such as age-related changes, long-standing hypertension, diabetes, or atheromatous disease of the renal vessels. They may have a raised premorbid serum creatinine level. However, this is not always the case. Often, what may seem to the clinician to be a relatively trivial insult that does not fully explain the onset of ARF in a normal patient is sufficient to indicate lack of renal functional reserve in another.

Postrenal ARF

Obstruction of urine outflow causes so-called postrenal renal failure, which is the most common cause of functional renal impairment in the community (nonhospitalized patients) and is secondary to prostatic hypertrophy. Typical causes of obstructive ARF include bladder neck obstruction from an enlarged prostate, ureteric obstruction from pelvic tumors or retroperitoneal fibrosis, papillary necrosis, or large calculi. The clinical presentation of obstruction may be acute or acute-on-chronic in patients with long-standing renal calculi. It may not always be associated with oliguria. If obstruction is suspected, ultrasonography can be easily performed at the bedside. However, not all cases of acute obstruction have an abnormal ultrasound, and in many cases, obstruction occurs in conjunction with other renal insults (e.g., staghorn calculi and severe sepsis of renal origin) such that the cause of renal dysfunction is a combination of factors.

Specific Syndromes

Hepatorenal Syndrome

This condition is a form of ARF that occurs in the setting of severe liver dysfunction and in the absence of other known causes of ARF. Typically, it presents as progressive oliguria with a very low urinary sodium concentration (<10 mmol/L). Its pathogenesis is not well understood but appears to involve severe renal vasoconstriction. However, in patients with severe liver disease, other causes of ARF are much more common.

These include sepsis, paracentesis-induced hypovolemia, raised intraabdominal pressure due to tense ascites, diuretic-induced hypovolemia, lactulose-induced hypovolemia, alcoholic cardiomyopathy, or any combination of these. The avoidance of hypovolemia by albumin administration in patients with spontaneous bacterial peritonitis was shown to decrease the incidence of renal failure in a randomized controlled trial. These causes must be searched for and promptly treated. Uncontrolled studies suggest that vasopressin derivatives (ornipressin or terlipressin) may improve GFR in this condition. The role of such agents is unclear.

Rhabdomyolysis-Associated ARF

This condition accounts for approximately 5% to 10% of cases of ARF in the ICU, depending on the setting. Its pathogenesis involves prerenal, renal, and postrenal factors. It is typically seen following major trauma, drug overdose with narcotics, vascular embolism, and in response to a variety of agents that can induce major muscle injury (e.g., combination of cyclosporine and statins). The principles of treatment are based on animal studies, retrospective data, small case series, and multivariate logistic regression analysis because no randomized controlled trials have been conducted. These principles include prompt and aggressive fluid resuscitation, elimination of causative agents, correction of compartment syndromes, the alkalinization of urine (pH > 6.5), and the maintenance of polyuria (>300 mL/hr). The role of mannitol is controversial.

PATHOGENESIS OF ACUTE RENAL FAILURE

The pathogenesis of obstructive ARF involves several humoral responses as well as mechanical factors. The pathogenesis of parenchymal renal failure is typically immunological. It varies from vasculitis to interstitial nephropathy and involves an extraordinary complexity of cell-mediated and humoral mechanisms, which are beyond the scope of this chapter. The pathogenesis of prerenal ARF, on the other hand, is of greater direct relevance to the intensivist. Several mechanisms appear to play a major role in the development of renal injury:

1. Ischemia of outer medulla
2. Activation of the tubuloglomerular feedback system (afferent arteriolar constriction)
3. Tubular obstruction from cell casts
4. Interstitial edema secondary to back diffusion of fluid
5. Inflammatory response to cell injury and local release of mediators
6. Disruption of normal cellular adhesion to the basement membrane
7. Radical oxygen species-induced apoptosis
8. Phospholipase A_2-induced cell membrane injury

It is important to realize that the previously mentioned mechanisms have been demonstrated to be operative in animal models of renal injury. Such models, however, bear only a very limited resemblance to the clinical scenarios in which ARF develops in humans. The relevance of these findings to human disease, therefore, remains speculative. Even if such experimentally proven mechanisms were operative in humans, their hierarchy and time sequence remain unknown, making the development of therapeutic targets difficult.

THE CLINICAL PICTURE

The most common clinical picture of ARF in the ICU is that of a patient who has sustained a major systemic insult. When the patient arrives in the ICU, fluid resuscitation is well under way or has already been completed. Despite such efforts, the patient is often anuric or profoundly oliguric, the serum creatinine is rising, and metabolic acidosis is developing. Potassium and phosphate levels may be rapidly rising as well. Accompanying multiple organ dysfunction (mechanical ventilation and the need for vasoactive drugs) is common. Ongoing or further fluid resuscitation is typically undertaken under the guidance of invasive hemodynamic monitoring. Vasoactive drugs are often used to restore mean arterial pressure (MAP) to "acceptable" levels (typically > 70–75 mm Hg). The patient may improve over time, and urine output may return with or without the assistance of diuretic agents. If urine output does not return, however, RRT needs to be considered.

If the cause of ARF has been removed and the patient has become physiologically stable, slow recovery may occur (from 4 or 5 days to 3 or 4 weeks). In some cases, once recovery occurs, urine output can be above normal for several days. If the cause of ARF has not been adequately remedied, the patient will remain gravely ill, the kidneys will not recover, and death from multiorgan failure will occur.

PREVENTING ACUTE RENAL FAILURE

The fundamental principle of ARF prevention is to treat its cause. If prerenal factors contribute, these must be identified and hemodynamic resuscitation quickly instituted. Intravascular volume must be maintained or rapidly restored, and this is often best done using invasive hemodynamic monitoring (central venous catheter, arterial cannula, pulmonary artery catheter, or a transpulmonary thermodilution continuous cardiac output system in some cases). Oxygenation must be maintained. An adequate hemoglobin concentration (at least >70 g/L) must be maintained or immediately restored. Once intravascular volume has been restored, some patients remain hypotensive (MAP < 70 mm Hg). In these patients, auto-regulation of renal blood flow may be lost. Restoration of MAP to levels closer to normal values may increase renal perfusion and GFR (Fig. 43.4). Such elevations in MAP typically require the addition of vasopressor drugs (Fig. 43.5). In patients with hypertension or renovascular disease, a MAP of 75 to 80 mm Hg may still be inadequate. The nephroprotective role of additional fluid therapy in a patient with a normal or increased cardiac output and blood pressure is unclear. Despite fluid resuscitation, adequate hemoglobin, and maintained MAP, ARF may still develop if cardiac output is inadequate. This may require a variety of interventions, from the use of inotropic drugs to the application of ventricular assist devices.

Following hemodynamic resuscitation and removal of nephrotoxins, it is unclear whether the use of additional pharmacological measures is of further benefit to the kidneys. Renal dose dopamine is still frequently used. Evidence of the efficacy of its administration in critically ill patients is lacking. However, this agent is a tubular diuretic and occasionally increases urine output. This may be incorrectly interpreted as an increase in GFR. Furthermore, a large phase III, double-blind, placebo-controlled, randomized trial in critically ill patients showed

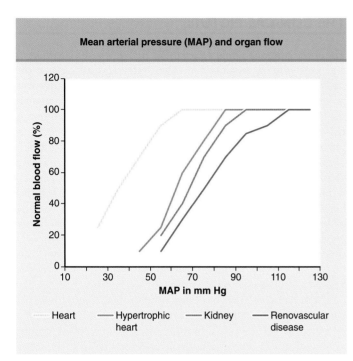

Figure 43.4. Mean arterial pressure (MAP) and organ blood flow. Graphic representation of the relationship between MAP and organ blood flow, highlighting the importance of perfusion pressure in maintaining renal blood flow.

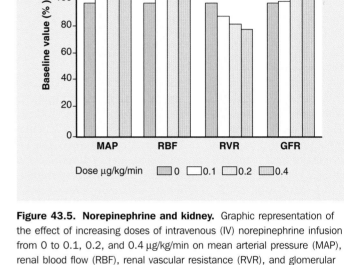

Figure 43.5. Norepinephrine and kidney. Graphic representation of the effect of increasing doses of intravenous (IV) norepinephrine infusion from 0 to 0.1, 0.2, and 0.4 μg/kg/min on mean arterial pressure (MAP), renal blood flow (RBF), renal vascular resistance (RVR), and glomerular filtration rate (GFR) in the dog.

low-dose dopamine to be no different from placebo in the prevention of ARF. In a patient with a low cardiac output, however, the administration of β-dose dopamine (as would dobutamine or milrinone) may increase cardiac output, renal blood flow, and GFR.

The effect of mannitol as a renal protective agent remains questionable. Loop diuretics may protect the loop of Henle from ischemia by decreasing its transport-related workload. Animal data are encouraging, as are ex vivo experiments. There are no double-blind, randomized controlled studies of suitable size to prove that these agents reduce the incidence of renal failure. However, there are several studies that support the view that loop diuretics may decrease the need for dialysis in patients with developing ARF. They appear to achieve this by inducing polyuria, which results in the prevention or easier control of volume overload, acidosis, and hyperkalemia, the three major triggers for RRT in the ICU. Because avoiding dialysis simplifies treatment and reduces cost of care, loop diuretics may be useful in patients with renal dysfunction, especially in the form of continuous infusion. On the other hand, an epidemiological study has linked the use of diuretics in these patients with increased mortality by means of multivariate analysis and propensity analysis. Thus, the role of diuretics in the management of ARF remains unclear.

Other agents, such as theophylline, urodilatin, and anaritide (a synthetic atrial natriuretic factor), have also been proposed as ways of protecting the kidney. However, studies performed to date have been experimental, too small, or have shown no beneficial effect.

Radiocontrast Nephropathy

Several randomized controlled trials have been conducted to test protective interventions in patients receiving radiocontrast agents. Studies have shown that the use of iso-osmolar radiocontrast agents reduces renal injury. A randomized controlled trial (RCT) suggested that in this setting, half-isotonic saline infusion to maintain intravascular fluid expansion is superior to the addition of mannitol or furosemide. Another study compared isotonic fluid to half-isotonic saline and found isotonic fluid to be superior. Several RCTs of similar patients have repeatedly demonstrated a beneficial effect of N-acetylcysteine (NAC) treatment before and after radiocontrast administration. These studies of NAC in the prevention of radiocontrast nephropathy have been meta-analyzed and indicate an approximately 50% reduction in the incidence of significant renal injury with the use of this agent. Since the previously mentioned preventive interventions have minimal toxicity and are not expensive, they should be considered whenever a patient with conditions that place him or her at risk (e.g., diabetes and chronic renal failure) is scheduled for the administration of intravenous radiocontrast.

DIAGNOSTIC INVESTIGATIONS

An etiological diagnosis of ARF must always be established. Such diagnosis may be obvious on clinical grounds. However, in many patients it is best to consider all possibilities and exclude common treatable causes by simple investigations. Such investigations include the examination of urinary sediment and exclusion of a urinary tract infection (most, if not all, patients), the exclusion of obstruction when appropriate (some patients), and the careful exclusion of nephrotoxins (all patients).

In specific situations, other investigations are necessary to establish the diagnosis, such as creatine kinase and free myoglobin for possible rhabdomyolysis. A chest radiograph, a blood film, the measurement of nonspecific inflammatory markers, and the measurement of specific antibodies (anti-GBM, antineutrophil cytoplasm, anti-DNA, anti-smooth muscle, etc.) are extremely useful screening tests to help support the diagnosis of vasculitis or of certain types of collagen disease or glomerulonephritis. If thrombotic–thrombocytopenic purpura is suspected, the additional measurements of lactic dehydrogenase, haptoglobin, unconjugated bilirubin, and free hemoglobin are needed. In some patients, specific findings (cryoglobulins and Bence–Jones proteins) are almost diagnostic. Rarely, a renal biopsy is necessary.

Managing ARF

The principles of management of established ARF are the treatment or removal of its cause and the maintenance of physiological homeostasis while recovery takes place. Complications such as encephalopathy, pericarditis, myopathy, neuropathy, electrolyte disturbances, or other major electrolyte, fluid, or metabolic derangement should never occur in a modern ICU. Their prevention may include several measures varying in complexity from fluid restriction to the initiation of extracorporeal RRT.

Nutritional support must be started early and must contain adequate calories (30–35 kcal/kg/day) as a mixture of carbohydrates and lipids. Adequate protein (approximately 1 or 2 g/kg/day) intake must be administered. There is no evidence that specific renal nutritional solutions are useful. Vitamins and trace elements should be administered at least according to their recommended daily allowance. The role of newer immunonutritional solutions remains controversial. The enteral route is preferred to the use of parenteral nutrition.

Hyperkalemia (>6 mmol/L) must be promptly treated with insulin and dextrose administration, the infusion of bicarbonate if acidosis is present, the administration of nebulized salbutamol (easily achieved without the need for intravenous access through the beta effect of the agent), or all of these in combination. If the serum potassium is more than 7 mmol/L or electrocardiographic signs of hyperkalemia appear, calcium gluconate (10 mL of 10% solution IV) should also be administered. The previous measures are temporary actions while RRT is being set up. The presence of hyperkalemia is a major indication for the immediate institution of RRT.

Metabolic acidosis is almost always present but rarely requires treatment per se. Anemia requires correction to maintain a hemoglobin of 70 g/L or more. More aggressive transfusion requires individual patient assessment. Drug therapy must be adjusted to take into account the effect of the decreased clearances associated with loss of renal function. Stress ulcer prophylaxis is advisable and should be based on H_2 receptor antagonists or proton pump inhibitors in selected cases. Careful attention should be paid to the prevention of infection.

Fluid overload can be prevented by the use of loop diuretics in polyuric patients. However, if the patient is oliguric, fluid overload can be avoided only by instituting RRT at an early stage. Marked azotemia ([urea] > 40 mmol/L or BUN > 112 mg/dL or

[creatinine] > 400 mmol/L or creatinine > 4.5 mg/dL) is undesirable and should probably be treated with RRT unless recovery is imminent or already under way and a return toward normal values is expected within 24 hours. It is recognized, however, that no randomized controlled trials exist to define the ideal time for intervention with artificial renal support.

Renal Replacement Therapy

When ARF is severe, resolution can take several days or weeks. In these patients, extracorporeal techniques of blood purification must be applied to prevent complications. Such techniques broadly fall under the term RRT and include continuous hemofiltration, intermittent hemodialysis, peritoneal dialysis, and, recently, so-called hybrid techniques, each with its technical variations.

All of these techniques rely on the principle of removing unwanted solutes and water through a semipermeable membrane. Such membrane is either biological (peritoneum) or artificial (hemodialysis or hemofiltration membranes) and offers several advantages, disadvantages, and limitations.

In the critically ill patient, RRT should be initiated early, prior to the development of complications. Fear of early dialysis stems from the adverse effects of conventional intermittent hemodialysis (IHD) with cuprophane membranes, especially hemodynamic instability (Fig. 43.6), and from the risks and limitations of continuous or intermittent peritoneal dialysis (PD). However, continuous renal replacement therapy (CRRT) or slow

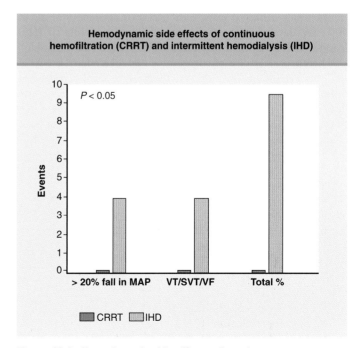

Figure 43.6. Hemodynamic side effects of continuous hemofiltration (CRRT) and intermittent hemodialysis (IHD). Graphic representation of the incidence of hypotension [decrease in mean arterial pressure (MAP)], arrhythmias [ventricular tachycardia (VT), supraventricular tachycardia (SVT), and ventricular fibrillation (VF)], and overall percentage of affected patients upon initiating conventional dialysis (IHD) in a cohort of 70 ICU patients compared to a similar group of patients treated with CRRT.

Box 43.3 Modern Criteria for the Initiation of RRT in the ICU

Anuria (no urine output for 6 hr)
Oliguria (urine output < 200 mL/12 hr)
BUN > 80 mg/dL or urea > 28 mmol/L
Creatinine > 3 mg/L or >265 µmol/L
[K$^+$] > 6.5 mmol/L or rapidly rising
Pulmonary edema unresponsive to diuretics
Uncompensated metabolic acidosis (pH < 7.1)
Temperature > 40°C
Uremic complications (encephalopathy, myopathy, neuropathy, pericarditis)
Overdose with a dialyzable toxin (e.g., lithium)

If one criterion is present, RRT should be considered. If two criteria are simultaneously present, RRT is strongly recommended.

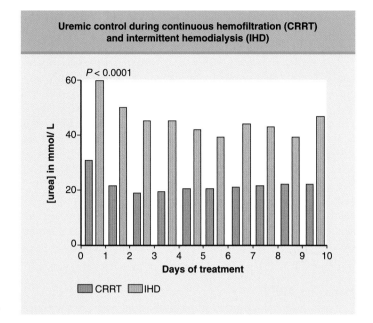

Figure 43.7. Uremic control during continuous hemofiltration (CRRT) and intermittent hemodialysis (IHD). Diagram illustrating the difference in uremic control over time in two cohorts of ICU patients treated with IHD or CRRT.

low-efficiency extended daily dialysis (SLEDD) (hybrid technique) minimizes these effects. The criteria for the initiation of RRT in patients with chronic renal failure may be inappropriate in the critically ill. A set of modern criteria for the initiation of RRT in the ICU is presented in Box 43.3.

There are limited data on what constitutes "adequate" intensity of dialysis once RRT is started with either IHD or CRRT. However, this concept should include the maintenance of homeostasis at all levels (water, electrolytes, blood pressure, and acid–base status), and better uremic control may translate into better survival. An appropriate target urea is 20 mmol/L, with a protein intake of at least approximately 1.5 g/kg/day. This can be easily achieved using CRRT at urea clearances of 30 to 40 L/day, depending on patient size and catabolic rate. If IHD is used, daily treatment and extended treatment are desirable.

There is a great deal of controversy regarding which mode of RRT is best in the ICU due to the lack of RCTs comparing different techniques. Trials of sufficient statistical power are difficult to conduct and may not be available for some time. In their absence, techniques of RRT may be judged on the basis of the following criteria:

1. Hemodynamic side effects
2. Ability to control fluid status
3. Uremic control (Fig. 43.7)
4. Avoidance of cerebral edema (Figs. 43.8 and 43.9)
5. Ability to allow full nutritional support
6. Ability to control acidosis (Fig. 43.10)
7. Ability to maintain electrolyte homeostasis (Figs. 43.11 and 43.12)
8. Ability to maintain phosphate and calcium homeostasis (Fig. 43.13)
9. Absence of specific side effects
8. Biocompatibility
10. Risk of infection
11. Cost

Using these criteria, CRRT and SLEDD offer many advantages over PD and conventional IHD (3 or 4 hours/day, three or four times/week). However, in some settings they may be more expensive. In order to make informed decisions, the intensive care physician needs to appreciate several technical and practical aspects of each approach to RRT.

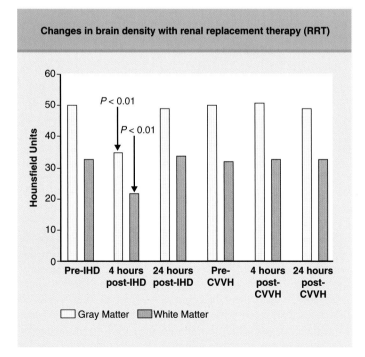

Figure 43.8. Changes in brain density with renal replacement therapy. Diagram representing changes in brain tissue density on CT scan with intermittent hemodialysis (IHD) or continuous venovenous hemofiltration (CVVH). IHD induced a significant decrease in brain tissue density (cerebral edema), whereas CVVH did not.

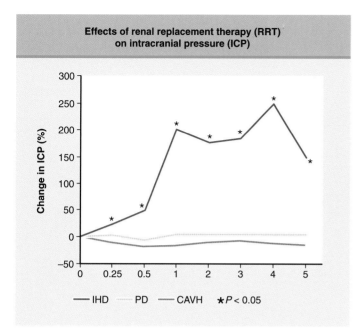

Figure 43.9. Effects of renal replacement therapy (RRT) on intracranial pressure (ICP). Illustration showing changes in ICP in patients with cerebral edema receiving different types of RRT. During continuous therapies [peritoneal dialysis (PD) or continuous arteriovenous hemofiltration (CAVH)], the ICP remained similar to preintervention values; during intermittent hemodialysis (IHD), it increased markedly.

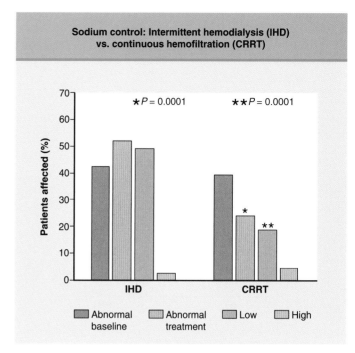

Figure 43.11. Sodium control: Intermittent hemodialysis (IHD) vs. continuous hemofiltration (CRRT). Illustration of the difference between sodium control during IHD and CRRT. Abnormal baseline values were seen in a high percentage of patients before treatment and decreased in prevalence after treatment (decreased "abnormal treatment") with CRRT, but not IHD; this was especially true for hyponatremia (asterisk).

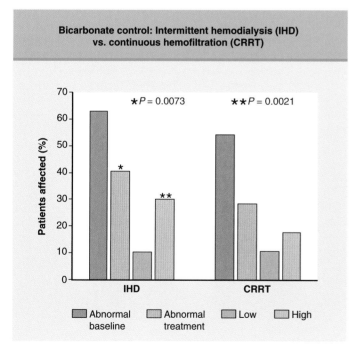

Figure 43.10. Bicarbonate control: Intermittent hemodialysis (IHD) vs. continuous hemofiltration (CRRT). Illustration of the difference between acid–base control during IHD and CRRT. Abnormal baseline values for serum bicarbonate were seen in a high percentage of patients before treatment and decreased in prevalence after treatment. However, the return to normal was greater with CRRT, especially for low values (asterisks), indicating superior correction of metabolic acidosis.

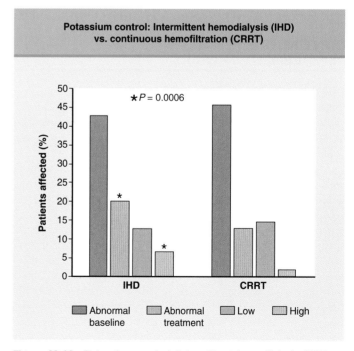

Figure 43.12. Potassium control: Intermittent hemodialysis (IHD) vs. continuous hemofiltration (CRRT). Illustration of the difference between potassium control during IHD and CRRT. Abnormal baseline values were seen in a high percentage of patients before treatment and decreased in prevalence after treatment. However, the return to normal (decreased "abnormal treatment") was greater with CRRT, especially for hypokalemia (asterisks).

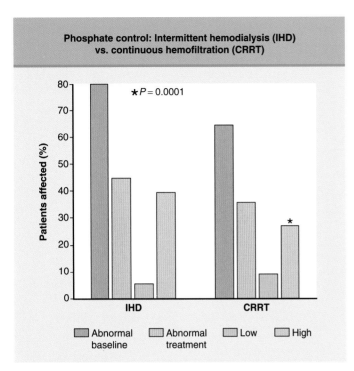

Figure 43.13. Phosphate control: Intermittent hemodialysis (IHD) vs. continuous hemofiltration (CRRT). Illustration of the difference between phosphate control during IHD and CRRT. Abnormal baseline values were seen in a high percentage of patients before treatment and decreased in prevalence after treatment. However, the return to normal (decreased "abnormal treatment") was greater with CRRT, especially for hyperphosphatemia (asterisks).

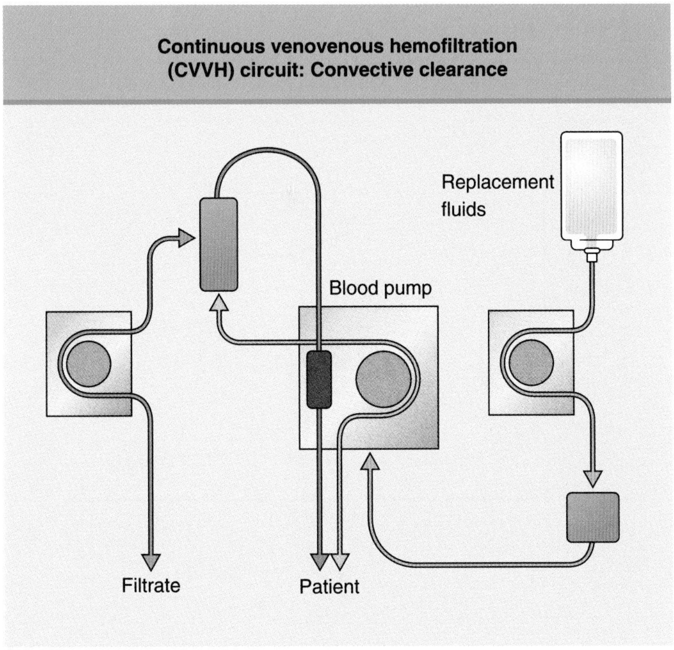

CONTINUOUS RENAL REPLACEMENT THERAPY

CRRT was initially performed as an arteriovenous hemofiltration therapy but is now typically performed with double-lumen catheters and peristaltic blood pumps in continuous venovenous hemofiltration (CVVH) (Fig. 43.14) mode with or without control of ultrafiltration rate (convective clearance).

Dialysate can also be delivered countercurrent to blood flow with or without replacement fluid (continuous venovenous hemodialysis/hemodiafiltration) (Figs. 43.15 and 43.16) to achieve either almost pure diffusive clearance or a mixture of diffusive and convective clearance (Fig. 43.17). Although all such therapies achieve solute, fluid, and acid–base control with ease, they mandate the presence of specifically trained nursing and medical staff 24 hours a day. Small ICUs often cannot provide such a level of support. If CRRT is only used 5 or 10 times per year, the cost of training may be unjustified and expertise may be difficult to maintain. Furthermore, depending on the organization of patient care, CRRT may be more expensive than IHD. Finally, the issues of continuous circuit anticoagulation and the potential risk of bleeding have been a major concern.

Anticoagulation during CRRT

Anticoagulants are frequently used during CRRT (Fig. 43.18). However, circuit anticoagulation increases the risk of bleeding. Therefore, the risks and benefits of more or less intense

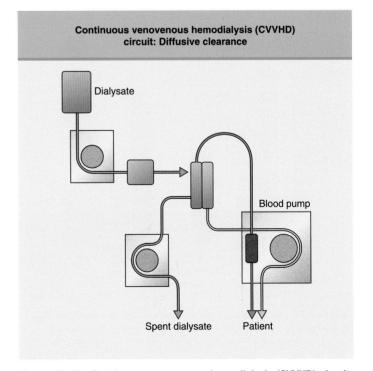

Figure 43.14. Continuous venovenous hemofiltration (CVVH) circuit: Convective clearance. Diagram representing the design of a CVVH circuit with predilution to achieve convective solute clearance.

Figure 43.15. Continuous venovenous hemodialysis (CVVHD) circuit: Diffusive clearance. Diagram representing the design of a CVVHD circuit to achieve diffusive solute clearance.

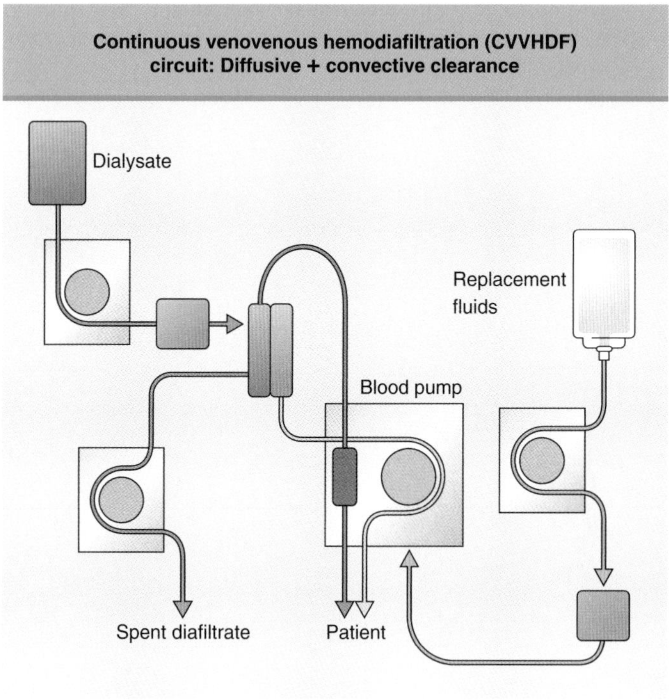

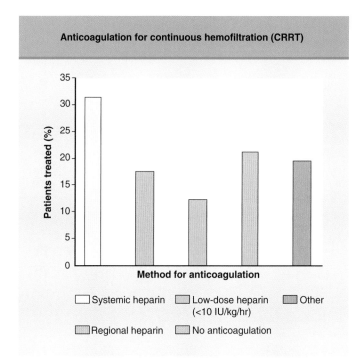

Figure 43.16. Continuous venovenous hemodiafiltration (CVVHDF) circuit: Diffusive + convective clearance. Diagram representing the design of a CVVHDF circuit with predilution to achieve mixed convective–diffusive solute clearance.

Figure 43.18. Anticoagulation for continuous hemofiltration (CRRT). Frequency of particular approaches to anticoagulation of CRRT circuits in Australia. As can be seen, different approaches are used according to local preference and patient needs.

anticoagulation and alternative strategies (Box 43.4) must be considered.

In the vast majority of patients, low-dose heparin (5–10 IU/kg/hr) is sufficient to achieve adequate filter life. It is also easy and cheap to administer, and it has almost no effect on the patient's coagulation tests. In some patients, a higher dose is necessary. In others (pulmonary embolism and myocardial ischemia), full heparinization may actually be concomitantly indicated. Regional citrate anticoagulation is very effective but requires a special dialysate or replacement fluid and the monitoring of ionized calcium (Fig. 43.19). Regional heparin/protamine anticoagulation is also somewhat complex but may be useful if frequent filter clotting occurs and further anticoagulation of the patient is considered dangerous. Low-molecular-weight heparin is also easy to give but more expensive. It must be used with caution because it accumulates in patients with renal failure. This is difficult to monitor. Heparinoids, prostacyclin, and citrate may be useful if the patient has developed heparin-induced thrombocytopenia and thrombosis. Finally, in 10% to 20% of patients anticoagulation is best avoided because of endogenous coagulopathy or recent surgery. In such patients, mean filter lives of more than 24 hours can be achieved

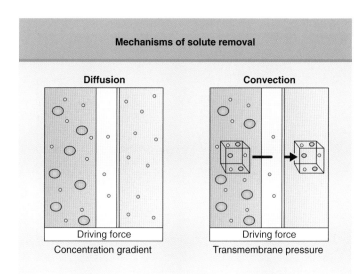

Figure 43.17. Mechanisms of solute removal. Diagram illustrating the principles of solute removal and their mechanisms of solute transport.

Box 43.4 Strategies Used for Circuit Anticoagulation during CRRT

No anticoagulation
Low-dose prefilter heparin (<500 IU/hr)
Medium-dose prefilter heparin (500–1000 IU/hr)
Full anticoagulation with heparin
Regional heparin/protamine anticoagulation
Regional citrate anticoagulation
Low-molecular-weight heparin
Prostacyclin
Heparinoids
Combination of prostacyclin and low-dose heparin

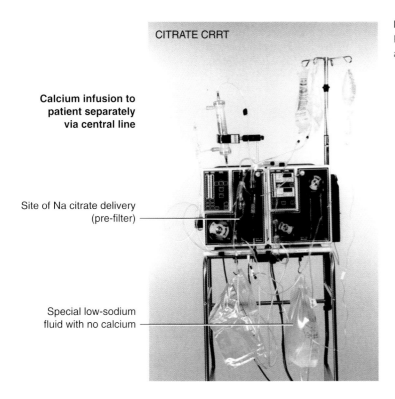

CITRATE CRRT

Calcium infusion to
patient separately
via central line

Site of Na citrate delivery
(pre-filter)

Special low-sodium
fluid with no calcium

Figure 43.19. Citrate continuous hemofiltration (CRRT) setup. Photograph illustrating the sites of infusion of special fluids for citrate anticoagulation.

provided that blood flow is kept at approximately 200 mL/min and vascular access is reliable. In the authors' opinion, patients who have had surgery in the past 24 hours should receive CRRT without anticoagulation or with citrate anticoagulation. Particular attention needs to be paid to the adequacy/ease of flow through the double-lumen catheter. Smaller (11.5 Fr) catheters in the subclavian position are a particular problem. Larger catheters (13.5 Fr) in the femoral position appear to function more reliably (Fig. 43.20). The choice of membrane is also a matter of controversy. There are several biosynthetic membranes on the market that have excellent biocompatibility (AN69, polyamide, polysulfone, and cellulose triacetate). There

are no controlled studies to show that one of them confers a clinical advantage over the others.

INTERMITTENT HEMODIALYSIS

Standard IHD uses high dialysate flows (300–400 mL/min), generates dialysate by using purified water and concentrate, and is applied for short periods of time (3–4 hr). These differences have important implications. First, volume has to be removed over a short period of time, which may be poorly tolerated, causing hypotension. Repeated hypotensive episodes may delay renal recovery. Second, solute removal is episodic, resulting in

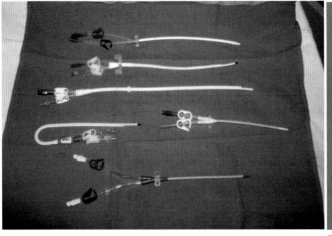

A

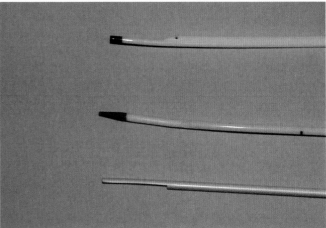

B

Figure 43.20. Catheters for renal replacement therapy. Array of different double-lumen catheters used for CRRT worldwide (A). Note the different tip designs (B).

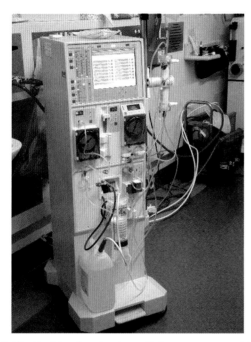

Figure 43.21. Machine for slow low-efficiency extended daily dialysis (SLEDD). The latest model (Fresenius ArRt plus 4008) for the performance of on-line fluid generation, extended, intermittent low-efficiency hemodiafiltration in the ICU.

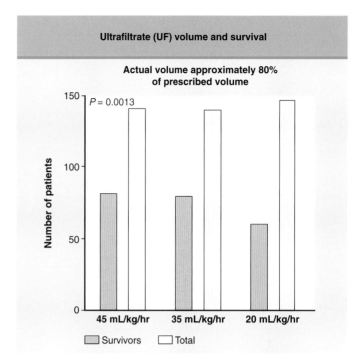

Figure 43.22. Ultrafiltrate (UF) volume and survival. Diagram illustrating the difference in survival from a randomized controlled trial between patients with acute renal failure treated with low-dose continuous hemofiltration (CRRT) (20 mL/kg/hr UF), higher dose CRRT (35 mL/kg/hr UF), and highest dose CRRT (45 mL/kg/hr UF). Patients treated with higher ultrafiltration rates had increased survival.

inferior uremic and acid–base control. Limited fluid and uremic control imposes limitations on nutritional support. Furthermore, rapid solute shifts increase brain water content and raise intracranial pressure.

The limitations of applying "standard" IHD to the treatment of ARF have led to the development of new approaches (so-called hybrid techniques) such as SLEDD (Fig. 43.21). These techniques seek to adapt IHD to the clinical circumstance and thereby increase its tolerance and its clearances. They operate by performing an intermittent therapy, which is of less intensity (lower dialysate flow), longer duration (8 hr or more), and greater frequency (daily). Early experience with SLEDD appears highly satisfactory.

The technique of peritoneal dialysis is now not commonly used in the treatment of adult ARF in developed countries. However, it may be an adequate technique in developing countries in which no other resources are available or in children for whom alternatives are considered too expensive or too invasive or are not available. A RCT from Vietnam demonstrated that in ARF, treatment with PD markedly increased mortality compared to CVVH.

The issue of "dose" in IHD or CRRT has become of greater importance because two single-center studies have suggested that daily dialysis may increase survival compared to dialysis every 2 days and that CRRT at 35 or 45 mL/kg/hr of effluent may increase survival compared to CRRT at 20 mL/kg/hr of effluent (Fig. 43.22). If multicenter RCTs confirm these findings, practice in this field will be altered to readjust the intensity of RRT.

BLOOD PURIFICATION TECHNOLOGY FOR NON-ARF INDICATIONS

There is growing interest in the possibility that blood purification may provide a clinically significant benefit in patients with severe sepsis/septic shock by removing circulating "mediators." A variety of techniques, including plasmapheresis, high-volume hemofiltration, very high-volume hemofiltration, and coupled plasma filtration adsorption, are being studied in animals and in phase I and II studies in humans. Initial experiments support the need to continue exploring this therapeutic option. However, no suitably powered RCTs have been reported. Also, blood purification technology in combination with bioreactors containing either human or porcine liver cells is under active investigation as a form of artificial liver support for patients with fulminant liver failure or for patients with acute-on-chronic liver failure. Finally, albumin-based dialysis with albumin recycling (so-called molecular adsorption recycling system) is also being tested in patients with acute or acute-on-chronic liver failure.

DRUG PRESCRIPTION DURING DIALYTIC THERAPY

ARF and RRT profoundly affect drug clearance. A comprehensive description of changes in drug dosage according to the technique of RRT, residual creatinine clearance, and other determinants of pharmacodynamics is beyond the scope of this

Renal and Metabolic Problems

Table 43.2 Drug Dosage during Renal Replacement Therapy[a]

Drug	CRRT	IHD
Aminoglycosides	Normal dose q36hr	50% normal dose q48hr 2/3 redose after IHD
Cefotaxime or ceftazidime	1 g q8–12hr	1 g q12–24hr after IHD
Imipenem	500 mg q8hr	250 mg q8hr and after IHD
Meropenem	500 mg q8hr	250 mg q8hr and after IHD
Metronidazole	500 mg q8hr	250 mg q8hr and after IHD
Cotrimoxazole	Normal dose q18hr	Normal dose q24hr after IHD
Amoxycillin	500 mg q8hr	500 mg daily and after IHD
Vancomycin	1 g q24hr	1 g q96–120hr
Piperacillin	3–4 g q6hr	3–4 g q8hr and after IHD
Ticarcillin	1–2 g q8hr	1–2 g q8hr and after IHD
Ciprofloxacin	200 mg q12hr	200 mg q24hr and after IHD
Fluconazole	200 mg q24hr	200 mg q48hr and after IHD
Acyclovir	3.5 mg/kg q24hr	2.5 mg/kg/day and after IHD
Gancyclovir	5 mg/kg/day	5 mg/kg/48 hr and after IHD
Amphotericin B	Normal dose	Normal dose
Liposomal amphotericin	Normal dose	Normal dose
Ceftriaxone	Normal dose	Normal dose

[a]The values represent approximations and should be used as a general guide only. Critically ill patients have markedly abnormal volumes of distribution for these agents, which will affect dosage. CRRT is conducted at variable levels of intensity in different units, also requiring adjustment. The values reported here relate to CVVH at 2 L/hr of ultrafiltration. Vancomycin is poorly removed by CVVHD. IHD may also differ from unit to unit. The values reported here relate to standard IHD with low-flux membranes for 3 or 4 hr every second day.

chapter and can be found in specialist texts. Table 43.2 provides general guidelines for the prescription of drugs that are commonly used in the ICU.

CONCLUSIONS

The areas of ARF and RRT have undergone remarkable changes during the past few years. Major advances have been made in the prevention of radiocontrast nephropathy. However, no drugs have been found to help patients with ARF due to other causes. CRRT is now firmly established as perhaps the most commonly used form of RRT in developed countries. Conventional dialysis, however, which was slowly losing ground, is reappearing in the form of SLEDD. Independent of technique, increasing the dose of RRT may improve survival in ICU patients. In the meantime, use of novel membranes, sorbents, and different intensities of treatment is being explored in the area of sepsis management and liver support.

SUGGESTED READING

ANZICS Clinical Trials Group; Low-dose dopamine in patients with early renal dysfunction: A placebo-controlled randomised trial. Lancet 2000; 356:2139–2143.

Bellomo R, Ronco C: Adequacy of dialysis in the acute renal failure of the critically ill: The case for continuous therapies. Int J Artif Organs 1996;19:129–142.

Birck R, Krzoosok S, Markowetz F, et al: Ecetylcysteine for prevention of contrast nephropathy: Meta-analysis. Lancet 2003;362:598–603.

Bonventre JV: Mechanisms of ischemic acute renal failure. Kidney Int 1993;43:1160–1178.

Cole L, Bellomo R, Silvester W, Reeves JH: A prospective, multicenter study of the epidemiology, management and outcome of severe acute renal failure in a "closed" ICU system. Am J Respir Crit Care Med 2000; 162:191–196.

Marshall MR, Golper TA, Shaver MJ, Chatoth DK: Hybrid renal replacement modalities for the critically ill. Contrib Nephrol 2001; 132:252–257.

Mehta R, Dobos GJ, Ward DM: Anticoagulation procedures in continuous renal replacement. Sem Dial 1992;5:61–68.

Mehta RL, McDonald B, Gabbai F, et al: A randomized clinical trial of continuous versus intermittent dialysis for acute renal failure. Kidney Int 2001;60:1154–1163.

Phu NH, Hien TT, Mai NT, et al: Hemofiltration and peritoneal dialysis in infection-associated acute renal failure in Vietnam. N Engl J Med 2002;34:933–935.

Ronco C, Bellomo R, Homel P, et al: Effects of different doses in continuous veno-venous haemofiltration on outcomes of acute renal failure: A prospective randomized trial. Lancet 2000;355:26–30.

Chapter 44

Hepatorenal Syndrome

Vicente Arroyo, Pere Ginès, Carlos Terra, and Aldo Torre

KEY POINTS

- Hepatorenal syndrome (HRS) is a functional renal failure that develops in patients with decompensated cirrhosis. It occurs in the setting of a severe circulatory dysfunction characterized by vasodilation in the splanchnic circulation, impaired cardiac function, marked stimulation of the sympathetic nervous and renin–angiotensin systems, and renal vasoconstriction.
- There are two types of HRS. Type I is characterized by a rapidly progressive impairment in renal perfusion and glomerular filtration rate. Type 2 is a moderate and steady type of functional renal failure.
- Without treatment, the median survival time after the onset of type 1 HRS is only 2 weeks. The probability of survival for type 2 HRS is between 6 months and 1 year. The most important problem for patients with type 2 HRS is refractory ascites.
- Treatment with vasoconstrictors and volume expansion with albumin reverses type 1 HRS and improves survival in a significant proportion of patients.
- Liver transplantation is the treatment of choice for HRS.

Hepatorenal syndrome (HRS) is a common complication of patients with cirrhosis, severe liver failure, and portal hypertension. It is characterized by renal vasoconstriction, very low renal perfusion and glomerular filtration rate (GRF), and intense reduction of the renal ability to excrete sodium and free water in the absence of significant histological renal lesions. HRS is the extreme expression of the circulatory dysfunction of cirrhosis, which has been classically considered to be secondary to an arterial vasodilation in the splanchnic circulation. However, data suggest that an impairment in cardiac function may also play a significant role. HRS may develop spontaneously during the course of the disease or be precipitated by factors that induce renal hypoperfusion, such as bacterial infections. The annual incidence of HRS in patients with cirrhosis and ascites has been estimated as 8%. Diagnosis of HRS relies on the exclusion of other potential causes of renal insufficiency in cirrhosis. HRS is the complication of cirrhosis associated with the worst prognosis, and for many years it has been considered as a terminal event of the disease. However, effective treatments for HRS that improve survival have been introduced, and a significant number of patients may now benefit from liver transplantation.

PATHOGENESIS

HRS occurs in association with a severe circulatory dysfunction characterized by vasodilation in the splanchnic circulation; vasoconstriction in the brain, liver, muscle and skin, and kidneys; and increased intrahepatic resistance to the portal venous flow. In addition, an impaired cardiac function with low cardiac output and the disappearance of the hyperdynamic circulation present in nonazotemic patients with cirrhosis has been reported in patients with type 1 HRS.

Renal Dysfunction

Chronologically, impairment in renal sodium metabolism is the first renal function abnormality in cirrhosis. It can be detected in patients with compensated cirrhosis (no ascites), who may be unable to escape from the effect of mineralocorticoids or to eliminate an acute sodium load normally. These features are observed in patients with significant portal hypertension and hyperdynamic circulation (high cardiac output and low systemic vascular resistance). As the disease progresses, the impairment in sodium metabolism increases and a critical point is achieved at which the patient is unable to excrete his or her regular sodium intake. Sodium is then retained with water and accumulates as ascites. GFR and the plasma concentrations of aldosterone and norepinephrine are normal. Sodium retention is therefore unrelated to the renin–aldosterone system and sympathetic nervous system, the two most important sodium-retaining systems identified. The plasma levels of natriuretic peptides are markedly increased, indicating that sodium retention is not due to reduced production of endogenous natriuretic substances. The most accepted mechanism of sodium retention at this early stage of decompensated cirrhosis is a decrease in the effective arterial blood volume secondary to splanchnic arterial vasodilation. This circulatory dysfunction, although greater than that in compensated cirrhosis, is not intense enough to stimulate the sympathetic nervous activity and the renin–angiotensin–aldosterone system. However, it would activate an unknown, extremely sensitive sodium-retaining mechanism (renal or extrarenal).

With the exception of alcoholic cirrhosis, in which renal function may improve after alcohol withdrawal, the degree of sodium retention increases with the progression of disease. When it is intense, the plasma renin activity and the plasma concentration of aldosterone and norepinephrine are invariably elevated. At this stage of the disease, the cardiac output and peripheral vascular resistance do not differ from those of the previous phase. Circulatory dysfunction, however, is greater since an increased activity of the sympathetic nervous and renin–angiotensin systems is needed to maintain the arterial pressure. Renal perfusion and GFR are also normal or only moderately decreased, but they are critically dependent on an increased renal production of prostaglandins and nitric oxide. These are vasodilators that antagonize the vasoconstrictor effect of angiotensin II and noradrenaline. A syndrome indistinguishable from HRS can be produced in patients with cirrhosis, ascites, and increased plasma renin activity following prostaglandin inhibition with nonsteroidal anti-inflammatory drugs. The renal ability to excrete free water is reduced due to a nonosmotic hypersecretion of antidiuretic hormone. However, only a few patients show significant hyponatremia (serum sodium concentration < 130 mEq/min). Water retention and dilutional hyponatremia develop when renal water metabolism is severely impaired (free water clearance after water load < 1 mL/min; normal, 6–12 mL/min), and this rarely occurs in cirrhosis in the absence of renal failure.

HRS develops at the latest phase of the disease when patients already have severe impairment of circulatory function, arterial hypotension, marked stimulation of the sympathetic nervous and renin–angiotensin systems, intense sodium retention, and hyponatremia. In fact, arterial hypotension, high plasma levels of renin and norepinephrine, and hyponatremia are important predictors of development of HRS. Impairment in GFR in HRS is due to renal vasoconstriction. Renal histology shows no lesions or lesions that do not justify the decrease in renal function. Since angiotensin II and norepinephrine are powerful renal vasoconstrictors, renal failure in HRS is thought to be related to the extreme stimulation of the endogenous vasoconstrictor systems. Urinary excretion of prostaglandin E_2 and 6-keto prostaglandin F_{1a} (a prostacyclin metabolite) is decreased in patients with HRS, which is compatible with a reduced renal production of these vasodilator substances. Renal vasoconstriction in HRS could therefore be the consequence of an imbalance between the activity of the systemic vasoconstrictor systems and the renal production of vasodilators. Finally, renal hypoperfusion in HRS may be amplified by the stimulation of intrarenal vasoconstrictors. For example, renal ischemia increases the intrarenal generation of angiotensin II, adenosine (which in addition to being a renal vasoconstrictor potentiates the vascular effect of angiotensin II), and endothelin. Other intrarenal vasoconstrictors implicated in HRS are leukotrienes and F_2 isoprostanes.

Sodium delivery to the loop of Henle and distal nephron, the site of action of furosemide and spironolactone, respectively, is very low in HRS due to low filtered sodium and increased sodium reabsortion in the proximal tubule. The delivery of furosemide and spironolactone to the renal tubules is also reduced due to renal hypoperfusion. It is therefore not surprising that patients with HRS respond poorly to diuretics.

Cardiocirculatory Dysfunction in Cirrhosis and HRS

Portal hypertension in patients with cirrhosis is associated with a circulatory dysfunction characterized by increased cardiac output and heart rate and reduced peripheral vascular resistance. This hyperdynamic circulation is a compensatory mechanism to maintain the effective arterial blood volume and arterial pressure. When it is insufficient to compensate the arterial vasodilation, arterial hypotension occurs, leading to activation of pressure receptors in the aorta and carotid sinus, reflex stimulation of the sympathetic nervous system, renin–angiotensin system and vasopressin release, and a compensatory increase in arterial pressure.

Splanchnic arterial vasodilation is a constant feature in portal hypertension and plays a major role in many abnormalities associated with this condition. It is the main determinant of hyperdynamic circulation in cirrhosis. There is a splanchnic resistance to the vasoconstrictor effect of angiotensin II, catecholamines, and vasopressin in cirrhosis. This explains why splanchnic arterial vasodilation and hyperdynamic circulation are maintained during the progression of the disease despite stimulation of the renin–angiotensin and sympathetic nervous systems and antidiuretic hormone. In contrast, these systems induce arterial vasoconstriction in other organs, such as the liver, kidneys, brain, muscle, and skin, in patients with cirrhosis and ascites. Nitric oxide is an important effector of splanchnic vasodilation in cirrhosis. The synthesis of this local vasodilator is increased in the splanchnic circulation in cirrhosis.

Investigations of circulatory function in cirrhotic patients with renal failure suggest that a decrease in cardiac output is also of major importance in the impairment of circulatory function that characterizes HRS. In 1967, Tristani and Cohn showed that cardiac output was normal or reduced in a significant number of patients with HRS. The peripheral vascular resistance in these patients (although below normal value) was higher than that reported by other authors in patients without HRS. In a study of patients with spontaneous bacterial peritonitis, the development of type 1 HRS was associated with a significant decrease in cardiac output, a feature not observed in patients who maintained serum creatinine within normal limits. At the end of treatment, mean arterial pressure and cardiac output were 10% and 30% lower, respectively, peripheral vascular resistance was 32% higher, and the plasma levels of renin and norepinephrine were 5 to 10 times higher in patients developing HRS compared with those without HRS. These studies suggest that the most likely mechanism of HRS is a combination of arterial vasodilation and a decreased cardiac output. Although there is a specific cardiomyopathy characterized by impaired ventricular contractibility in cirrhosis, the most likely mechanism of the impairment in cardiac output in HRS is central hypovolemia. Cardiopulmonary pressures are normal or reduced in HRS, and plasma volume expansion is associated with a marked increase in cardiac output. On the other hand, treatment with vasoconstrictors and IV administration of albumin, but not with vasoconstrictors alone, normalizes circulatory and renal function in HRS.

Influence of Systemic Circulatory Dysfunction on Hepatic Hemodynamics

A significant part of the increased intrahepatic vascular resistance in cirrhosis is unrelated to architectural changes, and there are data indicating that in decompensated cirrhosis the renin–angiotensin and sympathetic nervous systems may be involved in this functional component of portal hypertension. Angiotensin II and catecholamines reduce hepatic blood flow and increase intrahepatic vascular resistance and portal pressure. Impairment in circulatory function associated with HRS during spontaneous bacterial peritonitis is also associated with an increase in intrahepatic resistance to the portal venous flow and portal pressure and to a reduction in hepatic blood flow, a

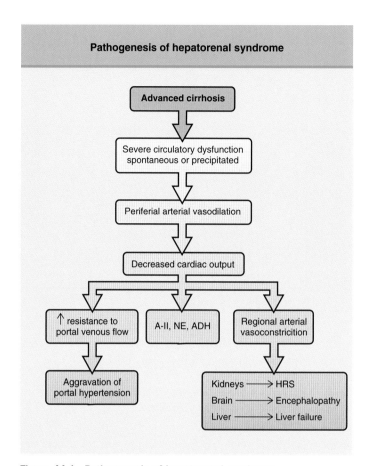

Pathogenesis of hepatorenal syndrome

Figure 44.1. Pathogenesis of hepatorenal syndrome.

The first step to diagnosis of HRS is the demonstration of a reduced GFR, and this is not easy in advanced cirrhosis (Box 44.1). The muscle mass is reduced in these patients, and they may present normal serum creatinine concentration in the setting of a very low GFR. Similarly, urea may be reduced as a consequence of hepatic insufficiency. Therefore, false-negative diagnosis of HRS is relatively common. There is consensus to establish the diagnosis of HRS when serum creatinine has risen above 1.5 mg/dL or creatinine clearance has decreased to less than 40 mL/min.

The second step is the differentiation of HRS from other types of renal failure. For many years, this was based on the traditional parameters used to diagnose a functional renal failure (oliguria, low urine sodium concentration and urine-to-plasma osmolality ratio greater than unity, normal fresh urine sediment, and no proteinuria). However, acute tubular necrosis in patients with cirrhosis and ascites usually courses with oliguria, low urine sodium concentration, and urine osmolality greater than plasma osmolality. On the contrary, a relatively high urinary sodium concentration has been reported in some patients with HRS. Therefore, diagnosis of HRS should be based on the exclusion of other disorders that can cause renal failure in cirrhosis. Acute renal failure of prerenal origin due to renal or extrarenal fluid losses should be investigated. If renal failure is secondary to volume depletion, renal function will improve rapidly after volume expansion, whereas no improvement occurs in HRS. Even if there is no history of fluid losses, renal function should be assessed after diuretic withdrawal and volume replacement (1.5 liters of isotonic saline) to rule out any subtle reduction in

feature not observed in patients who maintain serum creatinine within normal limits. These changes correlate closely with the increase in plasma renin activity and noradrenaline concentration. Circulatory dysfunction in HRS, therefore, affects not only the renal circulation and the circulation in other organs, such as the brain and muscle and skin, but also the intrahepatic circulation (Fig. 44.1). This may explain the rapid deterioration of hepatic function and the frequent development of hepatic encephalopathy in type 1 HRS.

DIAGNOSIS AND CLINICAL FEATURES

Type 1 and type 2 HRS show many differences from a clinical standpoint and probably also have a different pathogenesis. Renal failure in type 1 HRS is severe and rapidly progressive, whereas it is moderate and steady in type 2. Type 2 HRS develops insidiously, without an apparent precipitating factor, in patients without renal failure. In contrast, type 1 HRS frequently develops in patients who already have type 2 HRS in close association with a precipitating event, commonly an infection. The main clinical problem of type 1 HRS is the development of a rapidly progressive deterioration of circulatory function, severe hepatorenal failure, encephalopathy, and death. In contrast, in type 2 HRS the main clinical problem is refractory ascites. Survival is longer in patients with type 2 HRS. Type 2 HRS probably represents the genuine functional renal failure of cirrhosis secondary to splanchnic arterial vasodilation. In contrast, type 1 HRS is more likely an acute renal failure of circulatory origin similar to that which occurs in other diseases, such as sepsis, acute pancreatitis, and severe trauma.

Box 44.1 International Ascites Club's Diagnostic Criteria of Hepatorenal Syndrome

Major Criteria

- Chronic or acute liver disease with advanced hepatic failure and portal hypertension
- Low glomerular filtration rate, as indicated by serum creatinine of > 1.5 mg/dL or 24-hr creatinina clearance < 40 mL/min
- Absence of shock, ongoing bacterial infection, and current or recent treatment with nephrotoxic drugs; absence of gastrointestinal fluid losses (repeated vomiting or intense diarrhea) or renal fluid losses (weight loss > 500 g/day for several days in patients with ascites without peripheral edema or 1000 g/day in patients with peripheral edema)
- No sustained improvement in renal function (decrease in serum creatinine to 1.5 mg/dL or less or increase in creatinina clearance to 40 mL/min or more) following diuretic withdrawal and expansion of plasma volume with 1.5 liters of isotonic saline)
- Proteinuria > 500 mg/dL and no ultrasonographic evidence of obstructive uropathy or parenchymal renal disease

Additional Criteria

- Urine volume < 500 mL/day
- Urine sodium < 10 mEq/liter
- Urine osmolality greater than plasma osmolality
- Urine red blood cells < 50 per high power field
- Serum sodium concentration < 130 mEq/liter

491

plasma volume as the cause of renal failure. The presence of shock before the onset of renal failure indicates a diagnosis of acute tubular necrosis. Cirrhotic patients with infections may develop transient renal failure, which resolves after resolution of the infection. Therefore, for cirrhotic patients with bacterial infections, HRS should be diagnosed in those without septic shock and only if renal failure persists following infection resolution. Cirrhotic patients are predisposed to develop renal failure in the setting of treatment with aminoglycosides, nonsteroidal anti-inflammatory drugs, and vasodilators (renin–angiotensin system inhibitors, prazosin, and nitrates). Therefore, treatment with these drugs in the days preceding the diagnosis of renal failure should be ruled out. Finally, patients with cirrhosis can develop renal failure due to intrinsic renal diseases, particularly glomerulonephritis. These cases can be recognized by the presence of proteinuria, hematuria, or both.

Type 1 HRS is characterized by a severe and rapidly progressive renal failure, which has been defined as doubling of serum creatinine reaching a level greater than 2.5 mg/dL in less than 2 weeks. Although type 1 HRS may arise spontaneously, it frequently occurs in close relationship with a precipitating factor, such as severe bacterial infection, gastrointestinal hemorrhage, a major surgical procedure, or acute hepatitis superimposed on cirrhosis. The association of HRS and spontaneous bacterial peritonitis has been carefully investigated. Type 1 HRS develops in approximately 25% of patients with spontaneous bacterial peritonitis, despite a rapid resolution of the infection with nonnephrotoxic antibiotics. Patients with intense inflammatory response and high cytokine levels in plasma and ascitic fluid are especially prone to develop type 1 HRS after infection. Besides renal failure, patients with type 1 HRS after spontaneous bacterial peritonitis show signs and symptoms of severe liver insufficiency (jaundice, coagulopathy, and hepatic encephalopathy) and circulatory dysfunction (arterial hypotension and very high plasma levels of renin and norepinephrine) that worsen with the impairment in renal function. Type 1 HRS is the complication of cirrhosis with the poorest prognosis, with a median survival time after the onset of renal failure of only 2 weeks (Fig. 44.2).

Type 2 HRS is characterized by a moderate and steady decrease in renal function (serum creatinine < 2.5 mg/dL). Patients with type 2 HRS show signs of liver failure and arterial hypotension but to a lesser degree than patients with type 1 HRS. The dominant clinical feature is severe ascites with poor or no response to diuretics (a condition known as refractory ascites). Patients with type 2 HRS are specially predisposed to develop type 1 HRS following infections or other precipitating events. Median survival of patients with type 2 HRS (6 months) is worse than that of patients with nonazotemic cirrhosis with ascites.

TREATMENT

Type 1 HRS

Volume Expansion and Vasoconstrictors

The rationale for this treatment is the current concept of the pathogenesis of type 1 HRS. Vasoconstrictors are given to reverse the splanchnic arterial vasodilation and volume expansion to improve venous return and cardiac output. Vasopressin analogs (orniressin and terlipressin) were the initial drugs used for the treatment of type 1 HRS due to their preferential effect

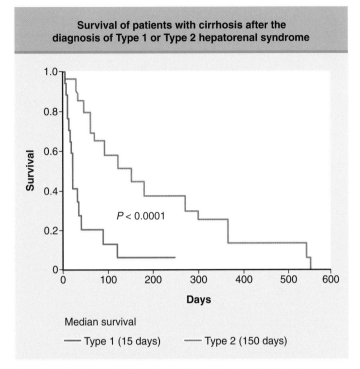

Figure 44.2. Survival of patients with cirrhosis after the diagnosis of Type 1 or Type 2 hepatorenal syndrome.

on the splanchnic circulation. Terlipressin has been the most frequently used drug. Ornipressin is also effective, but because it is given as a constant infusion, it frequently produces ischemic complications.

The administration of terlipressin (0.5–2 mg/4–6 hr IV) induces complete therapeutic response, as defined by a reduction of serum creatinine to less than 1.5 mg/dL, in 50% to 75% of patients (Table 44.1). This is associated with a marked suppression of renin and norepinephrine and a significant increase in mean arterial pressure. There is a lag between suppression of endogenous neurohormonal systems, which occurs within the first 3 days of treatment, and the decrease in serum creatinine, which starts 2 to 4 days later. Despite normalization of serum creatinine, renal function does not reach normal levels and there is persistence of low GFR, which ranges between 30 and 50 mL/min in most cases (normal, 120 mL/min). In most studies, treatment with terlipressin has been maintained until serum creatinine decreased to below 1.5 mg/dL or for a maximum of 15 days. It is unknown whether the continued administration of terlipressin after the end point of 1.5 mg/dL of serum creatinine has been reached may cause a larger increase in GFR. In responder patients, there is an improvement in urine volume within the first 24 hours. In some, but not all, patients, treatment also causes an increase in sodium excretion and improvement or normalization of serum sodium concentration. This latter effect is outstanding considering that terlipressin is a V2 vasopressin agonist. It suggests that impairment in free water clearance in type 1 HRS is related more to intrarenal mechanisms than to nonosmotic hypersecretion of antidiuretic hormone. In all studies, IV albumin has been given at variable doses for the duration of therapy with terlipressin. Some data indicate that the therapeutic response to terlipressin is very poor if given without the concomitant administration of albumin. A

Table 44.1 Rate of Response, Recurrence, Transplant, and Survival in Different Series of Patients with Cirrhosis and Hepatorenal Syndrome Treated with Vasoconstrictors and IV Albumin

Series	Response (%)[a]	Recurrence (%)[b]	Liver Transplantation (%)	1-Month Survival (%)
Angeli et al (1999)[c]	5/5 (100)	NR	2/5 (40)	4/5 (80)
Uriz et al (2000)	7/9 (77)	0/7 (0)	3/5 (60)	6/9 (67)
Mulkay et al (2001)	11/12 (92)	6/11 (55)	3/12 (25)	10/12 (80)
Moreau et al (2002)	53/91 (58)	NR	13/99 (13)	40/99 (40)
Colle et al (2002)	11/18 (61)	7/11 (64)	2/18 (11)	7/18 (40)
Halimi et al (2002)	13/18 (72)	NR	2/18 (11)	NR
Alessandria et al (2002)	8/11 (73)	8/8 (100)	NR	NR
Ortega et al (2002)	14/21 (66)	2/14 (14)	3/21 (14)	11/21 (52)
Duvoux et al (2002)[d]	10/12 (84)	0/10 (0)	3/8 (37)	11/19 (58)
Solanki et al (2003)	5/12 (42)	NR	NR	NR

[a]The definition of response varies among studies.
[b]Recurrence of hepatorenal syndrome after treatment withdrawal in responder patients. The definition of recurrence varies among studies.
[c]Vasoconstrictor used: midodrine.
[d]Vasoconstrictor used: noradrenalin.
NR, not reported.

recommended schedule for albumin administration is 1 g/kg during the first day followed by 20 to 40 g/day thereafter. The administration of albumin is interrupted if central venous pressure increases above 18 cm H_2O. Predictors of response to terlipressin include old age, severe liver failure (Child–Pugh score > 13), and lack of concomitant administration of albumin. The probability of survival in patients with type 1 HRS responding to terlipressin has been estimated to be 50% at 3 months and 30% at 1 year (Fig. 44.3). This is comparable to that reported in patients with type 2 HRS and considerably longer than that observed in untreated patients with type 1 HRS. A significant proportion of patients with type 1 HRS treated with terlipresin and albumin reach liver transplantation. Recurrence of HRS after discontinuation of treatment is uncommon (approximately 15% of patients). Treatment of HRS recurrence is usually effective. The incidence of ischemic side effects requiring discontinuation of terlipressin is low (5%–10%), although it has to be considered that most studies have excluded high-risk patients with ischemic heart or artery diseases.

Catecholamines are also effective for the treatment of HRS. Midodrine (an oral α-adrenergic agonist) was given by Angeli and colleagues in association with IV albumin and subcutaneous octreotide (to suppress glucagon) to five patients with type 1 HRS. The dose of midodrine (7.5–12.5 mg every 8 hr) was adjusted to increase mean arterial pressure by 15 mm Hg or more. Patients received treatment for at least 20 days in the hospital and continued treatment at home. There was a marked improvement in renal perfusion and glomerular filtration and suppression of renin, norepinephrine, and antidiuretic hormone to normal or near normal levels in all cases. Two patients were transplanted 20 and 64 days after inclusion while on therapy. One patient, who was not a candidate for liver transplantation, was alive without treatment 472 days after discharge from the hospital.

Duvoux and associates treated 12 patients with type 1 HRS with intravenous albumin and noradrenaline (0.5–3.0 mg/hr) for a minimum of 5 days. Reversal of HRS was observed in 10 patients in association with an increase in mean arterial pressure and a marked reduction in renin and aldosterone. There was an

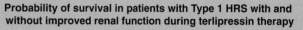

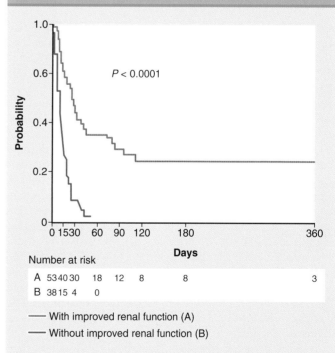

Probability of survival in patients with Type 1 HRS with and without improved renal function during terlipressin therapy

P < 0.0001

Number at risk

A	53 40 30	18	12	8	8		3
B	38 15 4	0					

—— With improved renal function (A)

—— Without improved renal function (B)

Figure 44.3. Probability of survival in patients with type 1 HRS with and without improved renal function during terlipressin therapy. (Data from Moreau R, Durand F, Poynard T, et al: Terlipressin in patients with cirrhosis and type 1 hepatorenal syndrome: A retrospective multicenter study. Gastroenterology 2002;122:923–930.)

episode of reversible myocardial hypokinesia. Three patients were transplanted and 4 others had prolonged survival (>6 months).

Transjugular Intrahepatic Portocaval Shunt

Four studies assessing transjugular intrahepatic portocaval shunt (TIPS) in the management of type 1 HRS have been reported.

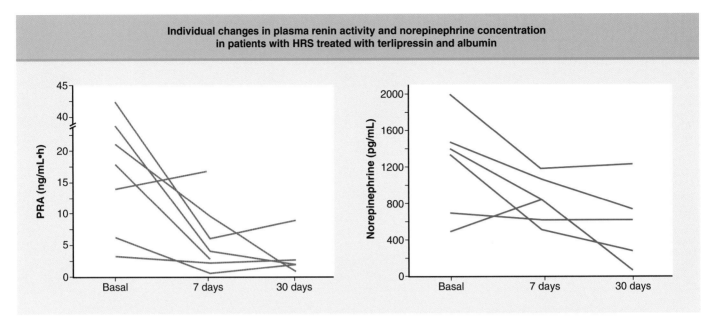

Figure 44.4. Individual changes in plasma renin activity (PRA) and plasma norepinephrine concentrations in patients with HRS treated by TIPS, in baseline conditions and 7 and 30 days after TIPS. (Data from Guevara M, Ginès P, Bandi JC, et al: Transjugular intrahepatic portosystemic shunt in hepatorenal syndrome: Effects on renal function and vasoactive systems. Hepatology 1998;28:416–422.)

In total, 30 patients were treated. In two series, no liver transplantation was performed, whereas in the other two series 3 of 9 patients underwent transplantation 7, 13, and 35 days after TIPS. TIPS insertion was technically successful in all patients. Only 1 patient died as a consequence of the procedure. GFR improved markedly within 1 to 4 weeks after TIPS and stabilized thereafter. In one study specifically investigating the neurohormonal systems, improvement in GFR and serum creatinine was related to a marked suppression of the plasma levels of renin and antidiuretic hormone. The suppression of plasma norepinephrine is lower than that of renin, a feature also observed in refractory ascites treated by TIPS (Fig. 44.4). Follow-up data concerning hepatic function were obtained from 21 patients. De novo hepatic encephalopathy or deterioration of preexisting hepatic encephalopathy occurred in 9 patients, but in 5 it could be controlled with lactulose. Survival rates based on the 27 patients without early liver transplantation at 1, 3, and 6 months were 81%, 59%, and 44%, respectively. These studies strongly suggest that TIPS is useful in the management of type 1 HRS. Studies comparing TIPS with pharmacological treatment in type 1 HRS are needed.

As indicated previously, one of the intriguing issues regarding the treatment of type 1 HRS with vasoconstrictors and IV albumin is the observation that despite a marked suppression of renin and norepinephrine, indicating a significant improvement in circulatory function, there is persistence of low GFR. The reason for this lack of normalization of renal function is not known but could be due either to the existence of a component of renal failure unresponsive to changes in circulatory function or to the fact that the effective arterial blood volume, although improved, is not normalized with pharmacology therapy. Results from one study are consistent with this hypothesis. Treatment with TIPS in patients responding to pharmacological treatment (midodrine, octreotide, and albumin) was associated with normalization in GFR in most cases. Whether the effect of TIPS in

the normalization of GFR was due to the correction of the arterial vasodilation, an increase in cardiac preload and ventricular function, or both remains to be investigated.

Liver Transplantation

Liver transplantation is the treatment of choice for HRS. Immediately after transplantation, a further impairment in GFR may be observed, and many patients require hemodialysis (35% of patients with HRS compared with 5% of patients without HRS). Because cyclosporine or tacrolimus may contribute to this impairment in renal function, it has been suggested to delay the administration of these drugs until a recovery of renal function is noted, usually 48 to 72 hours after transplantation. After this initial impairment in renal function, GFR starts to improve and reaches an average of 30 to 40 mL/min by 1 or 2 months postoperatively. This moderate renal failure persists during follow-up, is more marked than that observed in transplantation patients without HRS, and is probably due to a greater nephrotoxicity of cyclosporine or tacrolimus in patients with renal impairment prior to transplantation. The hemodynamic and neurohormonal abnormalities associated with HRS disappear within the first month after the operation, and patients regain a normal ability to excrete sodium and free water.

Patients with HRS who undergo transplantation have more complications, spend more days in the intensive care unit, and have a higher in-hospital mortality rate than transplantation patients without HRS. However, the long-term survival of patients with HRS who undergo liver transplantation is good, with a 3-year probability of survival of 60%. This survival rate is only slightly reduced compared to that of transplantation in patients without HRS (70%–80%).

The main problem of liver transplantation in type 1 HRS is its applicability. Due to their extremely short survival, most patients die before transplantation. The introduction of the MELD score, which includes serum creatinine, bilirubin, and the

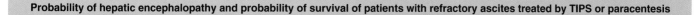

Probability of hepatic encephalopathy and probability of survival of patients with refractory ascites treated by TIPS or paracentesis

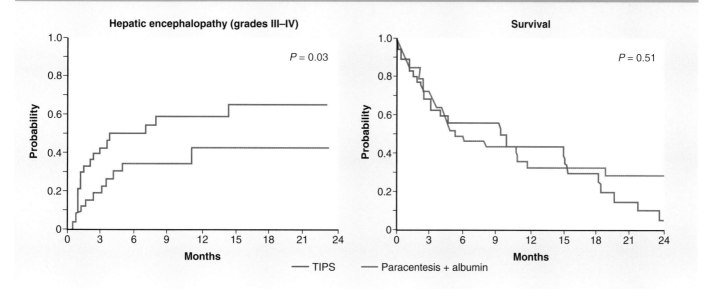

Figure 44.5. Probability of hepatic encephalopathy and probability of survival of patients with refractory ascites treated by TIPS or paracentesis. (Data from Ginès P, Uriz J, Calahorra B, et al: Transjugular intrahepatic portosystemic shunting versus paracentesis plus albumin for refractory ascites in cirrhosis. Gastroenterology 2002;123:1839–1847.)

international normalized ratio, for listing has partially solved the problem since patients with HRS are generally allocated to the top of the waiting list. Treatment of HRS with vasoconstrictors and albumin increases survival in a significant proportion of patients and, therefore, the number of patients reaching living transplantation, decreases early morbidity and mortality after transplantation, and prolongs long-term survival.

Other Therapeutic Methods

Hemodialysis is frequently used in the management of type 1 HRS in many centers, particularly in patients who are candidates for liver transplantation, with the aim of preventing the complications associated with renal failure and maintaining patients alive until transplantation. However, the beneficial effects of this procedure in type 1 HRS have not been convincingly demonstrated. Complications during hemodialysis in these patients are common and include arterial hypotension, bleeding, and infections. On the other hand, clinical or biochemical features indicating the need for renal replacement therapy, such as heart or respiratory failure, severe acidosis, or severe hyperkalemia, are uncommon in type 1 HRS. Extracorporeal albumin dialysis, a system that uses an albumin-containing dialysate that is recirculated and perfused through charcoal and anion-exchanger columns, has been reported to improve renal function and survival in a small series of patients with HRS. Further studies are required.

Type 2 HRS

Survival of patients with type 2 HRS is relatively prolonged, and many cases reach liver transplantation. The main clinical problem while patients are on the waiting list is refractory ascites. Total therapeutic paracentesis associated with IV albumin infusion is the treatment of choice in these patients. It is rapid, effective, and safe. TIPS is another effective therapy,

and four randomized controlled trials have compared this treatment with paracentesis in refractory ascites. Their main conclusion was that although TIPS markedly reduces the number of episodes of ascites in comparison to paracentesis, it increases the frequency of hepatic encephalopathy and does not improve survival (Fig. 44.5). TIPS dysfunction and the high cost of this treatment were also important problems.

There is limited information on the use of vasoconstrictors in the treatment of patients with type 2 HRS, but some reports suggest that, as in type 1 HRS, the administration of vasoconstrictors and IV albumin improves renal function in these patients. However, renal failure recurs after therapy is stopped in most patients.

PREVENTION

Two randomized controlled studies of large series of patients have shown that HRS can be prevented in specific clinical settings. In the first study, the administration of albumin (1.5 g/kg IV at infection diagnosis and 1 g/kg IV 48 hr later) to patients with cirrhosis and spontaneous bacterial peritonitis markedly reduced the incidence of circulatory dysfunction and type 1 HRS (10% incidence of type 1 HRS in patients receiving albumin vs. 33% in the control group). Hospital mortality rate (10% vs. 29%) and the 3-month mortality rate (22% vs. 41%) were lower in patients receiving albumin (Fig. 44.6). In the second study, the administration of tumor necrosis factor inhibitor pentoxyfilline (400 mg three times per day) to patients with severe acute alcoholic hepatitis reduced the occurrence of HRS (8% in the pentoxyfilline group vs. 35% in the placebo group) and the hospital mortality (24% vs. 46%, respectively). Because bacterial infections and acute alcoholic hepatitis are important precipitating factors of type 1 HRS, these prophylactic measures may decrease the incidence of this complication.

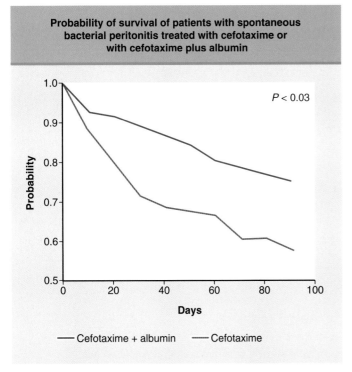

Probability of survival of patients with spontaneous bacterial peritonitis treated with cefotaxime or with cefotaxime plus albumin

$P < 0.03$

Figure 44.6. Probability of survival of patients with spontaneous bacterial peritonitis treated with cefotaxime or with cefotaxime plus albumin. (Data from Sort P, Navasa M, Arroyo V, et al: Effect of intravenous albumin on renal impairment and mortality in patients with cirrhosis and spontaneous bacterial peritonitis. N Engl J Med 1999;341:403–409.)

Box 44.2 Controversies

1. Which is the true predominant mechanism of HRS—progression of splanchnic arterial vasodilation or an impairment in cardiac function?
2. Clinically, type 1 and type 2 HRS are very different. Do they have a similar pathogenesis?
3. Which is the predominant mechanism of cardiac dysfunction in HRS—a reduced cardiac preload due to central hypovolemia or the so-called cirrhotic cardiomyopathy?
4. TIPS and vasoconstrictors plus albumin are effective treatments for type 1 HRS. Could therapeutic efficacy be increased by the simultaneous or repeated use of both treatments?
5. TIPS and total paracentesis plus albumin are effective treatments for refractory ascites in patients with type 2 HRS. Is there a specific indication for each treatment?
6. Morbidity and early mortality after liver transplantation are high in patients with HRS. Should HRS be treated prior to the transplantation?

SUGGESTED READING

Angeli P, Volpin R, Gerunda G, et al: Reversal of type 1 hepatorenal syndrome with the administration of midodrine and octreotide. Hepatology 1999;29:1690–1697.

Arroyo V, Ginès P, Gerbes AL, et al: Definition and diagnostic criteria of refractory ascites and hepatorenal syndrome in cirrhosis. International Ascites Club. Hepatology 1996;23:164–176.

Arroyo V, Guevara M, Ginès P: Hepatorenal syndrome in cirrhosis: Pathogenesis and treatment. Gastroenterology 2002;122:1658–1676.

Duvoux C, Zanditenas D, Hezode C, et al: Effects of noradrenalin and albumin in patients with type I hepatorenal syndrome: A pilot study. Hepatology 2002;36:374–380.

Moreau R, Durand F, Poynard T, et al. Terlipressin in patients with cirrhosis and type 1 hepatorenal syndrome: A retrospective multicenter study. Gastroenterology. 2002;122:923–930.

Ortega R, Gines P, Uriz J, et al: Terlipressin therapy with and without albumin for patients with hepatorenal syndrome: Results of a prospective, nonrandomized study. Hepatology 2002;36:941.

Ruiz-del-Arbol L, Urman J, Fernandez J, et al: Systemic, renal, and hepatic hemodynamic derangement in cirrhotic patients with spontaneous bacterial peritonitis. Hepatology 2003;38:1210–1218.

Schrier RW, Arroyo V, Bernardi M, et al: Peripheral arterial vasodilation hypothesis: A proposal for the initiation of renal sodium and water retention in cirrhosis. Hepatology 1988;8:1151–1157.

Chapter 45

Acute Endocrine Disorders

Yves Debaveye, Björn Ellger, and Greet Van den Berghe

Endocrine and metabolic adaptations to acute severe stress are essential for survival. Diseases of the endocrine system are commonly encountered in the intensive care unit (ICU) and can severely impair recovery from illness. Because early recognition and initiation of adequate treatment are crucial, ICU clinicians should be familiar with the presentation of a variety of acute endocrine disorders. This chapter focuses on the emergency management of the most frequent life-threatening endocrine disorders.

LIFE-THREATENING THYROTOXICOSIS: THYROID STORM

Thyrotoxicosis is the hypermetabolic state that results from increased levels of circulating thyroid hormone (Box 45.1). In the ICU setting, of greatest concern is thyroid storm (TS), a life-threatening decompensation of hyperthyroidism that develops in a setting of untreated or undertreated hyperthyroidism.

Clinical Features and Diagnosis

TS is characterized by an acute onset of severe symptoms of hyperthyroidism and is frequently triggered by precipitating events, including infections, (thyroid) surgery, withdrawal of antithyroid drugs, radioiodine therapy or iodinated radiocontrast dyes, trauma, and labor and delivery. It is important to recognize that TS remains a clinical diagnosis since thyroid function tests do not distinguish between symptomatic hyperthyroidism and TS. Because TS carries a mortality of 10% to 75%, early recognition and initiation of adequate therapy are crucial.

The clinical hallmarks of TS include severe thermoregulatory dysfunction (fever > 38.5°C), sinus or supraventricular tachycardia (out of proportion to the fever), congestive heart failure, gastrointestinal symptoms (nausea, vomiting, diarrhea, and, rarely, jaundice), and mental status changes (confusion, delirium, and coma). Thyroid function tests reveal undetectable thyroid-stimulating hormone (TSH) (<0.001 mU/L) and elevated total and free T4 and T3 levels. Typically, the increase of T3 is more dramatically pronounced than that of T4 due to concomitant enhanced peripheral thyroid hormone conversion of T4 to T3. Because of the high risk of concurrent adrenal insuf-

---

Box 45.1 Causes of Thyrotoxicosis

Endogenous Hyperthyroidism

Graves' disease
Toxic multinodular goiter
Toxic autonomous nodule
Thyroiditis (transient thyrotoxicosis)
    Subacute (granulomatous) thyroiditis
    Acute (bacterial) thyroiditis
    Postpartum thyroiditis
    Painless thyroiditis
    Riedel's thyroiditis
Struma ovarii
Iodine-induced hyperthyroidism
    Medications (iodinated radiocontrast dyes, amiodarone, antiseptic dressings)
    Postradioiodine thyroiditis
    Dietary supplements (e.g., kelp)
TSH-mediated
    Pituitary tumors
    Pituitary resistance to TSH
Metastatic follicular thyroid cancer

Exogenous Thyrotoxicosis

Iatrogenic thyrotoxicosis
Factitious use of thyroid hormone
Dietary supplements containing thyroid hormone

ficiency and the common use of corticosteroids in the acute management of TS, it is advisable to obtain a serum sample for measurement of circulating cortisol before initiation of therapy.

Treatment

The treatment of TS is complex and generally requires intensive care monitoring. The therapeutic endeavors may be grouped as follows: (1) interventions to decrease thyroid hormone synthesis and release, (2) strategies to reduce peripheral effects of thyroid hormone, (3) treatment to prevent systemic decompensation, (4) cure of the precipitating illness, and (5) definitive cure of the underlying thyroid dysfunction (Box 45.2 and Fig. 45.1).

A nearly complete and rapid blockage of de novo thyroid hormone synthesis is achieved by the thionamide drugs propylthiouracil (PTU) and methimazole (MMI). These agents are not available for parenteral administration and are therefore given orally or by nasogastric tube. Due to the substantial mortality associated with TS and the possibly concurrent gastrointestinal dysfunction, high doses are appropriate. PTU is the first-line thionamide because it supplementally blocks peripheral conversion of T4 to T3. However, using the more potent drug MMI in combination with other drugs that block the T4-to-T3 conversion is an alternative.

Blocking the release of thyroid hormone from stores in the colloid is achieved by iodine and lithium carbonate. The iodine preparation of choice is the oral contrast agent iopanoic acid. It has an extremely high iodine content and inhibits thyroid hormone release as well as T4-to-T3 conversion. Iodine administration should be delayed until at least 1 hour after thionamide administration in order to prevent iodine-induced thyroid hormone synthesis. Use of lithium is limited by its renal and neurologic toxicity and should only be considered in patients with contraindications for iodine and thionamide.

Beta blockers play a major role in the symptomatic antiadrenergic treatment of TS, although known contraindications of beta blockers are to be taken into account. Propanolol is used most frequently because it also suppresses peripheral thyroid hormone conversion. Reserpine and guanethidine can also be used as antiadrenergic agents, but these are a second choice after beta blockers because of side effects.

Glucocorticoids also play a major role in therapy of TS. They reduce T4-to-T3 conversion, may have a direct effect on the underlying autoimmune process of Graves' disease, and apparently improve outcome. Cholestyramine binds to thyroid hormones in the gastrointestinal tract, resulting in a modest reduction of circulating thyroid hormone levels. Hemodialysis, plasmapheresis, and charcoal hemoperfusion should be considered only if progression occurs despite aggressive therapy.

Hyperthermia must be treated aggressively with antipyretics and peripheral cooling. Acetaminophen is the first-choice antipyretic agent since salicylates displace thyroid hormone from serum binding sites, increasing bioavailability. Gastrointestinal and insensible fluid losses can be immense in TS and should be adequately replaced to prevent cardiovascular collapse. Because of rapid depletion of hepatic glycogen stores during TS, IV fluids containing 5% to 10% glucose should be used to avoid hypoglycemia in addition to the required electrolytes. Thiamine supplements are advisable to replace a possible concomitant deficiency. For patients with underlying

---

Box 45.2 Treatment of Thyroid Storm

Interventions to Decrease Thyroid Hormone Synthesis and Release

Inhibition of new hormone synthesis
Propylthiouracil (PTU): load 600–1000 mg, then 200–300 mg po q4–6 hr
Methimazole: load 60–100 mg, then 20–30 mg po q6–8 hr
Inhibition of thyroid hormone release
Inorganic iodine
Saturated solution of potassium iodide: 5 drops (250 mg) po q6–12 hr
Lugol's solution: 4–8 drops po q6 hr
Iopanoic acid: 1 g q8 hr on day 1, then 500 mg po q12 hr
Lithium carbonate: 300 mg po q6 hr (serum level <1 mEq/L)
Inhibition of T4 to T3 conversion
PTU
Corticosteroids: hydrocortisone 100 mg IV q6–8 hr (or equivalent)
Propanolol
Iopanoic acid

Strategies to Reduce Peripheral Effects of Thyroid Hormone

Beta-adrenergic blockade
    Propanolol: 0.5–1.0 mg IV q2–3 hr or 40–80 mg po q4–8 hr
    Esmolol: load 250–500 µg/kg, then 50–100 µg/kg/min IV
Corticosteroids
Reserpine: 2.5–5 mg IM q4 hr
Guanethidine: 30–40 mg po q4 hr
Removal of excess circulating thyroid hormone
    Gastrointestinal clearance
        Cholestyramine
    Blood clearance
        Hemodialysis
        Hemoperfusion
        Plasmapheresis

Prevention of Systemic Decompensation

Treatment of hyperkinesis: benzodiazepines, barbiturates
Antipyretics (acetaminophen)
Cooling
Correction of dehydration
Nutrition, vitamins
Oxygen, mechanical ventilation
Treatment of congestive heart failure

Cure of Precipitating Illness

Etiology-dependent therapy

Definitive Cure of the Thyroid Dysfunction

Standard medical therapy
Radioactive iodine
Surgical thyroidectomy

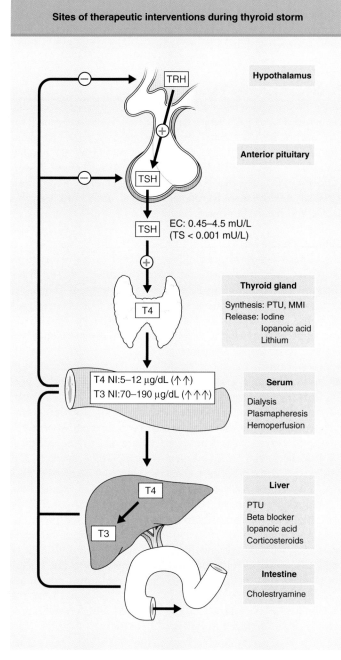

Sites of therapeutic interventions during thyroid storm

Figure 45.1. Sites of therapeutic interventions during thyroid storm. The potential sites of therapeutic interventions on the hypothalamic–pituitary–thyroid axis during thyroid storm. Serum values of T4, T3, and TSH are given for euthyroid conditions (EC) and during thyroid storm (TS; in parentheses). MMI, methimazole; PTU, propylthiouracil; TRH, thyrotropin-releasing hormone; TSH, thyroid-stimulating hormone.

cardiac disease, invasive monitoring is necessary. When sedation is required, phenobarbital may be preferred over benzodiazepines in the setting of TS because it stimulates hepatic clearance of thyroid hormone.

In most patients, clinical improvement is expected within the first 12 to 24 hours of adequate therapy. Once the acute event is controlled, long-term control of hyperthyroidism should be addressed. Note that the use of iodine in the emer-

gency management of TS will necessitate an appropriate delay before institution of radioactive iodine therapy, should this be required.

CRITICAL HYPOTHYROIDISM: MYXEDEMA COMA

Myxedema coma represents the most exaggerated form of thyroid hormone deficiency and is again often triggered by precipitating factors. Although it is indeed a clinical state of critical hypothyroidism, the term is often a misnomer since most patients with severe hypothyroidism reveal neither myxedema nor a comatose state. Instead, critical hypothyroidism is characterized by progressive parallel dysfunction of the cardiovascular, respiratory, and central nervous systems. If not recognized rapidly and treated adequately, myxedema coma may carry a 60% risk of mortality.

Clinical Features and Diagnosis

Myxedema coma is classically encountered in patients, mostly elderly, who have a known history of hypothyroidism. The diagnosis is based on the presence of three key diagnostic features: altered mental status, defective thermoregulation, and a precipitating illness or event. Altered mental status is revealed as disorientation, lethargy, frank psychosis, and, rarely, coma. Additional neurological features include seizures and delayed reflex relaxation. Defective thermoregulation may be expressed by either absolute or relative hypothermia. An example of the latter would be a septic patient with an inappropriately normal body temperature. Hypothermia in the absence of shivering is also indicative of the diagnosis. The presence of one or more precipitating factors is the final cardinal clinical feature (Box 45.3). Of all events listed, pulmonary or urinary infection should be considered as the presumptive cause until proven otherwise. In this regard, it is important to note that severe hypothyroidism blunts the normal leukocyte response to infection so that even a small alteration in infectious parameters must be considered

---

Box 45.3 Factors Precipitating Myxedema Coma

Severe infection, sepsis
Surgery
Trauma
Myocardial infarction
Cerebrovascular accident
Gastrointestinal bleeding
Cold exposure
CO_2 narcosis
Medication
    Analgesics
    Sedatives
    Tranquilizers
    Anesthetics
    Amiodarone
    Lithium carbonate
    Narcotics
    Diuretics
    Beta blockers

as highly suspicious for sepsis. Additional clinical features include bradycardia, hypotension, hypoventilation, constipation, paralytic ileus, megacolon, and bladder atony.

The clinical diagnosis requires confirmation by low or undetectable serum levels of T4 and T3. TSH levels are usually elevated, but they may be normal (or even low) in the case of hypothalamic–pituitary disease or advanced critical illness (e.g., nonthyroidal illness). Because the degree of abnormality of the thyroid function tests does not correlate with the level of consciousness, rapid treatment must be instituted on the basis of clinical suspicion without awaiting laboratory confirmation. Additional laboratory hallmarks include hyponatremia, hypoglycemia, and normocytic anemia.

Treatment

The treatment of myxedema coma includes (1) general supportive measures, (2) treatment of metabolic complications and infections, and (3) thyroid hormone replacement. The overall goal is to resuscitate and stabilize the patient in the first 24 to 48 hours, the time required for thyroid hormone therapy to start reversing the underlying metabolic state of hypothyroidism.

Importantly, ventilatory support is indicated at the first sign of respiratory failure, and hemodynamic deterioration must be treated aggressively. Since vasopressors in combination with thyroid hormone preparations may induce severe arrhythmias, they should be used only with extreme caution. Passive rewarming with blankets is preferred to active warming because the latter induces peripheral vasodilation and may thus precipitate cardiovascular collapse. Until coexisting adrenal insufficiency is excluded, every patient should be treated concomitantly with glucocorticoids in stress doses, after taking the necessary blood samples for later confirmation of the diagnosis.

Since a bacterial infection is the most probable event precipitating myxedema coma, all patients must be screened and empirically treated with broad-spectrum IV antibiotics until culture results are reported. Monitoring and treatment of hyponatremia must be considered. However, since hyponatremia in hypothyroidism is mediated by antidiuretic hormone (ADH), the restoration of free water clearance with thyroid hormone treatment usually suffices to normalize sodium levels. Importantly, hypoglycemia, which is seen more often in secondary than in primary hypothyroidism, should be treated with IV glucose infusion. Seizures should be treated with standard anticonvulsants after correction of hyponatremia, hypoglycemia, and hypoxia.

There is controversy regarding the optimal mode of initiating thyroid hormone therapy in myxedema coma, particularly with regard to drug selection and dosing. It is generally agreed that patients should be treated with a parenteral form of thyroid hormone. Many clinicians prefer a loading dose of up to 300 to 500 µg IV T4 in order to quickly restore circulating levels of T4 to approximately 50% of the euthyroid value, followed by 50 to 100 µg of IV T4 daily until oral medication can be given. The administration of T3 may be useful because of its greater biologic activity and the inability of the body to convert T4 into T3 during severe hypothyroidism. Because T3 has the potential to induce myocardial infarction and arrhythmias, monotherapy is not recommended. We prefer the combination of T4 and T3, using a loading dose of T4 (200–300 µg IV bolus) and T3 (5–20 µg slow IV injection) followed by a maintenance dose of

T4 (50–100 µg bolus daily) and T3 (7.5–30 µg per day via continuous IV infusion) until oral therapy is initiated. During the treatment of myxedema coma, hemodynamics and diuresis typically improve within 24 hours, whereas the restoration of body temperature takes 2 or 3 days.

PHEOCHROMOCYTOMA

Pheochromocytoma is a rare catecholamine-secreting neoplasm that occurs in less than 0.2% of patients with hypertension. Pheochromocytoma is also known to occur in certain familial syndromes (e.g., multiple endocrine neoplasia type 2, von Hippel–Lindau disease, and von Recklinghausen's neurofibromatosis) and other endocrinopathies (e.g., ACTH-excess syndrome and hyperparathyroidism).

Clinical Features

The clinical manifestations of pheochromocytoma result from excessive catecholamine secretion by the tumor, either intermittently or continuously, and thus are highly protean. The most common set of symptoms comprises attacks of headache, palpitations, and diaphoresis (Table 45.1). Although this classic triad has a high specificity of 94%, most patients show only two of these three classic symptoms.

Upon admission to the ICU, the clinical picture is dominated by endocrine and metabolic consequences such as hyperglycemia, hypercalcemia, and lactic acidosis; by surgical complications such as acute abdomen; by cardiovascular symptoms such as shock, myocarditis, dilatative cardiomyopathy, arrhythmias, pulmonary edema, and heart failure; and by neurological consequences such as altered mental status, stroke, seizures, and focal neurological pathology. Diagnosis thus is often missed. Features that should raise suspicion of pheochromocytoma include a paradoxical response to antihypertensive therapy, particularly beta blockers or guanethidine, a hypertensive response to anesthesia, naloxone, metoclopramide, thyrotropin-releasing hormone (when used as a diagnostic agent), tricyclic antidepressants, glucagon, and micturation or pregnancy. The differential diagnosis, including other clinical conditions associated with increased plasma catecholamine and urinary catecholamine metabolites in the range of those observed with pheochromocytoma, is summarized in Box 45.4.

Table 45.1 Common Clinical Manifestations of Pheochromocytoma	
Manifestation	**%**
Severe headache	80
Palpitations	60
Diaphoresis	60
Tremulousness	50
Anxiety	50
Hypertension	
Paroxysmal	50
Sustained	30
Orthostatic hypotension	40
Weight loss	30
No symptoms	8

Diagnosis

Diagnosis of pheochromocytoma is based on documenting catecholamine overproduction by measuring plasma catecholamine concentrations and urinary levels of total metanephrine, vanillylmandelic acid, and norepinephrine. Repeated testing is recommended because trade-offs between test sensitivity and specificity are a recurrent problem. This could lead to a false-positive diagnosis in the case of catecholamine secretion secondary to stress. After pheochromocytoma has been confirmed by biochemical testing, the next step is magnetic resonance imaging (MRI) in order to confirm the diagnosis and localize the tumor (Fig. 45.2). If MRI fails to localize the tumor, a meta-iodobenzylguanidine scan is helpful. An octreotide scan, arteriography, and vena cava sampling are rarely indicated. Finally, provocative tests carry a high risk of complications and thus are not recommended.

Treatment

Resection is the only definitive treatment for pheochromocytoma. The perioperative management should be orchestrated in order to prevent hypertensive crises and associated complications and also to reduce the incidence and severity of postoperative hypotension. However, the exact choice of drugs remains controversial. Phenoxybenzamine (POB), a long-acting nonspecific alpha blocker, is most widely recommended. The initial dose of 10 mg po twice a day should be increased every other day, usually up to 20 to 40 mg two or three times daily until the patient's blood pressure and other symptoms are under control. A beta blocker is indicated in order to overcome reflex tachycardia only after adequate alpha blockade, since it otherwise may precipitate a hypertensive crisis. Because of the adverse effects of nonspecific, prolonged alpha blockade, POB is now often replaced by selective α_1 blockers, such as prazosin, terazosin, and doxazosin. As an alternative approach, calcium channel blockers can be used to control blood pressure and other adrenergic symptoms.

To treat acute hypertensive crises, nitroprusside (0.5–10 µg/kg/min IV, not to exceed 800 µg/min) or phentolamine (5–15 mg IV), administered by continuous infusion, are the drugs of choice. If tachycardia or tachyarrhythmia is prominent, concomitant administration of a beta blocker (esmolol, 50–200 µg/kg/min IV) or lidocaine (50–100 mg IV) is indicated.

Adequate fluid replacement is crucial to avoid postoperative hypotension, keeping in mind that pheochromocytoma patients frequently require large amounts of volume after tumor resection. Additionally, stress doses of glucocorticoids should be administered if bilateral adrenalectomy is planned. Since the inhibitory effect of catecholamines on insulin secretion is suddenly removed after surgery, hypoglycemia occurs in up to 15% of patients. Be aware that beta blockers may mask the clinical manifestations of hypoglycemia; hence, all patients should be monitored for blood glucose levels for at least 48 hours postoperatively.

HYPERGLYCEMIA, KETOACIDOSIS, AND NONKETOTIC HYPERGLYCEMIA

Pathogenesis

Hyperglycemia often occurs in diabetic patients with poor treatment compliance. Severe hyperglycemia in diabetes mellitus, however, is most frequently induced by precipitating events such as overeating, use or abuse of drugs, trauma, infections, and severe illness. In the latter three, a physiological stress reaction is evoked by the release of catecholamines, cortisol, inflammatory cytokines, growth hormone, and glucagon. This jointly leads to insulin resistance, increased gluconeogenesis, glycogenolysis, and relatively insufficient pancreatic insulin production, leading to increased blood and low intracellular glucose levels in insulin-dependent tissues. In adipose tissue, this lack of intracellular fuel supply induces lipolysis, resulting in an increased release of free fatty acids. These are metabolized by the hepatocytes into ketones, which are responsible for the clinical picture of ketoaci-

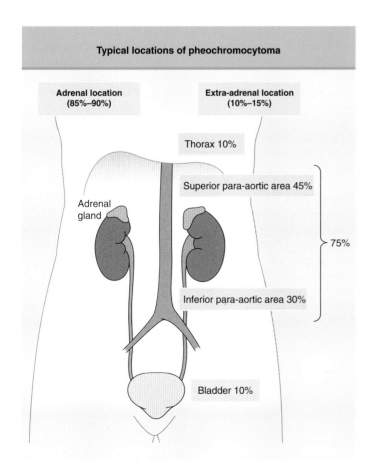

Typical locations of pheochromocytoma

Adrenal location (85%–90%)

Extra-adrenal location (10%–15%)

Thorax 10%

Superior para-aortic area 45%

Adrenal gland

Inferior para-aortic area 30%

75%

Bladder 10%

Figure 45.2. Typical locations of pheochromocytoma.

dotic hyperglycemia (KAH) in diabetic (type 1) patients. Moreover, profound insulin resistance in the liver and muscle cells further increases blood glucose through gluconeogenesis. In situations in which plasma insulin levels are high enough to prevent lipolysis but insufficient to ensure cellular glucose uptake, blood glucose level may slowly exceed 1000 mg/dL without noteworthy ketosis. When the reabsorption capacity of the kidneys (±180 mg/dL) is exceeded, glucosuria occurs, leading to osmotic diuresis, electrolyte loss, and severe hyperosmolar dehydration. This is the main mechanism behind the neurologic symptoms and complications in nonketotic hyperglycemia (NKH).

Clinical Features

Besides evidence of an underlying precipitating event, early clinical signs of hyperglycemia include polyurea, polydypsia, and weight loss. Patients frequently complain of nausea, vomiting, or abdominal pain. Symptoms of dehydration vary from dry mucosa to decreased skin turgor and hypovolemic shock. KAH patients often reveal the typical fruity odor of ketosis and Kussmaul respiration to compensate for the metabolic acidosis by respiration. Neurological alterations become obvious when plasma osmolarity rises above 320 mOsmol/kg.

Diagnosis

Hyperglycemia is diagnosed whenever fasting blood glucose levels exceed 110 mg/dL or a random blood glucose level exceeds 150 mg/dL. When this coincides with hyperosmolarity, severe electrolyte disorders, and dehydration, the patient is at risk of cardiac malfunction.

Diagnostic criteria to differentiate KAH from NKH are discussed in Chapter 46. To diagnose complications or underlying precipitating diseases, electrocardiogram, bacteriological investigations, and chest x-ray are required.

Treatment

Shock and respiratory distress require resuscitation, mechanical ventilation, and extended monitoring. Most important, fluid replacement with saline solution should be promptly initiated. The fluid deficit is typically 4 to 10 L and thus about 2 L should be infused in the first hour, followed by several hours of 1 L per hour in adult patients. In the case of pronounced hypovolemia with hemodynamic instability, the amount of fluids during the first hours may be even higher. The target of the aggressive fluid therapy is to compensate for the presumed fluid loss within a time frame of 24 hours. To decrease the blood glucose level, insulin is started in a continuous IV infusion of 0.1 IU/kg/hr after a bolus of 0.15 IU/kg IV. The use of a bolus is not recommended in states of hypokalemia, however. The rate of insulin infusion should be adjusted by at least hourly measurements in order to achieve a decrease of blood glucose of approximately 100 mg/dL per hour. Once blood glucose level reaches 250 mg/dL, the decrease in glucose levels should be slowed in order to prevent cerebral edema caused by a rapid change in osmotic gradient. The goal is to achieve a normalized glucose level (80–110 mg/dL) within 24 hours. As soon as normoglycemia is reached in a diabetic ketoacidosis patient, IV infusion should be switched to glucose 10%, with the insulin dose continued until ketones become negative. In all type 1 diabetic patients, a maintenance dose of insulin should be continued at all times. Acid status and electrolytes, mainly potassium and

sodium, must also be monitored frequently and corrected if necessary. Acidosis and other symptoms should disappear within hours after initiation of therapy. Meanwhile, the therapy of a potential underlying disease should not be forgotten.

Complications

KAH carries a mortality of 1% to 10% and NKH of 14% to 58%, depending on severity of the derangements. In cases of severe dehydration, myocardial ischemia and kidney failure are frequently encountered. Respiratory distress may occur due to embolism or pulmonary edema. Mainly in younger patients, brain edema, induced by a rapid change in plasma osmolarity, is a major concern.

Hyperglycemia in Critically Ill Patients

Hyperglycemia is uniformly present in critically ill patients independent of the underlying disease or a history of diabetes. The immediate adjustment of normoglycemic levels of 80 to 110 mg/dL in fed conditions by intensive intravenous insulin therapy is crucial. With this intervention, it is possible to reduce the overall mortality of ICU patients by 40%, mainly due to a reduced incidence of infectious complications and multiple organ dysfunction.

HYPOGLYCEMIA

Pathophysiology

Hypoglycemia occurs in patients with diabetes mellitus when insulin or oral antidiabetic drugs are overdosed and/or after inadequate feeding. Hepatic dysfunction, alcohol intoxication, an insulin-producing tumor (insulinoma), and excessive fasting are less frequent causes. Because the central nervous system is unable to generate glucose, severe neurological dysfunction may occur. Counterregulatory loops mediated by glucagon, cortisol, and catecholamines are initiated in an attempt to antagonize insulin effects, suppress insulin secretion, and stimulate gluconeogenesis and glycogenolysis. As in diabetic patients or patients undergoing certain medicinal treatments (e.g., beta blockers), those regulation loops may be altered, and severe complications can result.

Clinical Features

Neuronal fuel deficiency results in neurologic symptoms such as confusion, drowsiness, difficulty with speech and vision, hemiplegia (Todd's palsy), seizures, and, ultimately, coma. Sweating, palpitations, tremor, and hunger reflect functional counterregulation.

Diagnosis

Hypoglycemia is generally defined arbitrarily as a blood glucose level below 50 mg/dL (2.8 mmol/L) with neuroglycopenic symptoms or below 40 mg/dL (2.2 mmol/L) in the absence of symptoms. Clinically significant hypoglycemia is characterized by Whipple's triad: symptoms of neuroglycopenia, simultaneous blood glucose lower than 40 mg/dL (2.2 mmol/L), and relief of symptoms with the administration of glucose. This blood glucose cutoff corresponds to a plasma glucose level of 45 mg/dL (2.5 mmol/L). All three criteria should be met to establish a diagnosis of hypoglycemia, at least outside the ICU, because a precipitous fall from hyperglycemia to euglycemia in diabetes can produce hypoglycemic symptoms, and because asymptomatic hypoglycemia with glucose levels as low as 30 mg/dL (1.7 mmol/L) can occur during fasting in normal women and during pregnancy. In the ICU, however, sedation may mask symptoms of neuroglycopenia, and counterregulatory responses may be impaired, which complicates the diagnosis of hypoglycemia in this setting. Furthermore, asymptomatic patients may have artifactual hypoglycemia due to in vitro consumption of glucose by blood cell elements.

A blood sample for HbA1c, insulin, and C-peptide should be taken before glucose administration for adequate differential diagnosis (e.g., insulinoma).

Treatment

In conscious patients, the oral application of 20 g glucose (e.g., glucose tablets or juice) is recommended. If oral intake is impossible, IV administration of 10 to 25 g glucose is sufficient to cure symptoms within minutes. Special care must be taken when the hypoglycemia is caused by oral antidiabetic drugs because they may induce a more pronounced organ dysfunction due to their long-lasting action. In such cases, as well as with excessive fasting or if insulinoma is suspected, a continuous glucose infusion must be started and adjusted by frequent glucose measurement. Parenteral glucagon (1 mg IM) is also an effective therapy, but patients with depleted glycogen stores or alcohol intoxication may not respond.

Complications

Cerebral edema must be expected when unconsciousness lasts longer than 30 minutes after normalization of blood glucose. In these cases, steroids, diuretics, and mannitol may be considered. If hypoglycemia is severe and prolonged, it can lead to severe permanent disability or death.

ACUTE ADRENAL CRISIS

Pathogenesis

Acute adrenal insufficiency (AI) occurs when the adrenal glands are not able to cope with the body's current physiological needs. This can be due either to an acute manifestation of a chronic process or to the acute onset of a new pathology. In both conditions, the secretory inability leads to a deficiency of the steroid hormones glucocorticoids, mineralocorticoids, and androgens. The former two are of importance in acute crisis.

Glucocorticoids are crucial for homeostasis within the immune and cardiovascular systems and for carbohydrate metabolism. Mineralocorticoids play a predominant role in water and electrolyte balance through regulation of renal fluid and sodium reabsorption and potassium excretion (Figs. 45.3 and 45.4).

Functionally, underlying reasons for acute adrenal crisis can be divided into primary and secondary AI (Fig. 45.5). Mainly in patients undergoing chronic glucocorticoid treatment who are

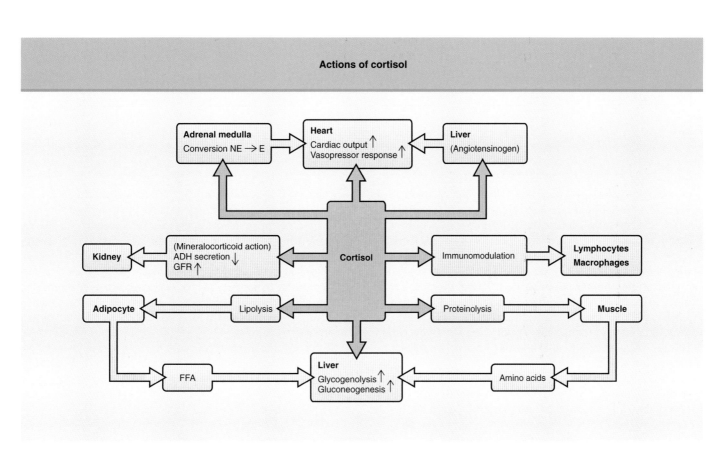

Figure 45.3. Actions of cortisol. Schematic overview of cortisol action. Actions in parentheses are only induced by higher cortisol levels. ADH, antidiuretic hormone; E, epinephrine; FFA, free fatty acids; GFR, glomerular filtration rate; NE, norepinephrine.

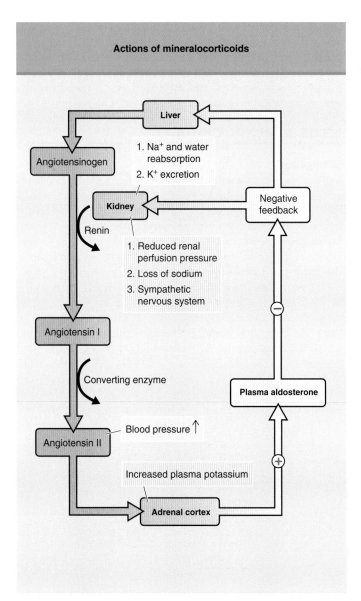

Figure 45.4. Actions of mineralocorticoids. Schematic illustration of mineralocorticoid action. Note that glucocorticoids at high doses also possess mineralocorticoid properties. Stimuli of the cascade are shown in orange and the resultant effects in green.

Actions of mineralocorticoids

Liver

Angiotensinogen

1. Na$^+$ and water reabsorption
2. K$^+$ excretion

Kidney

Renin

1. Reduced renal perfusion pressure
2. Loss of sodium
3. Sympathetic nervous system

Negative feedback

Angiotensin I

Converting enzyme

Plasma aldosterone

Angiotensin II

Blood pressure ↑

Increased plasma potassium

Adrenal cortex

subjected to major stress, such as a febrile illness, trauma, or surgery, adrenal hormone production may become insufficient to meet the current elevated needs. Additionally, rapid withdrawal of glucocorticoid treatment can evoke an adrenal crisis.

Clinical Features

The clinical presentation is dominated by dehydration, fever, myalgia, joint or back pain, and nonspecific neurological (from weakness to coma) and gastrointestinal (diarrhea, vomiting, and abdominal pain) symptoms. This can develop slowly over days or acutely, leading to potential life-threatening hemodynamic instability and shock.

In a critically ill patient, the clinical presentation of an adrenal crisis may mimic that of septic shock with vasoplegia, hypotension, and relatively impaired cardiac output, oliguria and vasopressor dependency, or even total resistance to vasopressors.

Diagnosis

Hemodynamic alterations, caused by a decrease in vascular resistance accompanying a normal cardiac function, and therapy-resistant shock may raise suspicion for the diagnosis of acute AI. Indeed, in the absence of glucocorticoids, large amounts of fluid and high doses of catecholamines may be inadequate to reverse shock. Further diagnostic hints arise from a history of glucocorticoid treatment, the presence of chronic infections, the use of anticoagulants, or known hypoadrenalism. Suspicion is increased when hyponatremia, increased serum potassium, and eosinophilia are present. The blood glucose level in adrenal crisis is usually low, but it can rise dramatically after initiation of glucocorticoid treatment.

To confirm the diagnosis of acute AI, blood tests are required, followed by imaging modalities to visualize lesions, infarctions, or bleeding in the hypothalamus, pituitary, or adrenal glands. Whenever a diagnosis is suspected, a blood sample should be drawn for plasma cortisol and corticotropin (or ACTH), and a short ACTH (250 μg IV) stimulation test should be performed before administration of glucocorticoids. A baseline cortisol level below 3 μg/dL (83 nmol/L) confirms the diagnosis of AI. Patients with primary AI do not respond to exogenous ACTH and have plasma ACTH concentrations that invariably exceed

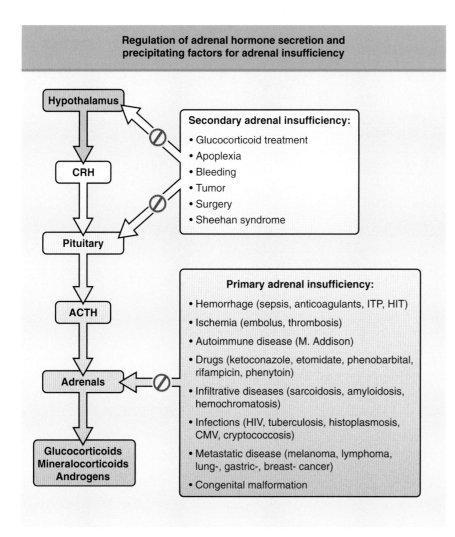

Regulation of adrenal hormone secretion and precipitating factors for adrenal insufficiency

Secondary adrenal insufficiency:
- Glucocorticoid treatment
- Apoplexia
- Bleeding
- Tumor
- Surgery
- Sheehan syndrome

Primary adrenal insufficiency:
- Hemorrhage (sepsis, anticoagulants, ITP, HIT)
- Ischemia (embolus, thrombosis)
- Autoimmune disease (M. Addison)
- Drugs (ketoconazole, etomidate, phenobarbital, rifampicin, phenytoin)
- Infiltrative diseases (sarcoidosis, amyloidosis, hemochromatosis)
- Infections (HIV, tuberculosis, histoplasmosis, CMV, cryptococcosis)
- Metastatic disease (melanoma, lymphoma, lung-, gastric-, breast- cancer)
- Congenital malformation

Hypothalamus → CRH → Pituitary → ACTH → Adrenals → Glucocorticoids / Mineralocorticoids / Androgens

Figure 45.5. Regulation of adrenal hormone secretion and precipitating factors for adrenal insufficiency. ACTH, adrenocorticotropic hormone; CMV, cytomegalovirus; CRH, corticotropin-releasing hormone; HIT, heparin-induced thrombocytopenia; ITP, idiopathic thrombocytopenic purpura.

100 pg/mL (22 pmol/L). In secondary AI, plasma cortisol increases after administration of ACTH, but this increase may be minor or even absent due to adrenocortical atrophy.

However, in critically ill patients with septic shock, the concept of "relative adrenal insufficiency" may complicate the diagnosis. In relative AI, plasma cortisol levels, despite being high in absolute terms (mostly > 15 µg/dL or 414 nmol/L), are insufficient to control the inflammatory response. Although controversial, the short ACTH test is advisable since an increase in plasma cortisol of less than 9 µg/dL (250 nmol/L) is associated with an increased risk of death.

Treatment

Acute adrenal failure is a life-threatening event accompanied by severe hemodynamic alterations. Therapy must be started before laboratory or diagnostic imaging results are available. The first line of therapy is rapid administration of saline solution— at least 3 liters for an adult—to correct fluid and sodium deficiency. The second line comprises administration of 100 to 200 mg IV bolus hydrocortisone followed by 50 to 100 mg every 6 hours on the first day, 50 mg every 6 hours on the second day, and 25 mg every 6 hours on the third day, tapering to a maintenance dose of approximately 12 to 15 mg hydrocortisone/m² by the fourth or fifth day. If the patient remains critically ill due to underlying disease, the dose should be maintained at two or three times the normal maintenance dose for as long as the critical state persists. During therapy, potassium and glucose levels must be carefully monitored and corrected.

Patients who are under chronic corticoid therapy or have a known AI require additional glucocorticoids when they undergo stressful procedures or suffer from a significant medical illness (Fig. 45.6).

Special attention should be paid to patients with concomitant diabetes insipidus because lack of cortisol prevents polyuria since cortisol is needed for free water clearance. Hence, glucocorticoid therapy may induce or aggravate diabetes insipidus in these patients. Another specific condition is the posthypophysectomy phase of Cushing's disease, characterized by a high vulnerability to Addison-like crisis. Drugs such as phenytoin, barbiturates, and rifampicin can accelerate glucocorticoid metabolism by induction of microsomal enzyme activity and can increase the glucocorticoid replacement dose requirement. If this increased requirement is not met, adrenal crisis may occur.

Complications

If the diagnosis of acute AI is overlooked, severe life-threatening shock, not responding to catecholamines and fluid resuscitation, may result. On the other hand, if the diagnosis is appropriate and adequate treatment is initiated promptly, acute

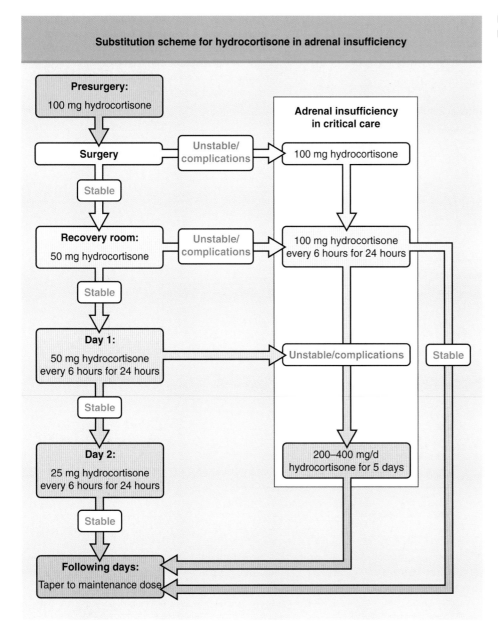

Figure 45.6. Substitution scheme for hydrocortisone in adrenal insufficiency.

AI has no major additional impact on the morbidity and mortality of the underlying disease.

SUGGESTED READING

Bravo E: Evolving concepts in the pathophysiology, diagnosis, and treatment of pheochromocytoma. Endocr Rev 1994;15:356–368.

Bravo E, Tagle R: Pheochromocytoma: State-of-the-art and future prospects. Endocr Rev 2003;24:539–553.

Burch H, Wartofsky L: Life-threatening thyrotoxicosis. Thyroid storm. Endocrinol Metab Clin North Am 1993;22:263–277.

Cooper M, Stewart P: Corticosteroid insufficiency in acutely ill patients. N Engl J Med 2003;348:727–734.

Kitabchi A, Umpierrez G, Murphy M, et al: Hyperglycemic crises in diabetes. Diabetes Care 2004;27:S94–S102.

Nicoloff J, LoPresti J: Myxedema coma. A form of decompensated hypothyroidism. Endocrinol Metab Clin North Am 1993;22:279–290.

Oelkers W: Adrenal insufficiency. N Engl J Med 1996;335:1206–1212.

Ringel M: Management of hypothyroidism and hyperthyroidism in the intensive care unit. Crit Care Clin 2001;17:59–74.

Shakir K, Amin R: Endocrine crises. Hypoglycemia. Crit Care Clin 1991;7:75–87.

Van den Berghe G, Wouters P, Weekers F, et al: Intensive insulin therapy in critically ill patients. N Engl J Med 2001;345:1359–1367.

Chapter 46

Diabetic Ketoacidosis and Hyperosmolar Nonketotic Coma

Ken Hillman

KEY POINTS

- Rapid correction of airway, breathing, and circulation.
- Slow correction of blood glucose with IV insulin infusion according to regularly measured levels, not inflexible formulae.
- Replacement of electrolytes and fluids according to regular measurement and assessment.
- Exclude reversible course of diabetic ketoacidosis (DKA) and hyperosmolar nonketotic coma (HONC), such as infection.
- Patient education is crucial for the prevention of DKA and HONC.

Diabetes is becoming more common throughout the Western world. This trend will continue as diabetics become better controlled, live longer, and their gene pool becomes larger. Diabetic ketoacidosis (DKA) and hyperosmolar nonketotic coma (HONC) are acute life-threatening presentations of a decompensated chronic disease. Both feature serious metabolic disturbances as well as abnormalities of vital cardiorespiratory function. Rapid resuscitation and careful correction of metabolic disturbances are required.

EPIDEMIOLOGY, RISK FACTORS, AND PATHOPHYSIOLOGY

Epidemiology

Diabetic ketoacidosis is the most common cause of mortality in individuals with type I diabetes younger than age 40 years. Both DKA and HONC can occur in either type I or type II diabetes. Mortality for DKA remains between 0% and 9% and for HONC between 36% and 46%. The annual incidence of DKA is increasing; it ranges between 4.6 and 8 episodes per 1000 diabetic patients and accounts for 4% to 9% of all hospital discharges.

Risk Factors

Although infection is commonly cited as being the major precipitating factor of DKA, inadequate insulin treatment and noncompliance are probably more common (Box 46.1). This becomes important when considering patient education strategies. Up to 20% of patients may present to the emergency department (ED) without a previous diagnosis of diabetes. The most common precipitating infections are pneumonia and urinary tract infection. Drugs, myocardial infarction (MI), trauma, alcohol abuse, cerebrovascular accidents (CVAs), pulmonary embolism (PE), and pancreatitis can also precipitate DKA and HONC. Insulin resistance as a result of endocrine diseases such as Cushing's syndrome, acromegaly, and thyrotoxicosis can also result in HONC and DKA.

Pathogenesis

Intermediary Metabolism

Fat, liver, and muscle cells are particularly insulin sensitive and are the key to the production of hyperglycemia and ketosis in DKA (Fig. 46.1). The metabolic disturbances are a result of the lack of effective insulin as well as increases in the levels of counterregulatory hormones, such as cortisol, growth hormone, adrenaline, and noradrenaline. The counterregulatory hormones are released in high levels as a result of hypovolemia and shock. Interestingly, because the brain cells are insulin-insensitive tissue, they continue to utilize glucose. Hyperglycemia is a result of decreased cellular uptake as well as gluconeogenesis and glycogenolysis occurring in the liver cells.

Lipolysis occurs as a result of decreased insulin levels as well as counterregulatory hormones (Fig. 46.2). The resulting free fatty acids (FFA) are transformed into β-hydroxybutyric acid

---

Box 46.1 Precipitating Causes of DKA and HONC

Newly diagnosed cases of diabetes
Inadequate insulin treatment or noncompliance
Infection (urinary tract and pneumonia most common)
Concomitant cardiovascular disease (especially myocardial infarction, cerebrovascular accident, and pulmonary edema)
Drugs (corticosteroids, sympathomimetic agents, thiazide diuretics, phenytoin, calcium channel blockers, chlorpromazine, cimetidine, ethacrymic acid, L-asparaginase, immunosuppressive agents, diazoxide)
Other causes—trauma, pancreatitis, intestinal obstruction, peritoneal dialysis, heat stroke, severe burns, mesenteric thrombosis, renal failure
Insulin resistance, Cushing's syndrome, acromegaly, thyrotoxicosis

Biochemistry of hyperglycemia in DKA

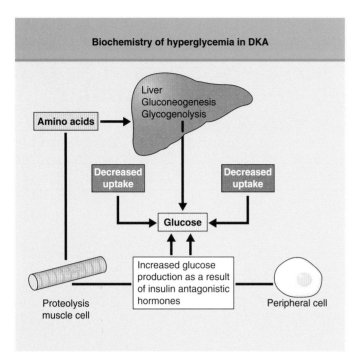

Figure 46.1. Biochemistry of hyperglycemia in DKA. Hyperglycemia is a result of abnormal biochemical pathways, precipitated by inadequate insulin action and exacerbated by hormones antagonistic to the action of insulin. The liver produces glucose as a result of gluconeogenesis and glycogenolysis, peripheral cells have a decreased uptake and increased production of glucose, and amino acids become incorporated in liver gluconeogenesis as a result of proteolysis.

Biochemistry of ketoacidosis in DKA

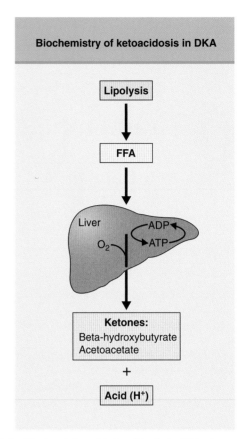

Figure 46.2. Biochemistry of ketoacidosis in DKA. Increased lipolysis occurs as a result of decreased insulin levels, forming free fatty acids, which are broken down in the liver, forming ketones and acid. ADP, adenosine diphosphate; ATP, adenosine triphosphate; FFA, free fatty acids.

and acetoacetic acid in the liver. Collectively, these are known as ketoacids. At the same time, there is also an increase in triglyceride synthesis as a result of the increased FFA load to the liver, resulting in hyperlipemia. There is little ketone production in HONC, probably related to reduced concentrations of FFA, cortisol, glucogen, and growth hormone, together with higher insulin levels. It may be that patients with HONC have enough insulin to inhibit lipolysis but not enough to facilitate peripheral glucose uptake and optimal carbohydrate metabolism.

Fluid and Electrolyte Losses and Metabolic Acidosis

The abnormal metabolism, as a result of the lack of effective insulin, has some devastating secondary effects, including fluid loss, electrolyte losses and shifts across body fluid compartments, as well as metabolic acidosis.

The major cause of fluid loss is an osmotic diuresis, secondary to glycosuria. Although urinary ketone excretion on a molar basis is generally less than half that of glucose, the excretion of ketones presents a further osmotic load, resulting in further electrolyte loss (sodium, potassium, and ammonium). As with any osmotic diuresis, it is fixed by biochemical principles; the kidney has little control over the amount of water lost or the electrolyte concentration in the urine. The urine is isotonic: Sodium accounts for approximately 70 mmol/liter, approximately half the concentration of isotonic saline, which is important when considering the most appropriate fluid for replacement. Potassium concentration is slightly less. Other

ions, such as chloride, magnesium, and phosphate, are lost in relatively fixed amounts as well. The average fluid loss in DKA is between 5 and 10 liters; the average sodium loss is 400 to 700 mmol, and potassium loss is between 250 and 700 mmol.

The fluid and electrolyte losses occur almost equally from the three body fluid compartments: intravascular space (IVS), interstitial space (ISS), and intracellular space (ICS) (Fig. 46.3). Initially, fluid moves osmotically from the cells (ICS) into the ISS and IVS, which collectively make up the extracellular fluid (ECF). Fluid loss can also occur as a result of insensible water losses, especially if there is an underlying infection and fever, as well as from the high tidal volumes as a result of compensating for the underlying metabolic acidosis (Kussmaul breathing). Fluid losses as a result of glycosuria are higher in patients with HONC, in which water deficits are reported to be between 6 and 19 liters. Serum sodium levels are greater than 150 mmol/liter in more than half of all patients on presentation. This is a result of greater loss of water compared to sodium. This is exacerbated in patients with HONC, especially in the latter stages.

Although fluid loss occurs from all three body compartments, most life-threatening signs and symptoms are related to hypovolemia and shock (i.e., depletion of IVS). The shock in turn causes high levels of counterregulatory hormones. These exacerbate hyperglycemia and ketone production.

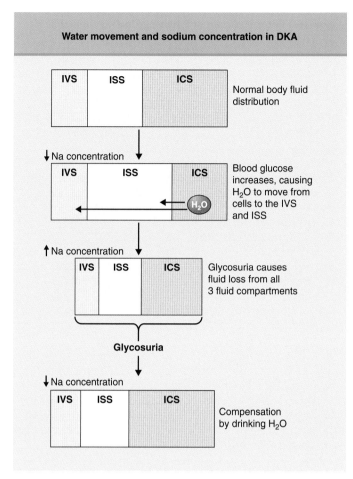

Figure 46.3. Water movement and sodium concentration in DKA. ICS, intracellular space; ISS, interstitial space; IVS, intravascular space.

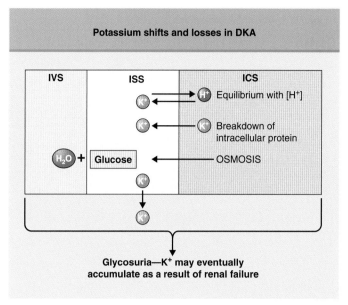

Figure 46.4. Potassium shifts and losses in DKA. Potassium moves from the cell to the ECF as a result of increased extracellular glucose and osmosis. The ion also moves from the cell as a result of the breakdown of intracellular protein and in exchange for increasing levels of hydrogen ion. Finally, potassium is lost in large amounts through the urine. The end result is a large total body loss of potassium but usually a relatively normal serum level on admission. If renal failure supervenes, serum potassium levels may be elevated. ICS, intracellular space; ISS, interstitial space; IVS, intravascular space.

Sodium levels can also appear erroneously low as a result of elevated lipid levels displacing water. This degree of lipidemia can be easily recognized on visual inspection. The serum sodium concentration on admission in patients with DKA varies (see Fig. 46.3). In early presentations, the patient usually compensates for the glycosuria by drinking water. Although the glycosuria has a relatively low concentration of sodium compared to serum, it does not result in a high concentration of serum sodium as a result of increased water intake. However, in patients who present late, the glycosuria continues without adequate fluid replacement, resulting in hypernatremia. As the hypovolemia becomes more severe, the glomerular filtration rate (GFR) decreases and less electrolytes and water are excreted.

Potassium (Fig. 46.4) is also lost in large amounts as a result of the glycosuria (total loss is approximately 10 mmol/kg). Initially, however, the plasma potassium concentration remains normal as a result of water and potassium moving osmotically from the cells to the ECF in response to high blood glucose levels. The potassium movement is enhanced by the breakdown of intracellular protein in muscle and by the increased amount of hydrogen ions moving into cells, displacing potassium in an attempt to maintain electroneutrality. Potassium losses may be enhanced by hyperaldosterone related to sodium depletion as well as by potassium following the urinary excretion of negatively charged ketoanions. As hypovolemia and decreased GFR

supervene, there may be decreased potassium excretion. Large amounts of chloride, phosphate, magnesium, and calcium are also lost as a result of polyuria.

The ketoacids produced in DKA easily dissociate at physiologic pH, resulting in high serum levels of ketosis and hydrogen ion, which is buffered extracellularly (predominantly HCO_3) and intracellularly. Lactic acidosis can also accompany hypovolemia as a result of decreased tissue perfusion. In the latter stages of DKA and HONC, there may be decreased acid loss in the urine as a result of renal insufficiency. The ketoanions contribute to the plasma anion gap, which in most patients is equivalent to the decrease in plasma HCO_3 concentration. As hypovolemia supervenes, GFR decreases and both glucose and ketone are increasingly retained. During treatment with insulin, hydrogen ions are consumed as ketoanion metabolism is facilitated.

CLINICAL FEATURES

There is a typical history over days or weeks of polyuria, polydipsia, and lethargy (Box 46.2). Nausea and vomiting are common, and diffuse abdominal pain is prominent in approximately 25% of patients. The cause is associated with the unstable metabolic state, especially in DKA, but a separate underlying abdominal pathology is more common in HONC.

End-stage presentations of DKA and HONC are usually obvious. The major features are related to fluid loss and acidosis. Hypovolemia is the major threat to life and accounts for hypotension and tachycardia in the later stages. Decreased tissue perfusion, resulting in features such as renal insufficiency and

---

Box 46.2 Clinical Assessment

- Screen for history of polyuria, polydipsia, and lethargy, together with symptoms of concomitant infection
- Assess level of consciousness and airway patency
- Assess adequacy of oxygenation, especially in obese, obtunded, and older patients
- Assess circulation status (e.g., peripheral perfusion, systemic blood pressure, and heart rate)
- Assess total body fluid status (e.g., weight loss and tissue turgor)
- Assess extent of metabolic acidosis, especially tidal volume, air hunger, respiratory rate, and smell of acetone on breath
- Exclude precipitating infection—history and extensive physical examination

---

Box 46.3 Interpretation of Pathology in DKA and HONC

Blood glucose: Does not correlate well with qualitative urine dipstick testing, especially at levels > 20 mmol/liter.

Acetone/acetoacetate: Determined semiquanitatively in the blood with the nitroprusside reaction and in the urine by ketosticks or acetest tablets, which also use nitroprusside.

β-Hydroxybutyrate: The major ketone cannot be determined by the nitroprusside reaction. Many hospitals now use a direct measurement technique that provides a more accurate estimation of ketoacidosis.

Blood count and differential: Leukocytosis (usually < 20,000/mm^3) may be secondary to hypovolemia alone.

Serum amylase and lipase: Can be nonspecifically elevated and may not indicate pancreatitis.

Severe hyperlipidemia: Visible on inspection at levels high enough to reduce serum glucose and sodium. This can be corrected by removing the lipemic component before measurement or using ion-specific electrodes with undiluted samples.

Creatinine: Can be falsely elevated as a result of acetoacetate interference.

---

even decreased level of consciousness, is a life-threatening late complication. Fluid loss from ICS and ISS results in decreased tissue turgor, weight loss, and dry mucosa. The acidosis that accompanies DKA stimulates the respiratory center in an attempt to compensate, causing Kussmaul's breathing—typically very large tidal volumes and air hunger rather than tachypnea. Despite these obvious signs and symptoms, the diagnosis can be delayed, particularly in elderly patients with HONC, in whom it may be confused with conditions such as a cerebrovascular event or sepsis.

Approximately 50% of patients with HONC and many patients with DKA present with concomitant medical problems (see Box 46.1). In the presence of an infection, there may or may not be an accompanying fever. In fact, many patients are hypothermic on admission as a result of heat loss.

It is important that the physical examination and history include possible sites of infection, including the urinary and respiratory tracts, nasal turbinates, sinuses, and palate, as well as other potential accompanying infections, such as meningitis, appendicitis, diverticulitis, and pelvic inflammatory disease. Patients may present with MI without pain, and obstetric patients may present after hyperemesis or as a result of β-adrenergic drugs.

DIAGNOSIS

The history and examination usually make the diagnosis obvious. A finger stick positive for high blood glucose or a strongly positive urine dipstick for glucose, together with a positive keto-diastix, strongly suggests the diagnosis of DKA. Confirmation is usually made with arterial blood gases and a low arterial pH.

The extent of laboratory abnormalities is estimated by measuring blood glucose, serum osmolality, plasma electrolytes, arterial blood gases, and blood and urine ketones, and by determination of the anion gap: $(Na^+ + K^+) - (Cl^- + HCO_3)$ (see Chapter 41). Some of the possible problems with interpreting laboratory tests are outlined in Box 46.3. Serum lactate should be measured if there is renal insufficiency or hypovolemia in order to differentiate lactic acidosis from ketoacidosis. Many patients with diabetes have underlying disease, such as diabetic nephropathy, that makes them more vulnerable to insults such as hypotension. Measurement of blood urea and creatinine will

give some indication of renal function. A 12-lead electrocardiogram (ECG), cardiac enzymes, and a chest radiograph may indicate myocardial ischemia. A cerebral computed tomography (CT) scan may be indicated if there are focal neurological signs or a persistent decrease in the level of consciousness.

Investigations for precipitating factors obviously overlap with possible complications of acute diabetic emergencies. Possible MI or cerebral events can be the cause or result of the disease, especially in elderly patients with HONC.

Infection is a very common major precipitating factor, especially in DKA. Blood, urine, and sputum cultures and a white cell count and differential need to be performed. A chest radiograph can indicate pneumonia. A CT scan and possibly a lumbar puncture may be indicated if meningitis is suspected. Cultures from wounds and facial radiographs to exclude sinusitis may have to be performed. A CT and/or ultrasound of the abdomen may be indicated, as well as serum amylase.

Possible alternative diagnoses of DKA are listed in Box 46.4. A rare manifestation of diabetic deterioration, euglycemic ketoacidosis, can occur, especially in young patients and often during a concurrent infection. Plasma glucose is relatively normal (<15 mmol/liter) and the patient may still be administering insulin. Symptoms such as nausea, vomiting, and clouding of the level of consciousness may occur, and ketoacidosis rapidly supervenes. This rare presentation highlights the importance of measuring urinary ketones as well as glucose in diabetic patients. A further diagnostic trap can occur, although rarely, when there is little acetate or acetone. In these cases, plasma levels of the other ketone, β-hydroxybutyrate, need to be specifically requested.

TREATMENT

Diabetic ketoacidosis and HONC are life-threatening emergencies in patients who often have compromised organ dysfunction. For many years, medical textbooks and review articles have sug-

---

Box 46.4 Differential Diagnosis of DKA

Acute or chronic alcoholic abuse: Alcoholic ketoacidosis usually presents with normal or low plasma glucose levels and a higher β-hydroxybutyrate-to-acetoacetate ratio

Starvation ketoacidosis: Usually mild ketoacidosis, little hyperglycemia, and relatively high bicarbonate levels

Other causes of high anion gap (e.g., shock and renal failure): Usually differentiated by high serum lactate

Salicylate overdose: Usually mixed acid–base disorder (primary respiratory alkalosis and increased anion gap metabolic acidosis)

Methanol overdose: Differentiated on history and methanol level

Ethylene glycol overdose: Diagnosis suggested by high serum osmolality, high anion gap acidosis and ketonemia, as well as neurological (e.g., seizures) and cardiovascular (e.g., shock) signs

Eugylcemic acidosis: Rare manifestation of diabetic patient when blood glucose is normal or only slightly raised. Routine blood and urine ketones, as well as specific plasma β-hydroxybutyrate levels, need to be tested for.

Box 46.5 Principles of Management in DKA and HONC

- Airway: Secure the airway if required.
- Breathing: Correct oxygenation and manage respiratory failure.
- Circulation: Restore the intravascular volume rapidly.
- Slowly correct body water defects with 5% dextrose.
- Measure and correct electrolyte levels (K^+, Na^+, Mg^{2+}, $PO4^{2-}$).
- Simultaneously exclude precipitating causes.
- Slowly correct blood glucose levels to normal with insulin (at a maximum rate of <5 mmol/hr).
- Closely monitor cardiorespiratory status.
- Regularly measure blood glucose, plasma electrolytes, arterial blood gases, and ketone levels.

---

gested management strategies primarily aimed at giving insulin to reduce blood glucose levels. The following management plan (Box 46.5) is based on the generic principles of resuscitation. Although insulin is part of this strategy, lowering of blood glucose is not the most urgent therapy.

All but the most minor cases of DKA and HONC should be managed in a carefully monitored environment, such as an ED or intensive care unit (ICU), with staff who have experience in caring for seriously ill patients.

Airway

Patients with a HONC often present obtunded, usually as a result of the underlying metabolic disturbance. Patients with both DKA and HONC can also have a decreased level of consciousness as a result of concomitant disease, such as generalized sepsis, a CVA, or meningitis. Usually, the airway is compromised when the Glasgow Coma Scale is approximately

---

Box 46.6 Causes of Hypoxia in DKA and HONC

- Elderly, obese, obtunded patient with HONC: Collapsed lung bases and/or aspiration
- Concomitant chronic lung disease secondary to smoking, especially in patients with HONC
- Pulmonary edema secondary to MI
- Raised intraabdominal pressure secondary to pathology such as pancreatitis causing basal lung collapse
- Precipitating infection (e.g., pneumonia)
- Acute lung injury secondary to remote infection (e.g., generalized sepsis or shock)
- Pulmonary embolism secondary to hypovolemia, coma, and immobility

---

9 or less, and intubation should be considered in order to control the airway and to safely sedate the patient before performing investigations such as CT scan.

Breathing

Patients with DKA are usually hyperventilating and generating very low levels of $PaCO_2$. Interestingly, levels of PaO_2 are usually very high, partly because of the space created in the alveolus by low levels of CO_2, but also because the lungs become very efficient gas exchangers due to the decreased space between the alveolus and capillary as a result of dehydration. As the patient becomes more hypovolemic, lung perfusion can decrease and degrees of hypoxia can occur, as it does with any form of shock.

Hypoxia (Box 46.6) is most common in elderly, obese, and obtunded patients with HONC who present with bilaterally collapsed lung bases and/or aspiration. All patients with shock should be given supplemental oxygen. Depending on the degree of hypoxia, patients may also require artificial ventilation, either noninvasively or after intubation.

Occasionally, patients with DKA develop extraalveolar air, such as pulmonary interstitial emphysema, mediastinal emphysema, subcutaneous emphysema, and even pneumothoraces. The mechanism is related to alveolar overexpansion as a result of large tidal volumes, decreased pulmonary circulation, and decreased interstitial fluid. The result is volutrauma, the same as that which occurs when excessive positive pressure ventilation is used. It is very common to observe large black lung fields on the initial chest radiograph in patients with DKA, but it is relatively uncommon for patients to develop alveolar disruption and volutrauma. Nevertheless, signs such as subcutaneous emphysema and pneumothorax should be searched for.

Circulation

Hypovolemia is a feature of most presentations of DKA and HONC and should be corrected as a matter of urgency. Many sources still recommend inflexible fluid replacement recipes based on average losses as a result of DKA or HONC. These must be avoided, and each patient's fluid circulatory status needs to be individually assessed and fluid titrated against measured responses to resuscitation, as for any other cause of shock (Box 46.7).

Simple measures, such as blood pressure, pulse rate, and peripheral skin perfusion, should be used initially. History and

Box 46.7 Guidelines for Fluid Replacement

- Rapidly resuscitate the intravascular space with colloid according to estimations such as systemic blood pressure, pulse rate, and peripheral perfusion.
- Slowly replace total body water losses with 5% dextrose according to estimated dehydration levels (50 mL/hr, mild; 100 mL/hr, moderate; 150 mL/hr, severe).
- If no or little circulatory compromise, replace fluid losses with a fluid containing a sodium concentration of approximately 70 mmol/liter.
- Fine-tune serum sodium levels by adjusting 5% dextrose infusion rate.
- Aim for rapid restoration of the patient's own spontaneous oral intake and normal renal function.

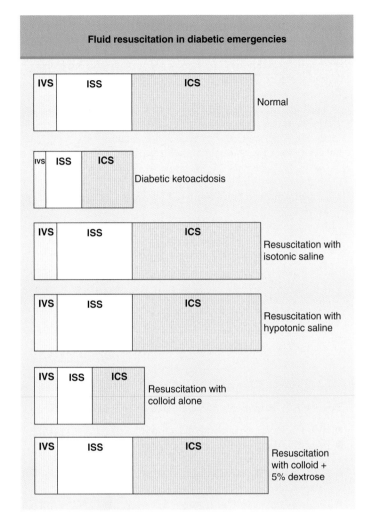

Figure 46.5. Fluid resuscitation in diabetic emergencies. The top of the diagram represents normal body fluid distribution. The nature of fluid and electrolyte loss in DKA is such that there is equal fluid loss from each compartment. When these losses are replaced with isotonic saline alone, it can be seen that although IVS is restored, there is gross expansion of ISS and no replacement of ICS. Because hypotonic saline is similar to the fluid lost, there is accurate replacement of all compartments. However, because of the large distribution volume of hypotonic saline, IVS is not resuscitated rapidly enough. To overcome this disadvantage, colloid may be given initially to reverse the hypovolemic shock and 5% dextrose given concurrently to replace the other two spaces. (Adapted with permission from Hillman K: Fluid resuscitation in diabetic emergencies—a reappraisal. Intensive Care Med 1987;13:4–8.) ICS, intracellular space; ISS, interstitial space; IVS, intravascular space.

the degree of other fluid compartment losses, such as tissue turgor, may also give some idea of total fluid losses.

The most appropriate fluid to replace losses is one that is approximately the same as that lost, with a sodium concentration of approximately 70 mmol/liter (Fig. 46.5). Many centers successfully use this type of regimen. Not only does the sodium concentration match that of the fluid lost but also it prevents excessive chloride administration associated with isotonic saline predisposing to hyperchloremic metabolic acidosis. The major problem with using this hypotonic fluid initially is that it does not rapidly correct hypovolemia and shock, which is the major priority in initial resuscitation. Other centers use isotonic saline and similar crystalloids, such as Hartmann's solution. However, these fluids are confined to the extracellular space (see Fig. 46.5). Moreover, isotonic saline and similar crystalloids are mainly distributed to the interstitial, not the intravascular, compartment in a ratio of approximately 3:1.

Rapid resuscitation of the circulation is not just a basic principle in acute medicine; it is even more important for diabetic patients because they may have underlying organ dysfunction, such as renal and cardiac disease, which makes them even more vulnerable to inadequate circulatory flow and pressure. The most efficient fluid to resuscitate the circulating volume is one that is mainly distributed to that space—a colloid (see Fig. 46.5).

However, even more important than the type of fluid used is the rapidity with which circulatory volume is restored. Initially, rapidly infused fluid challenges of 300 to 500 mL should be used to correct the shock, and then a rate of between 50 and 200 mL/hr should be used to replace the circulatory volume. Initially, simple bedside monitoring of the circulation, such as pulse rate and blood pressure and peripheral perfusion, should be used. Later, measurements such as serum lactic acid levels, central venous pressure, and hourly urine output may be useful in fine tuning the circulatory volume.

Correction of Other Body Fluid Compartments

If a colloid or crystalloid is used to initially correct the circulatory volume, there is no free water available to replace the largest compartment in the body—the ICS. This becomes important when insulin is commenced, as water moves from the ECF to ICS following glucose as it enters the cell (Fig. 46.6).

When a colloid is being used to resuscitate the circulation, the most efficient way of initially replacing total body water is with 5% dextrose. The total amount of glucose in this fluid is minimum and can easily be controlled with appropriate rates of insulin infusion. As with most fluid replacement to the ICS, the volume required can only be empirically estimated (see Box 46.7). Fluid resuscitation should be ceased once the patient's vital signs are stable and an adequate urine output (without significant glycosuria) has been established, and 5% dextrose replacement can cease when the patient's oral intake is adequate and the plasma sodium is within normal limits.

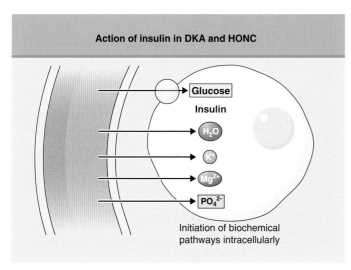

Action of insulin in DKA and HONC

Figure 46.6. Action of insulin in DKA and HONC. In reducing blood glucose to normal levels, insulin causes water to move from the ECF, exacerbating hypovolemia as well as potentially causeing cell swelling, hypokalemia, hypophosphatemia, and hypomagnesemia if blood glucose is not reduced slowly.

Electrolytes

The plasma sodium level is usually determined by the severity and stage of the disease (see Fig. 46.3). As a general rule, increased serum sodium indicates decreased total body water, and a low serum sodium indicates excessive total body water.

Resuscitation with a crystalloid alone will result in excessive sodium, which may result in an expanded ISS, with relatively normal serum concentrations. If the patient is rehydrated with colloid and appropriate quantities of 5% dextrose, the sodium from the colloid solution should be sufficient to replace total body levels. As the patient recovers, sodium levels should be measured and the 5% dextrose infusion titrated against them (i.e., less fluid if the sodium remains low and more if it remains high). The best way to achieve final sodium balance is to restore the patient's natural thirst and normal renal function.

Other electrolytes, such as potassium, magnesium, phosphate, chloride, and calcium, are also lost as a result of the glycosuria. Electrolytes undergo shifts between fluid compartments, as well as being lost in the urine. As a result, a new equilibrium has been established, often over days and weeks. Replacing electrolytes has to respect this metabolic chaos. The best guideline for electrolyte replacement is frequent measurement (initially every hour) and then appropriate doses to restore normal values.

Potassium levels are particularly volatile and affected by many factors. As the patient is resuscitated and insulin commenced, potassium moves back into the cell. Less important are the continuing losses as a result of the osmotic diuresis and dilution as a result of fluid replacement. Potassium should be intravenously replaced and not added to other IV fluids. The measurement and replacement of potassium should be independent of IV fluid replaced, using different end points and appropriate rates. If the initial serum levels are between 4.0 and 5.5 mmol/liter, the renal function is normal, and the patient is passing urine, an infusion of 10 mmol/hr should be commenced. If the potassium levels are less than 4.0 mmol/liter, then a rate

of 20 mmol/hr should be commenced. Potassium levels should be remeasured after 1 hour. Often, the rate will need to be increased. Hourly measurement should continue for approximately 6 hours and/or until a relatively stable level has been achieved, and then every 2 to 6 hours as clinically indicated.

Both phosphate and magnesium are also lost as a result of polyuria. Phosphate should be measured on admission and replaced. If KH_2PO is used, there will be 10 mmol of K^+ for every 10 mmol of PO_4^{2-}. As such, the potassium infusion rate should be reduced by approximately one third while the KH_2PO_4 is administered as 10 mmol aliquots over approximately 60 minutes. Regular measurements (as for potassium) need to be performed, and phosphate should be replaced as necessary to achieve normal levels. Phosphate can also be delivered as a sodium combination (13.4 mmol of phosphate in each ampoule) if the potassium levels are too high. Magnesium levels should also be measured. Initially, magnesium should be replaced as aliquots of approximately 10 mmol over 60 minutes, and levels should be monitored closely, as for other electrolytes.

Bicarbonate

Bicarbonate is no longer routinely recommended for treatment of DKA and HONC. The acid–base status usually returns to normal levels during resuscitation. Sodium bicarbonate can exacerbate an already hyperosmolar state. There are also potential dangers associated with exacerbating hypokalemia, causing paradoxical intracellular acidosis, and precipitating a rebound metabolic alkalosis as ketones are oxidized. A stat dose of 0.5 mmol/kg should be considered if the pH is less than 6.9 or when the cardiovascular system is not responsive to vasopressors and inotropes.

Some patients have a prolonged metabolic acidosis due to acids other than ketoacids, such as lactic acid. Direct measures of lactate and β-hydroxybutyrate should be made in these cases.

Exclude and Treat Precipitating Causes

As with any form of emergency management, resuscitation, diagnosis, and further management need to occur simultaneously. A thorough history, physical examination, and appropriate investigations should exclude most possible precipitating causes, such as infection, MI, cerebrovascular events, and pancreatitis (see Box 46.1).

Insulin

Insulin is not a high priority in the initial management of DKA and HONC. Obviously, in the management of chronic diabetes, insulin and education are the mainstays of treatment. However, the principles of acute medicine and the underlying metabolic chaos in DKA and HONC necessitate a different approach. Restoration of the intravascular volume alone decreases the levels of cellular regulatory hormones, reducing hyperglycemia and increasing vital organ perfusion. Equally important, the doses of insulin required to normalize metabolic disorders is much lower if there is adequate peripheral tissue perfusion. Moreover, the high glucose by itself is not the threat to life that the resultant fluid electrolyte and acid–base disturbances are. The rigid doses and rates still recommended in some texts should be avoided. When managing DKA and HONC with insulin therapy, it is crucial to understand what the insulin is doing to fluid and electrolyte shifts as well as general cellular

Renal and Metabolic Problems

well-being (see Fig. 46.6). Most patients develop DKA and HONC over days to weeks. It is potentially dangerous to rapidly correct blood glucose levels because this could lead to hypovolemia, cell swelling, cell membrane potential changes, hypokalemia, hypophosphatemia, and hypomagnesemia. Insulin should be delivered as an IV insulin infusion, without a loading dose. Like any IV infusion, initial rates should be low—0.5 U/hr for HONC and 1.0 U/hr for DKA. Although blood glucose levels are usually higher in HONC, the required insulin infusion rates are lower. The rate should be increased according to regularly increased end points, such as blood glucose, serum potassium, ketone levels, bicarbonate levels, arterial pH, and clinical state. Although small amounts of insulin are adsorbed onto the plastic of intravenous giving sets, this has little clinical relevance because the rate is determined by easily measured clinical end points. The insulin infusion rates required to eventually restore normality may eventually be high (e.g., 20–30 U/hr). However, this is unusual, and other factors, such as renal failure, severe infection, and untreated hypovolemia, should be considered.

The reduction of blood glucose should occur smoothly and slowly over 24 to 48 hours and at no more than 5 mmol/hr. Intravenous insulin has a short half-life (approximately 5 min), so care has to be exercised when changing to a subcutaneous regimen after metabolic stabilization in order to avoid rebound hyperglycemia. A combination of short- and long-acting insulin similar to the patient's regular regime should be initially commenced. For newly diagnosed diabetics, an initial total insulin dose of approximately 0.6 U/kg/day, divided into at least three doses, in a mixed short- and long-acting combination should be commenced.

Monitoring

The patient's vital signs—level of consciousness, systemic blood pressure, heart rate, respiratory rate, peripheral perfusion, urine output, and temperature—should be measured at least every hour. Patients should be managed in an environment in which they can be observed by staff familiar with seriously ill patients (e.g., ED and ICU) for all presentations apart from those with no hypovolemia and relatively low blood glucose levels.

Continuous ECG monitoring and oxygen saturation are minimum continuous monitoring requirements. Continuous arterial blood pressure recording may be indicated in severe cases or when there are complications.

Continuing Investigations

Biochemistry such as blood glucose, serum electrolytes, and arterial blood gases should be measured at least hourly for the first 6 hours and then every 2 to 6 hours, as clinically indicated. Other investigations, such as hematology, further imaging, as well as renal and liver function tests, should be repeated as required. Because of frequent investigations, including arterial blood gases, it is more comfortable for the patient to have an arterial line inserted for frequent sampling.

Clinical Course and Prevention

The reported mortality for DKA is approximately 5% and for HONC between 30% and 50%. This is much higher than that for cardiac surgery, which is routinely managed in an ICU environment, and emphasizes the need for patients with DKA and

HONC to also be managed in an appropriate environment. Most patients with DKA recover within 48 hours with a good outcome if care is appropriate. Patients with HONC often require 4 or 5 days for the coma to resolve and also require more complex support in order to reduce reported high mortalities.

Approximately 5% of the population in Western countries is diabetic. Because patients are surviving longer and having children, the incidence is increasing. There is now a greater emphasis on patient education and primary physician awareness.

All patients who have been admitted to a hospital for DKA or HONC should be referred to an effective education program if they have not previously participated in one.

PITFALLS, COMPLICATIONS, AND CONTROVERSIES

Pitfalls
The major life-threatening pitfalls are related to inadequate and delayed resuscitation, especially fluid replacement and overzealous use of insulin (Box 46.8).

Complications
The major complications (Box 46.9) are a result of inappropriate resuscitation, such as hypoperfusion and damage to organs such as the kidneys and heart. Acute respiratory distress syndrome is a rare but life-threatening complication related to delayed treatment of shock and excessive use of crystalloids. It needs to be differentiated from pulmonary edema as a result of a MI.

Box 46.8 Pitfalls in the Management of DKA and HONC

- Delayed diagnosis
- Delayed and inappropriate fluid resuscitation
- Rapid reduction of blood glucose
- Failure to detect precipitating cause of DKA and HONC
- Failure to manage in an appropriate environment with staff familiar with resuscitation of the seriously ill
- Incorrect interpretation of laboratory investigations
- Underestimation of the importance of history and physical examination

---

Box 46.9 Complications in the Management of DKA and HONC

- Organ failure as a result of hypovolemic shock
- Hypoglycemia and hypokalemia
- Hyperchloremic metabolic acidosis
- Thromboembolic complications (e.g., myocardial and cerebral infarction and pulmonary embolism)
- Hypothermia, usually as a result of hypovolemia, coma, and tachypnea
- Persistent vomiting, gastric dilatation, and abdominal pain
- Adult respiratory distress syndrome
- Cerebral edema
- Rhabdomyolysis and pressure areas as a result of coma

Cerebral edema is common during the resuscitation of DKA, but usually at a subclinical level. It is a rare but devastating complication when clinically apparent, occurring more commonly in children. It accompanies treatment and is thought to be related to factors such as rapid reduction of blood glucose and excessive crystalloid use. Other complications can occur as a result of prolonged coma, such as pressure areas, rhabdomyolysis, thromboembolic complications, and hypothermia.

Controversies

Many of the controversies in the management of DKA and HONC arise as a result of lack of consistency and agreement between endocrinologists, who usually care for diabetic patients in an ambulatory setting, and acute care physicians such as emergency physicians and internists, who are trained in acute medicine and resuscitation.

Endocrinologists primarily possess expertise in areas such as education, primary physician awareness, and long-term control. When treating a patient with DKA or HONC, they concentrate on giving insulin, whereas acute care physicians emphasize rapid stabilization of the airway, breathing, and circulation. Acute care physicians titrate therapeutic interventions such as fluid and electrolyte replacement and blood glucose levels on an individual basis. Endocrinologists, on the other hand, often use fixed formulae for fluid and electrolyte replacement and insulin doses. Acute care physicians manage DKA and HONC patients in a closely monitored environment, often with invasive monitoring and with staff focused on resuscitation. Endocrinologists usually

do not work in these settings and may not be aware of advances in resuscitation and acute care medicine. The trend to separate chronic diabetic stabilization from resuscitation of patients with DKA and HONC may also explain the paucity of research by endocrinologists in the acute aspects of these diseases.

A separate set of skills is required for acute management of DKA and HONC. These skills overlap with those of the endocrinologist as the patient becomes more stable. It is important that the two specialties work closely together at this interface.

SUGGESTED READING

American Diabetes Association: Hyperglycemic crises in patients with diabetes mellitus. Diabetes Care 2001;24:1988–1996.

Berger W, Keller U: Treatment of diabetic ketoacidosis and non-ketotic hyperosmolar diabetic coma. Baillière's Clin Endocrinol Metab 1992; 6:1–22.

Fish LH: Diabetic ketoacidosis. Treatment strategies to avoid complications. Postgrad Med 1994;96:75–96.

Gonzalez-Campoy JM, Robertson RP: Diabetic ketoacidosis and hyperosmolar nonketotic state. Gaining control over extreme hyperglycaemic complications. Postgrad Med 1996;99:143–152.

Hillman K: Fluid resuscitation in diabetic emergencies—A reappraisal. Intensive Care Med 1987;13:4–8.

Hillman K: The management of acute diabetic emergencies. Clin Intensive Care 1991;2:154–162.

Kitabchi AE, Wall BM: Diabetic ketoacidosis. Med Clin North Am 1995; 79:9–37.

Kitabchi AE, Kreisberg RA, Umpierrez GE, et al: Management of hyperglycaemic crises in patients with diabetes. Diabetes Care 2001;24:131–153.

Chapter 47
Gastrointestinal Bleeding

Josep M. Bordas, Àngels Escorsell, Faust Feu, and Antoni Mas

Gastrointestinal bleeding (GIB) is a common cause of emergency consultation and hospital admission. In our hospital, it has been found to be more common than coronary disease. For practical purposes, it is very important to distinguish between upper GIB (UGIB), when the source of bleeding is above the Treitz angle, or lower GIB (LGIB), when it is below.

Portal hypertension (PH), usually caused by cirrhosis of the liver, is a cause of UGIB and clearly differs from other causes of bleeding in patients without PH (mainly peptic ulcers). In fact, hemorrhage from ruptured gastroesophageal varices is one of the most frequent and severe complications of cirrhosis.

In recent years, an increase in the frequency of LGIB has been observed. In most cases, the source of bleeding is located in the colon and rectum (80%), and in only 10% of cases is the source of bleeding in the small bowel. In approximately 10% of patients, the origin is unknown.

EPIDEMIOLOGY, RISK FACTORS, AND PATHOGENESIS

The average incidence of UGIB in the general population ranges from 67 to 172 cases per 100,000 people per year. In older people, the incidence has been reported to be as high as 500 cases per 100,000 people per year. The frequency of LGIB is approximately one fourth that of UGIB. Despite advances in the management of GIB, mortality related to this complication has remained unchanged in recent years (approximately 10% in UGIB not caused by PH), probably due to the presence of comorbidity and older age in the most recently published series. Mortality from LGIB varies from 2% to 4% and is also related to age and associated diseases.

Causes of UGIB are shown in Table 47.1. Gastric and duodenal peptic ulcers are the main causes of bleeding in patients without PH. *Helicobacter pylori* infection and nonsteroidal anti-

Table 47.1 Etiology of Upper Gastrointestinal Bleeding	
Etiology	**%**
Esophagus	
Esophageal varices	10
Erosive esophagitis	2
Mallory–Weiss tear	5–15
Infectious esophagitis	≤1
Esophageal carcinoma	≤1
Others (pharmacological or caustic lesions, etc.)	≈1–2
Stomach	
Peptic lesions	15–20
Dieulafoy's disease	≤1
Fundal varices	1–3
Portal hypertensive gastropathy	10–15
Vascular lesions	≤1
Neoplastic lesions	≤1
Duodenum	
Peptic ulcer	30–35
Vascular lesions	≤1
Others (aortoenteric fistula, pancreatitis, etc.)	≈1–2

inflammatory drug intake are the etiological factors in 98% of peptic ulcers, which bleed when a vessel present in the ulcer is eroded.

Hemorrhage from ruptured gastroesophageal varices due to PH accounts for 80% of the bleeding episodes in cirrhotic patients. PH is defined as a pathological increase in portal pressure. It is initiated by an increased resistance to portal blood flow (due to both disruption of the liver vascular architecture and active contraction of different hepatic cells) and aggravated by an increased portal venous inflow (caused by an increased release of local endothelial factors, such as nitric oxide and humoral vasodilators). Approximately 5% to 8% of patients who develop variceal bleeding die from uncontrolled hemorrhage within 48 hours. The rate of mortality is 20% 6 weeks after the acute event, with the most important death risk indicators being the severity of liver disease, the presence of renal failure, and the persistence and recurrence of bleeding. Once varices have developed, the risk of their rupture and bleeding increases with the increase in the pressure and the size of the varices and the decrease in the thickness of the variceal wall.

Frequent causes of LGIB are diverticulosis, angiodysplasia, tumors, Crohn's disease, ulcerative colitis, ischemic colitis, and Meckel's diverticulum. Diverticulosis and angiodysplasia are the most frequent causes of LGIB of colonic origin, whereas angiodyplasia is the lesion found in most bleeding episodes in the small bowel.

CLINICAL FEATURES

Exteriorization of blood from the digestive tract is the most important diagnostic feature of GIB. In UGIB, hematemesis alone, hematemesis and melena, or melena alone can occur. Passage of bright red blood or clots per rectum (hematochezia) is usually due to LGIB. However, UGIB may sometimes be manifested by red blood per rectum and, conversely, melena may be due to LGIB.

In cases of massive hemorrhage, GIB may be associated with hypovolemic shock or frank signs of hypovolemia, and these patients should be treated unquestionably in an intensive care unit setting. Taking into account that GIB is an intermittent event, the management of less dramatic situations should also

---

Table 47.2 Classification of Liver Failure According to the Child–Pugh and MELD Scores

Child–Pugh score[a]

Parameter	1 point	2 points	3 points
Bilirubin (mg/dL)	<2.0	2.0–3.0	>3.0
Albumin (g/100 mL)	>3.5	2.8–3.5	<2.8
Prothrombin index (%)	>50	30–50	<30
Presence of ascites	No	Mild	Moderate–severe
Hepatic encephalopathy (grade)	No	1–2	3–4

MELD score[b]

$$MELD\ score = 10 \times [0.957 \times \log_e (creatinine\ mg/dL)$$
$$+ 0.378 \times \log_e (bilirubin\ mg/dL)$$
$$+ 1.120 \times \log_e (INR)$$
$$+ 0.643]$$

[a]**Child–Pugh score** = sum of all the points derived from the five items evaluated. **Child–Pugh class:** A, 5 or 6; B, 7 to 9; C, 10 to 15.
[b]If the patient received dialysis twice within the week prior to calculation, then the score has to be calculated with a serum creatinine value of 4.0 mg/dL despite the "real" value.

---

be very cautious, especially in cases with associated diseases. Risk factors associated with an increase in mortality in GIB are shown in Box 47.1.

The presence of cirrhosis and the degree of liver insufficiency are especially important in UGIB due to PH. In this situation, once a patient is diagnosed, a complete evaluation should be performed in order to assess the prognosis of the bleeding episode according to liver function, assessed by the Child–Pugh classification or the Model for End-Stage Liver Disease (MELD) (Table 47.2); renal function, assessed by blood urea nitrogen or creatinine; age; active alcohol abuse; the presence of concomitant bacterial infection; active bleeding on endoscopy and hepatic hemodynamic study, if available; as well as the presence of hepatocellular carcinoma and the permeability of the portal vein by Doppler ultrasound examination.

DIAGNOSIS

In UGIB, endoscopy is the first diagnostic procedure to be undertaken because of its diagnostic and therapeutic capabilities. Cardiovascular and respiratory stabilization must be obtained before performing the endoscopic procedure. The risk induced by endoscopy should be weighed in patients with recent myocardial infarction, recent abdominal surgery, or respiratory insufficiency. Previous orotracheal intubation is mandatory in patients with alterations in consciousness and/or encephalopathy.

Emergency endoscopy during acute bleeding is not simple and requires an experienced examiner. When active bleeding is detected, endoscopic accuracy is similar in PH and non-PH patients. However, in the remaining cases (lesions without active bleeding), endoscopic accuracy decreases significantly in PH patients while remaining higher than 90% during 24 hours in non-PH patients. Thus, in patients with suspicion of PH, endoscopy should be performed as soon as possible after patient stabilization. In patients with non-PH, the Forrest classification is widely used, given its important relationship with prognosis of the hemorrhage (Fig. 47.1).

Variceal bleeding is also diagnosed on emergency endoscopy (Fig. 47.2). Diagnosis is based on the observation of blood spurt-

---

Box 47.1 Prognostic Factors for Adverse Outcome in Nonvariceal Upper Gastrointestinal Bleeding

Clinical Factors

Age > 60 years
Comorbidity: ischemic cardiac disease, cardiac failure, chronic obstructive pulmonary disease, chronic renal failure, cirrhosis, diabetes mellitus, neurological diseases, malignancy, coagulation abnormalities
Hypovolemic shock

Endoscopic Factors

Source of bleeding: peptic ulcer
Ulcer > 2 cm in diameter
Ulcer located in duodenal posterior wall, lesser gastric curvature
Presence of stigmata of recent hemorrhage

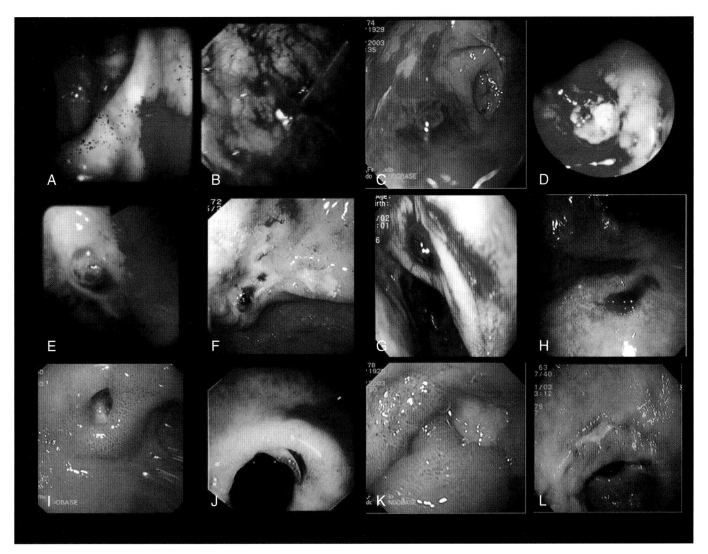

Figure 47.1. Forrest classification of lesions found in nonvariceal, upper gastrointestinal bleeding. *A*, Forrest Ia: Spurting bleeding lesion near GI anastomosis (Billroth I). *B*, Forrest 1a: Jet in Dieulafoy lesion. *C*, Forrest Ib: Oozing active bleeding gastric ulcer. *D*, Forrest Ib: Oozing bleeding from an ulcer with visible arterial vessel. *E*, Forrest IIa: Large ulcer with visible arterial vessel. *F*, Forrest IIa: Arterial visible vessel in the margin of gastric ulcer. *G*, Forrest IIb: Red clot in a duodenal ulcer. *H*, Forrest IIb: Red clot on a lesion located in the upper part of the stomach. *I*, Forrest IIc: Black spot (hematin) on the ulcer surface. *J*, Forrest IIc: Hematin on the ulcer surface. *K*, Forrest III: Ulcer without hemostasia signs. *L*, Forrest III: Antral clean gastric ulcer.

ing from a varix (approximately 20% of patients), white nipple or clot adherent on a varix, or varices without other potential sources of bleeding.

Colonoscopy is the first-choice examination in the study of LGIB. Diagnostic yield increases if polyethylene glycol/electrolyte bowel cleansing is performed before examination. The procedure should also be performed after hemodynamic stabilization. After cessation of the hemorrhage, the accuracy of colonoscopy is approximately 50%. If no active bleeding is found, colonoscopy may provide information on potential bleeding lesions, thereby allowing other diagnostic procedures or treatments to be undertaken. Diverticulosis is the most prevalent finding, present in more than 35% of patients.

Endoscopic examination of the small bowel may be performed in two different situations. In self-limited bleeding with negative upper and lower endoscopy, push enteroscopy allows the examination of the upper portion of small bowel and the

application of hemostatic therapy if indicated. Intraoperative enteroscopy is performed during emergency surgery of those patients with nondiagnosed active bleeding.

Angiography is usually performed in patients with massive or recurrent bleeding and in those with severe self-limited bleeding. Active bleeding may be observed if extravasation is a minimum flow of 0.5 to 1 mL/min. Angiodysplasia and tumors may be diagnosed by angiography.

In recent years, capsule endoscopy has been increasingly used in the evaluation of patients with LGIB after negative upper and lower endoscopy, allowing examination of the small bowel. The diagnostic yield is higher than that of push enteroscopy and barium intestinal series. In fact, small bowel barium examination with the conventional follow-through technique or by enteroclysis is of limited utility in the study of LGIB.

Isotopic studies are of limited value because of their low sensitivity and specificity. Studies using ^{99}Tc-labeled red blood cells

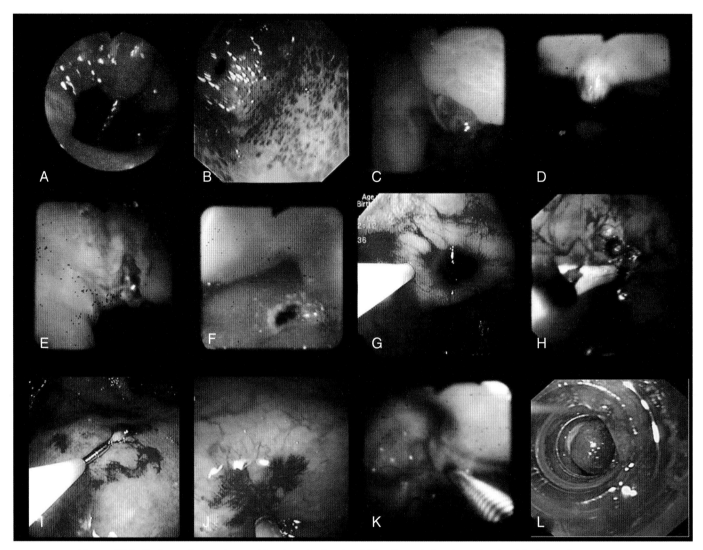

Figure 47.2. Endoscopic imaging and treatment of variceal bleeding. *A,* Esophageal variceal jet hemorrhage. *B,* Severe portal hypertension gastropathy in the antrum. *C,* Recent hemostasis (red clot) on the esophageal varice. *D,* Recent hemostasis (fibrin clot) on the esophageal varice. *E,* Cardial tear with recent hemostasia. *F,* Superficial lesion (erosion) showing recent hemostasia (hematin) (Forrest IIc). *G,* Sclerotherapy in a duodenal ulcer, using injection needle catheter. *H,* Treatment of the bleeding lesion using heater probe. Note the holes induced by the pressure. *I,* Hemostatic clip. *J,* Colon angiodysplasia treated by sclerotherapy. *K,* Variceal sclerotherapy. *L,* Variceal ligation (note entrapped esophageal varice).

are frequently performed to diagnose active bleeding because repeated, dynamic, continuous imaging may be achieved for up to 24 hours without reinjection. The study of heterotopic gastric mucosa using ^{99}Tc-pertechnectate in young patients is very useful and may allow Meckel's diverticulum to be ruled out as a cause of bleeding.

Other imaging techniques have been introduced. Computed tomography has a high diagnostic yield for angiodysplasia located in the large bowel and for intestinal lesions such as tumors, inflammatory bowel disease, and diverticuli. Magnetic resonance imaging may also be useful for the study of LGIB in select cases.

Taking into account these considerations, the diagnostic approach in LGIB is as follows: In patients with no massive bleeding or with stable hemodynamic status, colonoscopy is the first diagnostic procedure. However, 10% to 15% of the episodes of bleeding presenting with hematochezia have an upper source; therefore, upper endoscopy should be the first examination

performed in these cases. Most of these patients present with a stable hemodynamic status or with self-limited bleeding, which allows additional studies to be performed. If the source of bleeding is not found with endoscopy, two different options may be considered: In persistent or recurrent bleeding, an angiographic study is indicated, whereas in self-limited hemorrhage the small bowel should be investigated using capsule endoscopy or a combination of push enteroscopy and barium small bowel series. Angiography is indicated if the source of bleeding remains unknown. Surgery must be indicated in cases of persistent or recurrent undiagnosed bleeding, but additional examinations (scintigraphy, computed tomography, and repeated examinations) can be considered in patients with a more stable condition and/or associated diseases.

In patients with massive bleeding, emergency angiography is mandatory. If no diagnosis is achieved, surgery should be performed with intraoperatory enteroscopy if needed.

TREATMENT, CLINICAL COURSE, AND PREVENTION

General Management

This includes the treatment of hypovolemic shock, when present, and of anemia with packed red cell transfusion, according to the general standard procedures. In patients with UGIB due to PH, it is very important to avoid hypervolemia because it may cause a rebound increase in portal pressure and a consequent risk of further bleeding or subsequent rebleeding. Coagulopathy and thrombocytopenia should also be treated according to standard protocols. Recombinant activated factor VII has been shown to correct prothrombin time in cirrhotic patients. Its use in patients with cirrhosis or in other situations with coagulation disturbances and GIB is under investigation. Antibiotic prophylaxis should be instituted in patients with cirrhosis and UGIB from admission and maintained for 7 days. Early administration of antibiotics has been shown to reduce the rate of bacterial infections and to improve survival in these patients. Oral norfloxacin (400 mg/12 hr) is the drug of choice.

Therapeutic Approach in UGIB Not Due to PH

Several controlled trials have demonstrated that endoscopic hemostatic therapy reduces recurrence, need for emergency surgery, and mortality. Endoscopic therapy is useful in active bleeding ulcers, arterial visible vessels, and lesions with an adhered blood clot (see Fig. 47.2). Bleeding cardial tear, esophageal ulcers, and angiodysplasia are also indications for endoscopic hemostasis. Endoscopic sclerotherapy with adrenaline (1/10,000) alone or associated with irritants (1% polydocanol) is the simplest hemostatic treatment. Other hemostatic techniques (bipolar or multipolar electrocoagulation, heater probe, and argon plasma coagulation) obtain similar results. Hemostatic clips (mechanical hemostasis) are useful in arterial bleeding. Primary hemostasis is obtained in more than 95% of patients. Recurrence appears in 10% to 15% of patients. A second endoscopic treatment can then be performed. After retreatment, significant bleeding recurrence is an indication for emergency surgery. Less hemostatic efficacy is obtained in large ulcers and in lesions with difficult endoscopic access.

Antagonists of H_2 receptors and proton pump inhibitors (PPIs) have been widely used in the treatment of nonvariceal UGIB. It is known that the physiological mechanisms of hemostasis are completely abolished when gastric pH values are lower than 5. The aim of pharmacological treatment should be to achieve a sustained increase in gastric pH above 6.

A meta-analysis of randomized clinical trials assessing the efficacy of H_2 antagonists (cimetidine, ranitidine, and famotidine), including a total of 2670 patients, showed no beneficial effect of H_2 antagonists in achieving hemostasis or preventing rebleeding.

A greater decrease in gastric acid secretion may be achieved with the use of PPIs. The best results are obtained with 80 mg of omeprazole or pantoprazole given as an intravenous bolus, followed by a continuous intravenous infusion of 8 mg/hr. Gastric pH values increase above 6 during more than 90% of the infusion time. The efficacy of omeprazole has been assessed in two randomized controlled trials with contradictory results. Several small studies have suggested that omeprazole infusion may decrease the incidence of rebleeding after endoscopic therapy

of peptic ulcers with stigmata with a high risk of rebleeding (active bleeding, nonbleeding visible vessels, and adherent clots). In this setting, large randomized controlled trials have shown that intravenous (infusion of 8 mg/hr for 3 days after a bolus of 80 mg) or oral (40 mg/12 hr for 3 days) omeprazole decreases the incidence of rebleeding to 5% compared to 20% for patients receiving placebo.

Somatostatin has been used in the treatment of UGIB not due to PH because it decreases gastric acid secretion and causes splanchnic vasoconstriction. Somatostatin is given as a continuous intravenous infusion of 250 µg/hr after a bolus of 250 µg. The beneficial effect of somatostatin is controversial because some studies have shown a reduction in rebleeding, whereas others failed to demonstrate any beneficial effect. A meta-analysis showed a reduction in rebleeding and need for surgery in patients receiving somatostatin in comparison to patients receiving placebo.

Persistent or recurrent UGIB may be defined as the presence of hematemesis or signs of bleeding (blood in gastric aspirate and melena) with hypovolemia (systolic pressure < 100 mm Hg and/or heart rate > 100 bpm) and/or a decrease in hemoglobin level of more than 2 g/liter within 12 hours.

First-choice treatment for the first episode of rebleeding is endoscopic therapy, which controls rebleeding in 75% of patients without impairing prognosis. Figure 47.3 shows an algorithm for the therapeutic approach to patients with rebleeding. Indications of emergency surgery are massive bleeding, active arterial bleeding that is not stopped by endoscopic therapy, and failure of endoscopic therapy.

Therapeutic Approach of UGIB Due to PH

The management of variceal bleeding should be undertaken in an intensive care setting by a team of experienced medical staff, including well-trained nurses, clinical hepatologists, endoscopists, interventional radiologists, and surgeons. Once acute bleeding has been satisfactorily treated, secondary prophylaxis should be started to prevent episodes of recurrent bleeding (Fig. 47.4).

Initial therapy should be aimed at both achieving hemostasis at the bleeding site and preventing bleeding-related complications, such as renal failure, infection, and hepatic decompensation.

Specific therapy to stop bleeding is usually given following initial resuscitation and diagnostic endoscopy, but pharmacological therapy can be started earlier in the course of the bleeding episode. Hemostatic treatment for variceal bleeding includes the use of vasoactive drugs to decrease portal pressure, endoscopic procedures, and portosystemic shunts, either surgical or the transjugular intrahepatic portosystemic shunt (TIPS).

The current recommendations for hemostatic treatment are to initiate drug treatment as soon as possible and to undertake endoscopic therapy at the time of diagnostic endoscopy. This approach has a success rate of approximately 75% at 5 days (drugs should be maintained for 5 days to reduce early rebleeding).

Esophagogastric varices and PH gastropathy are the most common sources of bleeding in cirrhotic patients (see Fig. 47.2). Intravenous vasoactive drugs can obtain primary hemostasis or a significant reduction in bleeding, thereby facilitating endoscopic procedures. Terlipressin should be the first option, since it is the

521

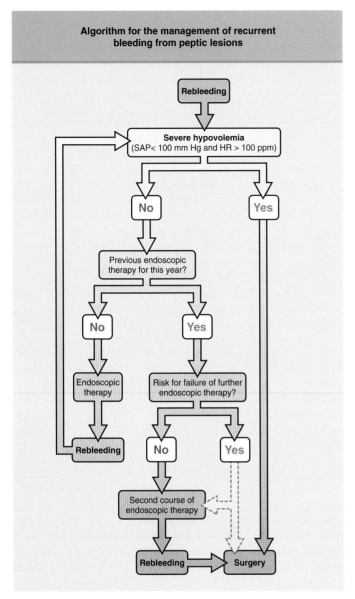

Figure 47.3. Algorithm for the management of recurrent bleeding from peptic lesions.

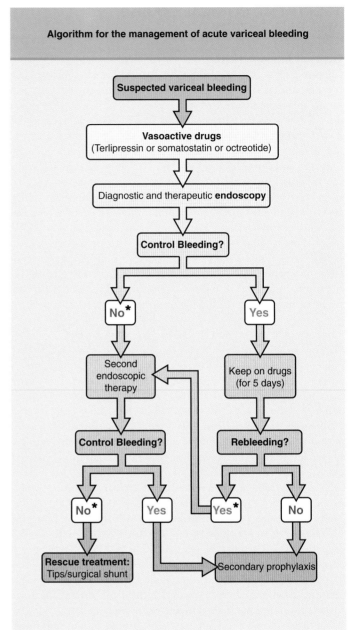

Figure 47.4. Algorithm for the management of acute variceal bleeding.

only vasoactive drug shown to improve survival to date. Somatostatin is the second choice. If these drugs are not available, octreotide and vasopressin plus transdermal nitroglycerin are acceptable options.

Esophageal and related subcardial varices can be treated by sclerotherapy or variceal band ligation (VBL). Sclerotherapy induces thrombosis, local edema, and smooth muscle spasm and facilitates hemostasia. VBL is more difficult to perform in active bleeding patients, and after the diagnostic procedure a second procedure is required following the placement of the ligation applicator. In unselected cases, primary hemostasis is achieved in more than 95% of patients. The proportion of final hemostasis decreases in patients with advanced liver failure or portal vein thrombosis.

VBL cannot be used on gastric varices because of the risk of partial drawing of the selected variceal channel into the ligator chamber, with the risk of massive bleeding if the scar tissue is

removed. Case series have suggested that injection with cyanoacrylate lipiodol is effective in achieving acute hemostasis and ultimately variceal obliteration in bleeding gastric varices. This technique can also be affective in treating esophageal varices.

Many randomized controlled trials have demonstrated that the early administration of a vasoactive drug facilitates endoscopy and improves control of bleeding and decreases 5-day rebleeding. Even if drug therapy is started after endoscopic treatment, it still improves the results. Concomitant endoscopic therapy improves the efficacy of vasoactive treatment alone, both in low- and in high-risk patients. If early recurrent bleeding occurs, a single endoscopic retreatment may be undertaken if bleeding does not compromise the patient.

The role of balloon tamponade is limited to obtain temporary hemostasis by direct compression of the bleeding varices.

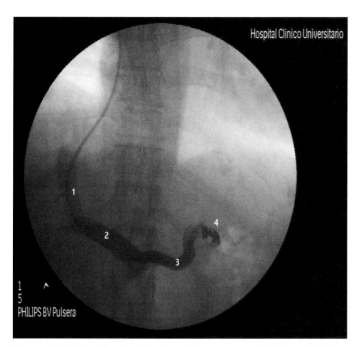

Figure 47.5. Transjugular intrahepatic portosystemic shunt (TIPS) and embolization of the gastric varices with coils. 1, TIPS; 2, portal vein; 3, splenic vein; 4, coils.

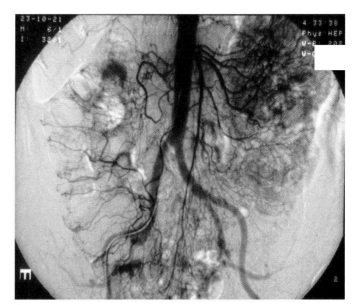

A

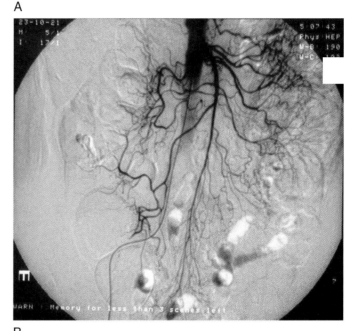

B

Figure 47.6. Angiographic image of colonic angiodysplasia before (A) and after (B) embolization.

In experienced hands, it provides bleeding control rates up to 90%. It should only be used by skilled staff in intensive care facilities because fatal complications may occur in 6% to 20% of cases and aspiration pneumonia in 10%. The double-balloon Sengstaken–Blakemore tube is used in patients bleeding from esophageal varices. The Linton–Nachlas tube is used for gastric variceal bleeding. Although temporarily effective, the use of balloon tamponade should be restricted to patients with massive bleeding not controlled by initial pharmacologic and endoscopic therapy, as a bridge to other treatment.

Both TIPS and surgical shunts are effective in controlling variceal bleeding (control rate of approximately 95%), but invasiveness and side effects (encephalopathy and worsening of liver function) result in a high mortality. Therefore, these procedures should be restricted to those cases of esophageal variceal bleeding not responding to the previously mentioned measures. TIPS is the treatment of choice in patients with moderate to advanced liver failure, associated with a high surgical mortality. Shunt surgery, preferably an H-graft mesocaval shunt, may be an option in Child A patients with persistent or recurrent bleeding refractory to the other therapeutic measures.

Patients with gastric variceal bleeding may warrant an earlier decision for TIPS than patients bleeding from esophageal varices. TIPS is very effective in the treatment of bleeding gastric varices, with more than a 90% success rate for initial hemostasis and a low rebleeding rate. TIPS also allows embolization of the collateral vessels that feed the varices (Fig. 47.5). Other derivative and devascularization surgical therapies are also effective but have limited applicability in advanced cirrhosis.

Therapeutic Approach to LGIB

Colonic diverticulosis is found in more than 35% of patients with LGIB, but it is considered the source of bleeding only if stigmata of recent hemorrhage are present in the lesion, which occurs in only 3% to 5% of patients. In most cases (up to 70%), the source of bleeding is located in the right colon. Colonoscopy may allow the application of hemostatic therapy. Most patients have a self-limited episode of bleeding, but hemorrhage will recur in up to 25% of patients. Surgery is reserved for persistent bleeding and for cases with several recurrent episodes of bleeding.

Angiodysplasia is a frequent cause of LGIB in older patients, usually diagnosed by angiography and, rarely, by colonoscopy or other techniques such as computed tomography. In most cases, lesions are located in the right colon, but it is common to find diffuse angiodysplasia involving the large and small bowel. Bleeding from angiodysplasia may present as overt or occult bleeding. Acute bleeding episodes are frequently self-limited, but hemorrhage will recur during admission in approximately 15% of patients. No medical treatment has proven to be effective to stop or prevent further bleeding. Transcatheter arterial

---

Box 47.2 Pitfalls, Complications, and Controversies

Patients with portal hypertension must be distinguished at admission because endoscopy, management, clinical course, and prognosis may vary greatly.

Clinical features and endoscopy are able to distinguish between severe and nonsevere bleeders.

Upper GI bleeding should be controlled by continuous automated monitoring of beats per minute and arterial pressure or by period assessment of the gastric aspirate using a NG tube.

Early upper GI endoscopy provides a high diagnostic accuracy but not in all cases. In this situation, emergency surgery, other diagnostic procedures, or new endoscopy after hemostasis should be considered, depending on the severity of bleeding.

Emergency endoscopy is difficult and involves some risk.

Intubation is mandatory for endoscopy in patients with consciousness disorders.

Therapeutic endoscopy may be repeated once, but after one retreatment surgery should be considered.

Significant rebleeding is defined as the presence of hematemesis or rebleeding with hypovolemia (<100 mm Hg of systolic pressure and/or heart rate > 100 bpm) and/or decrease in hemoglobin level > 2 g/liter within 12 hr.

Portal hypertension bleeders need early clinical, ultrasonographic, and endoscopic evaluation for treatment and prognosis.

Antibiotherapy should be considered early and maintained for 7 days in bleeding portal hypertension patients.

Acute active variceal bleeding should be treated by vasoactive drugs and therapeutic endoscopy.

The association of endoscopic therapy and vasoactive drugs improves the final hemostatic results in portal hypertension patients.

TIPS and surgery are considered to be rescue treatment in uncontrolled variceal bleeders, after drugs and therapeutic endoscopy.

Endoscopy in LGIB is difficult and has limited diagnostic accuracy.

Other diagnostic tools in LGIB are angiography, isotopic studies, push endoscopy, and the endoscopic capsule. Their use depends mainly on the bleeding activity rate and the general condition of the patient.

A high percentage of patients with LGIB remain undiagnosed despite all the additional examinations.

---

embolization is reserved for select cases with active bleeding during examination (Fig. 47.6). Rebleeding and perforation are complications of embolization. Surgery is indicated for persistent or recurrent episodes of bleeding. With no therapy, rebleeding occurs in 40% of patients during follow-up.

Meckel's diverticulum is a common congenital abnormality of the gastrointestinal tract containing heterotopic gastric mucosa, pancreatic tissue, or a combination of both. Bleeding may occur if acid secretion causes ulceration of the mucosa. Since most cases have heterotopic gastric mucosa, this may be detected using ^{99}Tc-pertechnetate scintigraphy. Meckel's diverticulum should be considered as the cause of LGIB in patients younger than 35 years old. Surgical resection is the treatment of choice.

PITFALLS, COMPLICATIONS, AND CONTROVERSIES

Box 47.2 presents the pitfalls, complications, and controversies regarding gastrointestinal bleeding.

SUGGESTED READING

Bordas JM, Terés J: Upper G.I. haemorrhage in portal hypertension. Clinical and endoscopic diagnosis. In Bosch J, Rodés J (eds): Recent Advances in Pathophysiology and Therapy of Portal Hypertension, Serono Symposia Review No. 22. Rome, SEDAL, 1989, pp 275–286.

Bosch J, Burroughs AK: Clinical manifestations and management of bleeding episodes in cirrhotics. In Bircher J, Benhamou P, McIntyre N, Rizzetto M, Rodés J (eds): Oxford Textbook of Clinical Hepatology, 2nd ed. Oxford, Oxford University Press, 1999, pp 671–693.

Cook DJ, Guyatt GH, Salena BJ, Laine LA: Endoscopic therapy for acute nonvariceal upper gastrointestinal hemorrhage: A meta-analysis. Gastroenterology 1992;102:139–148.

de Franchis R: Updating consensus in portal hypertension: Report of the Baveno III Consensus Workshop on definitions, methodology and therapeutic strategies in portal hypertension. J Hepatol 2000;33:846–852.

Escorsell A, Rodés J. Drug therapy in portal hypertension. In Farthing M, Ballinger A (eds): Drug Therapy for Gastrointestinal and Liver Diseases. London, Martin Dunitz, 2001, pp 289–312.

Feu F, Brullet E, Calvet X, et al: Recomendaciones para el diagnóstico y el tratamiento de la hemorragia digestiva alta aguda no varicosa. Gastroenterol Hepatol 2003;26:70–85.

García-Pagán JC, Escorsell A, Bosch J: The rational basis for the use of TIPS in the treatment of variceal bleeding, ascites and hepatorenal syndrome. In Arroyo V, Bosch J, Bruguera M, Rodés J, Sánchez Tapias JM (eds): Therapy in Liver Diseases. The Pathophysiological Basis of Therapy. Barcelona, Masson, 1999, pp 13–18.

Laine L, Peterson WL: Bleeding peptic ulcer. N Engl J Med 1994;331: 717–727.

Lingenfelser T, Ell C: Lower intestinal bleeding. Best Practice Res Clin Gastroenterol 2001;15:135–153.

Zuckerman GR, Prakash C, Askin MP, Lewis BS; American Gastroenterological Association Clinical Practice and Practice Economics Committee: AGA technical review on the evaluation and management of occult and obscure gastrointestinal bleeding. Gastroenterology 2000;118:201–221.

Chapter 48

Pancreatitis

John C. Marshall

Acute pancreatitis is a relatively uncommon disease that presents a spectrum of clinical severity from self-limiting abdominal pain to a devastating systemic inflammatory disorder associated with substantial morbidity and mortality. The pancreas is a retroperitoneal organ. Its anatomic relationships define the local complications of the disease—for example, gastric and colonic ileus, splenic vein thrombosis or pseudoaneurysms of the splenic or hepatic arteries, and focal necrosis of the colonic mesentery. The systemic evolution of severe pancreatitis reflects the consequences of leakage of activated pancreatic digestive enzymes into the pancreatic parenchyma and retroperitoneum, producing, in essence, a chemical burn of the retroperitoneum, and activating an innate host systemic inflammatory response.

Successful treatment of more severe cases typically necessitates admission to an intensive care unit, and the ICU stay is often lengthy and complicated. Approaches to the patient with severe pancreatitis have evolved substantially over the past two decades, and mortality has declined, reflecting an improved understanding of the pathophysiology of the disease and generic advances in the care of the critically ill patient.

EPIDEMIOLOGY, RISK FACTORS, AND PATHOPHYSIOLOGY

Epidemiology

It is estimated that the annual incidence of acute pancreatitis in the United States is approximately 40 cases per 100,000 population and that 210,000 patients are hospitalized with the disease each year. Approximately 20% of these episodes are severe pancreatitis, associated with a mortality rate of 10% to 25%, depending on whether infected pancreatic necrosis is present. Patients with severe pancreatitis experience prolonged hospitalizations and often are admitted to an intensive care unit.

Risk Factors

The most common causes of acute pancreatitis are gallstones and alcohol, which together account for approximately 80% of all cases. However, a large number of factors have been implicated as causes of pancreatitis (Box 48.1), and familiarity with these is of importance in removing the precipitating cause and preventing recurrent attacks. Obesity is associated with greater disease severity, likely because of a greater degree of fat necrosis. Genetic factors have been inconsistently linked with disease severity; polymorphisms in the IL-1 signaling complex show the most consistent association with disease severity.

Box 48.1 Causes of Acute Pancreatitis

Gallstones
Alcohol abuse
Anatomic abnormalities of the pancreatic ductal system
    Pancreas divisum
    Duodenal diverticulum, choledochocele
Trauma to the pancreatic ductal system
Metabolic abnormalities
    Hypertriglyceridemia
    Hypercalcemia
Toxins
    Drugs—thiazide, corticosteroids
    Scorpion venom
Infectious agents
    Mumps
    Salmonellosis
    Ascariasis
Familial pancreatitis

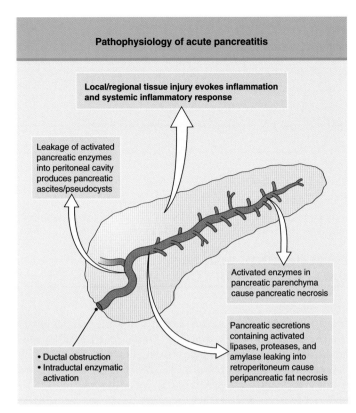

Figure 48.1. Pathophysiology of acute pancreatitis. Acute obstruction of the pancreatic duct or altered permeability of the ductal epithelium permits back-diffusion of activated pancreatic enzymes into the parenchyma of the gland, into the surrounding retroperitoneal fat, and into the free peritoneal cavity. Regional tissue injury activates an innate immune response, producing a hyperdynamic circulatory state and a diffuse increase in microvascular permeability.

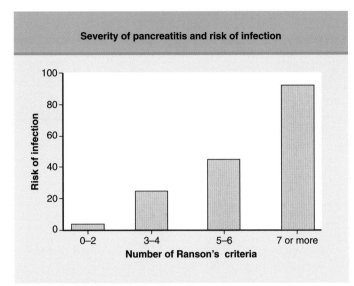

Figure 48.2. Severity of pancreatitis and risk of infection. The risk of infection of peripancreatic fluid collections or necrotic tissue increases over time, reaching a maximum at 2 to 3 weeks after the onset of the illness; infectious risk is a function of the initial severity of the acute episode, measured in this series using Ranson's criteria. (Adapted from Beger HG, Bittner R, Block S, Buchler M: Bacterial contamination of pancreatic necrosis: a prospective clinical study. Gastroenterology 1986;91:433–438.)

Pathogenesis

The predominant exocrine secretions of the pancreas are enzymes involved in the digestion of carbohydrates (amylase), fat (lipase), and proteins (proteases). These enzymes are released as inactive zymogens and become activated following their secretion into the pancreatic ductal system. Retrograde diffusion into the pancreatic parenchyma as a result of increased intraductal pressure (e.g., in gallstone pancreatitis), altered permeability of the ductal epithelium (e.g., in alcoholic pancreatitis), or ductal disruption (e.g., following pancreatic trauma) results in autodigestion of the pancreas and leakage of activated enzymes into the surrounding peripancreatic tissues (Fig. 48.1).

The evolution of the episode depends on the extent of leakage and the path taken by the pancreatic secretions. Disruption of the pancreatic duct posteriorly results in the diffusion of pancreatic enzymes throughout the retroperitoneal fat, causing fat necrosis that may extend through the perirenal fat into the pelvis. When the pancreatic duct is disrupted anteriorly, pancreatic juices leak into the lesser sac or free peritoneal cavity, causing pancreatic ascites and, occasionally, tracking through the diaphragm and producing a pleural effusion. The presence of irritant pancreatic secretions within the peritoneal space evokes an inflammatory response and fibrin deposition, which walls off the pancreatic fluid collection, creating a pseudocyst.

Tissue injury by activated pancreatic secretions activates a systemic inflammatory response of variable degree, depending on the extent of injury. The systemic response is characterized by increased capillary permeability and disseminated peripheral vasodilatation, producing clinical findings of intravascular volume deficit with tachycardia and hypotension and of increased pulmonary capillary permeability, resulting in tachypnea. The relative intravascular volume deficit is often large, a consequence of the combined effects of peripheral vasodilatation and increased capillary permeability, extravasation of fluid into the injured peripancreatic tissues, and losses into the adjacent gastrointestinal tract as a result of ileus. Pyrexia and leukocytosis may be present and, early in the course of the disease, result from the activation of a host inflammatory response to injured tissues rather than from bacterial infection.

Infection is a common complication of severe pancreatitis, its prevalence increasing with the severity of the initial episode (Fig. 48.2). While bacteria may reach devitalized peripancreatic tissue by bacteremic spread, or retrograde passage up the pancreatic duct, the most important route of infection appears to be the translocation of organisms from the adjacent gastrointestinal tract; the most common infecting species are enteric organisms (Table 48.1). Passage of bacteria and bacterial products into the mesenteric lymph can lead to systemic activation of an innate immune response, with further systemic sequelae—endothelial injury, increased microvascular permeability, microvascular thrombosis and shunting, tissue ischemia, and neutrophil-mediated tissue injury. Anaerobic bacteria do not translocate, and

Table 48.1 Microbiologic Causes of Pancreatic and Peripancreatic Infection	
Organism	**Percentage of Isolates (%)**
Escherichia coli	35
Klebsiella	24
Enterococcus	24
Staphylococcus	14
Pseudomonas	11
Proteus	8
Enterobacter	7
Bacteroides	6

Table 48.2 Ranson's Criteria in Acute Pancreatitis	
On Admission	**Over First 48 Hours**
Age > 55 yr	P_{O_2} < 60 mm Hg
White cell count > 16,000/μL	Estimated fluid sequestration > 6 L
Blood sugar > 11.1 mmol/L (200 mg/dL)	Calcium < 2.00 mm/L (8 mg/dL)
LDH > 350 IU/L	Hematocrit fall < 10%
AST > 250 IU/L	BUN rise > 1.8 mmol/L (5 mg/dL)
	Base excess > −4 mEq/L

Table 48.3 Balthazar Grading of CT Findings in Acute Pancreatitis	
Grade	**Finding**
A	Normal pancreas
B	Pancreatic edema only
C	Peripancreatic inflammation
	Pancreatic necrosis involving < 30% of gland
D	Single peripancreatic collection
	Pancreatic necrosis involving 30%–50% of gland
E	Two or more pancreatic collections and/or retroperitoneal air
	Necrosis > 50% of gland

the isolation of anerobic organisms in necrotic pancreatic tissue is highly suggestive of focal ischemic perforation of the colon.

Heterogeneity in the pathologic features of acute pancreatitis reflects the fact that the disease represents a spectrum, with varying degrees of fluid and solid tissue changes, inflamed viable and nonviable tissue, infected and sterile necrosis, intraperitoneal and retroperitoneal involvement, and pancreatic and peripancreatic injury, all of which evolve over time. Moreover, the severity of the systemic disease is only weakly correlated with the nature of the anatomic injury.

CLINICAL FEATURES AND DIAGNOSIS

Abdominal pain, maximal in the epigastrium, is almost invariably present in the patient with acute pancreatitis; the pain is commonly experienced as radiating to the back. Nausea and vomiting are common symptoms. Physical findings are variable. Abdominal tenderness is common but may be minimal because of the retroperitoneal location of the pancreas. Retroperitoneal bleeding is suggested by Cullen's (periumbilical ecchymosis) or Grey-Turner's (flank ecchymosis) signs, although these are relatively uncommon. The severity of the episode is suggested by the degree of acute physiologic instability reflected in tachypnea, tachycardia, hypotension, and oliguria.

Serum levels of amylase and lipase are typically elevated. Hyperamylasemia is not specific for pancreatitis but may occur during other acute abdominal disorders including acute cholecystitis or bowel obstruction. Moreover, the degree of elevation does not correlate with the clinical severity of the disease. Computed tomography (CT) can confirm the diagnosis and establish the anatomic extent of tissue involvement.

A number of systems have been used to quantify the early severity of the episode and thus to aid in decisions regarding triage and in predicting the likelihood of later complications. Generic severity-of-illness measures such as APACHE II have proved effective in quantifying disease severity. Ranson's criteria (Table 48.2), or the Glasgow-Imrie modification of these, have been widely used in clinical reports and have the advantage of greater face validity, although their prognostic capacity is not superior to that of APACHE. The severity of the disease can also be graded radiologically (Table 48.3); necrosis involving more than 30% of the gland is associated with greater disease severity.

With a careful history and physical examination, supplemented by the results of laboratory and radiologic investigations, the diagnosis of acute pancreatitis can usually be established with confidence. The differential diagnosis includes acute cholecystitis, perforated peptic ulcer, rupture of an abdominal aortic aneurysm, intestinal ischemia, and myocardial infarction.

MANAGEMENT

Initial Resuscitation and Triage
The first priority in the management of the patient with acute pancreatitis is fluid resuscitation and hemodynamic stabilization. Because third space fluid losses are substantial in severe pancreatitis, large volumes of fluid must typically be given over the first 24 hours, and as resuscitation proceeds, it is not uncommon for the patient to develop respiratory failure, necessitating intubation and mechanical ventilation. The patient with moderately severe or severe pancreatitis (three or more Ranson's criteria) is best managed in an adequately monitored environment, either a stepdown unit or an ICU.

Supportive Care in the ICU
Beyond physiologic management and support, there is no compelling evidence to support any specific therapy for the patient with severe acute pancreatitis. The role of antibiotic prophylaxis is controversial. Pooled data from small clinical trials suggest that the administration of systemic prophylactic antibiotics results in reduced rates of infectious complications and improved survival. However, the individual trials that form this meta-analysis are of variable quality, and the apparent benefit is driven by the results of the weakest studies. Moreover, indiscriminate antibiotic exposure is associated with superinfection and the

emergence of resistance; it also facilitates the translocation of enteric bacteria and renders the diagnosis of infection more difficult. The author's practice, consistent with the recommendations of a recent consensus conference, is to withhold antibiotic prophylaxis until more compelling evidence of efficacy has been established through randomized trials. Selective digestive tract decontamination—a mode of infection prophylaxis based on the administration of topical, nonabsorbed antibiotics with activity against gram-negative aerobes and fungi—has shown promise in two studies; however, its routine use also awaits further confirmation of efficacy.

An alternative strategy to reduce infectious risk is the early initiation of enteral feeding; by promoting gut motility and supporting the integrity of the intestinal mucosa, enteral nutrition can reduce rates of bacterial translocation and so may prevent infection of necrotic peripancreatic tissues. Five small randomized trials show enteral nutrition to be safe and suggest benefit in reducing the severity of the inflammatory response and in improving survival. Enteral feeding is safe, cost-effective, and biologically rational, and it obviates the complications associated with parenteral nutrition; it should be instituted in the absence of compelling contraindications. As a result of gastric ileus secondary to retroperitoneal inflammation, it may be necessary to decompress the stomach with a nasogastric tube, while enteral feeds are delivered to the duodenum or jejunum, and radiologic placement of feeding tubes is commonly required.

Multiple adjuvant therapies for the patient with severe pancreatitis have been studied, including protease inhibitors, fresh-frozen plasma, somatostatin, and platelet-activating factor inhibition; however, none has shown any evidence of benefit. Following resuscitation and the establishment of physiologic organ system support, the management of the patient with severe acute pancreatitis is entirely supportive.

Source Control

Surgical intervention is indicated for early diagnostic uncertainty or for the management of the complications of severe acute pancreatitis—intestinal ischemia, bleeding, and infection. With improvements in diagnostic imaging techniques, diagnostic uncertainty is uncommon, and early exploratory laparotomy is rarely indicated. Mesenteric venous thrombosis—a consequence of prolonged underresuscitation—is an uncommon early complication of severe acute pancreatitis; even with surgical intervention, the mortality is prohibitive. Significant bleeding requiring early intervention is also an uncommon complication but may arise as a result of erosion of the inflammatory process into a major artery.

Infection of necrotic retroperitoneal fat or collections of pancreatic fluid, on the other hand, is a relatively common complication. Peripancreatic infections develop gradually, with the majority presenting 2 or 3 weeks after the onset of illness. The diagnosis is challenging. Signs of a systemic inflammatory response, including persistent organ dysfunction, are often present and lack specificity for a diagnosis of infection. The CT scan may suggest infection; however, accurate discrimination of infected from noninfected necrosis is unreliable. Although biochemical markers such as procalcitonin or C-reactive protein have been suggested to have diagnostic utility in discriminating sterile from infected pancreatic necrosis, the gold standard

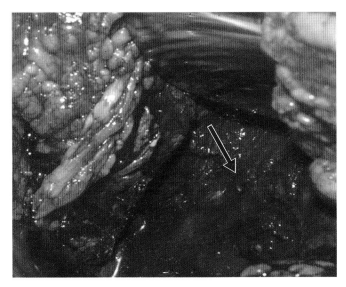

Figure 48.3. Operative findings early in the course (day 10) of acute necrotizing pancreatitis. Tissues are hemorrhagic (arrow) and bleed when débridement is attempted; areas of necrosis are not well demarcated. The need for repeat débridement to excise necrotic tissue, or packing to control retroperitoneal bleeding, often results in the need for open-abdomen approaches, with their attendant morbidity.

diagnostic technique is fine-needle aspiration under CT scan guidance. The sensitivity and specificity of fine-needle aspiration exceed 80%.

Evolving clinical experience reported in case series and a single randomized, controlled trial suggests that outcomes are best when surgical intervention is delayed. Early in the course of peripancreatic necrosis, there is no clear demarcation between viable, inflamed, bleeding tissue and adjacent areas of necrosis. Surgical intervention at this time, therefore, is often complicated by uncontrolled retroperitoneal bleeding or incomplete débridement of areas of infected necrosis, and open abdomen approaches become necessary (Fig. 48.3). On the other hand, by 3 to 4 weeks after the onset of the disease, a clear demarcation of viable from nonviable tissues has occurred. At the time of surgery, necrotic material can be evacuated from a well-delineated cavity; complications are rare, and primary closure is usually possible.

The challenge for the surgeon is to establish the optimal time for intervention in the patient with infected pancreatic necrosis, balancing the risks of early intervention with the adverse consequences of delayed management of infection. The author's experience has been that infected pancreatic necrosis is usually tolerated without significant further physiologic deterioration and that surgery can be performed electively for the indication of persistent failure to resolve organ dysfunction, generally 3 to 4 weeks after admission to the ICU. Narrow-spectrum systemic antibiotics selected on the basis of data from fine-needle aspiration are administered. Percutaneous drainage may aid as a temporizing measure by decompressing infected fluid collections, although it is not generally definitive (Fig. 48.4). The area of infected necrosis may be approached through a midline or

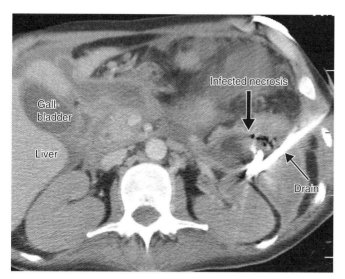

Figure 48.4. Percutaneous CT-guided drainage of the fluid component of a complex pancreatic infection can serve to temporize until definitive surgical management can be safely performed, even though necrotic, infected solid tissue remains.

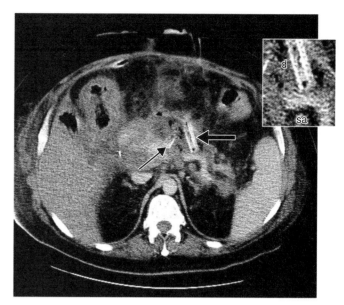

Figure 48.5. Massive upper gastrointestinal bleeding developed in a 38-year-old man, 24 days after laparotomy and placement of two drains *(arrows)* in an area of infected retroperitoneal necrosis. At laparotomy, he was found to have a linear tear of the splenic artery (sa), resulting from erosion of the drain tip (d), seen in the inset image, into the vessel.

bilateral subcostal incision, or, when it is predominantly localized to one side of the abdomen, through a flank incision. Intraoperative decision making is facilitated by the availability of a preoperative CT scan. When fat necrosis is extensive and involves the mesentery of the colon, the probability of undetected microperforation of the colon increases, and proximal diversion by loop ileostomy should be considered.

Minimally invasive approaches to source control for pancreatic infections, including laparoscopic CT-guided débridement, have been described and will play an increasing role in the future management of these complex infections.

When delayed intervention has successfully removed all necrotic infected tissue, there is no need for the use of drains larger than soft flexible closed suction drains that permit egress of pancreatic juice from the injured pancreas. Large-bore rigid drains increase the risk of colonic perforation or bleeding; moreover, they are ineffective in evacuating necrotic solid tissue (Fig. 48.5).

Other Adjuvant Therapies

Early endoscopic retrograde cholangiopancreatography (ERCP) has been reported to reduce late complications of acute pancreatitis, although the results of clinical trials are inconsistent. Activated protein C should be considered for the patient with infected pancreatic necrosis and organ dysfunction, and corticosteroids are indicated for the patient with prolonged vasopressor dependence and an inadequate cortisol response to ACTH stimulation.

CLINICAL COURSE AND PROGNOSIS

Late complications of pancreatitis include endocrine and exocrine insufficiency (both of which are surprisingly uncommon) and sequelae of surgical management such as fistulas

---

Box 48.2 Controversies

- The role of antibiotic prophylaxis—either systemic or topical
- The potential role of therapies targeting mediators of systemic inflammation
- Nonoperative management of infected necrosis and surgery for sterile necrosis
- The role of minimally invasive source control measures
- The role of ERCP in gallstone pancreatitis

---

and abdominal wall hernias. Surgical management of these complications is best delayed until the patient has been discharged from the hospital and has convalesced. Cholecystectomy for the patient with gallstone pancreatitis—if not performed at the time of surgical débridement—is best deferred until the patient has recovered.

The ICU course of the patient with severe acute pancreatitis is characteristically prolonged and complicated (Boxes 48.2 and 48.3). However, long-term quality of life for survivors is excellent and fully justifies the extraordinary efforts that are often required to manage these patients.

529

Box 48.3 Pitfalls
■ The severity of the fluid deficit during the early evolution of severe acute pancreatitis is frequently underestimated; monitoring of volume status by frequent evaluation of vital signs, urine output, or central pressures is key to early recognition of fluid deficits. ■ Pancreatitis is the prototypical example of a disorder that results in a systemic inflammatory response in the absence of infection; decisions regarding antibiotic therapy should be guided by the results of culture rather than by clinical manifestations of a systemic inflammatory response. ■ Source control intervention is almost never an emergency, and significant morbidity and mortality can result from injudicious early surgical intervention. Decisions regarding the optimal timing of source control should involve a surgeon with interest and experience in the management of patients with pancreatitis, and it is, as a general rule, preferable to err on the side of continuing conservatism. ■ Although patients with severe pancreatitis present enormous management challenges and commonly develop significant degrees of organ dysfunction, with ICU support and well thought out surgical intervention, the probability of survival to a good long-term quality of life fully justifies an aggressive approach to continued care, and decisions to limit support should be made only when source control has failed and patient preferences dictate a switch to compassionate care.

SUGGESTED READING

Baron TH, Morgan DE: Acute necrotizing pancreatitis. N Engl J Med 1999;340:1412–1417.

Beger HG, Bittner R, Block S, Buchler M: Bacterial contamination of pancreatic necrosis: a prospective clinical study. Gastroenterology 1986;91:433–438.

Mier J, Leon EL, Castillo A, et al: Early versus late necrosectomy in severe necrotizing pancreatitis. Am J Surg 1997;173:71–75.

Nathens AB, Curtis JR, Beale RJ, et al: Management of the critically ill patient with severe acute pancreatitis. Crit Care Med 2004;32: 2524–2536.

Swaroop VS, Chari ST, Clain JE: Severe acute pancreatitis. JAMA 2004; 291:2865–2868.

Uhl W, Warshaw A, Imrie C, et al: IAP Guidelines for the surgical management of acute pancreatitis. Pancreatology 2002;2:565–573.

Werner J, Feuerbach S, Uhl W, Buchler MW: Management of acute pancreatitis: from surgery to interventional intensive care. Gut 2005;54: 426–436.

Chapter 49

Acute Liver Failure

Timothy Cross, James O'Beirne, and Julia Wendon

KEY POINTS

- Early discussion with and referral to regional liver transplant centers is essential to optimize patient outcome in acute liver failure (ALF).
- Antibiotic prophylaxis reduces the incidence of infection in ALF patients.
- Criteria for poor prognosis allow identification of patients unlikely to survive without liver transplantation.
- Patients with grade 3 encephalopathy and above are at risk of intracranial hypertension and cerebral herniation and should be managed in specialized centers.
- The use of moderate hypothermia and mild hypernatremia reduces the incidence of sustained rises in intracranial pressure in ALF.

Acute liver failure (ALF) is a life-threatening illness defined by the coexistence of progressive coagulopathy, hepatic encephalopathy, and biochemical evidence of liver dysfunction in a patient with no previous history of liver disease. The prognosis of the syndrome is variable, dependent on the etiology, mode of presentation, and the age of the patient. The care of ALF patients in intensive care units (ICUs) with modern organ support techniques and the advent of liver transplantation has revolutionized the management of the syndrome such that many patients can be supported until spontaneous hepatic recovery or liver transplantation occurs. However, a significant number of patients will die from refractory hypotension and intracranial hypertension, making ALF one of the most challenging medical conditions encountered in the ICU.

EPIDEMIOLOGY, ETIOLOGY, AND PATHOGENESIS

The term fulminant hepatic failure (FHF) was first used in 1970 when Trey and Davidson described an acute liver disease complicated by encephalopathy within 8 weeks of the onset of symptoms in a patient without previous liver disease. However, this definition did not reflect the diverse outcome of patients with ALF of different etiologies. After recognizing that patients with a very florid presentation may paradoxically have the best outcome, O'Grady and colleagues (1993) proposed a definition of ALF that better reflects the contribution of etiology to outcome. In this classification, liver failure in patients with a jaundice-to-encephalopathy time of less than 7 days is termed hyperacute, jaundiced patients who present with encephalopathy from 7 to 28 days are defined as having acute liver failure, whereas those who present with encephalopathy up to 3 months after becoming jaundiced are defined as having subacute liver failure. Using these definitions, it is possible to gain insight into the pathological process and the likely outcome (Table 49.1).

In the United Kingdom, the leading cause of ALF is poisoning with paracetamol (acetaminophen), whereas in the United States and Europe, ALF from viral and seronegative causes predominates, although the incidence of acetaminophen poisoning is increasing in the United States. The principal causes of ALF are outlined in Box 49.1. Important geographical differences exist, and these are highlighted in Figure 49.1.

PROGNOSIS

There is no doubt that the advent of liver transplantation has transformed the outcome of ALF, with 1- and 5-year survival rates of 65% and 59%, respectively, post-liver transplantation compared to less than 20% survival with medical management alone. However, due to the liver's remarkable ability to regenerate and recover from acute injury, the rate of survival with optimal medical management can be surprisingly high in some patients, especially those with a hyperacute presentation. Therefore, the challenge facing clinicians who care for these patients is the early identification of those patients who will not survive with medical management so that they may undergo timely transplantation, while avoiding transplantation in those who may have a favorable outcome with medical management alone.

Table 49.1 Subclassification of Acute Liver Failure and Impact on Prognosis[a]

Jaundice to Encephalopathy	Classification	Example	Chance of Spontaneous Survival (%)
<7 days	Hyperacute	Acetaminophen toxicity	40
7–28 days	Acute	Viral hepatitis, drug reactions	<20
28 days–3 months	Subacute	Seronegative hepatitis	<20

[a]Despite having the highest incidence of severe prolongations of prothrombin time and the highest incidence of cerebral edema, patients with hyperacute liver failure have the best chance of spontaneous survival.

A number of systems have been developed to aid the clinician in these decisions, the most widely used of which is the Kings College Hospital (KCH) criteria, which were developed using a cohort of 588 ALF patients and subsequently prospectively validated in a further cohort of 175 patients. The criteria distinguish between ALF due to acetaminophen and other causes, reflecting the quite different natural history of these patients (Box 49.2). In the original study, the criteria were accurate in predicting death in 84% and 98% of the acetaminophen and nonacetaminophen groups, respectively. The percentage of patients who did not fulfill the criteria and subsequently survived was 86% for the acetaminophen and 82% for the nonacetaminophen group. The KCH criteria have been subjected to validation in other cohorts in Europe and the United States and have been found to have acceptable specificity; however, they have been shown to have rather limited sensitivity in some studies (i.e., nonfulfillment of the criteria does not guarantee survival). Furthermore, in patients who fulfill the criteria, there is a high rate of deterioration that often precludes transplantation; hence, there is a need for criteria that can identify patients with a poor prognosis at an earlier point in the evolution of the syndrome. The KCH criteria for acetaminophen-induced ALF have been combined with serum lactate, and this combination results in an increased sensitivity and specificity for the identification of patients with a poor prognosis at an earlier time point than the standard criteria and should be validated in a further cohort of patients.

Other centers use different criteria that perform reasonably well in terms of sensitivity and specificity. For instance, the Clichy criteria (Box 49.3) use the percentage activity of factor V, patient age, and encephalopathy to determine poor prognosis. These criteria were derived from a cohort of 115 patients with hepatitis B infection and hence may not be applicable in more heterogeneous groups. Nonetheless, they are used in many centers, especially in northern Europe.

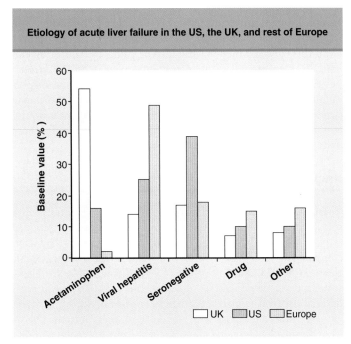

Etiology of acute liver failure in the US, the UK, and rest of Europe

Figure 49.1. Etiology of acute liver failure in the United States, United Kingdom, and the rest of Europe. Note the high incidence of acetaminophen toxicity in the United Kingdom. Studies suggest that the incidence of this etiology is increasing in the United States. The "other" category includes etiologies such as Budd–Chiari syndrome, Wilson's disease, and pregnancy-induced ALF.

Box 49.2 King's College Hospital Criteria for Poor Prognosis in ALF

In Nonacetaminophen-Induced Liver Failure

Prothrombin time > 100 sec (INR > 6.5)
Or
pH < 7.3
Or any three of the following:
    Age < 10 years
    Age > 40 years
    Seronegative hepatitis (non-A to E), halothane, or other
      drug reaction
    Duration of jaundice > 7 days before hepatic
      encephalopathy
    Prothrombin time > 50 sec (INR > 6.5)
    Bilirubin > 300 μmol/L

In Acetaminophen ALF

pH < 7.3 (after fluid resuscitation)
Or all three of the following in a 24-hr period
    Prothrombin time > 100 sec (INR > 6.5)
    Creatinine > 300 μmol/L
    Grade 3 or 4 hepatic encephalopathy

Box 49.1 Causes of Acute Liver Failure

Infective	Drugs	Poisoning	Immune and Metabolic	Other
Hepatitis A	Acetaminophen	Acetaminophen	Autoimmune hepatitis	Budd–Chiari syndrome
Hepatitis B[a]	Halothane	Ecstasy	Wilson's disease	Ischemic hepatitis
Hepatitis E	NSAIDs[b]	Amanita phalloides	Reye's syndrome	Malignant infiltration
Herpes simplex (1 + 2)	Isoniazid	Herbal remedies	Acute fatty liver of pregnancy	Heat stroke
Varicella zoster	Rifampicin			Trauma
Parvovirus B19	Valproate			
Coxsackie B viral	Carbamzepine			
hemorrhagic fevers				

[a]and delta agent superinfection.
[b]Nonsteroidal anti-inflammatory drugs.

Box 49.3 Clichy Criteria in Viral Fulminant Hepatic Failure
Coma or confusion And Factor V < 20% if younger than 30 years of age Or Factor V < 30% if older than 30 years of age

Other criteria in clinical practice are a liver volume less than 1000 mL on computed tomography (CT) scan, which, although specific for a poor outcome, is logistically difficult because of the risks involved in transporting these patients to the radiology department; likewise, the use of liver biopsy to define the degree of necrosis is practically difficult. Patients with ALF often have a low serum phosphate, possibly reflecting substrate utilization by the regenerating liver. In 125 ALF patients, a serum phosphate more than 1.2 mmol/L was found to be sensitive and specific for a poor outcome, with an overall accuracy of 98%. However, in a larger cohort of ALF patients, the criteria did not perform as well.

Special Circumstances
The existing criteria for the identification of patients with a poor prognosis are not applicable to certain patient groups, mainly because these patients are rare in practice. Budd–Chiari syndrome is one such condition resulting from hepatic venous thrombosis that has a heterogeneous presentation ranging from ascites to the full-blown syndrome of ALF. Because the presentation is so heterogeneous, there is no consensus on the correct management of these patients. Different therapies have been proposed, ranging from hepatic vein repermeation and transjugular intrahepatic stent shunts to liver transplantation. No randomized data exist to guide the clinician in these decisions; however, using the coexistence of renal failure and encephalopathy as criteria for emergent liver transplantation, the current 5-year survival for patients undergoing transplantation for acute Budd-Chiari syndrome (BCS) is approximately 70%.

Acute Wilson's disease is also very uncommon and can present as a de novo illness or due to noncompliance with copper chelation therapy in a patient already diagnosed with the disease. The disease presents in childhood or early adulthood with jaundice, which may be hemolytic, and coagulopathy; usually the signs of chronic liver disease are already present. In the adult population, an acute presentation tends to lead to a poor prognosis, and therefore most adult patients with acute Wilson's disease will undergo liver transplantation.

Acute fatty liver of pregnancy and preeclamptic liver disease can cause ALF; most patients recover with medical management. Although liver transplantation may be needed in selected cases, there are no guidelines on liver transplantation in these conditions.

DIAGNOSIS

The patient with ALF may present in a number of ways, ranging from mild encephalopathy to rapidly deteriorating course with multiple organ failure and intracranial hypertension. The key points in the management of these patients are the early

Box 49.4 Guidelines for the Referral and Transfer of Patients with ALF to Regional Specialist Centers	
Acetaminophen	**Nonacetaminophen**
Arterial pH < 7.30	pH < 7.30
INR > 3.0 on day 2 or > 4.0 thereafter	INR > 1.8
Oliguria and/or elevated creatinine	Oliguria/renal failure
Altered conscious level	Encephalopathy
Hypoglycemia	Hypoglycemia
	Shrinking liver size
	Na < 130 mmol/L
	Bilirubin > 300 μmol/L

identification of those patients with a poor prognosis who may benefit from urgent listing for transplantation and the prevention or treatment of the multiple organ complications of the syndrome, allowing survival of liver transplantation or hepatic regeneration.

The clinical course of patients with ALF is extremely rapid; hence, all patients should be discussed with a regional liver unit to determine priority for transfer before the development of complications such as intracranial hypertension that may make subsequent transfer hazardous (Box 49.4).

As with any illness, a thorough history and examination should be undertaken. Often, the patient will be unable to give an accurate history due to encephalopathy, and a collateral history should be sought from relatives, caregivers, paramedical staff, and the patient's primary care physician. Important points to cover in the history are the speed of onset of encephalopathy after the appearance of jaundice, drug use (either illicit or prescribed), use of herbal remedies or mushroom ingestion, alcohol use, recent travel, and possible exposures to blood-borne viruses. In patients with ALF secondary to deliberate overdose, special attention should be given to obtain a full psychiatric history, preferably from the patient's own psychiatrist or primary care physician, because important background information such as this may be important in deciding whether a patient is a suitable candidate for liver transplantation.

The physical examination of the patient with ALF reveals information about the severity of the syndrome and the possible etiology. The patient may or may not be jaundiced; this is a relatively rare initial finding in hyperacute liver failure. The signs of chronic liver disease are characteristically absent, but it is worth noting that patients with a subacute presentation of ALF may have ascites, and patients with ALF secondary to Wilson's disease or autoimmune cirrhosis may have splenomegaly and spider nevi. It is important to accurately note the grade of encephalopathy (Table 49.2) because this has prognostic importance. Intracranial hypertension is common in these patients; therefore, it is vital to examine the pupils for size and reactivity as well as to perform a general neurologic examination, which may reveal increased tone and hyperreflexia in patients with cerebral edema.

In patients with a suspected diagnosis of Wilson's disease, it is useful to obtain an opthalmological opinion, and slit lamp examination is useful to search for Kayser–Fleischer rings, which are almost pathognomonic in this clinical setting. General examination may also reveal other signs, such as lymphadenopathy, that may point to malignant infiltration as a cause of ALF.

Table 49.2 Grading of Hepatic Encephalopathy[a]

Grade	Conscious Level	Personality and Intellect	Neurology
0	Normal	Normal	None
Subclinical	Normal	Normal	None
1	Inverted sleep, restless	Forgetful, mild confusion	Tremor, apraxia, impaired handwriting
2	Lethargy, slow responses	Disorientation, inappropriate behavior	Dysarthria, ataxia, asterixis (liver flap)
3	Somnolence, confusion	Aggression, agitation	Hyperreflexia, muscle rigidity, clonus
4	Coma	None	Cerebral herniation

[a]Patients with advanced grade encephalopathy (grade 3/4) have a worse outcome overall and are at high risk for the development of cerebral edema.

INVESTIGATIONS

The initial blood investigations of a patient with ALF are directed toward the diagnosis, prognosis, and identification of complications. Hence, the minimum data set should include arterial blood gases; serum lactate; full blood count; urea and electrolytes; liver function tests; immunoglobulins; coagulation screen and more specific blood tests, such as viral markers (A, B, C, and E, as appropriate); copper studies; and autoantibodies. Other tests that may be helpful are a blood film, split bilirubin, ammonia, and 24-hour urine collection for creatinine clearance and copper estimation. When transplantation is being considered, tests for HIV, cytomegalovirus, and Epstein–Barr virus status are valuable.

HEMATOLOGICAL CHANGES IN ALF

One of the hallmarks of ALF is the profound coagulopathy that accompanies the syndrome. It comprises a prolongation in the prothrombin time (PT), activated partial thromboplastin time, and thrombocytopenia. In addition, patients may have other coagulation abnormalities, such as hyperfibrinolysis or disseminated intravascular coagulation (DIC).

The serum fibrinogen level is often low in ALF due to deficient production by the failing liver or concomitant DIC. Even when the fibrinogen level is normal, the thrombin time may be prolonged due to the presence of dysfibrinogenemia. Hyperfibrinolysis can also occur in ALF and is suggested by shortened whole blood euglobulin clot lysis times, elevated levels of fibrin degradation products, and typical appearances on thromboelastography. Thrombocytopenia is almost universal in patients with ALF and, when severe, is a marker of poor prognosis. The cause of the thrombocytopenia is probably due to deficient thrombopoiesis and increased peripheral consumption of platelets; certainly, there is no relation to thrombopoetin, the production of which is either normal or increased in ALF.

In practice, most patients with ALF will have a coagulopathy that is multifactorial in origin, and it is often difficult to distinguish patients with hyperfibrinolysis from those with DIC.

BIOCHEMICAL CHANGES IN ALF

There are a number of important biochemical abnormalities that occur in ALF, and certain patterns may be observed that have important prognostic and therapeutic implications. Spontaneous hypoglycemia is often present in the advanced stages of liver failure, hypoglycemia makes interpretation of the grade of encephalopathy difficult, and evaluation of the grade of hepatic encephalopathy should only be done if the serum glucose is in the normal range, which may require continuous infusion of 20% to 50% glucose. Glucose levels should be maintained within the normal range in all patients, and this may require insulin therapy in some.

Serum sodium is often decreased below the normal range in ALF patients, and this may be a factor in precipitating cerebral edema by lowering the osmotic gradient across the blood–brain barrier (BBB). Hyponatremia is often worsened by the inappropriate administration of glucose infusions as volume replacement and can be corrected by the administration of hypertonic sodium infusions. Most patients with hyperacute and acute liver failure are not sodium overloaded, and therefore the routine use of sodium restriction is not advised. Low levels of other electrolytes, such as potassium, magnesium, and phosphate, are often observed; of these, serum phosphate deserves special mention because hyperphosphatemia is associated with a poor prognosis, possibly reflecting decreased substrate utilization by regenerating hepatocytes and renal impairment.

Evaluation of standard liver function tests is often not helpful in the initial assessment of ALF. Transaminase (AST and ALT) levels may be very high, but this carries no prognostic importance other than the fact that the association of a falling transaminase level with a rising INR heralds a poor prognosis. The transaminase levels tend to be highest in hyperacute and acute liver failure, whereas there may be only modest elevations of transaminase in the subacute group. Conversely, the bilirubin level may be normal in hyperacute liver failure and very high in those with subacute liver failure. In some cases of hyperbilirubinemia, it is often valuable to determine the amounts of conjugated and unconjugated bilirubin present. A very high level of unconjugated bilirubin suggests a hemolytic process, as can often be seen in the acute presentation of Wilson's disease and in patients with glucose-6 phosphate dehydrogenase deficiency.

The alkaline phosphatase (ALP) level is often only mildly elevated and is not helpful in the majority of cases. However, if it is very low, this may indicate Wilson's disease as the cause of ALF. In contrast, when it is significantly elevated, an infiltrative etiology is suspected.

Hyperlactatemia is common in liver failure, representing decreased hepatic clearance in addition to potential overproduction by peripheral tissues. The serum lactate level is a useful guide to the adequacy of intravascular volume replacement and cardiac output. In patients who are well resuscitated, the serum lactate level has prognostic importance, as can be shown when used in combination with the KCH criteria for the identification of patients with acetaminophen toxicity who have a poor prognosis.

The role of ammonia in the pathogenesis of hepatic encephalopathy (HE) is discussed later, but its measurement in the initial evaluation is helpful because levels greater than

150 µmol/L are associated with an increased risk of cerebral herniation.

OTHER TESTS

Blood tests for the common hepatitis viruses are performed in all cases of ALF. Viral hepatitis A is suggested by the presence of hepatitis A virus IgM and a typical history. Hepatitis B infection is a relatively common cause of ALF, accounting for up to 41% of cases from a single center in a U.S. study, but due to vaccination the incidence of ALF caused by hepatitis B virus (HBV) is decreasing in the Western world. The presence of anti-hepatitis B core IgM is highly suggestive of HBV as the cause of the ALF; HBV surface antigen may or may not be present. Results for hepatitis A and B serology should be available within a few hours of the admission of the patient to the hospital, whereas hepatitis C virus is almost never a cause of ALF; therefore, it is not mandatory to have these results in the first few hours. Hepatitis E IgM should be evaluated, especially in those returning from an endemic area such as the Indian subcontinent.

Serum immunoglobulins and liver autoantibodies should be requested on admission. Elevated immunoglobulin G or the presence of antismooth muscle or antinuclear antibodies should lead to the consideration of autoimmune hepatitis as the underlying diagnosis. In this situation, the timely administration of corticosteroids may be life saving.

Acute pancreatitis is not uncommon in patients with ALF, in which it represents a possible contraindication to transplantation. Hence, it is recommended to check the serum amylase in all patients.

IMAGING IN ACUTE LIVER FAILURE

All patients with ALF should have a baseline liver ultrasound scan aimed at evaluation of the liver texture and hepatic vasculature. Doppler ultrasound of the liver vasculature may reveal abnormalities such as hepatic vein thrombosis in Budd–Chiari syndrome or portal vein thrombosis that may complicate subsequent liver transplantation. The liver texture is often normal but may be heterogeneous in cases of malignant infiltration or preexisting chronic liver disease, in which splenomegaly and ascites may also be present. It is important to remember that the presence of ascites, a small nodular liver, and splenomegaly can also be features of Wilson's disease and ALF running a subacute course; therefore, care is required in the interpretation of the ultrasound results. Ultrasound scanning is cheap and convenient but is often not accurate enough when there is uncertainty about the diagnosis (e.g., in cases of suspected malignant infiltration or when an accurate assessment of liver size is needed). CT of the liver gives information about liver volume (Fig. 49.2) and can help to define the vasculature, including the portal and mesenteric systems, and to rule out complications such as pancreatitis. However, transporting a patient with ALF, who may be hemodynamically unstable with cerebral edema, to the CT scanner is potentially hazardous and therefore should not be undertaken unless the results are likely to change management.

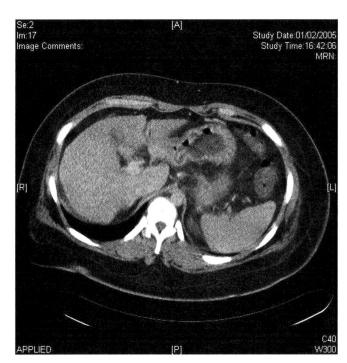

Figure 49.2. CT scan of liver in ALF. CT scan of the liver from a patient with subacute liver failure. The liver is small and collapsed. Liver size by volumetry has been used to define poor prognosis in ALF.

PATHOLOGY

In most cases of ALF, histological examination of tissue lends little to the diagnosis because the findings are often similar irrespective of etiology. There is almost total loss of hepatocytes, whereas connective tissue remains intact, leading to a collapsed appearance microscopically and a small pale liver macroscopically (Fig. 49.3). Areas of regeneration may be apparent both macroscopically and microscopically, giving rise to a nodular appearance to the liver that may be mistaken for cirrhosis.

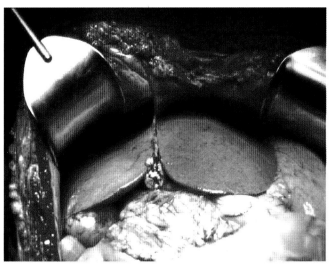

Figure 49.3. The macroscopic appearance of the liver in a patient with ALF. The liver is small and characteristically pale.

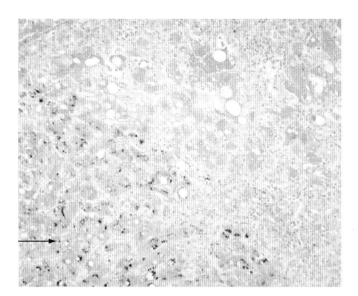

Figure 49.4. The microscopic appearances of ALF induced by Wilson's disease. Microscopic appearance of the explant of a patient transplanted for ALF due to Wilson's disease. The arrow indicates deposits of copper-associated protein. (Orcein stain, magnification × 400.)

In some circumstances (i.e., malignant infiltration, Budd–Chiari syndrome, and Wilson's disease), the histological features are typical (Fig. 49.4). However, other than in cases of suspected malignant infiltration, biopsy of the liver does not routinely inform management or prognosis.

MANAGEMENT

Sepsis, Systemic Inflammatory Response Syndrome, and the Role of Prophylactic Antibiotics

Patients with ALF are prone to sepsis and the systemic inflammatory response syndrome (SIRS), with up to 80% of patients developing positive cultures at some point during their illness. This increased propensity to bacterial and fungal infections is due to a number of interrelated factors. First, the severity of the multiple organ failure seen in advanced ALF mandates the use of invasive ventilation and several intravascular monitoring devices that, despite the use of scrupulous aseptic technique and microbiological surveillance, result in a number of infections. Second, in ALF the liver is unable to produce components of the innate immune system, such as those required for the function of the complement system and acute phase proteins, resulting in an immunodeficient state. Finally, the liver's normal important role in filtering bacteria from portal blood is lost, leading to an increased level of bacteremia.

Thus, the issue of infection is of critical importance not only because sepsis-induced multiple organ failure (MOF) is the most common cause of death in ALF but also because infection and SIRS are thought to have a central role in the progression of encephalopathy. For instance, the acquisition of infection precedes the development of deeper stages of encephalopathy, suggesting a link between SIRS and encephalopathy. This notion is supported by the observation that SIRS can cause increases in cerebral blood flow and may also act synergistically with ammonia to cause increases in intracranial pressure (ICP). Apart

from effects on hepatic encephalopathy, infection-induced MOF may also render a patient too sick for transplantation, and in those that do undergo transplantation, increased severity of MOF at the time of transplant is independently associated with a poorer prognosis.

The high prevalence of positive cultures during the first few days of admission, coupled with the fact that up to 30% of patients may not manifest the typical signs of infection (fever and leukocytosis), has led many centers to employ antibiotic prophylaxis regimens in ALF patients with progressive organ failure or those who fulfill liver transplant criteria. Prospective data suggest that such an approach is successful in reducing documented instances of infection in treated patients; however, there is no evidence suggesting that this approach reduces mortality.

There is a high incidence of gram-positive infections in patients with ALF. Therefore, any prophylactic antibiotic regimens should ensure broad-spectrum coverage of these and gram-negative organisms.

Prospective studies have also documented an incidence of fungal infection of up to 30% in ALF patients. Fungal infection is suggested by the presence of ongoing fever and leukocytosis despite antimicrobial therapy. The most common isolate is *Candida*, but *Aspergillus* species are also frequently found. Most patients who develop fungal sepsis will already be undergoing treatment or have had recent treatment for bacterial infection. There is a high mortality even if the infection is treated appropriately; hence, many centers use antifungal prophylaxis in liver transplant candidates, but there is no evidence supporting the use of this approach.

HEPATIC ENCEPHALOPATHY, INTRACRANIAL HYPERTENSION, AND CEREBRAL EDEMA

By definition, patients with ALF have some degree of HE. This may not progress above grade 1/2 in some patients, but many will progress to the deeper stages of encephalopathy often within a few hours. Patients with higher grades of encephalopathy (grade 3/4) are at risk for the complications of cerebral edema, intracranial hypertension, cerebral herniation, and death in up to 35% of patients. Therefore, the correct management of this complication is central to the optimal management of ALF (Fig. 49.5).

The pathogenesis of intracranial hypertension (IH) in ALF is centered on three components that contribute to increased brain volume within the skull: cerebral blood volume, astrocyte swelling, and extracellular fluid volume.

Cerebral Edema

The first step in the pathogenesis of cerebral edema is thought to be the development of hyperammonemia. Ammonia levels have been correlated with the degree of encephalopathy, and ammonia levels greater than 150 µmol/L are associated with an increased risk of subsequent death from cerebral herniation, supporting a direct pathogenic role of ammonia in ALF. Patients with ALF exhibit net production of ammonia from the splanchnic circulation, with variable uptake across the brain. The site of ammonia metabolism within the brain is the astrocyte, in which ammonia is converted by the enzyme glutamine synthetase to glutamine. This enzyme is exclusively located within

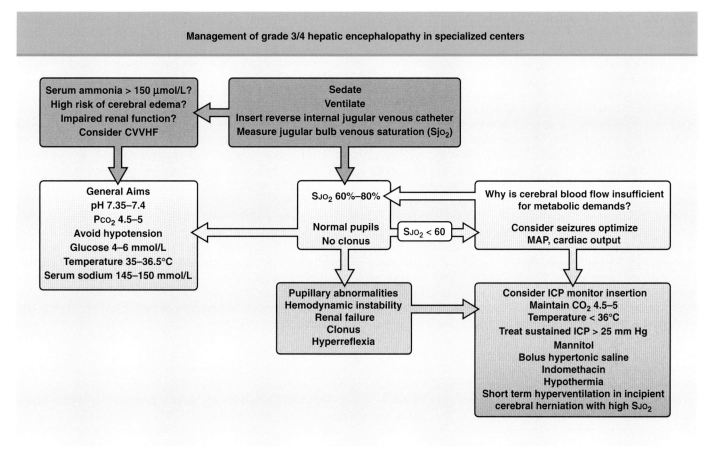

Figure 49.5. Management of grade 3/4 hepatic encephalopathy in specialized centers.

the astrocyte; hence, intracellular concentrations of glutamine in hyperammonemia are high, leading to osmotic swelling of astrocytes. This effect can be reproduced in animal models in which an ammonia load can be shown to induce astrocyte swelling acutely. Not only may hyperammonemia induce astrocyte swelling and hence increase brain volume, but also ammonia may disrupt neurotransmission, affect mitochondria, and cause oxidative stress, all of which add to the direct cytopathic effect and edema formation.

The generation of edema in ALF is also contributed to by changes in other molecules. Normally, the BBB tightly controls the passage of proteins and other small molecules maintaining the osmotic homeostasis. In ALF, however, there is a degree of dysfunction of the BBB, and an increased flux of water across the BBB can be observed. In this situation, the osmotic gradient across the BBB is critical to the flux of water and the subsequent development of cerebral edema. One important osmolyte in this situation is sodium, the levels of which are reduced in up to 65% of ALF patients.

Cerebral Blood flow

Cerebral blood flow (CBF) is highly variable in patients with ALF and, when increased, is thought to contribute to the development of intracranial hypertension by increasing cerebral blood volume and hence pressure, resulting in increased edema formation by means of hydrostatic Starling forces.

The determinants of CBF are mean arterial pressure (MAP), cerebral metabolic demands, and the partial pressure of CO_2. In

health, CBF is maintained within a relatively constant range, despite wide variations in arterial pressure, by the process of autoregulation. One of the cardinal features of ALF is loss of autoregulation to the MAP, and thus in ALF the CBF varies in parallel with the MAP. Hence, increases in MAP can cause increases in CBF and therefore ICP. Likewise, a reduction in MAP can cause a reduction in the cerebral perfusion pressure (MAP–ICP), and this may result in brain ischemia, which may also predispose to endothelial dysfunction and worsening edema formation.

Role of Infection and SIRS in the Pathogenesis of Intracranial Hypertension

As noted previously, the vast majority of ALF patients develop some form of infection during their illness and as many as 50% to 60% will manifest at least one SIRS criterion. In patients with chronic liver disease, the link between infection and encephalopathy is well established and there is accumulating evidence that a similar association exists in ALF.

In large studies, the presence of SIRS is associated with a poorer outcome and progression to deeper stages of encephalopathy. Likewise, acquisition of infection in ALF is associated with progression of HE.

Monitoring of Advanced Hepatic Encephalopathy

The high incidence of IH in advanced HE and its complications mandate the utilization of some form of monitoring in these patients. Clearly, the most effective way to monitor these patients for the development of IH is by the direct measurement of ICP. A number of devices to measure ICP are available, ranging from epidural monitors to intraparenchymal devices, and they are able to give accurate reproducible results in real time. Despite the obvious benefit of having a direct measure of ICP, their use has been controversial because of the risks of insertion in coagulopathic patients and the lack of evidence to suggest they improve mortality.

One of the first studies to directly address this issue found no mortality benefit in patients who underwent monitor insertion, but that the use of such monitors was associated with more interventions to treat elevations in ICP. Therefore, the use of these monitors allows the identification of asymptomatic episodes of IH that may have clinical relevance. The safety of these devices appears to be acceptable, especially the epidural monitors, which have a reported fatal hemorrhage rate of approximately 1% and a morbidity of 5%. The use of ICP monitors may also have indirect benefits other than identifying episodes of IH requiring treatment, such as allowing the reduction of sedation and routine nursing interventions such as tracheal suction to take place in those with a normal ICP.

It is possible to measure CBF, but these techniques are often cumbersome and have not entered routine clinical practice, although middle cerebral artery blood flow can be monitored at the bedside. Therefore, the use of jugular venous bulb catheters to sample the oxygen saturation of jugular bulb blood has become commonplace as a means of estimating the adequacy of CBF in relation to metabolic demands. Jugular bulb catheters may be helpful in determining which patients may benefit from insertion of an ICP monitor [i.e., those with a high (>80%) or low (<55%) jugular venous saturation]. In addition, jugular bulb saturation monitoring allows the effect of interventions such as manipulation of MAP, CO_2, and temperature to be evaluated along with ICP.

MANAGEMENT OF CEREBRAL EDEMA AND INTRACRANIAL HYPERTENSION

The management of cerebral edema and IH in ALF can be divided into strategies to prevent the development of IH and those that are aimed at treating established IH.

Prevention of Cerebral Edema and IH

All patients with grade 3/4 encephalopathy are at risk of developing cerebral edema and IH. Therefore, patients who reach this stage of encephalopathy should be electively intubated, sedated, and mechanically ventilated.

The patient should be placed in the 20-degree head-up position to facilitate venous drainage, thus reducing as much as possible the venous contribution to cerebral blood volume and hence ICP. Nursing interventions that may increase ICP, such as tracheal suction, should be minimized. However, suctioning is necessary to ensure clearance of secretions in some patients.

Sedation is routinely used to reduce cerebral metabolic demands and hence CBF. Of the sedating agents available, propofol is the most rational choice for routine sedation because a small uncontrolled study has demonstrated that propofol is able to control ICP in selected patients. In addition, most patients will also receive a low-dose opiate infusion. A concern in the sedated patient is subclinical seizure activity, which

has been proposed as a contributing factor in the subsequent development of IH. However, two controlled studies using prophylactic phenytoin have confirmed that the routine use of anticonvulsants does not improve outcome and therefore cannot be recommended.

As noted previously, up to 50% of patients admitted to an ICU with ALF and grade 3/4 encephalopathy will exhibit hyponatremia, which reduces the osmotic gradient across the BBB and may be a risk for the development of cerebral edema. On this basis, a small randomized study of hypertonic (30%) saline infusion to maintain serum sodium levels between 145 and 155 mmol/L was performed to test the hypothesis that mild hypernatremia can prevent cerebral edema and the development of IH in ALF patients. In the treated patients, serum sodium levels were higher than those of controls and there was a significant reduction in the baseline ICP and cumulative incidence of sustained increases in ICP greater than 25 mm Hg compared to standard of care. In addition to the induction of mild hypernatremia, the use of mild hypothermia has been shown to be effective in the reduction of ICP. The induction of mild hypothermia (35°C) was effective at reducing baseline ICP in patients with grade 4 encephalopathy, and this effect was still observed 24 hours after the induction of hypothermia. Decreased cerebral ammonia uptake was also demonstrated.

The association between the development of cerebral hyperemia and subsequent rise in ICP is well documented, and in patients at risk of IH prevention of cerebral hyperemia is an important goal. Maintenance of a partial pressure of CO_2 between 4.5 and 5.0 kPa will help to prevent increases in CBF due to CO_2-induced vasodilation.

Renal failure is very common in patients with ALF, and the use of continuous venovenous hemofiltration (CVVHF) may have added benefits other than replacement of renal function. The use of CVVHF as opposed to intermittent forms of renal replacement is associated with more hemodynamic stability and less acute fluid shifts, making changes in CBF less likely. Furthermore, the use of CVVHF may aid in the cooling of the patient, removal of ammonia, and the maintenance of serum sodium levels.

The routine use of N-acetyl cysteine in ALF is controversial; however, this agent has been shown in a controlled trial to reduce the incidence of cerebral edema in patients with acetaminophen-induced ALF. As discussed previously, patients who develop sepsis or SIRS have an increased propensity toward progression to encephalopathy and IH. Whether this can be altered by the use of prophylactic antibiotics or immunomodulatory agents is unknown; however, the case will be difficult to prove because most patients will already be receiving prophylactic antibiotics.

Treatment of Established Intracranial Hypertension

The treatment of sustained IH (ICP > 25 mm Hg for 10 min) was revolutionized by the introduction of osmotherapy with mannitol in the 1980s. At a dose of 0.5 g/kg as a rapid intravenous bolus, this drug is effective at reducing the ICP in the majority of patients. Single doses can be repeated if the serum osmolarity does not rise above 320 mOsm/mL. In order to prevent fluid overload, 500 mL of crystalloid should be removed from the circulation by hemofiltration or spontaneous diuresis after mannitol therapy. In addition to preventing IH, osmotherapy using bolus hypertonic saline may be effective in the treatment of sustained IH.

In patients who are refractory to the previously discussed treatment, further decreases in core body temperature to 32 or 33°C can control the ICP for prolonged periods, apparently without adverse effects. Care must be taken, however, when rewarming the patient because rebound increases in ICP can occur.

Reductions in CBF and cerebral metabolism can also be effected by the administration of thiopentone, which has been used in ALF but has not been subjected to controlled clinical trials. The use of thiopentone can be associated with reductions in cardiac output and blood pressure and is therefore not an ideal drug to use when there are concerns about cerebral perfusion pressure. However, where there has been no response to conventional therapy, a dose of 185 to 500 mg may be effective in controlling ICP.

Intravenous indomethacin at a dose of 0.5 mg/kg induces cerebral vasoconstriction and hence reduces cerebral blood volume. It very rapidly lowers the ICP, but the effect may not be sustained.

In patients with incipient cerebral herniation, short-term hyperventilation can be used to reduce cerebral blood volume by vasoconstriction. This mode of therapy should not be used routinely because the vasoconstriction induced may compromise CBF and result in ischemia. In addition, CBF "resets" at the lower CO_2.

Patients who undergo transplantation are also at risk of surges of ICP at critical points during the operation, such as at reperfusion. It is therefore important that the patient continue to be monitored appropriately during the operation and measures such as mild hypernatremia, hypothermia, and CVVHF continue if this does not interfere with the safe conduct of the operation. A management algorithm for ALF patients at risk of cerebral edema and IH is presented in Figure 49.5.

CARDIOVASCULAR EFFECTS OF ACUTE LIVER FAILURE

ALF is accompanied by profound changes in systemic hemodynamics. Systemic vascular resistance is lowered and there is resulting hypotension that in some patients is refractory to treatment and ultimately leads to death.

Hypotension and lowered systemic vascular resistance lead to a rise in the cardiac output and the development of a hyperdynamic circulatory state. It is likely that the pathophysiology is multifactorial, with SIRS, endotoxin, NO, and proinflammatory cytokine release from the necrotic liver all likely to have a role.

Patients with septic shock have been demonstrated to display abnormalities in adrenal function, and this has been related to severity of shock and vasopressor resistance. A similar profile exists in ALF patients, with a study showing abnormal short synacthen test (SST) results in 62% of patients. Furthermore, patients who were hemodynamically unstable had a significantly lower increment and peak cortisol after SST than hemodynamically stable patients, indicating a direct role for adrenal dysfunction in patients with circulatory failure and ALF.

The cardiovascular management of ALF patients follows standard lines. All patients with hepatic encephalopathy grade 3 or above should have invasive hemodynamic monitoring with at least central venous and arterial access. Measurement of cardiac preload and cardiac output is also helpful in the management of unstable patients. Pressor agents are often needed to maintain an adequate MAP and noradrenaline is the agent of choice. The cardiac index is often supranormal and does not need augmentation in the majority of patients. However, if the cardiac index falls and inotropic support is needed, milrinone or dobutamine is preferred over adrenaline because these have a less detrimental effect on hepatosplanchnic blood flow.

RENAL FAILURE

Between 30% and 80% of patients with ALF will develop renal failure severe enough to require extracorporeal renal replacement therapy. The most common causes of renal failure in ALF are hypovolemia-induced acute tubular necrosis (ATN), sepsis, and direct nephrotoxicity from drugs such as acetaminophen. Hepatorenal syndrome (HRS) is a relatively rare cause of renal failure in ALF because the strict diagnostic criteria are rarely fulfilled (Box 49.5).

The development of renal failure is associated with a poorer prognosis in ALF patients compared to those who retain renal function. Regardless of the etiology, the approach to patients is similar. The patient must be rendered volume replete and the

---

Box 49.5 Diagnostic Criteria for Hepatorenal Syndrome in Acute and Chronic Liver Disease

Major Criteria (in Advanced Liver Disease and Portal Hypertension)

1. Low glomerular filtration rate as evidenced by serum creatinine greater than 133 μmol/L or a 24k-hr creatinine clearance < 40 mL/min
2. Absence of shock/ongoing bacterial infection/fluid losses/treatment with nephrotoxic drugs
3. No sustained improvement in renal function (decrease in serum creatinine to less than 133 μmol/L or less or increase in 24-hr creatinine clearance to 40 mL/min or more) following diuretic withdrawal and volume expansion with 1.5 liters of plasma expander
4. Proteinuria less than 500 mg/day and no ultrasonographic evidence of obstructive uropathy or parenchymal renal disease

Additional Criteria

1. Urine volume lower than 500 mL/day
2. Urine sodium less than 10 mmol/liter
3. Urine osmolality greater than plasma osmolality
4. Urine red blood cells less than 50 per high-power field
5. Serum sodium concentration lower than 130 mmol/liter

All major criteria must be present for the diagnosis of hepatorenal syndrome. Additional criteria are not necessary for the diagnosis but provide supportive evidence.

Reproduced from Arroyo V, Ginès P, Gerbes AL, et al: Definition and diagnostic criteria of refractory ascites and hepatorenal syndrome in cirrhosis. Hepatology 1996:23;164.

MAP should be adequate to sustain renal perfusion. In patients who do not respond to volume expansion, a pressor agent should be considered if hypotension persists. The use of terlipressin, which is commonly used in HRS in chronic liver disease, should be avoided because this drug was shown to cause cerebral hyperemia in ALF in one study.

Despite the presence of severe coagulation defects in ALF patients, the majority of patients undergoing renal replacement therapy will require anticoagulation for the extracorporeal circuit. This can be safely achieved with low-dose heparin or prostacyclin infusions (2.5–5 ng/kg/min).

The natural history of renal failure complicating ALF is dependent on the restoration of normal liver function, whether by spontaneous recovery or transplantation. In each case, the chances of recovery of renal function are excellent. However, renal dysfunction prior to liver transplantation is associated with a decreased survival at 2 years and also significantly increased morbidity.

RESPIRATORY SUPPORT

The main indication for elective endotracheal intubation in ALF patients is to protect the airway in advanced grades of encephalopathy (grade 3/4). There is no specific respiratory management applicable in ALF as opposed to other conditions requiring mechanical ventilation. The principles of a high positive end-expiratory pressure and low tidal volume protective ventilation strategy apply to those who develop acute respiratory distress syndrome, although the use of permissive hypercapnia may be problematic in patients with cerebral hyperemia and IH. Intraabdominal hypertension is underrecognized in ALF and may be a factor in the development of respiratory compromise.

COAGULATION DISORDERS

Despite the severity of the coagulopathy associated with ALF, the incidence of severe bleeding complications is low. For this reason, routine correction of clotting factors is unnecessary, unless there is evidence of bleeding or invasive procedures are planned. Routine correction of the PT is also inadvisable because this negates its use as a prognostic marker. It is good practice to administer vitamin K intravenously to all patients to ensure they are replete in this vitamin because mild deficiency states seen in patients who are malnourished may cause an erroneously prolonged PT. When the PT needs to be corrected, such as when it is very high in patients who have already fulfilled poor prognosis criteria or prior to invasive procedures, 15 mL/kg of fresh frozen plasma can be administered.

Recombinant factor VII has been used to correct the coagulopathy of liver disease. This drug was initially developed to treat hemophilia A and works by augmenting the initial step of the coagulation cascade, namely the interaction of factor VIIa and tissue factor. Theoretically, because tissue factor is required, augmentation of factor VIIa will enhance coagulation only at the site of tissue injury and therefore systemic activation of coagulation can be avoided.

Recombinant factor VII can be shown to normalize the PT in patients with liver disease for a time, dependent on the dose given. For instance, with a dose of 80 µg/kg the PT is normalized for up to 12 hours. Recombinant factor VII also has the added benefit of augmenting platelet function. Recombinant factor VII has been used to correct the PT in patients prior to liver biopsy and intracranial pressure monitor insertion.

Correction of thrombocytopenia is undertaken in the presence of bleeding, prior to invasive procedures, or when the platelet count is less than 10,000/mm^3.

OTHER THERAPIES

N-acetylcysteine infusion is used as the antidote to acetaminophen poisoning and is also effective when given to patients who have presented late following poisoning. A number of studies have suggested that N-acetylcysteine also has a beneficial role in ALF of all etiologies by virtue of positive effects on systemic hemodynamics and oxygen transport. Adverse events related to N-acetylcysteine are rare when given at a dose of 150 mg/kg over 24 hours. The routine use of N-acetylcysteine has been questioned, and further studies are awaited before it can be recommended routinely in patients with non–acetaminophen-induced ALF.

ARTIFICIAL LIVER SUPPORT

A successful liver support system would revolutionize the management of ALF, allowing patients to survive until hepatic regeneration occurs or a liver becomes available for transplantation. The different approaches to liver support can be broadly categorized into detoxification strategies, cellular systems, or hybrid systems that comprise cellular and detoxification components.

Detoxification

The first attempts at detoxification involved the use of charcoal hemoperfusion, which, despite showing biocompatibility in ALF, was ineffective at reducing mortality in a randomized controlled study. Similarly, hemodiasorption using the Biologic DT system showed no clinical benefit in randomized clinical trials in ALF.

Many of the proposed toxins in liver failure are protein bound and therefore not removed by conventional hemodialysis. Plasmapheresis and albumin dialysis are effective at removing protein-bound toxins and have been evaluated in ALF. Albumin dialysis using the Molecular Adsorbents Recirculation System has shown improvement in encephalopathy and hemodynamics in ALF patients, but controlled data showing improvement in mortality are lacking. High-volume plasmapheresis has not been examined in controlled trials, but uncontrolled studies have shown improvement in the grade of encephalopathy and in systemic hemodynamics in ALF patients.

Bioartificial and Hybrid Devices

Bioartificial liver support devices contain a cellular component in an attempt to replace the synthetic function of the liver in addition to detoxification. The Extracorporeal Liver Assist Device (ELAD) was one of the first bioartificial devices to undergo trials in ALF. This device utilizes a bioreactor containing the C3A hepatoblastoma cell line. In a randomized controlled clinical trial, patients treated with ELAD showed no improvement in mortality, although there was an increase in galactose elimination, suggesting the device had metabolic activity.

Table 49.3 Characteristics of Current Liver Support Systems and Effects on Mortality in ALF Patients

Detoxification Technique	Mechanism	Effect on Mortality	Other Effects
Charcoal hemoperfusion	Toxin absorption	No benefit in controlled studies	Improvement in encephalopathy in uncontrolled studies
Biologic DT system	Hemodiasorption	No benefit in controlled studies	Improvement in encephalopathy
High-volume plasmapheresis	Toxin removal	No controlled studies	Improvement in systemic hemodynamics and encephalopathy
Molecular adsorbents Recirculation system	Albumin dialysis	No controlled studies	Improvement in systemic hemodynamics and encephalopathy
BAL[a]	**Cellular Component**		
ELAD	C3A hepatoblastoma cells	No benefit in controlled studies	Improved galactose elimination Delayed progression in encephalopathy grade
Performed BAL	Cryopreserved human hepatocytes	No controlled studies	ALF patient successfully bridged to liver transplantation
Modular extracorporeal liver support device	Human hepatocytes	No controlled studies	Two ALF patients bridged to liver transplantation
Amsterdam Medical Centre, BAL	Porcine hepatocytes	No controlled studies	Three ALF patients bridged to liver transplantation
Hepatassist, BAL	Porcine hepatocytes	Prolonged survival in ALF patients but not in primary graft nonfunction	Contains charcoal column

[a]BAL, bioartificial liver.

Other bioartificial liver devices have used porcine hepatocytes, cryopreserved hepatocytes, or fresh hepatocytes from unused donor livers, with either charcoal detoxification or albumin dialysis. One such device is the Hepatassist bioartificial liver, which uses porcine hepatocytes in combination with a charcoal column and has been evaluated in ALF and primary nonfunction of hepatic allografts. This study enrolled 171 patients—24 with primary liver allograft nonfunction and 147 with acute or subacute liver failure. Patients were randomized to standard of care or treatment with the bioartificial liver, with treated patients receiving an average of 2.9 treatments. The most common reason for the cessation of treatment was a liver becoming available for transplantation. The overall survival between the treated and nontreated groups was not significantly different, although when the data were analyzed to account for the impact of transplantation on survival, there appeared to be a survival benefit for acute and subacute liver failure patients at 30 days and a prolongation of survival for those patients with acute liver failure and defined etiologies. The characteristics of liver support techniques and their effect on mortality are presented in Table 49.3.

LIVER TRANSPLANTATION

Liver transplantation has had a remarkable impact on the outcome of patients with ALF, such that patients transplanted for ALF now have a survival of 65% at 1 year compared to less than 20% with standard medical management. The current success of liver transplantation owes much to developments in surgical technique and better postoperative management in dedicated ICUs.

The standard orthotopic liver transplant (OLT) operation with a graft matched for size and blood group is most frequently performed for patients with ALF. The quality of the graft has a major impact on outcome. Transplantation with poor quality grafts due to fatty infiltration or other factors, such as prolonged cold ischemic time, is associated with excess morbidity and early mortality. Patient factors that adversely affect outcome are age (>50 years) and severity of MOF prior to transplant. During the operation, intracranial hypertension and hemodynamic instability can still be problematic, especially at the time of reperfusion of the graft. Hence, all monitoring should remain in place for the duration of the operation.

Auxiliary Liver Transplantation

Auxiliary liver transplantation has recently been employed in the management of ALF (Fig. 49.6). In this technique, a whole or partial graft is transplanted, leaving a remnant of native liver in situ. The advantage of auxiliary liver transplantation is that the native liver can regenerate, regaining function over time. When this occurs, immunosuppression can be withdrawn and the transplanted liver undergoes atrophy. Although auxiliary liver transplantation is technically more demanding than standard OLT, patients who receive these grafts are able to discontinue all immunosuppressive drugs, thus reducing the long-term risk of side effects and complications, such as renal impairment and infection (Box 49.6 and Table 49.4).

Box 49.6 Current Controversies in the Management of ALF

- The use of intracranial pressure monitors
- Routine use of N-acetyl cysteine in nonacetaminophen-induced ALF
- Use and application of liver support devices

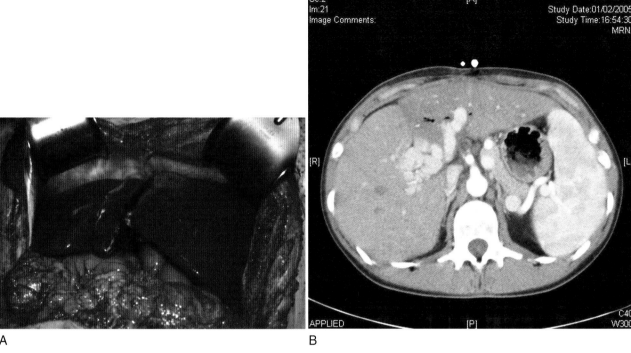

A

B

Figure 49.6. Auxiliary liver transplantation in ALF. *A,* Auxiliary liver transplantation: A healthy lobe of liver is implanted alongside the diseased liver (following partial hepatectomy). *B,* Postoperative appearance: Note the difference in arterial perfusion between the two segments.

Table 49.4 Pitfalls in the Management of ALF

Pitfall	Consequence
Delayed discussion with specialist liver centers	Patients with ALF may deteriorate rapidly, making transport of patients with advanced ALF potentially hazardous.
Patients with subacute liver failure can be mistakenly diagnosed as having chronic liver disease	Patients with subacute liver failure may have ascites and nodular liver on ultrasound scanning. Mistaking this condition for chronic liver disease may deny a patient life-saving transplantation.
Inappropriate administration of dextrose solutions	Hyponatremia is common in ALF and may contribute to the development of cerebral edema.
Failure to appreciate tiredness and lethargy as being early stages of encephalopathy	This may lead to underestimation of the severity of the condition.

SUGGESTED READING

Bernuau J, Goudeau A, Poynard T, et al: Multivariate analysis of prognostic factors in fulminant hepatitis B. Hepatology 1986;6:648–651.

Jalan R, Olde Damink SW, Deutz NE, et al: Moderate hypothermia prevents cerebral hyperemia and increase in intracranial pressure in patients undergoing liver transplantation for acute liver failure. Transplantation 2003;75:2034–2039.

Jalan R, Olde Damink SW, Deutz NE, Hayes PC, Lee A: Moderate hypothermia in patients with acute liver failure and uncontrolled intracranial hypertension. Gastroenterology 2004;127:1338–1346.

Kjaergard LL, Liu J, Als-Nielsen B, Gluud C: Artificial and bioartificial support systems for acute and acute-on-chronic liver failure: A systematic review. JAMA 2003;289(2):217–222.

Murphy N, Auzinger G, Bernel W, Wendon J: The effect of hypertonic sodium chloride on intracranial pressure in patients with acute liver failure. Hepatology 2004;39(2):464–470.

O'Grady JG, Alexander GJ, Hayllar KM, Williams R: Early indicators of prognosis in fulminant hepatic failure. Gastroenterology 1989;97:439–445.

O'Grady JG, Schalm SW, Williams R: Acute liver failure: Redefining the syndromes. Lancet: 1993;342(8866):273–275.

Ott P, Larsen FS: Blood brain barrier permeability to ammonia in liver failure: A critical reappraisal. Neurochem Int 2004;44:185–198.

Rolando N, Wade J, Davalos M, et al: The systemic inflammatory response syndrome in acute liver failure. Hepatology 2000;32:734–739.

Trey C, Davidson LS: The management of fulminant hepatic failure. In Popper H, Schaffer F (eds): Progress in Liver Dsease. New York, Grune and Stratton, 1970, pp 282–298.

Chapter 50

Coagulation Overview

Patricia C. Y. Liaw and Jeffrey I. Weitz

KEY POINTS

- Hemostasis is a complex, tightly regulated process that includes physical, biochemical, and cellular events.
- The major components involved in hemostasis include platelets, coagulation factors and their inhibitors, fibrinolytic enzymes and their inhibitors, and the vascular endothelium.
- Unexpected or excessive bleeding is common in the intensive care setting, especially after trauma or surgery; medical history and physical examination are important to identify congenital bleeding disorders and determine whether there is a systemic or localized defect in hemostasis.
- Diagnosis of venous thromboembolism is problematic in the intensive care setting; vigorous thromboprophylaxis is indicated to prevent the disorder.
- Disseminated intravascular coagulation (DIC) is a common coagulation abnormality in the ICU setting, occurring as a complication of a variety of disorders; the mainstay of DIC treatment is management of the underlying disease.

OVERVIEW OF HEMOSTASIS

Hemostasis depends on a dynamic balance between coagulation and fibrinolysis. The coagulation system is poised to rapidly generate a hemostatic plug at sites of vascular injury, thereby limiting blood loss from rents or tears in blood vessels. Intricately connected to coagulation pathways, the fibrinolytic system degrades fibrin, the primary matrix protein of venous or arterial thrombi, into soluble components. Solubilization of thrombi restores blood flow and prevents ischemia in downstream organs and tissues. Perturbation of the balance between coagulation and fibrinolysis can lead to thrombosis or bleeding. Thus, excessive activation of coagulation or impaired fibrinolysis can result in thrombosis, whereas enhanced fibrinolysis can lead to bleeding.

Thrombosis can occur in veins or in arteries. Typically, venous thrombosis starts in the deep veins of the calf or in the sinuses of the calf muscle. Some of these thrombi propagate proximally, where they may embolize to the lungs, a process that can be fatal. Venous thrombi also can originate in the veins of the upper extremities, particularly in patients with central venous catheters.

Arterial thrombi are often superimposed on disrupted atherosclerotic plaques. If they occur in the coronary arteries, these thrombi can transiently or permanently block blood flow to the myocardium, resulting in unstable angina or myocardial infarction, respectively. In contrast, thrombi in cerebral vessels produce transient ischemic attacks or ischemic stroke, depending on the duration of vascular occlusion. Transient ischemic attacks or stroke can also occur when clot fragments embolize from the heart into the brain arteries. Cardiac thrombi can develop in the left atrium and left atrial appendage in patients with atrial fibrillation as a consequence of sluggish blood flow, or they can form on heart valves in patients with mechanical valves or in those with diseased native valves. Finally, arterial thrombi or emboli in the arteries to the lower limbs can cause critical limb ischemia, a process that can lead to gangrene.

A simplified schematic of the sequence of events that occurs at sites of vascular damage is shown in Figure 50.1. After damage to the endothelium, the cell monolayer lining the lumen of blood vessels, there is immediate and transient vasoconstriction. The resultant reduction in blood flow promotes exposure of shed blood to subendothelial components, such as von Willebrand factor (vWF) and collagen. Platelets adhere to these subendothelial matrix proteins, where they become activated. Activated platelets release substances that recruit and activate nearby platelets and induce platelet aggregation. This results in the formation of a platelet plug at the site of injury, a structure that provides initial arrest of bleeding. The process of platelet plug formation is called *primary hemostasis*. Subsequent steps, which occur simultaneously, serve to stabilize the platelet plug, a process known as *secondary hemostasis*.

Disruption of the endothelium also exposes tissue factor (TF), a membrane-bound procoagulant factor found on subendothelial cells. Exposure of blood to TF triggers the coagulation cascade, a highly regulated series of reactions that involve the sequential conversion of proenzymes (also called zymogens) and procofactors into their active forms. Coagulation is amplified by several positive feedback loops. Activated platelets accelerate coagulation by providing surfaces onto which coagulation enzymes and cofactors bind to form efficient enzyme complexes. Through these amplifying pathways, the coagulation system has the ability to translate a small initiating signal into an explosive process that results in rapid fibrin formation. Secondary hemostasis is achieved when polymerized fibrin stabilizes the platelet plug.

Removal of the fibrin clot occurs through activation of another cascade system, the fibrinolytic system. Central to the fibrinolytic system is conversion of plasminogen, a zymogen, into

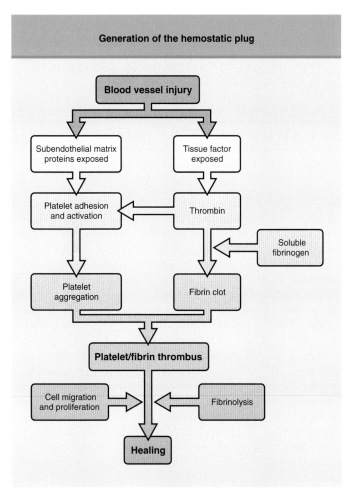

Figure 50.1. Generation of the hemostatic plug. Generation of the hemostatic plug in response to vascular injury depends on closely linked interactions between platelets, the coagulation cascade, the fibrinolytic system, and the endothelium.

plasmin, an enzyme that degrades the fibrin matrix of the clot into soluble fragments. Thus, the hemostatic response to injury depends on closely linked interactions between platelets, the coagulation cascade, the fibrinolytic system, and the endothelium, each of which is described in more detail.

COMPONENTS OF THE HEMOSTATIC SYSTEM

Platelets

Platelets play a critical role in hemostasis by aggregating to form a mechanical plug at sites of blood vessel injury. The platelet plug is sufficiently stable to stop bleeding from small wounds, even in the absence of effective fibrin formation. Thus, hemophiliacs do not exhibit excessive bleeding from superficial cuts despite impaired thrombin generation as a result of deficiency of coagulation factors VIII or IX.

Circulating platelets are anucleated, smooth, disc-shaped cells that do not adhere to normal vascular endothelial cells. *Platelet adhesion* at sites of vessel injury is a multistep process involving interactions between various platelet receptors and subendothelial adhesive ligands. Under high shear conditions,

such as occur in arterioles or in stenotic arteries, the initial tethering of platelets to exposed subendothelial collagen is mediated by vWF, a large multimeric protein secreted by activated endothelial cells and platelets. By binding simultaneously to collagen and platelets, vWF acts as a bridge between platelets and the damaged vessel wall. The interaction of vWF with platelets is mediated by glycoprotein (GP) Ib-IX-V, a vWF receptor that is constitutively expressed on the platelet membrane. Once tethered, stable platelet adhesion is effected by the interaction of GP IIb-IIIa, another platelet receptor, with vWF. Other adhesive proteins, such as fibronectin, vitronectin, and thrombospondin, also help bridge platelets to the injured vessel wall.

Adherent platelets become activated and undergo a *shape change*, becoming spherical and extruding long filopodia that enhance platelet-platelet interactions. Activated platelets secrete stored ADP from their dense granules and synthesize and release thromboxane A_2. Released ADP and thromboxane A_2, both of which are potent platelet agonists, bind to distinct receptors on nearby platelets and activate them, thereby recruiting additional platelets to the site of injury. Thrombin, whose generation is triggered by tissue factor exposed at the site of vascular damage, also serves as a potent platelet agonist. In fact, thrombin may be the most important platelet agonist because mice lacking the platelet thrombin receptor exhibit reduced thrombus formation at sites of arterial injury despite the fact that their platelets respond normally to other physiological agonists, such as ADP, collagen, and epinephrine.

Binding of agonists to platelet receptors triggers outside-inside and inside-outside signaling pathways. Outside-inside signaling results in the mobilization of calcium. The increase in intracellular calcium leads to cytoskeletal reorganization that provides the contractile forces necessary to effect platelet shape change and granule secretion. At the same time, inside-outside signaling pathways trigger functional activation of GPIIb/IIIa on the platelet surfaces. As the most abundant integrin, with about 80,000 copies per platelet, activated GPIIa/IIIa binds fibrinogen, a bivalent molecule that bridges adjacent platelets together. These platelet-platelet interactions result in platelet aggregation and formation of the platelet plug.

Substances released from activated platelets help solidify the platelet plug and may contribute to wound healing. Thus, adhesive proteins released from platelet alpha granules, such as thrombospondin, fibronectin, and fibrinogen, are involved in platelet-vessel wall and platelet-platelet interactions. Alpha granules also release platelet-derived growth factor, which together with acid hydrolases released from platelet lysosomal granules, may modulate wound healing.

Finally, activated platelets also promote coagulation at sites of vascular injury. As another example of inside-outside signaling in response to agonist binding, the activated platelet membrane undergoes a flip-flop such that negatively charged phospholipids such as phosphatidylserine, which are normally found on the inside of the membrane, move to the outside. Clotting factors bind to negatively charged phospholipids and assembly of these clotting factor complexes on the activated platelet surface results in explosive generation of thrombin.

Currently available antiplatelet agents target various steps in these pathways. Their sites of action are illustrated in Figure 50.2.

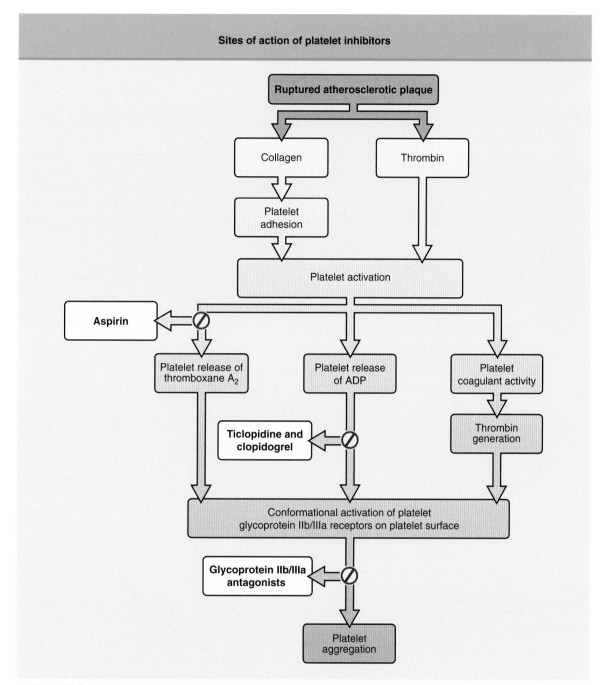

Figure 50.2. Sites of action of platelet inhibitors. By irreversibly acetylating cyclooxygenase, aspirin blocks synthesis of thromboxane A$_2$ by platelets. In contrast, ticlopidine and clopidogrel irreversibly block a key ADP receptor, thereby inhibiting ADP-induced platelet aggregation. Glycoprotein IIb/IIIa antagonists block platelet aggregation by inhibiting fibrinogen or vWF binding to activated glycoprotein IIb/IIIa receptors. (Adapted from Hirsh J, Weitz JI: New antithrombotic agents. Lancet 1999;353:1431–1436.)

Coagulation Cascade

The second component of the hemostatic response is the coagulation cascade. A fundamental principle of blood coagulation is the sequential conversion of zymogens to enzymes, a process that terminates in thrombin generation and subsequent conversion of soluble fibrinogen into insoluble fibrin. Traditionally, coagulation has been divided into the *extrinsic* and *intrinsic* pathways. The *extrinsic* pathway is initiated when TF is exposed as a result of injury to blood vessels. This pathway is termed "extrinsic" because it depends on exposure of TF, which is not normally found within the vessel but is constitutively expressed by subendothelial cells, such as fibroblasts and smooth muscle cells. In contrast, the intrinsic pathway is initiated when blood contacts negatively charged prosthetic devices, including mechanical heart valves, stents, and grafts. In vitro, the intrinsic pathway can be triggered by foreign substances, such as celite or kaolin. This pathway is termed "intrinsic" because all the necessary coagulation factors are found within the blood.

545

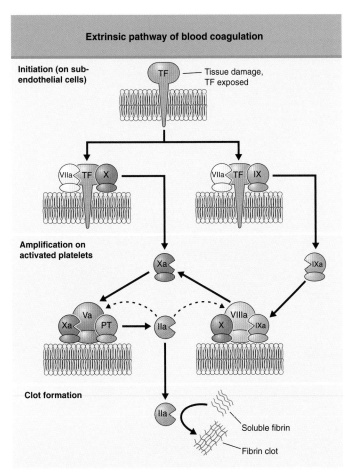

Extrinsic pathway of blood coagulation

Initiation (on sub-
endothelial cells) — TF — Tissue damage,
TF exposed

Amplification on
activated platelets

Clot formation

Soluble fibrin
Fibrin clot

Figure 50.3. Extrinsic pathway of blood coagulation. The extrinsic pathway of blood coagulation is initiated by the exposure of tissue factor (TF) on subendothelial cells. Once exposed, TF binds to factor VIIa and can initiate coagulation by converting either factor X to Xa or factor IX to IXa. Factor IXa together with its cofactor, factor VIIIa, converts factor X to Xa. The amplification phase of coagulation occurs on the surface of activated platelets. Here, factor Xa binds to its cofactor, factor Va, to convert small amounts of prothrombin (PT) to thrombin (IIa). Thrombin amplifies the coagulation process by activating factors V and VIII (dashed lines) and by activating platelets. The generation of thrombin leads to the conversion of fibrinogen to fibrin.

Blood coagulation can be divided into three stages: initiation, amplification, and fibrin formation. Amplification of coagulation occurs on the surface of negatively charged activated platelets and results in explosive generation of thrombin, the enzyme responsible for fibrin formation, the last step in this process.

Physiologically, initiation of coagulation usually occurs at sites of vascular injury where TF is exposed (Fig. 50.3). Once exposed, TF binds tightly to the active form of factor VII, termed factor VIIa. Normally, factor VIIa is found in trace amounts in blood (about 1% of total circulating factor VII). TF also can bind factor VII. Once bound, factor VII can be activated by factor Xa or thrombin.

The TF:VIIa complex, which is termed extrinsic tenase, triggers coagulation in two ways. First, it converts factor X to factor Xa. Although factor X is the preferred substrate of the TF:VIIa complex, the TF:VIIa complex can also activate factor

IX. Factor IXa then becomes the enzymatic component of the "intrinsic tenase" complex, composed of factor IXa, cofactor VIIIa, Ca²⁺, and a negatively charged membrane surface. The intrinsic tenase complex serves as the convergence point between the extrinsic and intrinsic pathways of blood coagulation.

Once factor Xa is formed, it assembles within the "pro-thrombinase" complex, which consists of factor Xa, cofactor Va, Ca²⁺, and a negatively charged membrane surface. Prothrombinase efficiently converts small amounts of prothrombin to thrombin. This small amount of thrombin serves as the spark to amplify coagulation by activating platelets and by activating factors V and VIII, key cofactors in coagulation. Thrombin also activates factor XIII to XIIIa, the enzyme that covalently cross-links fibrin. Cross-linking stabilizes the fibrin network and renders it more resistant to lysis.

Regulation of the Coagulation Cascade

The potentially explosive nature of the coagulation cascade is tightly regulated by three natural anticoagulant systems: antithrombin, the protein C pathway, and tissue factor pathway inhibitor.

Antithrombin

Antithrombin, a plasma serine protease inhibitor synthesized and secreted by the liver, has broad inhibitory activity for enzymes of the coagulation cascade, especially thrombin and factor Xa. To inhibit these enzymes, antithrombin forms a 1:1 covalent enzyme-inhibitor complex. These complexes are then rapidly cleared from the circulation by the liver.

The rate of enzyme inhibition by antithrombin is slow but is accelerated 1000-fold in the presence of negatively charged polysaccharides such as heparin. The physiologic counterpart of medicinal heparin is heparan sulfate, a glycosaminoglycan found on the vessel wall. The stimulatory effect of heparin and heparan sulfate is mediated by a unique pentasaccharide sequence that binds antithrombin with high affinity. Binding of this pentasaccharide sequence evokes a conformational change in the reactive center loop of antithrombin that facilitates its interaction with factor Xa but not with thrombin. To accelerate thrombin inhibition by antithrombin, heparin must bind simultaneously to antithrombin and thrombin, a process that bridges the enzyme and the inhibitor together to form a ternary complex. Only pentasaccharide-containing heparin chains composed of at least 13 additional saccharide units (which corresponds to a molecular weight of 5400) are of sufficient length to effect this bridging function. In contrast, pentasaccharide-containing chains of any length promote factor Xa inhibition by antithrombin. With a mean molecular weight of about 5000, at least half of the chains of low-molecular-weight heparin are too short to bridge thrombin to antithrombin. However, these shorter chains retain their capacity to catalyze factor Xa inhibition. Consequently, low-molecular-weight heparin has greater capacity to promote factor Xa inhibition by antithrombin than thrombin inhibition as reflected by its anti-factor Xa to anti-thrombin (IIa) ratio that ranges from 2:1 to 4:1. In contrast, with a mean molecular weight of 15,000, all the chains of unfractionated heparin are of sufficient length to bridge thrombin to antithrombin. By definition, therefore, heparin has an anti-factor Xa to anti-IIa ratio of 1:1.

The physiologic importance of antithrombin is highlighted by the consequences of congenital or acquired antithrombin deficiency. Individuals lacking antithrombin are prone to thrombosis that is confined to the venous system. There are three types of antithrombin deficiency. Type I deficiency is defined as a parallel reduction in both functional and antigen levels to 50% of normal. This defect results from reduced antithrombin production by hepatocytes. Type II deficiency results from the production of mutant antithrombin molecules with abnormal activity. These patients have reduced functional levels of antithrombin but normal antithrombin antigen. Type III deficiency is characterized by defective heparin binding to antithrombin. Patients with this type of antithrombin deficiency have normal levels of antithrombin antigen but reduced antithrombin activity in the presence of heparin.

Homozygous antithrombin deficiency has not been reported, suggesting that absence of this inhibitor is incompatible with life. Acquired antithrombin deficiency occurs in conditions where there is excessive activation of coagulation. This could include sepsis, trauma, malignancy, burns, and extracorporeal circulation.

Protein C Pathway

The second natural anticoagulant is activated protein C (APC), a plasma enzyme that provides an "on site" and "on demand" anticoagulant response whenever thrombin is generated (Fig. 50.4). APC circulates in blood as the inactive zymogen protein C, a vitamin K–dependent protein synthesized and secreted by the liver. The signal that triggers the conversion of zymogen protein C to APC is thrombin. Briefly, vascular injury, endotoxin, or inflammatory cytokines initiate the coagulation cascade, ultimately resulting in thrombin generation and blood clot formation. Excess thrombin then complexes with thrombomodulin (TM), a receptor found on the surface of vascular endothelial cells. The thrombin-TM complex rapidly converts protein C to APC. The binding of thrombin to TM is critical for efficient protein C activation because this interaction induces a structural change in thrombin that abolishes its procoagulant properties and accelerates the rate at which thrombin activates protein C more than 1000-fold compared with thrombin alone. The conversion of protein C to APC is augmented by endothelial cell protein C receptor (EPCR), another endothelial cell surface receptor. EPCR binds circulating protein C and presents it to the thrombin-TM complex. Once formed, APC, in combination with its cofactor, protein S, limits the amplification and progression of the coagulation cascade by degrading and inactivating factors Va and VIIIa, key cofactors in prothrombinase and intrinsic tenase, respectively.

The importance of the protein C anticoagulant pathway is highlighted by the fact that patients with congenital or acquired deficiencies in this pathway are prone to venous thrombosis. Homozygous protein C deficiency, a rare and life-threatening condition, manifests at birth as thrombosis in the small vessels, most notably as purpura fulminans. This disorder can be treated acutely with protein C concentrate, with or without concomitant heparin or low-molecular-weight heparin. Vitamin K antagonists can be used for long-term treatment, but a therapeutic anticoagulant response must be maintained to prevent recurrent skin necrosis.

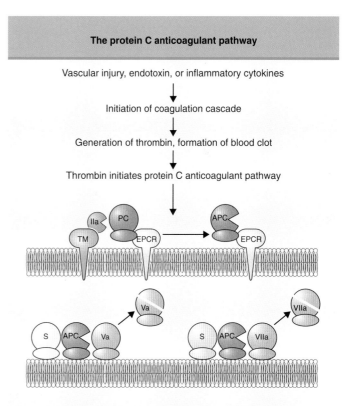

The protein C anticoagulant pathway

Vascular injury, endotoxin, or inflammatory cytokines

Initiation of coagulation cascade

Generation of thrombin, formation of blood clot

Thrombin initiates protein C anticoagulant pathway

Figure 50.4. The protein C anticoagulant pathway. Activated protein C (APC), a physiologic anticoagulant, is generated from the inactive precursor protein C "on demand" in response to thrombin formation. Briefly, vascular injury or endotoxin/inflammatory cytokines initiates the coagulation cascade, ultimately resulting in thrombin generation and blood clot formation. Excess thrombin then triggers the protein C pathway, which provides feedback inhibition of coagulation. The protein C pathway is initiated when thrombin (IIa) binds to thrombomodulin on the endothelial cell surface. The thrombin-thrombomodulin complex rapidly converts zymogen protein C (PC) to its active form, APC. Protein C activation is augmented by the endothelial cell protein C receptor, which binds circulating protein C and presents it to the thrombin-thrombomodulin complex. APC then dissociates from EPCR and, in combination with its cofactor protein S (S), acts as an anticoagulant by degrading factors Va and VIIIa, key cofactors in coagulation.

Heterozygous protein C deficiency, which occurs in approximately 0.2% of the general population and accounts for approximately 6% of familial thrombophilia, usually manifests later in life as deep vein thrombosis in the lower extremities, with or without associated pulmonary embolism. Patients with this disorder respond normally to conventional anticoagulant therapy.

The most common abnormality in the protein C pathway is APC resistance, a disorder found in about 4% to 6% of Caucasians. APC resistance is not a disorder of APC. Instead, it is usually caused by the factor V Leiden mutation, a point mutation in the factor V gene that results in the synthesis of a factor V molecule that, once activated, is relatively resistant to proteolytic degradation by APC. Consequently, inhibition of thrombin generation is delayed in patients with this disorder, thereby explaining their propensity for thrombosis. Although common

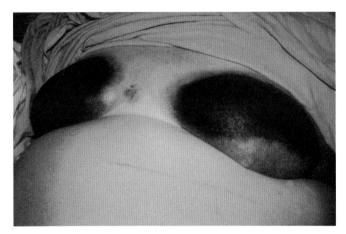

Figure 50.5. Warfarin-induced skin necrosis. (Reprinted from Warkentin TE, Sikov WM, Lillicrap DP: Multicentric warfarin-induced skin necrosis complicating heparin-induced thrombocytopenia. Am J Hematol 1999;62:44–48.)

in Caucasians, the factor V Leiden mutation is rare in Asians and Africans.

Patients with congenital or acquired protein C or protein S deficiency are prone to skin necrosis when started on treatment with vitamin K antagonists, such as warfarin. These drugs block the posttranslational modification of four procoagulant factors (factors VII, IX, X, and prothrombin) and two anticoagulant factors (protein C and protein S). This posttranslational modification, which occurs in the liver, is essential for the interaction of these proteins with negatively charged membranes. Consequently, when this step is blocked, nonfunctional proteins are produced.

The antithrombotic effects of warfarin depend on a reduction in the functional levels of factor X and prothrombin. Because these factors have half-lives of 48 and 72 hours, respectively, it takes some time to lower their levels into the therapeutic range. In contrast, protein C and protein S have relatively short half-lives (12 and 24 hours, respectively). Consequently, if the levels of these anticoagulant proteins are low to start, a precipitous fall can occur when warfarin therapy is initiated, particularly if large loading doses are administered. Reduction in the levels of these anticoagulant proteins can trigger thrombosis in the small vessels of the skin and underlying subcutaneous tissue (Fig. 50.5). This results in skin necrosis, a process that resembles the purpura fulminans seen in patients with homozygous protein C deficiency.

Acquired protein C deficiency can occur in any condition where there is excess activation of the coagulation system. Thus, it is a common finding in clinical conditions associated with disseminated intravascular coagulation, such as sepsis (see also Chapter 51.).

Tissue Factor Pathway Inhibitor
The third natural anticoagulant, tissue factor pathway inhibitor (TFPI), is a potent inhibitor of the tissue factor–mediated extrinsic pathway. TFPI forms a quaternary complex with tissue factor, factor VIIa, and factor Xa, thereby preventing further production of factor Xa and IXa by the TF:VIIa complex and blocking additional generation of thrombin by factor Xa. Con-

genital deficiency of circulating TFPI has not been clearly demonstrated in humans, possibly reflecting the fact that TFPI is found in at least four pools. TFPI is primarily synthesized by endothelial cells and approximately 75% of the intravascular TFPI is bound to glycosaminoglycans on the endothelium. About 20% of TFPI circulates in blood bound to lipoproteins, whereas 2.5% is free in the plasma and 2.5% is stored in platelet alpha granules.

Intravenous or subcutaneous administration of heparin or low-molecular-weight heparin displaces TFPI bound to glycosaminoglycans on the endothelial cell surface. It is uncertain whether the released TFPI contributes to the antithrombotic effects of these agents. Heparin-induced TFPI release from the endothelium is only effected by longer heparin chains. Thus, fondaparinux, a recently introduced synthetic analog of the pentasaccharide sequence that mediates heparin's interaction with antithrombin, does not cause TFPI release. Despite the lack of TFPI release, fondaparinux is effective for prevention and treatment of venous thromboembolism, suggesting that released TFPI does not contribute to the antithrombotic activity of heparin-like anticoagulants.

Fibrinolytic System
The third component of the hemostatic response is the fibrinolytic system (Fig. 50.6). This system counteracts fibrin deposition, thereby preventing excessive fibrin accumulation at sites of vascular injury and restoring normal blood flow. Plasmin, the enzyme that dissolves fibrin clots, is formed from zymogen plasminogen in the presence of tissue plasminogen activator (tPA) or urokinase plasminogen activator (uPA). tPA, which is synthesized and released by vascular endothelial cells upon stimulation with agonists such as thrombin, initiates intravascular fibrinolysis. Fibrin serves as a tPA cofactor by binding both

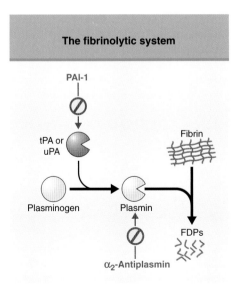

Figure 50.6. The fibrinolytic system. Plasmin is the enzyme that converts insoluble fibrin clots to soluble fibrin degradation products (FDPs). Plasmin is formed from its inactive precursor plasminogen in the presence of plasminogen activators, tissue plasminogen activator (tPA), and urokinase plasminogen activator (uPA). The principal inhibitors of plasmin and tPA are α_2-antiplasmin and plasminogen activator inhibitor type 1 (PAI-1), respectively.

plasminogen and tPA, thereby accelerating tPA-mediated conversion of plasminogen to plasmin. Once formed, plasmin degrades fibrin to generate soluble degradation products. uPA, the other endogenous plasminogen activator, is found in urine and in low concentrations in plasma. By binding to receptors on leukocytes, uPA converts cell-bound plasminogen to plasmin. Cell-surface plasmin allows passage of these cells through the extracellular matrix into the tissues.

The fibrinolytic system is regulated at two levels. Type 1 plasminogen activator inhibitor (PAI-1) controls plasminogen activation by inhibiting tPA and uPA. In contrast, α_2-antiplasmin is the primary inhibitor of plasmin. Although α_2-antiplasmin rapidly inhibits circulating plasmin, fibrin-bound plasmin is relatively protected from inhibition. This phenomenon allows fibrin degradation to proceed unchecked, while preventing systemic plasmin activity.

Impaired fibrinolytic activity, e.g., due to increased circulating levels of PAI-1 in acute inflammatory states, may contribute to thrombus growth by delaying clot lysis. Conversely, excessive fibrinolytic activity, due, for example, to α_2-antiplasmin deficiency, can result in renewed bleeding complications. Fibrinolytic therapy represents a pharmacologic approach to vascular reperfusion. Such therapy involves administration of plasminogen activators that serve to convert plasminogen to plasmin. These can be delivered systemically or can be administered directly into thrombi using a catheter-directed approach. Plasminogen activators also can be used in low doses to restore blood flow in catheters that are blocked by thrombi.

Endothelium

The fourth component of the hemostatic response is the endothelium, the monolayer of cells that lines the lumen of blood vessels. The endothelium is not simply a passive barrier that separates blood cells and plasma proteins from the thrombogenic components of the vessel wall. Instead, the endothelium plays an active role in maintaining hemostasis and has thromboresistant properties that reflect the synthesis and secretion of many molecules (Fig. 50.7). These properties include (1) the production of nitric oxide, prostacyclin, and ADPase, substances that inhibit platelet activation and promote vascular relaxation; (2) expression of thrombomodulin (TM) and endothelial cell protein C receptor (EPCR), key components of the protein C anticoagulant pathway; (3) expression of heparan sulfate, a heparin-like molecule, which catalyzes the inactivation of coagulation enzymes by antithrombin; (4) synthesis of TFPI, which limits TF-induced activation of coagulation on the vessel surface; and (5) constitutive and regulated secretion of tPA, an enzyme that promotes fibrinolysis by converting plasminogen into plasmin.

Under pathophysiologic conditions, e.g., upon exposure of the endothelium to bacterial lipopolysaccharide (LPS), proinflammatory cytokines, or thrombin, endothelial cells rapidly acquire a prothrombotic phenotype (Fig. 50.8). Perturbed endothelial cells not only shed surface TM, EPCR, and heparan sulfate but also exhibit decreased synthesis of tPA and increased synthesis of procoagulant and antifibrinolytic molecules, such as TF and PAI-1, respectively. Once activated, endothelial cells also express adhesion molecules that tether monocytes, neutrophils, and platelets onto their surface. Tethered monocytes are a source of TF, whereas adherent neutrophils can compound

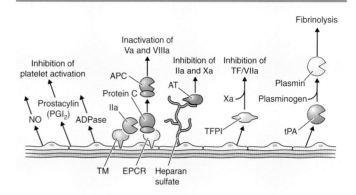

Figure 50.7. Thromboresistant properties of endothelial cells. Schematic illustration of the antiplatelet, anticoagulant, and profibrinolytic activities of endothelial cells. These activities include (1) production of nitric oxide, prostacyclin, and ADPase, substances that inhibit platelet activation and promote vascular relaxation; (2) expression of thrombomodulin (TM) and endothelial cell protein C receptor (EPCR), critical components of the protein C anticoagulant pathway; (3) expression of heparan sulfate, which catalyzes the inactivation of thrombin and factor Xa by antithrombin; (4) expression of tissue factor pathway inhibitor (TFPI), a potent inhibitor of the tissue factor (TF)–mediated extrinsic pathway; and (5) constitutive and regulated secretion of tissue plasminogen activator (tPA), an enzyme that promotes fibrinolysis by converting plasminogen to plasmin. APC, activated protein C.

endothelial injury by secreting free radicals and by releasing hydrolytic enzymes. Bound platelets become activated and promote coagulation. Finally, endothelial cell activation results in transbilayer movement of phosphatidylserine to the exterior surface, thereby providing another negatively charged surface onto which coagulation enzymes and cofactors can bind. Thus, both activated platelets and activated endothelial cells can promote coagulation.

BLEEDING PROBLEMS IN THE CRITICALLY ILL

Unexpected or excessive bleeding is common in the intensive care setting, especially after trauma or surgery. Bleeding may result from platelet defects or from impaired blood coagulation. Acquired and inherited risk factors for bleeding are listed in Box 50.1. A detailed medical history along with a clinical examination to determine the nature and sites of bleeding are essential. The history helps to identify congenital bleeding disorders, whereas the physical examination is important to determine whether there is a systemic or localized defect in hemostasis. Thus, the following questions need to be addressed:

Is the bleeding hereditary or acquired?

Is the bleeding the result of pharmacologic interventions?

Are there comorbid conditions that may exacerbate the bleeding tendency?

Is immediate treatment required, or is this an evaluation to assess the nature of the bleeding disorder for pending surgical procedures?

Are laboratory tests required to assess hemostatic function?

549

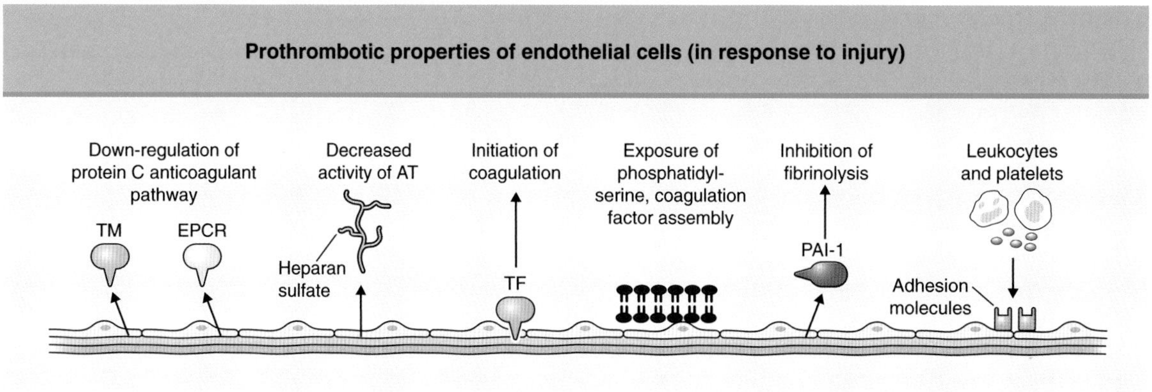

Figure 50.8. Prothrombotic properties of endothelial cells (in response to injury). Endothelial cells acquire a prothrombotic phenotype upon exposure to bacterial lipopolysaccharide or proinflammatory cytokines. Prothrombotic properties of injured endothelial cells include (1) shedding of cell-surface thrombomodulin (TM) and endothelial cell protein C receptor (EPCR), which results in down-regulation of the protein C anticoagulant pathway; (2) shedding of heparan sulfate moieties, which decreases the activity of antithrombin (AT); (3) increased synthesis of tissue factor (TF), which initiates coagulation; (4) exposure of phosphatidylserine, a negatively charged phospholipid onto which coagulation enzymes and cofactors assemble; (5) increased synthesis of plasminogen activator inhibitor–1 (PAI-1), an inhibitor of fibrinolysis; and (6) expression of adhesion molecules, which tether circulating leukocytes and platelets onto the endothelial surface.

Laboratory Assessment of the Bleeding Patient

Hemostatic function can be assessed with simple laboratory tests. The screening tests most commonly used for this purpose are the platelet count, prothrombin time, activated partial thromboplastin time, and thrombin clotting time. Abnormalities in platelet number or function or abnormalities in the coagulation tests help pinpoint the nature of the bleeding disorder (Table 50.1).

Platelet Count

The normal platelet count ranges from 150 to 400×10^9/L. Bleeding due to thrombocytopenia alone is unusual unless the platelet count is less than 50×10^9/L. Clinical findings suggestive of bleeding due to thrombocytopenia include petechiae, ecchymosis, and blood blisters in the mouth. Gastrointestinal and genitourinary bleeding also can occur in patients with thrombocytopenia. If these manifestations are found in a patient

with a platelet count over 100×10^9/L, a qualitative platelet defect or von Willebrand's disease should be considered. In either case, treatment of patients who are bleeding usually involves administration of platelet concentrate, or in the case of von Willebrand's disease, the administration of vWF.

Box 50.1 Acquired and Inherited Risk Factors for Bleeding

Acquired Risk Factors	Inherited Risk Factors
Trauma	von Willebrand's disease
Surgery	Quantitative or qualitative
Disseminated intravascular	platelet disorders
coagulation (DIC)	Deficiency in factor VIII
Dilution of blood constituents	(hemophilia A)
(e.g., blood transfusion,	Deficiency in factor IX
acellular fluid resuscitation)	(hemophilia B)
Immune-mediated platelet	Deficiency in factor VII
destruction in AIDS	Deficiency in factor X
Liver disease	Deficiency in factor V
Vitamin K deficiency	Deficiency in prothrombin
Anticoagulant therapy	Deficiency or abnormality
	in fibrinogen

Table 50.1 Platelet and Coagulation Tests Used to Diagnose Bleeding Disorders

Low Platelet Count

Dilution of blood constitutents (e.g., acellular fluid resuscitation)
Disseminated intravascular coagulation (DIC)
Immune-mediated platelet destruction

Coagulation Tests Abnormalities
Prolongation of PT only

Deficiency of factor VII

Prolongation of APTT only

Deficiency of factor VIII (Hemophilia A)
Deficiency of factor IX (Hemophilia B)
Deficiency of factor XI

Prolongation of both PT and APTT

Warfarin
Liver disease
Vitamin K deficiency
Disseminated intravascular coagulation
Deficiency of factor X, factor V, prothrombin, or fibrinogen

Prolonged thrombin clotting time

Use of heparin
Deficiency or abnormality of fibrinogen
Disseminated intravascular coagulation

Prothrombin Time

The prothrombin time (PT) assesses the integrity of the extrinsic system (factor VII) as well as factors involved in the common pathway (factors X, V, prothrombin, and fibrinogen). The PT measures the time for clot formation when tissue thromboplastin (either a tissue extract containing TF or relipidated recombinant TF) and calcium are added to citrated plasma. The time for clotting of normal plasma is approximately 12 to 15 seconds. Results are expressed as an international normalized ratio (INR), which is a calibration scheme based on the ratio of the patient's PT and the mean normal plasma PT corrected for the "sensitivity" of the thromboplastin used in the test. The sensitivity of the thromboplastin, a measure provided by the manufacturer, reflects its sensitivity to reductions in the levels of the vitamin K–dependent clotting factors. Thus, the INR allows more accurate interlaboratory comparisons.

Activated Partial Thromboplastin Time

The activated partial thromboplastin time (APTT), which assesses the integrity of the intrinsic and common coagulation pathways, measures the time for clot formation when phospholipid, calcium, and a surface activator (e.g., kaolin) are added to citrated plasma. The surface activator is added first to activate the contact factors. Thus, factor XII is converted to factor XIIa and this, in turn, activates factor XI. Factor XIa then activates factor IX. Factor IXa accumulates because it cannot trigger subsequent activation of coagulation factors in the absence of calcium. After a preincubation step, calcium is added and the accumulated factor IXa then triggers the generation of factor Xa and thrombin with resultant fibrin formation. The normal APTT is 30 to 35 seconds.

Thrombin Clotting Time

The thrombin clotting time (TCT) measures the time to clot formation after the addition of thrombin and calcium to citrated plasma. The TCT may be prolonged by (1) inhibitors of thrombin activity, such as heparin or low-molecular-weight heparin; (2) factors that impair fibrin polymerization, such as fibrin and fibrinogen degradation products; or (3) a deficiency or abnormality of fibrinogen. The presence of heparin-like substances can be identified by repeating the test after addition of protamine sulfate or polybrene, substances that neutralize heparin. Fibrin degradation product levels can be measured directly using tests such as D-dimer assays. Likewise, the fibrinogen concentration also can be determined antigenically or using a clot-based assay system.

Plasma Mixing Tests

In patients with prolongation of the PT and/or APTT, the plasma mixing test serves as a simple method to determine whether the prolongation is due to deficiency of a coagulation factor or inhibition of coagulation. Studies are performed by mixing patient plasma with reference control plasma. If the clotting time normalizes with mixing, a factor deficiency exists. Subsequent assays are then performed to identify the deficient clotting factor. Incomplete or minimal correction of the clotting time with mixing indicates the presence of an inhibitor. Inhibitor assays, which often are done with incubation, are performed to identify the target and titer of the inhibitor. Inhibitors most commonly develop in severe hemophiliacs; these inhibitors are

antibodies directed against the clotting factor used to treat their deficiency. Autoantibodies also can develop against specific clotting factors, such as factor VIII. Nonspecific inhibitors, the so-called lupus anticoagulant, are phospholipid-directed antibodies that prolong the APTT and/or PT. Paradoxically, patients with these types of inhibitors are prone to thrombosis, which can occur in either the arterial or the venous system.

Treatment of Bleeding in Critically Ill Patients

Bleeding may also reflect acquired abnormalities in coagulation. Liver disease or trauma can result in decreased synthesis of coagulation factors. Although vitamin K is often given, it may not be effective if the synthetic function of the liver is impaired. Fresh-frozen plasma (FFP) can be used as a source of clotting factors. If fibrinogen is low, cryoprecipitate is also given. Patients with life-threatening bleeding can be treated with recombinant factor VIIa.

Patients receiving anticoagulants are at increased risk of bleeding. The anticoagulant effects of heparin can be completely reversed with protamine sulfate. This agent also partially reverses the anticoagulant effects of low-molecular-weight heparin. Vitamin K antagonists, such as warfarin, can be reversed with vitamin K, a process that can take up to 24 hours. If there is bleeding, FFP should also be administered. Warfarin-treated patients with life-threatening bleeds should be given prothrombin complex concentrates or recombinant factor VIIa.

Thrombocytopenia can contribute to bleeding. The most common causes of thrombocytopenia encountered in critical care medicine are dilution of blood constituents, immune-mediated platelet destruction in patients with AIDS, and disseminated intravascular coagulation (described below).

THROMBOSIS IN THE CRITICALLY ILL

Venous thromboembolism encompasses deep vein thrombosis (DVT) and pulmonary embolism (PE). Acquired and inherited risk factors for venous thromboembolism are listed in Box 50.2. Patients are predisposed to venous thromboembolism during their stay in intensive care because of immobilization, indwelling catheters, use of mechanical ventilation, and sepsis. The estimated prevalence of DVT in critically ill patients ranges from 22% to almost 80%, depending on patient characteristics and the sensitivity of the tests used for diagnosis. Among patients who died while in the ICU, PE has been reported in 7% to 27% of those undergoing autopsy, and approximately 3% of the PEs were thought to have contributed to death. Because diagnosis of venous thromboembolism is problematic in the intensive care setting, vigorous thromboprophylaxis is indicated to prevent the disorder.

Laboratory Assessment of Thrombophilia

Screening for thrombophilic defects should be reserved for patients with thrombosis in an unusual site (e.g., mesenteric vessels), those with recurrent thrombosis, those with a family history of thrombosis, and patients in whom a first episode of unprovoked thrombosis occurred at age 45 or younger.

Thrombophilic defects can be identified using laboratory tests that include (1) functional assays for protein C and antithrombin, (2) assays for total and free protein S, (3) clotting assays to detect APC resistance with confirmation of abnor-

Box 50.2 Acquired and Inherited Risk Factors for Venous Thromboembolism

Acquired Risk Factors	Inherited Risk Factors
Disseminated intravascular coagulation (DIC)	Protein C deficiency
Trauma	Antithrombin deficiency
Malignancy	Protein S deficiency
Surgery	Factor V Leiden mutation
Immobilization	Prothrombin G20210A mutation
Use of central venous catheters	Hyperhomocysteinemia attributable to inherited deficiency of cystathione-β-synthase, methionine synthase, methylenetetrahydrofolate reductase
Mechanical ventilation	
Increased age	
Pregnancy	
Estrogens	
Heparin-induced thrombocytopenia	Dysfibrinogenemia
Warfarin-induced skin necrosis, warfarin-induced limb gangrene	
Antiphospholipid antibodies	
Hyperhomocysteinemia attributable to deficiency of folic acid, vitamins B₆ and B₁₂	

Box 50.3 Clinical Conditions That May Be Associated with DIC

- Sepsis/Severe infection (any microorganism)
- Trauma (e.g., polytrauma, neutrotrauma, fat embolism)
- Organ destruction (e.g., severe pancreatitis)
- Malignancy
  Solid tumor
  Myeloproliferative/lymphoproliferative maliganancies
- Obstetrical calamities
  Amniotic fluid embolism
  Abruptio placentae
- Vascular abnormalities
  Kasabach-Merritt syndrome
  Large vascular aneurysms
- Severe hepatic failure
- Severe toxic or immunologic reations
  Snake bite
  Recreational drug use
  Transfusion reaction
  Transplant rejection

Reprinted from Tayor FB, Toch CH, Hoots WK, et al: Towards definition, clinical and laboratory criteria, and a scoring system for disseminated intravascular coagulation. Thromb Haemost 2001;86:1327–1330.

mal results with DNA testing for the factor V Leiden mutation, (4) DNA analysis to detect the prothrombin G20210A mutation, and (5) phospholipid-based clotting tests to detect the lupus anticoagulant and immunoassays for antiphospholipid antibodies.

Treatment of Venous Thromboembolism in Critically Ill Patients

Although venous thromboembolism contributes to the morbidity and mortality associated with critical illness, thromboprophylaxis is underused in the ICU setting. Based on the results of randomized trials, either low-dose unfractionated heparin or low-molecular-weight heparin are effective means of prophylaxis. For patients at high risk for bleeding, mechanical methods of prophylaxis can be used. These include graded compression stockings and intermittent pneumatic compression.

DISSEMINATED INTRAVASCULAR COAGULATION

A common coagulation abnormality in the ICU setting is disseminated intravascular coagulation (DIC). DIC is an acquired syndrome characterized by systemic activation of coagulation, which can ultimately result in thrombotic occlusion of small and mid-sized vessels. DIC is not a disease in itself but rather occurs as a complication of a variety of disorders (Box 50.3). Intravascular coagulation can contribute to multiple organ failure as well as to severe bleeding because of consumption of platelets and coagulation factors. Thus, DIC can present as a thrombotic disorder, as a bleeding disorder, or with both thrombosis and bleeding.

DIC is associated with high morbidity and mortality. Prospective clinical studies in patients with trauma and sepsis indicate that the development of DIC increases the risk of death two- to fourfold. The estimated incidence of DIC in sepsis is about 83%, although it ranges in severity. The Scientific and Standardization Committee of the International Society on Thrombosis and Haemostasis has proposed a diagnostic algorithm to determine a DIC score, which can be calculated using routine laboratory tests. A score equal to or greater than 5 is consistent with DIC, whereas a score of less than 5 may indicate subclinical DIC.

Pathogenesis of DIC

The mainstay of DIC treatment is management of the underlying disorder. For example, in patients with sepsis and hypotension, appropriate antibiotic therapy is given along with measures to restore the blood pressure. However, DIC often persists despite aggressive treatment of the underlying disease. Although DIC has traditionally been defined as systemic activation of coagulation, a beneficial effect of anticoagulants such as heparin or antithrombin has not been shown in controlled clinical trials. The failure of these anticoagulants in the treatment of DIC has forced a reexamination of the assumption that the coagulopathy is the main determinant of clinical outcome in DIC. Indeed, current thinking is that the pathogenesis of DIC reflects intimate linkages between inflammation (see Chapter 51) and coagulation. Consequently, an imbalance in these pathways can lead to widespread thrombosis, inflammation, cell death, organ failure, and ultimately death.

Sepsis and Activated Protein C

The most common clinical condition associated with DIC in the ICU setting is sepsis, the leading cause of death in noncoronary ICU patients. Sepsis is initiated by a focus of infection from which microbes or microbial toxins released into the bloodstream trigger systemic and uncontrolled activation of inflammatory and coagulation pathways. Severe sepsis, defined as sepsis associated with at least one dysfunctional organ, is a disease that affects about 700,000 people in the United States annually and has a mortality rate of 30% to 50%.

Recently, a large phase III clinical trial (the PROWESS study; see Bernard and colleagues, 2001) demonstrated the efficacy and safety of recombinant APC (drotrecogin alfa, activated) for severe sepsis. This study randomized patients with severe sepsis to receive either recombinant APC or saline for 4 days by continuous intravenous infusion. Compared with placebo, recombinant APC produced a reduction in the relative risk of death of 19.4% and an absolute reduction in the risk of death of 6.1% ($P = 0.005$).

The protective effects of therapeutic APC in patients with severe sepsis likely reflects the ability of APC to modulate multiple pathways. As mentioned earlier, APC is a physiologically important anticoagulant. In addition to its anticoagulant properties, APC has profibrinolytic activity because it inactivates PAI-1. APC also possesses antiinflammatory properties. Thus, in cell culture systems, APC inhibits production of proinflammatory cytokines by monocytes and suppresses endothelial cell expression of leukocyte adhesion molecules, presumably by inhibiting nuclear factor kappa B (NF-κB), a gene regulatory protein that activates specific inflammatory genes. In laboratory animals challenged with bacterial endotoxin, APC blocks the production of inflammatory cytokines and inhibits leukocyte adhesion. The precise mechanisms by which APC exerts its antiinflammatory effects remain unclear.

Using cultured endothelial cells, APC has been shown to inhibit apoptosis, or programmed cell death. This may be important because apoptotic endothelial cells lose their anticoagulant properties and acquire a proinflammatory phenotype by releasing interleukin 1β. The antiapoptotic effects of APC are presumed to be mediated by the binding of APC to its cell surface receptor EPCR. Current thinking is that once bound to EPCR, APC cleaves protease activated receptor–1 (PAR-1), a cell surface receptor linked to intracellular signaling events, thereby up-regulating antiapoptotic genes.

SUMMARY

The hemostatic response is essential to stop bleeding at sites of blood vessel injury while maintaining vascular integrity. Hemostasis is a complex, tightly regulated process that includes physical, biochemical, and cellular events. The major components involved in hemostasis include platelets, coagulation factors and their inhibitors, fibrinolytic enzymes and their inhibitors, and the vascular endothelium. Therapeutic interventions must be carefully chosen to correct hemostatic defects without disrupting the delicate balance between procoagulant and anticoagulant mechanisms.

SUGGESTED READING

Aird WC: The role of the endothelium in severe sepsis and multiple organ dysfunction syndrome. Blood 2003;101:3765–3777.

Attia J, Ray JG, Cook DJ, et al: Deep vein thrombosis and its prevention in critically ill adults. Arch Intern Med 2001;161:1268–1279.

Bernard GR, Vincent J-L, Laterre P-F, et al: Efficacy and safety of recombinant human activated protein C for severe sepsis. N Engl J Med 2001;344:699–709.

Colman RW, Clowes AW, George JN, et al: Overview of hemostasis. In Colman RW, Hirsh J, Marder V, et al (eds): Hemostasis and Thrombosis: Basic Principles and Clinical Practice, 4th ed. Philadelphia, Lippincott Williams and Wilkins, 2001.

Esmon CT: The protein C pathway. Crit Care Med 2000;28(9 suppl): S44–S48.

Furie B: Presentation of bleeding disorders. In Furie B, Cassileth PA, Atkins MB, Mayer RJ (eds): Clinical Hematology and Oncology: Presentation, Diagnosis, and Treatment. Philadelphia, Churchill Livingstone, 2003.

Geerts W, Cook D, Selby R, Etchells E: Venous thromboembolism and its prevention in critical care. J Crit Care 2002;17:95–104.

Marino PL: The ICU Book, 2nd ed. Philadelphia, Lippincott Williams and Wilkins, 1998.

Taylor FB, Toh C-H, Hoots WK, et al: Towards definition, clinical and laboratory criteria, and a scoring system for disseminated intravascular coagulation. Thromb Haemost 2001;86:1327–1330.

Tripodi A, Mannuci M: Laboratory investigation of thrombophilia. Clin Chem 2001;49:1597–1606.

Chapter 51

Interaction of Coagulation and Inflammation

William C. Aird

KEY POINTS

- Despite new information about the pathophysiology and treatment of severe sepsis, it continues to be associated with an unacceptably high mortality rate.
- The endothelium is key in initiating, perpetuating, and modulating the host response to infection.
- Endothelial dysfunction occurs in the absence of reliable circulating markers, and the endothelium is a highly complex organ; therefore isolated endothelial cells cannot be relied on for a full understanding of the endothelium in health and disease. The endothelium is largely overlooked in clinical practice, a bench-to-bedside gap.
- Enormous resources have been expended on sepsis trials; most therapies failed to reduce mortality in patients with severe sepsis, but at least five phase 3 clinical trials demonstrated improved survival in critically ill patients or patients with severe sepsis.

The innate immune response involves the concomitant activation of inflammation and coagulation (see Chapter 50 for an overview of coagulation). Indeed, it may be argued that inflammation and coagulation *always* occur together. Although usually an adaptive mechanism, the innate immune response may lead to disease. Severe sepsis is the leading cause of death among hospitalized patients in noncoronary intensive care units. An important goal is to develop improved therapeutic strategies that will have a favorable impact on patient outcome. Sepsis is invariably associated with activation of coagulation and inflammation. Recent studies have pointed to a critical role for the endothelium in orchestrating the host response in severe sepsis. This chapter provides a conceptual framework for understanding the pathophysiology of sepsis, emphasizes the importance of the cross-talk between inflammation and coagulation, and underscores the potential value of the endothelium as a target for sepsis therapy.

SEPSIS PATHOPHYSIOLOGY

Sepsis pathophysiology may be described according to the following themes (Box 51.1). First, the host response—rather than the identity of the pathogen—is the primary determinant of patient outcome. Second, monocytes and endothelial cells serve to initiate and perpetuate the host response to infection. Third, sepsis is characterized by systemic activation of the inflammatory and coagulation cascades.[1] Fourth, the inflammatory and coagulation pathways interact with one another to further amplify the host response. Finally, the host response inflicts collateral damage on normal tissues, resulting in pathology that is not diffuse but remarkably focal in its distribution. Each of these themes has been previously reviewed in detail (Aird, 2003).

The pathophysiology of sepsis may be simplified according to the scheme shown in Figure 51.1. Monocytes and tissue macrophages engage pathogens through pattern recognition receptors (e.g., toll-like receptors). Ligand-receptor interactions result in the activation of both inflammatory and coagulation pathways. On the inflammatory side, the monocyte releases many inflammatory mediators—including tumor necrosis factor (TNF)–α and interleukin (IL)-1—which then bind to receptors in the presence of monocytes and endothelial cells, resulting in autocrine and paracrine activation, respectively. On the coagulation side, activated monocytes and macrophages express tissue factor (TF) on their cell surface, which in turn triggers the clotting cascade.

Box 51.1 Themes in Sepsis Pathophysiology

1. Host response is a primary determinant of pathology
2. Monocytes initiate host response to infection
3. Endothelial cells perpetuate the host response
4. Inflammatory and coagulation pathways are always activated
5. There is cross-talk between inflammatory and coagulation pathways
6. Host response may inflict focal "collateral damage" (organ dysfunction) on the host

---

[1]On the inflammatory side, IL-6 levels are increased in virtually every patient with severe sepsis, and TNF-α levels are increased in the majority of patients. On the coagulation side, D-dimers are elevated in all patients with severe sepsis, protein C levels are decreased in up to 90% of such patients, and antithrombin III levels are below 60% in more than half of patients. Although the operational definition varies among studies, disseminated intravascular coagulation (DIC) is estimated to occur in 15% to 30% of patients with severe sepsis, including those with septic shock.

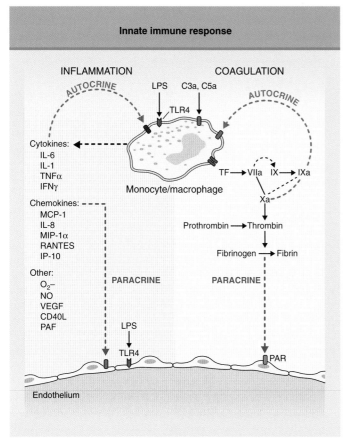

Innate immune response

INFLAMMATION   COAGULATION

Figure 51.1. Innate immune response. Circulating monocytes or tissue macrophages bind to lipopolysaccharide (LPS) via toll-like receptor 4 (TLR4), resulting in activation of inflammatory and coagulation pathways. Components of each pathway participate in autocrine and paracrine loops, which in turn lead to additional activation of monocytes and endothelial cells, respectively. At the level of the endothelium, input may arrive directly via LPS or indirectly via monocyte-derived inflammatory/coagulation mediators. The innate immune response may also be activated in nonsepsis states such as trauma and surgery.

Importantly, the inflammatory and coagulation cascades engage in significant cross-talk. For example, TNF-α and IL-1 (inflammatory cytokines) induce expression of TF on monocytes and possibly subsets of endothelial cells. In the other direction, serine proteases in the clotting cascade bind to protease-activated receptors on the surface of several cell types (including monocytes and endothelial cells), resulting in a proinflammatory phenotype.

ENDOTHELIUM IN SEPSIS

Bench-to-Bedside Gap in Endothelial Biomedicine

The endothelium, which lines the inside of all blood vessels, is a highly metabolically active organ. Despite a robust literature on endothelial cells (tens of thousands of published articles), the endothelium is largely overlooked in clinical practice. There are several possible explanations for this bench-to-bedside gap (Box 51.2). First, the endothelium is hidden from view and is poorly

---

Box 51.2 Bench-to-Bedside Gap in Endothelial Biomedicine

1. The endothelium is inaccessible
2. The endothelium displays emergent properties
3. The endothelium is tightly coupled to native microenvironment

---

accessible in the patient. Indeed, the endothelium does not lend itself to inspection, palpation, percussion, or auscultation. Although certain other organs such as the pancreas and kidney are also difficult to examine at the bedside, they are spatially confined and thus amenable to diagnostic imaging. Moreover, whereas disease of these latter organs is associated with changes in blood chemistry (e.g., amylase, blood urea nitrogen, and creatinine), endothelial dysfunction occurs in the absence of reliable circulating markers. Second, the endothelium—like other organs in the body—is highly complex. Most endothelial cell biologists study specific aspects of endothelial cell function in tissue culture and in doing so tend to overlook critical levels of organization that are essential to a full understanding of the system. Just as one could never predict the behavior of an ant colony by studying an individual ant in isolation, one cannot rely solely on isolated endothelial cells to fully understand the endothelium in health and disease. Third, the endothelium, more so than most other tissues in the human body, is extraordinarily adaptive and flexible. It is like a chameleon, "marching to the tune" of the local microenvironment. Indeed, so tightly coupled is the endothelium to the extracellular milieu that when it is removed from its native environment and grown in tissue culture, it undergoes phenotypic drift. Therefore, any results from in vitro studies must be interpreted with caution and ultimately validated in vivo.

Endothelial Cell Function and Dysfunction

The two most commonly used terms or descriptors in endothelium-based diseases are endothelial cell activation and endothelial cell dysfunction (Box 51.3). Both terms were coined in the 1980s, and their meaning has changed over the years. Endothelial cell activation was originally used to describe the proadhesive function of cultured endothelial cells treated with

---

Box 51.3 Definitions

Endothelial cell activation: Phenotypic response of the endothelium to inflammatory mediators (as occurs in sepsis, trauma, and surgery), usually consisting of some combination of proadhesive surface, procoagulant activity, altered vasomotor tone, increased apoptosis, and change in barrier function. Note: the phenotype may be functional (adaptive) or dysfunctional (nonadaptive)

Endothelial cell dysfunction: Phenotypic response of the endothelium that poses a net liability to the host. Note: the phenotype may be activated or nonactivated.

inflammatory mediators. Today, the term most commonly refers to the phenotypic response of the endothelium to inflammation or infection. An important caveat is that the so-called "activation phenotype" differs between different sites of the vasculature. For example, activated endothelial cells in culture have been shown to express decreased levels of thrombomodulin (TM) on their cell surface (in theory, resulting in reduced capacity to activate protein C). However, the human brain expresses very little, if any, TM. That does not mean that the blood-brain barrier is in a chronic state of activation. Rather, the brain must rely on other natural anticoagulants to balance local hemostasis. As another example, P-selectin (a cell adhesion molecule) is considered an activation marker for endothelial cells. However, endothelial cells in uninflamed skin constitutively express P-selectin. In summary, the state of activation must be judged in an appropriate spatial context.

Endothelial cell dysfunction is most often used to describe the abnormal endothelial phenotype in atherosclerosis (most notably, changes in endothelium-mediated vasomotor tone). However, the term may be applied more broadly to other disease states. Indeed, endothelial cell dysfunction occurs when the endothelial phenotype—whether or not it meets a definition for activation—represents a net liability to the host. This may occur locally (e.g., coronary artery disease) or systemically (e.g., sepsis).

Endothelial Response in Severe Sepsis

Each endothelial cell in the body is analogous to a miniature adaptive input-output device (Fig. 51.2). Input is derived from the extracellular environment and may include biochemical or biomechanical forces. Output represents the phenotype of the endothelium and may include changes in proliferation, cell sur-

vival, vasomotor tone, permeability, hemostatic balance, and/or release of inflammatory mediators. In sepsis, there are many changes in the input signals, including components of the bacterial wall, complement, cytokines, chemokines, serine proteases, fibrin, activated platelets and leukocytes, hyperglycemia, and/or changes in oxygenation or blood flow. Endothelial phenotypes in sepsis include both structural alterations (e.g., nuclear vacuolization, cytoplasmic swelling, cytoplasmic fragmentation, denudation, and/or detachment) and functional changes (e.g., shifts in the hemostatic balance, increased cell adhesion and leukocyte trafficking, altered vasomotor tone, loss of barrier function, and programmed cell death). Finally, the "set point" of the endothelium—as determined by the influence of epigenetic processes, age, comorbidity, and genetic polymorphisms—may alter the phenotype and/or transduction capacity (input-output coupling) of the endothelial cell.

Endothelial Dysfunction in Severe Sepsis

The host response to sepsis involves a complex orchestra of cells (e.g., leukocytes, platelets, and endothelial cells) and soluble mediators (e.g., components of the inflammatory and coagulation cascades). Normally, these mechanisms are highly coordinated with one another to defend host against pathogen. However, if the host response is disproportionate to the nature of the threat, i.e., it is excessive, sustained, or poorly localized, then the balance of power shifts in favor of the pathogen, resulting in the sepsis phenotype—namely, dysfunction of subsets of organ systems. Many hypotheses have been proposed to explain the cause of organ dysfunction. However, at this time, our understanding of the precise pathophysiologic processes is unclear.

Available evidence suggests that severe sepsis is associated with excessive, sustained, and generalized activation of the endothelium. Without artificial organ support, virtually all patients with severe sepsis would die of their disease. In other words, most of these individuals have crossed the threshold from an adaptive to a maladaptive response. Insofar as the endothelium contributes to the severe sepsis phenotype, its behavior may be characterized as dysfunctional. An important goal for the future is to learn how to identify the transition from function to dysfunction, before the onset of significant (and perhaps irreversible) organ damage. Importantly, the endothelium is an attractive therapeutic target.

SEPSIS THERAPY

Enormous resources have been expended on sepsis trials, with more than 10,000 patients enrolled in over 20 placebo-controlled, randomized phase 3 clinical trials. Most of these therapies have failed to reduce mortality in patients with severe sepsis, including antiendotoxin, anticytokine, antiprostaglandin, antibradykinin and antiplatelet activating factor (PAF) strategies, antithrombin III (ATIII), and tissue factor pathway inhibitor (TFPI). At the time of this writing, a total of five phase 3 clinical trials have demonstrated improved survival in critically ill patients or patients with severe sepsis. These include the use of low tidal volume ventilation, activated protein C, low-dose glucocorticoids, intensive insulin therapy, and early goal-directed therapy.

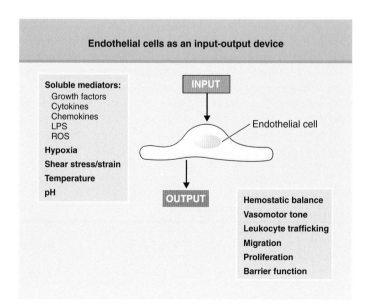

Endothelial cells as an input-output device

Soluble mediators:
Growth factors
Cytokines
Chemokines
LPS
ROS
Hypoxia
Shear stress/strain
Temperature
pH

INPUT

Endothelial cell

OUTPUT

Hemostatic balance
Vasomotor tone
Leukocyte trafficking
Migration
Proliferation
Barrier function

Figure 51.2. Endothelial cell as an input-output device. Each endothelial cell in the body (there are about 60 trillion of them) behaves like a miniature adaptive input-output device sensing changes in the extracellular environment and responding via altered phenotype. LPS, lipopolysaccharide; ROS, reactive oxygen species.

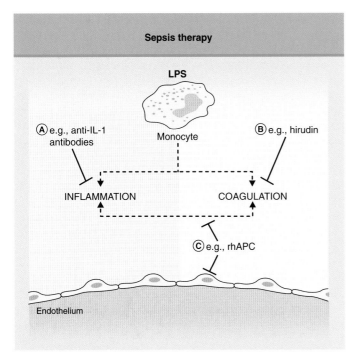

Figure 51.3. Sepsis therapy. Shown are components of the innate immune response. Circulating monocytes or tissue macrophages bind to lipopolysaccharide (LPS), resulting in activation of inflammatory and coagulation cascades (compare Figure 51.1). These pathways then operate in autocrine and paracrine pathways to activate monocytes and endothelial cells, respectively. As a general rule, neither the selective targeting of an inflammatory mediator *(A)* nor thrombin generation *(B)* improves survival in severe sepsis. In contrast, therapies that target both inflammatory and coagulation pathways and/or attenuate endothelial cell dysfunction *(C)* show more promise.

There are several lessons to be learned from these clinical trials. First, the use of single modality therapy aimed at inhibiting endotoxin or inflammation is ineffective (Fig. 51.3). These data are consistent with the notion that the inflammatory cascade, while certainly an important contributor to sepsis morbidity and mortality, is sufficiently redundant, pleiotropic, and interdependent as to preclude single modality therapy. Second, preclinical studies with selective thrombin inhibitors suggest that fibrin ablation has little or no effect on organ dysfunction or mortality. One interpretation of these findings is that clotting in and of itself is nonlethal in sepsis. Third, the combination of antiinflammatory and anticoagulant appears more promising. For example, TFPI, ATIII, and recombinant human activated protein C (rhAPC) have each been shown to inhibit inflammation and coagulation in vitro and in vivo and to yield improved survival in nonhuman primate models of sepsis and phase 2 clinical trials of severe sepsis. Of these three agents, only rhAPC reduced mortality in phase 3 clinical studies.

A common theme of the five successful treatments in severe sepsis is their capacity to attenuate endothelial cell dysfunction. The effect of rhAPC on the endothelium was discussed above. Low-volume ventilation would be expected to reduce barotraumas to the pulmonary endothelium. Low-dose glucocorticoids

may reduce the activity of proinflammatory transcription factors in endothelial cells, while intensive insulin therapy may reduce the deleterious effects of high glucose on the endothelium. Finally, early goal-directed therapy is predicted to maintain flow and hence shear stress at the level of the blood vessel wall. The extent to which these therapies exert their benefit through the endothelium remains unknown.

There are many other possible strategies for attenuating endothelial cell dysfunction (Aird, 2003). One may target the input signals, the coupling mechanism inside the cell, or the cellular phenotype (output). Examples of extracellular signals as targets include endotoxin, TNF-α, IL-1, and PAF. Examples of coupling mechanisms include receptors, such as cellular adhesion molecules and protease-activated receptors; signaling pathways such as p38 MAPK or novel/atypical PKC isoforms; and transcription factors, including NF-κB, GATA-2, and the Ets family of transacting proteins. Potential target outputs include endothelial control of hemostasis, inflammation, vasomotor tone, permeability, and leukocyte trafficking.

Although the failure of antiendotoxin and TNF-α antibodies to improve mortality in patients with severe sepsis is consistent with the complexity of the host response, these findings do not exclude a role for single target ("smart bomb") therapy. The host response, while unquestionably redundant and pleiotropic, is likely to contain certain component parts—whether an extracellular mediator, a cell surface receptor, a signal intermediate, or a transcription factor—that are so highly connected as to render that component (and the entire system) vulnerable to therapeutic targeting. A key challenge is to identify these so-called hubs in the sepsis cascade and to target those factors accordingly.

CONCLUSIONS

Despite new information about the pathophysiology and treatment of severe sepsis, this disorder continues to be associated with an unacceptably high mortality rate. Future breakthroughs will require a conceptual shift that emphasizes relationships between the various mediators (inflammatory and coagulation) and cells involved in host response. The endothelium is key in initiating, perpetuating, and modulating the host response to infection. Additional studies promise to provide new insight into the endothelium, not as an isolated mechanism of sepsis pathophysiology but rather as the coordinator of a far more expansive, spatially and temporally orchestrated response.

SUGGESTED READING

Aird WC: The role of the endothelium in severe sepsis and the multiple organ dysfunction syndrome. Blood 2003;101;3765–3777.

Annane D, Sebille V, Charpentier C, et al: Effect of treatment with low doses of hydrocortisone and fludrocortisone on mortality in patients with septic shock. JAMA 2002;288:862–871.

ARDSNET: Ventilation with lower tidal volumes as compared with traditional tidal volumes for acute lung injury and the acute respiratory distress syndrome. The Acute Respiratory Distress Syndrome Network. N Engl J Med 2000;342:1301–1308.

Bernard GR, Vincent JL, Laterre PF, et al: Efficacy and safety of recombinant human activated protein C for severe sepsis. N Engl J Med 2001; 344:699–709.

Cohen J, Guyatt G, Bernard GR, et al: New strategies for clinical trials in patients with sepsis and septic shock. Crit Care Med 2001;29:880–886.

Eichacker PQ, Parent C, Kalil A, et al: Risk and the efficacy of antiinflammatory agents: retrospective and confirmatory studies of sepsis. Am J Respir Crit Care Med 2002;166:1197–1205.

Rivers E, Nguyen B, Havstad S, et al: Early goal-directed therapy in the treatment of severe sepsis and septic shock. N Engl J Med 2001;345:1368–1377.

Van den Berghe G, Wouters P, Weekers F, et al: Intensive insulin therapy in the critically ill patients. N Engl J Med 2001;345:1359–1367.

KEY POINTS

- Whole blood is processed to produce components that should be used selectively to preserve these precious resources.
- The threshold for transfusion of red blood cells is generally accepted as 7 g/dL in the critically ill.
- The threshold for transfusion of red blood cells is generally 10 g/dL in patients with ongoing myocardial ischemia.
- Oxygen therapeutics is an increasingly interesting and active area of research in an effort to replace the dwindling blood pool.

In 1665, Richard Lower performed the first recorded blood transfusion in animals. Two years later, the French physician Jean-Baptist Denis transfused a teenage boy suffering from persistent fever with lamb's blood. It was not until 1795 that the first human-to-human blood transfusion was performed by a Philadelphia physician, Philip Syng Physick.

The idea of using blood transfusion to preserve life made its way into literary works of the time. Bram Stoker's famous novel *Dracula* (1897) describes a young maiden, Lucy, who is slowly drained of blood every night by Dracula during her sleep. Her fiancé, Arthur, is recruited by Professor Van Helsing to donate his own blood to her:

> She was ghastly, chalkily pale; the red seemed to have gone even from her lips and gums, and the bones of her face stood out prominently; her breathing was painful to see or hear. Van Helsing's face grew set as marble, and his eyebrows converged till they almost touched over his nose. . . . There is no time to be lost. She will die for sheer want of blood to keep the heart's action as it should be. There must be transfusion of blood at once. Is it you or me. . . . As the transfusion went on, something like life seemed to come back to poor Lucy's cheeks, and through Arthur's growing pallor the joy of his face seemed absolutely to shine.

It was not until 1914 when, almost simultaneously, Albert Hustin of Brussels and Luis Agote of Buenos Aires discovered that adding sodium citrate to blood would prevent clotting, giving birth to blood banking. The field of transfusion medicine has subsequently evolved to become an integral part of the surgeon's practice.

Most of today's blood pool is collected from voluntary donors (92%, allogenic). "Autologous" transfusions refer to those trans-fusions in which the blood donor and transfusion recipient are the same. This is typically used in the preoperative donation of blood for possible reinfusion into the donor during elective surgery. The percentage of total donations represented by autologous donations in the United States increased from 0.25% of total donations in 1980 to 8.5% in 1992. "Directed" or "designated" donation refers to blood obtained from relatives or friends of the recipient. These donor-directed units undergo the same rigorous screening methods as allogenic donor blood following studies that reported an increased frequency of hepatitis markers in the blood of these donors.

BLOOD COMPONENTS

K.C. is a 19-year-old female college student who, after a motor vehicle crash, presents with a Glasgow Coma Scale of 15, systolic blood pressure of 90 mm Hg, heart rate of 130, and respiratory rate of 26. She appears to have bilateral femoral fractures and abdominal tenderness. After receiving 2 L of fluid, her systolic blood pressure increased to 100 mm Hg and her heart rate decreased to 100. An abdominal ultrasound revealed a significant amount of blood in Morrison's pouch and the pelvis. Her initial chest and pelvic x-rays showed no evidence of significant pathology. Despite the initial response to fluids, she became more hypotensive with increased tachycardia. She received 2 units of uncrossmatched O-negative blood immediately and was given additional crystalloid fluid during transport to the operating room for an exploratory laparotomy. An exploration of her open abdomen revealed a large amount of hemoperitoneum and all four quadrants were packed. After removal of the packs, the liver began to bleed actively and the patient became increasingly hypotensive and tachycardic. With a Pringle maneuver applied, the bleeding decreased, allowing time to repack the liver. The anesthesiologists continued to transfuse her with packed red blood cells, platelets, and fresh frozen plasma to maintain her systolic pressure no higher than 90 mm Hg.

Although whole blood can be stored in refrigeration units for 21 to 35 days, its component function is significantly altered after a short time in storage. Platelet and granulocyte function is lost after 24 hours because of the storage temperature (1–6°C) necessary to maintain red blood cells' function. Further storage (14 days) will decrease the levels of "labile" coagulation factors V and VIII. A whole blood unit is usually separated into red blood cells, platelet concentrate, and fresh frozen plasma (FFP). The plasma can be further processed into cryoprecipitate and supernatant plasma. Separation permits the selective use of blood products. This methodology minimizes the infusion of harmful elements of blood and improves the availability of this precious resource.

Red Blood Cells

The hematocrit level of a whole blood unit reflects that of circulating blood and is approximately 40%. Packed red blood cells (PRBCs), the most frequently administered blood component, have a hematocrit of 70% to 80%. PRBCs were initially stored in a citrate–phosphate–dextrose–adenine solution, which increased the storage life to 35 days. Blood is now routinely stored for 42 days with the addition of preservative solutions that increase the volume to 300 mL and decrease the hematocrit to 60%. RBC viability is defined as the capability of RBCs to survive 24 hours after being transfused and their function as an oxygen carrier. Both of these factors change according to storage modalities (e.g., temperature). Blood is usually stored at a temperature of 4°C; lower temperatures will cause freezing. Higher temperatures increase metabolism and decrease pH, 2,3-DPG, and ATP levels. The reduction of 2,3-DPG levels contributes to the increase in oxygen affinity of hemoglobin and therefore shifts the dissociation curve to the left, decreasing oxygen availability. Twenty-five percent recovery of 2,3-DPG levels is expected within 8 hours and full recovery within 24 hours after transfusion. There is no evidence, however, that 2,3-DPG reduction and recovery have any clinical significance. During storage, there is also an accumulation of lactate and pyruvic acid from glucose metabolism. Osmotic fragility increases and pH decreases (from 7.16 at donation to 6.73 at the end of shelf life). RBCs in storage tend to lose potassium and accumulate sodium during refrigeration because the Na^+-K^+-ATPase pump function is impaired at low temperatures. Each unit of blood supplies an average of 7 mEq/L of potassium, which is easily tolerable. RBCs can be frozen for 10 to 21 years.

Indications for Transfusion

The optimal threshold for transfusion remains controversial. In a multi-institutional, randomized, controlled trial, more than 800 critically ill patients received blood for anemia targeted to maintain their hemoglobin levels at 7.0 g/dL (restricted group) versus 10 g/dL (liberal group). In this trial, the 30-day mortality rates were similar in both groups. Alternatively, hematocrit levels lower than 28% may contribute to perioperative myocardial ischemia in the elderly. A retrospective study (78,974 patients) showed that blood transfusion was associated with a lower short-term mortality rate among elderly patients (older than 65 years) with acute myocardial infarction if the hematocrit on admission was 30% or more.

Seven grams per deciliter hemoglobin is a well-established threshold in critically ill patients, with 10 g/dL appropriate for those with ongoing myocardial ischemia. There is no clinical evidence to support the assumption that RBC transfusion contributes to wound healing, recovery from surgical intervention, or resistance to infection.

Platelets

Each unit of platelets contains at least 5.5×10^{10} in 50 mL of plasma. Platelet pheresis (single-donor platelets or apheresis

platelets) are obtained from one donor by cytopheresis during a 1.5- to 2-hour procedure on an automated device producing 6 to 10 units of platelet concentrate. Platelets are stored at room temperature (20–24°C) and are constantly agitated to further improve their survival. The average shelf life of platelet concentrates is 5 days, during which they maintain their ability to promote hemostasis. ABO compatibility in platelet transfusion is recommended but not mandatory. Each unit of platelets is expected to raise the patient's platelet count by 10×10^9/L. The usual infusion is 6 units, or 1 unit per 10 kg of body weight. A 66% platelet recovery is expected in patients with an intact spleen, and a 100% response should be seen in asplenic patients. Thrombocytopenic patients will often yield 50% recovery, whereas levels of less than 50% reflect refractoriness.

Indications for Platelet Transfusion

Bleeding thrombocytopenic patients, those at high risk for bleeding because of severe thrombocytopenia, and those with platelet dysfunction are all candidates for platelet transfusions. Surgical patients with platelet counts greater than 50×10^9/L do not typically bleed. Other factors may change the likelihood of hemorrhage, such as uremia, sepsis, drugs, active bleeding, and foreign bodies (e.g., intraaortic pump balloon). A threshold of 10×10^9/L for platelet transfusion appears safe. However, only a few small randomized studies exist, and they deal primarily with the comparison of prophylactic versus therapeutic platelet transfusions. Bleeding time, a test that is increased as platelet counts are reduced, is a poor indicator of the risk of bleeding. Platelet transfusions in patients with thrombotic thrombocytopenic purpura, as well as in those with hemolytic uremic syndrome, are considered deleterious and, therefore, are reserved for life-threatening situations. The development of "refractoriness to platelets" transfusion is a serious event and usually seen in cases with splenomegaly, fever, disseminated intravascular coagulopathy, bone marrow transplantation, administration of amphotericin B or certain antibiotics, or when the units transfused were mismanaged before the transfusion.

Plasma Components

The plasma is frozen within 8 hours of its production at a temperature of −18°C and can be stored as FFP for 1 year. When needed, it is thawed in 98.6°F (37°C) in a hot water tub. The process of thawing usually takes approximately 30 to 40 minutes, after which it can be stored in the refrigerator for up to 24 hours. Plasma cryoprecipitate is formed by thawing FFP at a temperature of 4°C, at which the components of the fibrinogen (factor VIII, Von Willebrand factor, and fibrinonectin) are insoluble and can be separated. FFP contains all circulating plasma components, including stable and labile coagulation factors. Each FFP transfusion must be ABO compatible, but antibody cross-matching to the recipient is not necessary.

Indications for Transfusion of Plasma Products

FFP should be transfused to replace coagulation factors or plasma proteins to bleeding patients with acquired multiple coagulation factor deficiencies. It should not be used for volume expansion, wound healing, or as a nutritional source. FFP will not correct coagulopathy that is heparin induced. Prophylactic FFP administration does not prevent bleeding in cases of massive transfusion or after cardiac surgery. Most patients will not bleed from coagulation factor deficiencies when the prothrombin time/international normalizing ratio or activated partial thromboplastin time (PTT) are minimally prolonged (less than 1.5 times the normal laboratory mean). Prophylactic administration of FFP before most invasive diagnostic procedures to patients with a slight prolongation of their coagulation tests is not recommended.

The usual dose for cryoprecipitate transfusion is 10 units, followed by 6 to 10 units every 8 hours. The goal of transfusion is to elevate fibrinogen levels to 100 mg/dL. Since each cryoprecipitate unit carries the equivalent risk of disease transmission as 1 unit of blood, it is recommended to use recombinant factors in patients who are to be subjected to frequent plasma transfusions.

Immunoglobulin Preparations

The usage of immunoglobulin is variable and expanding. It is given as passive antibody prophylaxis in immune-deficient patients such as those with AIDS or bone marrow transplant. It may also be used in patients with idiopathic thrombocytopenic purpura, Guillain–Barré syndrome, chronic inflammatory demyelinating polyneuropathy, myasthenia gravis, and thrombotic thrombocytopenic purpura. The mechanism of action in these cases is yet to be defined.

Granulocyte Components

Once collected and suspended in 200 mL of plasma, white blood cells can be kept at room temperature for 24 hours only. Granulocyte concentrates are made from a single donor by cytopheresis methods. Each unit contains at least 10^{10} granulocytes and a significant amount of RBCs; therefore, cross-matching for the recipient is mandatory. Patients who may benefit from such transfusion are those with neutropenia ($<0.5 \times 10^9$/L) who do not respond to adequate antibiotic treatment and are expected to gain bone marrow recovery. A therapeutic course includes diurnal transfusion repeated for 4 to 7 days.

TRANSFUSION REACTIONS AND RISKS OF BLOOD TRANSFUSIONS

Hemolytic and Nonhemolytic Reactions

Fatal acute hemolytic reactions to transfusions still occur rarely (1/250,000 to 1/1,000,000 transfusions). The major cause is still ABO incompatibility resulting from administrative mistakes occurring at the bedside and in the laboratory. Other hemolytic and nonhemolytic reactions and their pathology, clinical manifestations, and treatment are listed in Table 52.1.

Transfusion-Mediated Immunomodulation

Allogeneic transfusions have immunosuppressive effects possibly related to leukocyte exposures. Prior sensitization remains of great importance in patients undergoing kidney transplantation and in women who have multiple miscarriages. The immunosuppressive effects of allogeneic blood have not been proven in other patient populations. Some retrospective studies revealed a relationship between exposure to allogeneic blood transfusion and early recurrence of cancer diseases. They also revealed increased rates of postoperative infections. Controversy exists as to the effect of various leukocyte-reduction techniques on the degree of immunosuppression.

Transfusion-Transmitted Viral Infection Risk from Blood Components

Despite routine screening of all blood units to HIV, human T-cell lymphocytic virus (HTLV) types I and II, hepatitis B virus (HBV), and hepatitis C virus (HCV), the risks for transmission still exist. Estimates for risk are listed in Table 52.2. There is no risk of HTLV transmission through acellular components since it is exclusively a cell-associated virus. The infectious potential is reduced by storage time, reaching zero after 14 days of storage. Other viral and protozoa infections may be transmitted via blood transfusion, but a very small estimated risk, combined with insufficient data and considerable cost, preclude them from being routinely screened on daily basis. A report of a likely prion transmission causing variant Creutzfeldt–Jacob disease from a blood transfusion has led to a greater awareness of the risk of transfer of previously unknown pathogens via blood.

Transfusion-Associated Graft versus Host Disease

Transfusion-associated graft versus host disease (TA-GVHD) is a severe immunologic complication resulting from transfusion of blood and blood components to severely immunocompromised patients. The mechanism involves the engraftment of the allogeneic lymphocytes and the recipient's tissue rejection due to the donor's active lymphocytes existing in the transfusion components. Patients considered to be at high risk for the condition are neonates, bone marrow and organ transplant recipients, leukemia and lymphoma patients, and those under chemotherapeutic therapy. The mortality rate in TA-GVHD is high, reaching 90% with no effective treatment. Prophylactic irradiation of the blood components with a dose of 25 Gy (2500 rad) eliminates lymphocytic mitogenic activity and, thus, the occurrence of this lesion. All blood components except FFP and cryoprecipitate should be irradiated prior to their transfusion to these high-risk patients.

Massive Blood Transfusion

Massive blood transfusion (MBT) is defined as transfusion of blood components exceeding one blood volume within 24 hours. MBT's unwarranted effects are related to the accumulation of blood bank-borne components or to the depletion of normal blood constituents resulting from dilution. The mortality among trauma patients receiving MBT approaches 50% and may even be higher in elderly patients. MBT, in the absence of coagulation factors, is commonly accompanied by "oozing coagulopathy" or diffuse microvascular bleeding (DMB). Less than 20% of massively transfused patients will develop clinical manifestation of DMB, but no laboratory test predicts which patients will develop this condition. The depletion of coagulation factors to 37%, as seen with the transfusion of 10 units of blood, still enables normal coagulation.

Hypothermia

Elective transfusion is usually well tolerated without prewarming, but body core temperature may significantly decrease with massive transfusion. Hypothermia has many hazardous effects on homeostasis, including increasing hemoglobin affinity to oxygen, thus reducing tissue oxygen delivery. Blood should always be warmed to body temperature (37°C) when transfusing at a rapid rate (>50 mL/min).

Table 52.1 Transfusion Reactions

Transfusion Reaction	Pathology	Clinical Manifestations	Diagnosis	Treatment	Other
Hemolytic reactions	ABO incompatibility Intravascular hemolysis Complement activation Release of inflammatory mediators and cytokines	Vasodilatation and vascular collapse Death DIC can be first presentation	Mismatch proved by blood bank	Supportive	Stop transfusion, keep or establish a good IV line, reidentify the patient and the blood unit (in order to prevent another patient from getting the wrong blood unit), inform the blood bank, keep urine output at high levels (prevent ATN).
Delayed hemolytic	Minor RBC antigens undiscovered during routine screening tests	Occurs 3–14 days after transfusion Fever, chills, and sudden decrease in hematocrit	Positive direct antiglobulin (Coombs') test	Supportive	Hemolysis is uncommon extravascularly and rarely causes renal failure or DIC.
Febrile non-hemolytic reactions (FNHR)	An inflammatory response provoked by leukocyte transfusion to a pre-alloimmunized (to leukocytes or platelets) recipient; transfusion of cytokines, pyrogens, and other inflammatory mediators accumulated during storage time; infusion of infected blood with bacteria or bacterial products	Increase in body temp > 1°C	Last no more than 8–12 hr	Discontinuation transfusion Reassuring the patient Antipyretic (acetaminophen) Chills (meperedine)	Susceptible populations are multiparous women and previously multiple times transfused patients. Antihistaminic drugs are not effective unless there are allergic signs such as pruritus or urticaria. Slow the speed of transfusion. Prophylactic premedication with acetaminophen or hydrocortizone (100 mg) should be performed a few hours before the transfusion.
Low anaphylaxis	Transfusion of an allergen from a previous sensitized recipient who acquired preexisting IgF transfusion of donor plasma containing IgA to an IgA-deficient recipient	Malaise, anxiety, flushing, dizziness, dyspnea, bronchospasm, abdominal pain, vomiting, diarrhea, and hypotension	Clinical	Transfusion termination Standard anti-anaphylactic treatment	Fever and hemolysis do not occur.
Allergic and urticarial reactions	Presence of certain antibodies to at least one component of the donor's plasma or even to a certain drug taken by the donor	Local or generalized urticaria	Clinical	Transfusion termination/ antihistamines administration	On the subsiding of hives, careful transfusion readministration might follow. Prophylactic premedication with antihistaminic drugs might be given in cases of repeated urticaria.
Transfusion-related acute lung injury (TRALI)	Blood donor antibodies with HLA or neutrophils antigenic specificity react with the recipient's neutrophils to causes an increase in microvascular permeability	Dyspnea and hypoxia	ARDS developing within 4 hr after transfusion	Supportive	90% of affected patients will undergo a complete recovery.
Microbial and endotoxin contamination	*Yersinia enterocolitica* causes most contaminations, but other gram-negative bacteria were identified	Signs start early during the transfusion and have a wide range of manifestations from a slight fever elevation to acute sepsis, hypotension, and death	Color changes of the unit bag compared to the adjunct tube	Antibiotics	The clinical mortality, which appears usually within 25 hr and might reach 26%, is closely related to contamination with *Staphylococcus aureus*, *Klebsiella pneumoniae*, *Serratia marcescens*, and *Staphylococcus epidermidis*, No current screening methods or devices identify blood components' contamination, and contamination must be suspected in any patient in whom fever develops within 6 hr of transfusion.

On removal of the packs, K.C.'s bleeding, although significantly decreased, persisted. Removing the Pringle restarted some bleeding from a now visualized vein in segment 5 that was controlled by ligation. The patient's liver continued to bleed slowly, and it was repacked with a hemostatic agent covered pack and given activated factor VII. The patient remained in the intensive care unit (ICU) for rewarming and correction of acidosis and coagulopathy. Upon arrival in the ICU her temperature was 35.0°C, her base deficit was −8 with a pH of 7.21, and her PT/PTT was 17/66 with a hematocrit of 18. Her platelet count was 81. She was rewarmed and given platelets, packed RBCs, and FFP administered with repeat PT/PTT of 15/35, hematocrit of 26, and platelet count of 110.

Table 52.2 Viral Infection/Risk per Units of Blood	
Viral Infection	**Risk Per Units of Blood**
HCV	1 : 813,000
HIV	1 : 971,000
HBV	1 : 81,000
HTLV	1 : 641,000
Hepatitis A virus (HAV)	1 : 10,000,000
Non-A–E hepatitis	Rare
Cytomegalovirus	Rare
Human herpesvirus-8	Rare
Parvovirus B19	Rare
Malaria	1 : 4,000,000
Babesia	1 : 9,600,000
Chagas disease	Rare
Variant Creutzfeldt–Jacob disease	One case reported

SPECIAL SITUATIONS REQUIRING TRANSFUSIONS

Autoimmune Hemolytic Anemia

Autoimmune hemolytic anemia (AIHA) is a clinical entity manifested by acute or chronic hemolysis and anemia. The definitive laboratory test for AIHA is a positive direct antiglobulin test. The initial and immediate treatment for the elusive autoantibodies causing a hemolytic crisis includes pharmacologic immunosuppression. AIHA is rarely experienced in the trauma or surgical critical care setting; however, it can pose difficult problems for transfusion of RBCs. The standard for detecting alloantibodies is the warm autoadsorption test. Once the alloantibodies are determined, the appropriate RBC unit can be selected. In addition to selecting units that do not contain the alloantibodies, it has also been suggested that attempting to completely match the phenotypes will improve the long-term outcomes.

Transfusion in Disseminated Intravascular Coagulation

Disseminated intravascular coagulation (DIC) spans a spectrum of disequilibrium between coagulation and fibrinolytic mechanisms. The first clinical observations of DIC were recorded in the 19th century. The manifestation of DIC ranges from diffuse bleeding to diffuse thrombus formation. Autopsy findings show small and medium-sized vessel thrombus, diffuse bleeding, and hemorrhagic tissue necrosis. Despite a lack of randomized clinical trials, some of the underlying causes have been identified in the past few years. Therapy should target the underlying etiology. There are four major themes in the pathophysiology of DIC: generation of thrombin in vivo, mechanisms of fueling and propagating thrombin, concomitant activation of the inflammatory cascade, and an endothelial microvasculature role. It is important to identify subtle signs of DIC in order to make the diagnosis early. The diagnosis of DIC can be made following several routinely used laboratory parameters. The efficacy of transfusing blood products and concentrates in an attempt to restore lost coagulation factors in bleeding patients with DIC has not been proven. The use of heparin to stop the formation of thrombin has been used with mixed results, but the safety of this algorithm is questionable in the bleeding patient.

Hepatic Failure

Patients with hepatic failure/cirrhosis may present with persistent coagulopathies that are recalcitrant to blood product replacement. The synthesis of coagulation factors may be severely impaired in hepatic failure. Blood products to replace these losses are mandatory if hemostasis is to be obtained. Other comorbidities (e.g., chronic DIC and renal failure) can exacerbate the severity of coagulopathy. The buildup of fibrin-split products and uremia, for example, can perpetuate platelet dysfunction. Concomitant splenomegaly will consume platelets, leading to thrombocytopenia. The blood component and factor replacement often have only a transient effect. However, blood product replacement may serve as a bridge to liver transplantation.

Uremia

The earliest recording of excessive bleeding associated with renal dysfunction comes from Morgagni in his *Opera Omnia*. The pathogenesis of uremic bleeding lies in the platelet–platelet and platelet–endothelial interactions. For more than 30 years, researchers have been attempting to identify the substance responsible for platelet dysfunction. When platelets from a uremic patient are placed in normal plasma, they function normally. Abnormalities of platelet α-granules, low levels of ADP and serotonin in uremic states, and defective arachidonate metabolism have been reported. Defective receptors impairing platelet binding to fibrinogen and von Willebrand factor (vWF) account for part of the dysfunction. Guanidinosuccinic acid induces dysfunctional platelets and also accumulates in uremic patients. A link between guanidinosuccinic acid and the excessive production of nitric oxide (NO) has been suggested. Normal subjects breathing NO demonstrate prolonged bleeding times. This NO-dependent inhibition of platelet aggregation may be linked to a decrease in fibrinogen binding to the platelet GP IIb/IIIa receptor. Levels of plasma concentrations of NO metabolites can be normalized in both rat models and humans by conjugated estrogens. Conjugated estrogens have been used to effectively reverse the coagulopathy associated with uremia. The use of desmopressin (DDAVP) has also been helpful by elaborating vWF from the endothelium and increasing the aggregation of platelets.

ALTERNATIVES TO TRANSFUSION OF BLOOD PRODUCTS

Approximately 12 million units of blood are transfused into approximately 4 million recipients in the United States each year. Due to the high demand on blood banks, shortages occur and can interrupt elective surgical schedules or delay needed transfusions. The limitations of blood transfusions include the following: Type- and cross-matching are time consuming, there is a limited shelf life, and there are risks of viral/bacterial infection contamination. In the United States, 35 patients per year die as a result of severe transfusion reactions or bacterial contamination. A diminishing blood supply, combined with the tremendous demand for blood transfusion and component therapy, has led to an increased interest in the development of new blood substitutes as oxygen therapeutic agents.

Box 52.1 Advantages and Disadvantages of HBOCs

Advantages	Disadvantages
Readily available	Short intravascular half-life (9–24 hr)
Do not require type and cross-match	Bind nitric oxide, leading to deleterious hypertension, esophageal dysfunction, and abdominal pain
Lower viscosity than blood	
Undergo extensive purification, filtration, and chemical cleansing, minimizing risk for bacterial/viral contamination	

Oxygen Therapeutics (Blood Substitutes)

The first hemoglobin solutions had fragments of the red cell membranes, which made them highly nephrotoxic. In the 1930s, animals were sustained with free hemoglobin and lactated Ringer's solution for a short period of time. Hemoglobin would quickly dissociate into dimers and accumulate in the nephron. This would cause direct obstruction, direct toxicity to nephrons secondary to the pigments and RBC membranes, and reduced renal blood flow secondary to vasoconstriction. The U.S. Army, in collaboration with Baxter Corporation, developed diaspirin cross-linked human hemoglobin. The Canadian military developed o-raffinose cross-linked human hemoglobin. The term "blood substitute" has been used by the layperson and in the medical literature incorrectly. The term "oxygen therapeutics" better fits the function and purpose of these synthesized products. Blood has several other properties, aside from volume expansion and oxygen delivery, that are not substituted by these synthesized compounds. However, there are other, nonoxygen transport properties or side effects of these compounds. These properties include the oncotic load and NO scavenging that leads to increased blood pressures. The NO scavenging increases vascular tone and thus increases afterload. The low viscosity and right-shifted p50 improve oxygen off-loading.

There are two major classes of oxygen therapeutic agents: hemoglobin-based oxygen carriers (HBOCs) and perfluorocarbons (PFCs). The HBOCs rely on the properties of hemoglobin to carry and off-load oxygen. HBOCs are derived from human, animal, and recombinant hemoglobin. The advantages and limitations are listed in Box 52.1. The second class of compounds are the PFCs. They are stable, concentrated emulsions of particles (0.2 μm) suspended in a water-based solution. The problems with these solutions are their short half-life and the need for high inspired oxygen concentration. Products under investigation are listed in Table 52.3.

Future applications vary from emergent trauma to elective surgical environments. Small particle size and low viscosity may allow these products to bypass vascular obstructions and oxygenate ischemic areas of brain or heart after stroke or myocardial infarction. Other applications may be in sickle cell disease or in donor organs prior to transplantation. Administration in septic shock may make use of the NO scavenging properties to provide hemodynamic stability. Sufficient clinical evidence of the safety of oxygen carriers is required prior to Food and Drug Administration approval and widespread use.

Desmopressin

DDAVP may be used to improve platelet function in uremic patients, mild hemophilia A, and type 1 von Willebrand's disease. The current dose for DDAVP is 0.3 μg/kg over 30 minutes, monitoring for tachyphylaxis (its main side effect). Its effects are related to its induction of vWF and factor VIII. It also improves platelet aggregation secondary to its effects on platelet–platelet interactions.

Antifibrinolytic Agents

The lysine analogs ε-aminocaproic acid and tranexamic acid block the binding of plasminogen and plasmin to fibrin, preventing fibrinolysis. They are commonly used in a setting of continued microvascular hemorrhage (e.g., post-cardiopulmonary bypass surgery, systemic fibrinolysis, or hemophilia). Activated recombinant factor VII has been shown to be effective in states of thrombocytopenia and states of acquired clotting factor inhibitors. It is undergoing trials in other bleeding disorders and as prophylaxis in surgery.

Aprotinin

Bovine serine protease inhibitor acts on plasma serine proteases, such as plasmin, kallikrein, trypsin, and some coagulation proteins. It has been shown to reduce blood loss in patients undergoing aortocoronary bypass grafting and has been used in liver transplantation.

Table 52.3 Current Oxygen Therapeutic Solutions			
Company	Product	Type	Clinical Trial Status
Northfield Laboratories	Polyheme	Human glutaraldehyde polymerized	Ongoing phase III multicenter trials in North America in aortic aneurysm surgery; initiating phase III in trauma with the U.S. Army
Biopure Corporation	Hemopure [hemoglobin glutamer-250 (bovine)]	Bovine glutaraldehyde polymerized	Completed phase III multicenter trail in the United States in orthopedic surgery and noncardiac elective surgery in Europe and South Aftrica; initiating phase III trauma trial with the U.S. Navy
Hemosol, Incorporated	Hemolink (hemoglobin raffimer)	Human o-raffinose polymerized	Completed phase III multicenter trial in coronary bypass patients in Canada and the United Kingdom; ongoing trials in cardiac surgery in the United States and United Kingdom; completed two phase II studies in cardiac surgery and two phase II studies in orthopedic surgery; also, one phase II study completed in patients with chronic renal failure undergoing dialysis

Vitamin K

Vitamin K is a substrate used by the liver to produce factors II, VII, IX, and X. Its administration may reverse coagulopathy secondary to oral anticoagulant therapy (warfarin) or liver disease. Its effects can usually be seen beginning 6 to 12 hours after administration.

Hematopoietic Growth Factors

Recombinant erythropoietin has dramatically reduced the need for red cell transfusions in chronic renal failure. Its uses are being expanded to perioperative care, bone marrow transplantation, anemias of prematurity, and chronic disease.

SUMMARY

Blood transfusion medicine is a complicated but necessary part of the surgeon's practice. An understanding of the advantages and disadvantages of transfusion therapy will help guide the practitioner to intervene in a safe manner. The evidence accrued over time has improved the safety and efficacy of these blood products. However, as our understanding improves, so does our understanding of other potential problems. The time of blood substitutes is quickly approaching and may solve some of the pitfalls of blood transfusions, but many more will remain. From the time of Van Helsing's fictional experiments on blood transfusion in victims of Dracula to the present-day advances, blood transfusion therapy has a long, vibrant history and a future filled with possibilities.

By the next morning, 16 hours after her initial operation, K.C.'s temperature was 37.8, the pH was 7.41, and her coagulopathy was reversed. She was taken to the operating room for a second-look procedure and to remove the packing. Observation of the patient following the pack removal revealed that her liver had ceased bleeding and there were

no other internal injuries identified. She was surgically closed and returned to the ICU for the remaining recovery time. K.C. received a total of 24 units of packed RBCs, 12 units of FFP, 20 units of cryoprecipitate, 12 units of platelets, and activated factor VII. The combination of the blood products and the coordinated care of the trauma team enabled K.C. to recover from the injuries sustained in the car accident and return home.

SUGGESTED READING

Cohn SM; Oxygen therapeutics in trauma and surgery. J Trauma 2003; 54:S193–S198.

Friedrich PW, Henny CP, Messelink EJ, et al: Effect of recombinant activated factor VII on perioperative blood loss in patients undergoing retropubic prostatectomy. A double-blind placebo-controlled randomized trial. Lancet 2003;361:201–205.

Goodnough LT, Brecher ME, Kanter MH, et al: Transfusion medicine. N Engl J Med 1999;340:438–447.

Herbert PC, Wells G, Blajchman MA, et al: A multicenter, randomized, controlled clinical trial of transfusion requirements in critical care. N Engl J Med 1999;340:409–417.

Innes G: Guidelines for red blood cells and plasma transfusion for adults and children: An emergency physician overview of the 1997 Canadian blood transfusion guidelines. Part 1: Red blood cell transfusion. Canadian Medical Association Expert Working Group. J Emerg Med 1998;16:129–131.

Kleinman S, Busch MP, Korelitz JJ, Schreiber GB: The incidence/window period model and its use to assess the risk of transfusion-transmitted human immunodeficiency virus and hepatitis C virus infection. Transfusion Med Rev 1997;11:155–172.

Remuzzi G, Minetti L: Hematological consequences of renal failure. In Brenner BM (ed): The Kidney. Philadelphia, Saunders, 1998.

Starr D: Blood magic. In Starr D: Blood. New York, Knopf, 1998, pp 3–31.

Stowell CP, Levin J, Speiss BD, Winslow RM: Progress in the development of RBC substitutes. Transfusion 2001;41:287–299.

Toh CH, Dennis M: Disseminated intravascular coagulation: Old disease, new hope. Br Med J 2003;327:974–977.

Chapter 53

Community-Acquired Pneumonia

Richard G. Wunderink

KEY POINTS

- Although unable to distinguish reliably between community-acquired pneumonia (CAP) and other diseases in the differential diagnosis or between causative etiologies of CAP, physical exam is critical to assessing the severity of CAP.
- One of the major differences in etiology between patients admitted to the intensive care unit and those managed in general wards is the incidence of gram-negative bacillary pneumonia, but *Legionella* and *Staphylococcus aureus* are also in the differential diagnosis.
- The backbone of antibiotic therapy of severe CAP is combination therapy with a cephalosporin and either a newer generation macrolide or a respiratory fluoroquinolone.
- The statistically significant survival advantage of drotrecogin alfa activated (activated protein C) in the CAP subgroup, with even greater benefit in patients with bacteremic pneumococcal pneumonia, suggests increased use may reduce mortality in severe CAP.

At one time called the "captain of the men of death," community-acquired pneumonia (CAP) remains one of the most common causes of admission to medical intensive care units (ICUs). Although CAP severe enough to require ICU admission represents only a small percentage of community-acquired respiratory tract infections, the persistent mortality and the economic and social burden of survivors warrant special consideration. In addition, the risk factors, etiology, and management differ from those of CAP treated in the outpatient or non-ICU setting.

EPIDEMIOLOGY, RISK FACTORS, AND PATHOGENESIS

Epidemiology

CAP is the seventh most common cause of death in the United States and is the most common infectious cause of death. One of the more disturbing facts about CAP is that the mortality in the United States has not changed significantly since penicillin became routinely available (Fig. 53.1). A large number of new antibiotic agents active against the pneumococcus, as well as other causes of CAP, has not lead to any further decrease in mortality.

Pneumonia is also one of the leading causes of severe sepsis. Pneumonia as a cause of sepsis is associated with the highest case fatality rate (Fig. 53.2). The majority of these cases of pneumonia-induced sepsis are CAP rather than hospital-acquired pneumonia (HAP), since HAP is significantly less likely to result in severe sepsis or septic shock.

Risk Factors

Age

Age is clearly a risk factor for both acquiring CAP and death from CAP (Box 53.1). CAP is often the final insult in a patient with multiple underlying chronic diseases. Further evidence of this association is the significant subsequent mortality in elderly patients who survive hospitalization for CAP (Fig. 53.3). Limitation of interventions, especially intubation and mechanical ventilation, in elderly patients with multiple underlying diseases may be a partial explanation for the increased inpatient mortality rates.

However, CAP is not just a disease of the elderly. Despite the higher case fatality rates in the elderly, more than 50% of deaths from bacteremic pneumococcal pneumonia occur in patients in the 18- to 65-year-old cohorts (Fig. 53.4). Some of these deaths in younger patients probably also reflect severe underlying diseases, such as sickle cell disease, but genetic risk factors probably also play a role.

Comorbid Conditions

The differential effect of age and comorbid conditions is very difficult to discriminate. Clearly, accumulating comorbid conditions increase the risk of death from CAP. The Pneumonia Severity Index (Table 53.1) was developed as a prediction model for CAP mortality and documents the additive effect of multiple comorbid conditions on CAP mortality. Interestingly, chronic obstructive lung disease is generally thought to be an increased risk factor for development of CAP but is not associated with increased mortality. Cardiac disease, cancer, and diabetes mellitus appear to exert a greater effect on mortality.

Preceding Upper Respiratory Infection

Many patients give a history of a preceding upper respiratory tract infection days to weeks prior to admission for CAP. The increased mortality associated with the worldwide pandemic of influenza of 1918 (see Fig. 53.1) and multiple smaller epidemics of influenza amply demonstrate that preceding viral infections may leave patients predisposed to CAP. The excess mortality found with patients who supposedly have polymicrobial CAP may also support this association. Most of these patients have

Infectious Disease Problems

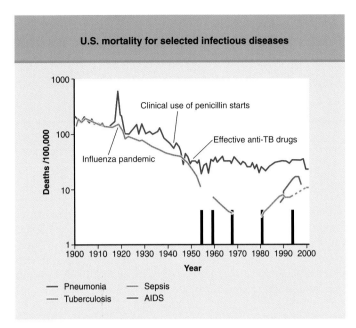

U.S. mortality for selected infectious diseases

Legend:
— Pneumonia
— Tuberculosis
— Sepsis
— AIDS

Figure 53.1. U.S. mortality for selected infectious diseases.
Unchanged mortality for CAP in the United States since routine availability of penicillin. CAP and tuberculosis were the two leading causes of death at the beginning of the 20th century. Both were declining before the availability of effective antimicrobial agents. In contrast to CAP, mortality from tuberculosis continued to decline with effective treatment. Persistent mortality of CAP was not due to either the epidemic of AIDS or the changing incidence of sepsis. The effect of influenza was especially evident in the preantibiotic era. Black bars indicate changes in definitions and reporting characteristics. Note log scale. (Data from www.cdc.gov/nchs/data.)

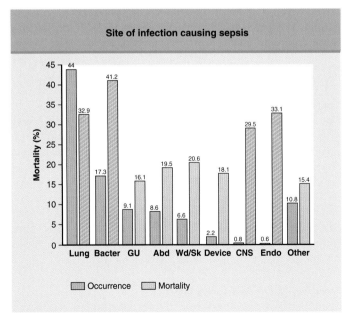

Site of infection causing sepsis

Legend: Occurrence / Mortality

Figure 53.2. Site of infection causing sepsis. Site of infection with associated mortality in patients discharged with a diagnosis of sepsis. Pneumonia is the leading cause of sepsis admissions and has one of the highest associated mortality rates. (Data from Angus DC, Linde-Zwirble WT, Lidiker J, et al: Epidemiology of severe sepsis in the United States: Analysis of incidence, outcome, and associated costs of care. Crit Care Med 2001; 29:1303–1310.)

Box 53.1 Risk Factors for Severe Community-Acquired Pneumonia

Extremes of age
Comorbid conditions
    Chronic obstructive pulmonary disease
    Congestive heart failure
    Diabetes mellitus
    Neoplastic disease
    Immunosuppressant therapy
    Sickle cell disease
    Asplenism
    Acute or chronic liver disease
    Cerebrovascular disease
    Renal disease
    Human immunodeficiency virus infection
Preceding upper respiratory tract infection
Alcoholism
Malnutrition
Obesity
Genetic

Table 53.1 Pneumonia Severity Index Score

	Points
Demographic	
Age	
Men	Age
Women	Age − 10
Nursing home resident	10
Coexisting conditions	
Neoplastic disease	30
Liver disease	20
Congestive heart failure	10
Cerebrovascular disease	10
Renal disease	10
Physical exam findings	
Altered mental status	20
Respiratory rate ≥ 30	20
Systolic BP < 90 mm Hg	20
Temperature < 35°, ≥ 40°C	15
Pulse rate ≥ 125	10
Other findings	
Arterial pH < 7.35	30
BUN > 30 mg/dL	20
Sodium < 130 mEq/liter	20
Glucose ≥ 250 mg/dL	10
Hematocrit < 30%	10
Po_2 < 60 mm Hg or O_2 sat < 90%	10
Pleural effusion on CXR	10
Risk class definition	
I	Age < 50, no coexisting conditions
II	< 71 points
III	71–90 points
IV	91–130 points
V	> 130 points

Data from Fine MJ, Auble TE, Yealy DM, et al: A prediction rule to identify low-risk patients with community-acquired pneumonia. N Engl J Med 1997;336:243–250.

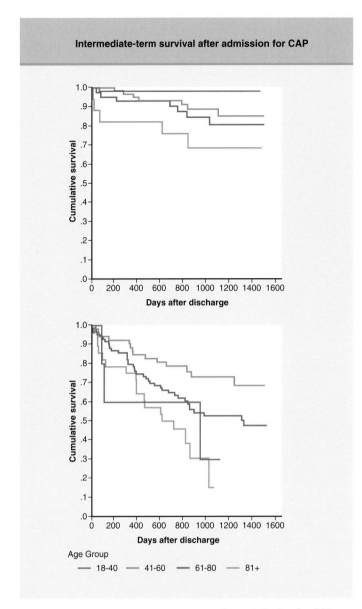

Figure 53.3. Intermediate-term survival after admission for CAP.
Effect of age and comorbid conditions on survival after hospital discharge.
(Top) Patients with no comorbidities; *(bottom)* patients with at least one
comorbidity. Subsequent mortality is increased with increasing age and
with the presence of underlying diseases. However, even 40- to 60-year-
old patients with no underlying diseases have significant subsequent
mortality after admission for CAP. (Data from Waterer GW, Kessler LA,
Wunderink RG: Medium-term survival after hospitalization with community-
acquired pneumonia. Am J Respir Crit Care Med 2004; 169:910–914.)

an atypical pneumonia agent diagnosed by serologic conversion
and a more typical bacterial agent diagnosed by culture. The
timing of serologic conversion cannot preclude a preceding
infection rather than a concomitant one.

Alcoholism
Alcohol appears to both predispose to CAP and increase the
mortality associated with CAP. Acute alcohol ingestion can
adversely affect pulmonary host defenses, not just by decreasing mechanical protection, such as the cough and gag reflexes,

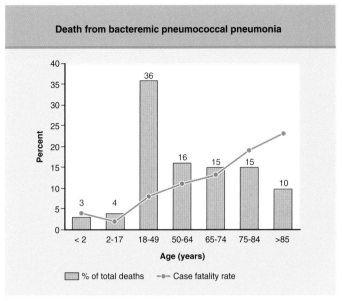

Figure 53.4. Death from bacteremic pneumococcal pneumonia.
Effect of age on mortality from bacteremic pneumococcal pneumonia.
Although the case fatality rate is clearly greater in the elderly population,
more than 50% of deaths from this well-defined type of CAP occur in 18-
to 65-year-olds. (Data from Feikin DR, Schuchat A, Kolczak M, et al:
Mortality from invasive pneumococcal pneumonia in the era of antibiotic
resistance, 1995–1997. Am J Public Health 2000;90:223–229.)

but also by markedly detrimental effects on polymorphonuclear
leukocyte function. In addition, early signs of severe sepsis,
including high fever, tachycardia, and mental confusion, may be
mistaken for delirium tremens and be treated inappropriately
with sedation. End-stage liver disease or cirrhosis also appears
to be associated with an increased case fatality rate.

Nutrition and Body Habitus
Malnutrition is well-known to predispose to infection, especially
pneumonia. This factor probably interacts significantly with both
age and alcoholism in predisposing to CAP. In contrast, obesity
also appears to be a risk factor for severe CAP. Pneumonia is one
of the most common causes of admission of morbidly obese
patients to a medical ICU. Whether morbid obesity is a risk
factor for CAP per se is unclear. However, pneumonia in the
morbidly obese is associated with a greater risk of mechanical
ventilation and a higher mortality compared to nonobese
patients.

Genetic
One of the most underappreciated risks for CAP is genetic.
Overt immune deficiencies, such as combined immunodeficiency syndrome or immotile cilia syndromes, are rare and
clearly do not explain the increased risk of death by themselves,
even in the younger age groups. Research has suggested that
more common polymorphisms in components of the antigen
recognition pathways, inflammatory and anti-inflammatory
response pathways, and the coagulation system may predispose
to increased risk of death from or complications of CAP specifically or from sepsis in general (Table 53.2). A careful family
history can sometimes elicit a significant familial pattern to
infectious death or complications (Fig. 53.5).

Table 53.2 Genetic Polymorphisms Associated with Risk of Infection

	Pneumonia	Sepsis	Other Severe Infections
Antigen recognition pathways			
Mannose-binding lectin	√		√
Toll-like receptors		√	√
CD-14		√	
Lipopolysaccharide-binding protein		√	
Immunoglobulin receptors	√		√
C-reactive protein	√		
Proinflammatory cytokines			
Tumor necrosis factor	√	√	√
Lymphotoxin-α	√	√	
Interleukin-1		√	√
Interleukin-6		√	
Heat shock protein	√		
Anti-inflammatory cytokines			
Interleukin-10	√	√	√
Interleukin-1 receptor antagonist		√	√
Effector mechanisms			
Angiotensin-converting enzyme	√	√	
Surfactant protein	√		
Plasminogen activator inhibitor-1			√
Factor V Leiden		√	

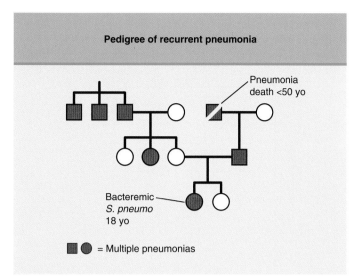

Figure 53.5. Pedigree of recurrent pneumonia. Pedigree of family with genetic predisposition to pneumonia. Two sentinel cases suggest potential risk: death from pneumonia in a patient younger than 50 years of age and bacteremic pneumonia in an 18-year-old. A careful family history in all patients presenting with CAP will not commonly uncover similar pedigrees.

Pathogenesis

Pneumonia is essentially the host response to uncontrolled proliferation of microorganisms in the alveolar space. The lungs are constantly challenged by the presence of microorganisms in the lower respiratory tree. The normal host defense mechanisms are able to handle the overwhelming majority of these invasions. Resident alveolar macrophages localize, engulf, and destroy the small numbers of microorganisms that may penetrate to the alveolar level. However, very pathogenic microorganisms, a large inoculum (usually via aspiration), or compromise in other components of the host immune system occasionally overwhelm the alveolar macrophages' ability to resist the proliferation of microorganisms. At this point, macrophages release a variety of cytokines, chemokines, and other inflammatory molecules.

This mediator release initiates the cascade of events that result in the clinical manifestations of pneumonia. Release of interleukin (IL)-8 and granulocyte colony-stimulating factor leads to both a systemic leukocytosis and a neutrophilic alveolitis. Tumor necrosis factor (TNF) and IL-1 induce fever and a localized capillary leak syndrome, resulting in alveolar flooding and a radiographically visible infiltrate. The capillary leak may be profound enough to allow red blood cells into the alveolar space, with rusty or frankly hemoptic sputum. The combination of the increased cellular response and alveolar fluid results in increased secretions and cough. Extension of the inflammatory response to the pleural surface can result in chest pain. Splinting from pain, hypoxemia, irritation of stretch receptors, decreased compliance from the alveolar edema, and increased airway resistance from secretions all combine to cause dyspnea.

The hypoxemia of pneumonia is predominantly due to ventilation perfusion mismatching. However, in some cases, especially with dense lobar infiltrates, the major mechanism of hypoxemia may be shunt. Release of a prostaglandin-like mediator by the bacteria prevents the normal hypoxemic vasoconstriction that would occur in response to alveoli with a low oxygen tension. Support for this concept is demonstrated by the benefit of nonsteroidal anti-inflammatory agents in reversing the hypoxemia.

Most of the pathophysiologic events noted previously are the appropriate inflammatory response to a microbiologic invasion. However, in some patients the inflammatory response does not remain localized. Spillover of inflammatory cytokines into the systemic circulation results in severe sepsis and septic shock, with attendant nonpulmonary organ dysfunction. The localized pulmonary inflammatory response may also break down, leading to a capillary leak syndrome even in uninfected areas of the lung. Although difficult to separate clinically from multilobar pneumonia, this acute respiratory distress syndrome (ARDS) is clearly associated with a systemic inflammatory response.

With certain notable exceptions, the majority of the bacteria that cause true CAP reach the lower respiratory tract via aspiration. Endemic cases of *Legionella* CAP are probably also caused by aspiration, whereas the namesake epidemic pattern often represents aerosol deposition. Deposition via inhalation of aerosols is also the mechanism of some unusual bacterial causes of CAP, such as *Coxiella burnetii*, viral pneumonias, acute histoplasmosis or blastomycosis masquerading as CAP, and cases of tuberculosis that present with an acute pneumonia syndrome.

Most patients with bacterial CAP are colonized, often chronically, with the typical pathogens prior to the onset of pneumonia. Child-to-parent transmission may be a component of the colonization, since childhood conjugate pneumococcal vaccination has been associated with a concomitant trend toward lower

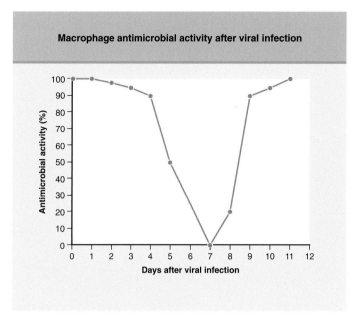

Figure 53.6. Macrophage antimicrobial activity after viral infection. Effect of preceding viral infection on macrophage antimicrobial activity. Many bacterial pneumonias appear to occur in this "vulnerable" period after preceding viral infection, particularly influenza. (Data from Jakab GJ, Warr GA, Sannes PL: Alveolar macrophage ingestion and phagosome-lysosome fusion defect associated with virus pneumonia. Infect Immunol 1980; 27:960–968.)

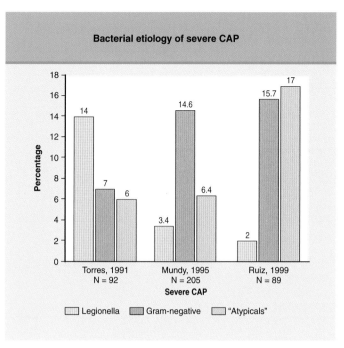

Figure 53.7. Bacterial etiology of severe CAP. Geographical and temporal variation in incidence of *Legionella*, other atypical pathogens, and gram-negative pathogens. Results from three studies with similar diagnostic aggressiveness. Torres and Ruiz studied CAP patients admitted to the same ICU in two different time periods. Note the significant variability in *Legionella* and emergence of gram-negative pathogens over time. Mundy used similar diagnostic techniques in a different locale and could not demonstrate a significant problem with *Legionella*. (Data from Torres A, Serra-Batlles J, Ferrer M, et al: Severe community-acquired pneumonia: Epidemiology and prognostic factors. Am Rev Respir Dis 1991; 144:312–318; Ruiz M, Ewig S, Torres A, et al: Severe community-acquired pneumonia. Risk factors and follow-up epidemiology. Am J Respir Crit Care Med 1999;160:923–929; and Mundy LM, Auwaerter PG, Oldach D, et al: Community-acquired pneumonia: Impact of immune status. Am J Respir Crit Care Med 1995;152:1309–1315.)

invasive infections in adults. A variety of insults then allow these bacteria to not only be aspirated more frequently but also to inhibit the ability of the alveolar macrophage to handle the microbial challenge. Prior respiratory tract infection is probably the most common. Usually this is viral, especially influenza in the adult (Fig 53.6; see Fig. 53.1), but it may also include other atypical pneumonia agents, such as adenovirus, *Mycoplasma*, and *Chlamydia*. Acute alcohol ingestion also appears to be a consistent antecedent event. In the majority of the other cases, worsening of underlying chronic illnesses, such as congestive heart failure, chronic bronchitis, or diabetes, is the triggering event.

Microbial Spectrum

Only a small number of microorganisms cause the overwhelming majority of cases of CAP. *Streptococcus pneumoniae* is by far the most common single cause in almost any series, including those of severe CAP. The documented incidence of the pneumococcus as the cause of CAP is directly proportional to the aggressiveness of the diagnostic workup. Because it is so common and is usually sensitive to antibiotics such as penicillin, the virulence of *S. pneumoniae* is often underestimated. It remains the single most common bacterial cause of death in the developed world.

In patients with CAP admitted to the ICU, *Legionella* is often an important pathogen. *Legionella* infection varies over both time and geography. Some locales rarely document *Legionella* as a cause of CAP despite using the same diagnostic tools as centers that report a high incidence of *Legionella* (Fig. 53.7). The incidence of *Legionella* in patients with severe CAP can vary from year to year in centers that routinely find *Legionella* pneumonia.

Probably the largest difference in etiologies between patients admitted to the ICU and those managed in general wards is the incidence of gram-negative bacillary pneumonia. Up to 20% of bacteremic cases of CAP are due to gram-negative bacilli. *Pseudomonas aeruginosa* and *Klebsiella pneumoniae* are the most common isolates, with *Acinetobacter* an important pathogen in warm, humid climates. Risk factors for *Pseudomonas* include exposure to antibiotics, severe chronic obstructive pulmonary disease (COPD), and HIV disease, whereas the major risk factor for *Klebsiella* and *Acinetobacter* pneumonias appears to be alcohol abuse.

The so-called atypical pathogens (other than *Legionella*) are less common causes of severe CAP. However, they can precipitate ICU admission not because the pneumonia is serious but because they are often associated with deterioration in the patient's underlying disease. Polymicrobial CAP, which usually involves seroconversion with one of these atypical microorganisms, is also associated with a complicated hospital course. Whether this is a real phenomenon or represents a preceding upper respiratory tract infection with these pathogens is unclear, but it may explain both the presence of these generally more

Table 53.3 Differential Diagnosis for Community-Acquired Pneumonia with Relative Frequency of Symptoms

Diagnosis	Cough	Dyspnea	Chest Pain	Hemoptysis	Sputum
Acute exacerbation of chronic bronchitis	++	++	±	±	++
Acute pulmonary embolus	±	+++	++	+	–
Bronchiectasis	+++	++	+	++	+++
Congestive heart failure	±	++	±	±	–
Vasculitis	+	++	±	++	+

benign pathogens in series of severe CAP and the associated mortality.

CLINICAL FEATURES

Symptoms

The cardinal symptoms of pneumonia are cough, fever, and dyspnea. These symptoms are not specific for pneumonia, even in combination. Many of the diseases that mimic or are confused with CAP, such as exacerbations of chronic bronchitis or pulmonary embolus, can have two or even three of the cardinal symptoms (Table 53.3). Symptoms of cough, fever, and dyspnea are not as prevalent in the elderly as in younger patients. Instead, the clinical presentation is frequently complicated by delirium and confusion, abrupt changes in functional capacity, or decompensation of a previously stable chronic illness. Several other symptoms are also seen with pneumonia. Hemoptysis is classically associated with pneumococcal pneumonia and possibly gram-negative pneumonia, whereas it is distinctly unusual in pneumonia due to atypical agents. Chest pain can result from either pleural inflammation or musculoskeletal discomfort secondary to protracted cough. Severe dyspnea and confusion portend a poor prognosis, whereas chest pain has been associated with a good prognosis.

Because of the lack of specificity of the cardinal symptoms of CAP, many patients ultimately found to have CAP may be admitted to the hospital under a variety of other diagnoses. Conversely, patients admitted with CAP are frequently found to have a different diagnosis once further information becomes available.

Physical Examination

Significant physical exam findings are usually limited to patients with lobar pneumonia. Only when the consolidation extends to the pleural surface with a patent bronchus are the classic findings of egophony, whispered pectoriloquy, and dullness to percussion found on exam. Rales or crackles are nonspecific, especially in the ill elderly patient. For this reason, physical exam can support the clinical suspicion of CAP but does not allow a definitive diagnosis. Ultimately, radiography is required to confirm the clinical suspicion of pneumonia.

Although unable to distinguish reliably between CAP and other diseases in the differential diagnosis or between causative etiologies of CAP, physical exam is critical to assessing the sever-

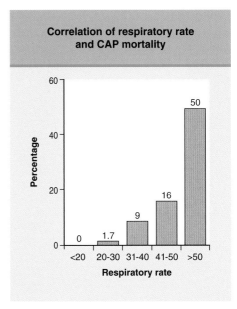

Figure 53.8. Correlation of respiratory rate and CAP mortality. Relationship between carefully measured respiratory rate and hospital mortality in patients with CAP. (Data from British Thoracic Society and the Public Health Laboratory Service: Community-acquired pneumonia in adults in British hospitals in 1982–1983: A survey of aetiology, mortality, prognostic factors and outcome. Q J Med 1987;62:195–230.)

ity of CAP. A major issue in improving outcome of severe CAP is appropriate placement of patients in the ICU. Initial admission to the floor with subsequent transfer to the ICU is associated with increased mortality. Careful measurement of the respiratory rate alone may be the most important component of the physical exam (Fig. 53.8). Visualization or palpation of either accessory inspiratory muscle use or paradoxical abdominal respirations suggests the patient is at risk for imminent respiratory failure. Three of the four criteria in modified British Thoracic Society guidelines for severe CAP are based on physical exam (mental confusion, respiratory rate, and blood pressure), and the Pneumonia Severity Index (PSI) score also gives great weight to vital sign abnormalities.

DIAGNOSIS

Chest Radiographs

Essentially, an infiltrate on chest radiograph is required for the diagnosis of CAP. A radiographic infiltrate is the major criteria distinguishing CAP from other diseases in the differential, such as acute bronchitis, exacerbations of chronic bronchitis, or bronchiectasis. However, the infiltrate may be fairly subtle, at least initially, and the need for a lateral view is often critical. Clinical compromise with a portable, single-view anteroposterior film is part of the reason for diagnostic confusion.

Given its pivotal role due to the nonspecificity of signs and symptoms for CAP, the fact that two radiologists agree with each other only 57.7% of the time on whether no infiltrate or possible, probable, or definite infiltrate is present is disconcerting. Even agreement on the number of lobes involved was only found in 75% of cases. The variability of radiographic interpretation adds to the diagnostic error rate and further explains why many patients initially admitted with CAP are discharged with a different diagnosis and vice versa.

As noted previously, the radiographic infiltrate results from a localized capillary leak syndrome. Fluid resuscitation can often make an infiltrate look significantly worse. This may be one reason why infiltrates may "appear" after admission in patients admitted with exacerbations of COPD or other diagnoses. A computed tomography (CT) scan can frequently pick up infiltrates in patients with a "normal" chest radiograph. Since pulmonary embolus is an important disease in the differential diagnosis, chest CT scans are not uncommonly ordered in patients ultimately found to have CAP.

Microbiologic Diagnosis

Although chest radiographs may be the pivotal (albeit flawed) test to confirm the presence of CAP, determining the causative etiology is even more difficult. Debate continues regarding the relative merits of most diagnostic tests in patients with CAP. One of the major issues driving the debate is the low yield of standard microbiologic specimens, especially blood and sputum cultures. The second issue is that even if an etiologic diagnosis is made, management often does not change, at least not in a positive manner. The incidence of false-positive blood cultures almost equals that of true positives in some studies. A false-positive blood culture, usually with coagulase-negative staphylococci, leads to significantly more vancomycin therapy and to approximately a 1-day longer average hospital stay than that of patients with negative blood cultures. For these reasons, the cost–benefit ratio is very high in patients with CAP. Proponents of aggressive diagnostic testing argue that a positive result can lead to important changes in individual patients. In addition, regular culturing is important for epidemiologic reasons, contact prophylaxis, and even for environmental investigation, such as for a *Legionella* outbreak.

Two factors make the issue of diagnostic testing less controversial in the critically ill patient with CAP. First, the diagnostic yield is increased in critically ill patients. Factors predicting a positive blood culture overlap almost completely with criteria for severe CAP (Box 53.2). Endotracheal aspirates have a higher yield than expectorated sputum and avoid some of the contamination issues that compromise reliability of sputum cultures. Second, the shift in causative microorganisms in severe CAP is toward bacteria that are more likely to grow on culture than the pneumococcus, even in the face of a dose or two of antibiotics. They are also less likely to be sensitive to the usual empiric antibiotic regimen.

The general consensus is therefore that all patients with CAP severe enough to require ICU admission should have blood cultures drawn. The yield of tracheal aspirates also appears high enough to warrant routinely obtaining both Gram stain and culture. Indications for the use of more invasive techniques, including bronchoscopy with protected specimen brush or bronchoalveolar lavage, are less clear.

Nonculture diagnostic techniques will probably play an increasing role in CAP. Already, a rapid urinary antigen test, appropriate for point-of-case testing, is available for both pneumococcus and *L. pneumophila*. Several types of rapid antigen detection kits for influenza are also available. A variety of new molecular techniques, including bacterial DNA detection, will become increasingly available. These technologies will likely

Box 53.2 Criteria for Severe Community-Acquired Pneumonia

Minor Criteria	Major Criteria
Respiratory rate ≥ 30 min	Invasive mechanical
$PaO_2/FIO_2 \leq 250$	ventilation
Multilobar infiltrates	Septic shock or the
Need for noninvasive ventilation	need for vasopressors
Mental confusion	
Hyponatremia	
Acute alcohol withdrawal	
Uremia (BUN ≥ 20 mg/dL)	
Unexplained metabolic acidosis	
Lactic acidosis	
Need for massive fluid resuscitation	
Neutropenia[a]	
Thrombocytopenia	
Hypothermia	
Hypoglycemia (in nondiabetic)	

[a]In the absence of chemotherapy.

replace any reliance on the serologic conversion testing, the standard for diagnosis of atypical agents in the past.

TREATMENT

The discussion of treatment of CAP is too often limited to a discussion of the appropriate antibiotic therapy. Although necessary, the limitations of antibiotics on mortality have already been noted (see Fig. 53.1). Other aspects of treatment will therefore also be discussed.

ICU Admission Criteria

One of the most critical decisions in the management of severe CAP is appropriate placement of the patient. As many as 40% of severe CAP patients are initially admitted to a non-ICU setting and require transfer in the first 24 hours. These patients with delayed onset of septic shock or respiratory failure have a higher mortality rate than those who present initially with these complications (Fig. 53.9). Therefore, identification of this subgroup of patients for more appropriate ICU admission may improve mortality.

Unfortunately, objective criteria to identify these patients are not available. The PSI score results in both false-positive and false-negative classification, with 27% of ICU admissions categorized into classes I to III. Other scoring systems, such as the British Thoracic Society score or the American Thoracic Society criteria, are similarly flawed (Fig. 53.10).

One of the problems with defining the optimal criteria is that validation studies have always included patients who present with septic shock or acute respiratory failure. These patients obviously need ICU admission. What is unclear is how the criteria function to identify the patient who will deteriorate and require subsequent ICU transfer. The other issue complicating validation of these criteria is the frequent occurrence of limitation of care in CAP patients with end-stage comorbid illnesses.

Infectious Disease Problems

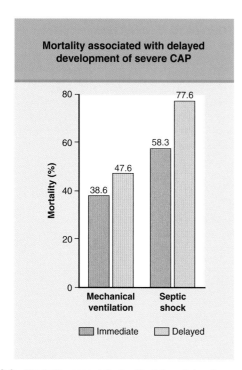

Figure 53.9. Mortality associated with delayed development of severe CAP. Excess mortality associated with delayed development of septic shock or respiratory failure in patients with severe CAP. Identification of patients at risk for these complications may improve mortality, especially when inappropriate admission to a non-ICU bed is avoided. (Data from Leroy O, Georges H, Beuscart H, et al: Severe community-acquired pneumonia in ICUs: Prospective validation of a prognostic score. Intensive Care Med 1996; 22:1307–1314.)

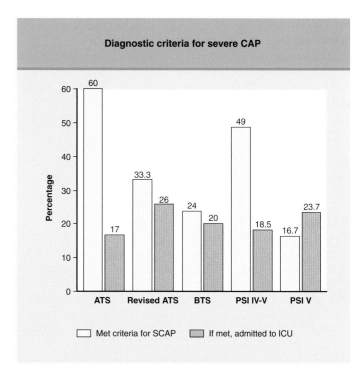

Figure 53.10. Diagnostic criteria for severe CAP. Operating characteristics of commonly used criteria for severe CAP. Most criteria are nonspecific, with a large percentage of the entire CAP population meeting the criteria, and overly sensitive, with only a small percentage of patients meeting criteria actually admitted to the ICU. ATS, American Thoracic Society; BTS, British Thoracic Society; PSI, pneumonia severity index; SCAP, severe CAP. (Data from Angus DC, Marrie TJ, Obrosky DS, et al: Severe community-acquired pneumonia: Use of intensive care services and evaluation of American and British Thoracic Society Diagnostic criteria. Am J Respir Crit Care Med 2002; 166:717–723.)

An intentionally conservative approach to these patients will skew the data regarding the accuracy of ICU admission criteria.

Box 53.2 lists other important factors associated with risk of death in CAP. Some of these risk factors may be interrelated. Tachypnea, hypoxemia, and need for noninvasive ventilation are obvious examples. However, other less obvious relationships also are known, such as the common occurrence of leukopenia and thrombocytopenia with alcohol abuse. Further study is needed to determine if each factor carries an equal risk and how many of the criteria are needed to define the patient who needs ICU care. Clearly, an increased number of these adverse risk factors probably does increase the risk of death and complications from CAP.

Antibiotic Therapy

Because of the broad spectrum of etiologies, definite recommendations for empiric therapy of severe CAP are difficult. Antibiotic recommendations for any infection are compromised by the constant evolution of antibiotic resistance. CAP is no different. Increasing resistance to β-lactams and macrolides in pneumococcal isolates is the most prominent example. To further complicate development of recommendations, almost all comparative studies of antibiotic treatment of CAP are pharmaceutical industry-sponsored trials that specifically exclude severe CAP patients. Therefore, most of the data on which recommendations are based are retrospective and not from randomized trials.

The backbone of antibiotic therapy of severe CAP is combination therapy with a cephalosporin and either a newer generation macrolide or a respiratory fluoroquinolone. Support for this recommendation derives from several types of data. The first is the etiologic spectrum of severe CAP. The pneumococcus and *Legionella* appear to be the most common single etiologies in some areas. Although a respiratory fluoroquinolone may adequately treat both agents, a study to validate this strategy has not been performed. Retrospective analyses of large databases, which mainly included nonsevere CAP, have also documented that the cephalosporin/macrolide combination was associated with a lower mortality than either alone. However, in most of these studies, fluoroquinolone monotherapy performed just as well.

The other reason to recommend combination therapy for severe CAP is the finding that mortality of bacteremic pneumococcal pneumonia is lower when two antibiotics are used compared to a single agent (Fig. 53.11). A prospective study from a single center has documented that this was true even before increasing penicillin resistance. Most studies have shown that the addition of a macrolide to a cephalosporin alone is superior. However, one demonstrated equivalent benefit from several combinations. Most have also found that the mortality benefit was only found in the more severely ill, such as those with a PSI score higher than 90. This latter data is the rationale for hesita-

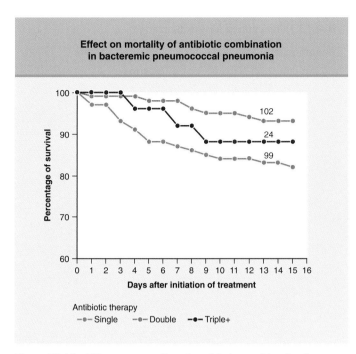

Figure 53.11. Effect on mortality of antibiotic combination in bacteremic pneumococcal pneumonia. Benefit of combination antibiotic therapy on survival in bacteremic pneumococcal pneumonia. Initial dual effective therapy had significantly lower mortality than monotherapy ($p = 0.02$). Even therapy with more than two agents had lower mortality than monotherapy despite significantly worse severity. The adverse effect of monotherapy was most pronounced in the more severely ill, for whom the predicted mortality-adjusted odds ratio for death was 6.4. (Data from Waterer GW, Somes GW, Wunderink RG: Monotherapy may be suboptimal for severe bacteremic pneumococcal pneumonia. Arch Intern Med 2001; 161:1837–1842.)

tion by most professional societies to recommend a broad-spectrum single agent, even the fluoroquinolones, for severe CAP in their guidelines.

A variety of additions or substitutions to this standard treatment regimen have been suggested to empirically treat the broader spectrum of etiologies in severe CAP. Addition of an aminoglycoside or substitution of ciprofloxacin for a respiratory fluoroquinolone has been recommended for patients with suspected gram-negative CAP. High-dose cephalosporins usually offer adequate temporary coverage of methicillin-sensitive *Staphylococcus aureus*, but the recent increase in methicillin-resistant isolates in patients with CAP has led to the addition of vancomycin to many regimens. Penicillin-resistant isolates of *S. pneumoniae* would also be covered. Clearly, superior treatment of ventilator-associated pneumonia (VAP) by linezolid compared to vancomycin and even better outcome in bacteremic *S. pneumoniae* compared to a cephalosporin suggest that linezolid may be a preferred agent in situations in which vancomycin has been used in the past.

Early infusion of the first dose of an antibiotic has been promoted as a means of lowering the mortality rate of CAP based on retrospective analysis of large databases, sometimes limited to elderly patients. However, several of these studies have specifically excluded patients admitted to the ICU. Even within

those studies, patients who received antibiotics in the first hour actually had a higher associated mortality. Severely ill patients are the group most likely to be recognized early and receive antibiotics within the first 4 hours of presenting to the emergency department. Conversely, a delay in antibiotic therapy may be a part of the problem in recognizing the severity of CAP, associated with a delayed transfer to the ICU and the attendant higher mortality. Therefore, although reducing the time to initial antibiotic dose is laudable, the likelihood that shorter times will by themselves lead to lower mortality is less clear.

Nonantibiotic Therapy

In contrast to early antibiotic therapy, early application of nonantibiotic treatment of severe CAP may indeed improve mortality. Aggressive fluid resuscitation and early goal-directed use of inotropes and blood products have been associated with a lower mortality for sepsis in general. CAP was the cause of septic shock in many of the patients studied. Again, one of the reasons for delayed ICU transfer of severe CAP patients may be inadequate fluid resuscitation before admission to the ward.

The other intervention shown to be associated with decreased mortality in CAP is the use of noninvasive ventilation (NIV). NIV for impending respiratory failure is associated with a lower incidence of endotracheal intubation and of subsequent nosocomial pneumonia. Since delayed respiratory failure was the major cause for late ICU transfer, early use of NIV may preclude this complication. Inability to expectorate did not appear to be a limitation to NIV in patients with severe CAP.

Hormone replacement of unrecognized relative adrenal insufficiency has also been associated with decreased mortality in septic shock. Not surprisingly, CAP was a common cause of sepsis in this study. Many of the underlying diseases predisposing to CAP, such as COPD, are treated with intermittent courses of corticosteroids, subsequently leaving the patient with mild adrenal suppression for a period of time after completion of the course.

The last non-antibiotic therapy that should be considered in severe CAP patients is the use of drotrecogin alfa activated [activated protein C (APC)]. Overall mortality was decreased in severe sepsis patients given APC compared to placebo. The survival advantage was even clearer in the more severely ill, as suggested by either more organ failure or higher acute physiologic scores. However, the survival advantage was statistically significant in the CAP subgroup, with even greater benefit in patients with bacteremic pneumococcal pneumonia. Preliminary trials of other agents active in the coagulation cascade suggest that CAP patients may be uniquely sensitive to the benefit of these agents.

Although a survival benefit has not been demonstrated, uncontrolled empyema or parapneumonic effusions are causes for failure of treatment for CAP. The microorganisms associated with severe CAP, including *S. pneumoniae*, *S. aureus*, and *P. aeruginosa*, are prone to pleural complications. Thoracentesis and/or chest tube placement is therefore an important component of nonantibiotic therapy of severe CAP.

CLINICAL COURSE AND PREVENTION

Clinical Course

The clinical course of severe CAP varies from that of the overwhelming majority of CAP patients, who either do not require admission or are admitted to the hospital for a relatively short period of time. Even in patients who survive, the time to reach clinical stability (i.e., resolution of fever, improvement in oxygenation, decrease in cough or chest pain, and normalization of the leukocyte count) is significantly longer in those with higher PSI scores.

The outcome of severe CAP can be analyzed in three phases. The first phase is roughly the initial 3 days of ICU admission. Many severe CAP patients have either rapid resolution of their organ dysfunction or rapid progression and death from fulminant sepsis. Death in this phase is principally cardiovascular. This is also the time span during which CAP patients initially admitted to the floor will deteriorate and require ICU transfer.

The second phase is the ensuing days to weeks. The primary determinant of mortality in this phase is the resolution of organ failure occurring in the initial time period. The principal organ failure of concern is respiratory failure and the need for mechanical ventilation. However, renal failure is another common and important issue. Nosocomial superinfection, especially ventilator-associated pneumonia, amplifies the injuries of the initial phase and prolongs the recovery period. An important factor in the mortality of this phase, especially in the aged patient with multiple underlying comorbid illnesses, is a decision to limit or withdraw care. The prospect of prolonged life support with dialysis and mechanical ventilation often precipitates invocation of living wills or family decisions to limit care.

The third phase is the recovery post-hospital discharge. Only recently has the importance of critical illness, such as severe CAP, on subsequent morbidity been appreciated. Severe CAP may be a life-altering illness for many patients, with a major shift in the level of independent functioning postdischarge (see Fig. 53.3). Need for a chronic care facility or high-level dependency even if discharged home is by itself associated with an increase in subsequent intermediate-term mortality. This is particularly true of patients with greater numbers of comorbid conditions, as demonstrated by PSI class V patients. However, even the loss of lean body mass and the deconditioning associated with severe illness may predispose to other complications, including recurrent pneumonia. Even interventions, such as the need for neuromuscular blockage in order to adequately ventilate a patient with ARDS from CAP, may result in prolonged neuromuscular weakness.

Prevention

With the significant associated mortality and the risk of long-term morbidity in survivors, prevention measures would appear to be a priority. Unfortunately, in practice this is often not true.

Part of the recalcitrance to use of prevention strategies is the perception that prevention strategies do not work for a large proportion of patients. Part of this misperception is due to a focus on prevention of pneumonia versus the more important issue of prevention of death or complications of pneumonia. Several examples illustrate this concept. The benefit of influenza vaccination is less in deaths from pneumonia but has an important benefit in preventing deaths from cardiovascular disease complicated by CAP. Active smokers have an increased risk of invasive pneumococcal disease, whereas former smokers do not. Active alcohol ingestion is a much greater risk of severe CAP than a history of alcohol abuse or even cirrhosis. Therefore, the

---

Box 53.3 Indications for Immunization

Pneumococcal Vaccine	Influenza Vaccine
All patients > 65 years of age	All patients ≥ 50 years
Patients 2–65 years with risk factors	High-risk persons 6 months to 49 years
Chronic cardiovascular, pulmonary, renal, or liver disease	Household contacts of high-risk persons
Diabetes mellitus	
Cerebrospinal fluid leaks	Health care providers
Alcoholism	Children 6–23 months old
Asplenia	Chronic cardiovascular or pulmonary disease (including asthma)
Immunocompromising conditions/medications	Chronic metabolic disease (including
Native Americans and Alaska Natives diabetes mellitus	Renal dysfunction
Long-term care facility residents	
Previous pneumonia[a]	Hemoglobinopathies
Active cigarette smokers[a] medications	Immunocompromising conditions/Pregnancy
	Residence in a long-term care facility
	Aspirin therapy in persons ≤ 18 years

[a]Indication not yet approved by the American Council of Immunization Practices.

---

benefit of prevention strategies should be viewed from the perspective of overall health rather than from the narrow focus on prevention of pneumonia.

Prevention can take two forms: vaccination or intervening in the predisposing condition. As discussed previously, smoking cessation and abstinence from alcohol are important prevention measures. Admission for pneumonia may be a window of opportunity to increase the quit rates from simple physician advice but also allow initial contact with support groups. Even improving control of congestive heart failure, COPD, and diabetes mellitus may prevent the development of CAP.

The indications for influenza and pneumococcal vaccination are listed in Box 53.3. Ideally, vaccinations should be given before the first episode of pneumonia for pneumococcal vaccination and yearly before the onset of illness for influenza. However, poor outpatient immunization practices have led to an emphasis on vaccination at the time of discharge for any hospitalization. Although patients who have experienced their first episode of CAP are appropriate candidates for immunization, the practice of immunization at the time of discharge for a CAP hospitalization has less clear benefit. Another important component of prevention of CAP is the use of chemoprophylaxis of patients at risk or active treatment of early influenza infection. Prevention or at least amelioration of subsequent pneumonia may be more important than the symptomatic benefit of the influenza. In addition, active treatment may shorten the duration of viral shedding, decreasing the risk of transmission to other susceptible people.

CONCLUSIONS

CAP remains an important cause of admission to medical ICUs. Recognition of the CAP patient who would benefit from ICU care is a critical issue in management. The spectrum of microorganisms causing severe CAP is different from that of less severe cases. This demands greater attention to an accurate diagnosis and frequent use of nonstandard antibiotic therapy. Aggressive resuscitation and consideration of immunomodulatory therapy may be more important to impact mortality.

SUGGESTED READING

American Thoracic Society: Guidelines for the management of adults with community-acquired pneumonia: Diagnosis, assessment of severity, antimicrobial therapy, and prevention. Am J Respir Crit Care Med 2001;163:1730–1754.

Angus DC, Linde-Zwirble WT, Lidiker J, et al: Epidemiology of severe sepsis in the United States: Analysis of incidence, outcome, and associated costs of care. Crit Care Med 2001;29:1303–1310.

Angus DC, Marrie TJ, Obrosky DS, et al: Severe community-acquired pneumonia: Use of intensive care services and evaluation of American and British Thoracic Society Diagnostic criteria. Am J Respir Crit Care Med 2002;166:717–723.

British Thoracic Society and the Public Health Laboratory Service: Community-acquired pneumonia in adults in British hospitals in 1982–1983: A survey of aetiology, mortality, prognostic factors and outcome. Q J Med 1987;239:195–220.

Feikin DR, Schuchat A, Kolczak M, et al: Mortality from invasive pneumococcal pneumonia in the era of antibiotic resistance, 1995–1997. Am J Public Health 2000;90:223–229.

Fine MJ, Auble TE, Yealy DM, et al: A prediction rule to identify low-risk patients with community-acquired pneumonia. N Engl J Med 1997;336:243–250.

Jakab GJ, Warr GA, Sannes PL: Alveolar macrophage ingestion and phagosome-lysosome fusion defect associated with virus pneumonia. Infect Immunol 1980;27:960–968.

Leroy O, Georges H, Beuscart H, et al: Severe community-acquired pneumonia in ICUs: Prospective validation of a prognostic score. Intensive Care Med 1996;22:1307–1314.

Mundy LM, Auwaerter PG, Oldach D, et al: Community-acquired pneumonia: Impact of immune status. Am J Respir Crit Care Med 1995;152:1309–1315.

Ruiz M, Ewig S, Torres A, et al: Severe community-acquired pneumonia. Risk factors and follow-up epidemiology. Am J Respir Crit Care Med 1999;160:923–929.

Torres A, Serra-Batlles J, Ferrer M, et al: Severe community-acquired pneumonia: Epidemiology and prognostic factors. Am Rev Respir Dis 1991;144:312–318.

Waterer GW, Kessler LA, Wunderink RG: Medium-term survival after hospitalization with community-acquired pneumonia. Am J Respir Crit Care Med 2004;169:910–914.

Waterer GW, Quasney MW, Cantor RM, et al: Septic shock and respiratory failure in community-acquired pneumonia have different TNF polymorphism associations. Am J Respir Crit Care Med 2001;163:1599–1604.

Waterer GW, Somes GW, Wunderink RG: Monotherapy may be suboptimal for severe bacteremic pneumococcal pneumonia. Arch Intern Med 2001;161:1837–1842.

Chapter 54

Pneumonia in the Immunocompromised Patient

Robert P. Baughman

KEY POINTS

- Identifying the type of immunosuppression will help guide diagnostic testing and empiric therapy.
- In the immunocompromised patient, classic signs and symptoms of pneumonia may be lacking. Therefore, a higher level of suspicion must exist.
- Bronchoscopy with bronchoalveolar lavage has proven useful in diagnosing a wide variety of organisms causing pneumonia.
- Supportive therapy such as hematologic growth factors and noninvasive ventilation will improve survival in some groups of immunosuppressed patients with pneumonia.

Pneumonia in the immunosuppressed patient represents a common problem in the intensive care unit (ICU). Changes in the host defense make the patient more susceptible to respiratory tract infection. The use of mechanical ventilation also increases the risk for pneumonia. The interaction of these two defects in host defenses leads to a high mortality for immunosuppressed patients with pneumonia.

EPIDEMIOLOGY, RISK FACTORS, AND PATHOGENESIS

The term immunosuppression is broadly applied in the ICU. A patient requiring admission to the ICU usually has one or more immune defects, either as a primary problem or as a result of therapy. This includes such common problems as alcoholism, malnutrition, and corticosteroid use. The immunity defects can lead to increased risk for several types of infections. However, not all immunosuppression is the same.

It is useful to think in terms of what specific immune deficit is present. This helps predict what organism could be the cause of pneumonia. The risk of more severe infection, such as dissemination, is also dependent on the level of immunosuppression. Table 54.1 lists the types of immunosuppression, examples of disease states, and types of infection. The table reflects the relative risks and highlights some of the standard examples. However, there are clearly overlaps. For the treating physician, examination of the risk factors for immunosuppression can help in deciding the diagnostic and therapeutic approach.

In the patient with a known immunodeficiency, prophylaxis strategies have been developed to reduce the risk of infection. It is important to recognize the effectiveness of these prophylaxis regimens in order to understand the underlying risk of infection.

For immunoglobulin deficiency, immunoglobulin replacement has been shown to be an effective method for reducing risk. In most cases, the patient will be on a routine intravenous infusion regimen of immunoglobulin, mostly IgG. The target for immunoglobulin infusion is to keep the IgG level at more than 500 mg/dL. During maintenance therapy, the level is checked prior the next infusion to determine if the lowest level is still more than 500 mg/dL. In the ICU setting, a patient with known IgG deficiency should have his or her IgG level checked. It may be necessary to increase infusion frequency to help the patient recover from his or her pneumonia.

The most common cause of neutropenia is the associated complication of chemotherapy. There are many studies demonstrating the increased risk for infection when the absolute neutrophil count declines below 1000 cells/mm^3. The risk increases as the neutrophil count declines below 500 cells/mm^3. Neutrophil dysfunction can be seen with various conditions. Patients with acute myelogenous leukemia may have a large number of neutrophils, but the cells are not functional and there is marked risk for infection. During the course of treatment, the patient will develop prolonged neutropenia. The duration of neutropenia increases the risk for infection. For many patients, infection is a constant problem, but the offending pathogen changes. Initially, the community-acquired bacteria such as *Streptococcus pneumoniae* are a problem. With antibiotic therapy, the patient develops infection with nosocomial bacteria, especially *Pseudomonas aeruginosa* and *Staphylococcus aureus*. With successful therapy for these bacteria, the patient develops infection with an *Aspergillus* species.

The T-cell defects can be either a part of the patient's medical problems, such as HIV infection or lymphoma, or a result of treatment, such as in the transplant patient. In either case, the key feature is the loss of the CD4 lymphocyte. Measurement of the CD4 count allows one to understand the risk for various infections. For example, HIV-infected patients who have a low CD4(+) lymphocyte count are at risk for various infections. For patients with CD4 counts between 250 and 500 cells/mm^3, the risk is for pathogens such as *Mycobacterium tuberculosis* and *Cryptococcus neoformans*. Once the CD4 count declines below 250 cells/mm^3, the risk increases for *Pneumocystis jiroveci* (for-

Table 54.1 Relationship Between Immunosuppression and Cause of Pneumonia			
	Immunoglobulin Defect	**Neutrophil Defect**	**T-Cell Defect**
Underlying conditions	Agammaglobulinemia Multiple myeloma Chronic lymphocytic leukemia	Chemotherapy–induced neutropenia Aplastic anemia Acute leukemia Bone marrow transplant Solid organ transplant < 30 days	AIDS Solid organ transplant > 30 days Lymphoma
Measurement of defect Respiratory infections	IgG < 400 mg/dL *S. pneumoniae* *H. influenzae*	Absolute neutrophil count < 1000 cells/mm^3 *P. aeruginosa* *S. aureus* *Aspergillus* species	CD4 lymphocytes < 500 cells/mm^3 *M. tuberculosis* *P. jiroveci*[a] *C. neoformans* *L. pneumophila* Cytomegalovirus

[a]Formerly known as *P. carinii*.

merly known as *P. carinii*). The prophylactic use of trimethoprim/sulfamethoxazole markedly reduces the risk for *P. jiroveci* pneumonia. A CD4 count of less than 50 cells/mm^3 is associated with an increased risk of recovery of *Mycobacterium avium* complex (MAC) from the lung. For the HIV-infected patient, the use of highly active antiretroviral therapy (HAART) has led to a reduction in the rate of *P. jiroveci* and MAC.

In solid organ transplants, a neutrophil and T-cell lymphocyte defect is present. During the first month after transplant, the patient is at higher risk for bacterial and *Aspergillus* infection. At approximately 6 weeks after the transplant, the risk is highest for *P. jiroveci* and cytomegalovirus. For the next year, the transplant team will be decreasing immunosuppression. With reduction of immunosuppression, the risk for pneumonia decreases. However, the transplant patient has a lifelong risk for *M. tuberculosis*, deep-seated fungal infections, and *Legionella pneumophila*. In addition, if the patient does develop acute rejection, increased immunosuppression may reintroduce the risk for *P. jiroveci*. Figure 54.1 summarizes the infections identified at four transplant centers using various diagnostic techniques. All four studies demonstrated an increased risk for bacterial infections, but various other pathogens could be encountered. The highest risk for pneumonia in these studies was the first year after transplant.

For the T-cell defect, various agents have been used as prophylaxis to prevent infection, including trimethoprim/sulfamethoxazole to prevent *P. jiroveci* pneumonia. This has been an extremely successful form of prophylaxis. However, this sulfa-based regimen is associated with renal toxicity when given with cyclosporine. Therefore, the drug is often discontinued 1 year after transplant, when the risk for *P. jiroveci* pneumonia has gone away. However, if a patient develops an acute rejection, prophylaxis should be reinstituted.

Cytomegalovirus (CMV) is a problem for both solid and bone marrow transplants. The risk is reactivation from either the host's own prior infection or new disease from the donated transplanted organ. New infection is associated with significantly higher morbidity and mortality. For the bone marrow transplant recipient who is CMV negative at the time of transplant, the use of CMV-negative blood products has been shown to eliminate this infection. For the patient who has CMV infection, it can lead to pneumonia and respiratory failure. Ganciclovir prophylaxis from the time of transplant is effective. Some groups

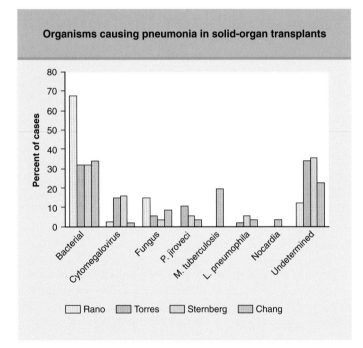

Figure 54.1. Organisms causing pneumonia in solid-organ transplants. Percentage of different pathogens as cause of pneumonia in solid organ transplants from four series throughout the world. (Adapted from Chang GC, Wu CL, Pan SH, et al: The diagnosis of pneumonia in renal transplant recipients using invasive and noninvasive procedures. Chest 2004;125:541–547.)

use intravenous drug for 4 to 8 weeks and then follow with oral ganciclovir for 1 year or longer. The prodrug valganciclovir is an oral agent with good absorption and appears to be as effective in preventing CMV pneumonia.

CLINICAL FEATURES

For the immunosuppressed patient, any suggestion of pneumonia will lead to a chest roentgenogram. There is a heightened awareness because the clinical features of pneumonia may be suppressed by the underlying condition. Changes in white blood count may not be present because of the immunosuppression and chemotherapy. Tachycardia may be part of the clinical con-

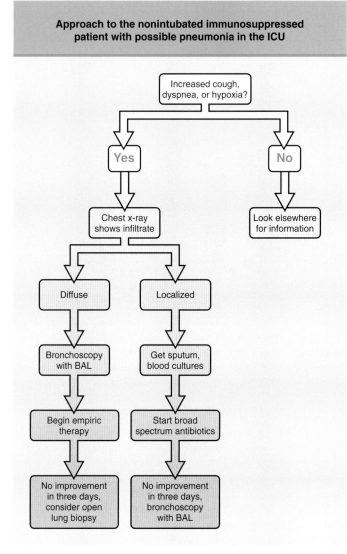

Approach to the nonintubated immunosuppressed patient with possible pneumonia in the ICU

Increased cough, dyspnea, or hypoxia?

Yes → No

Yes: Chest x-ray shows infiltrate

No: Look elsewhere for information

Chest x-ray shows infiltrate → Diffuse / Localized

Diffuse → Bronchoscopy with BAL → Begin empiric therapy → No improvement in three days, consider open lung biopsy

Localized → Get sputum, blood cultures → Start broad spectrum antibiotics → No improvement in three days, bronchoscopy with BAL

Figure 54.2. Approach to the nonintubated immunosuppressed patient with possible pneumonia in the ICU.

dition for the patient. The presence of fever should lead to evaluation for possible infection. However, fever is not specific for pneumonia.

The presence of new or worsening dyspnea or cough should be evaluated in all immunosuppressed patients. In the ICU setting, severe dyspnea is usually associated with hypoxia. Oxygenation is often monitored serially in these patients. The worsening of oxygenation is sensitive but not specific for pneumonia.

Although cough is often present, sputum production is unusual for many of the types of pneumonia encountered in immunosuppressed patients. If a patient does have purulent sputum, this would support the diagnosis of a bacterial pneumonia. Patients with *P. jiroveci* and CMV often have a nonproductive cough.

DIAGNOSIS

The immunosuppressed patient who has evidence of pulmonary infection usually undergoes chest roentgenogram. In the patient with an infiltrate, determining whether the infiltrate is localized

versus diffuse is a useful first step in deciding which procedure to perform. One proposed strategy for the nonintubated immunosuppressed patient is shown in Figure 54.2. In this situation, the patient with a localized infiltrate has a sputum (if available) and blood cultures, and empiric therapy is initiated. For the patient with diffuse infiltrates or localized plus diffuse infiltrates (Fig. 54.3), a bronchoscopy with bronchoalveolar lavage (BAL) is performed. The rationale is that infections such as *P. jiroveci* and CMV tend to cause diffuse infiltrates. However, this distinction is somewhat arbitrary, and clinical suspicion may lead to the use of bronchoscopy even in localized infiltrates. For example, an HIV-infected patient with a CD4 count of less than 200 and not on antipneumocystis prophylaxis should probably have a bronchoscopy. For the intubated patient with possible pneumonia, a bronchoscopy should be considered unless contraindicated.

For the patient with increased dyspnea or worsening oxygenation, a normal chest roentgenogram does not rule out pneumonia. Ten percent of patients with *P. jiroveci* have a normal film. In the ICU setting, the hypoxic patient with a normal chest roentgenogram needs further evaluation. This may include computed tomography pulmonary angiogram, which may demonstrate infiltrates not seen on the portable chest roentgenogram.

The role of bronchoscopy with BAL in the immunosuppressed patient is demonstrated in Figure 54.4. In a study from Barcelona, 200 immunosuppressed patients with possible pneumonia were evaluated. The figure shows the relative value of various techniques. Not all patients had all sampling. Blood cultures were obtained in most patients but had a very low yield. More important, the blood culture results rarely resulted in a change in therapy. On the other hand, BAL was performed in

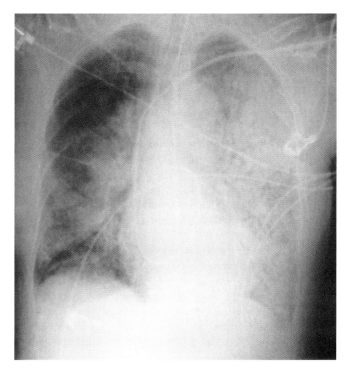

Figure 54.3. Ventilator-associated pneumonia. Chest roentgenogram of patient with both localized and diffuse infiltrates. BAL was performed in the lingual lobe. The patient grew *L. pneumophila*.

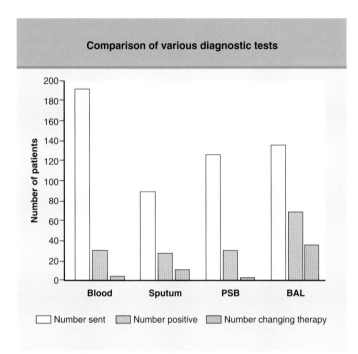

Figure 54.4. Comparison of various diagnostic tests. Results of evaluation of 200 non-HIV-infected, immunosuppressed patients. Although bronchoscopy with BAL was done on only two thirds of the patients, it led to the highest number of cases in which therapy was changed on the basis of the study results. (Adapted from Rano A, Agusti C, Jimenez P, et al; Pulmonary infiltrates in non-HIV immunocompromised patients: A diagnostic approach using non-invasive and bronchoscopic procedures. Thorax 2001;56:379–387.)

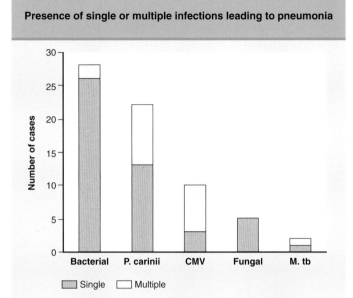

Figure 54.5. Presence of single or multiple infections leading to pneumonia. Results of one BAL performed on immunosuppressed mechanically ventilated patients. Patients could have more than one pathogen identified. (Adapted from Conrado CE, Rashkin MC, Baughman RP: Pneumonia in immunocompromised and immunocompetent patients requiring mechanical ventilation. J Bronchol 1999;6:78–83.)

approximately two thirds of patients. However, a positive result was seen in more patients. Therapy was changed due to BAL results more often than any other diagnostic test.

BAL yields a large sample that can be investigated for various types of pathogens: bacterial, viral, mycobacterial, and fungal. Patients often have more than one pathogen identified as the cause of their pneumonia (Fig. 54.5). At our institution, BAL samples are sent for semiquantitative bacterial, mycobacterial, viral, and fungal cultures. In addition, a BAL aliquot is sent for cytologic examination using Papinicolau and a silver stain. We send the bronchial wash for cytopathalogic, fungal, and mycobacterial studies. Compared to BAL, bronchial wash has a higher yield for mycobacteria.

The location of BAL can affect the results. For patients with localized disease, one should try to lavage the most affected area, such as the left lung in the patient shown in Figure 54.3. In patients with diffuse infiltrates, the tendency is to lavage the right middle lobe or the lingula since it is technically the easiest. However, if one suspects *P. jiroveci*, lavage of the upper lobes has a higher yield.

The lavage should be large enough to sample to alveolar space. This means the instilled volume should be at least 100 mL instilled fluid. If less than 10% of the instilled fluid is aspirated, a second lavage should be considered. If the patient becomes too hypoxic or otherwise unstable during the procedure, the second lavage may be aborted.

Bronchoscopy provides more than just a sample of the lower respiratory secretions. It can identify endobronchial changes.

Figure 54.6*A* shows an endobronchial lymphoma in an HIV-infected patient. This led to a localized infiltrate, which failed to respond to empiric therapy for bacterial pneumonia. Figure 54.6*B* demonstrates an obstructed bronchus in a renal transplant patient with presumed bacterial pneumonia in the right middle lobe. The patient failed to respond to empiric antibiotics and was transferred to the ICU for hyperglycemia and worsening respiratory distress. At bronchoscopy, the middle lobe was obstructed by necrotic material. Biopsy of the *P. carinii* to the right middle lobe revealed invasion of the tissue by mucor.

The diagnosis of CMV can be difficult. Patients with cytopathic changes in their tissue or in the BAL cytology are fairly straightforward. However, patients with disease advanced enough to have tissue changes may not respond to therapy. Early

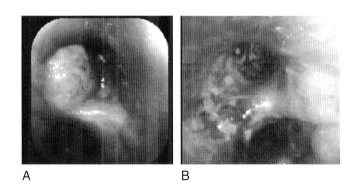

A   B

Figure 54.6. Endobronchial lesions in immunosuppressed patients. Endobronchial lesions identified during bronchoscopy of immunosuppressed patients with localized infiltrates. *A*, Endobronchial lymphoma. *B*, Necrotic material due to mucormycosis.

treatment is indicated in these patients; therefore, early diagnosis is recommended. Among the techniques employed are viral cultures and indirect fluorescent antibodies for early antigen. These techniques increase the sensitivity for identifying CMV in the lung. However, the clinician may be left with the difficulty of distinguishing between colonization and actual pneumonia in a patient who does not have cytopathic changes. This is the source of controversy in HIV-infected patients. In the patient with CMV isolated from the lung and for whom no other cause of the pneumonia can be identified, we treat for CMV pneumonia.

At the time of initial evaluation of the nonintubated patient, the intensivist has to decide whether to perform bronchoscopy. There is some risk involved with bronchoscopy. Worsening of oxygenation may lead to the need for intubation. As discussed later, avoiding intubation is associated with a better prognosis for immunosuppressed patients. Balanced against the risk of intubation is the risk of not knowing the cause of the infiltrate. In a prospective study of BAL for neutropenic patients being evaluated for respiratory failure, Gruson found that 49% had a positive BAL, similar to the experience in Barcelona shown in Figure 54.4. Of 51 patients not on mechanical ventilation at the time of bronchoscopy, only 2 required intubation as a direct result of bronchoscopy. For the nonintubated patient, one should consider aggressive use of bilevel positive airway pressure during and after bronchoscopy to avoid intubation. Bronchoscopy with lavage should not be performed in the patient whose level of oxygenation is not correctable. Bronchoscopy and lavage cause hypoxia, which can last for several hours. Our guideline is that the corrected oxygenation should be more than 95% saturation or a measured PO_2 of 60 torr.

Surgical lung biopsy is an alternative to making the diagnosis. Most commonly performed as video-assisted thorascopic surgery, it is associated with less morbidity than traditional open-lung biopsies. In a study of patient with acute respiratory distress syndrome undergoing open-lung biopsies, major complications were encountered in only 7% of cases, with no attributable mortality, but 8 of 57 cases were found to have infection. However, others have noted a much higher rate of morbidity and some 30-day mortality associated with surgical lung biopsy.

Regardless of the initial diagnostic procedure, one needs to start empiric therapy. The empiric therapy for each group of pathogens is summarized in Table 54.2. For all patients, one has to be concerned about bacterial infections, including gram-negative, gram-positive, and atypical bacteria. Several studies have demonstrated increased mortality for patients given inadequate empiric therapy for bacterial infections. The choice of treatment for gram-negative pathogens has to be based on the pathogen frequency and sensitivity normally seen in the particular ICU. Most immunosuppressed patients have received antibiotics within 3 months prior to arriving in the ICU. Therefore, one has to assume that all patients are at risk for resistant bacteria.

The need for empiric therapy for the other pathogens depends on the relative risk as summarized in Table 54.1. Not all patients will need coverage for all possibilities. In addition, not all possible infections require empiric therapy. In an analysis of 203 M. tuberculosis patients treated in one hospital in St. Louis, 57 died (28%). Of the 203 patients, 49 were treated in the ICU, including 26 on mechanical ventilation. More than two thirds of the patients were in the hospital for more than 7 days before starting therapy. However, early therapy was not associated with improved survival. Using multivariate logistic regression analysis, the underlying condition of the patient and severity of the disease were most important in determining survival. Immunosuppression was associated with an increased risk of mortality (odds ratio, 3.2). Thus, empiric therapy for M. tuberculosis does not seem warranted except in high-risk patients.

CLINCAL COURSE AND SUPPORTIVE THERAPY

Once empiric therapy has been given, it is critical to reassess the patient in 3 to 5 days. At this point, the results of the initial diagnostic material will be available. In addition, the clinical status of the patient is available. Within 72 hours, patients should begin demonstrating clinical evidence of response to therapy. The most reliable indicator of response is the improvement of oxygenation. Other parameters that can be assessed include temperature, chest roentgenogram, and white blood cell count. However, white blood cell count may be unreliable since this may be altered by the patient's underlying immunosuppression. The use of growth factors may increase the white blood cell count and may lead to an increase in the chest roentgenogram's infiltrates.

Table 54.2 Empiric Therapy for Potential Pathogens

Type of Microorganism	Important Pathogens to Consider	Empiric Therapy	Alternative
Gram-negative bacteria	P. aeruginosa	β-Lactam plus aminoglycoside or fluoroquinolone[a] with gram-negative coverage[b]	
Gram-positive organism	S. aureus	Vancomycin or linezolid	Quinupristin/dalfopristin
Atypical bacteria	L. pneumophila	Macrolide or fluorquinolone	
P. jiroveci[c]		Trimethoprim/sulfamethoxazole	Pentamidine Trimetrexate
Fungal	Aspergillus species	Liposomal amphotericin or voriconazole	Caspofungin
Cytomegalovirus		Ganciclovir	

[a]Ciprofloxacin or high-dose levofloxacin.
[b]For example, pipercillin tazobactam, ticarcillin salbactam, cefepmie, imipenam, merepenam, or aztreonam.
[c]Formerly known as P. carinii.

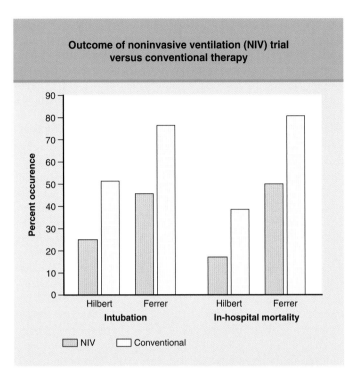

Figure 54.7. Outcome of noninvasive ventilation (NIV) trial versus conventional therapy. The results of two randomized trials of NIV versus conventional ventilation for immunocompromised patients with possible pneumonia and treated in the ICU. Both studies found that NIV therapy had a significantly lower rate of intubation and lower overall mortality.

Supportive therapy is an important feature of the management of the immunosuppressed patient with pneumonia. Specifically, one should try to avoid intubation. Figure 54.7 shows the results of two trials. Both were randomized trials investigating the utility of noninvasive ventilation (NIV) for immunosuppressed patients presenting to the ICU. Compared to conventional ventilation, NIV was associated with a significantly lower rate of intubation and lower mortality.

Other supportive therapy may be indicated for the specific immunosuppressive problem. As noted previously, for the patient with immunoglobulin deficiency, the use of IgG infusion should be considered if the IgG level is less than 500 mg/dL. For the neutropenic patient, growth factors such as granulocyte colony-stimulating factor should be used daily until the absolute neutrophil count is greater than 1000 cells/mm^3. For the transplant patient, decreasing immunosuppression may be necessary. For the HIV-infected patient, HAART therapy may have a relatively rapid onset of action. HAART reduces the mortality of severe *P. jiroveci* pneumonia in HIV patients. In another study, HAART therapy did not change ICU survival, but it reduced 3-month mortality.

PITFALLS, COMPLICATIONS, AND CONTROVERSIES

The major problem in the management of immunosuppressed pneumonia patients is the uncertainty of the causative agent. Even with the most aggressive diagnostic testing, many patients will have no specific diagnosis. It has been shown that patients without a specific diagnosis have a higher mortality. The

Table 54.3 Pitfalls

Pitfall	Comments
Bronchoscopy with BAL	Diagnositc yield approximately 50% Complications include worsening hypoxia, transient hyperthermia, and worsening infiltrates
Surgical lung biopsy	Higher diagnostic yield, but nonspecific findings common Yield for microorganism reduced because of prior antimicrobial therapy Complicaitons include need for intubation, worsening hypoxia, worsening infiltrates, chest wall pain, and risk for local infection
Isolation of potential nonpathogens	
Candida species	Unlikely to be cause of pneumonia; may be marker for systemic candidemia
Diphtheroids	Usually represent oral contamination during procedure; could be cause for pneumonia; very sensitive to conventional antibiotic therapy
Cytomegalovirus	Clearly a pathogen in bone marrow transplant patients; not clearly a pathogen in HIV-infected patients

increased mortality may be due to a noninfectious and uncorrectable problem. For example, pulmonary hemorrhage may look like pneumonia but is often a diagnosis of exclusion. The patient may also have worsening of his or her underlying condition. In these situations, no therapy may be available. This leaves the clinician with the difficulty of balancing more invasive procedures versus higher morbidity from the procedures. One problem patient is the one with no specific diagnosis but off mechanical ventilation. An open-lung biopsy will definitely lead to intubation, but it is not clear that it will increase survival.

A summary of the pitfalls in diagnostic testing and interpretation of these tests is given in Table 54.3. The isolation of *Candida* species and oral pharyngeal flora should be viewed with caution. The same holds for CMV from the HIV-infected patient. Although organisms can cause pneumonia, one should search for other potential pathogens.

Another pitfall is patient worsening during treatment. Table 54.4 lists the various factors that could cause deterioration. The patient may have more than one pathogen causing the initial problem. The patient remains susceptible to new problems, and the longer he or she is in the ICU, the more likely a second problem will arise. When a patient worsens during the first few days after evaluation, this may be due to the diagnostic

Table 54.4 Complications Encountered during Treatment of Pneumonia

Underlying Disease	Diagnostic Procedure	Therapy
More than one pathogen as initial problem	Worsening hypoxia	Allergic reaction to agent
Nosocomial infection during therapy	Need for mechanical ventilation	Renal failure
	Transient fever	Leukopenia Leukocytosis

Box 54.1 Controversies

- Need for invasive procedures as part of initial evaluation of nonintubated patient
- Role of open lung biopsy in patient failing empiric therapy
- When to add antifungal empiric therapy in neutropenic patient
- Role of CMV as a cause of pneumonia in HIV-infected patients
- Timing of intubation

procedure (e.g., the bronchoscopy). These effects are usually transient. Finally, the therapy may cause toxicity. Since patients may be on several agents for their underlying problem, drug interaction has to be avoided.

There are several controversies in the ICU (Box 54.1). The need for invasive procedures in nonintubated patients is a balance between the risk and the benefit. Although bronchoscopy is a common first step in evaluation, open-lung biopsy has been used as a definitive procedure by some groups to try to determine the diagnosis in all cases. It is associated with significant mortality. In addition, the findings of the open-lung biopsy are not always definitive, with nonspecific findings found in up to half of cases. One difficulty with regard to open-lung biopsies is that patients are usually already on antibiotics. Thus, the diagnosis of pneumonia may be made, but the pathogen may not be identified. The empiric treatment for fungal or viral etiologies depends on the underlying condition. The timing of intubation remains in flux. With studies stressing the value of noninvasive ventilation, fewer immunosuppressed patients will be intubated. However, the decision regarding when to intubate will always be based on the patient's condition.

SUGGESTED READING

Baughman RP: The lung in the immunocompromised patient: Infectious complications. Part 1. Respiration 1999;66:95–109.

Baughman RP, Dohn MN, Frame PT: The continuing utility of bronchoalveolar lavage to diagnose opportunistic infection in AIDS patients. Am J Med 1994;97:515–522.

Chang GC, Wu CL, Pan SH, et al: The diagnosis of pneumonia in renal transplant recipients using invasive and noninvasive procedures. Chest 2004;125:541–547.

Conrado CE, Rashkin MC, Baughman RP: Pneumonia in immunocompromised and immunocompetent patients requiring mechanical ventilation. J Bronchol 1999;6:78–83.

Ferrer M, Esquinas A, Leon M, et al: Noninvasive ventilation in severe hypoxemic respiratory failure: A randomized clinical trial. Am J Respir Crit Care Med 2003;168:1438–1444.

Hayner CE, Baughman RP, Linnemann CCJ, et al: The relationship between cytomegalovirus retrieved by bronchoalveolar lavage and mortality in patients with HIV. Chest 1995;107:735–740.

Hilbert G, Vargas F, Valentino R, et al: Noninvasive ventilation in acute exacerbations of chronic obstructive pulmonary disease in patients with and without home noninvasive ventilation. Crit Care Med 2002;30:1453–1458.

Maschmeyer G, Beinert T, Buchheidt D, et al: Diagnosis and antimicrobial therapy of pulmonary infiltrates in febrile neutropenic patients—Guidelines of the Infectious Diseases Working Party (AGIHO) of the German Society of Hematology and Oncology (DGHO). Ann Hematol 2003;82(Suppl. 2):S118–S126.

Rañó A, Agustí C, Jiménez P, et al: Pulmonary infiltrates in non-HIV immunocompromised patients: A diagnostic approach using non-invasive and bronchoscopic procedures. Thorax 2001;56:379–387.

Singh N, Gayowski T, Wagener MM, et al: Pulmonary infiltrates in liver transplant recipients in the intensive care unit. Transplantation 1999;67:1138–1144.

DEFINITIONS

Sepsis is defined in the abstract as the systemic host response to invasive infection (Fig. 55.1). However, it has proven very challenging to translate this concept into a clearly delineated clinical syndrome. Life-threatening infection may occur in the absence of a vigorous host response, and even more commonly, clinical manifestations of inflammation can occur in the absence of culture-proven infection. Moreover, the diagnosis of infection, particularly nosocomial infection, may be difficult, and the clinical features that define sepsis are highly variable from one patient to the next. The definitions presented here are those adopted by two consensus conferences meeting in 1991 and 2001.

Clinical signs and symptoms of acute inflammation can be elicited by infection but also by noninfectious stimuli, such as major surgery, massive hemorrhage, pancreatitis, burns, aspiration pneumonitis, or ischemia–reperfusion injury. *Systemic inflammatory response syndrome* (SIRS) refers to the presence of these signs, symptoms, and biochemical manifestations, independent of their cause (Box 55.1). The attribution of specific clinical manifestations is quite arbitrary, and no single pattern of signs and symptoms is diagnostic of a distinct pathologic process. Description of the clinical syndrome has been a source of considerable controversy, as reflected in the differing criteria recommended by the two consensus conferences. It is less important to define SIRS than to recognize that a compatible

Sepsis is the leading cause of death in patients admitted to the intensive care unit (ICU). This syndrome affects more than 750,000 people in North America every year and is responsible for more than 200,000 deaths annually. Its impact in Europe is comparable, and the number of patients who die of sepsis in the developed world rivals that of patients who die of acute myocardial infarction. As a complication of AIDS, malaria, tuberculosis, or gastrointestinal infection, sepsis has an extensive impact throughout the world, yet public awareness of it is limited.

The syndrome of sepsis arises from the innate response of the patient to an infectious insult. This response can be attenuated by timely resuscitation, control of infection, and judicious management in an intensive care setting. It can be further modified by the use of therapies that target its mediators.

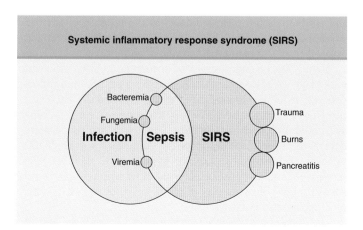

Figure 55.1. Systemic inflammatory response syndrome (SIRS). Not all patients with infection show evidence of an activated inflammatory response (SIRS), nor do all patients with SIRS have infection as the cause. When SIRS results from infection, sepsis is said to be present.

Box 55.1 Clinical Manifestations of Systemic Inflammation

Systemic Inflammatory Response Syndrome (SIRS)[a]

Tachycardia (heart rate > 90 beats/min)
Tachypnea (respiratory rate > 20 or mechanically ventilated)
Temperature < 36.0°C or > 38.0°C
White blood cell count > 11,000 or < 4000 or > 10% band forms

Diagnostic Criteria for Sepsis[b]

Infection—documented or suspected—and some of the following:
  General variables: Core temperature > 38.3°C or < 36°C, heart rate > 90, tachypnea, altered mental status, edema or positive fluid balance (> 20 mL/kg over 24 hr), hyperglycemia (glucose > 7.7 mmol/L) in the absence of diabetes
  Inflammatory variables: White count > 12,000/µL or < 4000/µL or > 10% immature forms, C-reactive protein > 2 SD above normal values, procalcitonin > 2 SD above normal
  Hemodynamic variables: Arterial hypotension (SBP < 90 mm Hg, MAP > 70, or an SBP decrease > 40), cardiac index > 3.5 L/min/m²
  Organ dysfunction variables: PaO_2/FIO_2 < 300, urine output < 0.5 mL·kg/hr for at least 2 hr, INR > 1.5, aPTT > 60 sec, ileus, platelet count < 100,000 µL, bilirubin > 70 mmol/L
  Tissue perfusion variables: Lactate > 1 mmol/L, decreased capillary refill or mottling

SIRS is defined as two or more of these criteria.
[a]From the ACCP/SCCM Consensus Conference 1991.
[b]From the SCCM/ESICM/ACCP/ATS/SIS Definitions Conference 2001.

Table 55.1 Differential Diagnosis of SIRS

Stimulus	Examples
Infection	Peritonitis and intraabdominal infection, pneumonia, mediastinitis, soft tissue infection, meningococcemia
Inflammation	Pancreatitis
Injury	Multiple trauma, burns
Ischemia	Ruptured aortic aneurysm, intestinal ischemia
Intoxication	Salicylate or arsenic poisoning
Immunologic	Autoimmune disease, blood transfusion, transplant rejection
Iatrogenic	Ventilator-induced lung injury, total parenteral nutrition, missed injury
Idiopathic	Heat shock, malignant hyperthermia, malignant neuroleptic syndrome, thrombotic thrombocytopenic purpura, hypoadrenalism

---

clinical presentation should trigger an aggressive search for a correctable cause. The differential diagnosis of SIRS includes a variety of insults (Table 55.1).

Microorganisms or their products are important triggers of SIRS. Although increased amounts of bacterial products such as endotoxin are present in a significant number of ICU patients, the diagnosis of infection is particularly important since it identifies a process that can be treated with source control measures and antibiotics. *Infection* is defined as the invasion of normally sterile host tissues by viable microorganisms; when bacteria are isolated from the blood, bacteremia is present.

Sepsis, the systemic response to infection (SIRS associated with evidence of infection), encompasses a continuum of illness severity from an appropriate adaptive response to a life-threatening and maladaptive process. *Severe sepsis* is sepsis associated with organ dysfunction (e.g., lactic acidosis, oliguria, decreased mental status, thrombocytopenia, prolonged INR, hypoxemia, liver dysfunction, or hypotension), whereas *septic shock* is defined as sepsis accompanied by hypotension despite adequate fluid resuscitation, resulting in compromised oxidative metabolism in the tissues.

The acute physiologic changes of SIRS and sepsis, and the measures required to support vital organ function in the ICU, contribute to a syndrome of persistent deranged organ function known as *multiple organ dysfunction syndrome* (MODS). Multiple organ dysfunction refers to impaired organ function in an acutely ill patient of a degree that homeostasis cannot be maintained without intervention. MODS can be primary or secondary. Primary MODS is a direct consequence of the acute insult (e.g., coma after head trauma or respiratory failure after pneumonia or chest trauma), whereas secondary MODS occurs as a consequence of the host response to the insult. Several scales are available to quantify the degree of organ dysfunction in critical illness, including the Multiple Organ Dysfunction score and the Sequential Organ Failure Assessment score (Table 55.2). Both are sensitive to changes in the patients' clinical status, are useful to assess changes induced by therapy, and correlate with mortality in critically ill patients.

EPIDEMIOLOGY AND RISK FACTORS

Incidence and Mortality

A large international study found that at least one episode of infection occurred during 27% of the admissions of 14,364 critically ill patients; others have reported incidence rates of infection of 21% to 58%, increasing with the duration of ICU stay. However, 18% to 44% of patients with infection do not meet SIRS criteria and thus do not meet criteria for sepsis. Conversely, not all patients who manifest SIRS criteria have infection as the cause. Rangel-Frausto and colleagues (1995) found that 2252 of 3708 patients with SIRS had concomitant infection, a 61% prevalence for all severities of sepsis.

Sepsis is a common indication for ICU admission. Sepsis is present at ICU admission in 10% to 30% of patients and has an incidence during the ICU stay of at least 22%. Among patients with sepsis at any time during the ICU stay, 47% to 58% have sepsis alone, 22% to 32% have severe sepsis, and 18% to 36% meet criteria for septic shock. At a population level, the incidence of sepsis ranges from 150 to 250/100,000 population and that of severe sepsis from 50 to 77/100,000 population; rates are even higher when non-ICU patients are included. In a study of eight U.S. university hospitals, Sands and associates recorded 2 cases of severe sepsis per 100 hospital admissions, 59% of which occurred in ICUs. In a 1-year study of 847 U.S. hospitals, Angus and coworkers (2001) found an incidence of severe sepsis of 2.3 cases per 100 hospital discharges. Rates appear to have been increasing over time (Fig. 55.2).

Incidence and prevalence rates for sepsis are confounded by the vagaries in establishing a diagnosis of infection. Between

Table 55.2 Multiple Organ Dysfunction (MOD) and Sequential Organ Failure Assessment (SOFA) Scores[a]					
	No. of Points				
System	**0**	**1**	**2**	**3**	**4**
Respiratory					
PaO_2/FiO_2 (MOD)	>300	226–300	151–225	76–150	≤75
PaO_2/FiO_2 (SOFA)	>400	301–400	201–300	101–200 (with support)	≤100 (with support)
Renal					
Creatinine (μmol/L) (MOD)	≤100	101–200	201–350	351–500	>500
Creatinine or urine output (SOFA)	<110	110–170	171–299	300–440, or urine output <500 mL/day	>440, or urine output <200 mL/day
Cardiovascular					
Pressure-adjusted rate[b] (MOD)	≤10.0	10.1–15.0	15.1–20.0	20.1–30.0	>30.0
Use of vasoactive agents[c] (SOFA)	No hypotension	MAP < 70 mm Hg	Dopamine < 5 μg	Dopamine > 5 μg or norepinephrine ≤ 0.1	Dopamine > 15 or norepinephrine > 0.1
Hematologic					
Platelets/mL × 10^{-3} (MOD)	>120,000	80,000–120,000	50,000–80,000	20,000–50,000	<20,000
Platelets/mL × 10^{-3} (SOFA)	>150,000	101,000–150,000	51,000–100,000	21,000–50,000	≤20,000
Hepatic					
Bilirubin (μmol/L) (MOD)	≤20	21–60	61–120	121–240	>240
Bilirubin (μmol/L) (SOFA)	<20	21–32	33–101	102–204	>204
Neurologic					
Glasgow Coma Score (MOD)	15	13–14	10–12	7–9	≤6
Glasgow Coma Score (SOFA)	15	13–14	10–12	6–9	<6

[a]The worst daily value is used in the calculation of the SOFA score. A representative value (usually the first of the day) is used for the calculation of the MOD score.
[b]The pressure-adjusted rate is the product of the heart and the central venous pressure (CVP), divided by the mean arterial pressure; in the absence of a central line, the CVP is imputed normal and assigned a value of 8.
[c]Doses of adrenergic agents are given in μg/kg/min and must have been administered for at least 1 hr.

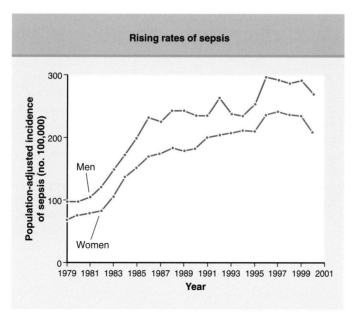

Figure 55.2. Rising rates of sepsis. Rates of sepsis have been increasing during the past decade, with men showing consistently higher rates than women. (Data from Martin GS, Mannino DM, Eaton S, Moss M: The epidemiology of sepsis in the United States from 1979 through 2000. N Engl J Med. 2003;348:1546–1554.)

one third and one half of patients classified as having sepsis do not have documented infection, and fewer than one third of patients with severe sepsis or septic shock have bacteremia. The most common sites of infection in ICU patients include the respiratory tract (40%–65%), abdomen (15%–30%), urinary tract (10%–15%), and bloodstream (2%–20%).

PATHOPHYSIOLOGY

Inflammation is a complex process that serves to recognize danger, to contain and eradicate its cause, and to initiate tissue repair. It is mediated through the coordinated action of hundreds of host-derived mediators, including protein cytokines such as the interleukins, tumor necrosis factor, and growth factors; acute phase reactants such as C-reactive protein and α_1 antitrypsin; the complement cascade; lipid mediators such as prostaglandins, leukotrienes, and platelet-activating factor; stress hormones such as cortisol and epinephrine; vasoactive substances such as histamine and bradykinin; intermediates of oxygen and nitrogen; and the coagulation cascade. Although a comprehensive consideration of these interacting elements is beyond the scope of this chapter, a conceptual understanding of its complexity and interdependence can be gained by considering the biologic processes activated during the cellular response to endotoxin.

Endotoxin or lipopolysaccharide (LPS) is an intrinsic component of the cell wall of all gram-negative bacteria and a prototypical trigger of the inflammatory response. Endotoxin enters the body during infection with gram-negative organisms or by absorption from the gastrointestinal tract, interacts with serum proteins, and engages a dedicated membrane receptor to activate cells of the innate immune system (Fig. 55.3A). Lipopolysaccharide-binding protein (LBP) and bactericidal permeability increasing protein (BPI) are lipid transfer molecules with high affinity for LPS. LBP is a plasma protein produced constitutively by the liver and released in increased amounts as an acute phase reactant. LBP binds free endotoxin and enables its recognition by host cells, serving to transfer endotoxin to a dedicated cell surface receptor, CD14. CD14, in turn, facilitates the interaction of endotoxin with a second receptor, toll-like receptor 4 (TLR4), whose engagement in association with an accessory protein, MD2, results in the activation of a cellular response. BPI, a cationic protein produced by polymorphonuclear neutrophils, is cytotoxic for gram-negative bacteria and inhibits LPS delivery to the CD14 receptor.

Engagement of TLR4 results in the recruitment of a number of adapter molecules to the intracellular portion of TLR4, and it activates an intracellular cascade that culminates in the expression or inhibition of more than 300 distinct genes and the release from the cell of the protein products of these genes (Fig. 55.3B). Central to this process is the activation of a cascade of intracellular enzymes called kinases, including the mitogen-activated protein kinases and phosphatidylinositol-3 kinase. These enzymes catalyze the attachment of a phosphate molecule to the amino acids tyrosine, serine, or threonine on their target molecules, a process known as phosphorylation, and, as a result, convey an activational signal through the cytoplasm to the nucleus. A critical step in this process is the phosphorylation of a protein known as IκB. Phosphorylation of IκB causes it to dissociate from the latent cytoplasmic transcription factor, NF-κB,

and enables NF-κB to translocate into the nucleus, where it binds to and activates early inflammatory genes.

The initial response to TLR4 engagement is the transcription of genes for proteins such as interleukin (IL)-1 and tumor necrosis factor, and these can be detected in the circulation within 90 minutes of endotoxin exposure. These early response mediators, however, evoke further cellular responses by engaging their own receptors. The resulting responses define key components of the inflammatory response. Upregulation of the gene for inducible nitric oxide synthase, for example, leads to increased generation of nitric oxide, a potent vasodilator that is responsible for the vasodilatation of sepsis, whereas increased expression of tissue factor on the surface of endothelial cells results in activation of the coagulation cascade, and release of IL-6 promotes the acute phase response in the liver, reflected in increased synthesis of C-reactive protein and reduced synthesis of albumin.

Each of the many hundreds of individual molecules whose expression is altered during the process of inflammation is a potential therapeutic target in sepsis, and in the highly artificial model of sepsis induced by injecting endotoxin in a mouse, manipulation of more than two dozen of these can be shown to alter survival (Table 55.3). Conversely, in established human sepsis, the consequences of manipulating any one of these are generally modest.

CLINICAL FEATURES

The clinical presentation of sepsis is highly variable, and the disorder is frequently difficult to recognize. Fulminant sepsis classically presents as decreased mental status, spiking fever, tachypnea, tachycardia, hypotension, and poor skin perfusion with livedo reticularis. However, its presentation may be subacute and include such signs and symptoms as tachypnea, tachycardia, and otherwise unexplained new organ failure (e.g., hyperbilirubinemia or renal failure). Other manifestations may be subtle and include an increased requirement for intravenous fluids to maintain hemodynamic stability, oliguria, unexplained hypotension, decreased mental status, new-onset arrhythmia, intolerance to enteral feeds, hyperglycemia and insulin resistance, or impaired coagulation manifested by prolongation of the INR or thrombocytopenia. Signs of tissue hypoperfusion may be identified in patients with severe sepsis or septic shock and include delayed capillary refill, mottling, decreased urine output, hypotension, acidosis, and hyperlactatemia.

Potentially reversible organ dysfunction is the hallmark of severe sepsis. Characteristic patterns of dysfunction are seen; their aggregate severity correlates with outcome.

Cardiovascular Dysfunction

The cardiovascular abnormalities of sepsis involve both the heart and the peripheral vessels; abnormalities of the peripheral circulation are particularly prominent. The combination of increased capillary permeability and peripheral vasodilatation results in hypovolemia. Small vessel vasodilatation results from increased release of endothelial cell nitric oxide (NO) and from opening of the K^+_{ATP} channels in vascular smooth muscle cells. NO is generated during the conversion of the amino acid arginine to citrulline, a reaction that is catalyzed by the enzyme NO synthase (NOS). An inducible form of this enzyme, iNOS, is upregulated in vascular smooth muscle cells and mononuclear

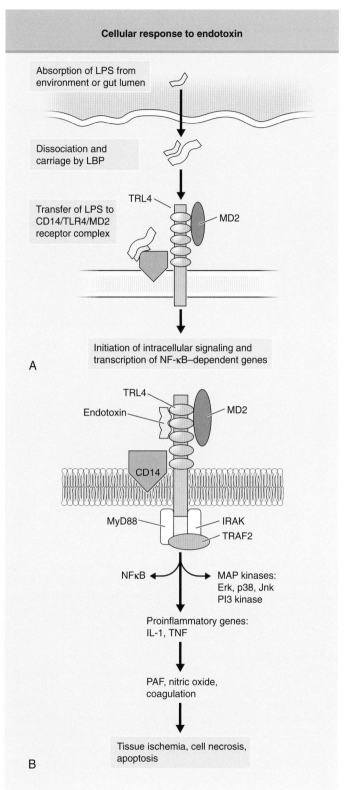

Cellular response to endotoxin

Absorption of LPS from environment or gut lumen

Dissociation and carriage by LBP

Transfer of LPS to CD14/TLR4/MD2 receptor complex

TRL4

MD2

Initiation of intracellular signaling and transcription of NF-κB–dependent genes

A

TRL4

Endotoxin

MD2

CD14

MyD88

IRAK

TRAF2

NFκB

MAP kinases: Erk, p38, Jnk PI3 kinase

Proinflammatory genes: IL-1, TNF

PAF, nitric oxide, coagulation

Tissue ischemia, cell necrosis, apoptosis

B

Figure 55.3. Cellular response to endotoxin. *A,* Either free or integrated into the cell wall of gram-negative bacteria, endotoxin is recognized by the host through its interactions with a network of host-based proteins. Endotoxin is carried in the circulation by a dedicated binding protein [lipopolysaccharide-binding protein (LBP)] that transfers the endotoxin molecule to the endotoxin receptor complex, which is composed of three proteins: CD14, Tlr4, and MD2. *B,* Engagement of the endotoxin receptor complex results in the aggregation of a series of intracellular adapter proteins and the activation of signaling cascades, including the mitogen-activated protein (MAP) kinases, and the nuclear transcription factor NF-κB. The result is the transcription of early proinflammatory genes, such as interleukin-1 and tumor necrosis factor. These protein cytokines then interact with their own receptors, triggering transcription of genes that mediate key components of the inflammatory response, such as inducible nitric oxide synthase, which catalyzes the production of nitric oxide and thus produces vasodilatation, and tissue factor, which initiates coagulation.

cells by endotoxin, tumor necrosis factor-α (TNF-α), and IL-1β, resulting in increased release of NO. NO from the endothelium and mononuclear cells stimulates the soluble guanylate cyclase in the smooth muscle, and cyclic GMP causes smooth muscle relaxation. K^+_{ATP} channels are opened by intracellular acidosis and reduced ATP stores, resulting in membrane hyperpolarization and muscle relaxation. Visualization of the sublingual microcirculation using reflectance spectrophotometry and orthogonal polarization spectral imaging reveals striking variability in patterns of microvascular flow, particularly an increased proportion of capillaries with no or intermittent flow. The consequence is a shunting of oxygenated blood which causes a decrease of cross-sectional area available for oxygen exchange.

Impaired myocardial function results from impaired myocardial contractility due to poorly characterized myocardial depressant factors and increased pulmonary vascular resistance. Prior

Table 55.3 Endogenous Molecules Whose Manipulation Alters Survival in Murine Endotoxemia		
	Activity Increases Lethality	**Activity Decreases Lethality**
Cytokines and other extracellular proteins	IL-1	IL-1 receptor antagonist
	IL-12	IL-4
	IL-18	IL-10
	Tumor necrosis factor (TNF)	IL-13
	Interferon-γ	IVIG
	Transforming growth factor-β	Interferon-α
	Macrophage inhibitory factor	Hepatocyte growth factor
	MIP-1α	Leukemia inhibitory factor
	Leukemia inhibitory factor	C-reactive protein
	High mobility group box-1	Kallikrein-binding protein
	MFP-14	MCP-1
	Lipopolysaccharide-binding protein	Bactericidal permeability increasing protein
	Parathyroid hormone-related protein	CAP-18
	Tissue factor	LL-37
		TSG-14
		Apolipoprotein E
		VLDL
		Complement components C3 and C4
		Melatonin
		Vasoactive intestinal peptide (VIP)
		Pituitary adenylate cyclase activation polypeptide
Cell surface receptors	IL-1 receptor	Macrophage FcγR
	TNF receptor	VIP receptor
	Platelet-activating factor receptor	Adenosine A3 receptor
	LDL receptor	
	CD11a	
	CD18	
	LFCAM-1	
	TREM-1	
Signal transduction molecules and other intracellular proteins	Hck	Stat-4, Stat-6
	Cyclooxygenase II	IκB
	Inducible nitric oxide synthase	Hemoxygenase
	Caspase-3	Heat shock protein 70
Miscellaneous	Platelet-activating factor	Vitamin B$_{12}$
		Vitamin D$_3$
		Oxidized phospholipids

to resuscitation, the cardiac index is reduced; however, restoration of adequate intravascular volume converts a low-output shock state to a high-output one, with increased cardiac index and a reduced systemic vascular resistance. Compensatory dilatation of the left ventricle results in an increase in stroke volume but a reduction in ejection fraction (the ratio between stroke volume and end-diastolic ventricular volume).

Once hypovolemia has been corrected by fluids, residual cardiovascular abnormalities contribute to the tissue hypoxia of sepsis (Fig. 55.4). Reduced peripheral vascular resistance leads to microvascular shunting, with the result that oxygenated arterial blood passes to the venous side of the circulation without entering capillary beds. Microvascular perfusion is further jeopardized by plugging of the capillaries with red cells and leukocytes whose deformability is reduced and by platelet thrombi resulting from increased intravascular coagulation. Unloading of oxygen in the tissues is a passive process, dependent on the gradient of hypoxia between the capillary and the cell and on the rate of flow through the microvasculature. Tissue edema increases the distance between the erythrocyte and cells in the tissues and thus reduces the gradient down which oxygen diffuses, whereas reduced resistance results in accelerated flow through the microvasculature: Both factors impede the unloading of oxygen from the red cell. Finally, abnormalities in oxygen

utilization by the cell, a state termed cytopathic hypoxia, have been described in sepsis. The net effect of these influences is to reduce the unloading of oxygen from red cells, and thus the oxygen saturation of blood returning to the venous side of the circulation is increased from its normal value of 70%.

Pulmonary Dysfunction

Endothelial injury, capillary hyperpermeability, interstitial edema, and increased recruitment of neutrophils into the lung all contribute to the pulmonary dysfunction of sepsis. Clinical manifestations range from mild ventilation/perfusion mismatch to acute lung injury (bilateral pulmonary infiltrates and PaO$_2$/FIO$_2$ ratio < 300) and full-blown acute respiratory distress syndrome (bilateral pulmonary infiltrates and PaO$_2$/FIO$_2$ ratio < 200).

Liver Dysfunction

Elevated transaminase levels are common following resuscitation from significant hypotension and reflect hepatic ischemia (shock liver). Other manifestations of hepatic dysfunction in sepsis include hyperbilirubinemia and coagulopathy. Activation of the hepatic acute phase response results in increased synthesis of acute phase reactants such as C-reactive protein and α$_1$ antitrypsin but reduced synthesis of albumin.

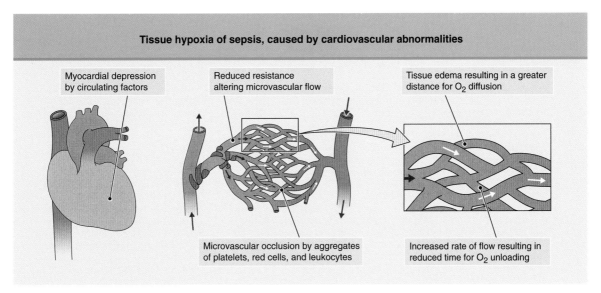

Figure 55.4. Tissue hypoxia of sepsis, caused by cardiovascular abnormalities. Multiple derangements in cardiovascular homeostasis result in impaired oxygen delivery to the tissues in sepsis, despite an increased cardiac output. Poorly characterized myocardial depressant factors reduce myocardial contractility. Reduced vascular tone, a result of vascular smooth muscle relaxation by nitric oxide, leads to reduced diversion of oxygenated blood into the microvasculature, whereas capillary plugging by red cells, leukocytes, and platelet thrombi results in maldistribution of flow within capillary beds. In addition, the rapid transit of red cells through the microvasculature and the increased distance between red cells and tissues due to edema impede the unloading of oxygen, a process that occurs by passive diffusion down a concentration gradient.

Gastrointestinal Dysfunction

The manifestations of gastrointestinal dysfunction in sepsis include ileus, mucosal ulceration and hemorrhage, and increased epithelial permeability, leading to absorption of bacterial endotoxin and the translocation of viable microorganisms from the gut lumen. Ileus, reduced bile flow, reduced levels of luminal nutrients, and the administration of broad-spectrum antibiotics all contribute to a reduction in the normal anaerobic flora and pathologic colonization by the typical pathogens of nosocomial infection, including fungi, gram-negatives such as *Pseudomonas* and *Enterobacter*, and gram-positives such as the *Enterococcus* and coagulase-negative staphylococci. Both aspiration and translocation contribute to the pathogenesis of infection with these organisms.

Renal Dysfunction

The spectrum of renal dysfunction ranges from mild reversible oliguria to established acute renal failure requiring renal replacement therapy. Adequate fluid resuscitation can minimize the early ischemia that leads to renal dysfunction; the mechanism of late renal insufficiency is uncertain but includes factors such as reduced renal perfusion, maldistribution of intrarenal blood flow, and the effects of nephrotoxins.

Metabolic Dysfunction

The metabolic changes of sepsis are extensive and include hypermetabolism, increased energy expenditure, and insulin resistance. Hypermetabolism is characterized by increased liver glycolysis, gluconeogenesis, and amino acid uptake. Splanchnic oxygen uptake and glucose output are increased. Increased glycolysis and gluconeogenesis give rise to hyperglycemia and hyperlactatemia. Enhanced gluconeogenesis is fueled by glycerol from increased lipolysis, amino acids from muscle proteolysis, and lactate and pyruvate from muscle glycolysis.

Nervous System

An altered level of consciousness is an early manifestation of severe sepsis, and persistent depression of central nervous system function is common in the septic patient. The causes are multifactorial and include the effects of medications, increased capillary permeability resulting in cerebral edema, and alterations in the production and release of cerebral neurotransmitters. Peripheral nervous system dysfunction is evident as peripheral sensorimotor polyneuropathy, and it presents as generalized weakness, muscle atrophy, hyporeflexia, and loss of peripheral sensation to light touch and pinprick but relative preservation of cranial nerve function.

Other Manifestations of Organ Dysfunction

Sepsis is typically accompanied by endocrine dysfunction, manifested by insulin resistance and hyperglycemia, occult adrenal insufficiency, and the sick euthyroid syndrome. Multiple abnormalities of immune function have been described, including profound inhibition of cell-mediated immunity, reflected in anergy to skin testing with common recall antigens. Wound healing is impaired, and skin breakdown is common.

STAGING OF SEPSIS

SIRS, sepsis, severe sepsis, and septic shock represent a continuum of disease severity. Mortality increases as the diagnosis progresses from SIRS to septic shock, from 7% for SIRS to 16% for

Table 55.4 The PIRO Model			
Domain	**Present**	**Future**	**Rationale**
Predisposition	Premorbid illness with reduced probability of short-term survival; cultural or religious beliefs	Genetic polymorphisms in components of inflammatory response (e.g., Tlr, TNF, IL-1, CD14)	In the present, premorbid factors impact on the potential attributable morbidity and mortality of an acute insult; deleterious consequences of insult are heavily dependent on genetic predisposition (future)
Insult	Culture and sensitivity of infecting pathogens; detection of disease amenable to source control	Assay of microbial products (LPS, mannan, bacterial DNA) or injurious autoantigens from host cells? Procalcitonin to detect infection	Specific therapies directed against inciting insult require demonstration and characterization of that insult
Response	SIRS, other signs of sepsis, shock, CRP	Nonspecific markers of activated inflammation (e.g., IL-6) or impaired host responsiveness (e.g., HLA-DR); specific detection of target of therapy (e.g., protein C, TNF, PAF)	Both mortality risk and potential to respond to therapy vary with nonspecific measures of disease severity (e.g., shock); specific mediator-targeted therapy is predicated on the presence and activity of mediator
Organ dysfunction	Organ dysfunction as number of failing organs or composite score (e.g., MODS, SOFA, LODS)	Dynamic measures of cellular response to insult—apoptosis, cytopathic hypoxia, cell stress	Response to preemptive therapy (e.g., targeting microorganism or early mediator) not possible if damage already present; therapies targeting the injurious cellular process require that it be present

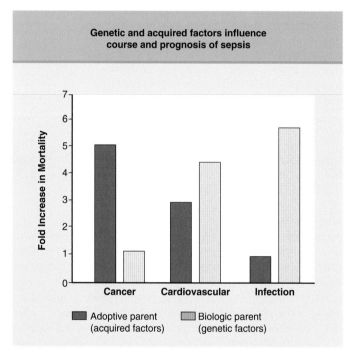

Genetic and acquired factors influence course and prognosis of sepsis

Figure 55.5. Genetic and acquired factors influence course and prognosis of sepsis. There is an increased risk of early death in adoptive children if an adoptive parent (dark blue bars) or a biologic parent (light blue bars) died before the age of 50 years of one of the three disease processes. An increased risk of death associated with that of an adoptive parent suggests environmental factors, and an increased risk of death associated with that of a biologic parent suggests genetic factors. (Data from Sorenson TI, Nielsen GG, Andersen PK, Teasdale PW: Genetic and environmental influences on premature death in adult adoptees. N Engl J Med. 1988;318:727–732.)

Table 55.5 Genetic Polymorphisms of Potential Relevance in Sepsis		
Gene	**Polymorphism**	**Association**
Lipopolysaccharide-binding protein (LBP)	Cys98 → Gly	Increased rates of sepsis
CD14	−159C → T	Increased rates and mortality
Tlr4	Asp299 → Gly, Thr399 → Ile	Increased gram-negative sepsis
TNF-α	−308G → A	Increased rates and mortality
TNF-β	252G → A	Increased mortality
IL-1ra	Tandem repeat, intron 2	Increased risk of death
IL-10	−1082G → A	Increased severity of illness
	−192 A allele	Increased mortality
HSP70	1538G → A	Increased morbidity

the syndrome may be stratified using a staging system analogous to those used in cancer (Table 55.4).

Predisposing Factors

Both genetic and acquired factors modify the course and prognosis of sepsis. Genetic factors play an important but counterintuitive role. A Scandinavian population-based study showed that adoptees having a biologic parent who died of infection before the age of 50 years had a 5.8-fold increased risk of dying of infection (Fig. 55.5).

Polymorphisms are conserved mutations in the DNA encoding a particular gene that result in variable expression of the resulting gene product. Polymorphisms have been described in a large number of genes involved in the inflammatory response that recognize danger, amplify the response to a perceived threat, and terminate the response and promote tissue repair (Table 55.5). The functional significance of many of these is controversial, and the establishment of causal relationships is confounded by problems of study power, selection of appropriate control groups, and definition of study end points, as well as by the phenomenon of linkage disequilibrium (increased risk associated with one polymorphism may actually result from the

sepsis, 20% to 35% for severe sepsis, and 46% to 60% for septic shock. Interestingly, mortality rates are not affected by the positivity of blood cultures within each category.

Determinants of outcome include factors related to the predisposition of the host, the infectious insult (site and type of infection), the response (magnitude of the inflammatory response), and the severity of organ dysfunction, suggesting that activity of another gene whose transmission is linked to the gene studied). Nonetheless, genetic variability is the hallmark of patients with sepsis, and as this variability becomes better understood, it will provide a basis for improved methods of therapeutic stratification.

Patients developing sepsis often have significant comorbid conditions that independently alter prognosis, including end stage organ failure, malignancy, diabetes, HIV/AIDS, and cardiovascular disease. Thus, survival in sepsis is independently impacted by factors such as age, race, McCabe score (a measure of comorbidity) higher than 0, and medical admission. Variable approaches to the continuation or withdrawal of ICU support can also influence the outcome of a disorder such as sepsis, whose prognosis is measured as mortality at an early time point (usually 28 days).

Insult

By definition, the inciting insult for sepsis is infection. However, noninfectious stimuli, such as pancreatitis, massive trauma, transfusion or drug reactions, or autoimmune disease, can evoke a clinical and biochemical response that is indistinguishable from sepsis. Moreover, infection in the hospitalized patient may be difficult to diagnose, and circulating bacterial products such as endotoxin are commonly detected in critically ill patients with systemic inflammation but no documented infection.

Although subtle differences have been described in the response to infection with gram-positive or gram-negative organisms, these differences tend to be of minor clinical significance. Urinary tract infections are typically associated with a lower mortality rate than pulmonary or intraabdominal infections, and certain organisms, notably *Pseudomonas* as a cause of pneumonia, are associated with higher mortality rates. Similarly, the mortality of nosocomial infection is greater than that of community-acquired infection: Bacteremias due to coagulase-negative staphylococci, *Enterococcus,* and *Candida* species have attributable mortality rates of 14%, 31%, and 38%, respectively. However, it is difficult to separate the independent influence of the organism or site of infection from the confounding factors that define a population at intrinsically increased risk of adverse outcome because of prolonged duration of mechanical ventilation, the presence of invasive devices, the use of broad-spectrum antibiotics, or other host comorbidities. Similarly, although it has been suggested that early administration of broad-spectrum antibiotics is associated with an improved outcome, it is unclear, particularly for the patient with nosocomial infection, whether this represents the therapeutic efficacy of antibiotics or systematic differences between patient populations.

Response

Since sepsis is defined as the host response to infection, it follows that the magnitude and nature of that response will be important determinants of outcome. Indeed, the distinction between sepsis, severe sepsis, and septic shock reflects increasing magnitude of the physiologic response and defines a spectrum of worsening prognosis. The host response variables that best segregate patients with regard to prognosis are many; however, the relative importance of each is poorly characterized.

Although fever and leukocytosis are cardinal manifestations of systemic inflammation, both hypothermia and leukopenia are associated with increased mortality in sepsis. Aggregation of

these abnormalities into one of several published sepsis scores identifies patients at increased risk of mortality. Also, generic severity of illness measures, such as APACHE II or SAPS, not only predict increasing mortality risk but also appear to identify patients more likely to benefit from therapeutic interventions such as activated protein C.

Multiple biomarkers of the septic response have been described, including microbial products such as endotoxin, measures of the acute phase response such as C-reactive protein, cytokines such as IL-6, and other markers such as procalcitonin (PCT). Although much has been written about the relative merits of these, their role in clinical management is less well defined. Each is able to stratify patients based on their risk of adverse outcome, but the rationale for doing so in the absence of a specific therapeutic decision is unclear; moreover, physiologic scales such as APACHE can accomplish the same objective. The more compelling role for biomarkers is in guiding therapy. Exposure to unnecessary empiric antibiotic therapy can be reduced when PCT levels are low since the probability of infection is minimal. Failure to respond to ACTH stimulation with a 30% increase in cortisol levels identifies patients who are more likely to benefit from corticosteroid supplementation.

Organ Dysfunction

Organ dysfunction is the embodiment of the sequelae of sepsis, and the magnitude of such dysfunction is a powerful determinant of survival. The severity of organ dysfunction at ICU admission and that developing over the entire ICU stay are both highly correlated with mortality risk. Using one of several organ dysfunction scales and calculating the difference between maximal scores over the ICU stay and that present at the time of admission provides a delta score that measures new organ dysfunction, developing after ICU admission, and thus potentially impacted by therapeutic intervention.

The degree of organ dysfunction at the time of intervention also influences the probability of response to treatment. Timely selection of the appropriate antibiotic regimen has the greatest impact in patients with minimal degrees of organ dysfunction. Conversely, patients with more advanced degrees of organ dysfunction appear to benefit more from intervention with activated protein C.

Staging systems have proven to be invaluable in the management of patients with cancer because they stratify patients into more homogeneous groups with respect to both their risk of adverse outcome and their potential to benefit from a particular treatment. The concept of staging sepsis is intuitively attractive but in its infancy.

DIAGNOSIS OF SEPSIS

The diagnosis of sepsis is directed toward identifying an inciting cause and characterizing the resulting physiologic derangements. The clinical signs and symptoms of sepsis are variable and non-specific; they suggest the possibility of infection as a cause, but proof requires the isolation of an infecting pathogen or the identification of a specific focus. Appropriate biologic samples should be obtained for culture before antibiotic therapy is initiated. At least two sets of blood cultures should be drawn—one or more by peripheral venipuncture and one through each vascular access device. Other samples, including cerebrospinal fluid, urine, wound exudates, or tracheal secretions, should be obtained as suggested by the clinical presentation. Imaging techniques such as computerized tomography are invaluable in identifying deep-seated foci of infection, such as an intraabdominal abscess or empyema; they also facilitate surgical planning and permit per-cutaneous drainage. Ultrasonography may be of value if the patient is too unstable to transfer to the radiology suite; ultra-sonography is of particular use in identifying infection in the biliary or urinary tracts. Occasionally, the diagnosis of infection can only be made at laparotomy.

As many as one fourth of all patients with septic shock have multiple sites of infection. Conversely, only one third have positive blood cultures, and 25% of patients presenting with a clinical picture of severe sepsis do not have culture-proven infection.

The results of a Gram stain or radiographic investigation can be obtained rapidly, whereas the results of culture and sensitiv-ity testing may not be available for 48 to 72 hours or more. Bio-chemical markers, such as procalcitonin, C-reactive protein, or endotoxin, and diagnostic scores, such as the Clinical Pulmonary Infection Score or the Infection Probability Score, may aid in establishing an infectious etiology.

MANAGAMENT OF SEVERE SEPSIS AND SEPTIC SHOCK

Severe sepsis and septic shock are medical emergencies. Early diagnosis and aggressive treatment are vital to minimize organ dysfunction and improve outcome. The initial priorities in the management of septic shock are to (1) establish adequate intravascular access and initiate fluid resuscitation, (2) assess the need for tracheal intubation and provide ventilatory support as needed, (3) administer appropriate antibiotics, and (4) deter-mine the source of the infectious process and undertake source control measures as appropriate.

Vascular Access Airway

Secure peripheral vascular access should be established using one or more large-bore intravenous catheters. A central venous catheter is invaluable to monitor central venous pressure (CVP) and superior vena caval oxygen saturation (ScvO$_2$) to aid in titrating resuscitation, as well as to facilitate the administration of medications, particularly vasoactive drugs. An arterial line should be placed to monitor blood pressure and obtain arterial blood gases and other blood samples. Placement of a central venous catheter or arterial line should not delay the initiation of the resuscitation once adequate peripheral access has been secured.

Arterial oxygen saturation should be monitored by pulse oximetry and supplemental oxygen administered by nasal prongs or face mask. Some degree of hypoxemia is evident in most patients, which is a consequence of increased pulmonary vascular permeability and ventilation–perfusion mismatch sec-ondary to atelectasis or an acute pulmonary problem such as pneumonia. Endotracheal intubation and mechanical ventilation should be considered if evolving respiratory distress is evident. Some patients require intubation for nonpulmonary reasons, such as a decreased level of consciousness or increased work of breathing secondary to fever in the face of diminished respira-tory reserve.

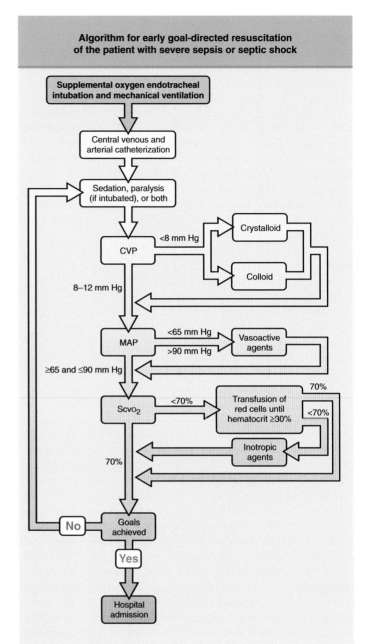

Figure 55.6. Algorithm for early goal-directed resuscitation of the patient with severe sepsis or septic shock. (Adapted from Rivers E, Nguyen B, Havstad S, et al: Early goal-directed therapy in the treatment of severe sepsis and septic shock. N Engl J Med 2001;345:1368–1377.)

Initial Resuscitation

The goal of fluid resuscitation is to restore tissue perfusion as rapidly as possible. Intravenous fluids are the mainstay of initial resuscitation. Optimal endpoints for resuscitation are not well defined; however, it has been shown that rapid and effective early resuscitation improves long-term survival. One such approach, early goal-directed therapy, sets as resuscitation targets a CVP of 8 to 12 mm Hg, mean arterial pressure higher than 65 mm Hg, urine output greater than 0.5 mL/kg/hr, and ScvO$_2$ more than 70%. If the proposed goals are not achieved by fluid infusion and blood volume is considered to be normal based on clinical signs and CVP measurements, packed red blood cells and infusion of dobutamine are administered (Fig. 55.6). Application of this intensive resuscitation protocol reduced the 28-day mortality of septic shock from 46% to 30% in a single center trial.

There is no clear advantage to the use of colloids over crystalloids in the fluid resuscitation of severe sepsis or septic shock. Both meta-analyses of clinical trials comparing crystalloids and colloids in sepsis and the results of a randomized clinical trial comparing albumin with saline resuscitation in a heterogeneous population of critically ill patients suggest that crystalloids and colloids are equally efficacious. In the latter study of 7000 patients, for the subgroup of patients with severe sepsis, mortality was 30.7% when albumin was used for resuscitation compared to 35.3% when saline was used [relative risk of death during the 28 days was 0.87 (95% confidence interval, 0.74–1.02, $P = 0.09$)]. However, this trend toward benefit was only observed in a subgroup analysis, and whether the use of natural colloids is associated with a better outcome in patients with severe sepsis remains unknown.

An initial fluid challenge should be given rapidly (i.e., 500–1000 mL of crystalloids or 300–500 mL of colloids over 30 min) and continued if hypotension or signs of tissue hypoperfusion persist; fluid requirements may be substantial—often as much as 5 to 10 L. In general, fluid resuscitation should be continued until there has been a satisfactory response, reflected in a urine output of more than 30 mL/hour, and normalization of the central venous and arterial pressures. Increased capillary permeability in the lung often results in increasing hypoxemia during fluid administration and necessitates intubation and mechanical ventilation.

Some patients do not respond to normalization of the blood volume alone but remain hypotensive and oliguric despite a normal or even elevated CVP; vasopressor therapy should be considered in these circumstances. The first-line agent of choice is either norepinephrine or dopamine. Norepinephrine is a more potent vasoconstrictor than dopamine, but it has less impact on cardiac output. There is no evidence that norepinephrine impairs renal function in sepsis but, rather, it increases renal perfusion pressure and urine output. At low doses, dopamine increases blood pressure by increasing cardiac output; at higher doses, it increases blood pressure by inducing vasoconstriction. Dopamine does not, however, prevent the development of acute renal failure, and it may cause more tachycardia than norepinephrine. Other vasopressor agents are occasionally used. Epinephrine has potent vasoconstrictor and inotropic activity; however, it may have adverse effects on splanchnic perfusion. Phenylephrine is the most selective alpha agonist and thus has the most specific vasoconstrictor effects; however, it may decrease cardiac output more markedly than other vasopressors. There has been interest in the use of low-dose vasopressin in the management of refractory hypotension in sepsis. Vasopressin is administered at a dose of 0.01 to 0.04 U/minute to correct a putative deficiency state, and it is not titrated to the blood pressure response. It should be used sparingly pending the results of a large, ongoing clinical trial to evaluate its efficacy and safety profile.

Inotropic Therapy

When signs of tissue hypoxia persist despite fluid resuscitation and optimization of blood pressure with pressor agents, the administration of inotropic agents such as dobutamine should be considered, particularly if the cardiac output remains low or

the superior vena cava or mixed venous oxygen saturation is reduced. Dobutamine has vasodilatory properties, and it may be necessary to add or increase the dose of a pressor agent if its administration aggravates hypotension. Whether the goal of resuscitation should be to augment oxygen delivery to higher than normal levels is unclear, although current consensus is that such a strategy is of limited, if any, benefit. Meta-analyses of studies of a deliberate strategy of supranormal oxygen delivery suggest that the therapy is not effective overall, although it may be of benefit in surgical or trauma patients. The addition of inotropic agents to attain a normal or above normal superior vena cava oxygen saturation is a component of the early goal-directed therapy regimen that has been shown to improve outcome in sepsis.

Antibiotics

Antibiotic treatment should be instituted within the first hour of the identification of sepsis, once appropriate cultures have been obtained. The initial empiric antibiotic regimen should be selected on the basis of its activity against the probable infecting pathogen(s), and the initial spectrum should be broad. Antibiotic treatment should be reassessed 48 to 72 hours later, adjusting the antibiotics on the basis of culture results to provide effective, narrow-spectrum therapy against the infecting species. If an infectious etiology is ruled out, antibiotics should be discontinued to limit the emergence of resistant microorganisms, decrease toxicity, and contain cost.

There is no convincing evidence that combination therapy is better than single-agent therapy, although most experts would use combination therapy in neutropenic individuals. Some experts recommend combination therapy for *Pseudomonas*.

Source Control

The term "source control" encompasses all physical measures directed toward eliminating a focus of infection and restoring optimal anatomy and function. Such measures include the drainage of abscesses (either percutaneously or surgically), the débridement of infected devitalized tissue or the removal of infected foreign bodies, and the definitive correction of an anatomic defect that has resulted in infection. The possibility of a focus of infection amenable to source control measures should be thoroughly assessed in all patients with sepsis and appropriate measures instituted in a timely manner using the simplest and safest approach possible.

Adjuvant Therapy
Corticosteroids

Septic shock commonly results in occult adrenal insufficiency, reflected by increased basal levels of circulating cortisol but an impaired response to ACTH stimulation. For such patients, identified by a basal cortisol level of more than 34 µg/dL and a response to ACTH stimulation of less than 9 µg/dL, replacement therapy that consists of 50 mg hydrocortisone four times daily and 50 µg fluorocortisone daily results in significantly greater shock reversal and an improved rate of survival. These findings are at odds with the results of two earlier studies showing no benefit for the administration of large doses of methylprednisolone to a more heterogeneous group of patients with sepsis. Meta-analyses of the published trials of corticosteroid therapy concluded that in studies that used small steroid doses (i.e., 300 mg of hydrocortisone per day) over a long period of time (i.e., 7 days), rather than large doses over short periods of time used in earlier trials (i.e., 400–1200 mg of prednisolone over 24 hr), survival in septic shock was improved. It is not clear whether baseline cortisol levels, response to ACTH stimulation, peak concentrations, or a combination of these criteria is the best way to identify occult adrenal insufficiency. Consequently, some experts recommend hydrocortisone supplementation in patients in septic shock regardless of the ACTH response. The optimal duration of therapy is also unknown.

Recombinant Human Activated Protein C

Severe sepsis is associated with activation of the coagulation and fibrinolytic systems and inhibition of fibrinolysis, resulting in a procoagulant state. Recombinant human activated protein C [drotrecogin alfa (activated)] is a recombinant form of the endogenous anticoagulant molecule, protein C. Protein C is synthesized in the liver and activated through interactions with thrombomodulin on endothelial cells. In patients with severe sepsis, hepatic synthesis of protein C is reduced, whereas its activation is inhibited as a consequence of shedding of endothelial cell-bound thrombomodulin; therapy with the recombinant protein corrects this defect. Activated protein C inhibits the activities of coagulation factors V and VIII, and its binding to the protein C receptor is associated with suppression of proinflammatory gene transcription.

In a multicenter randomized trial of patients with severe sepsis or septic shock, administration of drotrecogin alfa (activated) resulted in a significant survival benefit, reducing 28-day mortality from 30.8% in patients receiving placebo to 24.7% in patients receiving activated protein C. The mortality benefit was experienced primarily by patients whose illness severity was greater, reflected in increased APACHE II scores or two or more failing organ systems at study entry. Serious bleeding occurred more often in treated patients (3.5 vs. 2.0%, $P = 0.06$). Drotrecogin alfa (activated) has been approved for patients with severe sepsis at high risk of death (as assessed by an APACHE II score $\geq$ 25 in the United States or two or more failing organ systems in Europe). Contraindications of the drug are related to increased risk of bleeding.

Drotrecogin alfa (activated) is expensive; however, its cost utility profile compares favorably with other life-saving interventions such as coronary thrombolysis. The cost per year of life gained is US $16,000 to $30,000 in Canada, 15,000 euros in Germany, and $27,000 in the United States, and the cost-effectiveness profile improves if only patients with greater severity (APACHE II score $\geq$ 25 or more than one organ failure) are considered.

Other Supportive Measures

The ICU support of the patient with severe sepsis does not differ materially from that of any other critically ill patient, and principles are discussed in greater detail throughout this book. Secondary injury can be minimized by established approaches, such as the use of a lung-protective ventilation strategy, maintenance of tight glucose control, adoption of a lower transfusion trigger, and early initiation of enteral feeding. Prophylactic strategies to prevent deep venous thrombosis, stress ulceration, and ventilator-associated pneumonia should be employed.

MEDIATOR-TARGETED THERAPY FOR SEPSIS: THE FUTURE

The specific treatment of sepsis is largely limited to interventions that can control the inciting infection—source control measures and specific antimicrobial therapy. Strategies that can modulate the injurious host inflammatory response have shown tremendous promise in animal models but limited efficacy in human studies. Only corticosteroids and activated protein C have shown sufficiently convincing evidence of utility that they have been widely adopted in clinical practice. Other approaches, such as the use of intravenous immunoglobulins, plasmapheresis, granulocyte colony-stimulating factor (G-CSF), or antithrombin III, have their proponents; however, their benefits are not sufficiently well established that they can be recommended at this time.

Approximately 80 randomized trials have been performed evaluating a variety of therapeutic strategies for sepsis. Although individual results have been disappointing, they have provided some measure of insight into the complexity of managing patients with sepsis and have indicated approaches that may prove useful in the future.

Endotoxin Neutralization

A variety of strategies to neutralize circulating endotoxin have been evaluated, including the administration of polyvalent anti-LPS antiserum; broadly cross-reactive neutralizing antibodies (HA-1A and E5); a recombinant fragment of bactericidal permeability-increasing protein (rBPI); a soluble form of the CD14 receptor; recombinant HDL; taurolidine, an amino acid with antiendotoxic properties; and dextran-conjugated polymyxin B, an antibiotic with antiendotoxic properties. Although improved survival was shown in early trials of polyvalent antiserum and HA-1A, this apparent benefit could not be replicated in later studies and these strategies were abandoned. rBPI reduced major morbidity in a study of pediatric patients with meningococcemia but did not significantly improve survival and so was not licensed for therapeutic use. Extracorporeal techniques of endotoxin removal have been evaluated and appear to show promise; however, they have not been subjected to the rigors of a multicenter, randomized controlled trial with survival status as the primary endpoint.

Several other antiendotoxin strategies are under evaluation, including a nontoxic lipid A analog that serves as a competitive antagonist of TLR4, recombinant alkaline phosphatase to enhance the degradation of endotoxin, and a lipid emulsion with endotoxin-neutralizing capability.

Neutralization of Tumor Necrosis Factor

Two strategies to neutralize the activity of TNF have been evaluated—the administration of a neutralizing antibody and the use of a receptor construct consisting of one of the two TNF receptors fused to the Fc portion of an immunoglobulin molecule (yielding a high-affinity, immunoglobulin-like molecule). A single study of 2634 patients with sepsis demonstrated that an anti-TNF antibody could improve 28-day survival; pooled data from all completed studies support this conclusion, although the absolute mortality reduction is only 3%. Although a number of these molecules have been approved for the treatment of inflammatory bowel disease or rheumatoid arthritis, they have not been approved for the treatment of sepsis.

Pentoxifylline, a phosphodiesterase inhibitor, reduces TNF biosynthesis, and small studies have suggested potential benefit in patients with sepsis. However, definitive studies have yet to be performed.

Blockade of Interleukin-1

The biologic activity of IL-1 in vivo is attenuated through the release of a protein known as the IL-1 receptor antagonist (IL-1ra), a cytokine that binds to the IL-1 receptor but does not transduce a signal, and thus serves as a competitive inhibitor of IL-1. IL-1ra is normally released after the release of IL-1 and in much larger concentrations. Recombinant IL-1ra has been evaluated in three randomized controlled trials; in aggregate, these demonstrate a statistically significant 5% improvement in survival. Development of IL-1ra as a therapeutic, however, was curtailed because the two large phase III trials were unable to independently show survival benefit.

Inhibition of Bioactive Lipids

A number of lipid mediators have been implicated in the pathogenesis of an acute inflammatory response and have been evaluated as potential therapeutic targets. Neutralization of platelet-activating factor (PAF) has been accomplished using synthetic receptor antagonists and a recombinant form of the enzyme, PAF acetylhydrolase, that degrades PAF. Although one small trial showed a mortality reduction for patients treated with PAF acetylhydrolase, the effect could not be replicated in a larger study. Aggregated data from studies of three different synthetic receptor antagonists show a statistically insignificant 3% improvement in survival.

A trial evaluating a synthetic inhibitor of phospholipase A2 failed to show a mortality benefit. Prostaglandin inhibition with ibuprofen was shown to reduce temperature and heart rate but not to improve survival.

Granulocyte Colony-Stimulating Factor

Animal studies have shown that recombinant G-CSF can attenuate inflammation as well as augment the number of circulating neutrophils and thus accelerate bacterial clearance. However, clinical trials of G-CSF in patients with community-acquired or nosocomial pneumonia failed to show improvements in clinically important outcomes.

Neutralization of Nitric Oxide

Nitric oxide is generated during the conversion of arginine to citrulline, catalyzed by the enzyme iNOS. iNOS can be competitively inhibited using a methylated arginine analog, L-N-monomethylarginine (L-NMMA). L-NMMA is a potent vasopressor by virtue of its ability to block the generation of NO. In an international multicenter trial, however, administration of L-NMMA resulted in a significant increase in mortality, and the strategy has been abandoned.

Anticoagulant Molecules

Although recombinant activated protein C was shown to improve survival in sepsis, trials of two other key endogenous anticoagulants—tissue factor pathway inhibitor (TFPI) and

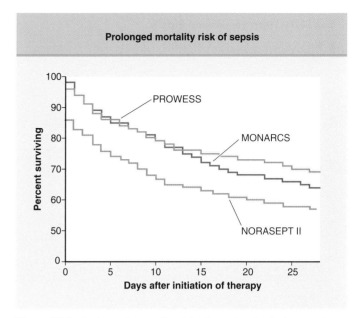

Figure 55.7. Prolonged mortality risk of sepsis. Survival curves for the placebo population in three large sepsis trials demonstrate that the mortality risk of sepsis arises early and remains elevated over a prolonged period. Natural history studies show that the elevated risk of acute mortality extends considerably beyond the 28-day time point traditionally used in clinical trials, and that survivors experience increased rates of mortality for years.

antithrombin III—failed to show a survival benefit for treated patients. A potentially detrimental interaction with heparin may have contributed to these disappointing results, and TFPI is undergoing evaluation in a separate study of patients with severe community-acquired pneumonia. Intriguingly, analysis of the placebo arms of large trials of all three anticoagulant strategies suggested that heparin alone may have salutary effects in patients with sepsis. This hypothesis has not been formally evaluated.

Large industry-sponsored trials of novel therapeutics for sepsis have generally yielded disappointing results, despite a strong biologic rationale and tremendous promise in preclinical studies. The reasons for this are many and include the challenges of identifying an appropriate at-risk population, stratifying that population to target those patients most likely to benefit, and detecting that benefit in a complex population exposed to multiple risk factors for morbidity and mortality.

PROGNOSIS

The mortality risk of sepsis is prolonged (Fig. 55.7). A fulminant and rapidly lethal course occurs rarely; typically, patients survive the initial resuscitative effort but die during the ensuing weeks to months of nonresolving organ dysfunction and supervening complications such as nosocomial infection. Ascribing a single cause of death is often difficult; rather, death occurs because of an acceptance of the improbability of survival and a conscious decision to limit life-sustaining therapy. Survivors of the acute illness experience significant longer term morbidity

Box 55.2 Controversies and Pitfalls

- Sepsis is not a single, well-defined disease but a syndrome with multiple causes and a highly variable clinical presentation. Successful treatment requires better stratification of patients into more pathologically homogeneous groups.
- The clinical manifestations of sepsis reflect alterations in host physiologic homeostasis and are not specific for the microbiology, or even the presence, of invasive infection.
- Rational management based on therapies that target the host-based changes in homeostasis that produce the syndrome are in their infancy, and strategies for optimal patient selection are still undefined.
- Successful management of a complex process such as sepsis is intrinsically multimodal, and the clinician must recognize that patient survival is maximized when all dimensions of this complex disorder are addressed.

in the form of neuromuscular weakness, physical limitations, and depression, and an elevated risk of dying that persists for years. Intensive rehabilitation and psychological support may be required.

Sepsis is a microcosm of the successes and limitations of contemporary critical care practice. Like other diseases that result in the need for prolonged intensive care, its morbidity is experienced not only by the patient but also by family and loved ones. Its profile as a modifiable cause of morbidity is much lower than that of cancer or cardiovascular disease, and its optimal management is correspondingly less well developed. However, improved insight into early resuscitation and an increased understanding of the pathogenetic mechanisms underlying the clinical syndrome promise to reduce the substantial toll of sepsis (Box 55.2).

SUGGESTED READING

Angus DC, Linde-Zwirble WI, Lidicker J, et al: Epidemiology of severe sepsis in the United States: Analysis of incidence, outcome, and associated costs of care. Crit Care Med 2006;29:1303–1310.

Annane D, Bellissant E, Bollaert PE, et al: Corticosteroids for severe sepsis and septic shock: A systematic review and meta-analysis. Br Med J 2004;329(7464):480.

Bernard GR, Vincent J-L, Laterre PF, et al: Efficacy and safety of recombinant human activated protein C for severe sepsis. N Engl J Med 2001;344:699–709.

Bone RC, Balk RA, Cerra FB, et al: Definitions for sepsis and organ failure and guidelines for the use of innovative therapies in sepsis. Chest 1992;101:1644–1655.

Dellinger RP, Carlet JM, Masur H, et al: Surviving sepsis campaign guidelines for management of severe sepsis and septic shock. Crit Care Med 2004;32:858–873.

Fink MP, Evans TW: Mechanisms of organ dysfunction in critical illness: Report from a Round Table Conference held in Brussels. Intensive Care Med 2002;28:369–375.

Hotchkiss RS, Karl IE: The pathophysiology and treatment of sepsis. N Engl J Med 2003;348:238–250.

Levy MM, Fink M, Marshall JC, et al: 2001 SCCM/ESICM/ACCP/ATS/SIS international sepsis definitions conference. Crit Care Med 2003;34:1250–1256.

Marshall JC: Such stuff as dreams are made on: Mediator-directed therapy in sepsis. Nature Drug Discovery 2003;2:391–405.

Marshall JC: Sepsis current status, future prospects. Curr Opin Crit Care 2004;10:250–264.

Minneci PC, Deans KJ, Banks SM, Eichacker PQ, Natanson C: Meta-analysis: The effect of steroids on survival and shock during sepsis depends on the dose. Ann Intern Med 2004;141:47–56.

Rangel-Frausto MS, Pittet D, Costigan M, et al: The natural history of the systemic inflammatory response syndrome (SIRS): A prospective study. JAMA 1995;273:117–123.

Rivers E, Nguyen B, Havstad S, et al: Early goal-directed therapy in the treatment of severe sepsis and septic shock. N Engl J Med. 2001;345:1368–1377.

Sands KE, Bates DW, Lanken PN, et al: Epidemiology of sepsis syndrome in 8 academic medical centers. JAMA 1997;278:234–240.

Van den Berghe G, Wouters P, Weekers F, et al: Intensive insulin therapy in the surgical intensive care unit. N Engl J Med 2001;345:1359–1367.

Chapter 56

Multitrauma, Including Peripheral Compartment Syndrome

Massimo Antonelli, Andrea Arcangeli, Maria Grazia Bocci, and Anselmo Caricato

Trauma is the leading cause of death and disability during the first four decades of life and the third leading cause of all deaths in Western countries, surpassed only by cancer and cardiovascular disease. Also, in underdeveloped countries, traumatic injury has become a significant and growing public health problem, in terms of both mortality and permanent disability. It has been predicted that by 2020, deaths from injury will probably increase to 8.4 million. Although injury is an uncommon cause of death in the elderly, death rates attributable to trauma in the elderly are greater than those in younger people. Moreover, disability caused by injury is often long-lasting. Thus, at all ages, trauma represents a major problem and a challenge for society. Early intensive care unit (ICU) therapy and interventions in patients suffering from severe trauma are characterized

by the stabilization of circulatory and respiratory function and control of hemorrhage.

EPIDEMIOLOGY

In 1990, approximately 5 million people died worldwide as a result of injuries. Annually in the United States, injury accounts for 37 million emergency department visits, 2.6 million hospital admissions, and approximately 600,000 people who are irreversibly disabled. Globally, it is estimated that millions suffer permanent disability each year, and it has been predicted that the total person-years of life lost will exceed worldwide the lives lost due to cardiovascular diseases and cancer combined.

Death from trauma occurs in a trimodal distribution, with three different peaks of mortality (Fig. 56.1). Immediate death usually occurs at the accident site or within the first hours. Injuries that cause death in this period include brain, heart, major vasculature, and high spinal cord injuries. In this period, victims are usually not able to reach the hospital alive. Nearly half of all traumatic deaths occur in this period. The second peak

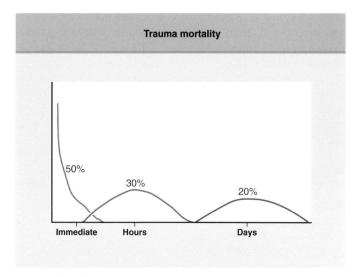

Figure 56.1. Trauma mortality. Trimodal distribution of trauma death. The first peak occurs immediately after an accident. The second peak occurs 1 to 4 hours later. The third peak occurs 1 to 5 weeks later.

occurs 1 to 4 hours after injury and accounts for 30% of deaths. During this period, the most common causes of death are severe hemorrhage, airway and breathing problems, and head injuries.

The primary goal of an efficient trauma care system should be to decrease the early deaths. The first hour after trauma is critical (the "golden hour") since the application of immediate and effective medical care may be crucial and life saving. Prevention of deaths at this stage represents the main goal of the trauma systems, and the application of Advanced Trauma Life Support (ATLS) protocols has been shown to effectively decrease the mortality rate. The first hour of care following trauma is characterized by rapid assessment and resuscitation, which are the fundamental principles of the ATLS program.

The third death peak, occurring at 1 to 5 weeks, is mainly due to sepsis and multisystem organ dysfunction. Early and best medical care applied during each phase may reduce the death rate.

ETIOLOGY

Trauma can vary from an isolated injury to multitrauma lesions. Traumatic injuries can be the consequence of exposure of the entire body to mechanical forces, heat, cold, electricity, chemical substances, and radiation. Usually, the resulting injuries can be classified as blunt or penetrating:

Blunt trauma is the result of the application of kinetic energy on a large area of the body. Usually, it is caused by concussion or deceleration. Damage can be related to tissue stretching, shearing, vascular disruption, and laceration caused by bone fractures. Blunt trauma is the result of vehicle accidents, falls, and blast injuries.

Penetrating traumas are usually a consequence of knife and gun wounds. They entail the application of forces restricted to a narrow area of the body that lead to a direct impact with lacerations and fractures.

In the case of gun wounds, the extent of damage is directly correlated to the kinetic energy of the missile at the site of impact. The major determinant of wounding potential is the speed of the bullet, which can exceed 2000 ft/sec. Weapons-related, hydrostatic pressure effect generates tissue compression and extensive damage with a cavity, whose hollow space can exceed up to 30 times the diameter of the missile. Knife injuries have no cavitation effect.

Injury patterns differ significantly between Europe and the United States. Road injuries with blunt trauma represent the great majority of deaths in Europe. In the United States, deaths related to penetrating injuries and gunshot wounds have exceeded those caused by motor vehicle accidents.

MANAGEMENT

In the late 1970s, the Committee on Trauma of the American College of Surgeons developed the standard of care for the acute trauma patient by introducing the ATLS course. ATLS protocols provide specific guidelines for the evaluation and treatment of trauma patients during the golden hour, when a rapid assessment and proper intervention can dramatically improve survival rates. These guidelines are used throughout the world. ATLS concepts imply several phases: primary survey, resuscitation, secondary survey, and definitive management. Primary survey includes the "ABCDE" approach. This abbreviation refers to

Airway with cervical spine stabilization
Breathing
Circulation and control of bleeding
Disability or neurological status
Exposure (undress) and environment (temperature control)

The patient should be rapidly monitored [electrocardiogram (ECG) and pulse oximetry]; urinary and gastric tubes should be placed; and instrumental examinations of the lateral cervical spine and chest and pelvic radiographs and sonography [focused assessment with sonography in trauma (FAST)] should be performed.

Once the primary survey has been completed, a secondary survey, which consists of a comprehensive physical examination, must be conducted. At this stage, specialized diagnostic tests, including additional radiographs, computed tomography (CT), and transesophageal echocardiography (TEE), may be performed. Once this first phase is completed, a definitive treatment should be instituted. Information obtained during the primary and secondary survey should lead to subsequent operative decisions.

The trauma patient must be continuously reevaluated during all these phases, and the primary survey should be performed several times, especially if the patient shows a deterioration of vital signs.

Primary Survey

The purpose of this phase is to seek and treat any life-threatening conditions. Each patient should be evaluated following the standardized sequence of actions listed previously.

Airway and Cervical Spine Control

The first priority in trauma management is to evaluate and secure the patient's airway while providing in-line cervical spine stabilization. An inspection for foreign bodies, facial fractures, and tracheal–laryngeal injuries should be rapidly performed to ensure the airway is clear and secure.

Airway and ventilatory management are summarized in Figure 56.2. Regardless of the type of injury, patients with a possible cervical spinal injury should be stabilized immediately with a semirigid cervical collar.

Breathing

Once airway patency is guaranteed, the next resuscitation step in the trauma patient is to evaluate breathing. The adequacy of breathing is assessed by physical examination of the chest along with continuous monitoring of pulse oximetry (SaO_2) (Fig. 56.3).

Life-threatening traumatic chest injuries should be detected and treated immediately. Common causes are pneumothorax (with or without tension), hemothorax, flail chest, pulmonary contusion, and rib fractures (Fig. 56.4).

Circulation and Control of Bleeding

Once airway and breathing status have been assessed, volume resuscitation and control of bleeding are mandatory. The most common cause of posttraumatic hypotension is hemorrhagic shock, which represents the first preventable cause of death

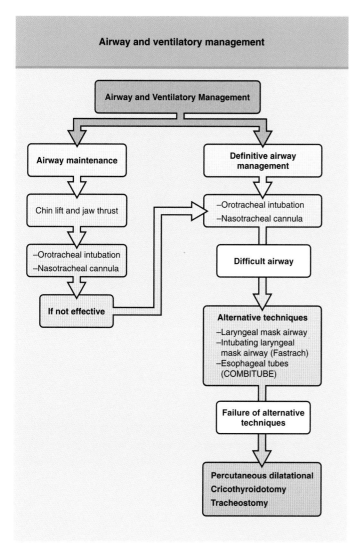

Figure 56.2. Airway and ventilatory management. The first approach may be conservative, but when ineffective or with a compromised level of consciousness, invasive airway management is mandatory.

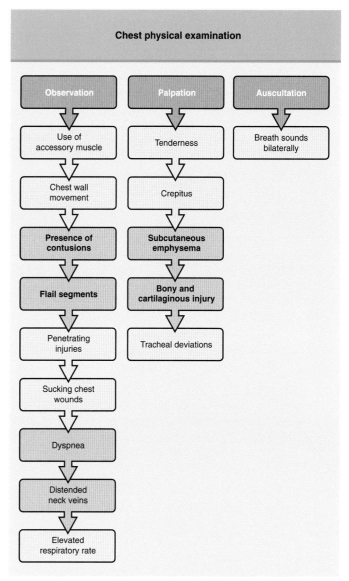

Figure 56.3. Phases of chest physical examination.

from injury. A classification system of the extent of hemorrhage has been developed by the American College of Surgeons based on patient hemodynamic status and clinical assessment (Table 56.1)

Treatment of hypovolemic shock aims to restore organ perfusion by fluid administration. Therefore, resuscitation of the trauma victim requires both blood and isotonic fluids (colloids and crystalloids) to reexpand the vascular spaces in order to ensure and maintain vital organ perfusion while awaiting definitive surgical hemostasis. During the past few years, a more discriminating approach to intravenous fluid infusion in trauma patients has evolved. The liberal use of fluid infusions for patients with presumed uncontrolled internal hemorrhage, such as that usually occurring after penetrating abdominal or thoracic injuries, is no longer advised. Attempts to restore blood pressure to normal values before the control of bleeding can exacerbate blood loss and reduce chances for survival. Ongoing

crystalloid resuscitation hemodilutes available red cells and clotting factors, inducing an increased risk of bleeding. Hypotension slows the blood flow within injured vessels, allowing for spontaneous hemostasis via the formation of platelet plugs. The restoration of a normal blood pressure risks dislodgement of the hemostatic clot. Therefore, "hypotensive resuscitation" should be the optimal way to manage victims with presumed anatomic sites of major bleeding from the thorax or abdomen, until surgical hemostasis is achieved. However, for patients with isolated limb and head injuries (blunt or penetrating), immediate support of blood pressure through fluid infusions should be considered because prolonged hypotension worsens neurological prognosis. Nonhypovolemic causes of shock may not be evident and should be taken into account in patients who do not respond to volume infusion after injury. Cardiogenic shock may be present in a patient with blunt myocardial injury, cardiac tam-

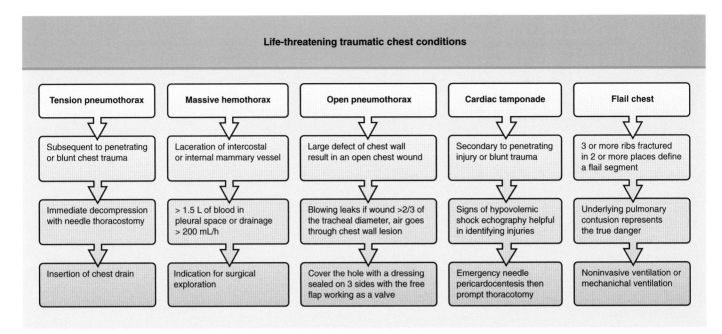

Figure 56.4. Life-threatening traumatic chest conditions. Therapeutic algorithm and main findings of principal severe chest injuries.

Table 56.1 Estimated Fluid and Blood Losses Based on Patient's Clinical Presentation[a]

	Class			
	I	**II**	**III**	**IV**
Blood loss (mL)	Up to 750	750–1500	1500–2000	>2000
Pulse rate (bpm)	<100	>100	>120	>140
Blood pressure	Normal	Normal	Decreased	Decreased
Respiratory rate (bpm)	14–20	20–30	30–40	>35
Urine output (mL/hr)	>30	20–30	5–15	Tiny
Mental status	Slightly anxious	Mildly anxious	Anxious and confused	Confused and lethargic

[a]Modified with permission from the American College of Surgeons Committee on Trauma: Advanced Trauma Life Support for Doctors: Student Course Manual, 6th ed. Chicago, American College of Surgeons, 1997, p 98.

Table 56.2 Grading the Serenity of Coma: The Glasgow Coma Scale[a]

Eye-opening response	**E**
Spontaneously	4
To voice	3
To pain	2
None	1
Best verbal response	**V**
Oriented	5
Confused	4
Inappropriate words	3
Incomprehensible sounds	2
None	1
Best motor response	**M**
Obeys commands	6
Localizes to a painful stimulus	5
Withdraws from a painful stimulus	4
Abnormal (spastic) flexion	3
Extension	2
None	1

[a]Score: E + V + M = 3–15.

ponade, or myocardial infarction, and it may require inotropic therapy. Neurogenic shock can intervene after spinal cord lesions. Tension pneumothorax may occur after blunt chest injury and requires immediate drainage. Other causes of shock in this setting include adrenal insufficiency and abdominal compartment syndrome.

Disability

At the end of "ABC," a brief neurological examination is performed to evaluate the level of consciousness and the integrity of brain function. This should be performed using the Glasgow Coma Score (Table 56.2).

Management should be directed toward rapid diagnosis and therapeutic intervention and to minimize the potential risk of secondary injury. Secondary brain injury can be generated by a combination of hypoxia, hypercarbia, hypotension, and raised intracranial pressure. Consequently, restoring respiratory and hemodynamic functions is paramount in the early management of the head-injured patient. Prompt endotracheal intubation and ventilation can effectively reduce the risk of hypoxia.

Box 56.1 Rewarming Techniques after Hypothermia

- **Passive external rewarming (mild hypothermia)**
  Insulation of the patient in a warm environment
  Application of warm, dry blankets
- **Active external rewarming (moderate or severe hypothermia)**
  Immersion, radiant heat, forced air, heating blankets
  Heated humidified air, warm intravenous fluids
  Gastric, peritoneal, or vescicle lavage
- **Extracorporeal warming (severe hypothermia)**
  Cardiopulmonary bypass, venovenous bypass, hemodialysis

Exposure and Environment

Injury often exposes the patient to the risk of hypothermia. Every patient should be undressed to permit a complete physical examination. However, during this procedure, heat loss may occur due to a cool environment in bad weather conditions. Hypothermia is detrimental to the coagulation system and can exacerbate blood loss. Therefore, a major effort must be made to maintain heat and prevent hypothermia (Box 56.1).

THORACIC TRAUMA

Thoracic injury accounts for 25% of all trauma deaths, with deaths on the scene caused by severe injuries of the great arteries, heart, and tracheobronchial tree. Thoracic trauma also accounts for an additional 25% of early, potentially preventable, deaths caused by cardiac tamponade, tension pneumothorax, or airway obstruction.

Once the primary survey and stabilization have been completed, a novel assessment should be done by careful physical examination and multiple diagnostic investigations.

Diagnostic Investigations

Chest x-ray is the most valuable imaging technique in both stable and unstable trauma patients and is essential for the evaluation of suspected chest trauma. Indeed, the most common injuries, including pneumothorax, hemothorax, or fractures of the ribs, clavicles, sternum, and thoracic spine, may be diagnosed by chest radiograph alone.

A widened mediastinum (>8 cm) may suggest rupture of the thoracic aorta and indicate that further investigations should be performed. Aortic rupture may also be evoked by the presence of obliteration of the aortic knob, deviation of the trachea to the right, the presence of pleural cap, fractures of the first and second ribs, elevation and rightward shift of the right mainstem bronchus, depression of the left mainstem bronchus, and deviation of the nasogastric tube. This last finding, if present, is the most reliable sign. Unfortunately, many cases of aortic disruption show normal radiographs. For this reason, the use of more sophisticated diagnostic methods, such as a helical chest CT or TEE, is mandatory to exclude a possible aortic injury.

Chest x-ray is also useful to diagnose rupture of the diaphragm; in this case, the presence of the nasogastric tube in the left thoracic cavity confirms the diagnosis. In the past few years, many centers have proposed dynamic helical chest CT as the first-line investigation for thoracic trauma. Using the proper software, it is possible to reconstruct three-dimensional CT images and investigate chest and neck great arteries by CT angiography. CT is more sensitive than standard chest x-ray for the diagnosis of a variety of thoracic injuries, such as atelectasis, pulmonary contusions, and diaphragmatic injuries. For this reason, whole body CT can be used as the primary evaluation of stable patients with blunt trauma.

TEE also may have a role in screening blunt chest trauma. It has the limitation of being operator dependent, but it is very useful for assessing injuries of the descending thoracic aorta and for evaluating cardiac structures and function. The application of percutaneous ultrasound to blunt chest trauma is more limited, but it can rapidly detect significant pericardial effusions due to cardiac injury. The early use of ultrasound by emergency medical staff for the evaluation of trauma has been recommended in the FAST protocol.

Management of Specific Injuries
Chest Wall
Rib fractures

Simple rib fractures are the most frequent injury of the thoracic cage. Anteroposterior compression of the chest produces fractures of the ribs on the lateral side, where they are bowed; a direct impact resulting in a rib fracture may cause dislocation of the fragments inward, causing pneumothorax or hemothorax. The presence of rib fractures indicates increased mortality and morbidity in older patients, and these rates rise with the number of ribs involved. Rib fractures can cause major physiologic harm, decreasing dynamic compliance, and coupled with lung contusion and chest pain can compromise ventilation and coughing, lead to atelectasis, and induce the onset of pneumonia. Fractures of the scapula and of the first and second ribs are potential markers of severe injuries, such as rupture of the great arteries, and prompt conventional or CT angiographic assessment is recommended.

Flail chest

Flail chest occurs when multiple rib fractures render the chest wall unstable. A flail chest usually develops when the victim has two sites of fractures in multiple adjacent ribs, resulting in a "floating" portion of the chest wall, paradoxically moving in and out during respiration. The physiopathologic effects of flail chest are an important decrease in vital capacity and functional residual capacity, always associated with pulmonary contusion and often with hemorrhage or edema. The basis of treatment is adequate pain relief, clearance of pulmonary secretions, and the eventual use of invasive or noninvasive mechanical ventilation.

Flail chest patients without respiratory impairment generally have a favorable evolution without ventilatory assistance. Intubation and ventilator support are often required for all patients with large flail segments and for any patient with underlying acute or chronic lung disease. Aggressive pulmonary physiotherapy with suctioning, incentive spirometry, early mobilization, and humidification is fundamental for all patients. Noninvasive ventilation, postural drainage, and fiberoptic bronchoscopy to treat atelectasis are indicated.

Pleural Space
Pneumothorax

Pneumothorax can be defined as the presence of air within the pleural cavity and is usually due to blunt rupture of the lung surface or to penetrating thoracic injuries. Accumulation of air within the pleural space may compromise respiration by interfering with lung expansion. Jugular vein distention, decreased unilateral breath sounds, shortness of breath, and hyperresonance at the percussion of the chest are the most common signs. Diagnosis is confirmed by chest x-ray, and treatment consists of the insertion of a tube in the chest to drain the air from the pleural cavity.

Tension pneumothorax

This injury can occur when an injured piece of tissue acts as a flap, creating a one-way valve mechanism: Air can enter but not leave the pleural space. Intrapleural pressure increases, inducing compression of mediastinal structures, a decrease in venous return, and significant hemodynamic instability. Hallmarks include decreased breath sounds on the affected side, deviation of the trachea away from the injured side, and marked hypotension. The diagnosis is generally clinical. Management consists of rapid evacuation of the air collected within the pleural space by the insertion of a chest tube. In emergency situations, this can be effectively done by needle decompression at the second intercostal space in the midclavicular line, before definitive drainage.

Open pneumothorax

Open pneumothorax usually results from a large defect of the chest wall that creates a communication between the pleural space and external environment. When the size of the lesion exceeds by two thirds the size of the trachea, air will flow preferentially through the lower resistance injured tract. This can severely affect oxygenation and ventilation. The affected lung is exposed to atmospheric pressure and collapses with a mediastinal shift toward the healthy side. The patient becomes cyanotic with serious respiratory distress due to the severe venoarterial shunting and ventilation–perfusion inequality.

The first-line treatment consists of the application of a sterile occlusive dressing firmly secured at three sites, with the fourth left free to act as a flapping, one-way valve. The second step consists of placing a chest tube distant from the wounded part. If needed, the patient can be intubated, starting positive pressure ventilation. Surgical repair is required as soon as possible.

Hemothorax

Bleeding into the pleural cavity causes a hemothorax and may induce respiratory failure and circulatory collapse with impairment of oxygenation and ventilation. Sources of bleeding include lung parenchyma, great arteries, and chest wall vessels such as the intercostal artery. After blunt trauma, the main causes of bleeding are direct lung injury and laceration of the intercostal vessels. Bleeding from these sources is usually moderate and self-limiting when the pleural space is drained. If the initial volume of blood is less than 1000 mL, the patient should be observed. If significant bleeding continues (>200 mL/hr), thoracoscopy or thoracotomy is recommended. Massive hemothorax is defined as a blood loss of more than 1500 mL in the thoracic cavity. It is generally observed after penetrating injury that has damaged large vessels. The presentation is characterized by circulatory shock associated with the absence of breath sounds at the affected side(s). Dullness to percussion may also be present, although this finding is difficult to elicit in most resuscitation

settings. A 1500- to 2000-mL hemothorax with persistent bleeding of more than 100 to 200 mL/hr is a stringent indication for emergency thoracotomy or thoracoscopy.

Lung

Pulmonary contusion

Pulmonary contusion usually derives from a strong impact against the chest that typically causes multiple fractures and a "missile blast effect." Histologically, a pulmonary contusion is depicted by intra-alveolar edema, hemorrhage, and inflammation, whose effect is ventilation–perfusion mismatching, increased physiologic dead space, and decreased pulmonary compliance. Hypoxemia and impaired ventilation frequently ensue. The chest x-ray shows opacity in the peripheral lung near to the injured chest wall. The chest x-ray may holdup 12 to 24 hours behind the clinical extent of the contusion. Blood gases may worsen for 2 or 3 days after trauma if edema increases in the lung. Stiffness of the lung causes dyspnea and elevated respiratory rate. Patients who cannot adequately maintain oxygenation and ventilation can be treated with noninvasive ventilation (NIV). If NIV is unsuccessful, it can be replaced with endotracheal intubation and controlled mechanical ventilation.

Tracheobronchial tree

Tracheal and tracheobronchial tree ruptures are unusual. They can be secondary to blunt or penetrating injury. The intimate anatomical relationship of the trachea with the great arteries, lungs, and heart explains the high incidence of serious injuries associated with blunt and penetrating trauma. The usual signs of a suspected tracheobronchial disruption are hemoptysis, dyspnea, and subcutaneous and mediastinal emphysema. The hallmark sign is the presence of a thoracostomic tube that fails to reexpand the lung, showing large and persistent air leak. The chest x-ray demonstrates pneumothorax, pleural effusion, pneumomediastinum, or subcutaneous emphysema. In the absence of indications for immediate thoracostomy, bronchoscopy represents the most reliable diagnostic tool and should be immediately carried out. The finding of a large tear (more than one third of the bronchial lumen) indicates prompt thoracotomy to attempt primary repair.

Heart

Blunt cardiac injury

Contusion of the myocardium results from the direct blunt insult to the anterior portion of the thorax with injury of the underlying myocardium. Major sequelae include regional wall motion abnormalities, pericardial effusion, and depression of cardiac function, sometimes in association with myocardial infarction and arrhythmia. In rare cases, intracardiac lesions such as ventricular or valvular rupture may be observed. The diagnosis of myocardial contusion may be difficult and implies ECG monitoring to detect the occurrence of arrhythmias, the measurement of cardiac enzymes to reveal myocardial injury, and the use of ultrasound to identify wall motion abnormalities or intracardiac injury. The current treatment is conservative and often similar to the management of myocardial infarction.

Traumatic aortic rupture

Rupture of the thoracic aorta is the most common cause of sudden death in blunt chest trauma and after crashes. Victims of penetrating aortic injuries usually die at the scene of trauma. Blunt traumatic tear of the aorta is typically seen when the mechanism of injury entails a high-impact collision with rapid deceleration, resulting in differential forces on the descending aorta between fixed and more mobile portions. Thus, the most common site of injury is located where the aorta is fixed by the ligamentum arteriosum.

In those patients who survive, the injury induces a tear of the intima with entrapment of the blood between the adventitia and the surrounding tissues. The result is a periaortic hematoma, often without active bleeding. The high diagnostic suspicion is basically founded on the mechanism of injury. The hallmark sign is a mediastinum enlargement on chest x-ray, which is the result of an adventitial hematoma. Patients with strong suspicion must be screened by TEE and CT scan. The treatment is immediate surgery. In patients with severe associated injuries, surgical repair may be delayed; in these cases, administration of beta blockers may decrease the risk of rupture. Endovascular techniques have been developed for the treatment of select cases. These techniques imply the percutaneous placement of intraluminal stents as an alternative to operative graft replacement.

Esophageal injuries

Traumatic rupture of the esophagus is very rare. Most injuries are related to penetrating wounds. Blunt rupture of the esophagus is usually quite uncommon. Esophageal trauma may be lethal if not recognized early because leakage of saliva, gastroesophageal secretions, and material into the thoracic cage, bronchial tree, and mediastinum may generate empyema pneumonia or mediastinitis. Clinically, the patient may complain of acute pain in the epigastrium with thoracic or abdominal irradiation; later, signs of sepsis from mediastinal and pleural contamination can occur. Chest radiographs may show widening of the mediastinum, subcutaneous emphysema, pneumothorax, hydrothorax, or a combination. Usually, the lower esophagus is affected and the rupture located into the left pleural cavity. The diagnosis can be confirmed by esophagoscopic visualization of an actual laceration or blood localized in the esophagus. Early surgical treatment is essential to minimize contamination of the mediastinum and pleura. Surgical repair and diversion are both possible; the choice depends on the esophageal conditions, the degree of contamination, and the time elapsed between injury and surgery.

Diaphragmatic injuries

Diaphragmatic ruptures are generally difficult to identify and are commonly observed on the left side because the right diaphragm is protected by the liver. The most common etiology of diaphragmatic injuries is a penetrating trauma that usually produces small perforations.

The defects observed in blunt trauma are rare, but generally serious, and larger, and they often result in an abrupt herniation of the abdominal contents related to the rapid increase in intraabdominal pressure. The stomach is the most common viscus involved, and nasogastric tube positioning may help the diagnosis by chest x-ray alone. The chest radiograph usually shows an opacity with air–fluid levels and mediastinal shift. CT is often nondiagnostic. If the insertion of a chest tube is needed, great attention is necessary to prevent the accidental perforation of the migrated intraabdominal organs. Possible complications

are related to strangulation and incarceration of herniated viscera that can be associated with high mortality. Treatment involves laparotomy for reduction of the herniated contents and diaphragm repair.

ABDOMINAL TRAUMA

Abdominal trauma is one of the primary causes of morbidity and mortality among multitrauma victims and should always be taken into account. Identification of serious intraabdominal pathology is often extremely difficult during the initial assessment. Signs suggestive of abdominal injuries include abrasion, contusion, abdominal pain and tenderness, and absent bowel sounds. Unfortunately, these findings are often absent and may be inaccurate in the presence of comorbid conditions such as mental obtundation, head trauma, shock, or intoxication. The etiology of abdominal trauma is of great importance in determining the correct diagnostic procedures. Penetrating injuries frequently require immediate surgical intervention.

Diagnostic Investigations
Diagnostic Peritoneal Lavage
Diagnostic peritoneal lavage (DPL) is a rapid and accurate diagnostic procedure that identifies the presence of intraabdominal bleeding after trauma and can be performed in the emergency room. The preferred technique implies an open or semiopen approach through the infraumbilical line. The peritoneum is incised under direct vision and a catheter for peritoneal dialysis is directed into the pelvis. In the unstable patient, abdominal surgical exploration is always indicated if 10 mL of blood or more is aspirated upon insertion. If no blood is drawn, infusion of 1 liter of normal saline into the peritoneum is recommended, followed by gravitational drainage and laboratory analysis of the collected fluid.

The finding of more than 100,000 red blood cells/mm^3 or more than 500 white blood cells/mm^3 is considered a positive test. DPL can be easily and rapidly performed by expert hands during resuscitation maneuvers in the emergency room. The sensitivity of this test is high, but it does not offer information on retroperitoneum status. False-positive results may occur in the presence of pelvis fractures, which may result in unnecessary laparatomies. For these reasons, patients who are hemodynamically stable can be better investigated by abdominal CT scan.

CT Scan
CT scan offers the best detailed images of traumatic pathology and may clarify whether a surgical operation is needed. CT scan can reveal the presence of blood in the peritoneal cavity or injuries of the abdominal organs and retroperitoneum. CT is also very useful for the diagnosis of pelvic fractures. Unfortunately, CT scan may miss diaphragmatic injuries and perforations of the gastrointestinal tract. Pancreatic injuries may not be identified on initial CT scans but are frequently found on follow-up of high-risk patients. The primary advantage of CT scanning is its high specificity for solid organ injuries. Disadvantages include the need to move the patient from the emergency area and the longer time required to perform the exam compared to FAST or DPL. As a consequence, only hemodynamically stable patients should be transported to the CT scanner. With the widespread diffusion of spiral CT scanners, the total body

examination has become faster and patients with multiple injuries can now be completely assessed in a short period of time.

FAST

Abdominal sonography is rapidly becoming the first-choice diagnostic procedure for early and rapid detection of intraabdominal bleeding. A complete FAST examination allows the visualization of Morrison's pouch (perihepatic), the perisplenic region, the pelvis (pouch of Douglas), and the pericardium (Fig. 56.5). Free fluid, generally assumed to be blood in the setting of abdominal trauma, appears as a black stripe. Sensitivity and specificity of FAST range between 85% and 95%. The high sensitivity, specificity, and accuracy of this approach justify immediate surgical intervention if abdominal free fluid is detected. In select stable cases, a CT scan may improve diagnostic accuracy. FAST is specifically indicated in patients with penetrating precordial wounds and in patients with blunt abdominal trauma and

hypotension. In these situations, the correct indication for early surgical intervention improves survival.

FAST is noninvasive and can be easily performed during resuscitation. The apparatus is compact and portable, and the exam can be repeated several times in any setting, if necessary.

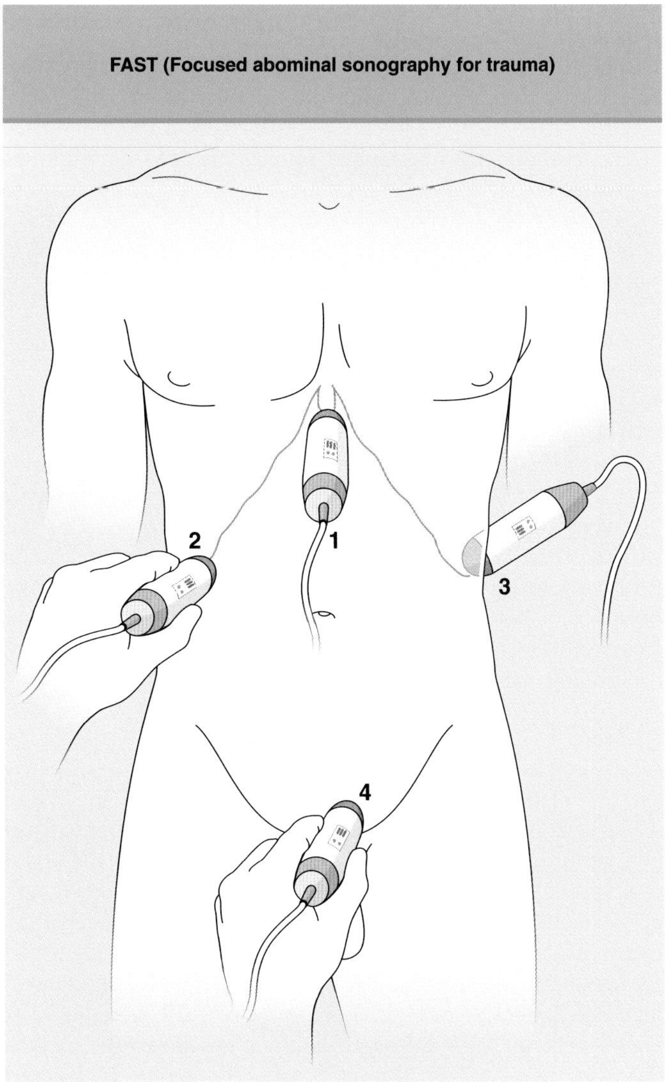

Special Procedures

Nonoperative treatment can be the first-line intervention for stable patients with low- or medium-grade liver, spleen, and kidney injuries. CT scan upon admission can identify these patients. The initial selective nonoperative management of blunt and penetrating abdominal trauma requires the patient to be located in an area where continuous evaluation and monitoring are possible and the eventual transfer to the operating theater is feasible and fast.

Damage control surgery (DCS) is an accepted method of minimal surgical management of unstable trauma patients with severe disorders (coagulopathy, hypotension, acidosis, poor response to fluid loading, and large blood losses). DCS consists of a three-phase approach:

- An initial, nondefinitive, surgical treatment for the control of visceral lesions, hemorrhage, and vascular injuries with simple temporary measures, including stapler intestinal sutures without anastomosis, sponge packing, and vascular shunts using plastic tubes
- A resuscitation phase in the intensive care setting
- A final definitive surgical intervention once homeostasis is restored

DCS is improving overall survival rates and is gaining acceptance among surgeons.

Special Problems

Pelvic Fractures

Pelvic fractures account for approximately 3% of all skeletal injuries. Mortality rates range from 5% to 20%, but open pelvic fractures may have a mortality rate of approximately 50%. Significant forces are required to produce a severe pelvic fracture; vast soft tissue and vessels injuries are often concomitant; and most patients have associated abdominal, thoracic, and head lesions. Hemorrhage is the principal life-threatening complication of pelvic trauma. Despite continuous and prolonged bleeding that is characteristic of retroperitoneal bleeding, severe hemorrhages are rare. Signs of retroperitoneal hematoma are variable and nonspecific.

Pelvic fractures are identified by clinical signs that include evidence of ecchymosis and contusion, limb shortening, and perineal wounds. Extensive ecchymosis of the external genital organs is specific but sometimes absent. Urethra (especially in men), bladder, and rectum are the structures most frequently involved in this kind of trauma. The incidence of urological lesions is 7%. Hematuria is considered the most important clinical sign following pelvic trauma and clinical investigations for urological lesions should be performed. Pain or instability revealed at anteroposterior (pubis and sacrum) or lateral compression (iliac wings) may induce suspicion of anorectal and vaginal lacerations, and rectal examination is mandatory. Diagnosis can be confirmed with an anteroposterior pelvis radiograph. More precise radiological information can be obtained by inlet and outlet views and CT scan.

Figure 56.5. FAST. Schematic diagram of the areas imaged by FAST. A complete FAST examination allows visualization of the pericardium (1), Morrison's pouch (perihepatic) (2), the perisplenic region (3), and the pelvis (pouch of Douglas) (4).

Hemodynamic instability is present in 60% of patients presenting with pelvic trauma. The management of these cases is difficult because hemorrhage may originate from fractures, damaged pelvic blood vessels, and abdominal or thoracic trauma. A complete patient evaluation to exclude extrapelvic source of bleeding should be performed. Once the presence of blood loss from pelvic injuries is confirmed, rapid hemostasis should be obtained. Venous hemorrhage is responsible for most of the pelvic bleeding. Immediate pelvic stabilization with an external fixation device can be applied, stabilizing the pelvic ring and interrupting venous bleeding in most cases. If stabilization is unsuccessful in controlling the hemorrhage, angiography must be performed to allow the localization of bleeding vessels and their embolization. If the bleeding point is identified, a high success rate can be achieved, but unsuccessful embolization may require hypogastric artery ligation.

Peripheral Compartment Syndrome

Acute compartment syndrome is an important clinical entity requiring prompt diagnosis and treatment. It can be observed when the interstitial pressure inside a myofascial compartment increases, equalizing the capillary perfusion pressure and compromising tissue flow. If this situation is not resolved, tissue necrosis with permanent functional impairment occurs, and renal failure and death are possible.

The underlying reason for the increase in interstitial pressure is an increased fluid content or a decreased compartment size. Peripheral compartment syndrome can localize wherever an anatomical compartment is possible: hand, forearm, upper arm, abdomen, buttock, and entire lower extremity. Almost any injury can cause this syndrome, including injury resulting from vigorous exercise (Box 56.2). The patient complains of severe pain, tenderness, hypoesthesia, and weakness, and the compartment is under tension on palpation. Paralysis and absence of pulse are late findings occurring with massive neuromuscular damage. The measurement of pressures by a transducer connected to a needle or a catheter introduced into the compartment is the gold standard for the diagnosis. If the compartment pressure is higher than 40 mm Hg, fasciotomy is mandatory. Patients with a pressure of approximately 30 mm Hg should be carefully observed and fasciotomy should be performed if this value persists for more than 6 hours. Fasciotomy consists of large longitudinal incisions of the affected compartments. Complications of the procedure include wound infections. In some cases, early administration of mannitol may contribute to relieve compartment pressure. Hyperbaric oxygen

---

Box 56.2 Etiologies of Compartment Syndrome

Tibial fractures
Reperfusion of acutely ischemic limbs
Muscle contusion
Intensive muscle use (tetany, strenuous exercise, seizures)
Tear of gastrocnemius muscle
Hemorrhage (exp. in anticoagulation therapy)
Burns
Malignant hyperthermia
Crush injuries
Extensive deep venous thrombosis
Electrical injury
Snakebite
Tourniquet application
Malignant neuroleptic syndrome
Malfunction of automated blood pressure cuff

---

has been advocated as adjunctive therapy and has been shown to be beneficial.

SUGGESTED READING

American College of Surgeons Committee on Trauma: Advanced Trauma Life Support for Doctors. Student Course Manual, 6th ed. Chicago: American College of Surgeons, 1997.

Bickell WH, Wall MJ, Pepe PE, et al: Immediate versus delayed fluid resuscitation for hypotensive patients with penetrating torso injuries. N Engl J Med 1994;331:1105–1109.

Blow O, Magliore L, Claridge JA, et al: The golden hour and the silver day: Detection and correction of occult hypoperfusion within 24 hours improves outcome from major trauma. J Trauma 1999;47:964–969.

FAST Consensus Conference Committee: Focused assessment with sonography for trauma (FAST): Results from an international consensus conference. J Trauma 1999;46:466–472.

Feliciano DV, Rozycki GS: Advances in the diagnosis and treatment of thoracic trauma. Surg Clin North Am 1999;79:1417–1429.

Gentilello LM: Advances in the management of hypothermia. Surg Clin North Am 1995;75:243–256.

Pepe PE: Current issues in resuscitative trauma management: An overview. Curr Opin Crit Care 2001;7:409–412.

Roberts I, Evans P, Bunn F, et al: Is the normalisation of blood pressure in bleeding trauma patients harmful? Lancet 2001;357:385–387.

Shapiro MB, Jenkins DH, Schwab CW, Rotondo MF: Damage control: Collective review. J Trauma 2000;49:969–978.

Whitesides TE, Heckman MM: Acute compartment syndrome: Update on diagnosis and treatment. J Am Acad Orthop Surg 1996;4:209.

Chapter 57

Burns, Inhalation, and Electrical Injuries

Ilkka Parviainen

KEY POINTS

- The main phases of burn care are initial evaluation and resuscitation, early wound excision and closure, and rehabilitation and reconstruction.
- Intensive care constitutes a significant part of the treatment and supports the recovery. The main threat during intensive care is burn wound sepsis, which may contribute to multiple organ dysfunction and death.
- After initial evaluation, the main focus of treatment is fluid resuscitation during the first and second days. The greatest amount of fluids is usually needed during the first 8 to 12 hours.
- Topical wound care decreases vapor loss and prevents desiccation and bacterial growth.
- Seventy percent of pediatric burns are caused by scalding.
- Inhalation injury from burns may lead to pulmonary edema, bronchospasm, and ventilation-perfusion mismatch, which in turn can lead to increased airway pressure, decreased compliance, and arterial hypoxemia.
- Electricity can cause injury in several ways, and some injuries may remain hidden. Particular attention must be paid to patients exposed to high-voltage injury, and deep electrical injuries to vital organs should be excluded.

burn wound sepsis, which may contribute to multiple organ dysfunction and death.

Epidemiology, Risk Factors, and Pathophysiology

In the United States, approximately 1.25 million people are burned, 50,000 are hospitalized, and 5500 die annually. In Europe, the incidence of burns admitted to hospitals is estimated to be 13 to 31 per 100,000 inhabitants annually. Seventy-five percent of hospitalized patients have burns over less than 10% of the body-surface area. Seventy percent of pediatric burns are caused by scalding. Children ages 0 to 4 years have the highest population-based scald and hot-object contact injury rate of all age groups, with an average annual incidence rate of about 36 per 10,000. Young adults are the most likely to be injured by flame and fire-related causes secondary to open fires. Terrorist attacks, natural disasters, and military operations are threats that may predispose large numbers of patients to burns.

Burn injury induces total or partial destruction of skin and, possibly, of underlying tissues. Burn injury of significant body-surface area and depth results in systemic responses (Fig. 57.2). Immediately after a burn, various inflammatory mediators (cytokines, kinins, histamine, thromboxane, free radicals) are released locally from platelets, macrophages, and leukocytes. In severe burns, affecting more than 15% to 20% of the body-surface area, the local injury triggers the release of circulating

BURNS

Over the past decades burn care has developed, leading to improved survival and long-term outcome. In-hospital mortality rates have declined to less than 5% in patients who are treated in specialized burn centers. However, mortality increases with increased percentage of burned body-surface area, increased age, and inhalation injury. Treatment of severely burned patients is complex and requires the expertise of an experienced multidisciplinary team. The American Burn Association has recommendations for who should be treated in burn units (Box 57.1). Treatment of patients in burn centers is associated with shortened length of hospital stay, better outcome, better quality of life, and lower costs. The main phases of burn care are initial evaluation and resuscitation, early wound excision and closure, and rehabilitation and reconstruction. Intensive care constitutes a significant part of the treatment and supports the recovery postburn (Fig. 57.1). The main threat during intensive care is

---

Box 57.1 Burn Unit Referral Criteria (American Burn Association)

1. Partial thickness burns greater than 10% of total body surface
2. Burns that involve the face, hands, feet, genitalia, perineum, or major joints
3. Third-degree burns in any age group
4. Electrical burns, including lightning injury
5. Chemical burns
6. Inhalation injury
7. Burn injury in patients with preexisting medical disorders that could complicate management, prolong recovery, or affect mortality
8. Any patient with burns and concomitant trauma
9. Burned children in hospitals without qualified personnel or equipment for the care of children
10. Burn injury in patients who will require special social, emotional, or long-term rehabilitative intervention

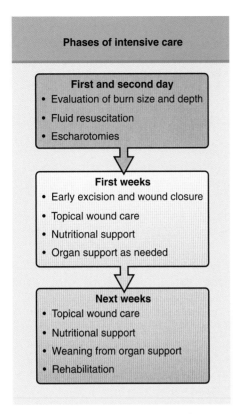

Figure 57.1 Phases of intensive care. Phases of treatment of a severe burn patient during intensive care.

inflammatory mediators, such as tumor necrosis factor α and different interleukins, leading to both local and systemic inflammatory responses. The systemic inflammatory response contributes to "burn shock," characterized by increased microvascular permeability, hypovolemia, and even myocardial dysfunction. Hypovolemia is a consequence of the fluid leakage from intravascular to extravascular compartments. When burns are treated aggressively, generalized burn edema is inevitable. Edema formation is most rapid during the first 6 to 8 hours and continues in major burns for 24 to 48 hours. If treatment of hypovolemia is insufficient or delayed, the risks of cardiovascular collapse and remote organ dysfunctions increase. The existence of myocardial dysfunction in burn patients is controversial. In a recent study, hypovolemia associated with persisting capillary leakage, rather than myocardial depression, affected myocardial performance during the early postburn period, as assessed by pulmonary artery catheter and echocardiography. After burn shock, a hyperdynamic cardiovascular response develops, characterized by high cardiac output and low systemic vascular resistance.

Circulating mediators, catecholamines, cortisol, possible bacterial byproducts from the gastrointestinal tract and wounds, and heat loss across burn wounds contribute also to a hypermetabolic state. In addition, there is accompanying muscle catabolism in response to injury. Energy expenditure increases markedly, and optimal nutritional support is required from the beginning of a burn injury to minimize catabolism.

Diagnosis

Initial Evaluation and Resuscitation

Initially, all severely burned patients should be evaluated as multiple trauma patients and each organ system should be studied. Airway security is the first priority, especially in patients with burns of the face and neck region. If delayed, intubation may be difficult or impossible as a result of marked edema. A burn patient with the risk of a compromised airway must be intubated before transport to another hospital. For fluid resuscitation, adequate vascular access is required. Peripheral vascular access may be difficult if deep burns are located in extremities, and central venous access may be the only route possible. An unburned area is preferable when choosing central venous access, but sometimes a central venous catheter must be inserted through the burned area. In unconscious patients, the possibility of carbon monoxide poisoning has to be kept in mind and the concentration of carboxyhemoglobin has to be measured. Patients with serious carbon monoxide poisoning are at risk for neurologic sequelae, and hyperbaric oxygen treatment can be considered. Tetanus prophylaxis is indicated in all patients with burns of greater than 10% of the total body surface area.

Evaluation of Burn Size and Depth

In major burns, loose necrotic skin parts should be removed and the burned area cleaned in a shower, followed by initial evaluation of the burned area. Wallace's "rule of nine" is a useful guide to evaluate the extent of the burn area in adults. Anatomic regions represent 9% of the total body surface area or a multiple thereof: head plus neck, and each arm, 9%; anterior trunk, posterior trunk, and each leg, 18% (Fig. 57.3). In children, body proportions are different from those of adults; an age-adjusted

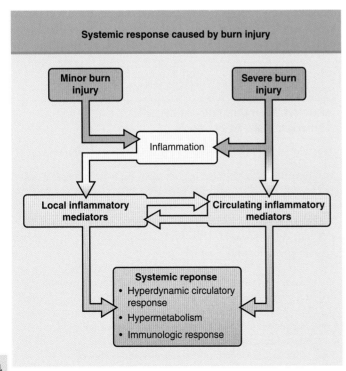

Figure 57.2 Systemic response caused by burn injury.

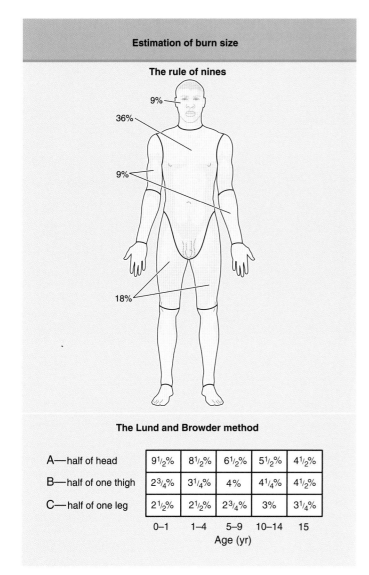

Figure 57.3 Estimation of burn size. Estimation of burn size, using the rule of nines *(top)* and the Lund and Browder method *(bottom)*.

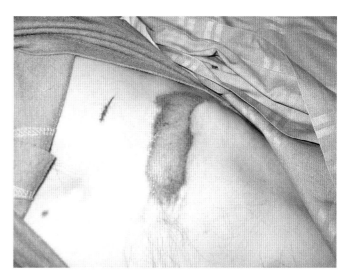

Figure 57.4 Superficial second-degree burn.

estimate can be made using the Lund and Browder chart (see Fig. 57.3). The initial assessment remains a general approximation and predicts fluid resuscitation requirements. The extent of deep burn injury may increase during the first days. Usually, depth of burns is underestimated initially. First-degree injury involves only the epidermis, leading to erythema and pain. Second-degree burns are categorized as superficial (Fig. 57.4) and deep burns (Fig. 57.5). In superficial injuries, all of the epidermis and a superficial part of the dermis are destroyed and are painful. In second-degree deep burns, most of the dermis is destroyed. Third-degree burns involve the entire thickness of the skin and require excision and grafting (Fig. 57.6). Fourth-degree injury extends to deep structures, such as tendon, muscle, and bone. Circumferential burns should be noted because soft-tissue edema within nonelastic compartments may compromise tissue perfusion. Extremities at risk should be examined serially, focusing on temperature, vessel pulsations, capillary refill, voluntary motion, and pain. If necessary, escharotomies can be performed at the bedside (Fig. 57.7). If deep cir-

cumferential burns are located in the thoracic or abdominal region, compartment syndrome may develop and worsen thoracic wall compliance, disturb ventilatory treatment, and decrease perfusion of abdominal organs. In these cases, escharotomies are required.

Treatment
Fluid Resuscitation
In patients with burns of more than 15% to 20% of the body surface, increased systemic capillary permeability leads to capillary leak and hypovolemia. Increased burn area, delay in fluid resuscitation, and inhalation injury increase fluid leak and requirements for fluids. Capillary leak peaks about 6 to 12 hours postburn and typically decreases 24 to 48 hours postburn. Therefore, the greatest amount of fluids is usually needed during the first 8 to 12 hours. The aim of fluid resuscitation is to preserve and ensure sufficient tissue perfusion.

Several fluid resuscitation formulas have been used (Table 57.1), but no formula accurately predicts the need for fluids. These formulas can be used initially to approximate the amount

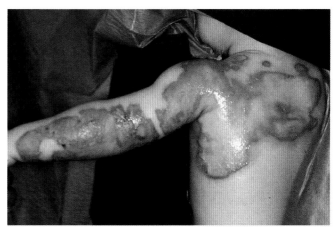

Figure 57.5 Deep second-degree burn.

Other Critical Care Problems

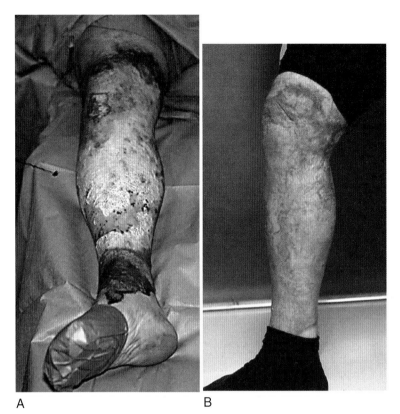

A   B

of fluids needed, but serial evaluations of volume status are necessary at the bedside in order to titrate fluid resuscitation. In clinical practice, titrating fluid resuscitation is seeking to avoid both hypovolemia (risk of hypoperfusion) and overresuscitation (which leads to massive tissue edema). The Parkland formula is mostly used to guide initial evaluation. The formula recommends isotonic crystalloid 4 mL/kg/% burn during the first 24 hours and one half of the total volume during the first 8 hours. Owing to capillary leak, the intravascular volume effect of colloids is not better than that of crystalloids, and colloids are therefore not recommended during the first 12 to 24 hours. Synthetic colloids are recommended after 12 to 24 hours. The use

of albumin has been challenged and is not recommended in fluid resuscitation. If initial fluid requirements are exceptionally high, slightly hypertonic crystalloids (sodium concentration 200 to 320 mmol/L) can be used. During the second day postburn, fluid requirements are usually approximately half of the requirements of the first 24 hours.

The response to fluid resuscitation is assessed by clinical and laboratory examinations (Box 57.2). Approved clinical end points are mean arterial pressure over 60 to 65 mm Hg, warm periphery and normal capillary refill, and urine output of 0.5 to 1 mL/kg/hr. Normal base deficit and lactate concentration suggest sufficient tissue perfusion. If the response to fluid

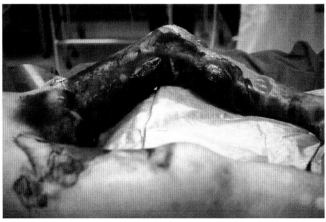
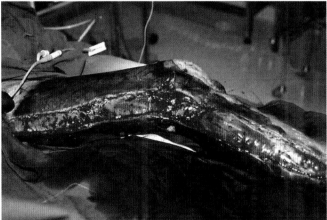

A   B

Figure 57.7 Insufficient *(A)* and sufficient *(B)* escharotomy of limb.

Table 57.1 Fluid Resuscitation Formulas (First 24 Hours)	
Adults	**Recommendations**
Parkland formula	Lactated Ringer's 4 mL/kg/% burn/24 hr
	Half of total amount in first 8 hr, second half in the next 16 hr
Modified Brooke formula	Lactated Ringer's 2 mL/kg/% burn/24 hr
Hypertonic saline	Fluid containing 250–310 mmol Na/L (risk for hypernatremia)
Children	**Recommendations**
Galveston formula	Lactated Ringer's 5000 mL/m^2 burn + 2000 mL/m^2 TBSA
	Half of total amount in first 8 hr, second half in the next 16 hr

TBSA, total body surface area.

Box 57.2 End Points of Initial Hemodynamic Resuscitation

- Mean arterial pressure 60–65 mm Hg
- Warm peripheral temperature of limbs
- Urine output 0.5–1 mL $\times$ kg^{-1} $\times$ h^{-1}
- Base deficit > −5 (−2)
- Lactate concentration ≤ 2 mmol $\times$ l^{-1}

resuscitation is not sufficient and the amount of fluids is increased, invasive monitoring using a pulmonary artery catheter is recommended. It has to be emphasized that, in major burns, so-called "normal" filling pressures cannot usually be reached and are not the goal of fluid resuscitation because of increased capillary leak. The most common hemodynamic problem in a burn patient is hypotension, which requires evaluation of filling pressures and cardiac output. If filling pressures and cardiac output are low, an effort should be made to increase fluid resuscitation. If the response to fluid increase is poor, inotropes are the next step. In a hyperdynamic state, the patient is hypotensive and cardiac output is high; in this case, vasopressors are indicated. In major burns, the heart rate is always increased and β-adrenergic vasoactive agents may worsen tachycardia.

As a result of primary fluid resuscitation, the amount of sodium administered is high and hypernatremia may develop. Therefore, after the primary resuscitation, the administration of sodium-free fluids (free water) is recommended.

Early Wound Excision and Closure
Topical wound care decreases vapor loss and prevents desiccation and bacterial growth. Silver-containing creams and dressings are useful in burn wounds. In major burns, early excision and closure of deep burn wounds decreases colonization and risk for infection. In major full-thickness burns, early excision and closure during the first 48 hours is recommended, with the aim of operating on all wounds by the end of the first week postburn (Fig. 57.8). In burns of greater than 30% to 40% of the body surface, it is often impossible to reach immediate autograft closure, and allografts and other skin substitutes are needed (Fig. 57.9). Wounds are later replaced with autografts when donor sites have healed.

Sedation and Pain Management
Sedation and pain management in burn patients is challenging. Burn patients experience severe pain that consists of background and procedural pain. During the early postburn period, sedatives

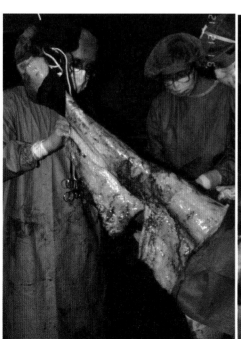
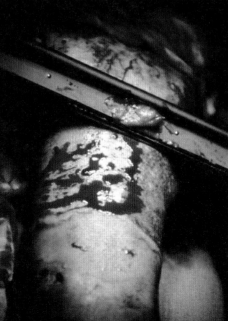

A   B

Figure 57.8 Fascial excision *(A)* and tangential excision of burn injury *(B)*.

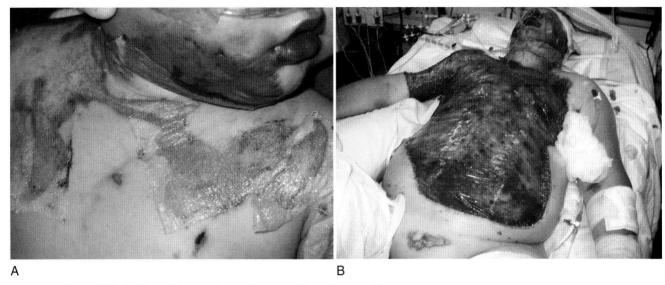

Figure 57.9 Artificial skin substitutes: Trancyte (A) and Integra (B).

and opioids are administered, usually as a continuous low-dose infusion. Additional doses of analgesia are provided for painful procedures. Sedative agents used mostly in continuous infusions are midazolam and propofol. Long-acting benzodiazepines—such as lorazepam and diazepam are usually used as repetitive boluses. Morphine and other opioids (e.g., fentanyl, oxycodone) are used for pain management. The combination of sedative and opioid infusion results in a synergy that usually decreases the need for both drugs. After excision and closure of burn wounds, efforts to gradually decrease the doses of sedative and opioid agents may prevent the development of severe withdrawal syndrome. In order to titrate adequate levels of sedation and pain control and to avoid oversedation, clinical scoring systems should be routinely used.

Nutritional Support

Metabolic rate is increased by as much as 100% to 150% after major burns, and hypermetabolism continues at least until wound closure. Hypermetabolism associated with muscle catabolism leads inevitably to muscle loss and weakness. Fever, pain, heat loss, and infections increase the metabolic rate, and efforts to prevent these factors are important. Measurement of metabolic rate by indirect calorimetry gives a satisfactory evaluation of caloric needs. Measurements made in the resting state should be increased by about 20% to estimate daily caloric needs. The need for proteins is 2 to 3 g/kg/day. Administration of enteral glutamine may be beneficial for burn patients, but the role of immunonutrition is controversial. Enteral nutrition should be started as soon as possible, and most patients tolerate it. If caloric needs cannot be met through enteral administration, combination with parenteral support will be necessary.

Efforts to decrease hypermetabolism have been studied intensively. To date, early wound excision and closure remain clinically the most important procedures to limit hypermetabolism.

Infections

Burn wound sepsis leading to organ dysfunctions is the mechanism of death in most burn patients. Burn wounds predispose

to bacterial growth and are easily colonized. Topical wound care aims to prevent wound infections. Silver sulfadiazine has a broad antibacterial spectrum, and silver-containing creams and dressings are widely used in topical care. Antibiotic prophylaxis is not routinely used. In major burns, the risk for wound infections remains until wound closure, and the need for antibiotic treatment is often inevitable. Bacterial growth in burn wounds does not necessarily lead to wound infections, and therefore only clinical infections are treated with systemic antibiotics. Long-term antibiotic treatment predisposes to antibiotic resistance.

Clinical Course

After initial evaluation, the main focus of treatment is fluid resuscitation during the first and second days. Owing to an increase in capillary permeability, general tissue edema develops. Inhalation injury in particular increases the requirement for fluids and predisposes to pulmonary edema. When hemodynamics are stable, early wound excision and closure are performed during the first days. In major burns, skin substitutes are usually needed in early closure. Until early excision and closure, patients usually need continuous infusion of sedative and analgesic drugs and ventilatory treatment. Weaning from mechanical ventilation is started while decreasing infusions of sedatives and opioids. Early tracheostomy should be considered for patients with severe burns; it provides a stable, secure airway and facilitates ventilatory treatment and weaning. As needed, other organ dysfunctions are supported. Rehabilitation should be started already during intensive care.

Survival after burn injury has improved over the past few decades. Pediatric patients with a burn injury of 90% to 95% of the body surface area have a 50% chance of survival. All severely burned children should be given a course of treatment before consideration of treatment futility. In adults, three risk factors are associated with increased risk of death: age over 60 years, burns of more than 40% of the body surface area, and inhalation injury. The mortality is estimated to be 0.7%, 14%, 39%, and 90% for patients with zero, one, two, and three risk factors, respectively. Participation in burn-center-based rehabilitation seems to be associated with satisfactory long-term quality of life after massive burn injury in childhood.

INHALATION INJURIES

Epidemiology, Risk Factors, and Pathophysiology
The incidence of inhalation injury is reported to be between 19% and 26% in burn patients; in nonsurvivors, even higher occurrence rates (up to 58%) have been reported. Direct thermal damage due to flame, liquid, or steam inhalation is rare. House fires, explosions, and other disasters increase the risk for smoke inhalation injury. Risk for inhalation injury increases with the extent of burn injury, so that two thirds of patients with flame burns over 70% of the body surface area have inhalation injury. Direct injury to the respiratory epithelium and pulmonary alveolar macrophages triggers the inflammatory response. After injury, bronchial blood flow and microvascular permeability increase. Increased nitric oxide production contributes to loss of hypoxic pulmonary vasoconstriction and increased pulmonary capillary leak. Inhalation injury impairs mucociliary transport and predisposes patients to accumulation of secretions. As a result, lung edema, airway obstruction, and ventilation-perfusion mismatch develop.

Clinical Features
Pulmonary edema, bronchospasm, and ventilation-perfusion mismatch may soon lead to increased airway pressure, decreased compliance, and arterial hypoxemia. After days, endobronchial debris causes small airway obstruction, alveolar flooding, and atelectasis.

Diagnosis
The diagnosis of inhalation injury is based on clinical and fiberoptic bronchoscopy findings. Facial burns, singed nasal hairs, and carbonaceous debris in the mouth and pharynx raise the suspicion of inhalation injury. Bronchoscopic findings involve mucosal edema, erythema, hemorrhage, and ulceration. A chest radiograph is usually normal immediately after burn injury, but pulmonary edema may occur soon.

Treatment
Ventilatory support, pulmonary toilet, and bronchoscopic removal of secretions are the main components of management. In general, early endotracheal intubation is indicated in order to avoid difficult intubation and respiratory failure. Ventilation with low tidal volumes and airway pressures is recommended to prevent ventilator-induced lung injury. Therapeutic interventions, such as specific inhibitors of inducible nitric oxide synthase (iNOS) and aerosolized anticoagulants, have been studied in the treatment of smoke inhalation injury but are not yet part of clinical routine.

Clinical Course
In mild injury, healing requires 2 to 3 weeks. In diffuse injury, pulmonary infection is often severe, requiring long-term ventilatory treatment. Inhalation injury remains a major cause of death.

ELECTRICAL INJURIES

Electricity can cause injury in several ways, and some injuries may remain hidden. Particular attention must to be paid to patients exposed to high-voltage injury, and deep electrical injuries to vital organs should be excluded.

Epidemiology and Risk Factors
Electrical injuries are almost always accidental. The majority of high-voltage accidents are work-related and affect mostly construction and electrical workers. In children, most electrical injuries take place at home, in association with electrical and extension cords and with wall outlets. It is estimated that 3% to 4% of all admissions to burn units are caused by electrical injuries. Electrical injuries account for more than 500 deaths every year in the United States, and an average of 100 are caused by lightning. Lightning is the third most common cause of nature-related deaths.

Principles of Electricity and Pathophysiology
The variables that affect the extent of electrical injury are voltage, resistance, amperage, type of current, current pathway, and duration of contact. Voltage is the force that causes electrons to flow and is measured in volts (V). Voltage in high-tension transmission lines exceeds 100,000 V. Voltage is reduced to 120 V (US) or 220 V (Europe, Australia, Asia) before delivery to homes. Current is the flow of electrons per second and is measured in amperes (A). Electrical current exists in two forms: alternating current (AC) and direct current (DC). In alternating current, the electrons flow back and forth through a conductor in a cyclic fashion, whereas in direct current, electrons flow only in one direction. AC is most commonly used in households and is three times more dangerous than DC of the same voltage. AC causes tetanic muscle contractions that prolong the contact. Lightning can generate peak DC of 200,000 A for a span of 1 to 3 msec.

The current is proportional to the voltage of the source and inversely proportional to the resistance of the conductor. Therefore, exposure of different parts of the body to the same voltage will generate a different current because resistance varies between various tissues. The most important resistor against electrical current is the skin. Bone, fat, and tendons have higher resistance than dry skin, whereas muscle, blood vessels, and nerves exhibit lower resistance. The pathway traveled by current in the body determines the organs affected and the severity of injury. A vertical pathway, parallel to the body's axis, is dangerous, with a high incidence of respiratory arrest, ventricular fibrillation, and central nervous system complications. In both electrical and lightning injuries, arcs may generate extremely high temperatures (3000–5000°C) that cause severe thermal injuries from high voltage. A salient feature of electrical injury is the presence of extensive deep injuries with only minimal superficial evidence.

Lightning strikes the victim in a different way than does low or high voltage. A direct strike results in maximum damage. Side flash occurs when the current moves from an object to a nearby victim. In stride potential, the lightning hits the ground and then enters the victim from one foot and exits from the other foot.

Electrical Injury to Specific Tissues

Electrical injury may affect the heart by causing direct necrosis of the myocardium or by causing cardiac dysrhythmias. Relatively low currents with hand-to-hand transmission can precipitate ventricular fibrillation, whereas high-voltage currents most often cause ventricular asystole. Electric current may cause direct and indirect effects on blood vessels, which owing to their high water content are excellent conductors. The high temperature produces coagulation necrosis and occlusion in small vessels. In large vessels, rapid flow dissipates the heat, but medial necrosis may cause delayed thrombosis. Vascular injury in extremities predisposes to compartment syndrome. Loss of consciousness, confusion, and poor recall after high-voltage injury are common. Nearly half of patients who have high-voltage injury have loss of consciousness immediately after injury, but full recovery is common unless there is associated anoxia. The most serious central nervous system complication is respiratory arrest caused by depression of the respiratory center. This can result in secondary cardiac arrest and death. Dysfunction of peripheral nerves may acutely cause motor and sensory deficits. The eyes and ears may be entry points for a lightning strike, and in half of the patients rupture of the tympanic membrane occurs.

Management of Electrical Injuries

Rescuers are also prone to electrical injury if the patient is still in contact with the source of the current. Immediate attention must be directed toward resuscitation of patients in respiratory or cardiac arrest. Treatment generally follows the same principles as any other traumatic injury. However, certain points should be kept in mind. The entire body should be examined for unsuspected wounds. Evaluation for hidden injuries and for blunt thoracic and abdominal trauma is important. Patients with high-voltage injury should be evaluated for rhabdomyolysis and myoglobinuria and for compartment syndrome of limbs, which may require fasciotomy. Ophthalmologic and otoscopic evaluations are also needed in high-voltage injuries. Patients who have serious burn injuries should be transferred to a specialized burn center.

The prognosis depends on the severity of the initial injury and the development and severity of subsequent complications. Because most electrical injuries are preventable, public education, careful inspection, and safe use of electric equipment are the best means of reducing mortality and morbidity associated with electrical injuries.

SUGGESTED READING

Garrel D, Patenaude J, Nedelec B, et al: Decreased mortality and infectious morbidity in adult burn patients given enteral glutamine supplements: a prospective, controlled, randomized clinical trial. Crit Care Med 2003; 31:2444–2449.

Gueugniaud P-Y, Carsin H, Bertin-Maghit M, et al: Current advances in the initial management of major thermal burns. Intensive Care Med 2000; 26:848–856.

Jain S, Bandi V: Electrical and lightning injuries. Crit Care Clin 1999;15:319–331.

Koumbourlis AC: Electrical injuries. Crit Care Med 2002;30(suppl):S424–S430.

Monafo WW: Initial management of burns. N Engl J Med 1996;335: 1581–1586.

Murakami K, Traber DL: Pathophysiological basis of smoke inhalation injury. News Physiol Sci 2003;18:125–129.

Ryan CM, Schoenfeld DA, Thorpe WP, et al: Objective estimates of the probability of death from burn injuries. N Engl J Med 1998;338: 362–366.

Saffle JR, Davis B, William P: Recent outcomes in the treatment of burn injury in the United States: a report from the American Burn Association patient registry. J Burn Care Rehabil 1995;16:216–232.

Sheridan RL: Burns. Crit Care Med 2002;30(suppl):S500–S514.

Spies M, Herndon DN, Rosenblatt JI, et al: Prediction of mortality from catastrophic burns in children. Lancet 2003;361:989–994.

Chapter 58

Hypothermia and Hyperthermia

Gordon Giesbrecht and Frank Hubbell

GENERAL THERMOREGULATION

A proper understanding of human thermoregulation is helpful in understanding the onset of and treatment for thermal disorders such as hypothermia and hyperthermia. Thermal inputs from the skin and core structures (including the spinal cord and the brain) converge at the hypothalamus, where an integrated thermal signal indicates the thermal status of the body. In response to deviations (normally from a core temperature of 37°C), autonomic responses are initiated that include peripheral vasoconstriction and shivering to prevent hypothermia during cold stress and also vasodilation and sweating to prevent hyperthermia during heat stress (Fig. 58.1).

HYPOTHERMIA

Epidemiology and Risk Factors

When heat loss exceeds heat gain, core temperature decreases to levels of mild (35–32°C), moderate (32–28°C), and severe (<28°C) hypothermia (Table 58.1). Hypothermia results from two primary conditions: (1) excessive cold stress in active healthy adults or (2) continued cooling in infants or the elderly, in whom thermal defense mechanisms are blunted or absent, or those affected by disease (Box 58.1).

Diagnosis

Moderate to severe hypothermia is generally indicated by waning or loss of shivering and consciousness, and core temperature (if available) below 32.0°C. The best noninvasive measure of heart temperature is esophageal temperature, and this is the preferred site. A careful history can help determine

if hypothermia is primary (excessive heat loss) or secondary (i.e., disease, age, etc.) or if symptoms are caused by other factors, such as trauma, drugs, and alcohol.

Treatment

The main priorities are to establish a safe rewarming rate while maintaining the stability of the cardiovascular system and providing sufficient physiological support (i.e., oxygenation, correction of metabolic and electrolyte imbalances, and intravenous volume replenishment). Patients should be primarily classified by level of consciousness and cardiovascular stability, with core temperature (preferably esophageal) used as an adjunct diagnostic tool. A cardiac monitor should be applied, intravenous catheters inserted, and a neurological exam conducted. The most informative blood tests include CBC, electrolytes, and

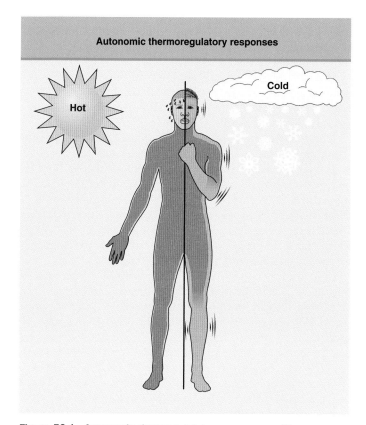

Figure 58.1. Autonomic thermoregulatory responses. Warm responses include peripheral vasodilation and sweating. Cold responses include peripheral vasoconstriction, shivering, and piloerection.

Table 58.1 Classifications of Level of Hypothermia

Classifications	Core Temp	Patient's Ability to Rewarm without External Heat Source	Clinical Presentation	
Normal	37°C (98.6°F)		• Cold sensation • Shivering	
Mild	35°C – 32°C (95°F – 90°F)	Good	Physical impairment	Mental impairment
			• Fine motor • Gross motor	• Complex • Simple
Moderate	32°C – 28°C (90°F – 82°F)	Limited	Below 30°C (86°F): • Shivering stops • Loss of consciousness	
Severe	Below 28°C (82°F)	Unable	**Rigidity** • Vital signs reduced or absent • Severe risk of mechanically stimulated ventricular fibrillation (VF) (rough handling)	
	Below 25°C (77°F)	Unable	• Spontaneous ventricular fibrillation (VF) • Cardiac arrest	

^aClassification is based primarily on status of the thermoregulatory system as well as mental and physical status and core temperature. **Bold text** shows the major thresholds between stages of hypothermia. VF, ventricular fibrillation.

Box 58.1 Risk Factors for Decreased Thermostability

Increased Heat Loss

Cold exposure (wet/wind, immersion)
Cold infusions
Pharmacology/toxins
Burns/dermatitis

Decreased Heat Production

Infants, elderly
Malnutrition/hypoglycemia
Endocrinologic failure
Fatigue/exhaustion/trauma

Impaired Thermoregulation

Neuropathies/spinal injury
Diabetes
CNS failure
Trauma
Shock

glucose. Arterial blood gases should not be corrected for temperature. Endotracheal intubation and ventilation are indicated unless protective airway reflexes are present. Monitoring end tidal CO_2 may be helpful. Nasogastric tube insertion is indicated in moderate or severe hypothermia and an indwelling bladder catheter should be used, and urine output should be monitored.

Do not sedate to suppress shivering because of concerns for patient comfort when hypothermia is the primary problem. Naloxone may reduce the severity of hypothermia in drug overdoses and in spinal shock.

If myxedema coma is suspected, thyroid function studies should be conducted and serum cortisol should be measured. Acid–base, fluid, and electrolyte imbalances should be corrected. A CVP line should be inserted to monitor fluid status. Intravenous D5W, NS, or D5NS can be administered with a 250-mL bolus (20 mL/kg for pediatric patients) and repeated as clinically indicated. It may be preferable to keep the patient at a lower range during resuscitation, especially during early stages. Intravenous fluid should be heated to 40 to 42°C.

In mild to moderate hypothermia, noninvasive heat sources may be sufficient. In severe cases in which cardiorespiratory activity is present, invasive measures such as arteriovenous fistula and body cavity lavage are warranted. In the case of cardiac arrest, cardiopulmonary bypass is preferred for rewarming. Defibrillation can be initially attempted with 2 W sec/kg up to 200 W sec. Two further attempts may be made at 360 W sec. If unsuccessful, the patient should be warmed, with CPR or cardiopulmonary bypass, to core temperatures above 32°C before further defibrillation attempts. Medications are generally contraindicated in the cold patient because increased protein binding and decreased metabolism render the drugs ineffective during hypothermia and predispose to overdose

following warming. Thus, pharmacologic intervention should await warming to core temperatures above 32°C.

Hypothermia compromises host defenses and may result in serious bacterial infections, which can be accompanied by minimal inflammatory responses. Bone marrow release and circulation of neutrophils are compromised for up to 12 hours. Children and the elderly are more prone to sepsis, and prophylactic antibiotics (e.g., aminoglycosides and broad-spectrum β-lactams) are recommended. Antibiotic prophylaxis is not normally indicated for previously healthy adults but is indicated if there is a failure to rewarm or any evidence of aspiration, myositis, chest x-ray infiltrate, bacteriuria, or persistent altered mental status.

Prevention

Healthy individuals who are active in cold environments should be knowledgeable about proper clothing, hydration, and nutrition. Care should be taken to avoid or prepare for cold, wet, and windy conditions or accidental immersion in cold water. Caregivers should be aware that infants do not possess adequate thermal defense mechanisms and that their large mass/surface ratio makes them prone to excessive heat loss or heat gain. Thus, care should be taken not to overinsulate them or to allow continued excessive heat loss. The very elderly should be regularly monitored and environmental conditions maintained at adequate temperatures (>22°C) to prevent slow but continued core cooling leading to significant hypothermia.

HYPERTHERMIA

Epidemiology and Risk Factors

Hyperthermia is a potentially life-threatening elevation in core temperature, with a broad and varied differential diagnosis (Box 58.2). Although many of the management principles pertain to any cause of hyperthermia, this section concentrates on environmental hyperthermia (i.e., heat stroke). Heat stroke is a true life-threatening medical emergency that requires immediate treatment. It is caused by a combination of dehy-

Box 58.2 Hyperthermia Differential Diagnosis

Environmental Heat Stress

Heat stroke

Hypermetabolic Disorders

Infection/sepsis: meningococcemia, *Plasmodium falciparum* malaria
Drug intoxication: cocaine, amphetamines, phencyclidine, theophylline, tricyclic antidepressants
Thyroid storm
Alcohol or drug withdrawal (hypersympathetic states)

Damage to the Thermoregulatory Center

Pontine or hypothalamic hemorrhage
Hypothalamic infarct

Iatrogenic Drug Reaction

Serotonin syndrome
Malignant hyperthermia
Neuroleptic malignant syndrome

and disseminated intravascular coagulopathy (DIC) is not uncommon. Alterations in serum proteins also change the blood oncotic pressure and encephalopathy ensues.

The liver is the first organ to suffer damage. Being a biochemical factory, the liver is usually 1°C warmer than the core organs (e.g., heart, lungs, and brain), predisposing it to heat injury. Renal failure is compounded by dehydration, myoglobinuria from rhabdomyolysis, and altered electrolyte concentrations. Muscle damage occurs from rhabdomyolysis.

Diagnosis

These patients are red, hot, and mad. In 80% of patients, the essentials of a clinical diagnosis are that they are very warm to the touch, have a core temperature higher than 41°C, have red skin, and have an altered level of consciousness (LOC) of sudden onset. The symptoms are the effect of the elevated core temperature and vasodilation in an effort to cool the blood. The altered LOC is secondary to a hot brain and the encephalopathy. Heat stroke patients will be disoriented, confused, combative, and hallucinating. They can rapidly progress to unconsciousness, coma, and death.

Many textbooks note that the hyperthermic's skin is red, hot, and dry. However, approximately 50% of these patients will be wet with sweat. If they were managed well by the prehospital teams, they may have been cooled and will not seem to be terribly hot on admission.

On evaluation, the lab results will show hyperkalemia, hypernatremia, hyperchloremia, and hemoconcentration. They typically are profoundly dehydrated and require IV rehydration with normal saline. They may have to be recooled multiple times.

Prehospital Treatment

Final outcome is highly dependent on proper prehospital care. Patients must be removed from the heat and sun. Remove clothing down to the skin layer. Cool the patient immediately by soaking with water and fanning to accelerate evaporative heat loss. Vigorously massage the limbs to increase the return circulation of cooled peripheral blood to the core. Note, however, that if cooling is too aggressive, shivering may occur, thus producing more heat and exacerbating the problem. Transport the patient to the hospital immediately.

Critical Care: Emergency Room Treatment and ICU Admission

As quickly as possible, bring the core temperature down to 39°C. The goal is to lower the core temperature 0.2°C/min. Active cooling should be discontinued when the core temperature reaches 39°C. Anticipate that patients will have to be recooled several times. Use a mist of water at approximately 80°F and fan the air to accelerate the evaporative heat loss. Circulating cooling blankets may be used, or the patient may be packed in ice, taking care to put towels, and so on, between the patient and the ice. With aggressive cooling, consider a paralytic agent to prevent the heat production of shivering.

Intravenous fluid resuscitation typically involves NS administered at 1 to 1.5 L per hour for the first 2 hours. Endotracheal intubation will maintain airway control with reduced LOC and allow supplemental oxygenation. Patients are frequently agitated, combative, or seizing. Benzodiazepines may be adminis-

dration, decreased electrolyte concentrations, and failure of thermoregulation, all of which result in end organ damage or failure. Untreated heat stroke has an approximately 70% mortality.

There are two forms of heat stroke: classic and exertional. In the case of classic heat stroke, the individual has "oversweated" by working hard and sweating profusely in a hot environment. Available fluid that could sweat onto the surface of the skin, for evaporative cooling of the peripheral blood, is exhausted. As the sweating mechanism fails, the body core temperature rises rapidly. Common risk factors for heat stroke are presented in Box 58.3.

With exertional heat stroke, which occurs during exercise in a hot and humid environment, the sweat produced to cool the skin, even though copious, cannot evaporate to keep the peripheral circulation cool. Sweat evaporation requires a water vapor gradient; thus, sweating in a humid environment (either in the ambient air or within protective clothing) will be ineffective because sweat does not evaporate and merely drips off the body or is absorbed in clothing.

Regardless of the cause, damage occurs to the internal organs as the core temperature rises. The extent of damage depends on how high the core temperature goes, and how long it remains elevated. The brain, liver, kidneys, muscles, and blood components are the most sensitive to heat injury.

Hyperthermia destroys platelets and the serum proteins that are responsible for coagulation. As a result, coagulopathies occur

Box 58.3 Risk Factors that Predispose to Heat Stroke

Poor acclimatization to heat or poor physical conditioning
Dehydration, febrile illness, chronic illness (DM, HTN), obesity
Medications—antihistamines, antipsychotics, antidepressants
Alcohol or other recreational drugs
Environment—high humidity, poor air circulation

tered intravenously, via endotracheal tube, or rectally. This will also help prevent shivering. An NG tube should be inserted to control vomiting.

Hyperkalemia is the most life-threatening early condition and should be managed appropriately. A Foley catheter should be inserted for monitoring urine output and urinalysis. Central venous or pulmonary artery catheters may be helpful to guide fluid management.

Laboratory studies are conducted primarily to detect end organ damage. Monitor the blood for DIC. Measure CBC, prothrombin time, activated partial thromboplastin time, fibrinogen, and platelets. Measure hepatic transaminases for acute liver damage, and reconsider the diagnosis if these are not elevated.

Evaluate for acute renal failure, uremia, acid–base disorders, and hyperkalemia. Measure serum electrolytes, blood urea nitrogen, and creatinine. Monitor blood sugar because hypoglycemia may occur as a result of impaired gluconeogenesis. Arterial blood gas readings are needed. Obtain a head computed tomography scan to determine the causes of altered LOC and to evaluate for the presence of cerebral edema or hemorrhage. Perform a chest x-ray to evaluate for aspiration, acute respiratory distress syndrome, or pneumonia. Monitor the ECG for cardiac status and hyperkalemia.

No medications will help lower the core temperature. Concentrate on fluid resuscitation to maintain peripheral circulation, where the blood can be cooled, and continue active surface cooling. Avoid salicylates because they will complicate coagulopathies, and also avoid acetaminophen because it can exacerbate hepatic injury.

With proper, aggressive cooling, survival rates are approximately 90%. Poor prognostic signs include coagulopathy, lactic acidosis, temperature higher than 42.2°C, acute renal failure, hyperkalemia, AST higher than 1000 U/liter, and coma.

Prevention

Outdoor enthusiasts or industrial workers in hot environments must stay well hydrated. They should be trained to drink to maintain normal urine output; the urine should be light in color. Cotton clothing is preferred, and the head should be protected from the sun. People should rest and rehydrate often in hot, humid environments. Salty food and electrolyte replacement fluids should be consumed.

SUGGESTED READING

Danzl DF, Pozos RS: Accidental hypothermia. N Engl J Med 1994; 331:1756–1760.

Danzl DF, Pozos RS, Hamlet MP: Accidental hypothermia. In Auerbach PS (ed): Wilderness Medicine: Management of Wilderness and Environmental Emergencies, 4th ed. St. Louis, Mosby, 2001, pp 51–103.

Giesbrecht GG: Cold stress, near drowning and accidental hypothermia: A review. Aviat Space Environ Med 2000;71:733–752.

Kunihiro A, Foster J: Heat exhaustion and heat stroke. www.emedicine.com, September 17, 2004.

Moran DS, Gaffin SL: Clinical management of heat-related illnesses. In Auerbach PS (ed): Wilderness Medicine: Management of Wilderness and Environmental Emergencies, 4th ed. St. Louis Mosby, 2001, pp 290–316.

U.S. Army Research Institute in Environmental Medicine. Heat acclimatization guide—Ranger and Airborne School Students. www.usariem.army.mil/download.htm.

U.S. Army Research Institute in Environmental Medicine. Heat stress control and heat casualty management. www.usariem.army.mil/download.htm, March 7, 2003.

Chapter 59

Pregnancy-Related Critical Care

Stephen E. Lapinsky

Assessment and management of critically ill pregnant patients are similar to those for nonpregnant patients, with some important differences. The cardiorespiratory changes that occur in pregnancy alter maternal physiologic requirements and affect normal laboratory and physiologic values. Furthermore, pregnant patients are at risk for a number of pregnancy-specific diseases that can produce critical illness with sudden onset (Box 59.1). The presence of a fetus may necessitate modification of some aspects of the diagnostic interventions and management of these patients.

MATERNAL PHYSIOLOGY IN PREGNANCY

Respiratory Physiology

Pregnancy affects the respiratory system by changes to the airways, thoracic cage, and respiratory drive (Fig. 59.1). The airway mucosa may become hyperemic and edematous, and extra care should be taken when inserting nasogastric tubes or nasotracheal tubes owing to the increased risk of bleeding. As the uterus expands, it displaces the diaphragm cephalad, reducing functional residual capacity (FRC) by 10% to 25% by term. The anteroposterior and transverse diameters of the thoracic cage widen to compensate for the volume loss. Vital capacity remains unchanged and total lung capacity decreases only minimally during pregnancy. Forced expiratory volume in one second (FEV_1) is not affected by pregnancy. Lung compliance is unchanged, but chest wall and total respiratory compliance are reduced in late pregnancy.

A significant augmentation in minute ventilation occurs, as a result of increased tidal volume, beginning in the first trimester and reaching 20% to 40% above baseline at term (Fig. 59.2). This is due to both the increase in metabolic CO_2 production as well as the increase in respiratory drive mediated by an increased serum progesterone level. The increased ventilation produces a respiratory alkalosis with compensatory renal excretion of bicarbonate. The arterial CO_2 pressure falls to a level of 28 to 32 mm Hg, with plasma bicarbonate decreased to 18 to 21 mEq/liter. Oxygenation usually is unaffected by pregnancy, but mild hypoxemia and an increased alveolar-arterial oxygen tension difference may develop in the supine position toward term. Oxygen consumption increases by 20% to 33% by the third trimester owing to the demands of the fetus and maternal metabolic processes. The combination of reduced FRC and increased oxygen consumption make pregnant patients particularly susceptible to development of hypoxia in response to hypoventilation or apnea.

In active labor, tachypnea due to pain and anxiety may produce a respiratory alkalosis, which can adversely affect fetal oxygenation by reducing uterine blood flow. Pain relief with narcotics or epidural analgesia reduces hyperventilation and can correct these gas exchange abnormalities.

Box 59.1 Common Causes of Admission of Pregnant or Postpartum Women to the ICU

Admission diagnoses vary considerably by geographic region.

Obstetric Complications

Preeclampsia and complications
    HELLP
    Eclampsia
    Pulmonary edema
Hemorrhage
Obstetric sepsis
    Chorioamnionitis
    Endometritis

Nonobstetric Conditions

Thromboembolism
Postanesthetic complications
Trauma
Respiratory failure
    Heart failure
    ARDS
    Pneumonia
Diabetic ketoacidosis

Pulmonary physiology in pregnancy

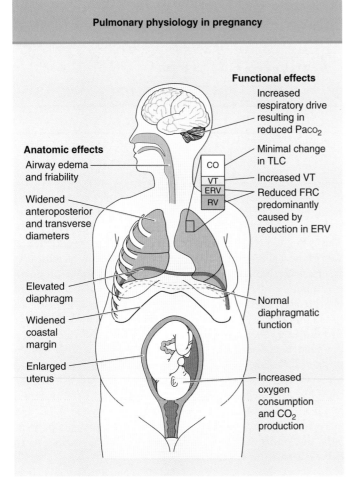

Anatomic effects

Airway edema and friability

Widened anteroposterior and transverse diameters

Elevated diaphragm

Widened coastal margin

Enlarged uterus

Functional effects

Increased respiratory drive resulting in reduced $Paco_2$

Minimal change in TLC

Increased VT

Reduced FRC predominantly caused by reduction in ERV

Normal diaphragmatic function

Increased oxygen consumption and CO_2 production

CO
VT
ERV
RV

Figure 59.1. Pulmonary physiology in pregnancy. Anatomic and functional effects of pregnancy that influence pulmonary physiology. ERV, expiratory reserve volume; FRC, functional residual capacity; IRV, inspiratory reserve volume; RV, residual volume; TLC, total lung capacity.

Physiologic changes of pregnancy

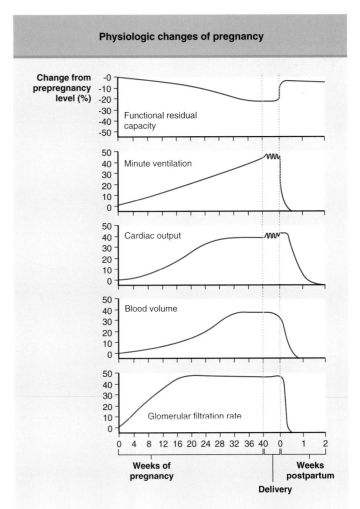

Figure 59.2. Physiologic changes of pregnancy. Schematic representation of some of the physiologic changes occurring during pregnancy and the postpartum period.

Cardiovascular Physiology

Maternal blood volume increases progressively throughout pregnancy, peaking at a level 40% above baseline by the third trimester. The increase in blood volume provides some protection against peripartum blood loss. The cardiac output increases from as early as 5 weeks' gestation, reaching 30% to 50% above baseline levels by 25 to 32 weeks (see Fig. 59.2). Heart rate rises to a level 10% to 30% above prepartum values by 32 weeks. Left atrial and left ventricular (LV) end-diastolic dimensions enlarge, and LV wall thickness and LV mass increase. Systemic blood pressure decreases slightly during pregnancy, with diastolic pressure falling 10% to 20% and reaching a nadir at 28 weeks. The decrease in systolic pressure is less marked, resulting in an increased pulse pressure. Blood pressure slowly increases throughout the third trimester but remains below prepregnancy values. Hemodynamic measurements by pulmonary artery catheter in the near-term patient reveal an increased cardiac output, with systemic vascular resistance and pulmonary vascular resistance decreased by 20% to 30%. The central venous pressure and pulmonary capillary wedge pressure are not different from nonpregnant values (Table 59.1).

Near term, the enlarged uterus may compress the vena cava in the supine patient, which can decrease venous return, causing

Table 59.1 Normal Hemodynamic Parameters in the Third Trimester[a]		
Parameter	**Mean Value**	**Change from Nonpregnant State**
Heart rate	83 ± 10/min	10% to 30% increase
Mean arterial pressure	90 ± 6 mm Hg	No change
Central venous pressure	4 ± 2.5 mm Hg	No change
Pulmonary capillary wedge pressure	7.5 ± 2 mm Hg	No change
Cardiac output	6.2 ± 1.0 L/min	30% to 50% increase
Systemic vascular resistance	1200 ± 260 dyne·cm·sec^{-5}	20% to 30% decrease
Pulmonary vascular resistance	75 ± 22 dyne·cm·sec^{-5}	20% to 30% decrease

[a]Mean (± SD) values and the change relative to the nonpregnant state are shown.

a drop in cardiac output, sometimes associated with reflex vasovagal effects. Further hemodynamic changes occur during labor and in the immediate postpartum period. Cardiac output increases by about 10% to 15% during labor, augmented further during contractions, due to the return of 300 to 500 mL of blood to the central circulation. Similarly, immediately after delivery there is an increase in preload, resulting in an increased cardiac output. Cardiac output remains elevated at the levels seen during pregnancy for about 2 days postdelivery.

Renal Physiology
Glomerular filtration rate increases early in pregnancy, reaching a value 50% above prepregnancy levels at 16 weeks, and remains elevated at this level throughout pregnancy. The normal serum creatinine level is therefore in the range of 0.5 to 0.7 mg/dL (45 to 60 μmol/L). As pregnancy progresses, the ureters dilate as a result of uterine compression and smooth muscle relaxation. A dilated collecting system does not therefore always indicate pathologic obstruction.

Gastrointestinal Physiology
Pregnancy is associated with a reduced lower esophageal sphincter pressure, probably mediated by progesterone levels, reaching a nadir at 36 weeks. As pregnancy progresses, the stomach is displaced, causing a further decrease in the effectiveness of the gastroesophageal sphincter and reducing gastric emptying. Pregnant women should always be considered at risk for aspiration of stomach contents, regardless of the time that has elapsed since the last meal.

Hematologic Changes
The increase in plasma volume associated with a lesser increase in red cell production causes a physiologic anemia with a hematocrit of 32% to 34% by the third trimester. The erythrocyte sedimentation rate (ESR) also rises related to increased levels of plasma globulins and fibrinogen in pregnancy. Increased coagulation factors may shorten prothrombin and partial thromboplastin times.

Determinants of Fetal Oxygenation
Oxygen delivery to the placenta and fetus is dependent on the maternal arterial oxygen saturation, hemoglobin concentration, and the uterine blood flow. The uterine vasculature is normally maximally dilated, and maternal hypotension, alkalosis, as well as endogenous or exogenous catecholamines can vasoconstrict the uterine artery. Uterine blood flow is also reduced by uterine contractions. Umbilical venous blood returning to the fetus has a low oxygen tension (Fig. 59.3), but a high fetal oxygen content is maintained by the left shift of the oxygen dissociation curve of fetal hemoglobin.

Interventions aimed at optimizing fetal oxygenation should be considered in the management of any critically ill pregnant patient. Depending on gestational age, delivery of the fetus may be the most appropriate intervention. Uteroplacental oxygen delivery can be optimized by increasing oxygen-carrying capacity by blood transfusion, improving maternal cardiac output or improving maternal oxygenation. The simple maneuver of tilting the patient to the left lateral position, to increase cardiac output, should always be considered.

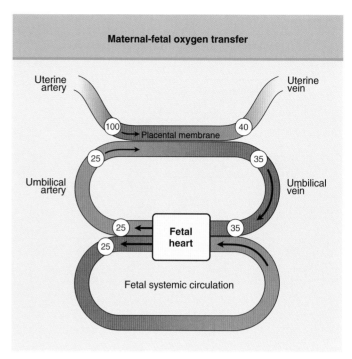

Figure 59.3. Maternal-fetal oxygen transfer. The encircled numbers represent approximate values of the partial pressure of oxygen (in mm Hg). (Adapted from Lapinsky SE, Kruczynski K, Slutsky AS: Critical care in the pregnant patient. Am J Respir Crit Care Med 1995;152: 427–455.)

PREGNANCY-SPECIFIC CONDITIONS

Amniotic Fluid Embolism
Epidemiology, Risk Factors, and Pathogenesis
Amniotic fluid embolism is an uncommon complication of pregnancy (between 1 in 8000 and 1 in 80,000 live births) but carries a mortality rate of 10% to 86%. It is usually associated with labor and delivery, but it may also occur with uterine manipulations or uterine trauma or in the early postpartum period. The mechanism involves the entry of amniotic fluid into the vascular circulation through endocervical veins or uterine tears (Fig. 59.4). Particulate cellular contents or humoral factors in the amniotic fluid produce acute pulmonary hypertension by obstructing the pulmonary vessels and by causing vascular spasm. Acute LV dysfunction mediated by cytokines may also occur. The cardiovascular changes of amniotic fluid embolism may resemble those of anaphylaxis, and sensitivity to amniotic fluid contents may be responsible.

Clinical Features
A pregnant woman will have the sudden onset of severe dyspnea, hypoxemia, and cardiovascular collapse, often accompanied by seizures. Less common presentations include hemorrhage caused by disseminated intravascular coagulopathy (DIC) or fetal distress. Almost half of the patients may die within the first hour, and cardiac arrest is common during this period.

Diagnosis
The diagnosis of amniotic fluid embolism is based on a typical clinical picture. Fetal squames in a wedged pulmonary capillary

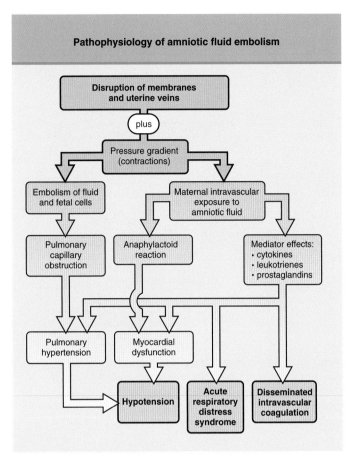

Figure 59.4. Pathophysiology of amniotic fluid embolism. Proposed pathophysiologic mechanisms for the development of circulatory shock and respiratory failure caused by amniotic fluid embolism.

aspirate have been suggested to confirm the diagnosis, but this is not a specific finding. The differential diagnosis includes septic shock, pulmonary thromboembolism, abruptio placentae, tension pneumothorax, and a myocardial ischemic event.

Treatment
Treatment involves routine resuscitative and supportive measures, including attention to oxygenation, mechanical ventilation, and inotropic support. No specific therapy has been shown to be effective, but a role for corticosteroids has been suggested. In view of the inconsistent hemodynamic findings, invasive monitoring may be considered.

Clinical Course and Prevention
Survivors of the initial hemodynamic collapse are likely to develop the complications of DIC or acute respiratory distress syndrome (ARDS). Late sequelae of neurologic damage caused by hypotension and hypoxemia are common.

Pitfalls, Complications, and Controversies
The predisposing factors, pathophysiology, and therapy of this condition are poorly understood. Since only supportive therapy can be undertaken, little can be done to prevent the condition or to reduce its morbidity or mortality.

Preeclampsia
Epidemiology, Risk Factors, and Pathogenesis
Preeclampsia is a pregnancy-induced disorder, characterized by hypertension, proteinuria, and edema. Presentation is almost always after 20 weeks' gestation and most frequently near term. Although preeclampsia usually resolves within a few days of delivery, postpartum onset of the disease occurs. The etiology of this condition is unclear, but there is a diffuse effect on maternal endothelium leading to reduced organ perfusion and multiple organ dysfunction. This is accompanied by arterial vasoconstriction and reduced plasma volume. Preeclampsia and its complications are an important cause of maternal morbidity and mortality. This syndrome accounts for 20% to 50% of obstetric admissions to the ICU and is responsible for 12% to 17% of all maternal deaths in the United States.

Clinical Features
The clinical features of early disease may be difficult to recognize, since the classical features of hypertension, proteinuria, and edema may not occur simultaneously and they are not individually specific for this condition. Patients may have one of the complications of this condition, including pulmonary edema, seizures (eclampsia), renal failure, or HELLP syndrome (see next page).

Diagnosis
The diagnosis is made clinically, based on the presence of hypertension, proteinuria, and edema. Signs suggestive of severe preeclampsia and impending complications include blood pressure higher than 160/110, oliguria, thrombocytopenia, abdominal pain, and visual or neurologic disturbances. Due to the multiorgan nature of this disease, patients may be admitted to the ICU without the typical clinical picture but with a variety of clinical or laboratory abnormalities. The intensivist should be aware of the differential diagnosis in pregnancy of laboratory abnormalities such as thrombocytopenia, hepatic dysfunction, and renal failure (Table 59.2).

Treatment, Clinical Course, and Prevention
From an obstetric perspective, management involves early recognition of the disease and well-timed delivery. Medical treatment is supportive, involving fluid management, control of hypertension, and prevention of seizures. No specific treatment is effective other than removal of the fetus and placenta. Management decisions may be difficult when gestation is at an early stage or when the mother is unstable, but delivery is almost always in the best interest of the mother.

Antihypertensive therapy is used to prevent maternal hypertensive vascular damage and does not alter the natural history of preeclampsia. Furthermore, the fetus does not benefit from lowering blood pressure. Commonly used regimens include small boluses of hydralazine (5–10 mg IV), boluses or infusion of labetalol, or calcium antagonists. A concern with the use of antihypertensives is the risk of reducing uteroplacental perfusion, and rapid decreases in blood pressure should be avoided. Sodium nitroprusside may be used in acute crises, but because of potential fetal toxicity, the duration of infusion should be minimized. After delivery of the fetus, these restrictions no longer apply.

tension requiring intravenous therapy, pulmonary edema, and persistent oliguria despite careful fluid challenge.

Pitfalls, Complications, and Controversies

Pulmonary edema occurs in about 3% of preeclamptic patients, most commonly in the early postpartum period. This is associated with aggressive intrapartum fluid replacement and return of blood to the central circulation as the uterus contracts. Pulmonary edema also occurs in chronically hypertensive, obese, pregnant patients who develop mild preeclampsia. Diastolic LV dysfunction results from both the hypertension and the obesity, and pulmonary edema is precipitated by volume overload of pregnancy and hemodynamic stresses of preeclampsia.

HELLP Syndrome

Epidemiology, Risk Factors, and Pathogenesis

The HELLP syndrome (*h*emolysis, *e*levated *l*iver enzymes, and *l*ow *p*latelet count) is a complication of preeclampsia characterized by multiorgan dysfunction, occurring in 4% to 12% of preeclamptic patients. The endothelial abnormality characterizing preeclampsia produces fibrin deposition and organ hypoperfusion, with the development of a microangiopathic hemolytic anemia and a consumptive thrombocytopenia. Reduced hepatic perfusion results in periportal and focal parenchymal necrosis, elevated liver enzymes, and, rarely, hepatic rupture.

Clinical Features

The clinical presentation is usually with epigastric or right upper quadrant pain, nausea, vomiting, or evidence of bleeding. Features of preeclampsia may be found but do not occur in all patients. Approximately 30% of patients with HELLP syndrome develop the disease only in the postpartum period.

Diagnosis

The diagnosis is made in the presence of thrombocytopenia (<100 × 10^9/L), moderate elevation of liver enzymes, and microangiopathic hemolytic anemia (increased LDH and bilirubin, abnormal blood smear). Severity may be inferred by the degree of thrombocytopenia. Many patients are found to have a more widespread coagulation defect than isolated thrombocytopenia. White blood cell count may be elevated and hypoglycemia is uncommon, in contrast to acute fatty liver of pregnancy. Other conditions that may present with similar multiorgan involvement should be considered (see Tables 59.2 and 59.3).

Table 59.2 Differential Diagnosis of the Features of Preeclampsia and Its Complications

Feature	Pregnancy-specific	Nonspecific
Hypertension	Preeclampsia	Essential hypertension
	Preeclampsia superimposed on chronic hypertension	Secondary hypertension (renal, pheochromocytoma)
Thrombocytopenia	Preeclampsia	TTP
	HELLP syndrome	ITP
	Acute fatty liver of pregnancy	Sepsis
		SLE
Elevated liver enzymes	Preeclampsia	Viral hepatitis
	HELLP syndrome	Drug-induced hepatitis
	Acute fatty liver of pregnancy	
	Cholestasis of pregnancy	
Renal dysfunction	Preeclampsia	Sepsis
	Acute fatty liver of pregnancy	Hypovolemia/hemorrhage
	Idiopathic postpartum renal failure	TTP/HUS
		SLE
Pulmonary edema	Preeclampsia	Valvular heart disease
	Peripartum cardiomyopathy	Ischemic heart disease
	Tocolytic pulmonary edema	ARDS
	Amniotic fluid emboli	Aspiration

ARDS, acute respiratory distress syndrome; HELLP, hemolysis, elevated liver enzymes, low platelets; HUS, hemolytic-uremic syndrome; ITP, idiopathic thrombocytopenic purpura; SLE, systemic lupus erythematosus; TTP, thrombotic thrombocytopenic purpura.

Seizure prophylaxis is with magnesium sulfate, using an initial intravenous bolus of 4 g over 10 to 20 minutes followed by an infusion of 1 to 3 g/hr for 24 hours. Clinical monitoring (patellar reflexes, respiratory status) and magnesium levels (therapeutic range 2–3.5 mmol/L), are essential, particularly in the presence of renal dysfunction. Toxic levels can cause respiratory muscle weakness and conduction defects. Hypocalcemia is common and should not always be treated—intravenous calcium will reverse the toxic and therapeutic effects of magnesium.

Patients with preeclampsia are intravascularly volume depleted and require volume expansion. However, excessive fluid administration can cause pulmonary or cerebral edema as a result of the reduced serum albumin and increased capillary permeability common in these patients. Pulmonary artery catheterization may be of value in the presence of severe hyper-

---

Table 59.3 Differential Diagnosis of Liver Disease in the Critically Ill Pregnant Patient[a]

Disease	Trimester	Clinical Features	Laboratory Values
Acute fatty liver of pregnancy	3	Abdominal pain, nausea, vomiting	ALT < 500 U/L, hypoglycemia, coagulopathy
Preeclampsia	2 or 3	Abdominal pain, hypertension, edema	ALT < 500 U/L, proteinuria
HELLP syndrome	3	Abdominal pain, vomiting, bleeding	ALT < 500 U/L, PLT < 100,000, increased LDH
Viral hepatitis	Any	Nausea, vomiting, fever	ALT > 1000 U/L, hyperbilirubinemia
Biliary tract disease	Any	RUQ pain, vomiting, fever	Hyperbilirubinemia, elevated alkaline phosphatase
Toxin-induced hepatic necrosis	Any	Nausea, vomiting, pain, jaundice	ALT > 1000 U/L, hyperbilirubinemia
Budd-Chiari syndrome	3	Abdominal pain, hepatomegaly, ascites	ALT < 500 U/L, rising bilirubin

ALT, alanine aminotransferase; LDH, lactate dehydrogenase; PLT, platelet; RUQ, right upper quadrant.
[a]Trimester of presentation and laboratory values are not absolute but serve to provide a comparison between conditions.

Other Critical Care Problems

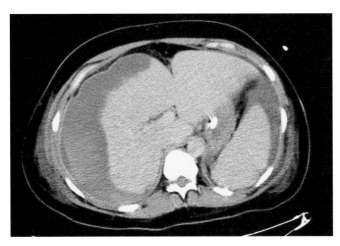

Figure 59.5. Hepatic subcapsular hemorrhage. Abdominal CT scan following intravenous contrast administration demonstrating a subcapsular hematoma in the right lobe of the liver of a patient with HELLP syndrome.

Treatment

Management includes blood product support and management of preeclampsia. Early delivery is indicated if the fetus is viable. Corticosteroid therapy begun prior to delivery (e.g., dexamethasone 10 mg every 12 hr) may produce more rapid maternal hematologic recovery. Delivery may require platelet support, and if operative delivery is necessary, hemorrhage should be anticipated and adequate drains should be inserted. Epidural anesthesia is contraindicated in the presence of thrombocytopenia.

Significant overlap between HELLP syndrome and other thrombotic microangiopathies exists, and a response to plasmapheresis is noted in some patients, possibly representing those with thrombotic thrombocytopenic purpura (TTP) or hemolytic-uremic syndrome (HUS). This procedure is recommended for patients with delayed postpartum resolution, when severe thrombocytopenia, massive hemolysis, or organ dysfunction persists for more than 72 hours after delivery.

Clinical Course and Prevention

The maternal mortality for patients with HELLP syndrome is reported as between 1% and 3% (but as high as 25%), with a high perinatal mortality at 8% to 60%. The maternal complications of HELLP syndrome include acute renal failure, ARDS, and hemorrhage. A rare but catastrophic consequence of HELLP syndrome is hepatic hemorrhage (Fig. 59.5), occurring in about 2% of patients, which can progress to hepatic rupture. This complication should be considered in any preeclamptic patient with sudden shock or acute abdominal pain, and management includes hemodynamic and blood product support, urgent delivery, and invasive control of the hemorrhage with embolization or immediate surgery with packing of the liver. Hemorrhage without rupture may be managed conservatively if the patient remains hemodynamically stable.

Pitfalls, Complications, and Controversies

HELLP syndrome may be difficult to differentiate from other conditions, including acute fatty liver of pregnancy, TTP, HUS,

and systemic lupus erythematosus (SLE). Management decisions can be difficult given the varying roles of therapeutic interventions such as platelet transfusion, corticosteroids, and delivery in these conditions.

Acute Fatty Liver of Pregnancy

Epidemiology, Risk Factors, and Pathogenesis

Acute fatty liver of pregnancy (AFLP) is an uncommon complication that affects about 1 in 15,000 pregnancies. Early reports described acute fulminant hepatic failure during the third trimester of pregnancy with a high maternal and fetal mortality rate, but the condition is now recognized at an earlier stage, allowing early delivery and an improved outcome. Maternal mortality has been reported at 0 to 18% with fetal loss of 23% to 60%. The etiology of this condition has not been established, but an association with an inborn error of metabolism in the fetus (LCHAD deficiency) has been suggested. The pathologic picture of AFLP is of diffuse fatty infiltration of the liver with necrosis and inflammation being mild or absent.

Clinical Features

Clinical presentation is usually toward the end of the third trimester but may occur as early as 30 weeks' gestation or in the puerperium. A prodromal phase of malaise, anorexia. and vomiting may precede the onset of jaundice by 1 to 2 weeks. Abdominal pain may occur, which may be diffuse or localized to the right upper quadrant.

Diagnosis

Laboratory investigations demonstrate a moderately elevated transaminase level (300–500 U), in contrast with higher levels in acute hepatitis. The white blood cell count is usually elevated, and thrombocytopenia and fragmented red blood cells may be demonstrated. Features of hepatic dysfunction, namely, hypoalbuminemia, hypoglycemia, and a coagulopathy, occur in more severe cases.

The differential diagnosis of liver disease in pregnancy is wide (see Table 59.3), and the multisystem effects of AFLP may resemble SLE, TTP, or HUS (see Table 59.2).

Treatment

Delivery of the fetus is the definitive treatment, and early delivery is responsible for the improved outcome in this condition. As the presentation is usually close to term, delivery carries little additional risk for the fetus. However, AFLP is associated with increased fetal loss due to placental insufficiency associated with fibrin deposition, which may be exacerbated by therapeutic coagulation factor replacement. Supportive therapy is similar to that for other causes of fulminant hepatic failure. Coagulation abnormalities and hypoglycemia must be appropriately corrected. Hepatic encephalopathy will require attention to airway protection, dietary protein restriction, bowel sterilization, and oral or rectal lactulose administration.

Clinical Course and Prevention

Although transient worsening of hepatic function may be observed in the puerperium, improvement begins within 2 to 3 days of delivery. A small subset of patients continue to deteriorate following delivery, and liver transplantation may be an appropriate consideration.

Complications such as hemorrhage, pancreatitis, renal failure, diabetes insipidus, and infection should be sought and treated.

Obstetric Hemorrhage

Epidemiology, Risk Factors, and Pathogenesis

The increased uterine blood flow near term (500 mL/min) puts pregnant patients at risk of devastating blood loss. Antepartum hemorrhage may occur from placenta previa or placental abruption. Fetal mortality is high, and maternal complications include a coagulopathy with postpartum hemorrhage and renal failure. Most obstetric hemorrhage occurs postpartum as a result of uterine atony, cervical or vaginal lacerations, or DIC. Uterine atony may result from prolonged labor, oxytocin augmentation, chorioamnionitis, operative delivery, or retention of placental fragments. DIC may occur as a result of preeclampsia/HELLP syndrome, amniotic fluid embolism, or placental abruption.

Clinical Features

The clinical features of massive hemorrhage are those of hypovolemic shock, but clinicians frequently underestimate blood loss, since patients may initially have relatively normal vital signs. Occasionally, antepartum hemorrhage may present initially with fetal distress.

Diagnosis

In addition to monitoring hemoglobin and coagulation factors, conditions that may aggravate hemorrhage should be sought, e.g., thrombocytopenia associated with HELLP syndrome. Obstetric consultation will guide diagnostic procedures to assess the cause of hemorrhage. These investigations may include ultrasound to exclude retained products of conception and examination of the genital tract for lacerations.

Treatment

Management of severe obstetric hemorrhage requires supportive measures as well as specific interventions to control bleeding. The initial management involves rapid volume replacement with crystalloid or blood products, supplemental oxygen administration, and blood product support for associated dilutional coagulopathy. Specific measures to improve uterine contraction are of value in the presence of uterine atony. These include uterine massage, the intramuscular administration of methylergonovine (0.2 mg) (which should be avoided in the presence of hypertension), and intravenous oxytocin infusion. Oxytocin is administered in a higher dose than used for augmentation of labor, using 20 to 40 U in 1000 mL normal saline at an infusion rate up to 100 mU/min (150–300 mL/hr). This dose may have a significant antidiuretic effect, causing hyponatremia. An analog of prostaglandin $F_{2\alpha}$ (carboprost tromethamine, Hemabate) given intramuscularly (0.25 mg) or intramyometrially has a high success rate in controlling hemorrhage after one or two injections. Reported side effects include vomiting, hypertension, bronchoconstriction, and increased intrapulmonary shunt. Recombinant factor VIIa has also been successfully used in the management of severe obstetric hemorrhage.

If pharmacologic methods fail, invasive approaches may be required. Radiologic transcatheter embolization of the internal iliac or uterine artery has been used to successfully control obstetric hemorrhage. If these measures fail, surgical exploration will be necessary to repair lacerations, reduce blood flow by arterial ligation, or remove the uterus.

Clinical Course and Prevention

Obstetric hemorrhage remains a frequent cause of maternal mortality, accounting for about a quarter of maternal deaths. Early aggressive treatment is essential, and although the patient's future childbearing needs to be considered, hysterectomy may be life-saving.

Pitfalls, Complications, and Controversies

Pregnant patients are at risk of hypoperfusion injury to the kidney, particularly when renal function is already compromised by preeclampsia, and acute tubular necrosis is a common sequela. Acute cortical necrosis, which carries a poor prognosis for recovery of renal function, may result from severe hemorrhagic shock in the presence of a hypercoagulable state. A high incidence of myocardial ischemia has been noted in pregnant women with hemorrhagic shock, and this should be considered in the management of these patients.

Obstetric Sepsis

Epidemiology, Risk Factors, and Pathogenesis

Antepartum infection leads to chorioamnionitis, but most obstetric sepsis occurs in the postpartum period. The most common location of infection is the placental site, leading to endometritis, which may spread to the parametrium and peritoneum. Less commonly, episiotomy sites or cesarean section wounds may become infected. Infections are often mixed, involving microorganisms that originate from the vagina or the intestine or from sexual transmission or that are blood-borne (Box 59.2). Pregnancy may be associated with a decreased cell-mediated immune response, which increases susceptibility to certain infections, including *Listeria monocytogenes*, disseminated herpesvirus, varicella, and coccidioidomycosis infections. Human immunodeficiency virus disease should be considered in any pregnant patient with pneumonia or unusual opportunistic infections.

Clinical Features

The clinical presentation is with fever (in the antepartum period or first 24 hours postpartum) associated with uterine tenderness, foul lochia, and sometimes vaginal bleeding. Persistent fever 2 to 4 days postpartum should suggest complications such as puerperal ovarian vein thrombosis or abscess formation.

Diagnosis

In addition to the usual diagnostic tests in the septic patient, amniocentesis (antepartum) or endometrial specimens (postpartum) should be obtained for culture. Adequate aerobic and anaerobic cultures should be taken, including the culture of tissue obtained from uterine aspiration or surgery. Ultrasound is essential to exclude retained products of conception.

Treatment

The management of obstetric sepsis follows the usual principles of care, and prompt hemodynamic resuscitation with volume expansion is essential for both maternal and fetal survival. If inotropic therapy becomes necessary in the antepartum situa-

631

Box 59.2 Source of Microorganisms Causing Obstetric Sepsis

Vaginal

Peptostreptococcus spp.
Group B streptococci
Bacteroides bivius
Gardnerella vaginalis
Mycoplasma hominis
Staphylococcus aureus

Intestinal

Escherichia coli
Enterococcus spp.
Enterobacter spp.
Clostridium perfringens
Clostridium sordelli
Bacteroides fragilis

Sexually Transmitted

Neisseria gonorrhoeae
Chlamydia trachomatis

Hematogenous

Listeria monocytogenes
Campylobacter spp.
Group A streptococci

tion, the effects of such drugs on uteroplacental perfusion must be considered.

Initial empiric antibiotic therapy should provide broad gram-negative, gram-positive, and anaerobic coverage. Chorioamnionitis in the presence of sepsis syndrome is usually treated with ampicillin and an aminoglycoside but is unlikely to respond to antibiotic therapy alone. Prompt stabilization and delivery are required, with close monitoring of the fetus. Commonly used regimens in the postpartum patient are ampicillin, gentamicin, and clindamycin; ampicillin/sulbactam; ticarcillin-clavulanate; piperacillin and gentamicin; or imipenem/cilastatin. Surgical intervention may be required and can be life-saving.

Clinical Course and Prevention

In the postpartum septic patient who deteriorates despite antibiotic therapy, a resistant organism (e.g., *Enterococcus*), localized abscess, myometrial microabscesses, or septic pelvic thrombophlebitis should be considered.

Pitfalls, Complications, and Controversies

Myometrial microabscesses present with an enlarged, tender uterus in patients who do not respond to adequate antibiotic therapy. Gas in the subcutaneous tissues or uterine walls on radiographic studies suggests clostridial gas gangrene. Patients at risk are those with devitalized tissue or retained placenta. If a Gram stain demonstrates gram-positive rods with spores, high-dose penicillin should be administered. Early surgical evacuation of the uterus is essential, and laparotomy with hysterectomy and wide excision of gangrenous areas may be required.

Puerperal ovarian vein thrombophlebitis usually presents with acute deterioration with fever, following postpartum endometritis. The diagnosis may be difficult to confirm, but computerized tomography (CT) or magnetic resonance imaging (MRI) of the pelvis is useful. Treatment is with broad-spectrum antibiotics and standard anticoagulation, but patients who remain ill may require surgical intervention with venous ligation or excision.

Necrotizing fasciitis, due to group A streptococci, manifests with local erythema and tenderness that rapidly progress to bullae formation and skin discoloration. This may be associated with streptococcal toxic shock syndrome. This condition often occurs unexpectedly following an uncomplicated pregnancy and delivery, with an influenza-like prodrome followed rapidly by profound shock. Management includes antibiotic therapy with penicillin and clindamycin and early surgical interventions. Intravenous immunoglobulin (2 g/kg) is thought to be beneficial. Toxic shock syndrome due to *Staphylococcus aureus* or *Clostridium sordelli* may rarely occur in puerperal infection, usually associated with instrumentation and septic abortion.

Tocolytic Pulmonary Edema
Pathogenesis and Clinical Features

β-Adrenergic agonists have been used to inhibit uterine contractions in preterm labor. A complication of β-agonist use in pregnancy is the development of pulmonary edema, the mechanism of which is unclear.

The clinical presentation is of acute respiratory distress with features of pulmonary edema. No specific features characterize this condition.

Diagnosis

The diagnosis is made in the presence of acute pulmonary edema occurring during or immediately after the administration of parenteral β-agonists. The differential diagnosis includes cardiogenic pulmonary edema, amniotic fluid embolism, and other conditions (Table 59.4). Failure of the pulmonary edema to resolve in 12 to 24 hours should prompt consideration of alternative causes.

Treatment, Clinical Course, and Prevention

The β-agonist must be discontinued and supportive treatment, including diuresis, provided. Early recognition and management should reduce the need for invasive, hemodynamic monitoring and mechanical ventilation.

Pitfalls, Complications, and Controversies

Use of β-agonists has decreased markedly following studies demonstrating that tocolysis does not improve the outcome in preterm labor. The condition remains of physiologic interest as the pathophysiology has not yet been clarified.

Gestational Trophoblastic Disease

Pulmonary hypertension and pulmonary edema may complicate benign hydatidiform mole as a result of trophoblastic pulmonary embolism. This most commonly occurs during evacuation of the uterus, and the incidence of pulmonary complications is higher in later gestations. Molar pregnancy may be associated with choriocarcinoma, which can produce multiple, discrete pulmonary metastases and occasionally pleural effusions.

Table 59.4 Differential Diagnosis of Acute Respiratory Distress in Pregnancy

Disorder	Distinguishing Features
Pregnancy-Specific	
Amniotic fluid embolism	Cardiorespiratory collapse, seizures, DIC
Pulmonary edema secondary to preeclampsia	Hypertension, proteinuria
ARDS secondary to obstetric sepsis	Evidence of obstetric sepsis, shock
Tocolytic pulmonary edema	Tocolytic administration, rapid improvement
Peripartum cardiomyopathy	Gradual onset, cardiac gallop, cardiomegaly
Trophoblastic embolism	Nodular infiltrate, molar pregnancy
Risk Increased by Pregnancy	
Aspiration pneumonitis	Vomiting, aspiration
Venous thromboembolism	Evidence of DVT, positive V/Q scan, Doppler ultrasound of leg, CT angiogram
Pneumomediastinum	Occurs during delivery, subcutaneous emphysema
Valvular heart disease	Pulmonary edema, cardiac murmur, cardiomegaly
ARDS secondary to sepsis	Evidence of obstetric or nonobstetric sepsis
Air embolism	Sudden hypotension, cardiac murmur
ARDS secondary to pyelonephritis	Associated pyelonephritis or other intra-abdominal sepsis
Unrelated to Pregnancy	
Asthma	Features similar to those seen in the nonpregnant patient
Pneumonia	

ARDS, acute respiratory distress syndrome; CT, computed tomography; DIC, disseminated intravascular coagulopathy; DVT, deep venous thrombosis; V/Q, ventilation-perfusion.

CONDITIONS NOT SPECIFIC TO PREGNANCY

Trauma

Epidemiology, Risk Factors, and Pathogenesis

The anatomic and physiologic changes of pregnancy may alter the severity and manifestation of trauma. Uterine injury can produce severe hemorrhage because of the prominent uterine circulation. Penetrating injury to the abdomen predominantly affects the uterus in later pregnancy. However, because intra-abdominal viscera are compressed in the upper abdomen, relatively minor injury may produce significant damage. Fractures of the pelvis may produce severe retroperitoneal hemorrhage owing to dilation of pelvic veins. Injury to the uterus may precipitate placental abruption or rarely uterine rupture, manifesting with maternal shock, abdominal pain, and palpable fetal parts.

Maternal trauma is associated with a significant increase in fetal loss, secondary to maternal shock or hypoxia, placental injury, or direct fetal injury. Direct fetal injury due to blunt trauma usually involves head injury secondary to maternal pelvic fracture. Other fetal injuries may occur following blunt or penetrating trauma, with minimal maternal injury. A high fetal mortality occurs with maternal burns to greater than 30% of the body surface area.

Placental abruption is an important cause of fetal demise and presents with vaginal bleeding, abdominal cramps, uterine tenderness, amniotic fluid leakage, and unexplained fetal distress or maternal hypovolemia. When fetus and mother are stable following partial abruption, expectant management can be considered. However, further placental separation can occur at any time and close observation is essential. Placental abruption is often complicated by DIC as a result of release of thromboplastin into the maternal circulation.

Clinical Features

The secondary survey should include a detailed abdominal examination, but physical signs may be affected by changing organ position and the reduced peritoneal sensitivity that occurs in pregnancy. Fetal evaluation includes heart rate assessment by auscultation (possible from 20 weeks) or Doppler probe. Obstetric consultation and continuous fetal cardiotocography are important when the fetus is at a viable gestation.

Diagnosis

Initial investigations include a complete blood count, blood typing with Rh, and coagulation studies. Ultrasound is a useful investigation for evaluation of the fetus for injury and biophysical profile and to assess intra-abdominal organ damage. Ultrasound-guided paracentesis or diagnostic peritoneal lavage (by open technique, above the uterus) may aid in detecting bowel perforation or intraperitoneal hemorrhage. The transplacental hemorrhage of fetal blood into the maternal circulation may complicate abdominal trauma and can result in fetal exsanguination and maternal Rh sensitization. Fetomaternal hemorrhage is detected by the Kleihauer-Betke test, which identifies fetal cells in the maternal blood smear. The volume of fetal hemorrhage can be calculated by the percentage of red cells of fetal origin, and the test is sensitive to about 5 mL of fetal blood.

Treatment, Clinical Course, and Prevention

Initial resuscitation follows usual management principles with efforts directed primarily at stabilizing the mother. It has been recommended that fluid replacement be given more rapidly than in nonpregnant women owing to the physiologic increase in plasma volume. Maternal blood pressure and heart rate may not be reliable predictors of the degree of hemorrhage. The fetus is vulnerable to hypotension and hypoxemia—uterine blood flow will be markedly reduced when maternal circulation is compromised. Signs of fetal distress may indicate impending maternal shock.

Management of shock in a woman beyond 20 weeks' gestation should include left lateral positioning to prevent supine hypotensive syndrome. In the unstable mother, management of maternal injuries should take precedence over fetal distress, since correction of maternal hemodynamics is beneficial to the fetus. If the mother is stable, cesarean section may be indicated if the fetus is considered viable, the limits of viability being largely dependent on the level of neonatal care available. Rh-negative mothers with abdominal trauma should receive Rh immune globulin even in the presence of a negative Kleihauer-Betke test. The dose of Rh immune globulin is related to the volume of fetal-maternal hemorrhage, ranging from 50 µg to 300 µg or more (50 µg per 5 mL of hemorrhage).

633

Table 59.5 Fetal Risk from Diagnostic Radiologic Procedures[a]

Investigation	Fetal Radiation Exposure (mGy)	Comment
Chest radiograph (abdomen shielded)	0.01–0.08	Minimal risk
Pelvis radiograph	0.4	Low risk
Ventilation-perfusion scan:		
Perfusion	0.1–1.0	Low risk; begin with perfusion scan
Ventilation	0.1–0.4	
Chest CT angiogram	0.1–0.9	Low-dose protocols can reduce exposure to 10% to 50%
Head CT	0.1–0.5	Low risk
Abdominal/pelvic CT	up to 50	Significant risk
Pulmonary angiogram:		
Brachial route	0.5	Perform if indicated
Femoral route	2.0–4.0	

[a]Estimated values based on the use of appropriate abdominal shielding and good collimation (1 mGy = 0.1 rad).

Care of the severely injured pregnant patient requires a multidisciplinary approach involving the emergency physician, trauma surgeon, obstetrician, intensivist, and neonatologist.

Pulmonary Thromboembolic Disease
Epidemiology and Pathophysiology
Pulmonary thromboembolism occurs in up to 1.3% of pregnancies, both during pregnancy and in the postpartum period. The increased incidence results from hypercoagulability that occurs in pregnancy, from hormonally mediated venous stasis, and from local pressure effects of the uterus on the inferior vena cava. Pulmonary embolism occurs more frequently in the early postpartum period than during pregnancy, particularly following cesarean section.

Clinical Features
The presentation is similar to that in patients who are not pregnant. A marked predilection for left-leg deep venous thrombosis occurs in pregnancy, likely the result of anatomic factors.

Diagnosis
Investigation of suspected pulmonary embolism follows a similar approach to that in patients who are not pregnant. Duplex ultrasound is useful for the diagnosis of deep venous thrombosis, although venous Doppler alone can give false-positive results owing to venous obstruction by the gravid uterus. Ventilation–perfusion scanning can be performed with less than 0.5 mGy radiation exposure to the fetus (<50 mrad) and, if necessary, a CT pulmonary angiogram may be carried out with similarly low fetal exposure (Table 59.5).

Treatment
Warfarin is usually avoided, since first-trimester use has been associated with development of an embryopathy, and central nervous system abnormalities have been described with second- and third-trimester exposure. Heparin does not cross the placenta, is not associated with adverse fetal outcome, and can be readily reversed. Low-molecular-weight heparins are both safe and effective in pregnancy but are less easy to reverse acutely. When administered with adequate precautions, streptokinase, urokinase, and tissue plasminogen activator have been used successfully without major hemorrhagic complications or significant adverse effects on the fetus or placenta, but they should be limited to life-threatening situations. Transvenous placement of an inferior vena cava filter can be performed, although there is some risk of dislodgement because of the dilated venous system and pressure effects during labor.

Clinical Course and Prevention
Women who have a known hypercoagulable state and those who have had a previous thromboembolism are at increased risk and should receive prophylaxis with anticoagulation throughout pregnancy.

Pitfalls and Controversies
The use of radiologic investigations during pregnancy remains a concern for the fetus. It is nevertheless important to establish the diagnosis because of the major implications if such a diagnosis is missed and because of the effects of unnecessary therapy on the health of mother and fetus.

Acute Respiratory Distress Syndrome
Epidemiology and Pathophysiology
Pregnant patients are at risk of developing ARDS from pregnancy-associated complications or other conditions (see Table 59.4). Iatrogenic factors such as excessive fluid administration and tocolytic therapy may contribute, as may the reduced albumin level occurring in pregnancy.

Clinical Features
The clinical features are similar to those in patients who are not pregnant.

Diagnosis
The diagnosis is by the usual criteria of hypoxemia in the presence of diffuse pulmonary infiltrates and in the absence of left ventricular failure. A detailed history is critical to identification of the underlying problem.

Treatment
There are no major differences in the management of pregnant patients who have ARDS compared with those who are not pregnant, other than the need for continuous assessment of the fetus. Ventilatory management includes consideration of the normal physiologic changes of pregnancy. Adequate maternal oxygen saturation is essential for fetal well-being. Fetal delivery may benefit both mother and fetus. Epidural anesthesia may reduce the increased oxygen demand produced by uterine contractions.

Clinical Course and Prevention
Survival appears to be similar or better than that in the general population, possibly because of the young age of the patients and the reversibility of many of the predisposing conditions.

Pitfalls and Controversies
Specific causes of ARDS that pertain to pregnancy should be sought when assessing patients who have this syndrome. When

women of childbearing age present with ARDS, the possibility of pregnancy should be considered.

Asthma

The hormonal changes of pregnancy can affect the asthmatic patient variably, with worsening, improvement, or no substantial change being noted. Since asthma is a common condition, acute deterioration represents an important cause of respiratory compromise in pregnancy. The normal PCO_2 in pregnancy of 28 to 32 mm Hg should be considered in the assessment of arterial blood gases. No significant modification of treatment is required; in particular, pregnancy is not an absolute contraindication to corticosteroid therapy. While there is a natural reluctance to prescribe drug therapy in pregnancy, uncontrolled asthma is more dangerous for the fetus than any of the recommended medications are. The management of the severe pregnant asthmatic should highlight the importance of adequate oxygenation, to avoid fetal compromise.

Heart Failure

Cardiac failure is commonly precipitated when cardiac output requirements increase in late pregnancy, in the presence of obstructive lesions (mitral stenosis, aortic stenosis, and pulmonary hypertension). Cardiac failure may occur in the absence of preexisting heart disease as a result of the hypertension of pregnancy, and from peripartum cardiomyopathy. This idiopathic condition presents in the last month of pregnancy or in the postpartum period and is associated with significantly increased mortality. During labor and the early postpartum period, tachycardia and increased cardiac output may precipitate pulmonary edema.

CRITICAL CARE MANAGEMENT

General Principles

Several aspects of the management of critically ill pregnant patients differ from routine care:

Positioning

In the supine position, the gravid uterus produces mechanical effects on the vena cava and aorta that reduce central venous return, causing a decrease in cardiac output and blood pressure. This "supine hypotensive syndrome" should be considered in hemodynamically unstable patients. The patient should be positioned on her left side, or at least with the right hip slightly elevated.

Nutrition

During starvation, maternal body stores are protected at the expense of the fetus and malnutrition may result in intrauterine growth retardation and fetal loss. Growth restriction before 26 weeks' gestation may lead to neurologic impairment. Caloric requirements in pregnancy increase by only about 300 kcal/day, and protein intake should be augmented by 20% to 50%. Nutrients with an increased requirement in pregnancy include iron, folate, and calcium. In patients for whom enteral nutrition is not possible, total parenteral nutrition (TPN) has been used successfully to provide nutritional support during pregnancy. Blood glucose should be measured frequently in view of the predisposition to hyperglycemia.

Box 59.3 Safety in Pregnancy of Common Drugs Used in the ICU

Classification of risk according to the FDA classification of drug safety in pregnancy. Column 1 (categories A and B) represents drugs for which no fetal risk has been demonstrated in human and/or animal studies in the first trimester. Column 2 (category C) represents drugs in which animal studies have demonstrated adverse effects or inadequate data exist. Column 3 represents drugs in which evidence of human fetal risk exists, but these drugs may be used in exceptional circumstances with serious diseases in which the expected benefit outweighs the risks (category D); and category X drugs, which should be avoided in pregnancy, since risks outweigh benefits.

Categories A and B	Category C	Categories D and X
Acyclovir	Aminoglycosides	ACE inhibitors
Amphotericin	Atracurium	Acetylsalicylic acid
Cephalosporins	Atropine	Benzodiazepines
Clindamycin	β-Blockers	Tetracyclines
Dalteparin	Digoxin	Warfarin (category X)
Dobutamine	Haloperidol	
Enoxaparin	Inotropes	
Erythromycin	Flumazenil	
Glycopyrrolate	Fluconazole	
Insulin	Furosemide	
Lidocaine	Heparin	
Magnesium sulfate	Labetalol	
Morphine	Metronidazole	
Naloxone	Pancuronium	
Penicillins	Phenytoin	
Prednisone	Prednisone	
Propofol	Suxamethonium	
Ranitidine	Vecuronium	
Terbutaline	Vancomycin	

Thrombosis Prophylaxis

Pregnancy increases the risks of venous thrombosis due to hypercoagulability and venous stasis. Antithrombotic precautions, including physical interventions and heparin prophylaxis, are important.

Drug Therapy

Pharmacotherapy during pregnancy requires consideration of the pharmacologic and teratogenic effects of drugs on the embryo (Box 59.3). Clearance and volume of distribution of drugs may be altered in pregnancy. The major risk period for teratogenesis is the first 10 weeks of gestation.

Catecholamines

Commonly used catecholamines including dobutamine, dopamine, norepinephrine, and epinephrine have the potential to reduce uterine blood flow. Animal studies and limited human data suggest that ephedrine increases maternal blood pressure as well as increasing uterine blood flow. The rapidity of correction of blood pressure may be more important than the specific inotropic agent used. The importance of nonpharmacologic maneuvers such as volume replacement and left lateral positioning must be stressed. If vasopressor therapy is required to support maternal hemodynamics, it should not be withheld out of concern for potential adverse effects on the fetus.

Sedation, Analgesia, and Paralysis

Few data on the preferred drugs for prolonged sedation, analgesia, and neuromuscular blockade exist. Sedation with benzodiazepines has been associated with a small risk of congenital malformations, mainly cleft lip and palate, when used in early gestation. Midazolam crosses the placenta to a lesser degree than diazepam does, which can accumulate in the fetus at levels greater than in the mother. No significant risk of congenital malformations has been demonstrated for narcotic analgesics such as morphine, meperidine, and fentanyl. The majority of nondepolarizing neuromuscular blocking agents have been shown to cross the placenta, including pancuronium, vecuronium, and atracurium, but transfer is unlikely to have clinical effects on the fetus in the short term. Nevertheless, the use of any of the above agents prior to delivery must be communicated to the neonatologist, who should anticipate the need for ventilatory support for the fetus.

Antibiotics

Similar antibiotic regimens to those used in the nonpregnant patient are appropriate, with a few precautions. Quinolones should probably be avoided because of the potential risk of arthropathy. Tetracyclines produce adverse effects on fetal teeth and bone, and aminoglycosides and sulfonamides should be used with caution.

Hemodynamic Monitoring

In general, the indications for use of the pulmonary artery catheter are similar to those in nonobstetric patients and pregnancy is not a contraindication to invasive monitoring. An awareness of the normal cardiovascular physiologic changes in pregnancy (discussed previously) is necessary to correctly interpret the hemodynamic data obtained.

Radiologic Procedures and Fetal Risk

Despite the potential risk of exposing the fetus to ionizing radiation, radiologic investigations are often essential for management of the critically ill pregnant patient. Fetal well-being depends on maternal recovery, and necessary radiologic procedures should not be avoided. Estimated fetal radiation exposure varies from less than 0.1 mGy (0.01 rad) for a chest radiograph to as high as 20–50 mGy (2–5 rad) for pelvic CT (see Table 59.5). Techniques such as shielding the abdomen with lead and using a well-collimated x-ray beam can effectively reduce exposure.

The potential adverse effects of uterine exposure to radiation include oncogenicity and teratogenicity. A twofold increased risk of childhood leukemia may occur with relatively low-dose fetal exposure (20–50 mGy). Teratogenicity is thought not to occur at these low radiation doses and likely to occur only after radiation exposure greater than 50 to 100 mGy (5–10 rad). Nonetheless, every effort should be made to minimize fetal exposure, particularly in the first trimester.

Cardiopulmonary Resuscitation

The management of cardiac arrest in pregnant patients should be according to standard protocols, with some modifications. Electrical cardioversion and defibrillation may be performed in pregnancy, after removal of fetal monitoring leads, to prevent arcing. Appropriate pharmacologic therapy should not be withheld when clinically indicated. Conventional CPR in the supine position may cause significant aortocaval compression, resulting in impaired venous return and inadequate cardiac output. The use of a table that provides a lateral tilt, a wedge under the right hip, or manual displacement of the uterus to the left is recommended. Perimortem cesarean section may be indicated when initial attempts at resuscitation have failed in a woman at 24 to 26 weeks or more of gestation. Data suggest that infant survival without neurologic sequelae is highest if the postmortem cesarean section is initiated within 4 minutes of cardiac arrest.

Ventilatory Support

Noninvasive Ventilation

Noninvasive ventilation has the potential benefit of avoiding the adverse effects of endotracheal intubation, which include airway trauma, an increased risk of nosocomial pneumonia, and the complications of sedation. Intubation in pregnancy can be associated with increased risk, making noninvasive support an attractive consideration. This modality is also ideally suited to short-term ventilatory support, which may be the case in many obstetric complications that reverse rapidly. The major concern of mask ventilation in pregnancy is the risk of vomiting and aspiration. Pregnant women may be at increased risk of reflux due to increased intra-abdominal pressure, delayed gastric emptying, and reduced lower esophageal sphincter pressure. Noninvasive ventilation should therefore be reserved for patients who are alert and protecting their airway and who have an expectation of a relatively brief requirement for mechanical ventilatory support.

Airway Management

Failed intubation in the obstetric population occurs at a significantly higher rate than in other anesthetic intubations. The reduced oxygen reserve, resulting from a diminished functional residual capacity and increased oxygen consumption, produces rapid desaturation in response to apnea or hypoventilation. Adequate preoxygenation with 100% oxygen is beneficial, while avoiding respiratory alkalosis. In view of the delayed gastric emptying and elevated intra-abdominal pressure, pregnant patients should always be considered to have a full stomach and appropriate precautions taken. Upper airway hyperemia and edema may reduce visualization and increase bleeding. The nasal route should be avoided, and a smaller endotracheal tube should always be available.

Mechanical Ventilation

The indications for mechanical ventilation in pregnancy are similar to those in the nonpregnant patient, but the normal $PaCO_2$ of about 30 mm Hg in late pregnancy should be considered in the interpretation of arterial blood gases. Data on mechanical ventilation in pregnancy are limited. Hyperventilation should be avoided, since it adversely affects uterine blood flow as a result of the resulting alkalemia and the effect of positive pressure ventilation in reducing cardiac output. The current ventilatory approach of avoiding excessive lung stretch by pressure limitation and permissive hypercapnia has not been assessed in pregnancy. While ventilatory strategies restricting alveolar distention limit plateau pressure to 35 cm H_2O, chest wall compliance is reduced in late pregnancy, and the transpulmonary pressures may not be elevated at a plateau pressure of 35 cm H_2O. Higher ventilatory pressure may be acceptable in pregnant patients near term. Regarding the level of acceptable $PaCO_2$, maternal hypercapnia up to 60 mm Hg in the presence of adequate oxygenation does not appear to be detrimental to the fetus, although fetal heart rate changes associated with fetal acidemia may be noted. If marked respiratory acidosis results from permissive hypercapnia, treatment with bicarbonate may improve maternal and fetal acidemia. Increased oxygen consumption may make adequate oxygen delivery difficult to achieve.

SUMMARY

Management of critically ill pregnant patients requires an awareness of the physiologic changes of pregnancy and the various pregnancy-specific complications that can result in ICU admission. The welfare of the fetus should always be considered, although improving maternal well-being is almost always beneficial to the fetus. Management is best carried out in a multidisciplinary environment, with input from specialists in critical care, obstetrics, anesthesia, and maternal-fetal medicine.

SUGGESTED READING

Briggs GG, Freeman RK, Yaffe SJ (eds): Drugs in Pregnancy and Lactation, 6th ed. Baltimore: Lippincott Williams & Wilkins, 2001.

Campbell LA, Klocke RA: Update in nonpulmonary critical care: implications for the pregnant patient. Am J Respir Crit Care Med 2001; 163:1051–1054.

Clark SL, Hankins GDV, Dudley DA, et al: Amniotic fluid embolism: analysis of the national registry. Am J Obstet Gynecol 1995;172:1158–1167.

Ginsberg JS, Greer I, Hirsh J: Use of antithrombotic agents during pregnancy. Chest 2001;119:122S–131S.

Hazelgrove JF, Price C, Pappachan VJ, et al: Multicenter study of obstetric admissions to 14 intensive care units in southern England. Crit Care Med 2001;29:770–775.

Lapinsky SE, Kruczynski K, Slutsky AS: State of the art: critical care in the pregnant patient. Am J Respir Crit Care Med 1995;152:427–455.

Lewin SB, Cheek TG, Deutschman CS: Airway management in the obstetric patient. Crit Care Clin 2000;16:505–513.

Rizk NW, Kalassian KG, Gilligan T, et al: Obstetric complications in pulmonary and critical care medicine. Chest 1996;110:791–809.

Intensive Care after Cardiac Surgery

Michael Hiesmayr and Daniel Schmidlin

Intensive care after cardiac surgery is one of the important elements that determines outcome in cardiac surgery and has to be conceptually viewed as one of four complementary periods: preoperative preparation, intraoperative management and events, intensive care, and postoperative care on the ward. The majority of patients are operated on electively. Approximately half of the admitting intensive care units (ICUs) are general surgical ICUs and the other half are ICUs that specialize in the care of cardiac patients. In a recent development, more specific facilities providing standard intensive care after surgery are identified by names such as *fast-track recovery area*, *postanesthetic care unit*, and *surgical recovery area*. Their main goal is to create sufficient intensive care resources to make elective surgery independent from traditional ICUs. To achieve their goal, these structures have focused on shortening length of stay and thus rapidly decreasing the level of care soon after surgery in "fast-track" programs. Increasingly more patients from other surgical disciplines are referred to these specialized structures if the duration of intensive care treatment is expected to be limited to 1 or 2 days. All these areas have to integrate knowledge about the preoperative cardiac pathology, the operative process, and typical complications into their treatment (Fig. 60.1).

Nevertheless, a significant percentage (5%–25%) of patients require prolonged intensive care after cardiac surgery. This percentage is likely to increase because the number of patients with significant comorbidities, older age, and who require complex surgery is likely to increase in the near future. Several of the issues presented in this chapter will also apply to patients with cardiac pathologies admitted to an ICU without prior cardiac surgery.

EPIDEMIOLOGY, RISK FACTORS, AND PATHOPHYSIOLOGY

Epidemiology

Cardiac surgery is performed in approximately 500 to 1500 per 100,000 population, or about 1 million people in Europe. Cardiac surgery services typically treat several patient groups with typical pathologies and different requirements for intensive care. Each group has a typical pattern of age, gender distribution, and comorbidities (Table 60.1). Resource utilization may vary among institutions (Fig. 60.2) and depends on patient characteristics, perioperative events, and structures. Namely, a high nurse:patient ratio decreases time to extubation, as does the use of written protocols for weaning. In addition, length of stay is dictated by the availability of specific competences in the wards.

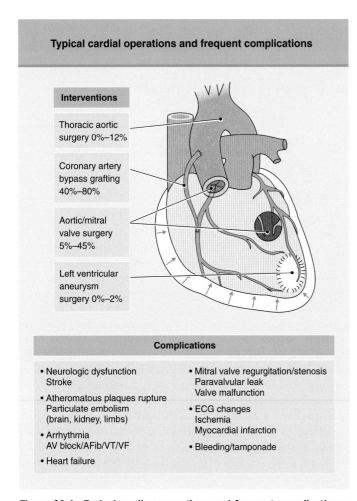

Typical cardial operations and frequent complications

Interventions

Thoracic aortic surgery 0%–12%

Coronary artery bypass grafting 40%–80%

Aortic/mitral valve surgery 5%–45%

Left ventricular aneurysm surgery 0%–2%

Complications

- Neurologic dysfunction Stroke
- Atheromatous plaques rupture Particulate embolism (brain, kidney, limbs)
- Arrhythmia AV block/AFib/VT/VF
- Heart failure

- Mitral valve regurgitation/stenosis Paravalvular leak Valve malfunction
- ECG changes Ischemia Myocardial infarction
- Bleeding/tamponade

Figure 60.1. Typical cardiac operations and frequent complications. The typical operations are given with their frequencies in different centers in Europe along with the major complications. Arrows indicate the effect of tamponade.

Risk Factors

The risk profile of cardiac surgery patients varies over time, and the relative weight of the individual risk factors also varies. Together, these factors determine outcome (Fig. 60.3). The patient's heart disease is the only factor that typically improves

with surgery. Improved heart function may not be immediate since previous heart disease may have profoundly modified the architecture as well as systolic and diastolic function of the heart. The manipulation of the heart for surgery and cardioplegia have reversible effects on function. Comorbidities will remain the same throughout hospitalization. The effect of anesthesia on organ function may continue into the early postoperative period.

Specific scores to evaluate outcome after cardiac surgery have been developed, including the EuroSCORE, which is in the public domain as an additive score for low- and moderate-risk patients and as a logistic score for a more precise evaluation of all risk categories. This score is applicable to continuous quality control.

Pathophysiology

Typical factors related to the intraoperative period are an inconstant cardiac output, intermittent reduction in organ perfusion, intense inflammatory response, hemodilution, and rapid changes in body temperature. The inconstant cardiac output is related to manipulation of the heart and great arteries, cardiopulmonary bypass (CPB), and unstable heart function after surgery. The inflammatory response appears to be related to the operation itself, to the use of the heart–lung machine, induced rapid temperature changes, and ischemia reperfusion phenomena from particulate or air embolism. The heart–lung machine induces a contact activation related to the foreign surfaces involving in a first step complement and thereafter multiple pro- and anti-inflammatory cytokines. A further element triggering inflammation is the large amount of tissue factor that directly enters the circulation via the cardiotomy reservoir, which is used to collect blood from the pericardium into the circuit. The temperature distribution within the body may be highly affected because, depending on the characteristics of the operation and preferences of the surgeon, the body temperature may be lowered to 15 to 18°C. Such a low temperature allows a complete circulatory arrest for approximately 1 hour. The main intention of lowering the temperature is to protect the brain and other organs during phases of inadequate or absent circulation. The consequences of such large temperature changes over a short period of time are an altered temperature regulation and tissue injury with edema.

Table 60.1 Profiles of Different Types of Cardiac Surgery						
Type of Surgery	Activity (%)	Urgent (%)	Female (%)	Diabetes (%)	Age, Years (SD)	Characteristics Features
Coronary artery surgery on CPB	65	5	24	20	65 (10)	High risk of perioperative ischemia, generalized atherosclerosis
Coronary artery surgery off-pump	8	3	22	19	64 (11)	Patient selection in evolution from low risk to high risk
Aortic stenosis	14	3	45	15	69 (11)	Left heart hypertrophy, afterload and volume crucial
Aortic regurgitation	8	5	31	10	62 (14)	Left heart dilated, poor volume tolerance
Mitral stenosis	2	10	72	12	64 (11)	Pulmonary hypertension frequent
Mitral regurgitation	9	6	49	11	64 (12)	Pulmonary hypertension frequent
Aneurysm ascending aorta	3	26	27	5	62 (12)	Risk of dissection, cerebral ischemia
Aorta descending aorta	1	25	16	2	64 (13)	Spinal cord perfusion at risk
Congenital heart defects	1	0	64	6	44 (17)	Pulmonary hypertension
Heart transplantation	1	100	35	17	55 (11)	Organ dysfunction as a consequence of left heart failure

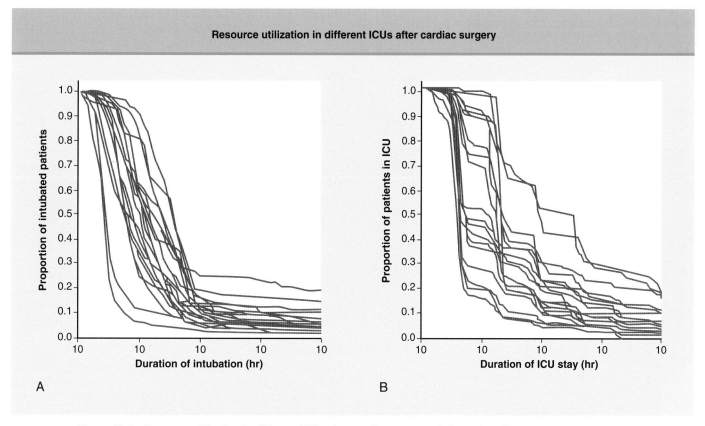

Figure 60.2. Resource utilization in different ICUs after cardiac surgery. *A,* Proportion of intubated patients in 21 European ICUs versus time. *B,* Proportion of patients still in ICU versus time. There is a major difference in resource utilization. (Data from Lassnigg A, Hiesmayr M, Bauer P, et al: Effect of centre-, patient-, and procedure-related factors on intensive care resource utilisation after cardiac surgery. Intensive Care Med 2002;28:1453–1461.)

Particulate emboli are delivered to the systemic circulation during cannulation of the aorta before cardiopulmonary bypass, at removal of the aortic cross-clamp, and during weaning from CPB. Air emboli are typically found after open procedures such as valve operations. The first manifestation of the inflammatory response is a strong postoperative febrile response that peaks approximately 6 hours after surgery.

An additional effect is related to hemodilution. With the onset of CPB, the blood of the patient is mixed with a volume of 1500 to 2000 mL of fluid (crystalloids and colloids in various proportions). Coagulation is prevented in general during CPB by a large dose of unfractionated heparin (300 IU/kg body weight) and reversed by protamine after separation from CPB. The pharmacokinetic profile is such that the half-life of protamine is shorter than that for heparin. Thus, adequate reversal may necessitate an additional dose of protamine within 1 or 2 hours. The use of protamine is convenient, but histamine release with bronchoconstriction and acute pulmonary hypertension with acute right heart failure may occur. All other methods to induce systemic anticoagulation for surgery, as applied in patients with heparin-induced thrombopenia, such as danaparoid and lepirudine, have no antidote. In addition, certain drugs have a short half-life only when renal function is preserved and are not eliminated with standard renal replacement therapy. The consequence is a highly increased risk of bleeding.

Another pathophysiologic factor is related to respiratory function. The lung is collapsed during surgery and reexpanded after CPB. Atelectasis is a frequent manifestation. In addition, the chest wall is subjected to stretch trauma during the surgical procedure by retractors that decrease chest wall compliance for more than 1 week.

The typical access is median sternotomy. The circulation to the sternum may be decreased after harvesting the internal mammary artery. This poor perfusion may be related to a prevalence of acquiring a deep sternal wound infection of 1.5% to 3%. Known risk factors for deep sternal wound infection are resternotomy, adipositas, diabetes, and hyperglycemia.

CLINICAL FEATURES

Timely reaction to deviations from normal is crucial after heart surgery, and action may be necessary before all information is available. Action sometimes may be based on an educated guess.

Each of the following clinical features should be considered according to the availability and robustness of the information. Typically, information about rhythm is most easily obtained, together with electrocardiogram (ECG), blood pressure, and blood gases including mixed venous or central venous saturation (SvO_2), followed by capnometry ($EtCO_2$), cardiac output (CO), and pulmonary capillary wedge pressure. Thus, the clinical decision-making process may greatly differ from a standard pathophysiological process. Decision trees should follow the clinical path, including first available information. Additional consideration has to be given to the likelihood of the event in

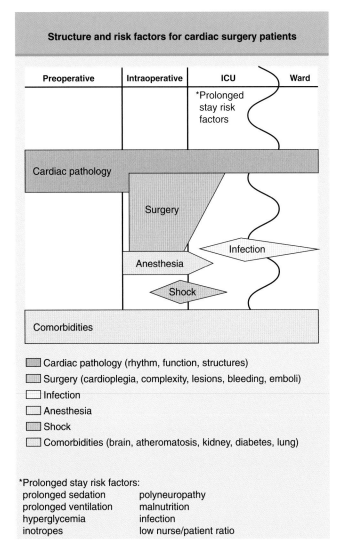

Structure and risk factors for cardiac surgery patients

Preoperative	Intraoperative	ICU	Ward

*Prolonged stay risk factors

Cardiac pathology

Surgery

Anesthesia

Infection

Shock

Comorbidities

▢ Cardiac pathology (rhythm, function, structures)
▢ Surgery (cardioplegia, complexity, lesions, bleeding, emboli)
▢ Infection
▢ Anesthesia
▢ Shock
▢ Comorbidities (brain, atheromatosis, kidney, diabetes, lung)

*Prolonged stay risk factors:
prolonged sedation   polyneuropathy
prolonged ventilation   malnutrition
hyperglycemia   infection
inotropes   low nurse/patient ratio

Figure 60.3. Structure and risk factors for cardiac surgery patients. The aim is to reduce the burden of cardiac disease, but success is determined by several other factors, such as the prolonged effects of anesthesia, surgery, shock, and management.

question. In a substantial number of units, rates may differ from those proposed in the literature based on case mix and local policy.

Monitoring

Standard monitoring is ECG, invasive arterial pressure, and the central venous pressure. Some institutions use pulmonary artery catheters (PACs) for all cases, but others are more restrictive. In cases of poor ventricular function, pulmonary hypertension, and multiple valve replacement, a PAC remains the standard of care. The combination of PAC with continuous mixed venous oximetry is useful in cases in which significant tricuspid regurgitation makes thermodilution measurements unreliable. In case of worsening cardiac function with increasing regurgitation, the monitor will indicate an increasing CO that is not real, whereas oximetry will clearly show a rapid decline. In cases in which only CO measurements are required, monitoring methods such as pulse contour measurements are used. The necessity to recalibrate these devices after significant hemodynamic changes makes their use in the early unstable postoperative phase more difficult.

Hypotension

Normal mean arterial blood pressure after cardiac surgery is 60 to 90 mm Hg. Hypotension may be caused by a decrease in either vascular resistance or CO or both. The differentiation may involve measurements or estimations (Tables 60.2 and 60.3).

Hypovolemia

In case of suspected hypovolemia bleeding, sequestration in the third space due to a capillary leak syndrome and intravascular pooling have to be considered. Typically, sequestration will be more pronounced if impaired heart function necessitates higher filling pressures because higher filling pressures are very likely to increase microvascular pressure at the capillary level. There is considerable debate regarding whether lowered colloid osmotic pressure, a uniform finding after cardiac surgery, also precipitates fluid sequestration. Typically, colloid is decreased by 50% after surgery (colloid osmotic pressure of

Table 60.2 Arterial Hypotension: Blood Pressure < 60 mm Hg[a]			
	Features		**Cause**
Cardiac output low (or indirect signs)	Low filling pressure	CVP < 10 mm Hg	Bleeding?
		PCWP < 12 mm Hg	Vasoplegia?
			Vasodilator drugs?
	Rhythm disturbance	Bradycardia	Use pacemaker
		Loss of sinus rhythm	Consider ischemia
		Bundle branch block	
		Tachycardia	
	High filling pressure	Increasing CVP	High intrathoracic pressure?
		CVP > 15 mm Hg	Patient shivering?
		Pulmonary hypertension	Tension/fighting the ventilator?
		Increasing PCWP	Heart failure?
		PCWP > 20 mm Hg	Myocardial ischemia?
			Tamponade
			Pneumothorax
Cardiac output high	Filling pressure normal or low	Low vascular resistance syndrome	

[a]The conditions are listed by decreasing probability.
CVP, central venous pressure; PCWP, pulmonary capillary wedge pressure.

Table 60.3 Arterial Hypertension: Blood Pressure > 100 mm Hg[a]			
Features			**Cause**
Cardiac output low (or indirect signs)	High filling pressure	Increasing CVP	Pain?
		CVP > 15 mm Hg	Stress?
		Pulmonary hypertension	Patient shivering?
		Increasing PCWP	Patient fighting the ventilator?
		PCWP > 20 mm Hg	Check for heart failure
			Check for myocardial ischemia
			Vasopressor overdose
	Rhythm disturbance	Bradycardia	Use pacemaker
		Loss of sinus rhythm	Consider ischemia
		Bundle branch block	
		Tachycardia	
Cardiac output high	Filling pressure high	Hypervolemia possible with good heart function	Drug overdose with positive inotropic properties
	Filling pressure normal or low		

[a]The conditions are listed by decreasing probability.
CVP, central venous pressure; PCWP, pulmonary capillary wedge pressure.

12–15 mm Hg) and increases rapidly during recovery. In standard care, no correction is instituted as long as values are higher than 12 mm Hg.

Vasoplegia

Vasoplegia is induced by hemodilution, drugs, and the vasculature response to rewarming after surgery. In certain phases of the inflammatory process that is common after surgery, vasoplegia is possible. Some drugs, such as vasodilators and certain inotropes with vasodilating properties, may have intended vasodilating properties whereas others, such as sedatives or narcotics, have unintended vasodilating properties.

Hypertension

The evaluation of postoperative hypertension can be divided into three major categories: stress, reaction to treatment, and recurrence of hypertension. All efforts have to be made to avoid hypertension. Especially the vulnerable ventricle after cardiac surgery will suffer from increased afterload (Figs. 60.4 and 60.5). The typical range for mean arterial blood pressure is 65 to 95 mm Hg (100/50 to 125/80).

Bradycardia

Change in heart rate is usually associated with a proportional change in CO. This will be the case when filling is limited by myocardial stiffness rather than by duration of diastole. In contrast to many other clinical situations in which an increase in heart rate may only be obtained with a drug or a new invasive procedure, after cardiac surgery wires sutured directly on the heart are available for temporary pacing.

Loss of Sinus Rhythm

The most frequent loss is due to atrial fibrillation, but nodal rhythm may have a similar effect on hemodynamics. Nodal rhythm is typically associated with canon waves on the central venous monitoring. If this change is uncertain from the ECG, a missing A wave on the transmitral Doppler flow interrogation is pathognomonic. The effect of the loss in sinus rhythm is most prominent due to diastolic dysfunction with a ventricle that requires a higher pressure to be filled during diastole. A return to sinus rhythm should be attempted with either a synchronized

electrical cardioversion or pharmacologic cardioversion with amiodarone:

Check potassium: K+ > 4.5 mmol/liter
Consider synchronized electrical cardioversion (anesthesia required)

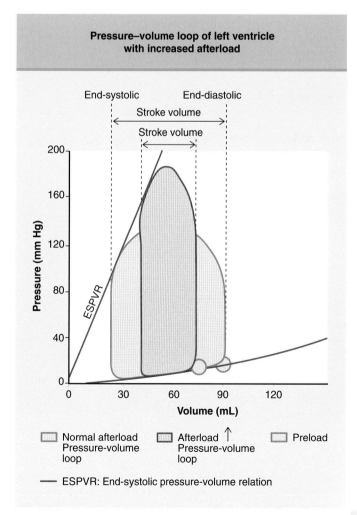

Figure 60.4. Pressure–volume loop of the left ventricle with increased afterload.

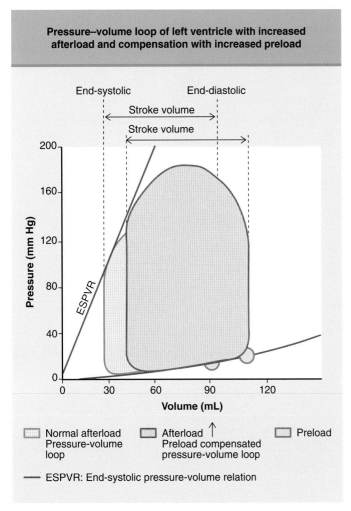

Pressure–volume loop of left ventricle with increased afterload and compensation with increased preload

Normal afterload Pressure-volume loop

Afterload ↑ Preload compensated pressure-volume loop

Preload

ESPVR: End-systolic pressure-volume relation

Figure 60.5. Pressure–volume loop of the left ventricle with increased afterload and compensation with increased preload.

Attempt pharmacologic cardioversion and prevention of recurring atrial fibrillation with amiodarone, β-adrenergic blocking agents

In all these interventions, an external pacemaker should be connected and checked for ventricular stimulation to allow maintenance of ventricular rate in case of bradycardia or cardiac arrest after treatment attempts. Patients with preoperative atrial fibrillation will not maintain a postoperative sinus rhythm unless a specific procedure to restore normal conduction, such as a Maze procedure, has been performed during surgery.

Tachycardia

Tachycardia has the following etiologies in order of frequency: stress, cardiac pathology, and drug effects. The desired heart rate is between 60 and 90 beats per minute (bpm). Typically, heart rate is increased after surgery by 10% to 20%, probably as an expression of the decreased compliance compensated for by an increased heart rate to obtain a satisfactory CO.

Any elevation above 100 bpm needs careful evaluation. In a large percentage (up to 30%) of patients, tachycardic atrial fi-

brillation occurs. In severe tachycardia (heart rate > 125–140 bpm) filling of the ventricle will be decreased because the diastole is too short. Furthermore, tachycardia may precipitate myocardial ischemia on its own because coronary perfusion is also related to the duration of diastole. Precipitating factors for tachycardia are stress, anxiety, disorientation, and pain in patients without beta blocking agents. In these cases, tachycardia is often associated with hypertension. It also has to be considered that in the case of poor heart function, heart rate may be the only factor that can be manipulated to maintain CO. Therapy should be prompt, especially in relation to stress and possible myocardial ischemia. Arrhythmia can be prevented by pharmacologic interventions such as maintaining high normal potassium, prophylactic amiodarone, and appropriate use of beta blocking agents.

Arrhythmia

Arrhythmia is a very common complication after cardiac surgery, occurring in 20% to 40% of patients. The most common rhythm disturbance is atrial fibrillation. All new rhythm abnormalities should direct attention to possible precipitating factors. The most frequent precipitating factors are preoperative atrial fibrillation, preoperative hypertension, male gender, poor cardiac preservation during surgery by cardioplegia, postoperative electrolyte abnormalities, side effects of inotropic drugs, and endogenous catecholamine liberation by stress and pain. In addition, a unit must have an overview of the rates of rhythm disturbances since several interventions have been shown to effectively prevent atrial fibrillation, for example.

After identifying the causes of rhythm disturbances, management will be determined by their effect on global cardiac performance and the chance of cure (Fig. 60.6). Patients with preoperative atrial fibrillation may have a period of sinus rhythm after surgery, but electric cardioversion often fails.

ECG Changes

Evaluation of ECG changes is an integral part of follow-up after cardiac surgery and focuses on ongoing or new ischemia. A baseline 12-lead ECG after surgery is the reference. Thereafter, observation of the ECG on the monitor, which may integrate automatic ST segment analysis, is typically done for leads II and V5 simultaneously in order to obtain maximal sensitivity for ST segment changes obtainable from two leads. ECG changes are frequent, especially with conduction changes. Bundle branch blocks and onset of pacemaker activity do not have a major impact on management, whereas ischemia requires prompt evaluation to prevent progressive loss of myocardium.

Any change on the 12-lead ECG must be related to the preoperative angiographic information and to the vessel that was operated on. The other elements that have to be sequentially addressed are hemodynamic changes and regional wall motion abnormalities (RWMAs) as detected by echocardiography (Fig. 60.7). RWMA abnormalities are typically reported with the 16-segment system proposed by the Society of Cardiovascular Anesthesiologists/National Board of Echocardiography. The first step in the therapeutic approach is to remove all factors that may induce ischemia. The second step is to discuss with the surgeon whether an intervention is possible. Four options are considered: reoperation, angiography, intraaortic balloon pumping, and medical treatment.

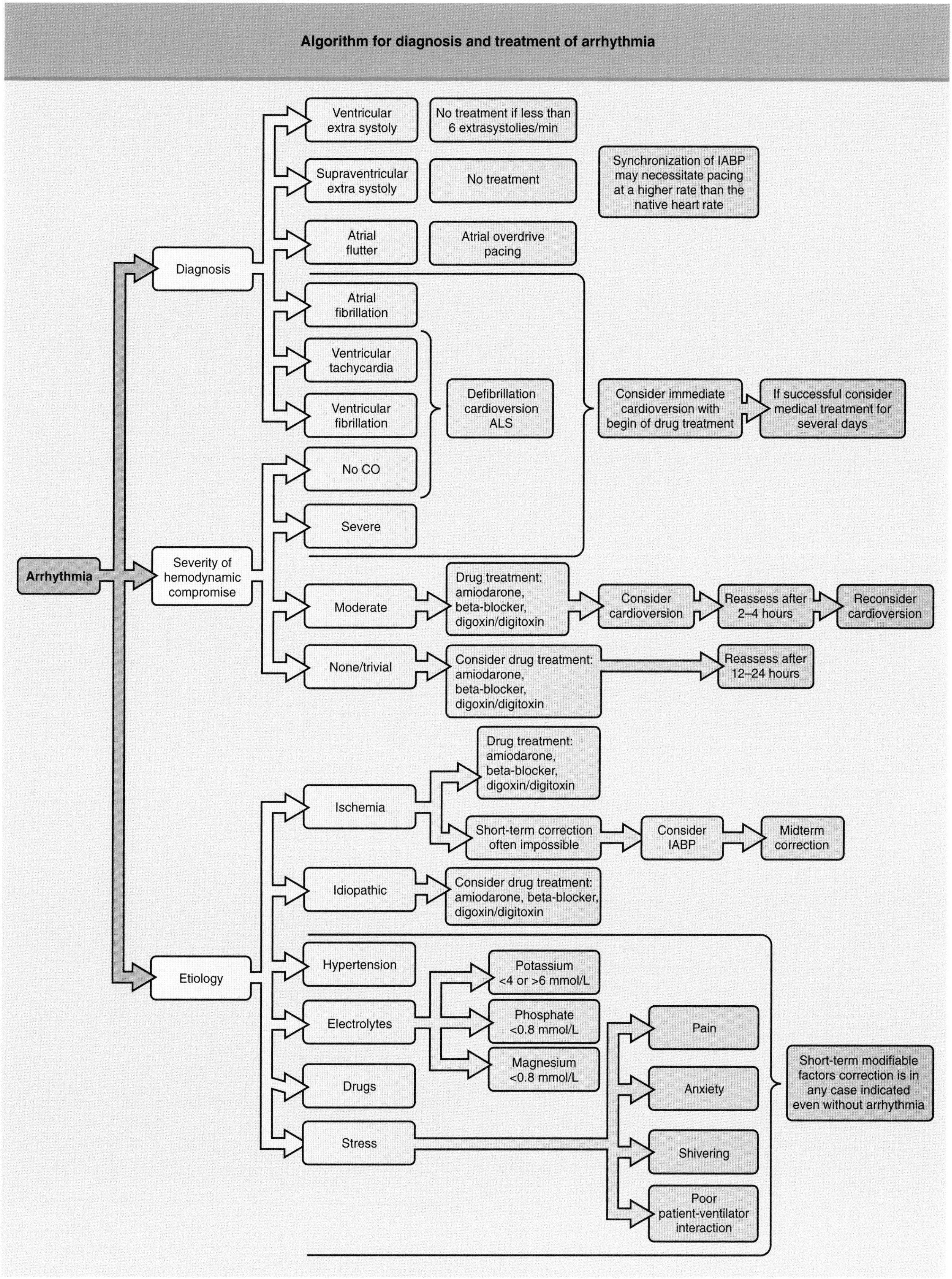

Figure 60.6. Algorithm for diagnosis and treatment of arrhythmia. In all cases in which ischemia is possible, the surgeon needs to be questioned about possible correctable lesions.

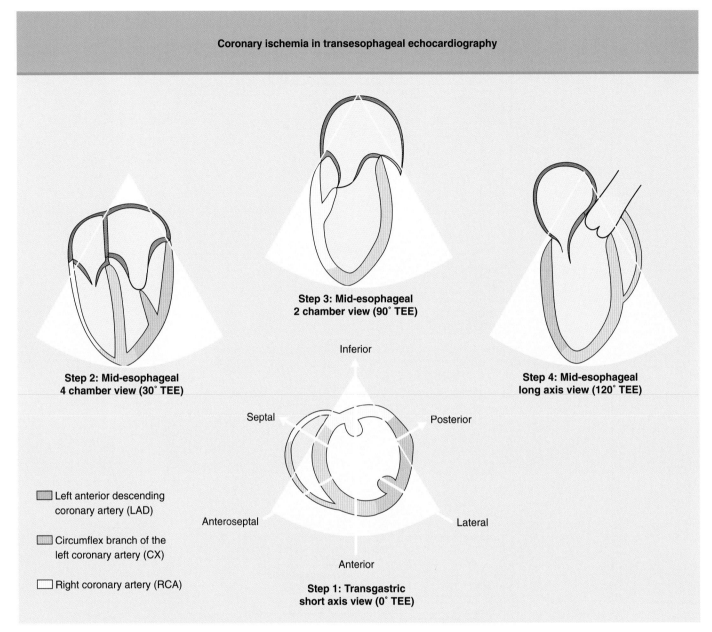

Coronary ischemia in transesophageal echocardiography

Step 3: Mid-esophageal 2 chamber view (90° TEE)

Step 2: Mid-esophageal 4 chamber view (30° TEE)

Step 4: Mid-esophageal long axis view (120° TEE)

Inferior

Septal

Posterior

Anteroseptal

Lateral

Anterior

Left anterior descending coronary artery (LAD)

Circumflex branch of the left coronary artery (CX)

Right coronary artery (RCA)

Step 1: Transgastric short axis view (0° TEE)

Figure 60.7. Coronary ischemia in transesophageal echocardiography. Identification of coronary ischemia in transesophageal echocardiography (TEE) and topographical attribution to individual coronary arteries. The arrows in the short-axis view (step 1) indicate the related longitudinal view (steps 2–4).

Tamponade

Tamponade is much rarer than bleeding, necessitating rethoracotomy because the operative field is drained. Suspicion rises when a previously notably bleeding patient has no further blood coming off the drains and becomes hemodynamically unstable. A further common risk situation is after drain or epicardial pacemaker wire removal and on days 5 to 10 after heart transplantation. Classical signs, such as the triad—tachycardia, high central venous pressure, and low blood pressure—are often missing and by no means pathognomonic. Even small fluid collections or clots can cause a severe impairment of cardiac function, especially if diastolic dysfunction coexists. The diagnosis is obtained by (transesophageal) echocardiography. If not readily available, it will be necessary to reopen the chest for inspection when an unexplained hemodynamic situation occurs early after surgery. The more chronic form is often characterized by clinical signs of decreased CO and decreased renal function.

Bleeding

Bleeding exceeding normal values (first hour, 400 mL; second hour, 200 mL; and third hour, 100 mL) should be checked for adequate heparin reversal and communicated to the surgeon. It is helpful to control the hematocrit of the drained fluid since values lower than one third of the systemic hematocrit are less likely to be surgical. In general, prompt surgical reintervention helps to reduce exposure to blood products.

Table 60.4 Typical Time Course of Median Laboratory Values after Cardiac Surgery in 3860 Surviving Patients

	Normal	Preop	Postop	POD 1	POD 2	POD 3	POD 4	POD 5	POD 6	POD 7
Hgb (g/dL)	12–16	13.50	11.20	10.80	10.30	10.00	10.20	10.50	10.60	10.75
Plt (10^3/μL)	150–350	227	132	131	126	124	153	205	209	259
WBC (10^3/μL)	4–10	7.0	12.5	10.5	11.3	10.2	8.9	8.2	9.2	9.7
CRP (mg/dL)	<1	<0.5	1.97	8.72	19.90	19.30	15.10	9.59	8.80	7.70
Albumin (g/liter)	34–48	40.0	25.2	25.1	25.2	24.6	25.0	26.9	26.1	26.6
Protein (g/liter)	65–85	75.2	45.5	47.0	51.1	52.3	54.1	57.6	57.4	58.7
CK (U/liter)	<70	28	189	260	208	136	87	49	38	28
CK-MB (U/liter)	<10 or <6% of CK	12	24	17	13	10	8	8	8	7
ASAT (U/liter)	<15	10.0	22.0	26.0	19.0	15.0	14.0	13.0	14.0	13.5
ALAT (U/liter)	<19	12.0	11.0	12.0	12.0	13.0	15.0	17.0	19.5	21.0

ALAT, alanineaminotransferase; ASAT, aspartateaminotransferase; CK, creatine kinase; CK-MB, creatine-kinase MB fraction; CRP, C-reactive protein; Hgb, hemoglobin; Plt, platelets; POD, postoperative day; Postop, at ICU arrival; Preop, before the operation; WBC, white blood cells.

Pneumothorax

Laceration of the lung is possible during thoracotomy or harvesting of the internal mammary. The anesthesiologist should inform the intensivist whether the pleura has been opened and drained. In cases of opened pleura that is not drained, the risk of pneumothorax is increased. The clinical presentation can be either ventilatory, with dyspnea and hypoxia, or hemodynamic, similar to a tamponade with a decreased venous return caused by the increased intrathoracic pressure.

Patients Sedated Too Much or Not Enough

Traditionally, after cardiac surgery patients have been heavily sedated as a stress prevention measure. However, the most important element is adequate pain relief with narcotics, acetaminophen, and eventually thoracic epidural analgesia with minimal sedation. The patient should be relaxed, arousable, with assisted spontaneous breathing 1 to 4 hours after surgery. Extubation is preferred over further sedation in all stable patients. In a few patients with severe uncontrolled heart failure, sedation may be necessary until stabilization of hemodynamics.

Confusion/Cerebral Dysfunction

The patient with confusion is a particular challenge. Communication is poor and adaptation to the ventilator or unassisted breathing impossible. A period of sedation until the confusion has abated is often necessary. In rare cases, adaptation may not be possible without a short phase of relaxation and deeper sedation. The risk for confusion is clearly increased by a history of neuropsychiatric abnormality after previous operations. The origin of confusion is much less clear than for cerebral dysfunction, in which particulate, atheromateous, and air emboli are considered etiologic factors. In confused patients, a particular susceptibility to certain hypnotics, participation of the brain in the inflammatory process, fever, and structural factors have been proposed as relevant factors.

Shivering

Shivering is an undesired effect related to disturbed temperature regulation and a changed set point due to the inflammatory process. Shivering is accompanied by a large increase in oxygen consumption and in muscle tension that impairs venous return.

Thus, a situation with inadequate oxygen supply to the tissues may ensue.

The incidence of shivering has decreased with a more appropriate temperature management aimed at maintaining or returning to normothermia soon after the operation has been performed. In addition, a prophylactic dose of pethidine at the end of surgery and parenteral paracetamol diminish the level of fever early after surgery and also provide pain relieve.

Fever

Fever in the range of 38.5 to 39.5°C between 4 and 8 hours after surgery is common and not completely suppressible. It is also unclear whether suppression would be beneficial or detrimental. Some patients have an even more extreme febrile reaction. In all patients, after the peak in body temperature a phase of peripheral vasodilatation occurs. Usually, it is preferable to counteract the vasodilating properties of anesthetics with a small dose of vasopressors rather than to give a large amount of fluid.

Lab Values

The typical lab values during the first week after surgery are given in Table 60.4.

TREATMENT AND CLINICAL COURSE

The general principle in the treatment of patients after cardiac surgery is to shorten ICU stay by a fast-track management, avoid periods of shock by carefully checking for complications of surgery, and treat heart failure appropriately.

Principles of Fast-Track Treatment

- Normothermia as soon as possible
- Treat shivering aggressively
- Good pain control
- Mild sedation until rewarming to normothermia (36–37°C)
- Early extubation 1 to 5 hours postsurgery (independently of moderate hemodynamic support)
- Tight control of glycemia to 90 to 110 mg/dL with continuous insulin

Other Critical Care Problems

Table 60.5 Checklist at Admission		
Preoperative information		
Reason for operation	Cardiac and general functional status	
Cardiac pathology	Rhythm	Chronic Afib, AICD
	Function	LV, RV
	Structure	Valves: stenosis/regurgitation
		Coronary arteries: localization and degree of stenosis
		Ventricle: aneurysm
Comorbidity	Vascular, brain, kidney, diabetes, lung	
Infection	Chronic/acute	
All chronic medications	Beta blocker, antihypertensives, ACE inhibitors, thrombolytics, antiparkinson, antidementia	
Intraoperative information		
ECG changes	Comparison pre- vs. postoperative	
Cardioplegia	Antegrade, retrograde	Retrograde preferred but higher rate of poor RV protection
		Poor cardioplegia related to postoperative heart failure
Revascularization	Which vessels?	To allow evaluation of ECG or function changes or TEE changes
	Complete or partial?	
	Arterial/venous grafts?	
	Central anastomosis?	
	RWMA after CPB?	
Valve surgery	Mechanical valve	Dimension limit CO
	Biological valve	Paravalvular leaks
	Reconstruction	Reconstruction success
Ascending aorta	Cannulation site	Site of bleeding
	Repair for dilatation	Risk of dissection
Rhythm	Cardioversion after CPB	Spontaneous sinus rhythm indicates good cardioplegia and improved function
	Sinus rhythm postoperatively	
Pacemaker	A or V or both	Function test
Drugs	What was necessary to wean from CPB?	In patients with difficult weaning, function may deteriorate for several hours before stabilization
Coagulation reversal	Protamine dose sufficient?	ACT or alternative measurement to document return to baseline (ACT 110–130")
Antibiotic prophylaxis	Duration limited to intraoperative or maximum 24 hr	Agent selected based on resistance pattern in the strains present in mediastinitis
Opioid used	Ultra short acting	Determines postoperative pain therapy
	Short acting	
Thoracic epidural	Drugs and dose	
Antishivering drug	Type and dose	Intraoperative start of treatment is more effective

- Give fluid only when necessary for hemodynamic stabilization (but consider low-dose vasopressors to counteract vasodilating side effects of sedatives)
- Drinking soon after extubation allowed
- Normal food on the morning after surgery

Checklists at admission (Table 60.5) and discharge (Table 60.6) are helpful to obtain all useful information for ICU care and provide information for subsequent ward care. The hemodynamic target values (Table 60.7) can only guide treatment and alert for deviations. It is of utmost importance to detect and treat postoperative heart failure according to the baseline pathology.

Baseline Cardiac Pathology

Three major categories should be distinguished:

1. Ischemic heart disease with coronary artery bypass grafting: Vulnerable to ischemia, avoid tachycardia, hypertension. Stunned myocardium may need several days until full recovery is achieved. Arterial grafts are generally preferred because of the good long-term results, but the flow in these grafts is lower postoperatively than in venous grafts.

2. Aortic stenosis with small hypertrophic left ventricle: Diastolic dysfunction is common, and careful filling and maintenance of systemic arterial pressure and sinus rhythm are essential. Subaortic stenosis can occur when an underfilled ventricle is stimulated with inotropes.

3. Aortic and mitral regurgitation: Ventricles are often large and recovery of function is not immediate. These patients often benefit from low-dose inotropes for several days after surgery. Intravenous inotropes should be withdrawn when chronic heart failure treatment has been reinstituted.

Heart Failure Following Cardiac Surgery
Essentials of Diagnosis: Clinical Signs

- Cold, pale/blue skin
- Dyspnea, rales, or signs of bronchoobstruction at auscultation
- Often, neurologic signs such as restlessness or extreme fatigue or both
- Especially in older people, loss of orientation and even consciousness
- Low urine output
- Arterial hypotension (not mandatory)

Table 60.6 Checklist at Discharge

Category	Intervention and Medication	Comments
Vulnerable organ function	Brain, heart, kidney, lung	Insist on continuity of treatment
Cardiac medications	Beta blocking agents	Ischemic heart in general
	Nitrates	Depending on level of revascularization or postoperative ECG changes
	ACE inhibitors (+ antihypertensives)	Heart failure
	Amiodarone	If arrhythmia was successfully converted to sinus rhythm
	Digoxin/digitoxin	Rate control in Afib and heart failure
	Diuretics	Heart failure/backshift?
	Aldosterone antagonist	Heart failure
Pacemaker	Treatment/standby	Based on ICU history
Thrombolytics	ASS low dose	According to surgeon in ischemic heart disease or atheromatosis
	Clopidogrel or analog	
Anticoagulants	Heparin	1. Prophylaxis against peripheral thrombosis
	LMWH	2. Therapy after valve replacement
	Coumadin	Only after chest tube removal
Pain treatment	Paracetamol	
	Cox-2 inhibitors	
	Thoracic epidural	Alternatives depending on institutional standards
	PCA	
Metabolism	Insulin sc	For diabetics and those with stress hyperglycemia that needed continuous IV insulin
Laboratory	Glucose, potassium, creatinine, and others	Define follow-up interval of assessment
Nutrition	Nutritional supplements	Malnutrition develops rapidly especially in heart failure

Table 60.7 Hemodynamic Target Values

	Low	High
Heart rate	>60	<90[a]
Mean arterial pressure	>60	<90[b]
CVP	—	<10[c,d]
PCWP	—	<12[c,d]
PAP	—	<25[e]
CI	>2	<3.5[f]
SvO$_2$	>65	<80

[a]Often manipulated to maintain cardiac output at higher levels.
[b]Myocardium may be extremely sensitive to afterload increases.
[c]No lower limit if hemodynamics stable and no direct or indirect signs of low cardiac output.
[d]Higher values are often necessary in patients with severely impaired heart function.
[e]High levels may indicate LV failure, myocardial ischemia, pulmonary hypertension, or hypervolemia.
[f]Lower limits may be appropriate in the elderly and in those at extremes of body mass index.

- Heart failure measured by NYHA classification from I to IV (dyspnea at rest)

Confirmation of Diagnosis
Measure what matters:
- Echocardiography (only method indicating the cause of heart failure) and/or
- Measurement of cardiac output (pulmonary artery catheter, arterial thermodilution, other)

Laboratory Parameters
- Low central or mixed venous saturation (<60% at hemoglobin levels > 9 g/dL)
- High lactate levels and acidosis
- Less specific: electrocardiography (transmural ischemia and volume overload)

- Signs of organ hypoperfusion (e.g., increased serum creatinine and oliguria, increased liver enzyme parameters, and hypoxemia in pulmonary edema)

Definition
Heart failure (HF) is defined as a failure of the cardiac pump to deliver enough blood at a sufficient pressure to organ systems that are demanding it. HF is always a consequence of a relative cardiac "fatigue"; it occurs after collapse of one or more compensation mechanisms. The more central organs are insufficiently perfused, the more severe is HF. In adults, a large majority of HF patients have insufficiently pumping left ventricles, and a minority have biventricular heart failure and, less commonly, isolated right heart failure. We primarily discuss left ventricular HF and a few aspects of right ventricular failure. Due to the fact that in adults coronary artery disease (CAD) is the most operated cardiac disease, it is not surprising that CAD and, most often, left ventricular failure after extended myocardial infarction remain the most common causes of global HF.

Pathophysiology/Compensation Mechanisms
- The major precipitating factors for heart failure are myocardial ischemia, hypertrophy, and rhythm disturbances such as atrial fibrillation. Except in CAD, ventricular hypertrophy is usually the first compensation mechanism in situations of increased afterload, such as aortic valve stenosis or arterial hypertension.
- Concentric if pressure overload (with subendocardial ischemia) or hypertrophic cardiomyopathy, consecutive diastolic dysfunction, or systolic dysfunction in late phase (decompensation)
- Eccentric if volume overload (aortic or mitral valve incompetence) or cardiomyopathy
- Asymmetrically eccentric in CAD (regional wall motion abnormalities)

649

Other Critical Care Problems

Compensation occurs with the help of
- Vasoconstriction if not anesthetized/heavily sedated
- Increased antidiuretic hormone secretion
- Increased circulating catecholamines
- Downregulation of myocardial and vascular β-adrenergic receptors (reduced sensibility to endogenic and exogenic β-adrenergic stimulation)

Causes of HF after cardiac surgery are shown in Figure 60.8: One must rule out very quickly any surgically correctable cause of HF (ongoing ischemia, valve problems, bleeding, and tamponade). In most cases, an urgent echocardiographic diagnosis is mandatory. In cases of nonsurgically treatable HF after cardiac surgery, therapy for HF (Fig. 60.9) first targets all extracardiac stressing factors (pain, anxiety, electrolyte disorders, infection, etc.), then optimize the loading conditions and, thus, also restore normocardic sinus rhythm or normocardic pacing, and, finally, application of inotropic drugs.

It is very difficult to treat severe HF after cardiac surgery without adequate monitoring and measuring methods. Frequent echocardiography and/or CO measurement with a method of sufficient accuracy are mandatory in such cases to allow optimization of inotropy and vascular resistance. One must also follow the changes of left ventricular preload, either with serial echocardiography or with other methods (double dye dilution,

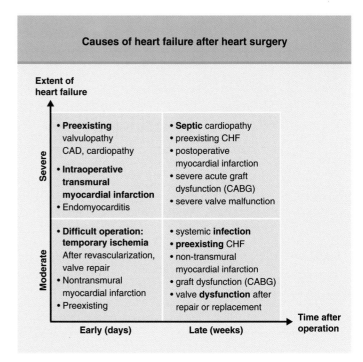

Figure 60.8. Causes of heart failure after heart surgery. Early and late causes of heart failure after cardiac surgery.

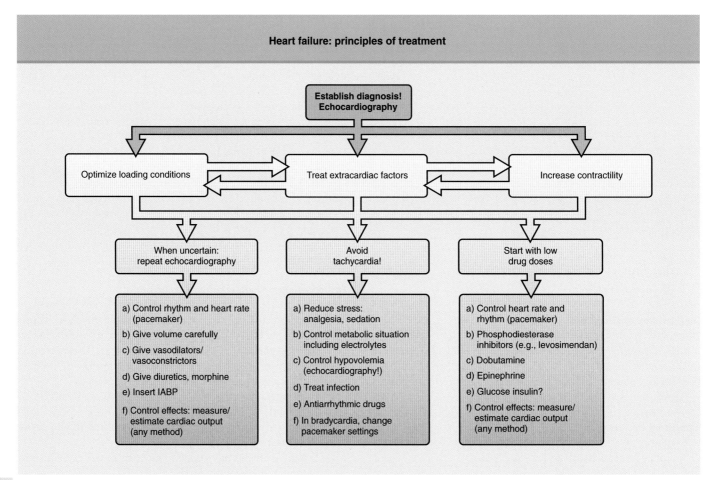

Figure 60.9. Heart failure: principles of treatment. Principles of heart failure treatment in a stepwise approach from diagnosis to basic choices.

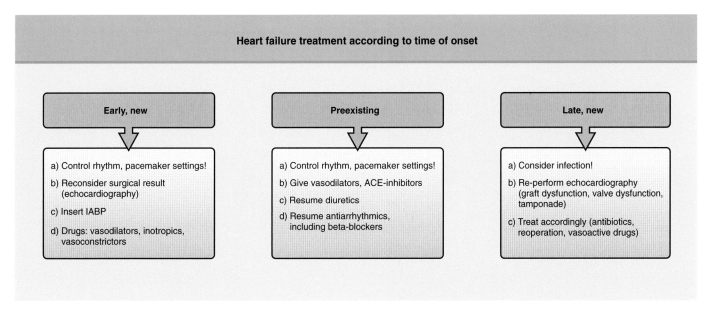

Heart failure treatment according to time of onset

Early, new	**Preexisting**	**Late, new**
a) Control rhythm, pacemaker settings!	a) Control rhythm, pacemaker settings!	a) Consider infection!
b) Reconsider surgical result (echocardiography)	b) Give vasodilators, ACE-inhibitors	b) Re-perform echocardiography (graft dysfunction, valve dysfunction, tamponade)
c) Insert IABP	c) Resume diuretics	
d) Drugs: vasodilators, inotropics, vasoconstrictors	d) Resume antiarrhythmics, including beta-blockers	c) Treat accordingly (antibiotics, reoperation, vasoactive drugs)

Figure 60.10. Heart failure treatment according to time of onset. Principles of treatment depending on baseline heart function and time of onset of heart failure.

pulmonary artery catheter filling pressures, etc.) during therapy. Clearly, for measuring the pure pump function of the ventricles, thermodilution CO measurement remains the standard method and is easy to perform to evaluate the success of drug therapy.

Drug therapy has to be prompt early after surgery to restore sufficient CO and arterial pressure without delay (Fig. 60.10). Crucial phases for patients with borderline or low CO are weaning from ventilator, tracheal extubation, mobilization, and the change from parenteral to oral drug therapy before transfer to the ward. Immediately following tracheal extubation, intrathoracic pressures change dramatically: There is no positive airway pressure anymore, and negative pressure during inspiration leads to an immediate and important influx of blood into the thorax, resulting in acute hypervolemia in the failing heart. It is essential that in this phase no inotropic and/or vasodilating drug is stopped or reduced.

A combination of angiotensin-converting enzyme inhibitors or angiotensin II receptor antagonists, loop diuretics, aldosterone, antiarrhythmic agents (beta blocking agents to suppress tachycardia, amiodarone), and nitroglycerin starting at very low doses followed by slowly increasing doses should recompensate the failing heart. In complex cases, one must consider the cardiologist's advice and/or studying the corresponding literature. Intermittent application of parenteral inotropic drugs or resynchronization therapy with dual-chamber pacemakers may be necessary.

Signs of Right Heart Failure
- Persistently increased central venous pressure and, clinically, extended neck veins
- Low CO and low left ventricular filling pressures
- High pulmonary artery pressures (not mandatory)
- Dilated, hypocontractile right ventricle with small left ventricle in echocardiography

Pathophysiology of Right Ventricular Failure
- The right ventricle is a volume and not a pressure pump.
- The maximal elastance line (dP:dV ratio) is flat (Fig. 60.11), showing that small increases in pressure (= afterload) result in large increases in volume.

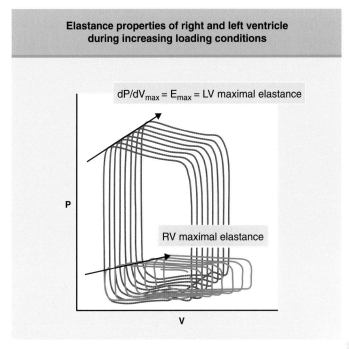

Elastance properties of right and left ventricle during increasing loading conditions

$dP/dV_{max} = E_{max} = $ LV maximal elastance

P

RV maximal elastance

V

Figure 60.11. Elastance properties of right and left ventricles during increasing loading conditions.

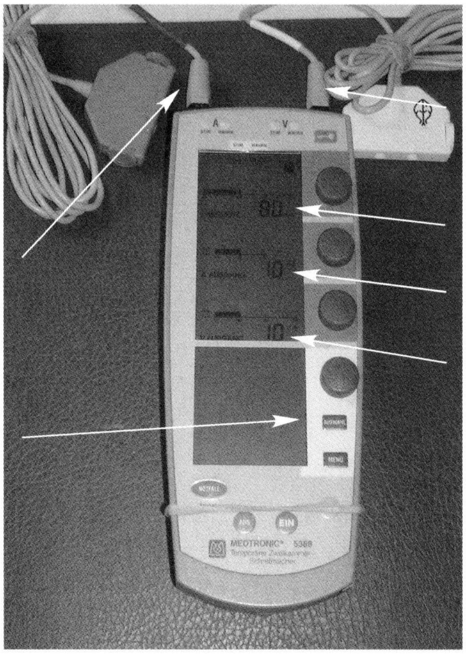

Figure 60.12. External pacemaker. A standard model of an epicardiac pacemaker with DDD pacing capacity.

Labels on figure:
- Ventricular cable/electrode
- Atrial cable/electrode
- Heart rate setting
- A output
- V output
- Additional menu (AV-interval, sensing A+V etc.)

Reasons for Right Heart Failure Following Cardiac Surgery

- Underlying chronic left heart failure, secondary pulmonary hypertension, and consecutive cor pulmonale (right ventricular hypertrophy)
- Insufficient cardioplegic protection of the right ventricle during extracorporeal circulation
- CAD with right heart infarction
- Acute increase in pulmonary vascular resistance (transfusion-related lung injury, histamine release due to any cause, adult respiratory distress syndrome, sepsis, and pulmonary embolism)

Therapy for the failing right ventricle is synonymous with reducing afterload, eventually increasing preload and secondary application of inotropic drugs, and/or insertion of an intra-aortic balloon pump (which also increases coronary perfusion pressure of the right ventricle) and monitoring normal systemic arterial pressure with vasopressors (to improve coronary perfusion pressure and maintain a normal shape of the interventricular septum). Pulmonary vascular resistance can be lowered with common vasodilating agents (nitroglycerin, calcium antagonists, nitroprusside, etc.), all of which do not selectively lower resistance in the pulmonary circulation. This effect is desired in most cases since isolated right HF is a rare condition in adult patients without congenital heart disease. In patients with proven isolated right HF, specific agents must be considered, such as inhaled nitric oxide (5–40 ppm) or inhaled prostaglandins.

In conclusion, HF following cardiac surgery has to be treated the same as HF in any patient with the difference that all relevant postoperative complications have to be ruled out and/or treated since they complicate the serious symptom complex of HF.

Pacing Following Cardiac Surgery

Rationale and Standard Procedures

Almost all surgeons fix provisional pacemaker wires (leads) at the epicardium of the right ventricle (V) and usually also at the right atrium (A) to permit pacing with an external pacemaker (Fig. 60.12). Conventionally, the V lead is pulled through the skin on the left hemithorax and the A lead to the patient's right side. Intraoperative pacemaker wire implantation is performed to allow easy and safe treatment of frequent bradycardic arrhythmia in the immediate post-CPB period or in the early period following revascularization without CPB bypass. Additionally, this provides the possibility of increasing heart rate (thereby usually CO as well) as required and/or to decrease heart rate and to suppress arrhythmia with antiarrhythmic drugs under the protection of a standby pacemaker.

The best ventricular filling is achieved with spontaneous conduction of excitation from sinus node or from atrial pacing down to the ventricles. If both A and V are stimulated to mimic sinus rhythm, the physiologic excitation path is interrupted. Thus, this sequential pacing of A and V (DDD mode) often results in a reduced SV that must be compensated by an increase in heart rate set on the pacemaker. Isolated ventricular stimulation has the most unfavorable effect on SV. For pacemaker settings, see Box 60.1 for coding conventions and Table 60.8 for troubleshooting. Briefly, pacing threshold means the minimal current needed to get the corresponding myocardial area excited (mV), sensing threshold—the minimal current sensed by the lead/pacemaker (mV) that inhibits pacing of the corresponding area (A or V). Try to pace only the atrium with the longest A–V interval possible (usually 300 msec). For details about pacemaker use, refer to standard textbooks.

Table 60.8 Troubleshooting in Epicardiac Pacemakers

Disturbance	Step 1	Step 2	Step 3	Step 4
No pacing possible at all	Change pacemaker/battery	Change all cables[a]	Give calcium,[b] check electrolytes	Resuscitation, other external pacing[c]
No sensing/pacing either A or V	Change polarity[d]	Change corresponding cable	Change pacemaker/battery	
Intermittent pacing only	Refix all connections	Change battery/pacemaker	Increase frequency	Check threshold values
DDD mode does not work correctly	Refix all connections	Check threshold values	Check if atrial fibrillation is present	Change mode (VVI)
A and V pacing do not work correctly	Check if A and V cables are confounded	Change both cables	Change pacemaker/battery	Change polarity of both cables
Very irregular heat rate	Check if atrial fibrillation is present	Check if many supraventricular premature beats	Antiarrhythmic drugs	
Sudden AV block II or III	Change to DDD pacing	Increase AV interval[e]	Decrease frequency	Decrease antiarrhythmic drugs
Pacing disturbed by **electrocautery**	Change mode to VOO (AOO ev.)	**Do not forget to switch to previous mode, after change**		
IABP: bad trigger signal	Change first lead on patient's monitor[f]	Decrease A output[f]	Fix additional ECG electrodes and recheck	Use transport cable directly to IABP console
Cross-talk with **internal pacemaker**[g]	Decrease output of external pacemaker	Stop external pacemaker	Let the internal pacemaker get checked[h]	
ECG is correct, low/no arterial pressure	Increase frequency	Diagnose cause of heart failure		

[a]Sometimes cable endings are not correctly fixed: They are completely loosened instead of completely fixed (small screw turned the wrong way). Thus, there is no contact.

[b]Hyperkalemia is a frequent disturbance in the ICU, either spontaneous or iatrogenic.

[c]Also try to take three electrodes together (2 A and 1 V) into the positive pole of the pacemaker's V connection and the remaining V electrode into the negative pole. Sometimes stimulation is possible again.

[d]In external epicardiac pacing, monopolar electrodes are used, one as positive and one as negative, with the current flowing from positive to negative across the epicardium. It does not matter in which direction the current flows; therefore, polarity can be changed without any danger.

[e]To give the heart a chance for "physiologic" AV conduction in AV block I.

[f]Very often, the first ECG lead on the patient's monitor is transferred via an analog exit to the IABP console. Changing the lead on the patient's monitor often increases R wave signal and triggering of the IABP is better.

[g]Sometimes the A signal of the pacemaker is sensed as "R wave" by the IABP console.

[h]Internal and external pacemaker intermittently inhibit each other.

Box 60.1 National Board Code (Shortened)

I	2	3	4
Stimulation	Sensing	Mode	Frequency adaptation
O = none	O = none	O = none	
A = atrium	A = atrium	T = triggered	
V = ventricle	V = ventricle	I = inhibited	
D = double (A + V)	D = double (A + V)	D = double (T + I)	R = frequency adaptation ("rate modulation")

Pacemaker Essentials at Admission in the ICU

- Check actual cardiac rhythm; pacing yes/no.
- Check threshold values (A + V) of sensing and pacing at a rate above that of the patient. Write down these values on patient's record.
- Check mode of (pre-)setting of the pacemaker (DDD, VVI, other).
- Pace with the double energy (mV) of the threshold value.
- Oversensing (too sensitive adjustment) is dangerous. If the pacemaker senses artifacts, muscle contractions, movements, or, in older models, the atrial pacing spike, V pacing is suppressed. Set sensing to 4 or 5 mV.

- If the patient does not need pacing, switch the pacemaker off.
- Record a 12-channel ECG (not necessary if A + V are paced; then you only see the pacemaker rhythm and a left bundle branch block).

Essentials during the Stay in the ICU

- Check the functioning of the pacemaker daily as described previously.
- Remember the possibility of using the pacemaker, for example, as protection in bradycardia following antiarrhythmic drug therapy.
- Remember that ventricular pacing (VVI) or sequential pacing (DDD) impedes the physiologic distribution of myocardial excitation and therefore reduces CO.
- Try as long as possible to stimulate only the atrium (with V on demand; e.g., set the longest possible A–V interval).
- As long as the epicardial pacemaker wires are not pulled out, have the pacemaker ready.

Complications of Pacemaker Implantation and Use, and Wire Withdrawal

- Rarely, epicardiac wires are not fixed correctly or have insufficient current flow to the corresponding myocardial area (reoperated patients and pericardiac disease).

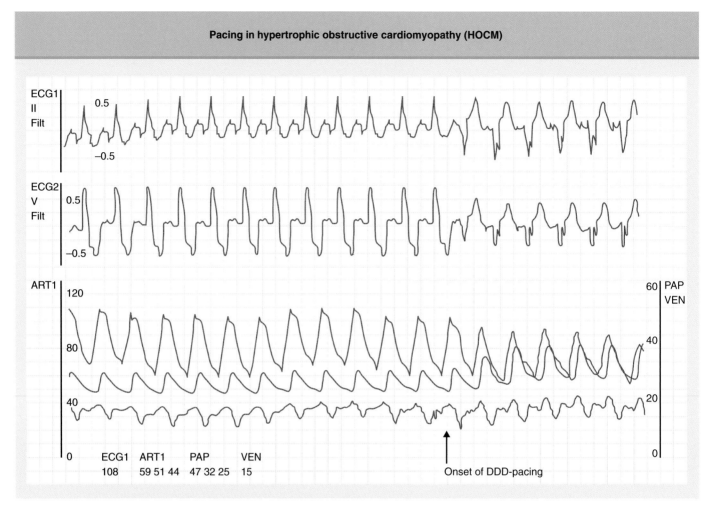

Figure 60.13. Pacing in hypertrophic obstructive cardiomyopathy. (From top to bottom) ECG channel II, V5, pulmonary artery pressure (PAP; with the corresponding scale on the right side), systemic arterial pressure (SAP; scale on the left side), and central venous pressure (VEN). From the beginning of DDD pacing, hemodynamics improve dramatically (PAP decreases and SAP increases significantly).

- Premature beats (supra- or ventricular) if sensing settings are not correct.
- Induction of severe arrhythmia with fixed pacing (no sensing, no inhibition, V00).
- Phrenic stimulation: The diaphragm sometimes contracts due to a high current of the A electrode. Change polarity and/or reduce output of the A channel.
- Electrocautery during surgery in the ICU causes severe pacing troubles; it requires a temporary change in the pacemaker mode (to V00).
- Pericardiac tamponade due to bleeding soon after removal of epicardial wires.

Difficulties during Pacemaker Use and Problem-Solving Propositions

In general, one must exclude simple technical problems, such as incorrectly attached wires, confounded or broken A or V electrodes, and dead batteries. It is extremely helpful to have exchange material in the proximity of postoperative cardiac surgical patients; this is true for patients in the ICU as well as for those on the ward. Relatively late postoperative bradycardic

arrhythmia is not rare and is promptly treated with temporary pacing.

Rare Cases

Pathophysiologically very interesting are concentric hypertrophic hearts with severe diastolic dysfunction (such as in severe aortic stenosis or in hypertrophic obstructive cardiomyopathy). Due to the hypertrophic interventricular septum, they can reveal significant subaortic stenosis in situations of hypovolemia and/or low peripheral vascular resistance. Sometimes, it may be helpful to interrupt the physiologic excitation pathway by introducing sequential pacing (DDD with a short A–V interval). When this is done, ventricular contraction is less effective, the high ejection fraction is reduced, and thus diastolic filling is improved (Fig. 60.13).

In conclusion, epicardiac pacing following cardiac surgery prevents life-threatening situations based on bradycardic arrhythmia. Furthermore, it may serve to increase CO in the failing heart simply by increasing heart rate. If the intensivist uses pacing with the necessary precautions, it is a very simple and powerful tool in the postoperative treatment of the cardiac surgical patient.

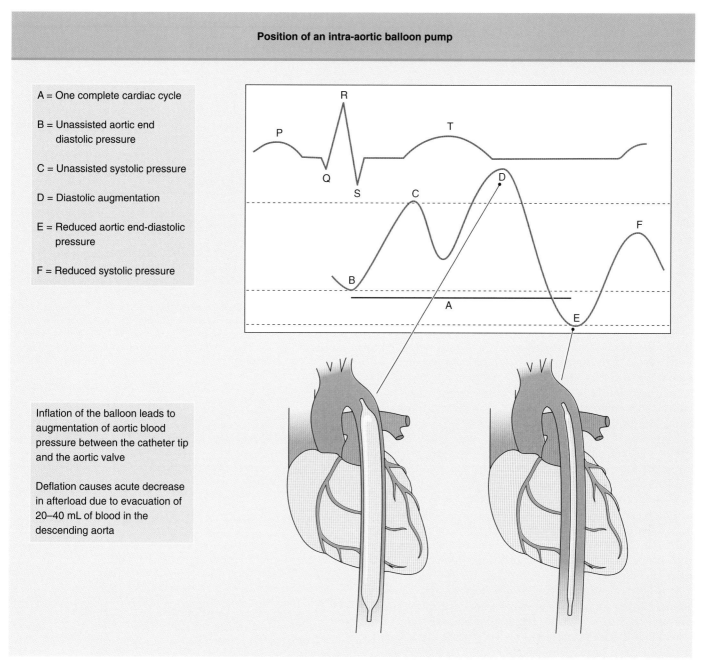

Position of an intra-aortic balloon pump

A = One complete cardiac cycle

B = Unassisted aortic end diastolic pressure

C = Unassisted systolic pressure

D = Diastolic augmentation

E = Reduced aortic end-diastolic pressure

F = Reduced systolic pressure

Inflation of the balloon leads to augmentation of aortic blood pressure between the catheter tip and the aortic valve

Deflation causes acute decrease in afterload due to evacuation of 20–40 mL of blood in the descending aorta

Figure 60.14. Position of an intra-aortic balloon pump in the aorta and typical pressure tracing.

Intra-aortic Balloon Pump in Cardiac Surgical Patients

Indications (Dependent on Individual Centers)

- Preoperative implantation
  Severe myocardial ischemia despite adequate therapy
  Low ejection fraction and catecholamine dependency
  Acute coronary artery occlusion and cardiogenic shock
  Critical coronary artery disease (left main stem stenosis)
- Intraoperative indication
  Impossible to wean the patient from CPB
  Persistent severe myocardial ischemia
  Need for high doses of catecholamines and difficulty weaning the patient off CPB

- Sudden deterioration in ventricular performance (either left or right ventricular function)
  New significant ischemia
  Acute problems with a mechanical valve (leak, otherwise disturbed function)
  Slow deterioration of a previously bad performing heart with low CO
  Evidence of a severe perioperative myocardial infarction

Contraindications

- Absolute: Severe aortic valve insufficiency
- Relative: Peripheral arterial atheromatosis with ischemia

655

Size, Position, and Monitoring of IABPs
- Balloon size according to patient's size (25, 34, 40, or 50 mL), usually 8-Fr catheters.
- Position immediately distal to left subclavian artery (echocardiographic and/or x-ray control).
- Always monitor arterial pressure upstream of the catheter tip (radial artery, tip of the catheter; never femoral arterial pressure for IABP timing).
- Control perfusion downstream of the catheter insertion site (foot pulse) regularly.
- Heparinize with standard heparin.

In the early 1970s, intra-aortic balloon counterpulsation (IABP) was a complicated procedure requiring large consoles and was dependent on regular cardiac rhythm. It consisted of a 30- to 40-mL helium-filled caoutchouc balloon inflated in diastole and deflated in systole. IABP therefore increased diastolic and, hence, coronary perfusion pressure and decreased afterload by instantaneous evacuation of a 30- to 40-mL volume from the descending aorta, necessitating no additional myocardial work. Since this method proved to be very effective in a variety of clinical situations, much effort led to improvements in the balloon, its introducing possibilities, its inflating and deflating speed, and, most important, its triggering capacities (fast response even in tachycardia and arrhythmia). The consoles also became battery driven, facilitating transportation within or even outside the hospital with dedicated ECG cables for trigger signal during transport.

Currently, IABP devices usually have an outer diameter of 7.5 to 8 Fr, are introduced percutaneously (with or without introducer sheath), and have balloons with a filling volume of 25 to 50 mL, according to the patient's weight and height.

Whereas IABP use (pre- and/or postoperatively) is common in some centers in patients with critical myocardial ischemia and/or very poor left ventricular function, other centers implant IABPs only as a last resort in otherwise untreatable patients due to the potentially dangerous complications (limb ischemia and infection).

It is easy to insert and use IABPs (Fig. 60.14). The most common errors are insufficient trigger signal, measuring arterial pressure downstream of the IABP tip, and missing a limb ischemia. In a noncardiac surgical ICU, physicians not used to handling IABP devices should ask for help by technicians and/or surgeons/cardiologists.

SUMMARY

Knowledge and understanding of the cardiac pathology is the basis for fast and safe treatment of these patients in the ICU. Prompt action in the case of hemodynamic impairment is necessary. Competence in invasive diagnostic monitoring and echocardiography is helpful. Most tasks can be defined in strict protocols, but treatment of severe heart failure requires time and specific expertise.

SUGGESTED READING

American College of Cardiology/American Heart Association: Guidelines for the Evaluation and Management of Chronic Heart Failure, 2005. Available at www.acc.org.

Barold SS, Stroobandt RX, Sinnaeve AF: Cardiac Pacemakers Step by Step: An Illustrated Guide. Armonk, NY, Futura, 2004.

Bolooki H: Clinical Application of the Intra-Aortic Balloon Pump, 3rd ed. Armonk, NY, Futura, 1998.

Bonow RO, Carabello B, de Leon AC, et al: ACC/AHA Guidelines for the management of patients with valvular heart disease. Executive summary. A report of the American College of Cardiology/American Heart Association Task Force on Practice Guidelines (Committee on Management of Patients with Valvular Heart Disease). J Heart Valve Dis 1998;7(6):672–707.

Eagle KA, Guyton RA, Davidoff R, et al: ACC/AHA 2004 guideline update for coronary artery bypass graft surgery: Summary article: A report of the American College of Cardiology/American Heart Association Task Force on Practice Guidelines (Committee to Update the 1999 Guidelines for Coronary Artery Bypass Graft Surgery). Circulation 2004;110(9):1168–1176.

Heart Failure Society of America: HFSA guidelines for management of patients with heart failure caused by left ventricular systolic dysfunction—Pharmacological approaches. Pharmacotherapy 2000;20(5):495–522.

Kirklin JW, Barratt-Boyes BG, Kouchoukos NT (eds): Cardiac Surgery. Edinburgh Churchill Livingstone, 2003.

Laffey JG, Boylan JF, Cheng DC: The systemic inflammatory response to cardiac surgery. Anesthesiology 2002;97:215–252.

Mathew JP, Fontes ML, Tudor IC, et al: A multicenter risk index for atrial fibrillation after cardiac surgery. JAMA 2004;291:1720–1729.

Moses HW, Moulton KP, Miller BD: A Practical Guide to Cardiac Pacing, 5th ed. Philadelphia, Lippincott Williams & Wilkins, 2000.

National Electronic Library for Health: Full-Text Guideline Collection. Pharmacological Therapy for Patients with Heart Failure, 2005. Available at www.nelh.nhs.uk.

Warkentin TE, Greinacher A: Heparin-induced thrombocytopenia and cardiac surgery. Ann Thorac Surg 2003;76(6):2121–2131.

Chapter 61

Intensive Care after Major Surgery

Peter M. Suter

KEY POINTS

- The objective of postoperative critical care is to prevent complications and surgical death.
- Vital organ function monitoring and support of failing organs/organ dysfunction are the major tasks for the intensive care unit (ICU) team.
- An obsessional attitude about prevention, recognition, and treatment of organ dysfunction and nosocomial infection is essential.
- Risks and benefits of invasive and aggressive diagnostic and therapeutic interventions have to be evaluated continuously.
- Indications for postoperative ICU admission should be based on perioperative risk factors for postoperative complications.

During the past 10 to 20 years, marked progress has been made in the management of surgical patients. This is due to all aspects of perioperative care, including better preoperative evaluation and management of coexisting chronic diseases, improved techniques and drugs for anesthesia, more appropriate surgical approaches and procedures preserving tissue integrity and function, and improved understanding and prevention of surgical and other perioperative complications. Special mention has to be given to nosocomial infection, which has lost much of its morbidity and mortality despite, or due to, shorter antibiotic therapy.

Postoperative critical care is a key factor involved in the improved results of surgery in high-risk patients. However, intensive care is less necessary today for a certain number of interventions for which patients were traditionally admitted to these services a few years ago. Such patients include those undergoing cardiac surgery, repair of thoracic and abdominal aortic aneurisms, and extensive liver or pancreatic surgery, as well as invasive and prolonged orthopedic cases. The advent of the "fast-track" approach, realizing extubation in the operative room, and subsequent admission to the postoperative recovery room have indeed been made possible with modern surgical and anesthetic techniques and can provide good long-term results.

However, care and management in the intensive care unit (ICU) are still indicated for certain categories of high-risk patients. The demography of the latter, in part because of the increasing age of the population offered complicated surgical procedures, seems to increase steadily in most areas of the world. There is evidence that an adequate provision of critical care support can save lives in this context (Goldhill, 2004).

Specific training and competence for the intensivist in postsurgical critical care allows better and professional management in this specific domain and has a positive effect on outcome in these patients.

EPIDEMIOLOGY, RISK FACTORS, AND PATHOPHYSIOLOGY

Epidemiology

With the advent of improved management of the majority of acute and chronic disabilities, the number of years lived with a good quality of life has increased steadily, and many more patients presenting with serious health problems such as cardiovascular diseases, chronic pulmonary or renal dysfunction, and metabolic problems such as diabetes or marked obesity are referred for surgical procedures. In parallel, improved anesthesia and surgical procedures, but also good postoperative management, have decreased perioperative morbidity and mortality, especially in cases with multiple morbidities.

To provide optimal perioperative support to patients at high risk, the best possible management has to be tailored according to the individual situation. This analysis must include pre-, per, and postoperative identification of factors responsible for possible complications and unfavorable outcome.

Postoperative admission to the ICU should be considered when a certain number of elements suggest a high probability or risk of postsurgical complications and vital organ dysfunctions. To achieve this goal, the ICU must offer not only the possibility of supporting the function of chronically or acutely failing vital organs but also, as important, skills and equipment for close surveillance and monitoring of physiological signs and more complex indicators of cellue, tissue, and systemic (patho-)physiology. For both diagnostic and therapeutic interventions, invasive and noninvasive technologies should be available.

Risk Factors

Preoperative Risk Factors

As mentioned previously, a number of preexisting health variables will determine intermediate and long-term outcome after surgery. A predominant factor is the physiological reserve of the patient, also called "biological age," which seems clearly more important than chronological age. Other elements include

Other Critical Care Problems

Box 61.1 Indications for Postoperative Admission to the ICU

Planned Preoperatively

Severe heart disease
  Congestive heart failure
  Ejection fraction <40%
  Functional NYHA class III or IV
  Unstable angina pectoris
  Recent myocardial infarction (<6 months)
Chronic obstructive pulmonary disease, with home oxygen
  Forced expiratory volume in 1 sec <1 liter
Other severe
  Acute or chronic respiratory diseases
  Chronic renal failure, dialysis dependent

Perioperative Events

Sustained hemodynamic instability
Cardiac ischemia, arrhythmia
Requirement for postoperative ventilation
Hypothermia <35°C
Transfusion >3 liters
Anaphylactic reaction
Significant inhalation of gastric content, blood, etc.

---

chronic health problems and acute or chronic physiological derangements of body functions (Box 61.1).

A number of risk or scoring systems have been proposed to define as precisely as possible the preoperative risk. Among the best known are the ASA classification, the Goldman cardiac risk index, and the surgical mortality score (Goldhill, 2004). All these tools facilitate preoperative assessment of surgical and anesthetic risks. However, the careful evaluation by experienced specialists is irreplaceable for decisions regarding special intraoperative monitoring and management and the requirement for postoperative intensive care.

Intraoperative Risks

Patient outcome is related to factors such as the procedure to be undertaken. In addition, unforeseen anesthetic or surgical problems can add substantial risk for the subsequent need for intensive care practices such as vital organ monitoring and/or support. Such events include bronchopulmonary inhalation of gastric content, anaphylaxis, uncontrolled hemorrhage, or accidental intestinal perforation. In addition, duration of surgery, marked hypothermia, and other factors known to influence the natural defense mechanisms against infection and the physiologic stress response can also justify close postoperative surveillance and possibilities for rapid intervention (see Box 61.1).

Postoperative Risks

Incidence and gravity of complications after surgical procedures are best predicted by age, ASA physical status, smoking status, serious chronic disease, and emergency surgery. In addition, acute physiological derangements during the first postoperative hours influence prognosis significantly. The APACHE or SAPS scoring systems can be used to estimate these derangements and

may indicate a need for specific surveillance and vital organ function support systems.

Pathophysiology

Requirement for postoperative intensive care can have its origin in potential or real disturbances of different organ systems, on the basis of the specific preoperative, intraoperative, and postoperative risk factors mentioned previously. Schematically, these can be represented by five major organ functions.

Central Nervous System

Directly disturbed during and after important neurosurgical procedures, the nervous system may also be affected by hemodynamic and metabolic problems arising from an acute perioperative dysfunction of other vital functions. The principles of management after neurosurgical interventions are summarized in Box 61.2.

Cardiocirculatory Dysfunction

Cardiocirculatory dysfunction is a frequent problem in those postoperative patients who have severely reduced adaptive capability of the myocardium and/or vasotonus to react to rapid changes in intravascular volume status. In addition, different types of surgical interventions or anesthetic agents can interfere with normal physiological response mechanisms to (post)surgical stress states.

Diminished cardiocirculatory physiologic reserves in the elderly, for instance, may lead to impairment of adequate systemic oxygen delivery resulting in decreased tissue perfusion and

---

Box 61.2 ICU Management after Important Neurosurgical Procedures

Basic Principles

Hemodynamics
  Mean arterial pressure 60–80 mm Hg **and** cerebral
    perfusion pressure > 60 mm Hg
  Normovolemia
Respiratory
  SaO_2, 95%
  $PaCO_2$, 35–40 mm Hg
ICP < 20 mm Hg, controlled by mannitol, hypertonic saline,
  CSF drainage
Head elevation 30–45°, unless contraindicated
Temperature, 37°C
Seizure prophylaxis
General measures
  Sedation and analgesia
  Plasma glucose < 180 mg/dL
  Early enteral nutrition
  Prophylaxis for stress ulcers and venous thromboembolism

Refractory Intracranial Hypertension

Consider
  Optimized hyperventilation (check SjO_2 or $PbiO_2$)
  Barbiturate coma
  Therapeutic hypothermia (33 to 25°C)
  Decompressive craniectomy

---

cellular hypoxia. Insufficient tissue and organ perfusion may also be the result of blood flow maldistribution whereby regional hypoxia can develop despite a normal or even increased cardiac output. Diagnosis of inappropriate cardiovascular function usually requires invasive functional hemodynamic monitoring. Of special importance is the surveillance of adequate intravascular volume and cardiac filling. Invasive and noninvasive methods for a functional hemodynamic monitoring are listed in Table 61.1.

Respiratory System

Together with cardiovascular dysfunction, respiratory problems are the most frequent complications requiring specific postoperative intensive care. The following are the most important risk factors and causes for respiratory failure in this phase:

- Previous acute or chronic severe respiratory disease
- Extensive abdominal or thoracic surgery, interfering with physiologic ventilatory movements due to disturbed chest wall excursions or pathologic neuromuscular function
- Decreased defense mechanisms for clearing of secretions and regular opening and ventilation of peripheral lung regions, thus leading to pulmonary superinfection and atelectasis formation predominantly in dependent areas
- Sepsis or severe hypotension or shock, leading to acute lung injury or acute respiratory distress syndrome, both characterized by acute severe lung parenchymal inflammation with interstitial edema (due to increased capillary permeability to proteins and cells), leukocyte accumulation, and increased tissue stiffness
- Pulmonary superinfection due to reflux of oropharyngeal or gastric content into the bronchial tree, which can be promoted by abnormal swallowing and cough reflexes, as well as an increased intraabdominal pressure

Due to the protracted course of a number of these pathophysiologic mechanisms, prolonged specific therapy (e.g., by oxygen administration and respiratory therapy including positive pressure ventilation) may be required to ensure adequate systemic oxygenation and CO_2 elimination.

Renal, Hepatic, and Other Metabolic Functions

Rapid changes in intravascular volume, arterial and venous vasomotor tone, as well as cardiac function can lead to dysfunction of other organs. These failures are more common and more important when chronic derangements in these organ functions preexist. The consecutive metabolic and blood coagulation abnormalities can influence not only distant organ function (e.g., the brain) but also the importance of complications such as superinfections and bleeding. The interplay of different system functions in the human organism determines the clinical relevance of the derangements, their duration, and their influence on outcome of surgery.

CLINICAL FEATURES: SPECIFIC SURVEILLANCE AND MANAGEMENT

ICU Care after Neurosurgery

The most frequent complications in this type of patient are neurological dysfunctions, including altered level of consciousness, sensitive or motor deficits, hemorrhage, and hydrocephalus. Second, medical complications are composed mainly of infections, respiratory failure, myocardial infarction and other cardiac problems, and thromboembolic events (Beauregard and Friedman, 2003).

Selective use of ICU management for high-risk patients and procedures seems to provide cost-effective care and good outcome in neurosurgical patients (Beauregard and Friedman, 2003). The aim of intensive care management after neurosurgical procedures is to anticipate, prevent, and treat secondary physiologic insults to the central nervous system. There has been a shift of emphasis from primary control of intracranial pressure to a multifaceted approach of maintenance of adequate cerebral perfusion pressure and brain protection. High-quality neurocritical care using targeted therapeutic interventions does have an impact not only on survival but also on the quality of survival.

Critical Care after Major Vascular Surgery

Several vascular diseases requiring surgical intervention are frequently associated with comorbidities and risk factors indicating the need for postoperative ICU care (Gopalan and Burrows, 2003). Comorbidities include widely disseminated atherosclerosis, ischemic heart disease, arterial hypertension, diabetes, chronic obstructive pulmonary disease, and renal insufficiency.

Postoperative decompensation of these preexisting health problems is common. Frequently observed postoperative complications are bleeding, thromboembolic events, myocardial ischemia, heart failure, cerebrovascular accidents, respiratory insufficiency, renal and gastrointestinal problems, and superinfection. Careful and precise surveillance of all vital organ functions and rapid therapeutic interventions may be necessary to give these patients the best possible chance for a good prognosis.

Table 61.1 Functional Hemodynamic Monitoring in the High-Risk Postoperative Patient	
Purpose	**Means, Tools**
Noninvasive	
Cardiac rhythm control	6- or 12-lead ECG
Peripheral pulse + oxygen saturation	Pulse oximetry
Systemic arterial pressure	Blood pressure cuff
Cardiac structure and function (contractility, PAP, cardiac output)	Echo-Doppler, transthoracic, or transesophageal
Tissue, PO_2, PCO_2	Transcutaneous devices assessment
Cerebral perfusion	Transcranial Doppler
Invasive	
Systemic arterial pressure	Indwelling arterial catheter
Central venous pressure	Central venous line
Pulmonary artery and capillary wedge pressure	Pulmonary artery catheter
Intracranial pressure	Intracerebral or intraventricular pressure sensor or catheter
Cardiac output	Pulmonary artery catheter with thermistor
Circulating and intrathoracic blood volumes	Intravascular catheters and thermodilution assessment

659

A selective policy for ICU admission of patients after vascular surgery is recommended. Early and smooth restoration of physiological homeostasis and rapid management of complications contribute to improve short- and long-term outcome in this population (Gopalan and Burrows, 2003).

Critical Care after Extensive Orthopedic Surgery

Important surgical interventions in orthopedics have similar indications for postoperative ICU management as other surgical procedures (i.e., pre-, intra-, and/or postoperative risk factors for serious physiologic derangements and complications). Procedure-specific problems include bone-cement cardiac events, fat embolism, and local complications (Nazon and colleagues, 2003). Particular attention must be given to prophylaxis of thromboembolism and superinfection in these patients.

ICU Care after Solid Organ Transplantation

Organ transplantation is used increasingly more frequently in end-stage organ failure, and the results have attained a very satisfactory level in most institutions. The judicious use of postoperative intensive care contributes to a better long-term prognosis. Indeed, complications occurring after transplantation have a significant impact not only on mortality but also on resource utilization and costs. The type of complications is related to the surgical procedure and the function of the new organ, on the one hand, and the typical spectrum of the most frequent complications seen in other critically ill patients, including nosocomial infection and vital system failures, on the other hand. General measures of good care, including aseptic techniques, early extubation and mobilization, enteral feeding, adequate cardiovascular, respiratory and renal monitoring and support, as well as preventive measures for thromboembolic disease and stress ulceration, are all part of an efficient prevention of complications and unfavorable outcome.

Critical Care after Major Abdominal, Cardiac, and Other Extensive Surgical Procedures

As mentioned previously, progress in preoperative care, surgery, and anesthesia has allowed for management of many patients after major surgery in postoperative recovery rooms. However, important risk factors, comorbidities, and intraoperative complications may require admission to the ICU for subsequent monitoring and therapy. This means that indications for the ICU track depend less on the type of surgical procedures per se and more on the other characteristics of the patient. For instance, bariatric surgery in the morbidly obese requires a delicate but not extraordinary surgical technique, whereas the obesity, if extreme, constitutes an important risk factor for physiological disturbances of several vital system functions in the postoperative period (Helling and associates, 2004).

FREQUENT POSTOPERATIVE COMPLICATIONS: DETECTION, PREVENTION, AND THERAPY

Nosocomial Infection

Nosocomial infections are a major cause of morbidity and mortality in the postoperative ICU patient. This complication occurs in general because ICU patients have decreased immune and other host defense mechanisms and because they require

invasive devices for surveillance and therapy, providing entry portals for infectious organisms (Craven and Steger, 1995) (Fig. 61.1). In addition, they receive therapies that increase the risk of infection (e.g., glucocorticoids and parenteral nutrition). For the global ICU population, approximately two thirds of these infections are localized in the upper and lower respiratory tracts (Vincent, 2003). Of particular importance is ventilator-associated pneumonia (VAP) due to its influence on length of ICU and hospital stay, costs, and mortality. Another infection with serious consequences is catheter-related bacteremia. These two problems are presented here in more detail. Both are relatively unique to ICU care and should be considered first for the differential diagnosis when signs and symptoms suggestive of infection are noted (see Fig. 61.1).

Ventilator-Associated Pneumonia

The requirement for endotracheal intubation and prolonged mechanical ventilation are important risk factors for VAP. The most adequate diagnostic tools include clinical symptoms and microbiology. The samples for the latter analysis should be obtained by an invasive technique such as bronchoalveolar lavage to obtain a reliable diagnosis. The mortality attributable to VAP ranges between 30% and 70%, depending on the type of microbes involved and concurrent risk factors.

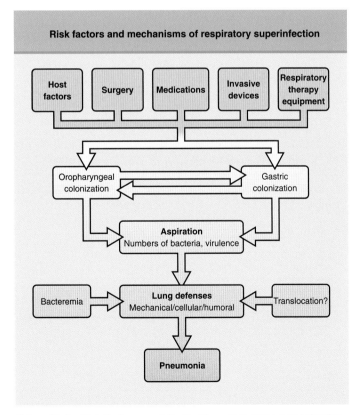

Figure 61.1. Risk factors contributing to colonization and infection of the lower respiratory tract. Important risk factors include the inoculum and virulence of infecting agents and the response of the pulmonary host defenses. (Adapted from Craven DE, Steger KA: Epidemiology of nosocomial pneumonia. New perspectives on an old disease. Chest 1995;108:1S–16S.)

Early onset VAP is defined as occurring within the first 48 to 72 hours after intubation, with late-onset VAP occurring thereafter. Frequently found organisms and the proposed empirical antibiotic therapy are summarized in Table 61.2.

Prevention

Interventions able to reduce the incidence of VAP include strict hand washing between patients, semirecumbent positioning of the patient, limitation of acid-suppression prophylactic therapies for gastric ulcers to high-risk patients, and subglottic aspiration of tracheal secretions. Selective digestive decontamination is a controversial method for VAP prophylaxis: Although it is efficient, the potential development of resistant strains of microbes remains an important concern.

Therapy

Appropriate and early antibiotic therapy is essential, as in any other serious infection (see Table 61.2). The adequate duration of this treatment is probably 6 to 8 days, provided that an adequate clinical response is observed.

Intravascular Catheter-Associated Infection

The Centers for Disease Control and Prevention's definition of this infection includes

- Clinical suspicion of catheter-related infection
- Positive culture of blood drawn from the catheter or a segment of it
- Matching positive blood culture drawn from another site

The incidence depends on conditions of catheter insertion; type, location, and duration of catheterization; and strict aseptic techniques. Mortality attributable to this complication is approximately 10%.

Microorganisms commonly responsible for catheter-related bacteremia include *Staphylococcus epidermidis* and *aureus*, enteric gram-negative bacteria, and, rarely, *Pseudomonas aeruginosa* or *Acinetobacter*.

Prevention

Preventive measures include sterile methods for insertion, use of antiseptic- or antibiotic-coated catheters (the latter have been more effective), and selection of the subclavian or internal jugular site for venous puncture.

Therapy

The responsible catheter should be removed and antibiotic treatment given for at least 7 days. Guidewire exchange of the catheter can be considered.

Other Nosocomial Infections

Sinusitis is a rare nosocomial infection, but this diagnosis has to be considered with the prolonged use of indwelling oral and nasal tubes. Radiographic signs of fluid in these cavities are very frequent with nasal intubation of 1 week's duration or longer. Approximately 10% of these are infected, mostly with the type of microbes seen in VAP (see Table 61.2). Prevention of sinusitis includes improvement of sinus drainage and avoidance of nasal intubation. Therapeutically, nasal decongestants, drainage by puncture and lavage, as well as appropriate antibiotic coverage must be considered.

Urinary tract infection is common in hospitalized patients requiring prolonged bladder drainage. Gram-negative bacteria are predominant. Preventive measures include careful aseptic techniques and minimization of catheterization duration. The benefit of silver alloy and antibiotic-coated catheters is controversial. Antibiotic therapy may be necessary if systemic signs of sepsis or severe sepsis are present.

Invasive fungal infections mainly caused by *Candida* species are increasingly common in the ICU. Risk factors include intravascular devices, neutropenia, parenteral nutrition, and prolonged use of broad-spectrum antibiotics, steroids, or other immunosuppressive treatments. Prevention must include avoidance of risk factors. Prophylactic therapy with fluconazole is effective in high-risk patients. Treatment of *Candida* bloodstream infection should include fluconazole (first-line treatment) or an alternative agent if resistance is present, and it should be continued for at least 2 weeks. Amphotericin B is generally reserved for refractory and life threatening infection because of its toxicity.

Postoperative Systemic Inflammation Response Syndrome

After major surgery, a significant number of patients present signs of systemic inflammation, such as fever, tachycardia, tachypnea, and leukocytosis, in the absence of significant microbial infection. This can be seen as an nonspecific physiologic response to surgical stress and as a part of a defense reaction facilitating metabolic and structural repair mechanisms. The etiology may be multifactorial, including direct response to tissue injury, activation of leukocytes and other parts of the immune system, and sympathicoadrenal outburst. Control of

Table 61.2 Empiric Therapy of Ventilator-Associated Pneumonia (VAP)

Frequent Microbes	Antibiotics
Early Onset of VAP	
Escherichia coli	β-Lactam/β-lactamase inhibitor combination, **or**
Enterobacter species	
Proteus species	Second-generation cephalosporin, **or**
Klebsiella species	Fluoroquinolone
Haemophilus influenzae	
Methicillin-sensitive *Staphylococcus aureus*	
Streptococcus pneumoniae	
Late Onset or Severe Early Onset of VAP	
Above, plus	β-Lactam/β-lactamase inhibitor combination, **or**
Pseudomonas aeruginosa	
Acinetobacter species	Third- or fourth-generation cephalosporin, **or**
Methicillin-resistant *Staphylococcus aureus* (MRSA)	Fluoroquinolone
	plus
	Aminoglycoside, **or**
	Second, structurally unrelated agent with anti-pseudomonal activity
	plus
	Vancomycin or linezolid (if likelihood of MRSA is high)

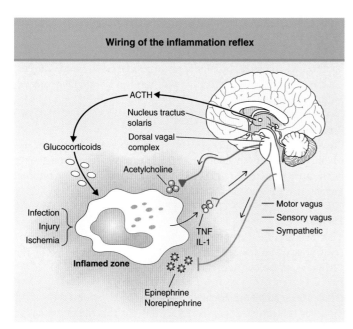

Wiring of the inflammation reflex

Figure 61.2. Wiring of the inflammation reflex. Inflammatory products produced in damaged tissues activate afferent signals that are relayed to the nucleus tractus solitarius: Subsequent activation of vagus efferent activity inhibits cytokine synthesis through the cholinergic anti-inflammatory pathway (the "inflammatory reflex"). Information can also be relayed to the hypothalamus and the dorsal vagal complex to stimulate the release of ACTH, thereby activating the humoral anti-inflammatory pathway. Activation of the sympathetic outflow by flight-or-fight responses or pain, or through direct signaling, can increase local concentrations of adrenaline and noradrenaline, which can further suppress inflammation. (Reproduced with permission from Tracey KJ: The inflammatory reflex. Nature 2002;420:853–859.)

the intensity and duration of the inflammatory response is ensured by the central nervous system through afferent and efferent nerve fibers belonging to the autonomous nervous system, mainly the vagus nerve (Tracey, 2002) (Fig. 61.2).

Management of the postoperative systemic inflammation response syndrome includes a careful infectious disease workup to diagnose or rule out significant infection, evaluation of the tolerance of the patient for fever and hyperdynamic state, and supportive therapy. Reduction of fever may be indicated depending on its level and the physiologic reserves of the patient. Anti-inflammatory drug therapy has not been shown to improve outcome in this situation.

Stress Ulcer and Gastrointestinal Hemorrhage

Gastric or duodenal stress ulcer can lead to severe blood loss and hemodynamic instability. The incidence of this complication has decreased markedly during the past 10 to 20 years from approximately 20% to less than 5% in high-risk patients due to earlier enteral nutrition and improvements in general postoperative care, including sedation, analgesia, and efficient prevention. Specific preventive measures should be taken in high-risk patients (i.e., those requiring mechanical ventilation or coagulopathies) and include acid production suppressive agents (H_2 blockers and proton pump inhibitors) and cytoprotective drugs (sucralfate) (Treggiari and Deem, 2005).

Venous Thromboembolism

The postoperative patient requiring ICU care is at high risk for developing thromboembolic complications. Major risk factors are summarized in Box 61.3. In addition to the classic lower extremity deep venous thrombosis, upper extremity localization is not rare in the ICU, probably due to the common presence of central venous catheters inserted via jugular or subclavian veins. Upper extremity venous thrombosis can result in pulmonary embolism in up to two thirds of cases and is also associated with a high rate of catheter-related infection and bacteremia (Box 61.3) (Treggiari and Deem, 2005).

High-risk patients without contraindications should receive prophylaxis with low-molecular-weight heparin, and patients with a low to moderate risk should receive low-dose unfractionated heparin. When contraindications to heparin are present, leg compression devices can be used. Diagnosis of venous thrombosis can be made by Doppler ultrasonography. Helical computerized chest tomography should be the primary test to diagnose pulmonary embolism. The mainstay of treatment in venous thrombosis and pulmonary embolism is heparin. When pulmonary embolism is associated with hemodynamic instability, thrombolytic therapy should be considered if no contraindications exist. When anticoagulation is not possible due to important risks, a vena cava filter can be placed.

Box 61.3 Risk Factors for Venous Thromboembolism
Strong Risk Factors (Odds Ratio, >10)
Fracture (hip or leg)
Hip or knee replacement
Major trauma
Spinal cord injury
Moderate Risk Factors (Odds Ratio, 2–9)
Arthroscopic knee surgery
Central venous lines
Chemotherapy
Congestive heart or respiratory failure
Hormone replacement therapy
Malignancy
Oral contraceptive therapy
Paralytic stroke
Pregnancy, postpartum
Previous venous thromboembolism
Thrombophilia
Weak Risk Factors (Odds Ratio, <2)
Bed rest >3 days
Immobility due to sitting (e.g., prolonged car or air travel)
Increasing age
Laparoscopic surgery (e.g., cholecystectomy)
Obesity
Pregnancy, antepartum
Varicose veins

From Treggiari M, Deem S: Critical care medicine. In Barash PG, Cullen BF, Stoelting RK (eds): Clinical Anesthesia, 5th ed. Philadelphia, Lippincott, Williams & Wilkins, 2005.

THE FUTURE OF POSTOPERATIVE INTENSIVE CARE

The evolution of extensive surgical procedures in the high-risk patient during the past 10 years allows prediction of future trends:

- The number of patients with significant preexisting diseases undergoing surgery will continue to increase.
- Progress in surgical and anesthetic management will keep the intraoperative mortality at acceptable low levels.
- Postoperative care, including recovery room and ICU management, will keep pace and contribute to the prevention of "surgical death."

A major challenge for the future will be the adequate recruitment, training, and retention of ICU personnel—physician–intensivists, nurses, and other well-trained specialists. In addition to training more people, alternative staffing models should be examined. The introduction of the hospitalist model for physicians, engaging patients and families in the care process, and providing critical care outside the ICU are possibilities to expand critical services and to meet the increased needs (Angus, 2005).

Intensive Care Outreach Services

To prevent late surgical death and ease the shortage of ICU beds, a number of hospitals have introduced an early warning and consultant system acting in traditional hospital wards. Staffed by ICU nurses and intensivists, such systems were introduced first in the United Kingdom and Australia. The main purpose of the system is early recognition of significant physiologic disturbances, and responsibility is given to the ICU team to prevent unexpected cardiac arrests and other life-threatening or serious effects.

These initiatives include education programs on the identification and appropriate management of critically ill patients on the ward and also interventions to expedite ICU admission when indicated. In addition, these teams can monitor discharged ICU patients and supervise the use of more invasive therapies and monitoring, such as continuous positive airway pressure, inotropic and vasoactive drugs, and central venous lines (Goldhill, 2004).

However, the basis of preventing surgical mortality in high-risk patients includes an adequate number of critical care beds to which appropriate surgical patients are admitted.

REFERENCES

Angus DC: The future of critical care. Crit Care Clin 2005;21:163–169.

Beauregard CL, Friedman WA; Routine use of postoperative ICU care for elective craniotomy: A cost–benefit analysis. Surg Neurol 2003;60:483–489.

Craven DE, Steger KA: Epidemiology of nosocomial pneumonia. New perspectives on an old disease. Chest 1995;108:1S–16S.

Goldhill DR: Preventing surgical deaths: Critical care and intensive care outreach services in the postoperative period. Br J Anaesth 2005;95:88–94.

Gopalan PD, Burrows RC: Critical care of the vascular surgery patient. Crit Care Clin 2003;19:109–125.

Helling TS, Willoughby TL, Maxfield DM, Ryan P: Determinants of the need for intensive care and prolonged mechanical ventilation in patients undergoing bariatric surgery. Obesity Surg 2004;14:1036–1041.

Nazon D, Abergel G, Hatem CM: Critical care in orthopedic and spine surgery. Crit Care Clin 003;19:33–53.

Tracey KJ: The inflammatory reflex. Nature 2002;420:853–859.

Treggiari M, Deem S: Critical care medicine. In Barash PG, Cullen BF, Stoelting RK (eds): Clinical Anesthesia, 5th ed. Philadelphia, Lippincott, Williams & Wilkins, 2005.

Vincent JL: Nosocomial infections in adult intensive-care units. Lancet 2003;361:2068–2077.

Chapter 62

Alcohol and Drug Ingestions

Santiago Nogué-Xarau and Eduardo Sanjurjo-Golpe

KEY POINTS

- Ethanol intoxication is the most frequent intoxication seen in emergency departments and may sometimes require intensive care unit admission when accompanied by deep coma or respiratory failure. In all inebriated patients, search for concurrent trauma, aspiration of gastric contents, or coingestion of drugs or other toxic ethanol substitutes. Treatment is supportive.
- Methanol poisoning should be suspected in all patients with severe metabolic acidosis and increased anion and osmol gaps, especially when accompanied by ocular or central nervous system impairment. Treatment is based on support measures, ethanol infusion, and hemodialysis.
- Cyclic antidepressants are inhibitors of the rapid sodium channels. Prolongation of QRS of more than 0.16 seconds or R_{aVR} greater than 3 mm are predictors of ventricular arrhythmias. Cardiogenic shock is possible. Sodium bicarbonate IV infusion is the treatment of choice for this cardiotoxicity.
- Paracetamol (acetaminophen) poisoning is a frequent cause of acute liver failure. Chronic heavy drinkers are at greater risk following overdose of paracetamol than light drinkers. Treatment is based on early administration of N-acetylcysteine.
- Central nervous system stimulation is the most prominent effect of cocaine, which may result in restlessness, excitement, increased motor activity, and tonic–clonic seizures. Arterial hypertension, dysrhythmias, myocardial ischemia, and infarction may occur after cocaine use. Sedative–hypnotics are uniformly successful in the treatment of cocaine toxicity and the prevention of mortality.

EPIDEMIOLOGY, RISK FACTORS, AND PATHOGENESIS

Severe poisonings constitute 5% to 10% of all the poisonings or overdoses attended by emergency departments. Depending on the risk to life (e.g., the ingestion of a lethal dose of paraquat), the presence of complications (pneumonia due to aspiration of gastric contents), or organ failure (deep coma) or multiorgan failure (arterial hypotension with renal failure), patients may require ICU admission. Severe intoxications represent 1% to 5% of ICU admissions. The most frequent causes of these poisonings are attempted suicides using therapeutic drugs and substance abuse overdoses and, less frequently, accidents due to domestic, agricultural, or industrial products. The average age of these patients is approximately 40 years, and men and women are usually equally represented. The type of toxic product involved in these poisonings is closely related to the sociological and cultural aspects of each country and to the toxic products available to the population. Attempted suicides are the most frequent cause (54%), followed by ethanol or substance abuse overdoses (31%) and occupational or domestic accidents. One third of these patients have a history of previous poisonings. The most frequent reasons for admission to the ICU are deep coma, respiratory failure and cardiovascular disorders, and, less frequently, hepatic or renal failure. The pathological mechanisms that lead to organ or multiorgan failure are detailed with the toxic products that cause them. Mortality is approximately 6%, being less in therapeutic drug poisonings (3% or 4%) than in other cases (9% or 10%).

CLINICAL FEATURES, DIAGNOSIS, AND PREVENTION

The signs and symptoms, diagnosis, clinical course, and prevention of these poisonings are detailed with the various toxins that are described in this chapter.

PRINCIPLES OF MANAGING THE POISONED OR OVERDOSED PATIENT

The patient admitted to the ICU due to acute poisoning or substance abuse overdose must be evaluated for the possible indication of four types of therapeutic actions: symptomatic or general support measures, measures to try to restrain the absorption of the toxin, measures to increase elimination, and measures to neutralize the toxic effect by the use of antidotes.

Acute poisonings constitute 3% of admissions to multipurpose intensive care units (ICUs). The prognosis of intoxicated patients is, in general, better than that of other patients with similar scores in severity indexes such as Apache II. The ICU stay is usually short (48–72 hr) but may be prolonged by complications, which are frequent in the respiratory system. The consumption of economic resources is also usually less than that of most ICU patients.

Other Critical Care Problems

For more than 40 years, support measures have been the fundamental tool in the treatment of severe acute poisoning and those that give the greatest guarantee of a good evolution. The measures basically consist of support for the organic or multiorgan failure that may be presented, using the most adequate methods and drugs to guarantee, when necessary, the permeability of the airways, alveolar ventilation, tissue perfusion and oxygenation, stabilization of the heart beat, conservation or substitution of the renal function, metabolic homeostasis (correction of metabolic acidosis or hypoglycemia, etc.), control of agitation and seizures, normalization of the temperature, etc.

The second group of therapeutic measures includes decontamination, especially gut decontamination, since in most poisonings the toxic product—usually a medicine—has been ingested orally. The efficacy of decontamination is closely related to its early use. Figure 62.1 shows a decision-making algorithm to determine the priority method of decontamination in the most frequent acute therapeutic drug poisonings. Of the two methods for gastric emptying, emetics and gastric lavage, only the second is relevant to critical care medicine. Efficacious and safe gastric lavage requires that the recommendations of the European Association of Poisons Centres and Clinical Toxicologists and the American Academy of Clinical Toxicology are followed. One of the most important recommendations is the protection of the airway in the case of coma.

Activated charcoal has great adsorbent capacity for many toxic products, constituting an alternative or a complement to gastric drainage maneuvers in recent ingestions (less than 2 hr)

of a toxic dose. It is administered orally if the state of consciousness permits or by a gastric tube after drainage of the stomach contents. Activated charcoal is ineffective or contraindicated in ingestions of ethanol, methanol, isopropanol, lithium, iron, and inorganic acids or alkalines. The initial, and normally only, dose usually recommended for adults is 1 g/kg. In some cases, the administration of repeated doses of 0.5 g/kg every 3 hours for a maximum of 24 hours or until the condition of the patient improves is necessary. These cases include ingestions of massive amounts of slowly absorbed toxic substances (e.g., aspirin); an ingestion accompanied by slowed intestinal peristalsis (e.g., opiates or hypnosedatives), the ingestion of retard pharmaceutical preparations (e.g., some presentations of verapamil), the ingestion of toxins with active enterohepatic recirculation (digitoxin, carbamazepine, meprobamate, indometacin, tricyclic antidepressants, and *Amanita phalloides*), and severe poisonings where it is proven that the toxin can be adsorbed by the charcoal from the capillaries of the intestinal mucosa (phenobarbital and theophylline). The most frequent side effect (7%) of the administration of activated charcoal is vomiting. Thus, the risk of broncoaspiration in patients with depressed consciousness must be anticipated. Repeated doses of activated charcoal produce constipation, and a dose of a cathartic is sometimes recommended.

The third objective of treatment is to evaluate the possibility of forcing renal or extrarenal elimination (hemodialysis, hemoperfusion, etc.) of the toxin. Table 62.1 shows the main toxins for which forced diuresis or dialysis techniques are

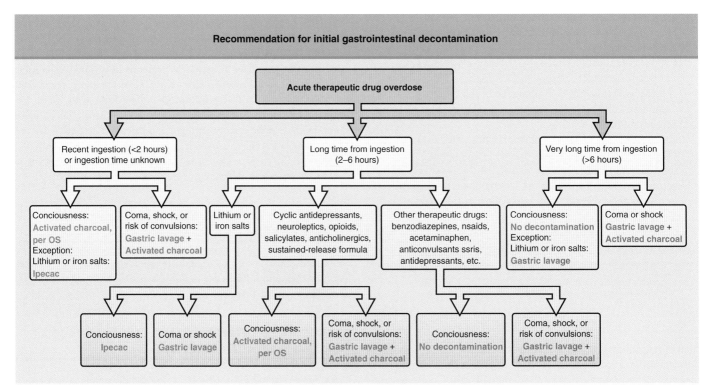

Figure 62.1. Recommendation for initial gastrointestinal decontamination. Algorithm to select the initial method of gut decontamination in the most frequently seen therapeutic drug overdoses. The algorithm must be adapted to the specific conditions of each case. If the patient is in a coma accompanied by loss of gag reflexes, gut decontamination should be carried out after intubation in order to avoid aspiration pneumonia. Patients with intoxications due to isoniazid, theophylline, and antimalarials and patients with previous seizures should be considered at high risk of seizures.

Table 62.1 Main Intoxications for Which Renal or Extrarenal Techniques May Be Indicated When Justified by Clinical Criteria

Toxic Agent	Blood or Plasma Level[a]	Type of Diuresis	Blood or Plasma Level[a]	Type of Elimination Technique
Long-acting barbiturates	7.5 mg/dL	Forced and alkaline	10 mg/dL	HD or HP (CI)
Medium- or short-acting barbiturates	—	Not indicated	5 mg/dL	HP (CI)
Salicylates	50 mg/dL	Alkaline	80 mg/dL	HD
Lithium	1.5 mEq/liter	Diuresis should be maintained	2–3 mEq/liter	HD or HDF
Methotrexate	100 µM/liter	Forced and alkaline	100 µM/liter	HP, HD/HP, or HDF (CI)
Theophylline	—	Not indicated	60 mg/liter	HP or HD
Carbamazepine	—	Not indicated	60 µg/mL	HP
Meprobamate	—	Not indicated	10 mg/dL	HP (CI)
Methaqualone	—	Not indicated	4 mg/dL	HP (CI)
Procainamide	—	Not indicated	20 µg/mL	HD, HP, or HDF
Quinidine	—	Not indicated	14 µg/mL	HP
Levothyroxine	—	Not indicated	Not definable	PE or HP (CI)
Digitoxin	—	Not indicated	60 ng/mL	PE or HP
Bromide	50 mg/dL	Diuresis should be maintained	100 mg/dL	HD
Thallium	0.3 mg/liter	Diuresis should be maintained	0.5 mg/liter	HD
2,4-Dichlorphenoxiacetic	3.5 mg/dL	Forced and alkaline	10 mg/dL	HD
Paraquat	0.1 mg/liter	Diuresis should be maintained	0.1 mg/liter	HD or HP (CI)
Isopropanol	—	Not indicated	1 g/liter	HD (CI)
Methanol	—	Not indicated	0.5 g/liter	HD
Ethylene glycol	—	Not indicated	0.5 g/liter	HD
Mecoprop	Not definable	Alkaline	—	Not indicated
Metahemoglobinemia-causing drugs	—	Not indicated	>40%	BE
Amatoxins	1 ng/mL	Diuresis should be maintained	1 ng/mL	HD or HP (CI)
Valproic acid	—	Not indicated	1 g/liter	HP or HD (CI)

[a]Concentration of toxic product in blood or plasma considered as justifying elimination technique according to clinical criteria.

BE, blood exchange; CI, controversial indication; HD, hemodialysis; HDF, hemodiafiltration; HP, hemoperfusion; PE, plasma exchange.

indicated, specifying the plasma or blood levels from which these techniques are usually justified on clinical criteria.

The fourth objective is the use of antidotes that, through various mechanisms, neutralize the toxic effects. Although there are a multitude of toxic products, there are only approximately 25 antidotes (Table 62.2). The most frequently used are naloxone and flumazenil due to their capacity to reverse coma and hypoventilation due to an overdose of opiates or benzodiazepines. Antidotes have some adverse effects, and their use must be justified by both the suspected diagnosis and the patient's condition. In some cases, the blood or plasma levels of a toxic (as in the case of acetaminophen or methanol poisoning) may be decisive in the initiation or suspension of treatment with antidotes.

ALCOHOL AND ETHYLENE GLYCOL POISONING

Ethanol

Ethanol intoxication is the most common intoxication seen in hospital emergency departments and may sometimes require ICU admission when accompanied by deep coma or respiratory failure. Ethanol is the main toxic component of alcoholic drinks, which may contain between 5% and 50% ethanol, but it is also found in perfumes, colognes, aftershaves, mouthwashes, liniments, and some rubbing alcohols.

The reported lethal ethanol dose is 5 to 8 g/kg for adults and 3 g/kg for children. Chronic alcoholics develop a marked tolerance to ethanol, even at blood levels considered potentially fatal to nontolerant individuals. Approximately 20% of the dose ingested is absorbed in the stomach and the remaining 80% by

the small intestine. In healthy adults, 80% to 90% of absorption occurs within 30 to 60 minutes, but food may delay complete absorption for 4 to 6 hours. The kidney and lungs excrete only 5% to 10% of an absorbed dose unchanged. The maximum rate of hepatic metabolism is 100 to 125 mg/kg/hr, although by enzymatic induction, tolerant individuals can increase their metabolic rates to 175 mg/kg/hr. The average adult metabolizes 7 to 10 g/hr and reduces the ethanol level 15 to 20 mg/dL/hr. Chronic alcoholics have metabolic rates as high as 30 to 40 mg/dL/hr. Alcohol dehydrogenase is the major pathway of ethanol oxidation in the body, converting the ethanol to acetaldehyde; the final step is conversion of acetate to acetyl-CoA and then to CO_2 and H_2O via the Krebs cycle.

The mechanism of action probably involves interference with ion transport at the cell membrane rather that at synapses, similar to the action of anesthesic agents. The frontal lobes are sensitive to a low concentration, resulting in thought and mood disturbances before changes in vision (occipital lobe) and coordination (cerebellum).

Ethanol is a generalized depressant in high doses (Table 62.3). A flushed face, dilated pupils, conjunctival hyperemia, excessive sweating, nausea, and vomiting may accompany central nervous system symptoms. Ethanol can produce dysrhythmias (e.g., atrial fibrillation) in nontolerant binge drinkers as well as in chronic alcoholics. Ethanol is a venodilator that produces decreased preload, afterload, and systemic vascular resistance in healthy adults after acute ingestion. Acute ingestion also has a myocardial depressant effect. In all acutely inebriated patients, one should search for concurrent trauma (Fig. 62.2), acute complications (i.e., gastric aspiration), and coingestion of drugs or more toxic ethanol substitutes (i.e., methanol). Death can occur

Other Critical Care Problems

Table 62.2 Antidotes Used in Intensive Medicine[a]			
Antidote	**Specific Poisoning**	**Usual Loading Dose**	**Usual Maintenance Infusions (When Necessary)**
Antidigoxin fab antibody fragments	Digoxin Digitoxin Cardiac glycosides present in plants	380–760 mg IV over 30 min; it must be administered as a bolus to patients in cardiac arrest	The same dose may be repeated after at least 1 hr if the first is not efficacious or if the clinical reasons for administration reappear.
Atropine	Cholinergic syndromes Organophosphate insecticides Carbamate insecticides Neurotoxic chemical weapons (sarin, tabun)	1 mg IV followed by further doses at 5- to 10-min intervals	Large doses of atropine (1 g/day) may be required in severe poisoning.
Calcium chloride	Calcium channel blockers Hydrofluoric acid	0.2 mL/kg of a 10% (w/vol) solution, IV, over 10 min	The dose may be repeated after 15 min.
Calcium disodium edetate	Lead	15 mg/kg IV every 12 hr, diluted with 250 liters of 0.9% (w/v) sodium chloride, for up to 5 days	After a rest period of 2 days, the same cycle of treatment may be repeated.
Deferoxamine	Iron	15 mg/kg/hr IV over 24 hr	The appropriate duration of deferoxamine infusion is unclear.
Dextrose	Hypoglycemia Insulin Oral hypoglycemic agents Coma of unknown origin	1 g/kg IV of a D_{50}W solution	Some patients may require 10% or 20% dextrose infusion with intermittent 50% dextrose boluses to maintain serum glucose > 100 mg/dL.
Dimercaprol (BAL)	Arsenic Lewisite Inorganic mercury Gold Lead	2.5 mg/kg by deep IM injection every 4 hr for 2 days, then 2.5 mg/kg every 12 hr on day 3, and once daily thereafter for 1–2 weeks	Dimercaprol has been largely superseded by DMPS and DMSA in many countries.
Ethanol	Methanol Ethylene glycol	See Table 62.5	See Table 62.5
Flumazenil	Benzodiazepines Coma of unknown origin	0.25 mg IV over 60 sec Wait 1 min and if the desired response is not obtained, repeat 0.25 mg IV over 60 sec Repeat to a maximum of 2 mg	0.50–1 mg/hr in 0.9% (w/s) sodium chloride or 5% (w/v) glucose, in patients who responded to the boluses
Folinic acid	Methanol	50 mg IV every 4 hr	Repeat while metabolic acidosis persists
Fomepizol	Methanol Ethylene glycol	15 mg/kg IV	10 mg/kg IV every 12 hr for four doses. Fomepizol should be administered every 4 hr during hemodialysis.
Glucagon	β-Adrenergic receptor antagonists Calcium channel antagonists	10 mg IV in 0.9% (w/v) sodium chloride	Intravenous boluses can be given every 20–30 min.
Hydroxocobalamin	Cyanide	5 g IV over 10 min; 10 g IV in case of cardiac arrest	The dose may be repeated in 30 min.
Methylene blue	Methemoglobinemia	1 mg/kg IV over 5 min in a 1% (w/v) aqueous solution	The dose may be repeated at 30-min intervals. Total dose should not exceed 7 mg/kg.
N-acetylcysteine	Acetaminophen (paracetamol) Carbon tetrachloride	150 mg/kg IV over 60 min	50 mg/kg IV over 4 hr + 100 mg/kg over 16 hr
Naloxone	Opiates and opioids Coma of unknown origin	0.2 mg IV over 30 sec Wait 1 min and if the desired response is not obtained, repeat 0.4 mg IV over 60 sec Repeat to a maximum of 4 mg	Infusion of two thirds of the bolus dose initially required to wake the patient could be given hourly, diluted in 0.9% (w/v) sodium chloride. Infusions should only be given to patients who respond to the boluses.
Obidoxime	Organophosphate insecticide Neurotoxic chemical weapons (sarin, tabun)	4 mg/kg IV over 10 min	4 mg/kg IV over 10 min repeated every 4 hr
Oxygen	Carbon monoxide Cyanide Hydrogen sulfide	100%, delivered at atmospheric pressure	Some cases of carbon monoxide poisoning may benefit from hyperbaric oxygen treatment.
Penicillin G sodium	Amatoxin mushrooms	1,000,000 IU IV every 2 hr	Efficacy is unproven.
Physostigmine (eserine)	Pure anticholinergic syndromes (*Datura stramonium*, *Atropa belladonna*)	1 mg IV over 2 min	1 mg IV over 2 min, every 15–30 min
Phytomenadione (vitamin k_1)	Coumarin and indandione anticoagulants	10 mg/IV slowly	Oral treatment may be needed for several weeks in case of superwarfarin poisoning.
Pralidoxime	Organophosphate insecticide Neurotoxic chemical weapons (sarin, tabun)	30 mg/kg IV over 10 min	8 mg/kg/hr in 0.9% (w/v) sodium chloride
Pyridoxine (vitamin B_6)	Isoniazid	5 g IV in 5% (w/v) glucose over 30 min	A second and final dose may be administered.
Silibinin	Amatoxin mushrooms	5–12.5 mg/kg IV in 500 mL 5% (w/d) glucose four times daily	Efficacy is unproven.
Sodium bicarbonate	Drugs blocking myocardial sodium ion channels (cyclic antidepressants, Ia antiarrhythmics, cocaine)	1 mEq/kg IV of hypertonic $NaHCO_3$ (1 mEq/mL) over 15 min	Additional boluses may be administered. Blood pH should be monitored and should not exceed 7.55.

[a]The doses described are for adults.

Table 62.3 Clinical Effects of Ethanol in Inexperienced Drinkers According to Serum Levels	
Serum Ethanol Concentration (g/liter)	**Clinical Effects**
0.2–0.5	Disinhibition, paradoxic excitation, emotional lability, euphoria
0.5–1	Increased reaction time, diminished judgment, fine motor incoordination, dysarthria
1–2	Diplopia, violence, disorientation, confusion, ataxia, stupor, vasodilatation
2–5	Respiratory depression, loss of protective airway reflexes, hypothermia, incontinence, hypotension, coma
>5	Shock, apnea, cardiac arrest

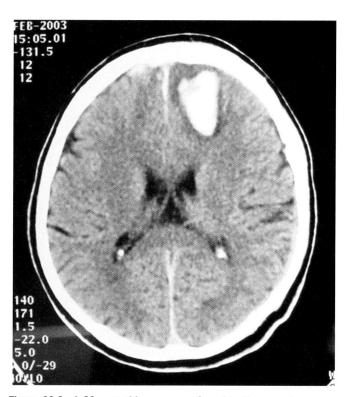

Figure 62.2. A 39-year-old man was referred to the emergency department due to agitation in the context of alcohol consumption accompanied by mild cranial trauma. On arrival, the patient smelled strongly of alcohol. Blood alcohol level was 3.22 g/liter. The patient was diagnosed with acute ethanol intoxication and placed under observation. Twelve hours later, the blood alcohol level was 0.41 g/liter, but the patient was confused and presented bradypsychia. A CT of the head showed a frontal left hematoma/contusion. The patient was admitted for observation and medical treatment. The evolution was good, and the patient was discharged without sequelae after 11 days.

from respiratory depression at ethanol levels exceeding 500 mg/dL.

Treatment is supportive, including venous access and fluids and maintenance of the airway and ventilation if required. Comatose patients should be treated with 100 mg of thiamine for potential Wernicke–Korsakoff syndrome, and hypoglycemia should be discounted. Nutritional deficiencies should be replaced in the chronic alcoholic (magnesium salts, 5 mg of folate, and 1 ampule of multivitamins). Activated charcoal should not be administered for pure ethanol intoxication, but it should be considered if coingestants are present. Aspiration of gastric contents may be reasonable if a very recent large ingestion has occurred; however, ethanol is absorbed rapidly, and lavage quickly becomes ineffective. Ethanol is easily removed by hemodialysis, but in most cases the minimal benefits of lowering the ethanol level quickly are outweighed by the risks of the procedure. No antidote is available for ethanol intoxication.

Isopropanol

Isopropanol is widely used in rubbing alcohol and as a disinfectant, antifreeze, and window cleaner. It is also abused as an inexpensive ethanol substitute. Its toxicity is of the same order of magnitude as ethanol. Although a dose of 240 to 250 mL has been proposed as lethal to humans, children and adults have survived much greater doses.

Isopropanol is rapidly and completely absorbed after ingestion. It is metabolized by ADH to acetone. It is also excreted by the kidneys and more slowly by the lungs. The serum elimination half-life ranges from 2.5 to 8 hours, depending on habitual ethanol consumption, but may be up to 16 hours if ethanol is coingested. Acetone is cleared much more slowly, with a variable half-life of more than 10 hours.

Isopropanol is primarily a CNS depressant. It is slightly more potent than ethanol, and its slower elimination contributes to prolonged toxicity after massive ingestion. Like ethanol, it commonly causes vasodilatation, hypotension, and gastritis.

The classic presentation is CNS depression and ketonemia without acidemia, due to its metabolism to acetone. The onset of toxicity is within 2 hours of ingestion and may be sudden. A fruity breath odor may be perceptible. Patients may present with hypotension and coma. A high osmolal gap is present due to isopropanol and acetone, and serum and urine ketone tests are strongly positive. The presence of a significant anion gap acidosis is rare and suggests tissue hypoperfusion or a coingestion.

Supportive care is the mainstay of therapy. Gastric aspiration may be useful in the unusual case of a large ingestion occurring just before hospital presentation. Activated charcoal should not be administered for pure isopropanol intoxication, but it should be considered if coingestants are present. Isopropanol is easily removed by hemodialysis, but in rare cases the use of hemodialysis may be reasonable because neither isopropanol nor its metabolites cause irreversible tissue damage. Some authors have proposed its use in patients with concentrations greater than 400 mg/dL who are in coma and are hemodynamically unstable despite support treatment. In most cases, the minimal benefits of lowering the isopropanol level quickly are outweighed by the risks of the procedure. No antidote is available for isopropanol toxicity.

Methanol

Methanol is produced from the destructive distillation of wood. Epidemics of methanol toxicity have resulted from the consumption of methanol-contaminated beverages. It is widely available as a solvent and in antifreeze, paint removers, and varnishes.

669

A minimal lethal dose is considered to be 30 mL. Adults have survived ingestions of 500 to 600 mL with aggressive medical care. Consumption of as little as 10 mL may cause blindness, but wide individual variations exist.

Methanol is well absorbed from the gastrointestinal tract, with peak levels occurring within 30 to 90 minutes. Hepatic metabolism in humans accounts for most elimination (90%–95%). Alcohol dehydrogenase oxidizes methanol to formaldehyde, which is rapidly converted by aldehyde dehydrogenase to formic acid. The folate-dependent pathway oxidizes formic acid to nontoxic carbon dioxide. Methanol is oxidized 10 times more slowly than ethanol and thus has a longer elimination half-life. Ethanol has 10 to 20 times greater affinity for alcohol dehydrogenase than methanol; therefore, ethanol is metabolized preferentially by alcohol dehydrogenase. Unchanged renal excretion accounts for 2% to 5% of methanol elimination. The serum half-life of methanol after mild toxicity is 14 to 20 hours and after severe ingestion 24 to 30 hours. Concurrent administration of ethanol increases the methanol half-life to 30 to 35 hours.

Toxicity results from the accumulation of two metabolites: formaldehyde and formic acid. Although formaldehyde previously was considered to be the primary toxic metabolite, it does not accumulate in methanol toxicity because of its rapid metabolism to formic acid. The accumulation of formic acid accounts for most of the metabolic acidosis that follows methanol ingestion and probably correlates better with clinical toxicity than serum methanol levels. Lactate may appear late in the course of severe methanol poisoning as a result of both formate-induced inhibition of mitochondrial respiration and tissue hypoxia, and it may contribute to metabolic acidosis and an increase in the anion gap. Methanol has inherent CNS depressant effects similar to those of ethanol.

Reports correlating blood methanol to clinical effects show variation of toxicity because of differences in sample timing, individual variation, concentration of toxic metabolites, and coingestion of ethanol. Peak methanol levels below 20 mg/dL are usually associated with asymptomatic individuals. Generally, CNS symptoms appear above 20 mg/dL, ocular symptoms appear above 100 mg/dL, and fatalities in untreated patients occur in the range of 150 to 200 mg/dL. The onset of symptoms varies between 1 and more than 24 hours. Coingestion of ethanol delays symptoms, and the absence of symptoms on initial presentation does not exclude serious toxicity. Symptoms and signs are usually limited to the CNS, eyes, and gastrointestinal tract (Table 62.4). Metabolic acidosis may produce dyspnea and tachypnea. Methanol poisoning causes a significant increase in the anion and osmolal gaps. Profound metabolic acidosis, bradycardia, bradypnea, shock, and anuria are bad prognostic indications. Severe intoxications may leave sequelae in the form of a permanent parkinsonian-like syndrome and visual defects.

Evaluate the use of support measures in all patients. Gastric lavage is indicated for any patient presenting within 2 hours of ingestion and may be useful up to 4 hours if coma or coingested drugs reduce gastrointestinal motility. There is no scientific evidence to substantiate the usefulness of activated charcoal or cathartics in methanol poisoning. All patients with metabolic acidosis should receive folinic acid (leucovorin) while the acidosis persists (see Table 62.2) because this cofactor accelerates

Table 62.4 Clinical Effects in Acute Methanol Poisoning

Target Organ	Manifestations
Central nervous system	Euphoria (little compared with ethanol)
	Headache, vertigo, lethargy, and confusion
	Coma and seizures (severe cases)
	Cerebral edema
	Necrosis of the putamen
Ocular	Blurred vision, decreased visual acuity, photophobia and feeling of being in a snowfield
	Constricted visual fields, fixed and dilated pupils, retinal edema, and hyperemia
Gastrointestinal	Nausea, vomiting, and abdominal pain
	Pancreatitis
	Elevation of hepatic aminotransferases

the metabolization of formic acid, which may lead to a reduction of ocular and neurologic sequelae. Forced diuresis is not effective, but hemodialysis effectively removes methanol (>100–150 mL/min clearance) as well as formaldehyde and formic acid. Indications for dialysis are shown in Table 62.5.

Administration of ethanol blocks the formation of formaldehyde and formic acid because of the preferential affinity of ethanol for alcohol dehydrogenase. Ethanol levels should be maintained between 100 and 150 mg/dL to inhibit toxic metabolite formation almost completely. Average dosages necessary to maintain a 70-kg patient in this blood ethanol range are listed in Table 62.5. An intravenous solution of 10% ethanol in D5W is optimal and is more reliable than oral administration. Blood must be drawn frequently before, during, and after dialysis until a steady-state ethanol level is confirmed. Ethanol infusion should be continued until the methanol level falls below 20 to 25 mg/dL. Ethanol indications are shown in Table 62.5.

Fomepizole has been shown to be a potent inhibitor of alcohol dehydrogenase and should prevent, or at least reduce, the further formation of toxic metabolites (see Table 62.2). However, this inhibition of hepatic metabolism results in a substantially decreased elimination rate of methanol. In some patients with slight or moderate intoxications, treatment with fomepizole may avoid the need for hemodialysis. The indications for the use of fomepizole are similar to those for ethanol (see Table 62.5). It has advantages over ethanol administration in that it can be administered to patients being treated with disulfiram or other acetaldehyde–dehydrogenase inhibitors, it causes no CNS depression or hypoglycemia, it is easier to administer, it has a longer duration of action, and serum levels do not have to be followed during its use. However, the cost of fomepizole is much higher than that of ethanol. There are no clinical data to confirm the superiority of fomepizole over ethanol in the treatment of methanol or ethylene glycol poisoning.

Ethylene Glycol

Ethylene glycol is a colorless, odorless, sweet-tasting, viscous liquid. It is primarily used as an automobile radiator antifreeze. Other uses include brake fluid and as a solvent. Ingestion of 1.5 mL/kg of ethylene glycol has been reported to be lethal. As with methanol, early aggressive treatment allows for survival after much larger ingestions.

Table 62.5 Indications for Hemodialysis and Ethanol Treatment in Methanol and Ethylene Glycol Poisoning[a]				
	Methanol Poisoning		**Ethylene Glycol Poisoning**	
Hemodialysis	Methanol level > 50 mg/dL		Ethylene glycol level > 50 mg/dL	
	Formate levels > 20 mg/dL		Glycolate level > 20 mg/dL	
	Metabolic acidosis (pH < 7.25) with increased anion gap		Metabolic acidosis (pH < 7.25) with increased anion gap	
	Visual impairment		Acute renal failure	
Ethanol	Methanol level > 20 mg/dL		Ethylene glycol level > 20 mg/dL	
	Ingestion > 0.4 mL/kg, pending confirmatory blood methanol levels		Ingestion > 0.2 mL/kg, pending confirmatory blood ethylene glycol levels	
	Any ingestion in a symptomatic patient, pending confirmatory blood methanol levels		Any ingestion in a symptomatic patient, pending confirmatory blood ethylene glycol levels	
	Osmol gap > 10 mOsm/kg H_2O		Osmol gap > 10 mOsm/kg H_2O	
	Metabolic acidosis (serum bicarbonate < 20 mEq/liter)		Metabolic acidosis (serum bicarbonate < 20 mEq/liter)	
	Any patient considered for hemodialysis		Any patient considered for hemodialysis	
		Loading Dose	**Maintenance Dose**	**Maintenance Dose during Dialysis**
Amount of ethanol needed to reach and maintain blood ethanol concentration of 100 mg/dL	Nondrinker	600 mg/kg IV in a 5% (w/v) glucose over 1 hr	66 mg/kg IV/hr in a 5% (w/v) glucose infusion	169 mg/kg IV/hr in a 5% (w/v) glucose infusion
	Chronic drinker	600 mg/kg IV in a 5% (w/v) glucose over 1 hr	154 mg/kg IV/hr in a 5% (w/v) glucose infusion	257 mg/kg IV/hr in a 5% (w/v) glucose infusion

[a]Ethanol doses calculated to achieve and maintain blood ethanol concentrations of 100 mg/dL in an adult.

Ethylene glycol is absorbed within 30 minute of ingestion. Hepatic metabolism occurs through successive oxidations by the alcohol and aldehyde dehydrogenase enzymes. The elimination half-life of ethylene glycol is 2.5 to 3 hours. If the alcohol dehydrogenase is blocked with ethanol or inhibited with fomezipole, the elimination half-life is increased to 17 to 20 hours. Like methanol, ethylene glycol is minimally toxic but is oxidized to more toxic acid metabolites, such as glycolic acid, glyoxilic acid, and oxalic acid. The complete oxidation of ethylene glycol also depresses the citric acid cycle, generating lactic acid. For this reason, metabolic acidosis with increased anion and osmol gaps is characteristic of this intoxication.

CNS inebriation is caused by ethylene glycol, but CNS depression, coma, and convulsions are due to the metabolites, especially glycolic acid. Cardiovascular effects, such as dysrhythmias and myocardial depression, are usually secondary to severe metabolic acidosis and hypocalcemia. Oxalate can crystallize in the presence of calcium, and these crystals are found in urine, kidney, myocardium, and other tissues. This may lead to both hypocalcemia and obstruction of the tubular lumen (Fig. 62.3).

Neurologic effects occur 1 to 12 hours postingestion and may be confused with ethanol intoxication. Once the ethylene glycol is metabolized, 4 to 12 hours after ingestion, a metabolic

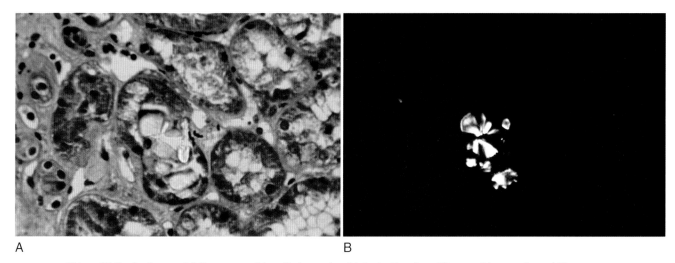

A   B

Figure 62.3. Acute renal failure caused by ethylene glycol intoxication in a 50-year-old man. A renal biopsy was performed 10 days after intoxication. *A,* Flattened, damaged renal tubules. The central tubule displays crystalline material surrounded by interstitial inflammation. *B,* The same section viewed under polarized light shows birefringent intratubular calcium oxalate crystals (Masson's trichrome, × 350).

671

acidosis develops and may cause CNS depression and coma. If the poisoning is severe, coma may be accompanied by hypotonia, hyperreflexia, seizures, cerebral edema, and papilledema. Cardiopulmonary effects occur 12 to 24 hours postingestion. Hypertension and tachycardia are common due to the severe metabolic acidosis. To compensate for this acidosis, hyperventilation occurs. Hypoxia, congestive heart failure, and acute respiratory distress syndrome have all been reported during this stage. Multiorganic failure and death are common at this time.

Renal insufficiency can be present as early as 16 hours postingestion, and overt renal failure is usually established by 48 hours. Calcium oxalate crystals may appear in the urine of the patient during this stage. Renal function often returns to baseline after 3 or more weeks.

Severe poisoning requires advanced intensive care support for optimal outcome. If chronic ethanol abuse is suspected, thiamine should be administered. Careful attention to fluid status is important because the patient may have renal failure. Systemic acidosis must be neutralized with IV sodium bicarbonate. If the patient develops cardiac dysrhythmias and is hypocalcemic, supplemental calcium must be administered. Activated charcoal binds ethylene glycol minimally and is not expected to be effective in preventing its toxic effects. Aspiration of gastric contents may be reasonable if a very recent large ingestion has occurred.

Hemodialysis effectively removes ethylene glycol and its metabolites from the blood, with a clearance rate of 145 to 230 mL/min. Indications for hemodialysis are shown in Table 62.5. Once hemodialysis is initiated, the goal of therapy is to decrease the ethylene glycol level to below 20 mg/dL. In addition, the patient should have normal serum pH and bicarbonate levels. Ethanol has been the traditional antidote for ethylene glycol. Ethanol and fomepizol have been shown to effectively block the formation of the toxic metabolites during ethylene glycol poisoning. Details on ethanol and fomezipole treatment were given in the section on methanol intoxication.

THERAPEUTIC DRUG INGESTION

Benzodiazepines
Benzodiazepine intoxications usually produce mild or moderate manifestations. Their severity depends mainly on the complications of CNS depression or the association with other toxic products with synergic actions.

By attaching to the polysynaptic terminals where GABA is released, benzodiazepines cause hyperpolarization and therefore potentiate the GABA effect, producing anxiolytic, hypnotic, miorelaxing, and antiepileptic effects. Their hepatic metabolism generates active metabolites that can have a sedative effect even greater than that of the original compound. Elimination of benzodiazepine metabolites occurs via renal clearance. The toxic dose and the clinical manifestations depend on the elimination half-life of the benzodiazepine and can vary due to simultaneous intoxication with other toxics, benzodiazepine tolerance in chronic consumers, and some underlying diseases (hepatic failure).

The clinical manifestations are secondary to CNS depression: dysarthria, ataxia, nystagmus, drowsiness, confusion, stupor, and coma. Generally, there is hypotonia with hyporeflexia and average or miotic pupils. There may be sinus bradycardia and

arterial hypotension. Alveolar hypoventilation is rare and affects mainly elderly patients and those with hepatic or pulmonary disease. The main complication and, in general, the cause of morbidity and mortality in pure benzodiazepine intoxications is bronchoaspiration, mainly due to the absence of cough reflex in the deepest comas and sometimes favored by gut decontamination maneuvers.

The toxicological diagnosis is usually made by enzyme immunoassay in plasma and urine. In some cases, the response to flumazenil in a coma of unknown origin confirms the diagnosis. Treatment is based on support measures. Gut decontamination is useful in the first hour postingestion. Renal or extrarenal techniques are not indicated. In patients with a low Glasgow Coma Score, flumazenil can be used (see Table 62.2).

Barbiturates
The most frequent intoxication is by phenobarbital, which is widely used, especially for the treatment of epilepsy. Barbiturates act on a specific chlorine channel receptor at the level of the CNS, producing depression of the neuronal function. To some degree, all barbiturates undergo metabolic degradation by the liver. Approximately 25% to 50% of a dose of phenobarbital is excreted unchanged in the urine. Barbiturates may have a short, intermediate, or long half-life, and the clinical effects observed depend on the dose, absorption, redistribution from tissue stores, the presence of active metabolites, and the hepatic and renal functions. Hence, the duration of action does not always correlate well with the elimination half-life.

Barbiturate intoxication produces coma, sometimes deep, with hypothermia, hypotonia, hyporeflexia, hypoventilation, and even apnea. There is a risk of bronchoaspiration with the posterior development of acute respiratory distress syndrome (ARDS). Arterial hypotension secondary to the inhibition of vascular smooth muscle tone and myocardial depression may also appear and give rise to a metabolic acidosis due to tissue hypoperfusion. There may also be cutaneous injuries due to bullous lesions and rhabdomyolysis with acute renal failure.

Toxicological analysis will confirm the diagnosis and allow evaluation of the severity. Treatment is based on support measures, gut decontamination (gastric lavage and repeated doses of activated charcoal), forced alkaline diuresis in long-acting barbiturate intoxications, and hemodialysis or hemoperfusion with activated charcoal in more severe cases (see Table 62.1).

Cyclic Antidepressants
Since the introduction of selective serotonin reuptake inhibitors, which are safer and have a higher therapeutic index, the prescription of cyclic antidepressants (CAs) has declined, and intoxications are now less frequent.

They act by inhibiting the reuptake of catecholamines at the cardiovascular and CNS levels, and they have a quinidine-like effect, inhibiting the rapid sodium channel in the myocardium, and also an alpha blocker effect. The metabolism is hepatic and the elimination half-life is prolonged. Serious acute intoxication results from a mean ingestion of 30 to 40 mg/kg and the mean fatal dose is 60 to 70 mg/kg.

Clinical manifestations are characterized by a reduced consciousness and the development of an anticholinergic syndrome with mydriasis, blurred vision, hyperthermia, dry skin and mucosa, delirium, tachycardia, paralytic ileus, myoclonias,

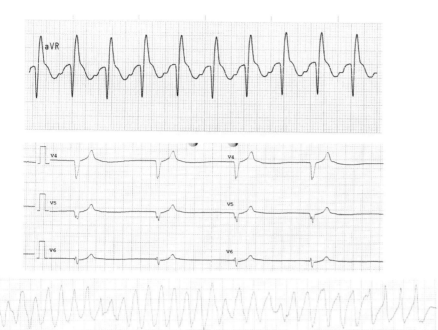

Figure 62.4. Different electrocardiographic patterns seen in cardiotoxicity. *Top,* An aVR derivation in an 18-year-old patient with severe maprotiline intoxication, with an R′ wave of 10 mm. *Middle,* Slow nodal rhythm in chronic digoxin intoxication. *Bottom,* A ventricular tachycardia in the form of torsades de pointes in a cocaine overdose.

and urinary retention. Seizures occur in 10% of patients. At the cardiac level, there is a sinus tachycardia with PR, QRS, and QTc prolongation. A Brugada electrocardiographic pattern mimicked by overdose of CAs has been reported. Severe cases may present ventricular arrhythmias including ventricular tachycardia and ventricular fibrillation. However, atrioventricular block and torsades de pointes are infrequent.

Diagnosis is made through the history and clinical and electrocardiographic findings, and it is confirmed by plasma CAs analysis. The prognosis is associated with the prolongation of the QRS since a QRS greater than 0.10 second is associated with a higher frequency of seizures, and if higher than 0.16, the risk of ventricular arrhythmias is high. The sensitivity of an R or R′$_{aVR}$ of at least 3 mm is 81% for predicting seizures or dysrhythmias (Fig. 62.4). Mortality generally occurs within the first 24 hours and is due to cardiovascular toxicity.

Treatment is based on gut decontamination measures such as gastric lavage and activated charcoal. In severe cases, repetition of active charcoal with the addition of a cathartic is advised if there is no paralytic ileus. Renal or extrarenal techniques are not indicated. If there is hypotension, R or R′$_{aVR}$ of at least 3 mm, or prolongation of the QRS, the treatment of choice is IV sodium bicarbonate (see Table 62.2). Care should be taken with regard to the fluid balance to avoid the appearance of acute pulmonary edema; hyperventilation may be useful to maintain the pH level at approximately 7.50. In the case of ventricular arrhythmias refractory to alkalinization, lidocaine is the safest, most effective agent. Benzodiazepines are the treatment of choice for seizures. Bradycardia or heart block requires alkalinization, isoprenaline, or a pacemaker. Hemodynamic collapse unresponsive to advanced life support measures may respond to femoral–femoral extracorporeal circulation, which can provide hemodynamic support until toxic cardiovascular effects abate.

Cardiac arrest requires prolonged resuscitation maneuvers with continuous administration of sodium bicarbonate.

Lithium

Lithium intoxications may occur in two circumstances: an acute intoxication due to attempted suicide or a chronic intoxication in a patient being treated with lithium in whom a drug interaction (thiazide diuretics, ibuprofen, and phenytoin) or an intercurrent process (dehydration) has triggered an accumulation of lithium.

Lithium is absorbed orally, is not bound to plasma proteins, and has a low volume of distribution. It is eliminated by glomerular filtration, and 80% of excreted lithium undergoes tubular reabsorption. The elimination half-life is 18 to 24 hours and may be prolonged in elderly patients, during chronic treatment, or in patients with renal failure. The toxic dose is estimated at 100 mg/kg for acute intoxication.

The initial symptoms are usually digestive (nausea, vomiting, or diarrhea). However, neurological symptoms are predominant. After a fine hand tremor is observed, the patient may develop muscular and reflex hyperirritability; spastic, dystonic, or choreiform movements; parkinsonism; and confusion and stupor progressing to coma. The clinical presentation is usually more severe in chronic intoxications than in acute ones, and often the recovery is slow. Other clinical manifestations, such as arterial hypotension or arrhythmias, are infrequent and are observed only in the most severe cases. In acute intoxications, the lithium level can only be evaluated 12 hours or more after ingestion due to the slow absorption and distribution of the drug.

In acute intoxications, ipecac or gastric lavage should be carried out since activated charcoal is not indicated because it has no adsorbent capacity for lithium. Some studies have shown that sodium polystyrene sulfonate and intestinal irrigation with polyethylene glycol are effective in reducing lithium absorption. Diuresis should be maintained, but forced diuresis does not significantly increase lithium clearance. Thiazidic diuretics are contraindicated because they reduce renal excretion of lithium.

The basic treatment of severe lithium intoxication is hemodialysis, which reduces lithium concentrations by 0.25 mEq/liter/hr. Hemodialysis should be prolonged until a lithemia less than 1 mEq/liter is achieved and should be restarted in case of rebound. The main indications for initiating hemodialysis are a lithemia more than 3.5 mEq/liter in acute intoxications, lithemia more than 2.5 mEq/liter in chronic intoxications, and in all the cases with lithemia higher than 1 mEq/liter and severe clinical manifestations. If hemodialysis is not possible, hemodiafiltration may be useful (see Table 62.1).

Acetaminophen (Paracetamol)

Acetaminophen is one of the most widely used drugs and may cause acute intoxication after attempted suicide or an involuntary subacute intoxication after treatment for pain. Acetaminophen is rapidly absorbed orally, reaching a plasma peak 1 hour after ingestion. The metabolism is hepatic, giving rise to approximately 20 metabolites. The two major pathways produce nontoxic sulfate and glucuronide conjugates. However, a reaction mediated by CYP2E1 results in a toxic metabolite (NAPQI) that is normally conjugated with glutathione to produce the nontoxic mercapturic acid excreted in the urine. After an overdose of acetaminophen, a large portion is oxidized to NAPQI, which reacts with more than 40 cellular components and leads to cell necrosis. Previously healthy, nonfasting patients who acutely ingest more than 150 mg/kg (children) or 7.5 g (adults) are at risk of developing toxicity. These toxic doses are smaller in patients with malnourishment, chronic alcoholism, hepatopathy, or habitual treatment with hepatic enzymatic inducers (rifampicin, phenobarbital, etc.).

Without treatment, clinical manifestations present in four phases. At 24 hours postingestion, anorexia, nausea, and vomiting are present. At 24 to 48 hours, analyses show hepatic cytolysis. At 48 to 96 hours, hepatocellular failure develops, with encephalopathy, hypoglycemia, and coagulopathy; extreme cytolysis and cholestasis; and possible acute renal failure due to tubular necrosis. In the final phase, the patient may develop multiorgan failure, which may be fatal without liver transplant.

Treatment is based on support measures, gut decontamination with gastric lavage and activated charcoal, and the administration of N-acetylcysteine, which increases the synthesis and availability of glutathione, which is combined with the toxic metabolite to inactivate it. This antidote is almost 100% effective if administered during the first 12 hours after ingestion, but it may also be effective if administered later, even when hepatic damage has been established. The antidote is indicated when the patient has ingested a toxic dose or when it is estimated that a plasma acetaminophen concentration in relation to the interval postingestion will result in hepatotoxicity. In general, the "150 treatment line" of the Rumack–Matthew nomogram is used (see Table 62.2).

Salicylates

Salicylates, like acetaminophen, are very frequently used drugs, and the intoxication can be acute or chronic in the context of pain treatment. Salicylates are well absorbed orally. Metabolism and elimination of salicylates are by hepatic and renal routes. Salicylates uncouple mitochondrial oxidative phosphorylation, causing an increase in oxygen consumption and CO_2 production, leading to respiratory alkalosis and metabolic acidosis. Disruption of the Krebs cycle metabolism and glycolysis leads to gluconeogenesis and lipolysis, with increased ketone formation. Hematologic effects include inhibition of platelet aggregation, a decrease in factor VII, and hypoprothrombinemia. The toxic acute dose is 150 mg/kg, with serious toxicity when 300 to 500 mg/kg is ingested. The toxic blood level is more than 30 mg/dL.

The clinical manifestations include nausea, vomiting, and epigastralgia, sometimes with upper digestive hemorrhage due to injury of the gastric mucosa, as well as tinnitus and vertigo in the mildest cases. The most severe cases present with tachycardia, tachypnea, fever, reduced consciousness, convulsions, rhabdomyolysis, acute renal failure, acute pulmonary edema, and hemorrhagic diathesis. Hypoglycemia or hyperglycemia may be present. Metabolic acidosis, together with respiratory alkalosis, is typical. All the manifestations are more severe in elderly patients.

Treatment is based on rehydration and the correction of the electrolyte balance, gut decontamination by gastric lavage and activated charcoal, and gastric protection (omeprazol). Urinary alkalinization enhances salicylate elimination and should be used when salicylate levels are greater than 40 to 50 mg/dL. Hemodialysis is indicated for serum salicylate levels higher than 100 to 120 mg/dL, intractable acidosis, renal failure, pulmonary edema, coma, or seizures (see Table 62.1).

Antiarrhythmic Drugs

Of the many antiarrhythmic drugs, only β-adrenergic receptor antagonists (BARAs), calcium channel antagonists (CCAs), and digoxin (DG) are considered here.

It is generally accepted that the mechanism of toxicity of BARAs involves excessive blockade of beta receptors, with decreased cyclic AMP and blunting of the metabolic, chronotropic, and inotropic effects of catecholamines, leading to myocardial depression, hypotension, and cardiovascular collapse. Slowing of the heart due to sinus node suppression and conduction abnormalities occurs in virtually all significant BARA intoxications. BARAs produce arterial hypotension, especially secondary to the depression of myocardial contractility and, to a lesser extent, the reduction of the heart rate and the inhibition of vascular smooth muscle tone. The QRS may be normal and asystole is possible. Heart failure with acute pulmonary edema may present as a consequence of myocardial depression, especially in elderly patients or those with underlying cardiopathy. Treatment is based on gastric lavage, activated charcoal, and support treatment. Glucagon has become the first-line pharmacotherapy for BARA toxicity, enhancing myocardial performance by increasing cyclic AMP concentration (see Table 62.2). Epinephrine may be beneficial in raising heart rate and increasing contractility through β receptor stimulation, as well as augmenting blood pressure through α-adrenergic receptor stimulation. Transvenous electrical or external pacing may be required to maintain heart rate when pharmacological measures fail.

Toxicity from CCA causes a decrease in mechanical contraction of heart and smooth muscle. Severe toxicity produces cardiogenic shock, characterized by bradycardia and hypotension. Because CCAs interfere with normal signaling of stimulatory hormones in the cardiovascular system, standard cardiotonic and vasopressor treatments for hypotension often produce minimal effects in patients with severe toxicity. The clinical presentation includes bradycardia and hypotension, altered mental status, metabolic acidosis, hyperglycemia, sinus arrest on electrocardiogram, and refractory shock. Treatment of CCA overdose consists of providing supportive care, decreasing drug absorption (activated charcoal), and augmenting myocardial function with cardiotonic agents: calcium chloride solution, glucagon, insulin/dextrose infusion, or epinephrine infusion (see Table 62.2). Electrical pacing should be employed for heart rate below 40 beats/min with shock.

Digoxin is the antiarrhythmic that most frequently gives rise to intoxications, especially chronic ones, in patients with cardiopathy and may be triggered by changes in the dose, pharmacological interactions, dehydration, renal failure, hypokalemia, hypomagnesemia, or hypercalcemia. However, acute intoxication is less frequent but much more severe, with 0.05 mg/kg considered to be a toxic dose. Clinical symptoms are characterized by nonspecific digestive symptoms, including nausea and vomiting. Patients often consult for symptoms derived from low cardiac output (syncope, fainting, and congestive heart failure). The electrocardiogram shows different types of arrhythmia (see Fig. 62.4) ranging from sinus bradycardia to different degrees of cardiac block or ventricular or supraventricular arrhythmias. Intoxicating digoxin levels are usually higher than 2 ng/mL, although there is not always a clinical–analytical correlation. Treatment of chronic intoxications is based on monitoring and the suspension of the drug, whereas acute intoxication requires gut decontamination (activated charcoal). Phenytoin may be used in cases of ventricular arrhythmias, whereas bradycardia may require atropine or the insertion of a pacemaker. Calcium salts and electrical cardioversion are contraindicated, and renal or extrarenal measures are not effective. In some severe cases, characterized by ventricular disorders of the cardiac rhythm refractory to conventional treatment, hemodynamic instability, and factors of a poor prognosis such as hyperkalemia higher than 6 mEq/liter, antidigital antibodies may be administered (see Table 62.2).

DRUGS OF ABUSE

Opioids

Opioids are naturally occurring or synthetic drugs that have opium or morphine-like activity and are used clinically for analgesia and anesthesia and illicitly for oral, inhalational, or parenteral abuse. Altering the structure of morphine produces many semisynthetic opioids, including heroin. Intravenous heroin consumption has decreased considerably during the past two decades, coinciding with the AIDS epidemic, leading to a decrease in the number of overdoses. Overdoses may occur independently of the route of administration, although intravenous injection makes overdose more likely. Fluctuations in drug purity and possibly decreased tolerance secondary to variable periods of voluntary or enforced abstinence increase the risk of overdose. Occasionally, opiate overdose is seen in patients with cancer or chronic pain treated with morphine, methadone, or fentanyl, especially when the dose is increased.

After intravenous injection, heroin is rapidly converted to acetylmorphine and then more slowly to morphine. Elimination is primarily by the kidneys, with 70% of the dose excreted in the urine as morphine. Opioids produce their effects by interacting with specific receptors distributed throughout the central and peripheral nervous systems and in the gastrointestinal tract. The lethal dose depends on individual tolerance but is usually approximately 120 mg for morphine, 20 mg for heroin, and 1300 mg for dextropropoxyphene.

The classic triad of opioid toxicity is a depressed level of consciousness, respiratory depression, and miosis, with the risk of respiratory failure and subsequent cardiac arrest. Hypotension, noncardiogenic pulmonary edema, aspiration pneumonitis, ileus, rhabdomyolysis, and arrhythmias may also present. Seizures may be associated with propoxyphene and meperidine overdose.

The diagnosis is clinical. The presence of opiates in urine may be confirmed by immunoassay screening tests, but plasma drug concentrations are not clinically useful. In some cases, a rapid response to naloxone corroborates opioid exposure in a patient with coma of unknown origin.

Treatment is based on support measures, especially respiratory and hemodynamic, when necessary. Decontamination is not useful in the majority of cases, except in oral ingestions (methadone and codeine). There is no role for forced diuresis, dialysis, or hemoperfusion. Naloxone is a competitive opioid antagonist with no opioid agonist properties. It is administered in an IV bolus (see Table 62.2). Its effect lasts approximately 20 to 30 minutes and the clinical manifestations of the overdose may reappear, especially for opioids with a prolonged half-life, such as methadone. In cases of renewed CNS depression, naloxone in continuous perfusion may be administered. Because naloxone is an opiate antagonist, its use may trigger withdrawal symptoms, characterized by anxiety, agitation, sweating, and piloerection.

Cocaine

Cocaine is a natural alkaloid found in *Erythroxylon coca*. Its use has reached epidemic proportions. Cocaine overdose may occur after recreational use through nasal, pulmonary, or endovenous routes. The digestive route is only used by body packers (swallowing of wrapped packages of cocaine in an attempt to smuggle the drug across national boundaries) (Fig. 62.5) and body stuffers (swallowing or concealing packets of cocaine in various body cavities when at risk of discovery).

Cocaine blocks fast sodium channels, stabilizing the axonal membrane, with a resultant local anesthetic effect. Due to blockade of myocardial fast sodium channels, cocaine has type I antiarrhythmic properties. Cocaine interferes with the uptake of neurotransmitters, such as epinephrine, norepinephrine, and dopamine. It acts as a vasoconstrictor agent and is rapidly absorbed through the nasal mucosa, gastrointestinal mucosa, pulmonary alveoli, and by direct intravenous injection. The half-life of cocaine is 1 hour. Benzoylecgonine and ecgonine methyl ester, the major metabolites of cocaine, have a half-life of 6 and 4 hours, respectively. Cocaine is hydrolized rapidly by liver and plasma esterases. Cocaethylene is a unique metabolite that results from the combined use of alcohol and cocaine. All these metabolites are excreted in the urine. A toxic dose is considered to be 50 to 100 mg by the intranasal route and 15 to 30 mg IV, and a lethal dose is 0.5 to 1 g.

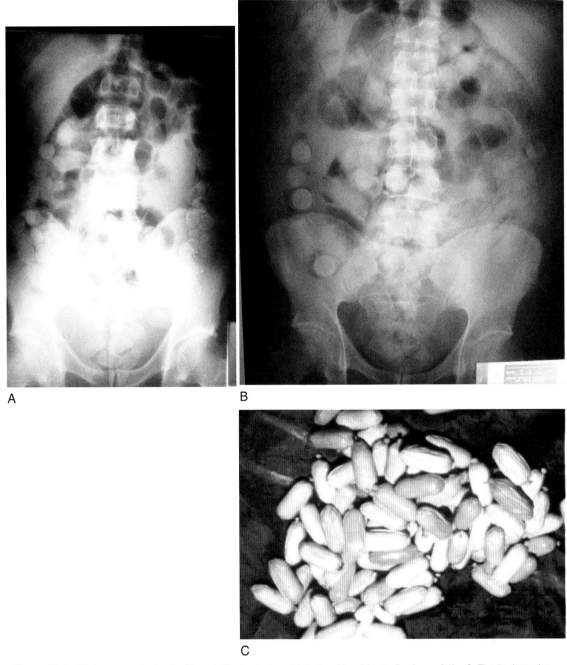

Figure 62.5. Abdomen radiographs (A and B) showing multiple foreign objects (body packs). *C,* The body packs after expulsion through the rectum.

Common CNS manifestations include dilated pupils, euphoria, anxiety, agitation, delirium, psychosis, and seizures. Cardiovascular manifestations include hypertension, arrhythmias, congestive heart failure, aortic dissection, and chest pain. Vasospasm and increased platelet aggregation can produce a myocardial infarction or ischemic cerebral infarcts, whereas severe hypertension can produce intracranial hemorrhage. Respiratory complications of cocaine include upper airway obstruction, status asthmaticus, pulmonary hypertension, and noncardiogenic or cardiogenic pulmonary edema. Other manifestations of cocaine abuse are rhabdomyolysis, bowel ischemia, and hyperthermia with muscle rigidity, disseminated intravascular coagulation, hepatic dysfunction, and renal failure resembling neuroleptic malignant syndrome. The differential diagnosis is established with amphetamine intoxication, which produces similar, although longer lasting, clinical manifestations.

Urine immunoassays for cocaine metabolites are screening tests that generally detect benzoylecgonine at concentrations higher than 300 ng/mL and are thus usually positive for 48 to 72 hours following use.

In body packers and body stuffers, activated charcoal followed by whole-bowel irrigation with a polyethylene glycol is a well-tolerated and safe method of rapid elimination of drug packets from the gastrointestinal tract. Contraindications to whole-bowel irrigation include gastrointestinal hemorrhage, ileus, and bowel perforation. Surgical removal of packages may be needed in patients with bowel obstruction or package perforation, whereas endoscopic removal is not recommended. There is no role for forced diuresis, dialysis, or hemoperfusion.

Support measures are necessary to control agitation, hypertension, and the complications derived from ischemia. Active and passive patient cooling, sedation with benzodiazepines, and muscle paralysis with nondepolarizing neuromuscular blockers may be necessary if the patient has hyperthermia. In cases of hypertension or thoracic pain due to myocardial ischemia, phentolamine, nitroglycerin, or nitroprusside may be used. Beta blockers should not be used in isolation because they can aggravate the myocardial ischemia by blocking the vasodilation mediated by the β_2-adrengergic receptors, although a combination of beta blockers with phentolamine or nitroprusside may be effective.

Amphetamines and Related Drugs

Amphetamines are a class of noncatechol sympathomimetic amines that produce CNS stimulation. A remarkable variety of amphetamine derivatives have been produced, the most important of which are methamphetamine and methylenedioxymethamphetamine (MDMA; Ecstasy). Ecstasy is the most widely used of the so-called "designer drugs" among young people. It increases empathy and self-esteem, verbal communication, and gives a profound feeling of well-being while reducing fatigue and the need for sleep.

Amphetamines exert their toxicity via CNS stimulation, peripheral release of catecholamines, inhibition of reuptake of catecholamines, and inhibition of monoamine oxidase. Ingestion is usually oral, but intranasal or intravenous consumption is also known. The usual dose is 100 mg MDMA per tablet. Onset of action is within 30 minutes, and peak serum levels are reached in 1 to 3 hours. The metabolism is hepatic and approximately one third is eliminated unchanged through the kidneys, although this may increase to 70% if the urine is acidified. The elimination half-life is 7 hours. The toxic dose depends on the amphetamine derivate and is between 5 and 20 mg for methamphetamine and between 100 and 150 mg for MDMA, although these doses may be lower based on individual tolerance or coingestion of alcohol.

In overdose, amphetamines cause anxiety, agitation, irritability, confusion, and tremor. Other features include mydriasis, arrhythmias, chest pain with myocardial infarction, sudden death, seizures, hypertension with intracranial hemorrhage, stroke, rhabdomyolysis and hyperthermia with muscle rigidity, disseminated intravascular coagulation, and renal failure. Occasionally, a fulminant hepatitis occurs. Most screening tests of urine for amphetamine-related compounds use an immunoassay technique. Confirmation is performed by a gas chromatography and mass spectroscopy analysis.

Digestive decontamination measures may be useful in recent ingestions. Extrarenal measures are not efficacious. Acidification of the urine increases renal elimination of amphetamines but may lead to acute renal failure when rhabdomyolysis is present and therefore is not recommended. There is no specific antidote, and treatment includes symptomatic and support measures. In cases of hypertension, labetalol, nitroprusside, or phentolamine may be used. Active cooling measures may become necessary in cases presenting with hyperthermia.

γ-Hydroxybutyrate (Liquid Ecstasy)

γ-Hydroxybutyrate (GHB) emerged in the 1990s as a drug of abuse. It is used for recreational purposes and results in disinhibition and euphoria and has empathetic and aphrodisiac properties. It may also be used for criminal purposes, including robbery and especially rape, due to its amnesiac effect.

GHB is derived from GABA and is thought to function as an inhibitory transmitter through specific brain receptors for GHB and possibly through GABA receptors. It is sold as a clear liquid with a slight smell of acetone, usually contained in 10-mL flasks.

Overdose is characterized by rapidly reduced levels of consciousness that frequently lead to deep, nonreactive coma. Pupil size varies, with a predominance of mydriasis. Overdose may be accompanied by hypothermia, bradycardia, hypotension, and alveolar hypoventilation. The patient normally recovers spontaneously and completely within 1 or 2 hours if there is no coingestion of alcohol or other drugs, but fluctuations of consciousness, agitation, convulsions, and ataxia may sometimes be present.

The diagnosis is clinical and the frequent coingestion of other drugs should be taken into account. Urine and serum tests for GHB are not routinely available. Confirmation is by gas chromatography and mass spectrometry analysis.

Treatment consists of symptomatic and support measures. Digestive decontamination measures are not used due to the rapid absorption, and renal or extrarenal elimination are contraindicated due to the short half-life. The use of physostigmine to reverse coma in GHB overdose is controversial since rapid recovery is the norm.

Phencyclidine (PCP or Angel Dust)

Phencyclidine (PCP) was initially developed as a general anesthetic but was abandoned due to side effects. In the 1970s, it was discovered as a drug of abuse. PCP has anticholinergic, opioid, dopaminergic, CNS stimulant, and α-adrenergic effects. The normal clinical manifestations include agitation, anxiety, irritability, violent behavior, and changes in the mental state, including coma. Patients may present vertical nystagmus and hypertension, sometimes severe, with stroke or intracranial hemorrhage. Abnormal analytical results include hypoglycemia, hepatic cytolysis, and rhabdomyolysis, sometimes accompanied by acute renal failure. The diagnosis is clinical, although PCP may be identified in the urine. Early digestive decontamination using activated charcoal may be useful. Acidification of the urine increases renal elimination but may lead to acute renal failure when accompanied by rhabdomyolysis. Agitation may be treated with benzodiazepines and psychosis with haloperidol. Nitroprusside or labetalol may be administered in cases of hypertension. There is no specific PCP antagonist.

Box 62.1 Controversies

- The use of naloxone and flumazenil in patients in coma of unknown origin
- The use of flumazenil in simultaneous ingestions of benzodiazepines and cyclic antidepressants
- The use of ipecac syrup and cathartics as digestive decontamination measures
- The use of multiple doses of activated charcoal as a method of accelerating the elimination of toxic agents
- The criteria for the indication of hemodialysis in severe lithium intoxications
- The role of hemoperfusion in acute poisonings
- Fomepizol *versus* ethanol in methanol or ethylene glycol poisoning

Box 62.2 Pitfalls

- In patients with organ failure due to severe acute intoxication, therapeutic priorities are usually the administration of general support measures rather than the use of an antidote.
- In patients in deep coma with loss of the gag reflex, gut decontamination measures without protection of the airways carry the risk of respiratory complications that outweigh the benefits of decontamination.
- In the majority of drug ingestions, the patient is seen when the toxic agent has been absorbed and therefore gut decontamination measures are ineffective.
- The indication of renal or extrarenal elimination techniques is based on the clinical state of the patient, the blood level of the toxic, and the pharmacokinetics and pharmacodynamics of the toxic agent.
- Activated charcoal is ineffective or contraindicated in ingestions of ethanol, methanol, isopropanol, lithium, iron, and inorganic acids and alkalines.
- Isopropanol poisoning increases the osmolal gap but usually not the anion gap.
- Ethanol infusion in methanol or ethylene glycol poisoning must be doubled during hemodialysis.

CONTROVERSIES AND PITFALLS

Controversies and pitfalls are listed in Boxes 62.1 and 62.2, respectively.

SUGGESTED READING

American Academy of Clinical Toxicology/European Association of Poisons Centres and Clinical Toxicologists: Position statement: Ipecac syrup, gastric lavage, single-dose activated charcoal, cathartics and whole bowel irrigation. J Toxicol Clin Toxicol 1997;35:699–762.

Barceloux DG, Bond GR, Krenzelok EP, Cooper H, Vale JA: American Academy of Clinical Toxicology. Practice guidelines on the treatment of methanol poisoning. J Toxicol Clin Toxicol 2002;40:415–446.

Barceloux DG, Krenzelok EP, Olson K, Watson W: American Academy of Clinical Toxicology. Practice guidelines on the treatment of ethylene glycol poisoning. J Toxicol Clin Toxicol 1999;37:537–560.

Dart RC: Medical Toxicology. Philadelphia, Lippincott Williams & Wilkins, 2004.

Flanagan RJ, Jones AL: Antidotes. London, Taylor & Francis, 2001.

Goldfrank LR, Flomenbaum NE, Lewin NA, et al: Toxicologic Emergencies. New York, McGraw-Hill, 2002.

Mokhlesi B, Leiken JB, Murray P, Corbridge TC: Adult toxicology in critical care. General approach to the intoxicated patient. Chest 2003;123:577–592.

Mokhlesi B, Leiken JB, Murray P, Corbridge TC: Adult toxicology in critical care. Specific poisonings. Chest 2003;123:897–922.

Nogue S, Munne P, Nicolas JM, Sanz P, Amigo M: Intoxicaciones Agudas. Protocolos de Tratamiento. Barcelona, Morales & Torre, 2003.

Proudfoot AT, Krenzelok EP, Vale JA: Position paper on urinary alkalinization. J Toxicol Clin Toxicol 2004;42:1–26.

Zimmerman JL: Poisonings and overdoses in the intensive care unit: General and specific management issues. Crit Care Med 2003;31:2794–2801.

Chapter 63

Carbon Monoxide Poisoning

Joshua Rucker and Joseph A. Fisher

KEY POINTS

- Carbon monoxide poisoning is the most common cause of poisoning morbidity and mortality in the world.
- Nonspecific symptoms frequently lead to misdiagnosis.
- The central nervous and cardiovascular systems are the most frequently affected.
- All patients should be treated with 100% oxygen.
- Severely poisoned patients should be considered for hyperbaric oxygen

Carbon monoxide (CO) is a colorless, odorless gas produced from the incomplete combustion of carbonaceous compounds. CO inhalation is the most common cause of poisoning in the industrialized world. Severe CO poisoning can cause multiorgan dysfunction, frequently necessitating admission to intensive care units.

EPIDEMIOLOGY, RISK FACTORS, AND PATHOGENESIS

In the United States, CO poisoning accounts for 40,000 to 70,000 emergency visits and between 3500 and 4000 deaths annually. The most common causes of severe CO poisoning are prolonged intentional or unintentional exposure to motor vehicle exhaust; indoor burning of wood, kerosene, or coal with inadequate ventilation; and combustion of fossil fuels in pipelines or containers. Risk factors for diagnosing CO poisoning include cold climate, the presence of an indoor gas heater, and cohabitants with influenza-like symptoms.

CO Kinetics

CO is inhaled into the lung and then diffuses into the blood, where it mostly binds to hemoglobin to form carboxyhemoglobin (COHb). (A small amount of CO remains dissolved in blood in equilibrium with that bound to hemoglobin.) The rate of uptake of CO into the blood is increased by higher ambient CO partial pressure and increased minute ventilation. The rise in COHb is also affected by the total body hemoglobin content. For a given rate of uptake of CO into the blood, anemic patients and those with reduced circulatory volumes (e.g., females and bleeding patients) will have a faster rise in COHb levels than large patients with high hemoglobin concentrations.

After absorbing into the blood, up to 15% of the CO will slowly diffuse into the tissues, where it is primarily bound to myoglobin and cytochrome oxidases. This intracellular binding is facilitated by conditions of hypoxia and hypotension. It can take several hours for equilibrium to be attained between the inhaled concentration and that in the blood and between the blood and the tissues. Removal of the victim from the elevated CO environment before equilibrium is established will limit the rise in COHb. Rapid elimination of COHb by early, vigorous treatment can help prevent the absorption of CO into the tissues and the resulting cellular toxicity.

CO is almost exclusively eliminated via the lungs. The rate of elimination varies with the partial pressure of oxygen (O_2) and minute ventilation (Fig. 63.1). The half-time of CO elimination when breathing room air ranges from 240 to 300 minutes. Breathing 100% O_2 reduces the half-time to 40 to 80 minutes. By raising the partial pressure of O_2 by two or three times, treatment with hyperbaric O_2 (HBO_2) reduces the half-time even further to 20 to 40 minutes. Although hyperventilation will accelerate the elimination of CO, the concomitant reduction in

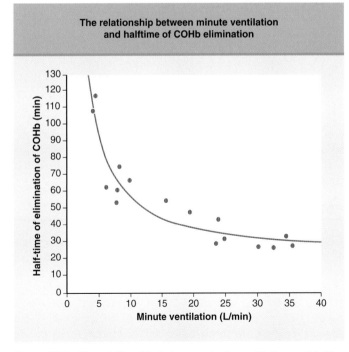

Figure 63.1. The relationship between minute ventilation and half-time of COHb elimination. (Adapted from Takeuchi A, Vesley A, Rucker J, et al: A simple "new" method to accelerate clearance of carbon monoxide. Am J Respir Crit Care Med 2000;161:1816–1819.)

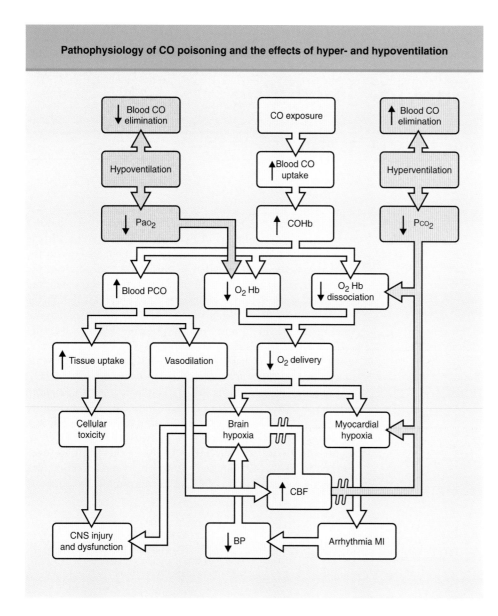

Pathophysiology of CO poisoning and the effects of hyper- and hypoventilation

Figure 63.2. Pathophysiology of CO poisoning and the effects of hyper- and hypoventilation. The multiple effects of CO poisoning ultimately result in CNS injury. $\frac{\perp}{\top}$ indicates an inhibitory effect.

the partial pressure of arterial carbon dioxide will reduce the blood flow to the brain and the heart. As such, hyperventilation without measures to prevent hypocapnia may be deleterious and is not recommended treatment for CO poisoning.

PATHOPHYSIOLOGY

CO has several pathophysiologic mechanisms; the importance of each remains unclear (Fig. 63.2). CO has long been known to bind tightly to hemoglobin with 240 times the affinity of oxygen. Not only does CO decrease blood O_2 content by preventing the binding of hemoglobin to O_2, but it also decreases oxygen delivery at the tissues by shifting the oxyhemoglobin dissociation curve to the left (Fig. 63.3). Hence, much of the cellular damage caused by CO is secondary to hypoxia. However, CO is also likely a direct cellular toxin. Intracellular CO can interfere with cellular respiration and when combined with hypotension can initiate a series of events resulting in

ischemia–reperfusion injury. Other postulated mechanisms of direct cellular toxicity include nitric oxide–mediated tissue injury, promotion of brain lipid peroxidation, hastening apoptosis, and interference with intracellular oxygen transport.

CLINICAL FEATURES

The symptoms of CO poisoning are nonspecific, frequently leading to misdiagnosis (Table 63.1). CO can affect multiple organ systems, but the central nervous system and cardiovascular system are the most severely affected due to their high oxygen requirements.

Central Nervous System Effects

Headache is the earliest and most common symptom of CO poisoning. Other common neurological symptoms include dizziness, lightheadedness, weakness, and confusion. Severely poisoned patients can have a decreased level of consciousness

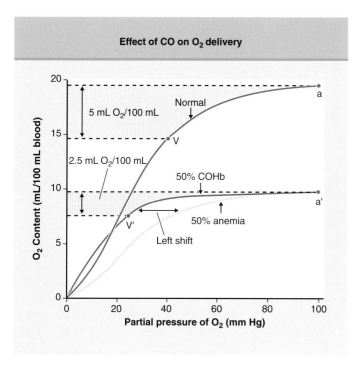

Figure 63.3. Effect of CO on O$_2$ delivery. The normal oxyhemoglobin dissociation curve and curves for 50% anemia and 50% carboxyhemoglobinemia are illustrated. The delivery of 5 mL/100 mL of blood delivered requires a decrease in the partial pressure of O$_2$ of approximately 60 mm Hg (from point a to point V on the normal curve). In the presence of 50% COHb, a delivery of only 2.5 mL/100 mL of blood delivered requires a decrease of 75 mm Hg (from point a' to point V'). (Modified from Bartlett RH, Allyn PA: Pulmonary Management of the burned patients. Heart Lung 1973;2(5):714–719.)

Table 63.1 Clinical Manifestations of CO Poisoning

Severity	Central Nervous System	Cardiovascular System	Other
Mild	Headache Dizziness		Nausea/vomiting
Moderate	Confusion Weakness Blurred vision Ataxia	Chest pain Tachycardia	Tachypnea Dyspnea Myonecrosis
Severe	Disorientation Seizures Coma Stroke	Palpitations Dysrhythmias Hypotension Myocardial ischemia	Pulmonary edema Renal failure

progressing to coma, seizures, and acute stroke. Brain computed tomography and magnetic resonance imaging of severely poisoned patients may reveal low density of the white matter and necrosis of the basal ganglia and cerebral gyri.

Cardiovascular Effects

Patients with CO poisoning may present with symptoms and electrocardiographic changes consistent with myocardial ischemia or infarction, especially if they have underlying coro-

nary artery disease. Cardiac troponin isoenzymes are often elevated even in the absence of electrocardiographic (ECG) changes. Supraventricular dysrhythmias and intraventricular conduction delay have also been observed. Early mortality in severely poisoned patients is often due to hypoxia-induced ventricular dysrhythmias.

Respiratory Effects

CO-induced hypoxia can result in a compensatory respiratory alkalosis that in severe cases is further fueled by the ventilatory response to lactic acidosis. Twenty percent to 30% of intubated CO-poisoned patients develop pulmonary edema. Presumably this is due to left ventricular failure because CO appears to have no direct pulmonary toxicity. Victims of smoke inhalation may develop airway compromise and/or acute lung injury independent of CO poisoning.

Renal Effects

Severely poisoned patients infrequently develop acute renal failure secondary to nontraumatic rhabdomyolysis. Although CO may have some direct toxicity to the renal tubules, nearly all reported cases of acute renal failure in CO poisoning have been accompanied by muscle necrosis.

Dermatologic Effects

Cutaneous blisters common in severe CO poisoning are likely secondary to pressure necrosis. The "classic" finding of "cherry-red skin" is a rare and usually postmortem observation likely due to the combination of CO-induced vasodilatation and tissue ischemia.

Delayed Neurologic Syndrome

Many patients with CO poisoning present with acute neurologic deficits; however, 1% to 10% of victims of CO poisoning will develop new neurologic symptoms after a lucid period of 2 to 40 days, described as delayed neurologic syndrome (DNS). These symptoms classically consist of mental deterioration (dementia, personality change, and appearance of primitive reflexes), urinary incontinence, and gait disturbance but can include a myriad of neurologic symptoms, such as parkinsonism, amnesia, mutism, psychosis, paralysis, tremor, peripheral neuropathy, and flaccid paralysis. The likelihood of DNS increases with severity of poisoning and the patient's age. Although up to 75% of patients with DNS will fully or partially recover, many victims of CO poisoning suffer permanent changes in personality, affect, and cognition.

DIAGNOSIS

CO poisoning is an often overlooked diagnosis because not only are the symptoms and signs nonspecific but also initial investigations can be misleading. Despite the decreased O$_2$ carrying capacity of CO-poisoned patients, pulse oximetry and arterial blood gasses will fail to reveal CO-induced hypoxia because the 660 and 940 nm diodes used in most pulse oximeters cannot differentiate COHb from oxyhemoglobin and the O$_2$ electrodes in blood gas analyzers respond only to the partial pressure of O$_2$ in plasma, which is often normal. The definitive diagnosis of CO poisoning can be made by measuring elevated levels of COHb in either arterial or venous blood with a CO oximeter. Normal

COHb levels are less than 3% (up to 10% in a recent smoker). The COHb level on presentation will depend on multiple factors related to the time course of exposure, rescue, and treatment and therefore may not correlate with the severity of symptoms. In some cases, the initial COHb level may even be normal and the diagnosis must be made on clinical grounds alone. Since cyanides can be produced during fires, victims of smoke inhalation should also be tested for cyanide poisoning.

TREATMENT

The prehospital management of CO poisoning is rapid removal of the patient from the CO environment and treatment with 100% O_2. Hyperoxia will both accelerate the elimination of CO and provide a modest increase in blood O_2 content. Since maximizing arterial PO_2 is crucial, we recommend that spontaneously breathing patients be treated with 100% O_2 via a tight-fitting self-inflating bag–valve–mask system. (Commonly available O_2 masks often provide far less than 100% O_2 because of obligatory entrainment of air from the side holes in the masks and because of leaks between the mask and the face.) If endotracheal intubation is indicated, then ventilation should continue with 100% O_2 while maintaining normocapnia. Intravenous access should be secured, and the patient should be monitored for dysrhythmias.

Upon arrival in the emergency room, vital signs, neurologic status cardiac rhythm, and urine output, should be monitored. Initial investigations should include an ECG, chest x-ray, complete blood count, electrolytes, blood glucose, creatinine, urinalysis including urine myoglobin, cardiac enzymes, creatinine kinase, arterial blood gas, and serial carboxyhemoglobin levels. Treatment should continue with 100% O_2 and supportive measures to maintain adequate blood pressure and urine output. Standard ACLS protocols should be followed for the treatment of serious dysrhythmias. Moderate acidemia can be tolerated since its effects on the oxyhemoglobin dissociation curve will improve O_2 unloading at the tissues. In contrast, even mild respiratory acidosis (i.e., $PCO_2 = 50$) may warrant mechanical ventilation to maximize oxygenation and accelerate COHb elimination. Given the deleterious effects of hyperglycemia on brain injury, euglycemia should be maintained with an insulin infusion if necessary. In cases of unintentional CO poisoning, it is important for the treating physician to ensure that the patient's cohabitants are alerted and evaluated.

Hyperbaric Oxygen

Hyperbaric oxygen therapy has long been considered standard therapy for CO poisoning. In addition to accelerating CO elimination, HBO_2 may also reverse some of the direct cellular toxicity of CO, such as lipid peroxidation. The major risks of HBO_2 are barotrauma and O_2 toxicity. The overall complication rate is approximately 2% or 3%. Although there has long been strong basic science research and numerous observational studies in support of HBO_2 therapy, only recently have large, well-designed randomized controlled trials investigated the efficacy of HBO_2 for CO poisoning.

Scheinkestel and colleagues (1999) randomized 191 CO-poisoned patients to be treated with either daily HBO_2 and intervening high-flow normobaric O_2 or only high-flow normobaric O_2 for 3 to 6 days. They found that patients treated with HBO_2

fared no better on neuropsychological tests following treatment or 1 month later. However, a high proportion (69%) of their patients had attempted suicide and half had ingested alcohol or drugs, which may have confounded their results. Furthermore, both the HBO_2 and the normobaric O_2 protocols did not conform to standard clinical practice, making it difficult to draw clinically relevant conclusions.

Weaver and associates (2002) randomized 152 acutely CO-poisoned patients to treatment with three sessions of either HBO_2 or normobaric O_2. At 6 weeks postpoisoning, cognitive sequelae were less frequent in the HBO_2 group (25 vs. 46%). However, patients randomized to normobaric O_2 in this study received only 4 to 10 hours of 100% O_2 compared to 3 days in Scheinkestel and colleagues's (1999) study, which may partially explain the difference in results.

Given the lack of consistency in the literature, it is not surprising that there are no universally accepted criteria for the treatment of CO poisoning with HBO_2 therapy. Based on expert opinion from senior members of the Undersea and Hyperbaric Medicine Society, patients with transient or persistent unconsciousness, neurologic or cardiovascular dysfunction, or severe acidosis should be treated with at least one session of HBO_2 at 2.5 to 3.0 atm if it can be provided within 24 hours of CO exposure. Patients with persistent neurologic symptoms can be considered for additional HBO_2 treatment. Regardless of whether a patient receives HBO_2, he or she should be treated with 6 to 12 hours of 100% normobaric O_2.

Many victims of CO poisoning are initially treated at hospitals without hyperbaric facilities, and often a decision must be made as to whether the patient should be transferred for HBO_2 treatment. Patients who are most likely to benefit from transport to a HBO_2 facility include those who can be transported a short distance by ground, will receive treatment within 6 hours of poisoning, and are at high risk for neurologic sequelae (i.e., history of neurologic dysfunction, cerebellar signs, loss of consciousness, and/or COHb > 25%).

Management of the CO-poisoned Pregnant Patient

CO poisoning poses significant risk to the fetus of a pregnant patient. Maternal CO poisoning (even minor exposures, without loss of consciousness) can result in fetal death, cerebral palsy, limb and cranial deformities, and a variety of mental disabilities. Animal studies in sheep have shown that fetal CO uptake is delayed for 2 or 3 hours. Nevertheless, extrication of the mother does not necessarily eliminate the risk to the fetus. Due to the greater affinity of fetal hemoglobin for CO compared to maternal hemoglobin, the fetus may continue to absorb CO from the maternal blood even as the maternal COHb is falling, and the fetus may eventually develop COHb levels exceeding maternal levels (Fig. 63.4).

Given the high toxicity of CO poisoning to the fetus, rapid treatment with HBO_2 therapy is generally recommended. It has been suggested that HBO_2 therapy may pose a risk of induction of labor or birth defects; however, several case series have demonstrated that HBO_2 therapy per se does not have significant adverse effects on the mother or fetus. Therefore, pregnant women who meet criteria should receive HBO_2 therapy, and since fetal COHb may rise significantly above maternal COHb, strong consideration should be given to treating even mildly poisoned, asymptomatic pregnant patients.

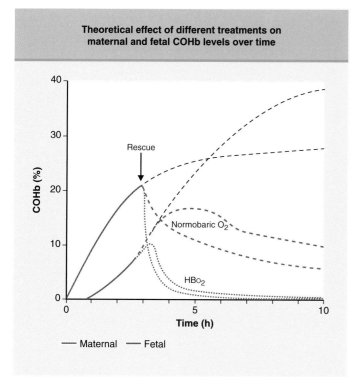

Theoretical effect of different treatments on maternal and fetal COHb levels over time

Rescue

Normobaric O$_2$

HBo$_2$

COHb (%)

Time (h)

—— Maternal —— Fetal

Figure 63.4. Theoretical effect of different treatments on maternal and fetal COHb levels over time. Although fetal CO uptake is delayed, fetal COHb levels will eventually far exceed maternal levels if the mother is not rescued from the CO environment. If the mother is rescued and treated with normobaric O$_2$, the prolonged CO elimination allows fetal levels to continue to rise; however, rapid elimination of CO with HBo$_2$ may prevent the delayed increase in fetal COHb. (Partially based on data from Longo LD: The biological effects of carbon monoxide on the pregnant woman, fetus, and newborn infant. Am J Obstet Gynecol 1977;129:69–103.)

SUGGESTED READING

Cobb N, Etzel RA: Unintentional carbon monoxide-related deaths in the United States, 1979 through 1988. JAMA 1991;266(5):659–663.

Elkharrat D, Raphael JC, Korach JM, et al: Acute carbon monoxide intoxication and hyperbaric oxygen in pregnancy. Intensive Care Med 1991;17:289–292.

Hampson NB: Emergency department visits for carbon monoxide poisoning in the Pacific Northwest. J Emerg Med 1998;16(5):695–698.

Hampson NB, Mathieu D, Piantadosi CA, et al: Carbon monoxide poisoning: Interpretation of randomized clinical trials and unresolved treatment issues. Undersea Hyper Med 2001;28(3):157–164.

Longo LD: The biological effects of carbon monoxide on the pregnant woman, fetus, and newborn infant. Am J Obstet Gynecol 1977; 129:69–103.

Scheinkestel CD, Bailey M, Myles PS, et al: Hyperbaric or normobaric oxygen for acute carbon monoxide poisoning: A randomized controlled clinical trial. Med J Aust 1999;170:203–210.

Thom SR, Weaver LK: Carbon monoxide poisoning. In Feldmeier J (ed): Hyperbaric Oxygen 2003: Indications and Results. Kensington, UK, Undersea and Hyperbaric Medical Society,2003, pp 11–17.

Tomaszewski C: Carbon monoxide. In Goldfrank L, Flomenbaum N, Lewin N, et al (eds): Goldfrank's Toxicologic Emergencies, 7th ed. New York, McGraw-Hill, 2002, pp 1478–1491.

Weaver LK, Hopkins RO, Chan KJ, et al: Hyperbaric oxygen for acute carbon monoxide poisoning. N Engl J Med 2002;347(14):1057–1067.

KEY POINTS

- No country is fully prepared to avert illness when large portions of the population are covertly exposed to a serious bioweapons agent; a moderate or large-scale intentional release of a serious pathogen will likely cause life-threatening illness in a large portion of exposed people.
- Intensivists will play a key role in the medical response to a bioterrorism event due to the clinical conditions caused by serious bioweapons pathogens, such as severe sepsis, septic shock, hypoxemic respiratory failure, and ventilatory failure.
- Compared with conventional disasters, bioterrorist attacks may not be readily recognized; thus, accurate clinical diagnoses and management on the basis of clinical suspicion are critical not only for appropriate care of individual patients but also for instituting an epidemiological investigation.
- Victims of a bioterrorist attack who require intensive care unit-level care may be more contagious than those who are less sick.
- Health care workers, accustomed to putting the welfare of patients ahead of their own in emergency situations, must be prepared for the proper use of personal protective equipment and trained in specific plans for the response to an infective or bioterrorism event.

INTRODUCTION

An intentional release of a biologic agent within a civilian population, exposing hundreds or thousands of people to a serious pathogen, is increasingly recognized as a plausible terrorism event. Unlike most mass casualty incidents, releases of bioweapons agents may be covert, thus providing additional security and public health challenges to the medical response beyond the generic burden of scores of casualties. An optimal medical response to a bioweapon attack will require all or most of the following: early diagnosis, rapid case finding, large-scale distribution of countermeasures for postexposure prophylaxis or early treatment, immediate isolation of contagious victims, and enhanced capacity for providing medical care to seriously and critically ill victims. No country is fully prepared to avert illness when thousands of people are covertly exposed to a serious bioweapons agent. Hence, after a moderate or large-scale intentional release of a serious pathogen, even one for which effec-

tive prophylactic countermeasures exist, a large portion of exposed people will likely develop life-threatening illness.

Although intensivists working in developed countries generally have little experience treating specific illnesses caused by serious bioweapon pathogens, these diseases result in clinical conditions that commonly require treatment in intensive care units (ICUs) (e.g., severe sepsis and septic shock, hypoxemic respiratory failure, and ventilatory failure). Therefore, intensivists will play a key role in the medical response to a bioterrorism event. Usual critical care practices will likely require modification for any event resulting in more than a few critically ill victims, and critical care specialists should participate in planning for such situations. Capabilities to provide medical care, especially critical care, services to large numbers of contagious patients are very limited in most countries. Local hospitals will be expected to care for seriously ill victims of a bioterrorist (BT) attack, and the ability to care for large numbers of critically ill patients will likely be a major determinant of the medical impact of such events.

Bioterrorism: Current Threat

Although the current risk of a large-scale BT event is uncertain, a number of groups throughout the world during past decades have deliberately exposed civilians to biologic agents. Fortunately, none of these prior events produced a large number of casualties because of the nonlethal nature of the pathogens released (e.g., *Salmonella typhimurium* in Oregon in 1984), the lack of technical expertise to successfully disseminate lethal pathogens (Aum Shinrikyo in Japan in 1994), or relatively limited exposure (the anthrax cases of 2001 in the United States). These limited exposures should not result in predictions of the numbers of potential casualties being reduced; rather, they simply reveal that an increasing number of groups throughout the world are willing to use biologic agents. The scope and effect of prior events could have been much greater if a contagious agent were used or if a lethal pathogen were widely disseminated. Despite the increased attention to biodefense, the risk of subsequent BT events may paradoxically be increasing. Rapid advancements in science are making synthetic and novel biologic agents more accessible and technologies to disseminate agents may no longer be restricted to only a few nations.

To reduce the medical effect of a BT event, the major determinants of morbidity and mortality must be understood (Fig. 64.1). The number of deaths from a BT event depends in part on the lethality and infectivity of the released agent, in addition to how effectively and widespread it is delivered. Many biologic agents could theoretically be used as weapons, but some are

Other Critical Care Problems

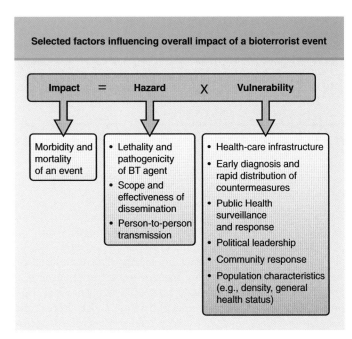

Selected factors influencing overall impact of a bioterrorist event

Impact = Hazard X Vulnerability

- Morbidity and mortality of an event

- Lethality and pathogenicity of BT agent
- Scope and effectiveness of dissemination
- Person-to-person transmission

- Health-care infrastructure
- Early diagnosis and rapid distribution of countermeasures
- Public Health surveillance and response
- Political leadership
- Community response
- Population characteristics (e.g., density, general health status)

Figure 64.1. Selected factors influencing the overall impact of a bioterrorist event.

Category	Definition	Agents
A	High-priority agents that can be easily disseminated or transmitted from person to person; result in high mortality rates and have the potential for major public health impact; require special action for public health preparedness	Anthrax Botulism Plague Smallpox Tularemia Viral hemorrhagic fevers
B	Second highest priority agents that are moderately easy to disseminate; result in moderate morbidity rates and low mortality rates	Brucellosis *Clostridium perfringens* epsilon toxin *Salmonella, Shigella, Escherichia coli* O157:H7 *Burkholderia* species Psittacosis Q fever Ricin toxin Staphylococcal enterotoxin B Typhus fever Viral encephalitis *Vibrio cholerae, Cryptosporidium parvum*
C	Third highest priority agents, including emerging pathogens that in the future could be engineered for mass dissemination secondary to availability, ease, or production and dissemination, and potential for high morbidity and mortality rates and major health impact	Emerging infectious diseases (e.g., Nipah virus and Hantavirus)

Table 64.1 Classification of Bioterrorist Agents[a]

[a]Data from www.cdc.gov (accessed October 25, 2004).

more lethal, more available, and more easily disseminated (Table 64.1). The agent's characteristics alone will not, however, determine the overall impact of the BT event. Population characteristics (i.e., vulnerabilities) will also affect the impact of a BT event (Fig. 64.1). Many agencies, professions, and community members must be involved in preparing and responding to a BT event. To optimally respond, hospital and public health cooperation, planning, and preparedness need to occur before the disaster.

The integration and coordination of all these responders is very important, and detailed operational descriptions are beyond the scope of this chapter (see Box 64.1). Instead, this chapter is intended to be an introduction to the medical response issues for a BT event, specifically the critical care medical response.

AGENTS OF BIOTERRORISM

The Centers for Disease Control and Prevention (CDC) has compiled a list of potential agents of bioterrorism and divided these into three categories, A–C (see Table 64.1). Category A agents are those believed to pose the greatest threat in terms of potential lethality, ability for widespread dissemination, ability for subsequent human-to-human transmission, and disruptive impact on the community and the public health system. These agents include *Variola major* (smallpox), *Bacillus anthracis* (anthrax), *Yersinia pestis* (plague), *Clostridium botulinum* (botulism), *Francisella tularensis* (tularemia), and viral hemorrhagic fevers (VHFs). This section provides a brief summary of the pathogenesis and diagnosis of each category A agent and also reviews current recommendations for treatment.

Anthrax

Bacillus anthracis is acquired from contact with infected animals or animal products and causes three forms of disease: cutaneous, inhalational, and gastrointestinal. Approximately

Box 64.1 Online Resources for Bioterrorism Information

www.acponline.org/bioterro
www.upmc-biosecurity.org
www.shea-online.org
www.cdc.gov

2000 cases of cutaneous anthrax occur annually worldwide. Inhalational anthrax has not occurred naturally within the United States since 1976; any case must therefore be considered a possible sentinel case of a bioterrorist event. Gastrointestinal anthrax is uncommon in developed countries and is not discussed here.

Cutaneous and inhalational anthrax are the forms expected following an aerosol release of spores, with the latter being the most lethal. A 1993 estimate by the U.S. Congressional Office of Technology Assessment predicted that an aerosolized release of 100 kg of "weaponized" anthrax over a populated city would cause 130,000 to 3 million deaths, similar to the mortality of a thermonuclear detonation. Inhalational anthrax results from spore particles 1 to 5 μm in diameter entering the alveolar spaces and being transported by macrophages to mediastinal lymph nodes. After an incubation period that ranges from 2 days to 7 weeks (median of 4 days during the 2001 cases and up to 60 days after the release of spores in Sverdlovsk in 1979), germination occurs, with the vegetative bacilli producing two toxins—lethal toxin and edema toxin. Initial symptoms of inhalational anthrax are nonspecific: fevers, chills, drenching sweats, nonproductive cough, dyspnea, nausea, vomiting, and fatigue. Hemorrhagic thoracic lymphadenitis and mediastinitis develop, and hemorrhagic pleural effusions with compressive atelactasis are common. Hemorrhagic meningitis may also occur. Patients may rapidly develop hemodynamic collapse, which typically has been refractory to treatment if it develops prior to antimicrobial administration.

Diagnosis is predicated on a high index of suspicion. In the 2001 attacks, all patients with inhalational anthrax had an abnormal chest radiograph or thoracic computed tomography scan. Mediastinal widening due to lymphadenopathy and large bilateral pleural effusions were the most common features (Figs. 64.2 and 64.3). These findings in the setting of a previously healthy patient with the abrupt development of sepsis should raise suspicion of anthrax infection. Sputum Gram stain and culture are rarely positive. Blood cultures may yield a diagnosis but require hours to days to grow the organism. As in many infections, blood cultures lose diagnostic utility if obtained after antibiotic administration. Hemorrhagic meningitis was common (50% of patients) during the Sverdlovsk incident but was only confirmed in 1 of 11 patients in 2001.

Patients suffering from inhalational anthrax are likely to require ICU care but do not require respiratory isolation. Antibiotics must be started as soon as possible without waiting for diagnostic confirmation. Treatment recommendations are summarized in Table 64.2. For adults, combination antimicrobial therapy with intravenous ciprofloxacin and one or two other agents is recommended. Given the potential for meningitis, agents with good central nervous system penetration, such as rifampin, penicillin, or chloramphenicol, are recommended. Clindamycin has been administered for the theoretical benefit of reducing toxin production by the vegetative bacilli, although

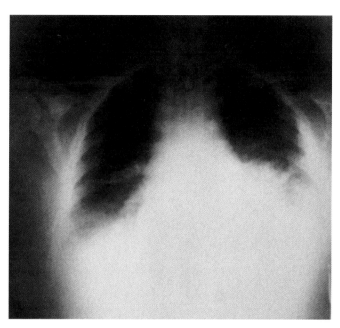

Figure 64.3. Chest radiograph of a patient with inhalational anthrax demonstrating bilateral pleural effusions. (Source: www.cdc.gov, Public Health Image Library, ID 1118.)

this has been done in too few instances to critically evaluate its effectiveness. A change to oral therapy is acceptable once the patient is stable. Therapy should continue for 60 days. The concomitant use of an anthrax vaccine in a modified dosing regimen (three doses within the first month) may be limited by availability. There is anecdotal evidence that drainage of pleural effusions carries some benefit. Whether the benefit is simply reduction of pleural fluid volume to improve oxygenation or actually helps to reduce toxin burden remains uncertain. During the 2001 outbreak, pleural drainage was accomplished via serial thoracenteses and tube thoracostomy. Optimal management may require tube thoracostomy due to the hemorrhagic nature of the fluid. Historically, inhalational anthrax had a mortality rate of approximately 90%. In the 2001 attacks, modern critical care interventions and use of multiple antimicrobial agents reduced mortality to 45%.

Cutaneous anthrax results after the inoculation of skin with anthrax spores. These patients are unlikely to require ICU-level care if they are treated promptly. Two exceptions are the possibilities of airway compromise due to a neck lesion with resulting edema or postoperative management of a compartment syndrome. Local edema is the first feature of the condition, with the subsequent appearance of a macule or papule that rapidly ulcerates and develops into a painless black eschar (Fig. 64.4). Systemic disease, including lymphadenopathy and lymphangitis, can follow. In the absence of antibiotic therapy, mortality has been reported to be as high as 20%; death is rare if adequate treatment is instituted.

Plague

Between 1347 and the early 1350s, *Y. pestis*, the causative agent of plague, swept through Europe, eventually killing 20 to 30 million people—one-third of the population. Plague continues to occur naturally as an insect-borne illness, infecting approxi-

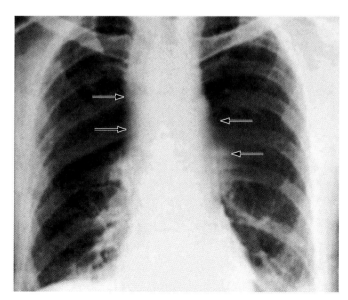

Figure 64.2. Chest radiograph of a patient with inhalational anthrax demonstrating mediastinal widening *(arrows)*. (Source: www.cdc.gov.)

Table 64.2 Specific Therapies for the Class A Bioterrorist Agents

Agent	Preferred Regimen	Alternate Regimen	Duration	Prophylactic Regimen
Anthrax				
Inhalational	Ciprofloxacin 400 mg IV q12 hr, or doxycycline 100 mg IV q12 hr, plus one or two of the following: clindamycin, rifampin, vancomycin, penicillin, ampicillin, chloramphenicol, imipenem, or clarithromycin	Same	60 Days	Ciprofloxacin 500 mg po q12 hr for 60 days, or doxycycline 100 mg po q12 hr for 60 days
Cutaneous	Ciprofloxacin 400 mg IV q12 hr, or doxycycline 100 mg IV q12 hr	Same	60 Days	Ciprofloxacin 500 mg po q12 hr for 60 days, or doxycycline 100 mg po q12 hr for 60 days
Plague	Streptomycin 1 g IM q12 hr, or gentamicin 5 mg/kg IV q day	Doxycycline 100 mg IV q12 hr, or ciprofloxacin 400 mg IV q12 hr	10 Days	Doxycycline 100 mg po q12 hr × 7 days, or ciprofloxacin 500 mg po q12 hr × 7 days
Tularemia	Streptomycin 1 g IM q12 hr, or gentamicin 5 mg/kg IV q day	Doxycycline 100 mg IV q12 hr, or ciprofloxacin 400 mg IV q12 hr	Streptomycin, gentamicin, or ciprofloxacin, 10 days; doxycycline, 14–21 days	Doxycycline 100 mg po q12 hr × 14 days, or ciprofloxacin 500 mg po q12 hr × 14 days
Botulism	Equine trivalent antitoxin	N/A	One dose	Equine antitoxin, if available
Smallpox	? Cidofovir		Uncertain	Vaccinia vaccine, within 4 days of exposure
Viral hemorrhagic fevers (unknown etiology or known to be caused by arenaviruses or bunyaviruses)	Ribavirin 30 mg/kg IV once, then 16 mg/kg IV q6 hr for 4 days; then 8 mg/kg IV q8 hr for 6 days	No therapy for filoviruses or flaviviruses	10 Days	None

Data from Inglesby TV, Dennis DT, Henderson DA, et al: Plague as a biological weapon. Medical and public health management. JAMA 2000;283:2281–2290; Inglesby TV, O'Toole T, Henderson DA, et al: Anthrax as a biological weapon, 2002. Updated recommendations for management. JAMA 2002;287:2236–2252; Dennis DT, Inglesby TV, Henderson DA, et al: Tularemia as a biological weapon. Medical and public health management. JAMA 2001;285:2763–2773; Arnon SS, Schechter R, Inglesby TV, et al: Botulinum toxin as a biological weapon: Medical and public health management. JAMA 2001;285:1059–1070; and Henderson DA, Inglesby TV, Bartlett JG, et al: Smallpox as a biological weapon: Medical and public health management. JAMA 1999;281:2127–2137.

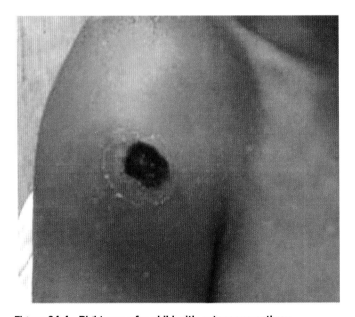

Figure 64.4. Right arm of a child with cutaneous anthrax demonstrating a painless black eschar. (Source: www.cdc.gov.)

mately 1700 people annually worldwide. In the United States, most cases occur in the rural states of the Southwest. Plague occurs in three forms: bubonic, septicemic, and pneumonic. Naturally occurring bubonic plague occurs when infected fleas bite a human and typically results in enlarged lymph nodes (bubo) and severe sepsis. A smaller percentage of patients may develop sepsis without bubo formation, and this is termed

primary septicemic plague. Rarely, patients with bubonic or septicemic plague develop pneumonia, and this is termed secondary pneumonic plague. Patients with pneumonic plague can transmit disease through respiratory droplets. Those who contract pneumonic plague from person-to-person transmission are considered to have primary pneumonic plague and do not develop buboes. Both primary and secondary pneumonic plague are transmissible from person to person.

The intentional release of aerosolized plague would result in primary pneumonic plague, a condition that is rare in naturally occurring plague. World Health Organization (WHO) estimates from 1970 predict that 50 kg of *Y. pestis* released over an urban area with 5 million inhabitants would cause pneumonic plague in 150,000, with 36,000 fatalities. Exposure is followed 1 to 6 days later by fever, dyspnea, and cough with bloody, watery, or purulent sputum. Gastrointestinal symptoms also occur. Cervical buboes are rare. Pneumonia progresses rapidly with unilateral or bilateral infiltrates or consolidation. Severe sepsis and septic shock develop with leukocytosis, multisystem organ failure, and disseminated intravascular coagulation. In the absence of therapy, irreversible shock and death occur 2 to 6 days after exposure. A bioterrorist attack with aerosolized plague would likely present as an outbreak of severe pneumonia and sepsis. Diagnosis depends on standard microbiologic studies, with confirmatory tests available only at select laboratories. Hence, unless epidemiologic clues alert health care workers that these patients do not have community-acquired pneumonia, the first group of patients will likely be cared for with the hospital's usual infection control policies for this condition. Unless droplet precautions are commonly used and strictly adhered to, a number of health care workers and additional patients may be exposed to plague early in the outbreak. Therapeutic recommendations for pneumonic plague appear in Table 64.2. Streptomycin and gentamicin are the first-line agents. Doxycycline, ciprofloxacin, and chloramphenicol are alternative choices. In the event of a mass casualty situation, or for postexposure prophylaxis, doxycycline or ciprofloxacin are the preferred agents for adults.

Tularemia

Francisella tularensis is an extremely infectious pathogen; exposure to as few as 10 organisms can cause tularemia. Naturally occurring throughout North America, Europe, and Asia, tularemia is transmitted to humans via arthropod bites, contact with small mammals or contaminated food, and inhalation. Tularemia can take many clinical forms (Box 64.2).

Disease manifestations depend on virulence, dose, and site of infection. The disease can begin in the skin, starting as a papule and resulting in an ulcer, and also involve regional lymph nodes (ulceroglandular). If contaminated water is ingested or contaminated droplets are inhaled, pharyngeal ulcers with cervical lymphadenitis can occur (oropharyngeal). The eyes can be the initial portal of entry leading to chemosis and lymphadenitis (oculoglandular). Sometimes, lymphadenitis may occur without ulceration (glandular).

Inhalational tularemia may also occur naturally due to aerosolization of contaminated materials. This clinical scenario is the most likely after an intentional release, since aerosol release would be the most likely method of dissemination. WHO estimated that 50 kg of aerosolized *F. tularensis* in a city of 5 million would affect 250,000 people and cause 19,000 deaths. After an incubation period of 1 to 21 days, abrupt fever develops, accompanied by influenza-like symptoms (headache, chills, rigors, myalgias, coryza, and pharyngitis). Bronchiolitis, pleuropneumonitis, and hilar lymphadenitis would be expected, although inhalational tularemia can often present as a systemic disease without respiratory features. Progressive weakness, fever, chills, malaise, and anorexia rapidly incapacitate victims. Hematogenous spread can lead to pleuropneumonia, sepsis, and meningitis. Sepsis due to tularemia may manifest as severe sepsis or septic shock. Mortality without antibiotic therapy can be as high as 30% to 60% for pneumonic and septic tularemia. Current antimicrobial therapy results in a mortality rate of less than 2%.

Rapid diagnostic testing for tularemia is not widely available. The constellation of atypical pneumonia, pleuritis, and hilar lymphadenopathy in association with the previously described symptoms should raise suspicion for tularemia. In the wake of a bioterrorist attack, until a number of patients present, initial diagnosis may be delayed. Most diagnoses are made serologically with a fourfold rise between acute and convalescent antibody

titers. Antibodies are slow to develop: Titers will usually be negative at 1 week, positive at 2 weeks, and peak in 4 to 8 weeks. Laboratories need to be specifically notified if tularemia is suspected, both to improve diagnostic accuracy and to protect laboratory workers. Polymerase chain reaction (PCR) and antigen detection are rapid and available at reference laboratories in the United States through the Laboratory Response Network. If the reference lab is alerted when specimens are sent, an answer can be given within hours.

Treatment recommendations for tularemia are presented in Table 64.2. In the event of a contained casualty situation, streptomycin is the preferred drug, with gentamicin as a first-line alternate. Doxycycline, chloramphenicol, and ciprofloxacin are acceptable alternates. For mass casualties and for postexposure prophylaxis, oral doxycycline and ciprofloxacin are the recommended agents. Treatment with aminoglycosides or fluoroquinolones should last 10 days; tetracyclines and chloramphenicol require a 14-day course.

Botulism

Botulinum toxin, produced by the bacteria C. *botulinum* and a few other *Clostridium* species, is the most potent known neurotoxin. Botulinum toxin inactivates proteins necessary for the release of acetylcholine into the neuromuscular junction. The toxin could be disseminated as an aerosolized agent or as a food contaminant.

Fewer than 200 naturally occurring cases of botulism occur annually in the United States. The use of botulinum toxin by terrorists would result in inhalational botulism or foodborne botulism, depending on the mode of dispersal. The neurologic signs are identical regardless of whether the toxin enters the body via the lungs or the digestive tract. Intestinal botulism may be preceded by gastrointestinal complaints. Symptoms appear approximately 12 to 72 hours after exposure.

Botulism presents as an acute, symmetric, descending flaccid paralysis. There is no associated fever, and the bulbar musculature is always affected first. Presenting complaints and findings are related to cranial nerve palsies and include diplopia, dysarthria, dysphonia, and dysphagia. Hypotonia and generalized weakness ensue. Loss of airway protection may necessitate intubation, and respiratory muscle paralysis may require mechanical ventilation. The course is variable and may require months of mechanical ventilation. During small outbreaks with sufficient medical resources, serial measurement of vital capacity can help identify patients with respiratory muscle weakness. Elevation of $PaCO_2$ is a late finding, and positive pressure ventilation should be instituted prior to frank ventilatory failure. Notably, cognitive function is not affected; patients are completely awake and alert. A fever should raise suspicion of secondary infection or an alternative diagnosis.

The diagnosis of botulinum intoxication is clinical and is classically described as the triad of symmetric cranial neuropathies with descending paralysis, clear sensorium, and lack of fever. Other diagnoses to consider are listed in Box 64.3.

In developed nations, the occurrence of a number of temporally related cases of acute paralysis points to botulinum intoxication. The edrophonium or "Tensilon" test may be transiently positive in botulism, although it still may be helpful in distinguishing it from myasthenia gravis. CSF is generally normal in botulism. An electromyogram demonstrating an incremental

Box 64.2 Forms of Tularemia
Glandular
Ulceroglandular
Oculoglandular
Oropharyngeal
Pneumonic
Septic

Box 64.3 Differential Diagnosis of Descending Paralysis

Miller–Fisher variant of Guillan–Barré syndrome
Myasthenia gravis
Tick paralysis
Atropine poisoning
Paralytic shellfish/puffer fish poisoning

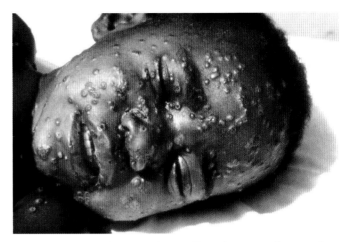

Figure 64.5. Face of a child with smallpox demonstrating pustular vesicles with uniform stage of development. (Source: www.cdc.gov, Public Health Image Library, ID #3.)

response with repetitive stimulation at 50 Hz may suggest botulism when the conduction velocity and sensory nerves are normal. Culture of stool or gastric contents (for foodborne exposure) may yield *Clostridium*. Confirmation usually requires the mouse bioassay (mice are exposed to samples and those given polyvalent and specific antitoxin survive) but takes several days. Samples for the mouse bioassay must be collected prior to the patient's receiving antitoxin. A clinician who suspects botulism must immediately notify local public health authorities to aid with epidemiologic and diagnostic investigations. Most laboratory testing cannot be performed at hospitals. Laboratories must be notified of suspicion regarding botulism, since samples can be potentially harmful to laboratory personnel.

Specific therapy consists of treatment with equine antitoxin (see Table 64.2), which will not reverse extant paralysis but may prevent progression. It must therefore be administered as early as possible. In mass casualty situations, when the antitoxin supply may be limited, patients with weakness but not yet requiring mechanical ventilation may be the most appropriate for antitoxin therapy. Supportive therapy is essential, with a specific focus on mechanical ventilation and efforts to prevent complicating events (e.g., ventilator-associated pneumonia, venous thromboembolism, and decubitus ulcers). Nonventilated patients should be placed in the reverse Trendelenberg position at 20 to 25 degrees to optimize respiratory muscle function and minimize the possibility of aspiration Aminoglycosides and clindamycin should be avoided because of the potential for exacerbating the neuromuscular blockade. Mortality for foodborne botulism averages 6%.

Smallpox

The last naturally occurring case of smallpox was identified in 1977, and the last case (due to a laboratory accident) was in 1978. Despite worldwide eradication, smallpox continues to concern biodefense experts due to uncertainties about available stocks of the virus. Despite the mortality rate of smallpox (30%) being considerably lower than those of other bioweapons agents, its potential for harm is still very high because those who survive may be severely deformed or blinded and no proven specific therapy exists once exposed people become symptomatic. In addition, with cessation of worldwide vaccination, entire populations and especially younger persons are susceptible to infection. The agent of smallpox, the *Variola* virus, belongs to the orthopoxvirus family. These viruses are quite stable in the environment, and hence an aerosol may be widely dispersed. Any case of smallpox would be an emergency and must be considered to be the result of a deliberate act.

The typical incubation period for smallpox is 7 to 17 days, with an average of 12 to 14 days for the majority of patients. Initial symptoms include fever, rigors, backache, and headache.

Vomiting and delirium may develop in this prodromal phase. Two or 3 days later, a nonspecific erythematous rash begins. The rash first appears in the mouth and throat, with red spots appearing on the buccal and pharyngeal surfaces. The usual dictum is that a person is not contagious until the rash begins. In most patients, the macular lesions become papular followed by vesicles. The lesions then become pustular, which umbilicate and are deeply seated in the dermis. The crops of lesions appear at the same time and are all at the same stage on the affected part of the body (Fig. 64.5). They usually begin and are more concentrated on the face and limbs rather than the trunk. This is in contrast to primary varicella, in which lesions on any given part of the body are in different stages of development (some macular, some vesicular, and some crusting) and in which the rash begins on the trunk and moves outward. After 8 to 10 days, scabs form at the sites of the pustules. In survivors, these become depressed depigmented scars. Smallpox lesions also occur on the palms and soles, which rarely occurs with chickenpox.

The previous description is seen in more than 90% of smallpox cases, but there are less common forms of smallpox as well. Hemorrhagic smallpox is uniformly fatal (it tends to affect pregnant women more frequently), and it typically has a shorter incubation period and does not lead to the classic rash. Instead, death follows development of a hemorrhagic rash. In the malignant or flat form of smallpox, the disease begins classically but does not progress to pustules. Instead, the rash is confluent and may desquamate. Also, *Variola minor* is a less severe form of smallpox.

Suspicion of smallpox must initially be based on clinical findings; the possibility of this disease must be considered in any patient displaying fever and a characteristic centrifugal and uniform rash. Definitive diagnosis requires specialized diagnostic techniques. Electron microscopy can determine whether the virus is an orthopox, and confirmatory PCR techniques require primers specific to *Variola*. Laboratory confirmation will likely be required for the sentinel cases of an outbreak. After initial cases are confirmed, additional case identification can be based on clinically consistent criteria.

If an exposure to smallpox is suspected but the patient is asymptomatic, administration of the *Vaccinia* virus within a few days from exposure can prevent or greatly diminish the severity of the illness. Once the disease develops, however, specific therapeutic options are limited (see Table 64.2). There is evidence that cidofovir may have activity against the *Variola* virus, although the evidence is based on alternative orthopox disease models and in vitro assays. Supportive care for critically ill patients may limit mortality, but since the last case occurred more than 25 years ago, it is uncertain what effect modern critical care will have on outcomes. Mortality is expected to be approximately 30%, with far greater rates of disfigurement or disability. Secondary transmission is most likely to occur through close contact with symptomatic patients (e.g., droplet and contact transmission), although fomite and airborne transmission have been documented. Patients with a cough may be more likely to transmit droplet nuclei (i.e., airborne transmission), and those with atypical disease courses (e.g., hemorrhagic and malignant) may be more difficult to identify, so unprotected exposure of health care workers may be more likely.

Viral Hemorrhagic Fevers

The viral hemorrhagic fevers believed to be possible agents of BT are listed in Box 64.4. The filoviruses and arenaviruses are transmissible from person to person. Although the limited information available suggests that transmission is primarily via infected body fluids, mucosal transmission has been documented in experimental animals and airborne or droplet transmission has been suggested in several outbreaks.

Clinical manifestations will vary with the particular virus. In general, the VHFs have an incubation period ranging from 2 to 21 days (commonly, 5–10 days). Initial symptoms are nonspecific and may last up to 1 week. Fever, malaise, headache, myalgias, arthralgias, nausea, and gastrointestinal complaints are prominent. A rash may be present. On exam, patients are typically febrile, relatively bradycardic, hypotensive, and tachypnic. As the disease progresses, hemorrhagic manifestations, such as petechiae, mucosal bleeding, hematuria, hematemesis, and melena, may appear. Eventually, disseminated intravascular coagulation, multiorgan system failure, and shock may develop. Mortality rates vary greatly, but in the case of Ebola virus they may be as high as 90%.

Confirmatory diagnosis of VHFs must be made at specialized laboratories. The diagnosis must be suspected in any patient presenting with acute fever, severe illness, and hemorrhagic manifestations. Any patient who presents with a VHF who does not have a travel, contact, or exposure history consistent with the known natural occurrence of these illnesses must be considered as the possible victim of a BT attack.

Unfortunately, VHFs have a high lethality and supportive therapy is the only treatment (see Table 64.2). There is evidence that ribavirin may have some effect against Arenaviridae and Bunyaviridae. No therapies have been shown to be effective against the filoviruses or flaviviruses. Additionally, there is no recommended agent or vaccine for postexposure prophylaxis to any of the VHFs.

CHALLENGES FOR THE MEDICAL RESPONSE TO BIOTERRORISM

Many of the operational functions for the response to bioterrorism events are similar to those for other disasters (intentional or natural), such as requiring coordination and communication among a number of government agencies, professions, citizens, and community stakeholders for the response. However, bioterrorism events pose specific challenges for the medical response that may be serious enough that if not addressed may shut down hospitals and leave many victims without adequate options for health care (Table 64.3).

Recognizing that a conventional disaster has occurred is usually immediate, and these events are limited both geographically and temporally. Casualties have traumatic injuries, and a large portion of the survivors are taken to the nearest health care facility. Within hours to a few days, the number of expected casualties is usually known. Immediate death rates may be high, especially with structural collapse, but typically only a small

---

Box 64.4 Viral Hemorrhagic Fevers
Filoviridae (Ebola, Marburg)
Arenaviridae (Lassa fever, New World arenaviruses)
Bunyaviridae (Rift Valley fever)
Flaviviridae (yellow fever, Omsk hemorrhagic fever, Kyasanur Forest disease)

Table 64.3 Comparisons of Common Characteristics of Conventional Disasters and Anticipated Characteristics of a Bioweapons Attack on Civilians

Characteristic	Conventional Disaster[a]	Bioterror Attack
Recognition that event has occurred	Usually immediate	May be delayed due to covert release
Time from event to victims' seeking medical care	Minutes to hours	May be days or longer
Number of victims who survive until initial medical evaluation	May be large, but most not critically ill (proportion of critically ill may be higher in confined space explosions)	May be very large, and for some pathogens the proportion of critically ill victims may be high
Affected geographic area and time to recovery	Usually geographically and temporally limited	May involve large regions and victims may continue to present for weeks to months or longer after the first case is recognized
Situational awareness of number of victims and scope of exposure	Minutes to hours	May be delayed by days or longer
Medical staff for response	Initially may be limited but usually remedied quickly	Likely to be limited if person-to-person transmission

[a]Characteristics for conventional disasters refer to events involving conventional explosives.

fraction of survivors are critically ill (injury severity score > 15). Enclosed space explosions may lead to higher proportions of survivors with critical injuries, but the absolute number of critically ill patients is usually less than 100. After the initial chaotic response period, medical staff and equipment are usually not in short supply. If local hospitals are overwhelmed, additional staff and resources can be transported to the disaster area, or patients can be evacuated to unaffected areas. The recovery plans for the affected health care facilities are usually initiated within the same day or a few days following a conventional disaster.

Unlike conventional disasters, a release of a bioweapons agent may go undetected. In such situations, exposed people would present for medical care after the incubation period has passed. Since people travel extensively in developed countries, and most incubation periods are days to weeks, patients are likely to present to a number of hospitals rather than to the facility located closest to the release. Having patients distributed to a number of hospitals may lead to delayed recognition that a BT event has occurred. In addition, most diseases resulting from serious bioweapons agents initially cause symptoms and signs that are commonly seen every day in hospital emergency departments and outpatient clinics. There may be no pathognomonic signs that a bioterrorist event occurred in the sentinel patients initially presenting with respiratory failure or hemodynamic collapse. No diagnostic tests are available to help clinicians rapidly diagnose most diseases, so a BT event may go unnoticed until scores of ill victims arrive at hospitals.

The presentation of multiple previously healthy patients with unusual and severe symptoms should prompt suspicion. Because of the specialized diagnostic techniques required for these organisms, and the biosafety precautions that are frequently beyond the capabilities of most hospital-based clinical laboratories, confirmatory diagnostic testing for the category A agents in the United States is handled at laboratories of the National Laboratory Response Network, which includes local and state labs as well as federal facilities, such as the U.S. Army Medical Research Institute of Infectious Diseases and the CDC. There will necessarily be a delay in final diagnosis because samples for confirmatory testing must be sent to off-site laboratories. This increases the importance of accurate clinical diagnoses and proceeding with management on the basis of clinical suspicion. Prompt diagnosis is critical not only for appropriate care of individual patients but also for instituting an epidemiological investigation. The community or nationwide response hinges on the results of this rapid investigation. Once the source, agent, and location of a BT attack have been deduced, other clinicians can be notified, resources can be mobilized, and the at-risk population can receive postexposure prophylaxis.

The difficulties of recognizing initial exposures to a BT attack have profound implications for hospital functionality, particularly if the pathogen is contagious. Health care workers (HCWs) and other patients without adequate infection control protections may be exposed to contagious patients. During an outbreak of severe acute respiratory syndrome (SARS), unprotected exposure of HCWs and hospitalized patients to patients with SARS was thought to be the major risk to a hospital remaining open.

Most victims of serious bioweapons attacks (e.g., anthrax, plague, smallpox, botulism toxin, tularemia, and VHFs) will develop illness that is rapidly progressive (ultimately requiring

mechanical ventilation, hemodynamic support, or other aggressive therapeutic interventions) if they do not receive early medical intervention or if no disease-specific medical countermeasures exist. These critically ill patients will also likely require extended critical care for survival. Few hospitals can provide even usual critical care services for an additional 100 critically ill BT victims, especially if the pathogen is contagious.

In the aftermath of a BT event, it may be very difficult to ascertain the extent of the exposure. Incubation periods have a range, so the first cases may simply represent the tails of the Gaussian distribution, and many more patients may require care in the following days. Some ill patients may go unrecognized as cases, and patients may arrive at hospitals in a larger geographical area than is typical after a conventional disaster. The initially affected area may be quickly overwhelmed because of shortages of critical care resources. The unaffected regions may choose to wait to offer help until the size of the event becomes better delineated so that they do not send staff and resources away until they are certain they were unaffected. Furthermore, if the pathogen is contagious, resources in affected areas may be more rapidly overwhelmed and unaffected regions may be even less likely to provide help.

BT attacks resulting in a disproportion of critically ill victims to available ICU beds are plausible. If such an event occurred today, many critically ill patients would have to forgo potentially life-sustaining critical care interventions. Hospitals can plan to give traditional standards of critical care to the few who are fortunate to arrive early during the event, or they can modify critical care so that more patients have access to some of the most important critical care interventions (e.g., mechanical ventilation). Methods to decide who should get critical care (e.g., triage algorithms), what critical care interventions should be provided, who should provide critical care, and where critical care should be provided need to be addressed before a BT event. Through such planning, hospitals may "gracefully degrade" services rather than ceasing to function when overwhelmed.

MANAGEMENT OF BIOTERRORISM AGENTS IN THE ICU

Disease-Specific Therapies

All efforts must be made to provide disease-specific therapies to victims of bioterrorism. Unfortunately, not all of the serious bioweapons agents have effective treatments, and for those with treatments there is concern about development of antimicrobial-resistant strains. Systems must be in place for testing new treatments during an outbreak so that effective treatments can be rapidly communicated to other clinicians and ineffective or harmful treatments can be rapidly withdrawn. Methodological issues, ethical concerns, skeleton protocol development, and information technology systems capable of making data rapidly available for analysis should all be developed and made functional before a disaster.

Supportive Critical Care

Patients seriously ill due to a bioweapons agent, regardless of whether a specific therapy exists, will likely require extensive supportive care, including interventions traditionally provided in ICUs. For small-scale events with few critically ill patients, traditional ICU care will likely be provided. For larger events, deci-

Box 64.5 Transmissible Bioweapons Agents
Smallpox
Viral hemorrhagic fevers
Pneumonic plague
Cutaneous anthrax

sions regarding which supportive care practices to continue and which to forgo will depend on the number of patients relative to the available resources. Supportive care that is deemed most important can be better maintained if advanced planning and preparedness are undertaken. ICU physicians should alert their hospitals to the potential need for rapid acquisition of additional mechanical ventilators, noninvasive respiratory aids, oxygen, palliative medications, and specialized staff in the event of a BT attack.

Infection Control

Perhaps the most critical aspect of caring for victims of a biologic attack or an emerging infective disease in an ICU is the prevention of secondary transmission. In the SARS outbreak of 2003, 77% of cases in Canada resulted from in-hospital exposure. In Taiwan, the percentage of hospital-acquired cases was 94%. These data include other patients in the hospital who contracted the disease as well as health care workers who suffered occupational exposures. Category A biologic agents that are transmissible from person to person are listed in Box 64.5.

Effective infection control measures are paramount in preventing the spread of disease through the hospital and, by extension, into the community. Infection control is particularly important in the ICU, in which a "perfect storm" for the rapid spread of an infection exists. Victims of a bioterrorist attack who require ICU-level care may be more contagious than those who are less sick due to higher levels of viremia or bacteremia. Invasive procedures with their attendant risks of splashing or aerosolization of blood, respiratory secretions, or other bodily fluids are more commonly performed on critically ill patients. Staff members in an ICU are often called on to rapidly complete a number of tasks in stressful conditions, a situation conducive to errors in infection-control practices. Since critically ill patients require a high level of frequent care, cumulative exposure to staff may be higher than in other areas of the hospital. Finally, other patients in the ICU are immunocompromised by virtue of their own critical illnesses, notwithstanding the disproportionate number of ICU patients who are immunosuppressed secondary to organ transplantation, oncologic conditions, or infection with the human immunodeficiency virus (HIV).

Decontamination of Patients

One of the mainstays of management of a chemical incident is rapid and effective decontamination of victims. Decontamination serves both to limit the total dose of chemical agent received by the victims and to protect health care workers from remnant chemicals on patient skin or clothing. Patients will not present for medical care after release of a biologic agent until the incubation period passes. Decontamination is not necessary for these patients, since they are not likely to be grossly conta-

minated at the time of presentation. For an overt attack, if the patient is grossly contaminated and there is concern about secondary aerosolization, it becomes reasonable to decontaminate the patient. Since T2 mycotoxin can be transdermally absorbed, decontamination of patients grossly contaminated with this agent is also warranted.

Isolation

If possible, symptomatic victims of a communicable bioterrorism agent should be placed in a private room to prevent exposure to other patients. In the case of smallpox or a viral hemorrhagic fever, rooms should be under negative pressure and equipped with high-efficiency particulate air (HEPA) filtration. The exhaust air from these rooms should be expelled directly to the outside, and the ventilation system should not be shared with other areas of the hospital. Documented cases of smallpox transmission have occurred through ventilation systems. Although the number of airborne infection isolation (AII) rooms in most hospitals is few, there are engineering modifications to increase modified AII capacity during an outbreak. Planning for these modifications before an event is critical.

Assuming a large outbreak of disease, patients should be grouped together not only with respect to location but also with respect to nursing staff, physicians, and equipment. If no diagnostic test exists, care must be taken to minimize exposure of uninfected patients with similar signs or symptoms who may be inadvertently housed in the same location.

Although friends and family undoubtedly bring much comfort and support to critically ill patients, in the face of an infectious disease they become both potential victims and potential vectors. Visitors of victims of bioterrorism with contagious agents, or victims of an emerging infectious disease, must be kept to an absolute minimum. They must be instructed and supervised in the use of proper protective equipment and notified that they must seek treatment immediately if they develop symptoms. In extreme circumstances, it may be necessary to completely preclude friends and family from visiting patients.

Health care providers are accustomed to putting the welfare of the patient ahead of their own; patient care, particularly in emergency situations, is often carried out without adequate protective equipment. This cannot be allowed in the case of extremely contagious agents, even in an emergency or "code" situation. A health care provider who has contact with a patient without suitable protective gear risks not only his or her own health but also the health of other patients, coworkers, visitors, and their own families. Individual patient care issues must be secondary to adequate infection control practices, lest an epidemic of smallpox, SARS, plague, or viral hemorrhagic fever spread unchecked.

Precautions

The CDC has developed categories of precaution that are to be applied to patients with potentially communicable diseases (Box 64.6). These categories have been described at length elsewhere but are summarized in the following sections, along with their applicability to the category A biological agents.

Standard

Standard precautions should be applied to all patients and include measures designed to prevent transmission of blood-

Box 64.6 Exposure Precaution Categories
Standard
Contact
Droplet
Airborne

borne illnesses such as HIV and hepatitis B/C. Most interactions with patients do not require any protective equipment, but gloves, gown, and face shield should be used for any activity that could potentially result in an exposure to blood or bodily fluids. Of the category A agents, anthrax, tularemia, and botulinum toxin require only standard precautions because these diseases are not transmissible from person to person. Cutaneous anthrax should perhaps be treated with contact precautions because transmission has been suggested following contact with the lesions of this type of anthrax.

Contact
Contact precautions are applicable to diseases that can be spread by touching the patient directly or indirectly by coming into contact with contaminated objects. Common examples include scabies, herpes, *Clostridium difficile*, and methicillin-resistant *Staphylococcus aureus*. Contact precautions must be used, if applicable, during all patient interactions, regardless of whether body fluid contact is expected. Protective equipment consists of gloves and gown, and a face shield is mandatory if splashing or spraying of body fluids is possible. Patients with smallpox and VHFs must be placed in contact precautions. Patient care equipment must also be dedicated to these patients and not used on patients not suffering from these diseases.

Droplet
Droplet precautions apply to diseases that are transmissible by large-particle droplets, defined as those greater than 5 μm. Due to the size of the droplets, transmission is highest over short distances (<1 m) and does not occur through ventilation systems. Necessary equipment includes a face shield or surgical mask with eye protection, gown, and gloves. Pneumonic plague requires droplet precautions.

Airborne
Airborne precautions are required for diseases that are spread via droplet nuclei, which are less than 5 μm. Tuberculosis is the most familiar of airborne infectious agents, but of the category A agents, both smallpox and VHFs fit into this category. Droplet nuclei may travel through ventilation systems, underscoring the importance of placing patients with these diseases in negative-pressure rooms with HEPA filters and exhaust of air to the outside. Required equipment includes gown, gloves, and adequate respiratory protection. Either an N95 respirator (specifications are described elsewhere) with eye protection or a powered air purifying respirator (PAPR) is acceptable.

Ventilator Expiratory Circuits
A misconception exists that once a patient is intubated and mechanically ventilated, both large droplets and droplet nuclei are no longer expelled into the air. This is true only if the ventilator expiratory circuit is fitted with a filter that meets HEPA guidelines. Unfortunately, many of the filters and heat/moisture exchanging filters commonly used do not meet HEPA criteria. This poses dangers to health care personnel, visitors, and other patients not only for bioterrorist agents but also for tuberculosis, SARS, and other emerging infections. Hospitals would be well advised to stockpile HEPA-grade filters for ventilator expiratory circuits.

Hand Washing
Correct hand washing is an essential component of hospital infection control in all circumstances. This is perhaps even more true in the circumstances of an outbreak of an emerging infectious disease or possible agent of bioterrorism. Hands must be washed after each patient contact even when protective gloves are used because a surprisingly high percentage of protective gloves contain microscopic holes, and holes may develop during the activities of routine patient care. Failure to thoroughly wash hands following patient contact places other patients and health care workers at risk. There has been an increase in the use of waterless alcohol rubs in ICUs rather than soap and water. Although these gels are generally effective against bacteria and viruses, they have been shown to be ineffective against bacterial spores such as anthrax. Soap and water, antimicrobial or not, are effective at removing anthrax spores from hands. Accordingly, we recommend the use of antimicrobial soap and water for the washing of hands after patient contact.

Prophylactic Vaccination or Treatment
Complete recommendations for postexposure prophylaxis are given in Table 64.1. In the case of anthrax and tularemia, postexposure prophylaxis with vaccination has not been proven effective. There is no need for prophylactic antibiotic therapy for health care workers unless they were potentially exposed in the initial attack. Vaccination does not confer protection against pneumonic plague. Health care workers caring for patients with pneumonic plague should, however, receive prophylaxis with 7 days of oral doxycycline. If symptoms such as fever develop, they should be aggressively treated with parenteral antibiotics.

Health care workers caring for patients with smallpox should be vaccinated as soon as possible because vaccination within 4 days of exposure can prevent or limit the severity of subsequent illness. Immediate isolation must follow the development of fever after exposure to smallpox. No postexposure prophylaxis exists for VHFs.

Environmental Decontamination
Although decontamination of victims of a biological attack is rarely necessary, the rooms in which they are treated can become contaminated with infectious organisms, particularly if sprays of bodily fluids or respiratory aerosols are produced. Virions of smallpox, in particular, can persist in linens for extended periods of time; documented cases exist in which laundry workers contracted smallpox from handling contaminated bedding and clothing. The causal agents of VHFs may also be transmitted via contaminated linens. Commercial hospital disinfectants and household bleach at a 1:10 dilution are effective at eliminating surface contamination with anthrax, smallpox, Ebola and Marburg viruses, tularemia, and plague. Linens from infected patients should be incinerated, autoclaved, or

washed with bleach. Contamination from SARS should also be handled in this manner.

Handling of Cadavers

The bodies of deceased patients with smallpox, plague, or VHFs continue to pose an infectious risk. Autopsies or postmortem examinations should be avoided if possible. The bodies of victims of smallpox should be cremated. People who have died of a VHF should preferably be cremated, although prompt burial without embalmment is a secondary option.

Personal Protective Equipment

Proper use of personal protective equipment is essential in order to protect staff from infectious disease. The equipment required depends on the particular disease, as described previously. Effort must be made to ensure that adequate supplies of equipment exist, and requirements will likely be far greater than expected. Calculations estimating the amount of equipment necessary for one nurse caring for four patients with a communicable disease are striking and sobering. During an 8-hour shift, one nurse would likely require 64 sets of personal protective equipment: 64 pairs of gloves; 64 gowns; 64 surgical masks, N95 masks, or PAPR hoods; and 64 face shields. Providing for the needs of physicians, respiratory therapists, and other ancillary personnel increases this equipment need markedly.

Beyond the availability of adequate stocks of equipment, health care workers must be adequately trained in their uses. N95 respirators require fit testing annually. The equipment must be used as designed, including donning and removing it correctly. Removing equipment in the proper order is particularly important: The gloves must be removed first to avoid contamination of the face or clothing when removing the gown, mask, and eye shield. Unfortunately, this correct sequence is not widely appreciated by health care workers.

Hospital and ICU-Specific Preparedness: A Broadly Applicable Paradigm

Given the complexity of caring for victims of a BT attack or an emerging infectious disease, early planning for such an incident must be carried out at the institutional and ICU levels. How will a hospital, or an ICU, care for a potentially massive influx of patients with communicable disease or specific requirements? Plans will differ in their specifics depending on each hospital and each ICU's architecture and capabilities. General principles include the following: Patients should be grouped according to infection, not necessarily by need. These patients should then be isolated from the remaining hospital population and staff. Dedicated physicians, nurses, ancillary personnel, and equipment should be used so as to prevent exposure to other patients and keep the numbers of exposed health care workers to a minimum.

The scale of a bioterrorist attack could potentially be enormous. As described previously, many of the category A agents could produce the same lethality as a nuclear explosion. The number of casualties could rapidly overwhelm any one hospital or even all of the hospitals in a community.

Staff safety must be paramount; if staff members believe themselves to be at risk, large numbers of nurses, physicians, and others may not show up to work, crippling or even forcing the closure of a hospital. Although all risk cannot be avoided, all possible provisions must be made. All staff members must be trained in the proper use of personal protective equipment. Beyond that, training should be provided in specific plans for the response to an infective or BT incident. Physicians and nurses in particular should be educated with regard to possible agents of BT and presented with disease-specific issues. Contingency plans must be made in advance for postexposure prophylaxis, either with antibiotics or vaccinations, as indicated. Given the critical and limited time windows to initiate effective prophylaxis, plans for distribution of medication or vaccine must be thought through in advance and not made in an ad hoc manner.

A large-scale bioterrorist incident could rapidly exhaust the resources of individual hospitals or even whole communities in a number of respects. The demand for personal protective equipment will be enormous. Beyond that, there will be a need for pharmaceuticals of all types. Antibiotics will be essential, but so will medications regularly employed in the ICU setting: vasopressors, sedatives, narcotics, and others. Mechanical ventilators may be at a premium for patients with acute respiratory distress syndrome, pneumonia, or ventilatory failure secondary to botulism. Although in the United States, and likely in other countries, the federal government has assembled stockpiles of antibiotics, smallpox vaccine, and mechanical ventilators, it will take time for these to be deployed, and they may not contain all essentials.

The prospect of bioterrorism is not an abstract one. It has been attempted before, and it will certainly be attempted again. That it has not happened is not reason for complacency. Adequate response to a bioterrorist incident is possible, but it requires careful and thoughtful preparation. Also, the preparation is hardly specific to the potential agents of bioterrorism. The principles of providing safe and effective care to victims of a BT incident are wholly applicable to the management of patients suffering from naturally acquired emerging infectious diseases. The age of bioterrorism is also that of SARS, coronavirus, avian influenza, Ebola virus, and, significantly, global travel. The potential for patients to present acutely ill with rare, unknown, and infectious diseases, whether naturally acquired or unleashed by criminals, has never been higher. Planning and preparation are essential.

SUGGESTED READING

Arnon SS, Schecter R, Inglesby TV, et al: Botulinum toxin as a biological weapon. Medical and public health management. JAMA 2001; 285:1059–1070.

Borio L, Inglesby T, Peters CJ, et al: Hemorrhagic fever viruses as biological weapons. Medical and public health management. JAMA 2002;287: 2391–2405

Dennis DT, Inglesby TV, Henderson DA, et al: Tularemia as a biological weapon. Medical and public health management. JAMA 2001;285: 2763–2773.

Grow RW, Rubinson L: The challenge of hospital infection control during a response to bioterrorist attacks. Biosecur Bioterror 2003;1:215–220.

Henderson DA, Inglesby TV, Bartlett JG, et al: Smallpox as a biological weapon. Medical and public health management. JAMA 1999;281: 2127–2137.

Inglesby TV, Dennis DT, Henderson DA, et al: Plague as a biological weapon. Medical and public health management. JAMA 2000;283:2281–2290.

Inglesby TV, O'Toole T, Henderson DA, et al: Anthrax as a biological weapon, 2002. Updated recommendations for management. JAMA 2002;287:2236–2252.

Index

Note: Page numbers followed by f indicate figures; t, tables; b, boxes.

A

ABCDE approach, to multiple trauma, 604–607, 605f, 606f, 606t, 607b
Abciximab, for myocardial infarction, 313
Abdomen, trauma to, 609–611, 610f, 633–634
Abdominal compartment syndrome, in nutritional support, 214t
Abdominal pain, in pancreatitis, 527
Abdominal pressure
  in ARDS, 243
  in obesity, 266, 266f, 271
Abscess, perivalvular, 360
Absence status epilepticus, 419
Acalculous cholecystitis, in nutritional support, 214t
Accelerating angina, 308
Acetaminophen
  for pain, 52, 53t
  for thyrotoxicosis, 498
  liver failure due to, 531–532, 532b
  poisoning from, 674
Acetazolamide, for metabolic alkalosis, 455
Acetoacetate
  in diabetic ketoacidosis, 507–509
  in hyperosmolar nonketotic coma, 507–509
Acetylcholine, in delirium, 55
N-Acetylcysteine
  as antidote, 668t, 674
  for kidney protection, 480
  for liver failure, 538, 540
Acid-base disorders, 445–457. *See also specific type, e.g.,* Metabolic acidosis.
  Boston "rules of thumb" in, 449, 449t
  carbon dioxide partial pressure/pH relationship in, 447–448, 448f
  compensation in, 449–450, 449t
  controversies in, 456b
  definitions of, 450t
  diagnosis of, 450–452, 450t–452t
  epidemiology of, 445, 446t
  Henderson-Hasselbalch equation in, 445
  hypokalemia in, 471, 471b
  kidney role in, 450
  mixed, epidemiology of, 446t
  pathophysiology of, 445–450
  physical chemistry of, 445–447, 446f, 447b, 447f, 448f
  potassium distribution in, 468
  primary, 449
  quantifying, 448–449
  renal replacement therapy effects on, 483f
  Stewart equations for, 445–450, 446f–448f, 447b
  strong ion concept in, 445–449
Acidemia, definition of, 450t
Acidosis
  lactic, 452–453, 454b
  metabolic. *See* Metabolic acidosis.
  renal tubular, 452, 453t, 454f
  respiratory. *See* Respiratory acidosis.
Acinetobacter pneumonia, 177, 177t, 182t

ACTH (adrenocorticotropic hormone)
  in stress response, 24, 27
  measurement of, in adrenal crisis, 504
  production of, after brain stem death, 442
Actin, in vascular smooth muscle mechanochemical cycle, 31, 32f
Activated charcoal, for poisoning, 666, 666f
Activated partial thromboplastin time, in bleeding, 550t, 551
Acute coronary syndromes, 301–318. *See also* Angina; Myocardial infarction.
  classification of, 307, 307f
  clinical features of, 306–308, 307b, 307f
  definitions of, 306–308, 307b, 307f
  diagnosis of, 308–312, 308b, 308t, 309b, 309f–312f
  epidemiology of, 301, 302f, 303f
  pathophysiology of, 304–306, 305f, 306f
  risk factors for, 301, 304, 304b, 304f
  risk stratification in, 308–312, 308b, 312f
  spectrum of, 301, 302t
  treatment of, 312–318, 313f–317f
Acute liver failure. *See* Liver failure.
Acute lung injury (ALI)
  ARDS as subset of, 245, 246t
  definition of, 245, 246t
  diagnosis of, 245–247, 247f
  gas exchange in, 244–245
  hemodynamics of, 371, 373f
  in inflammation, 6f, 7
  risk factors for, 247, 248t
  sponge model of, 240–242, 240f
  transfusion-related, 564t
  treatment of, 247–251, 248t, 249f, 249t
  ventilator-associated, 161–167
Acute Physiology and Chronic Health Evaluation (APACHE), 217–218
  in pancreatitis, 527
  in sepsis, 597
Acute renal failure. *See* Kidney failure.
Acute respiratory distress syndrome (ARDS), 2, 2t, 237–252
  airway resistance measurement in, 139
  as subset of acute lung injury, 245, 246t
  clinical features of, 245, 246t
  definitions of, 245, 246t
  diagnosis of, 245–247, 247f
  differential diagnosis of, 633t
  early phase of, 239f, 244–245, 245t, 251, 252f
  epidemiology of, 237, 237t
  gas exchange in, positioning and, 242–243, 243f
  hemodynamics in, 247, 371
  hypoxia in, 48–49
  in HELLP syndrome, 629
  in pneumonia, 572
  in pregnancy, 633t, 634–635
  in sepsis, 595
  intermediate phase of, 251–252
  late phase of, 245, 245t, 252, 252f
  mechanical ventilation in, alveolar distention in, 162

Acute respiratory distress syndrome (ARDS)—cont'd
  models of, 238, 239f, 240, 240f
  mortality in, 252
  nutritional support in, 210
  opening airway pressure in, 142, 144f
  partial ventilatory support in, 150, 151f, 152, 153
  pathophysiology of, 238–245, 238f
    chest wall compliance and, 243
    clinical course and, 251–252, 252f
    direct insult in, 238, 238f, 244–245
    gas exchange alterations, 244–245, 245t, 246
    indirect insult in, 238, 238f, 239f, 244
    models of, 238, 239f, 240, 240f
    positioning and, 242–243, 243f
    positive pressure mechanisms in, 241–242, 241f
    pulmonary circulation and, 243–244, 244f
    tidal volume distribution mechanisms in, 242, 242f
  treatment based on, 247, 249f, 249t
  positioning in, 242–243, 243f
  prevention of, 251–252, 252f
  risk factors for, 237–238, 247, 248t
  treatment of, 10, 247–251
    clinical course of, 251–252, 252f
    etiologic, 247–248, 248t
    pathogenic, 247, 249f, 249t
    symptomatic, 248, 250–251
  ventilator-associated pneumonia in, 176
Acute tubular necrosis, in hepatorenal syndrome, 492
Acutely unstable patient, 187–198. *See also* Subarachnoid hemorrhage.
  cardiopulmonary resuscitation in, 189, 189f
  epidemiology of, 187
  evaluation of
    airway, 189–191, 190b, 196–197
    cardiopulmonary, 189, 189f
    central nervous system, 195–197, 195t
    circulation, 191–195, 191b, 191f–194f, 193b, 194t, 197
    guidelines for, 188–189, 188b
    in sepsis and septic shock, 196
    pitfalls in, 196–197
    rapid systematic, 196, 197f
  failing to detect, 187–188, 188b
Acyclovir, dosage of, during dialysis, 488t
Adaptive support ventilation, modes of, 115–116, 115f
Adenosine
  for atrial tachycardia, 321
  in vascular tone control, 34, 36f
Adhesion, platelet, 544, 545f
Adhesion molecules, in inflammation, 6
Administrative controls, for infection control, 78
Admission, to ICU, criteria for, 217–218, 657–658, 658b
ADPase, in hemostasis regulation, 549, 549f

Adrenal gland
    function of, in stress response, 25
    insufficiency of
        acute, 503f–505f, 504–505
            hyponatremia in, 466
            pneumonia and, 577
    pheochromocytoma of, 500–501, 501f
Adrenocorticotropic hormone. See ACTH
        (adrenocorticotropic hormone).
Advance directives, 219
Advanced Trauma Life Support, in multiple
        trauma, 604
Afelimomab, for inflammation, 10
Afterload
    factors affecting, 355
    in left ventricular failure, 294–295
    in right ventricular failure, 291–293, 292f,
        293f
    intrathoracic pressure effects on, 380–381
    lung volume effects on, 374–375
    physiology of, 284, 284f, 286
Agitation
    assessment of, 53–54, 53t
    treatment of, 54–55, 55t
Air, in pleural space. See Pneumothorax.
Air embolism, 260–261
Airborne transmission
    in bioterrorism attack, 694
    of infections, 75, 75t, 76b
Airway management
    in acutely unstable patient, 189–191, 190b,
        196–197
    in diabetic ketoacidosis, 511
    in hyperosmolar nonketotic coma, 511
    in multiple trauma, 604, 605f
    in pregnancy, 636
    in sepsis, 598
    in spinal cord injury, 435
    in subarachnoid hemorrhage, 407
Airway obstruction
    in asthma. See Asthma.
    in COPD. See Chronic obstructive pulmonary
        disease.
Airway pressure
    cardiovascular effects of, 370–374,
        372f–374f
    opening. See Opening airway pressure.
Airway pressure release ventilation, 118, 118f,
        119f, 150, 151f, 152–153, 156t, 157
Airway resistance
    in COPD, 224
    in obesity, 264
    measurement of, 139
Albumin
    for dialysis, in liver failure, 540, 541t
    for hepatorenal syndrome, 492–493, 493t
Albuterol, for hyperkalemia, 470
Alcohol use
    as antidote, 668t, 670
    pancreatitis in, 525
    pneumonia in, 571
    poisoning in, 667, 669f, 669t
Alkalemia, definition of, 450t
Alkalosis. See Metabolic alkalosis; Respiratory
        alkalosis.
Alleles
    description of, 13
    segregation analysis of, 14
Allergic reactions, transfusion-related, 564t
Alpha blockers, for hypertensive crisis, 348t
Alpha-stat method, for arterial blood gas
        calculation, 450–451
Alveolar macrophages, antibiotic levels in, 67
Alveolar pressure, in dynamic hyperinflation,
        141, 141f
Alveolar–arterial oxygen tension gradient, in
        obesity, 264

Alveoli
    capillary failure in, in mechanical ventilation,
        163, 163f
    collapse of, in ARDS, 241, 241f
    overdistention of, in mechanical ventilation,
        162–163, 162f, 163f
Alveolitis, in pneumonia, 572
American Burn Association, burn unit criteria of,
        613, 613b
American College of Chest Physicians, on
        ventilator-associated pneumonia, 178,
        179, 180f
American College of Surgeons, blood loss
        estimation chart of, 605, 606t
American Spinal Injury Association classification,
        432, 433f
Amikacin, for ventilator-associated pneumonia,
        182t
Aminoglycosides
    dosage of, during dialysis, 488t
    for ventilator-associated pneumonia, 182t,
        661t
    host defenses and, 69
Aminophylline
    for asthma, 233–234
    for COPD, 229
Amiodarone
    for arrhythmias, 321b
    for atrial fibrillation, 328
    for electrical storm, 337
Ammonia, elevated, in liver failure, 534–537
Ammonium chloride, for metabolic alkalosis,
        455
Amnesia, in brain injury, 399
Amniotic fluid embolism, 260, 627–628, 628f
Amoxicillin
    dosage of, during dialysis, 488t
    for COPD, 230
Amphetamine poisoning, 677
Amphotericin B
    dosage of, during dialysis, 488t
    for postoperative infections, 661
    prophylactic, 89, 89t
Ampicillin, for bioterrorist agents, 688t
Ampicillin/sulbactam
    for obstetric sepsis, 632
    for ventilator-associated pneumonia, 182t,
        183t
Amylase, elevated, in pancreatitis, 527
Anabolism
    hypokalemia in, 468
    in repair, 24
Anaerobic metabolism, 48
Analgesia, in pregnancy, 636
Anaphylactic shock, tissue perfusion in, 194
Anaphylaxis, transfusion-related, 564t
Anemia
    autoimmune hemolytic, transfusions for, 565
    physiologic, in pregnancy, 627
Anemic hypoxia, 45
Anesthesia
    blood pressure variations in, 352
    for electrical storm, 337
    general, for seizures, 427
    in obesity, 266–270, 266f, 268t
    PEEP in, 270
Aneurysm, brain, subarachnoid hemorrhage in.
        See Subarachnoid hemorrhage.
Angel dust (phencyclidine), 677
Angina
    accelerating, 308
    new-onset, 308
    rest, 308
    unstable
        clinical features of, 306–308, 307f
        diagnosis of, 308–309, 308b, 309f

Angina—cont'd
    unstable—cont'd
        epidemiology of, 301, 302f
        pathophysiology of, 304–306, 305f, 306f
        risk factors for, 301, 304, 304b, 304f
        treatment of, 312–315, 312f
Angiodysplasia, bleeding in, 517, 523, 523f
Angiography
    cerebral, in brain death, 440
    computed tomography, in subarachnoid
        hemorrhage, 406, 406f
    coronary, in acute coronary syndromes, 311
    in gastrointestinal bleeding, 519
    pulmonary, in pulmonary embolism, 258
Angioplasty
    coronary, for acute coronary syndromes,
        315–317, 316f, 317f
    for subarachnoid hemorrhage, 413, 414f
Angiotensin II, in vascular tone control, 36
Angiotensin-converting enzyme inhibitors
    for hypertensive crisis, 348t
    for myocardial infarction, 318
Anion gaps, in acid-base disorders, 450, 450t,
        452t
Anorexia, supplements for, 213
Anoxia
    cellular, 42, 43f
    myoclonus after, 420t
Anthrax, 686–687, 687f, 688f, 688t
Antiarrhythmic drugs, poisoning from, 674–675
Antibiotics, 61–70. See also specific antibiotics.
    area under the inhibitory concentration-time
        curve for, 62–64, 62f–64f, 65t, 68f
    benefits of, 69b
    catheters coated with, 79, 80f
    dosage of
        during dialysis, 488t
        for resistance repression, 64, 64f, 65t
    for bioterrorist agents, 688t
    for burns, 618
    for COPD, 230
    for gastrointestinal bleeding, 521
    for hypothermia, 622
    for liver failure, 536
    for obstetric sepsis, 632
    for pancreatitis, 527–528
    for pneumonia, 576–577, 577f, 585, 585t
    for sepsis, 599
    for ventilator-associated pneumonia, 180–181,
        182t, 183t
    host defense influences on, 67–69, 68f
    in catheter locks, 79
    in pregnancy, 636
    killing rate of, 63, 64f
    minimum inhibitory concentration of, 62, 62f,
        64, 67–69
    mutant protective concentration of, 64,
        64f
    mutant selection window of, 64, 64f
    pharmacokinetics/pharmacodynamics of,
        62–64, 62f–64f, 65t
    programmed regular rotation of, 84
    prophylactic, 87–93
        benefits of, 92, 92b
        clinical experience with, 91–92
        controversies in, 92, 92b
        device-related reasons for, 87–88
        for ventilator-associated pneumonia, 184
        indications for, 89, 90t
        rationale for, 88–89, 88t
        regimen for, 89–92, 89t–90t
        resistance development in, 92–93
        risks of, 92, 92b
        systemic, 90
        topical, 90–91
    protein binding of, 64–66, 65f

Antibiotics—cont'd
  resistance to, 61
    prevention of, 64, 64f, 65t, 83–84, 83f
    prophylactic regimens and, 92–93
    repression of, 64, 64f, 65t
  risks of, 69b
  tissue level of, 66–67, 66t
  usage of, control of, 84
Anticholinergic agents
  for asthma, 233
  for COPD, 228
Anticholinesterase agents, for myasthenia gravis, 282
Anticoagulants
  bleeding due to, 551
  for atrial fibrillation, 327–328
  for continuous renal replacement therapy, 484–486, 485b, 485f, 486f
  for myocardial infarction, 314–315
  for pulmonary embolism, 258–259
  for sepsis, 557–558, 601
Antidepressants, poisoning from, 672–673, 673f
Antidigoxin fab antibody fragments, as antidote, 668t
Antidiuretic hormone. See Vasopressin.
Antidotes, for poisoning, 667, 668t
Antifibrinolytic agents, 566
Antihypertensive agents, 346–347, 348t
Antioxidants, supplementation with, 211
Antiphospholipid antibody syndrome, hypertensive crisis in, 353
α_2-Antiplasmin, action of, 548f, 549
Antiplatelet agents
  for myocardial infarction, 312–314, 313f, 314f
  mechanism of action of, 544, 545f
Antipsychotics, for delirium, 59
Antithrombin, 546–547
Antitoxin
  for botulism, 282, 690
  for myasthenia gravis, 282
Anxiety
  assessment of, 53–54, 53t
  in end-of-life care, 219
  treatment of, 54–55, 55t
Aorta
  balloon pump in, 356–357, 356f, 357f, 654–656, 655f
  dissection of, 308b, 365–368
    classification of, 366, 366f
    clinical features of, 366
    diagnosis of, 366–367, 367f
    in hypertensive crisis, 351
    pathogenesis of, 365–366
    predisposing factors for, 365, 365b
    prognosis for, 368
    treatment of, 367–368, 368f
  repair of, 367–368, 368f
  rupture of
    in dissection, 359–360
    traumatic, 608–609
Aortic outflow tract obstruction, cardiovascular failure in, 296
Aortic valve
  injury of, 359
  regurgitation of, 295–296, 362, 366
  stenosis of, 296, 362
APACHE (Acute Physiology and Chronic Health Evaluation), 217–218
  in pancreatitis, 527
  in sepsis, 597
Apoptosis, 22
  inhibitors of, 553
Aprotinin, for coagulopathy, 566
APTT (activated partial thromboplastin time), in bleeding, 550t, 551

Arachidonic acid, in vascular tone control, 22
ARDS. See Acute respiratory distress syndrome (ARDS).
Area under the inhibitory concentration-time curve, for antibiotics, 62–64, 62f–64f, 65t, 68f
Argatroban, for pulmonary embolism, 258
Arginine, for stress response, 29
Arrhythmias, 319–341
  after brain stem death, 442
  after cardiac surgery, 643–644, 645f
  bradycardia as, 337–341, 337f–340f, 339b
  classification of, 319, 320f
  in antidepressant poisoning, 673, 673f
  in carbon monoxide poisoning, 680
  in electrical injury, 620
  in hyperkalemia, 470
  in hypokalemia, 472
  in subarachnoid hemorrhage, 407
  supraventricular
    atrial fibrillation, 320f, 323–328, 325f–329f
    atrial flutter, 320f, 321–323, 324f, 325f
    atrial tachycardia, 319–321, 320f, 323f
    atrioventricular nodal reentrant tachycardia, 319–320, 320f, 322f, 328–329, 330f
    atrioventricular reciprocating tachycardia, 319–320, 320f, 322f, 328–329, 331f
    paroxysmal supraventricular tachycardias, 328–329, 330f, 331f
    Wolff-Parkinson-White syndrome, 329
  treatment of, 319, 321b, 674–675
  ventricular (wide-complex), 329–337
    drug-induced, 336
    electrical storm as, 337
    monitoring artifacts in, 336–337, 336f
    monomorphic ventricular tachycardia as, 331–333, 332b, 332f, 333f
    nonsustained, 330–331, 330b
    polymorphic ventricular tachycardia and fibrillation as, 333–335, 333b, 334f
    sustained, 331–335, 332b, 332f–336f, 333b
  types of, 329, 329t
Arterial blood gases
  in acid-base disorders, temperature corrections for, 450–451
  in acutely unstable patient, 190, 195
  in ARDS, correction of, 248, 250
  in asthma, 227
  in cerebral circulation regulation, 392
  in COPD, 227, 232f
  in mechanical ventilation, 146–148, 147f, 148t
  in pulmonary embolism, 256
  in seizures, 422
Arterial pressure, in cardiovascular failure, 283–290
Arterial pressure waveform analysis, 105–107, 105f, 106f
Artificial liver, 541, 541t
Ascites, in hepatorenal syndrome, 492
Aspergillus pneumonia, 581–582, 585t
Aspiration
  pulmonary
    in obesity, 267
    pneumonia due to, 572
  subglottic, in mechanical ventilation, 82, 83f
Aspirin
  for myocardial infarction, 312–313, 313f, 316, 318
  mechanism of action of, 544, 545f
  poisoning from, 674
Assist/control ventilation, 110, 111b, 111f, 142–146, 145f–147f, 149, 171t
Association constant, in antibiotic protein binding, 65, 65f
Association studies, in genetic studies, 14, 14f

Asthma
  airway resistance measurement in, 139
  clinical features of, 226–227, 226t
  controversies in, 235b
  diagnosis of, 227–228, 229f
  epidemiology of, 223
  in pregnancy, 635
  noninvasive ventilation for, 127
  pathogenesis of, 224–225
  pitfalls in, 235b
  risk factors for, 223–224
  severity of, 226, 226t
  treatment of, 233–234
  versus COPD, 223, 224t
Atelectasis
  after cardiac surgery, 641
  in ARDS, 241, 241f
  in obesity, 267, 269, 271, 271f
  in pulmonary embolism, 255
Atelectrauma, in mechanical ventilation, 163–164, 164f
Atherosclerosis
  as acute coronary syndrome risk factor, 304–305, 305f, 306f
  endothelial cell dysfunction and, 557
  thrombosis at, 543
A_{TOT} (nonvolatile weak acid), in acid-base balance, 445–448, 448f
ATP
  generation of, in mitochondrial respiration, 41–42, 42f
  in vascular smooth muscle mechanochemical cycle, 31, 32f, 34–35, 36f
ATP synthase, in mitochondrial respiration, 41–43, 42f
Atrial fibrillation, 320f, 323–328, 325f–329f
  after cardiac surgery, 644, 645f
  diagnosis of, 326, 326f–328f
  epidemiology of, 323–324, 326
  immediate recurrence of, 326–327
  pathogenesis of, 323–324, 326
  secondary causes of, 321b
  treatment of, 325f, 326–328, 329f
Atrial flutter, 320f, 321–323, 324f, 325f
Atrial tachycardia, 319–321, 320f, 323f
Atrioventricular block, 337, 339, 339b, 340f
Atrioventricular nodal reentrant tachycardia, 319–320, 320f, 322f, 328–329, 330f
Atrioventricular node disease, bradycardia in, 337, 338f
Atrioventricular reciprocating tachycardia, 319–320, 320f, 322f, 328–329, 331f
Atropine, as antidote, 282, 668t
A-type natriuretic peptide, in vascular tone control, 37
AUIC (area under the inhibitory concentration-time curve), for antibiotics, 62–64, 62f–64f, 65t
Autoimmune hemolytic anemia, transfusions for, 565
Automatic tube compensation ventilation, 116–117, 116f, 149, 156–157, 156t
Autonomic hyperreflexia, in spinal cord injury, 353
Autonomic nervous system
  function of, after brain stem death, 441
  in cerebral circulation autoregulation, 392–393
  in heart-lung interactions, 374
  in stress response, 25
  in thermoregulation, 621, 621f
Autonomy, 218–219
Autoregulation
  of cerebral blood flow, 343, 345f, 391–393, 392f
  of vascular tone, 38–39, 38f
Auxiliary liver transplantation, 541, 542f

Aztreonam, for ventilator-associated pneumonia, 182t

B

"Baby lung," in ARDS, 238, 239f, 240
Bacillus anthracis infections, 686–687, 687f, 688f, 688t
Bacitracin, prophylactic, 90
Bacteremia, catheter-related, 78–81, 78f, 80f, 80t, 81f
Bacterial translocation, in sepsis, 595
Bactericidal permeability increasing protein, in sepsis, 592–593, 592f
Balloon angioplasty, for subarachnoid hemorrhage, 413, 414f
Balloon fenestration, for aortic dissection, 367–368
Balloon tamponade, for gastrointestinal bleeding, 522–523, 523f
Balloon valvotomy
  for aortic stenosis, 362
  for mitral stenosis, 364
Balthazar grading, of CT findings in pancreatitis, 527, 527t
Band ligation, for gastrointestinal bleeding, 522
Barbiturates
  for seizures, 427, 428t
  poisoning from, 672
Barium studies, in gastrointestinal bleeding, 519
Barotrauma, in mechanical ventilation, 162–163, 162f, 163f
Bathtub model, of circulation, 286–288, 286f
Beneficence, 218
Benzodiazepines
  for agitation and anxiety, 54–55, 55t, 219
  for seizures, 427, 428t
  poisoning from, 668t, 672
Beta blockers
  for aortic dissection, 367
  for asthma, 233
  for atrial tachycardia, 320–321
  for COPD, 228–229
  for electrical storm, 337
  for hyperkalemia, 470
  for hypertensive crisis, 348t, 351
  for intracerebral hemorrhage, 351
  for mitral stenosis, 363–364
  for myocardial infarction, 315
  for pulmonary edema, 351
  for thyrotoxicosis, 498
  poisoning from, 674
Beta-lactam(s)
  for ventilator-associated pneumonia, 182t
  host defenses and, 67
  tissue levels of, 66–67, 66t
Beta-lactamases, bacteria producing, 73, 73f, 84–85
Bezold-Jarisch reflex, 339
Bicarbonate ion. *See also* Sodium bicarbonate.
  hyponatremia and, 465
  in acid-base disorders, Stewart equations for, 445–450, 446f–448f, 447b
  standard, 449
Bilevel pressure ventilation, 118, 119f
Bioartificial liver support devices, 540–541
Bioprosthetic heart valves, complications of, 364
Biopsy, lung, in pneumonia, 585, 586t
Bioterrorism agents, 685–695
  classification of, 686t
  current threat from, 685–686, 686b, 686t
  diagnostic laboratories for, 692
  information resources for, 686b
  management of, 692–695
    cadaver handling in, 695
    environmental decontamination in, 694–695

Bioterrorism agents—cont'd
  management of—cont'd
    hand washing in, 694
    infection control in, 693, 693b
    isolation in, 693
    patient decontamination in, 693
    personal protective equipment for, 695
    precautions in, 693–694, 694b
    preparedness paradigm for, 695
    supportive care in, 692–693
    vaccinations in, 694
    ventilator expiratory circuit filters in, 694
  medical response to, 691–692, 691t
  specific, 686–691
  versus conventional disasters, 691–692, 691t
Biotrauma, in mechanical ventilation, 164–166, 165f, 166f
Biphasic positive airway pressure ventilation, 150, 152–153, 156t, 157
Bispectral index, in agitation assessment, 54
Bleeding, 549–551. *See also* Hemorrhage.
  gastrointestinal. *See* Gastrointestinal bleeding.
  in multiple trauma, control of, 604–606, 606t
  in uremia, 565
  laboratory assessment of, 550–551, 550t
  risk factors for, 549, 550b
  treatment of, 551
Blindness, in methanol poisoning, 670, 670t
Blisters, in carbon monoxide poisoning, 680
Blood
  in pleural space (hemothorax), 608
  purification of, 487
Blood culture
  in infective endocarditis, 360
  in pneumonia, 575, 583–584, 584f
  in sepsis, 597
Blood flow
  cerebral. *See* Cerebral blood flow.
  evaluation of, in acutely unstable patient, 194, 194f
  in oxygen consumption, 43–45, 43f
  uterine, 627, 627f
Blood pressure
  high. *See* Hypertensive crisis.
  in hypovolemia, 192–193
  in pregnancy, 625
  measurement of, 343, 345f
Blood transfusions. *See* Transfusions.
Blood urea nitrogen, hyponatremia and, 465
Blood vessels, electrical injury of, 620
Blood volume, in pregnancy, 625, 626f
Blunt trauma
  cardiac, 608
  multiple, 604
  myocardial, 359–360
BMI (body mass index), 263
Body composition, 459–460, 460f
Body mass index, 263
Body temperature
  abnormal. *See* Hyperthermia; Hypothermia.
  control of, 29, 621, 621f
Boston rules of thumb, for acid-base disorders, 449, 449t
Botulism, 279, 281–282, 688t, 689–690, 690b
Bowel dysfunction, nursing interventions for, 202, 202b, 203f
Bradycardia, 337–341
  after cardiac surgery, 339, 643
  in atrioventricular node disease, 337, 338f
  in myocardial ischemia, 339
  medication-induced, 337
  pacing in, 339–341
  secondary causes of, 339, 339b, 340f
  sinus, 337, 338f
  terminology of, 337, 337f, 338f
  treatment of, 339–340

Brain. *See also* Encephalopathy.
  aneurysm of, subarachnoid hemorrhage in. *See* Subarachnoid hemorrhage.
  blood flow in. *See* Cerebral blood flow.
  carbon monoxide poisoning effects on, 680
  edema of
    in brain injury, 398–399
    in hypoglycemia, 502–503
    in liver failure, 536–538
  hemorrhage of, hypertensive crisis and, 350–351
  herniation of, 384, 399
  injury of. *See* Traumatic brain injury.
  ischemia of
    in hypertensive crisis, 350
    in injury, 398
  pressure on. *See* Intracranial pressure.
  renal replacement therapy effects on, 482f
  surgery on, ICP monitoring in, 385, 385t
Brain death, 439–443
  cautions in, 440
  confirmatory tests for, 440
  declaration of, 441
  definition of, 440
  determination of, 439–440
  diagnosis of, 440–441
  legal issues in, 439
  organ donor care after, 441–443, 441b, 442t
  pathophysiology of, 441–442, 441b, 442t
Brain natriuretic peptide
  in acute coronary syndromes, 310–311, 311f
  in pulmonary embolism, 256
  in vascular tone control, 37
Brain stem death, diagnosis of, 440–441
Breathing
  evaluation of, in acutely unstable patient, 189–191, 190b, 197
  heart interactions with. *See* Heart-lung interactions.
  inspiratory muscle dysfunction in, 275–277, 276f, 277f
  Kussmaul, in metabolic acidosis, 510
  management of, in multiple trauma, 604, 605f, 606f
  pursed lip, in COPD, 225–226
  spontaneous, mechanical ventilation interactions with. *See* Mechanical ventilation, partial support with.
  work of
    in obesity, 265
    in partial ventilatory support, 152
    measurement of, 144–145, 146f, 147f
Bronchi, injury of, 608
Bronchitis, chronic. *See* Chronic obstructive pulmonary disease.
Bronchoalveolar lavage, in pneumonia, 583–585, 584f, 586t
Bronchoconstriction, in obesity, 271
Bronchodilators
  for asthma, 233
  for COPD, 228–229
Bronchoscopy
  in pneumonia, 583–585, 584f, 586t
  noninvasive ventilation for, 127
Bronchospasm, in inhalation injury, 619
Brooke formula, modified, for burn resuscitation, 617t
B-type natriuretic peptide, in vascular tone control, 37
Bubonic plague, 688–689
Budd–Chiari syndrome, liver failure in, 533
Buffer base anions, in acid-base disorders, 446–447, 447b, 447f
Bulbar muscle dysfunction, respiratory failure in, 280

Burn(s), 613–619
circumferential, 615, 616f
clinical course of, 618–619
deep second-degree, 615
diagnosis of, 614–615, 615f, 616f
electrical, 619–620
epidemiology of, 613–614
first-degree, 615
fourth-degree, 615, 616f
hypertensive crisis in, 353
inhalation injury with, 619
mortality in, 613, 618–619
nutritional support in, 211t
pathophysiology of, 613–614, 614f
risk factors for, 613–614
second-degree, 615, 615f
shock in, 613–614, 614f
size and depth of, 614–615, 615f, 616f
superficial second-degree, 615
third-degree, 615, 616f
treatment of, 615–618
criteria for burn unit referral, 613, 613b
early wound care in, 617, 617f, 618f
fluid therapy in, 615–617, 617b, 617t
infection prevention in, 618
nutritional support in, 618
pain management in, 617–618
sedation in, 617–618

C
Calcitonin gene-related peptide, in vascular tone
control, 34, 36f
Calcium, in vascular tone control, 31–35,
32f–36f
Calcium channel blockers
for atrial tachycardia, 320–321
for hypertensive crisis, 348t
poisoning from, 674–675
Calcium chloride, as antidote, 668t
Calcium disodium edetate, as antidote, 668t
Calcium gluconate, for hyperkalemia, 470
Calmodulin, in vascular tone control, 31, 32f
Calories, in nutritional support, 208, 208f
Calorimetry, indirect
in burns, 618
in hemodynamic monitoring, 107
Camino system, for ICP monitoring, 386t, 387
Candidate genes, 14–16, 15f, 15t, 16f
Candidiasis, in liver failure, 536
Canonical response, to stress, 22–29, 24f–28f
Capacitance, in cardiovascular system, 287, 289
Capillary(ies)
alveolar, mechanical ventilation effects on,
163, 163f
oxygen delivery to, 43–44, 43f
Capillary refill rate, 191–192, 192f
Capnometry, in mechanical ventilation, 147–148,
147f
Capsule endoscopy, in gastrointestinal bleeding,
519
Carbapenems
for ventilator-associated pneumonia, 182t
host defenses and, 67
Carbicarb, for metabolic acidosis, 453
Carbon dioxide. See also Hypercapnia;
Hypocapnia.
elimination of, 44
partial pressure of
in acutely unstable patient, 190
in ARDS, 252
in cerebral circulation regulation, 392
in mechanical ventilation, 146–148, 147f,
148t
in obesity, 264
in pregnancy, 625

Carbon dioxide—cont'd
partial pressure of—cont'd
in pulmonary embolism, 256
in tissue hypoxia, 44–45, 44f
normal, 450t
pH relationship with, 445, 446f, 447–448,
448f, 452t
Carbon monoxide poisoning, 679–683
clinical features of, 679–680, 680t
diagnosis of, 680–681
elimination in, 679, 680f
epidemiology of, 679
gas kinetics and, 679, 680f
in pregnancy, 682, 683f
pathophysiology of, 679, 681f, 682f
risk factors for, 679
treatment of, 681–682, 683f
Carboprost, for obstetric hemorrhage, 631
Carboxyhemoglobin, 679, 680f–682f, 681
Cardiac arrhythmias. See Arrhythmias.
Cardiac function, in cardiovascular failure
curve plateau in, 290
determinants of, 284–286, 284f, 285f
failure of, 289–290
left heart, 293, 293f, 294f
return function interactions with, 288, 288f
right heart, 289f, 290–291, 292f
testing of, 289f, 290–291, 292f
Cardiac output
after cardiac surgery, 640, 642, 642t, 643t,
651, 651f
in acutely unstable patient, 191–192, 192f
in cardiovascular failure, 284
in hepatorenal syndrome, 490
in pregnancy, 625, 626f, 627
in sepsis, 594
in subarachnoid hemorrhage, 412–413
lithium dilution method for, 107
Cardiac surgery
bradycardia after, 339
cardiovascular failure after, 296–297
checklists for, 648t, 649t
postoperative care in, 639–656, 659–660
baseline cardiac pathology and, 648
clinical features of, 641–647
duration of, 639, 640f
fast-track principles in, 647–648, 648t,
649t
in arrhythmias, 643–644, 645f
in bleeding, 646
in bradycardia, 643
in cardiac tamponade, 644, 646
in confusion, 647
in electrocardiographic changes, 644,
646f
in fever, 647
in heart failure, 648–652, 650f, 651f
in hypertension, 642, 642t, 643, 643f, 643t,
644f
in hypovolemia, 642
in loss of sinus rhythm, 643–644
in pacemaker use, 652–654, 652f, 652t,
653t, 654f
in pneumothorax, 646–647
in sedation excess or deficiency, 647
in shivering, 647
in tachycardia, 644
in vasoplegia, 643
intra-aortic balloon pump for, 654–656,
655f
laboratory values in, 647, 647t
monitoring in, 642
pathophysiology of, 640–641
risk profile in, 640, 642f
statistics on, 639–640, 640f, 640t
types of, 642t

Cardiac tamponade, 364–365, 364b
after cardiac surgery, 644, 646
in aortic dissection, 366
Cardiogenic pulmonary edema, noninvasive
ventilation for, 122–124
Cardiogenic shock, 355–356, 356b. See also
specific causes.
in hemothorax, 608
lung interactions with, 369–370, 370f
Cardiomyopathy
dilated, 359
hypertrophic, 358–359
ventricular tachycardia in, 332b
Cardiopulmonary bypass
for hypothermia, 622
hemodilution in, 641
Cardiopulmonary resuscitation. See
Resuscitation.
Cardiovascular emergencies, 355–368
aortic dissection. See Aorta, dissection of.
aortic regurgitation, 362
aortic stenosis, 362
cardiac tamponade, 364–365, 364b
cardiogenic shock, 355–356, 356b
cardiomyopathy, 358–359
infective endocarditis, 360–362, 360b, 361b,
361f
intra-aortic balloon pump for, 356, 356f,
357b, 357f
left ventricular free wall rupture, 358
mitral regurgitation, 362–363, 362b, 363f
mitral stenosis, 363–364, 364f
prosthetic valve complications, 364
trauma, 359–360
ventricular septal rupture, 357–358
versus seizures, 421t
Cardiovascular failure, 283–299. See also Heart
failure.
backward, 283, 295
cardiac function in
determinants of, 284–286, 284f, 285f
failure of, 289–290
return function interactions with, 288,
288f
cardiac output in, 284
causes of, 295–298
clinical features of, 283
forward, 283, 295
in acute coronary ischemia, 297
in cardiac surgery, 296–297
in myocardial dyskinesia, 297
in sepsis, 296
in valvular disease, 295–296
left heart, 293, 293f, 294f
"pseudocardiac" failure and, 297–298, 297f
return function in
cardiac function interactions with, 288,
288f
determinants of, 286–288, 286f, 288f
failure of, 288–289, 289f
right heart
cardiac function curve in, 290
preload paradoxical effects in, 291–293,
293f
right ventricular afterload in, 291, 292f
tests for, 290–291, 291f, 292f
shock in, treatment of, 298, 298f
systemic vascular resistance in, 284, 284b
versus heart failure, 283
Cardiovascular system
carbon monoxide poisoning effects on, 680
dysfunction of. See also Arrhythmias;
Cardiovascular emergencies;
Cardiovascular failure; Heart failure.
in sepsis, 594–595, 594f
postoperative care in, 658–659, 659t

Cardiovascular system—cont'd
lung interactions with. *See* Heart-lung
interactions.
partial ventilatory support effects on, 152
physiology of, in pregnancy, 625, 626t, 627
support of, in organ donors, 442–443
Cardioversion
for atrial fibrillation, 326, 328, 329f
for ventricular fibrillation, 335
for ventricular tachycardia, 332, 332f
in pregnancy, 636
Carotid pulse, assessment of, 189, 189f
Carrier state, in infections, 88–89, 88t
Catabolism
evaluation of, 206, 206f
in stress response, 24, 27
Catecholamines. *See also specific catecholamines.*
excess of, in pheochromocytoma, 500–501,
500b
for hepatorenal syndrome, 493
hypertensive crisis due to, 352, 353f
in pregnancy, 635–636
in stress response, 23–24, 27
in vascular tone control, 36
Catheter(s)
urinary, infections due to, 661
vascular
infections due to, 78–81, 78f, 80f, 80t, 81f,
661
pulmonary artery. *See* Pulmonary artery
catheter.
thrombi formation in, 253
ventricular, for ICP monitoring, 385–387,
386f, 386t
Catheter tip transducer system, for ICP
monitoring, 386t, 387
Cation exchange resins, for hyperkalemia,
471–472
CC chemokines, in inflammation, 8
CD-40 ligand, soluble, in acute coronary
syndromes, 304
Cefazolin, for ventilator-associated pneumonia,
182t, 183t
Cefepime, for ventilator-associated pneumonia,
182t
Cefotaxime, dosage of, during dialysis, 488t
Ceftazidime
dosage of, during dialysis, 488t
for ventilator-associated pneumonia, 182t
Ceftriaxone
dosage of, during dialysis, 488t
for ventilator-associated pneumonia, 183t
prophylactic, 89t, 90
Cefuroxime
for ventilator-associated pneumonia, 183t
prophylactic, 90
Centers for Disease Control, on transmission
prevention, 75
Central nervous system. *See also* Brain; Spinal
cord injury.
carbon monoxide poisoning effects on, 680
evaluation of, in acutely unstable patient,
195–197, 195t
Central venous pressure waveform analysis,
105–107, 105f, 106f, 598
Cephalosporins
for pneumonia, 576–577
for ventilator-associated pneumonia, 182t,
661t
host defenses and, 67
prophylactic, 90
Cerebral angiography, in brain death, 440
Cerebral arteries, vasospasm of, 412b
Cerebral blood flow, 387–393
autoregulation of, 343, 345f, 391–393, 392f
circulation of, 387–388

Cerebral blood flow—cont'd
in brain injury, 401
in liver failure, 537
measurement of
computed tomography in, 388–389, 388t,
391
jugular bulb venous oxygen saturation in,
388t, 389
Kety-Schmidt technique in, 388, 388t
magnetic resonance imaging in, 388t, 391,
391f
near-infrared spectroscopy in, 388t, 390–391
photon emission tomography in, 388t, 389
single-photon emission computed
tomography in, 388t, 389
transcranial Doppler sonography in, 388t,
389–390, 390f
Cerebral perfusion pressure
as intracranial pressure determinant, 384
autoregulation of, 343, 345f
cerebral blood flow relationship with,
391–393, 392f
in brain injury, 398, 401
Cerebral salt wasting syndrome, 412
Cerebrospinal fluid
physiology of, 383–384, 384f
pressure of. *See* Intracranial pressure.
Cerebrovascular resistance, 391–393, 392f
Cervical spine, stabilization of, in multiple
trauma, 604
Cervical spine clearance algorithm, 435–436,
436f
Charcoal hemoperfusion, for liver failure, 540,
541t
Chemokines and receptors
in inflammation, 8
in sepsis, 555–556, 556f
Chemotherapy, immunodeficiency in, pneumonia
in, 581
Chest pain. *See also* Angina.
differential diagnosis of, 308b
in pneumonia, 574, 574t
in pulmonary embolism, 254, 254t
Chest physiotherapy, in organ donors, 443
Chest tube, for pneumothorax, 608
Chest wall
compliance of
in ARDS, 243
in obesity, 264, 271
injury of, 607
resistance of, measurement of, 139
Child-Pugh classification, of liver failure, 518,
518b
Chloramphenicol, for bioterrorist agents, 688t
Chlorhexidine, catheters coated with, 79, 80f
Cholecystitis, acalculous, in nutritional support,
214t
Cholestyramine, for thyrotoxicosis, 498
Chorioamnionitis, 631–632, 632b
Choroidal artery, vasospasm of, 412b
Chronic obstructive pulmonary disease (COPD),
223–235
airway resistance measurement in, 139
clinical features of, 225–226, 226b
conditions associated with, 230
controversies in, 235b
diagnosis of, 227, 228f
epidemiology of, 223, 224f
mechanical ventilation for, weaning from, 172,
172f
noninvasive ventilation for, 121–122, 123f
partial ventilatory support in, 152
pathogenesis of, 224–225, 225f
prognosis for, 224, 225f
respiratory failure in, precipitants of, 226,
226b

Chronic obstructive pulmonary disease—cont'd
risk factors for, 223
severity of, 227
treatment of, 228–233, 230t, 231f, 232f,
235b
versus asthma, 223, 224t
Ciaglia tracheostomy technique, 131, 133f
Cidofovir, for bioterrorist agents, 688t
Cimetidine, for gastrointestinal bleeding, 521
Ciprofloxacin
dosage of, during dialysis, 488t
for bioterrorist agents, 688t
for pneumonia, 576–577
for ventilator-associated pneumonia, 180, 182t
host defenses and, 67, 68, 68f
prophylactic, 92
Circulation
cerebral, 387–388
evaluation of, in acutely unstable patient,
191–195, 191b, 191f–194f, 193b, 194t,
197
restoration of. *See* Fluid therapy.
ventilation interactions with. *See* Heart-lung
interactions.
Cirrhosis
hepatorenal syndrome in. *See* Hepatorenal
syndrome.
portal hypertension in. *See* Portal
hypertension.
Citrate, for continuous renal replacement
therapy, 485, 486f
Clarithromycin, for bioterrorist agents, 688t
Clichy criteria, for liver failure, 532, 533b
Clindamycin, for bioterrorist agents, 688t
Clinical pulmonary infection score, 178–179,
180b
Clinical trials, severity of illness measures in, 99
Clonic seizures, 418
Clonidine, for hypertensive crisis, 352
Clopidogrel
for myocardial infarction, 313, 313f
mechanism of action of, 544, 545f
Clostridium botulinum toxins (botulism), 688t,
689–690, 690b
Coagulation cascade, 545–546, 546f
Coagulopathy. *See also* Bleeding; Thrombosis.
causes of, 550–551, 550t
in HELLP syndrome, 629–630
in hyperthermia, 623, 624
in liver failure, 534, 540, 565
in massive blood transfusions, 563
in pregnancy, 627
in sepsis, 595
inflammation interactions with, 555–557,
556b, 556f, 557f
laboratory assessment of, 550–551, 550t
obstetric hemorrhage in, 631
plasma transfusion for, 562–563
Cocaine poisoning, 675–677, 676f
Codman system, for ICP monitoring, 386t, 387
Coefficient shrinkage, in severity of illness
measures, 98
Cognitive impairment
after cardiac surgery, 647
assessment of, delirium and, 57–59, 58b, 58t,
59f
Colloids
for burns, 616, 617t
for diabetic ketoacidosis, 512, 513
for hyperosmolar nonketotic coma, 512, 513
for sepsis, 598, 598f
Colon, bleeding in. *See* Gastrointestinal bleeding,
lower tract.
Colonization
nosocomial infections and, 72, 88–89, 88t
of catheter surfaces, 78–79, 78f

Colonization—cont'd
  of digestive tract, 88–89, 88t
  outbreaks related to, 91
  pneumonia and, 572
  prevention of, 91
  ventilator-associated pneumonia due to,
      176–177, 176f, 177f
Colonoscopy, in bleeding, 519–520
Coma
  brain death and, 439–440
  hyperosmolar nonketotic. See Hyperosmolar
      nonketotic coma.
  myxedema, 499–500, 499b, 622
Communication, interventions for, 201, 201f
Compartment syndrome
  abdominal, in nutritional support, 214t
  peripheral, in multiple trauma, 611, 611b
Compensation, in acid-base disorders, 449–450,
      449t
Complex partial status epilepticus, 419
Complex seizures, 418
Compliance
  cardiovascular, 284, 284f, 289
  chest wall, in obesity, 271
  intracranial, 383–384
  respiratory system, in obesity, 264
Compression devices, for deep venous
      thrombosis, 260
Computed tomography
  in abdominal injury, 609–610
  in aortic dissection, 367
  in ARDS, 238, 239f, 240, 240f, 243f,
      246–247
  in brain injury, 399
  in cerebral blood flow measurement, 388t,
      391
  in COPD, 227, 228f
  in gastrointestinal bleeding, 520
  in liver failure, 535, 535f
  in pancreatitis, 527, 527t, 529, 529f
  in pulmonary embolism, 256–257, 257f
  in seizures, 422
  in spinal cord injury, 434–435, 434f
Computed tomography angiography, in
      subarachnoid hemorrhage, 406, 406f
Conduction system, anatomy of, 337, 337f
Confusion, after cardiac surgery, 647
Confusion Assessment Method for the ICU,
      58–59, 58t, 59b
Congestive heart failure. See Heart failure.
Consciousness alterations
  in acutely unstable patient, 195–197, 195t
  in brain death, 440
  in brain injury, 399
  in hyperthermia, 623, 624
  in hypothermia, 621, 622t
  in sepsis, 595
  in subarachnoid hemorrhage, 406
Constipation
  in nutritional support, 214t
  nursing interventions for, 201
Constriction, of vascular smooth muscle, 31–32,
      32f. See also Vasoconstriction and
      vasoconstrictors.
  autoregulation of, 38–39, 38f
  calcium and, 31–35, 32f–36f
  circulating factors in, 35–38, 36t
  membrane potential and, 34–35, 34f–36f
Contact transmission
  in bioterrorism attack, 694
  of infections, 75, 75t, 76b
Continuous positive airway pressure (CPAP),
      149, 151f, 152–153, 156t
  delivery of, 130, 130f
  for acute hypoxemic respiratory failure, 124
  for cardiogenic pulmonary edema, 122

Continuous positive airway pressure—cont'd
  for COPD, 232–233
  for heart failure, 374
  for intubation, of obese patients, 268
  for weaning, 171, 171t
  postoperative, in obesity, 271
  systemic venous return and, 377–378, 378f
Continuous renal replacement therapy, 481–482,
      482f–486f, 484–486, 485b
Continuous venovenous hemofiltration, 481–482,
      482f–486f, 484–486, 485b, 538
Contrast agents, kidney failure due to, 480
Contrecoup injury, 395, 396f
Control mode, for mechanical ventilation, 110,
      110f, 111f
Contusion
  brain, 395, 396f
  myocardial, 359, 608
  pulmonary, 608
Cooling, for hyperthermia, 623
COPD. See Chronic obstructive pulmonary
      disease.
Copenhagen school, acid-base disorder index of,
      448–449
Cor pulmonale
  in COPD, 227
  in pulmonary embolism, 255
Coronary angiography, in acute coronary
      syndromes, 311
Coronary artery(ies)
  blood flow in, 294
  blunt trauma to, 359
  oxygen extraction in, 293–294
  thrombosis in, 543
Coronary artery bypass surgery
  for acute coronary syndromes, 315, 315f
  nutritional support in, 211t
Coronary artery disease. See Acute coronary
      syndromes.
Corticosteroids
  deficiency of, 503f–505f, 504–505
  for asthma, 233
  for COPD, 229–230
  for HELLP syndrome, 629
  for inflammation, 10
  for sepsis, 557–558, 599
  for thyrotoxicosis, 498, 498b
  for ventilator weaning, 173
  in stress response, 24–25, 27
Cortisol, in stress response, 23–24, 24, 27
Costochondral pain, versus acute coronary
      syndromes, 308b
Cough
  in COPD, 227
  in pneumonia, 574, 574t, 583
Counterregulatory hormones, in stress response,
      27
Coup injury, 395, 396f
CPAP. See Continuous positive airway pressure.
CPR (cardiopulmonary resuscitation)
  in acutely unstable patient, 189, 189f
  in pregnancy, 636
Cranial neuropathy, in botulism, 689–690
C-reactive proteins
  in acute coronary syndromes, 304
  in inflammation, 1
Creatine kinase, in myocardial infarction, 310,
      310f
Creutzfeldt–Jacob disease, transfusion-related,
      563, 565t
Crisis
  adrenal, 503f–505f, 504–505
  hyperglycemic, 502. See also Diabetic
      ketoacidosis; Hyperosmolar nonketotic
      coma.
  hypertensive. See Hypertensive crisis.

Crisis—cont'd
  hypoglycemic, 502–503
  hypothyroid, 499–500, 499b
  thyroid storm as, 497–499, 497b, 499f
Critical illness polyneuropathy and myopathy,
      29–30, 29t, 279, 282
Cryoprecipitate, transfusion of, 562–563
Crystalloids
  for burns, 616, 617t
  for sepsis, 598, 598f
CT. See Computed tomography.
C-type natriuretic peptide, in vascular tone
      control, 37
Cullen's sign, in pancreatitis, 527
Culture
  blood
    in infective endocarditis, 360
    in pneumonia, 575, 583–584, 584f
    in sepsis, 597
  in ventilator-associated pneumonia, 180
Cushing response, 351
CXC chemokines, in inflammation, 8
Cyanosis, in acutely unstable patient, 190
Cyclic adenosine monophosphate, in vascular
      tone control, 32, 33f
Cystatin C, in kidney failure, 476–477
Cytochrome c oxidase, in mitochondrial
      respiration, 42f, 43
Cytochrome P450, polymorphisms of, drug
      response and, 18, 18t, 19t
Cytokine(s)
  anti-inflammatory, 17–18
  genes of, with promoter variations, 15–16, 16f
  in coronary artery disease, 305
  in inflammation, 7–8, 7t
  in pneumonia, 572–573
  in sepsis, 555, 556f, 593, 593t
Cytomegalovirus pneumonia, 582, 583f, 584,
      586t
Cytopathic hypoxia, 595

D

Damage control surgery, in abdominal injury,
      610
D-dimer, in pulmonary embolism, 256
Death. See also Mortality.
  brain, 439–443
  care at. See End-of-life care in ICU.
DeBakey classification, of aortic dissection, 366,
      366f
Decerebrate posturing, 419
Decompression, in spinal cord injury, 437
Decontamination
  gut
    for antidepressant poisoning, 673
    for poisoning, 666, 666f
  in bioterrorism attack
    environment, 694–695
    patient, 693
Decorticate posturing, 419
Deep venous thrombosis
  postoperative, 662
  prevention of, 260
  pulmonary embolism in, 258
  risk factors for, 551, 552t
  upper extremity, 258–259
Deferoxamine, as antidote, 668t
Defibrillation
  for atrial fibrillation, 326, 328, 329f
  for hypothermia, 622
  for ventricular fibrillation, 335
  in pregnancy, 636
Dehydration
  in hyperthermia, 623
  in severe hyperglycemia, 502

Delayed ischemic deficit (vasospasm), in subarachnoid hemorrhage, 410–413, 411f, 412b, 412t, 413f, 414f
Delayed neurologic syndrome, in carbon monoxide poisoning, 680
Delirium, 55–59
  assessment of, 57–59, 58b, 58t, 59f
  criteria for, 55, 55b
  hyperactive type, 55
  hypoactive type, 55
  in end-of-life care, 219
  nursing interventions for, 200
  outcomes and, 56–57, 56f, 57f
  pathophysiology of, 55
  risk factors for, 55–56, 56b
  treatment of, 59
Dendritic cells, in inflammation, 4t, 5
Deotrecogin-α, for inflammation, 11, 11f
Desmopressin, for bleeding, 566
Detoxification, for liver failure, 540, 541t
Dexamethasone
  for HELLP syndrome, 629
  for ventilator weaning, 173
Dextropropoxyphene, poisoning from, 675
Diabetes insipidus, 461, 461f, 505
Diabetes mellitus
  as cardiovascular risk factor, 304, 304f
  hyperglycemic crisis in, 502. See also Diabetic ketoacidosis; Hyperosmolar nonketotic coma.
  hypoglycemia in, 502–503
Diabetic ketoacidosis, 502
  clinical course of, 514
  clinical features of, 509–510, 510b
  complications of, 514–515, 514b
  controversies in, 514b, 515
  diagnosis of, 510, 510b, 511b
  differential diagnosis of, 510, 510b
  epidemiology of, 507
  pathogenesis of, 507–509, 508f, 509f
  pitfalls in, 514, 514b
  prevention of, 514
  risk factors for, 507, 507b
  treatment of, 510–514, 511b, 512b, 512f, 513f
Dialysis
  for ethylene glycol poisoning, 671t, 672
  for hepatorenal syndrome, 495
  for hyperkalemia, 471
  for lithium intoxication, 674
  for liver failure, 538, 540, 541t
  for methanol poisoning, 671t
  for poisoning, 666–667, 667t
  intermittent, 482f, 483f, 486–487, 487f
  peritoneal, 481, 482, 487
  slow low-efficiency extended daily, 481–482, 487, 487f
Diaphoresis, in pheochromocytoma, 500
Diaphragm
  displacement of, in obesity, 266, 266f
  dysfunction of, in mechanical ventilation, 280
  injury of, 609
Diarrhea
  in nutritional support, 214t
  nursing interventions for, 201, 202b
Diazepam
  for agitation and anxiety, 55, 55t
  for burns, 618
  for seizures, 428t
  in obesity, perioperative, 270
Diets, for nutritional support, 213, 214t
Diffuse axonal damage, 351, 396, 397f, 398
Digoxin poisoning, 668t, 675
Dilated cardiomyopathy, 359
Diltiazem, for aortic dissection, 367
Dimercaprol, as antidote, 668t

Disability, evaluation of, in multiple trauma, 606, 606t
Disorientation, nursing interventions for, 200
Dissection, aortic. See Aorta, dissection of.
Disseminated intravascular coagulation, 552–553, 552b
  after brain stem death, 442
  in liver failure, 534
  in pregnancy, 631
  transfusions for, 565
Dissociation constant, in antibiotic protein binding, 65, 65f
Diuresis and diuretics
  for kidney failure, 481
  for poisoning, 666–667, 667t
  in diabetic ketoacidosis, 508, 509f
  in hyperosmolar nonketotic coma, 508, 509f
  osmotic, 461–462, 461t
  water, 460–461, 461t
Diverticulosis, bleeding in, 517, 523
Diverticulum, Meckel's, 524
DO₂. See Oxygen delivery.
Dobutamine
  for organ donors, 442
  for sepsis, 598, 599
  for subarachnoid hemorrhage, 413
  in pregnancy, 635–636
Dolor, in inflammation, 9
Donnan phenomenon, in acid-base balance, 448
Donors, for transplantation, 441–443, 441b, 442t
Dopamine
  for delirium, 55
  for kidney protection, 479–480
  for organ donors, 442
  for sepsis, 599
  in pregnancy, 635–636
Dopamine agonists, for hypertensive crisis, 348t
Doppler studies
  in cardiac function, 290
  in hemodynamic monitoring, 107, 107f
  in increased ICP, 401
  in subarachnoid hemorrhage, 410–411
  transcranial, in cerebral blood flow measurement, 388t, 389–390
Doxycycline
  for bioterrorist agents, 688t
  prophylactic, 90
Drainage, of cerebrospinal fluid, in subarachnoid hemorrhage, 409–410, 410f
Dressings, for vascular catheters, 79
Driving pressure, in mechanical ventilation, for ARDS, 250–251
Droplet transmission
  in bioterrorism attack, 694
  of infections, 75, 75t, 76b
Drotrecogin alfa
  for disseminated intravascular coagulation, 553
  for pneumonia, 577
  for sepsis, 599–600
Drug(s)
  bradycardia due to, 337
  brain death declaration and, 440
  kidney failure due to, 478, 478b
  prescription of, during dialysis, 487–488, 488t
  response to, genetic factors in, 18, 18t, 19t
  seizures due to, 417
  ventricular arrhythmias due to, 336
Duodenum
  bleeding in. See Gastrointestinal bleeding, upper tract.
  stress ulcers of, 662
Dying, care during. See End-of-life care in ICU.
Dynamic hyperinflation, 139–141, 139f–141f
  in asthma, 234
  in COPD, 233

Dynamic intrinsic positive end-expiratory pressure, 143–144, 145f
Dyskinesia, myocardial, 297
Dyspnea
  in acutely unstable patient, 190
  in amniotic fluid embolism, 627
  in ARDS, 245
  in COPD, 227
  in pneumonia, 572, 574t, 583
  in pulmonary embolism, 254, 254t
  treatment of, in end-of-life care, 219
Dysrhythmias. See Arrhythmias.

E

Echocardiography
  in acute coronary syndromes, 311
  in aortic dissection, 367, 367f
  in aortic regurgitation, 362
  in atrial fibrillation, 327–328
  in cardiac tamponade, 365
  in hemodynamic monitoring, 107, 107f
  in infective endocarditis, 360, 361f
  in mitral regurgitation, 363, 363f
  in pulmonary embolism, 257, 257f
  in thoracic trauma, 607
Eclampsia, hypertensive crisis in, 352–353
Ecstasy
  hyponatremia due to, 466
  poisoning from, 677
Edema
  cerebral
    in brain injury, 398–399
    in hypoglycemia, 502–503
    in liver failure, 536–538
  in burns, 614
  in preeclampsia, 628–629, 629t
  in right heart failure, 292–293
  in sepsis, 595
  pulmonary. See Pulmonary edema.
EEG. See Electroencephalography.
Elastance
  in cardiac function, 284, 284f
  in respiratory function, 141–142, 142f, 243
Elderly persons
  delirium in, 56
  pneumonia in, 569, 571f
Electrical gaps, in acid-base disorders, 450, 450t, 451t
Electrical injuries, 619–620
Electrical storm, 337
Electrocardiography
  after cardiac surgery, 644, 646f
  artifacts in, 336–337, 336f
  in acute coronary syndromes, 308–309, 309b, 309f
  in antidepressant poisoning, 673, 673f
  in aortic dissection, 366
  in atrial fibrillation, 326, 326f–328f
  in atrial flutter, 322, 324f
  in atrial tachycardia, 320, 323f
  in atrioventricular nodal reentrant tachycardia, 330f
  in atrioventricular reciprocating tachycardia, 331f
  in carbon monoxide poisoning, 680
  in cardiac tamponade, 365
  in cardiomyopathy, 359
  in COPD, 227
  in infective endocarditis, 360
  in long QT syndrome, 333, 333b, 334b, 335
  in mitral stenosis, 363, 364f
  in myocarditis, 358
  in pulmonary embolism, 255
  in subarachnoid hemorrhage, 407
  in supraventricular arrhythmias, 319, 322f

Electrocardiography—cont'd
  in ventricular tachycardia, 332, 332f, 333, 334f, 335, 335f
  with intra-aortic balloon pump, 357
Electroencephalography
  in agitation assessment, 54
  in brain death, 440
  in seizures, 422, 423f–426f, 429, 429f
  patterns in, 422–423, 423f–425f
Electromyography, in neuromuscular respiratory failure, 280
Electron transport system, in mitochondrial respiration, 41–42, 42f
Embolectomy, for pulmonary embolism, 259–260
Embolism
  air, 260–261
  amniotic fluid, 260, 627–628, 628f
  fat, 260
  gas, from intra-aortic balloon pump, 357
  in cardiac surgery, 640–641
  in infective endocarditis, 360
  pulmonary. See Pulmonary embolism.
Embolization
  for gastrointestinal bleeding, 523f, 524
  for obstetric hemorrhage, 631
Emergencies. See Cardiovascular emergencies; Crisis.
Emotional support, management of, 219–220
Emphysema. See also Chronic obstructive pulmonary disease.
  in diabetic ketoacidosis, 511
  subcutaneous
    in asthma, 227–228, 229f
    in mechanical ventilation, 163
Enalaprilat, for hypertensive crisis, 348t
Encephalopathy
  hepatic, 533, 534t
    cardiovascular management in, 539
    cerebral blood flow in, 537
    cerebral edema in, 536–538
    diagnosis of, 533, 534t
    grading of, 533, 534t
    ICP monitoring in, 385, 385t
    increased intracranial pressure in, 537–539
    monitoring of, 537–538
    treatment of, 536–540, 537f
  hypertensive, 346, 350
End-expiratory lung volume, measurement of, 139–141, 139f–141f
Endocarditis, infective
  native valve, 360–362, 360b, 361b, 361f
  prosthetic valve, 364
End-of-life care in ICU, 217–221
  components of, 219–220, 219b, 220b, 220f, 220t
  ethical issues in, 218–219, 218b
  legal issues in, 218–219, 218b
  prognostication in, 217–218
  versus hospice care, 217
Endogenous infections, 88, 88t
Endometritis, obstetric, 631–632, 632b
Endoscopy, in gastrointestinal bleeding, 518–519, 519f, 520f
Endothelial cell protein C receptor
  action of, 547, 547f
  in hemostasis regulation, 549, 549f, 550f
Endothelin, in vascular tone control, 37
Endothelium and endothelial cells
  activation phenotype of, 556–557, 556b
  function and dysfunction of, 556–557, 556b
    in hemostasis, 549, 549f, 550f
    in sepsis, 556–557, 556b, 557f
    mediators in, 557
    overlooking significance of, 556–557, 556b

Endothelium and endothelial cells—cont'd
  injury of, thrombosis in, 543, 549, 549f, 550f
  set point of, 557
Endotoxin (lipopolysaccharide)
  cytokine actions on, 18–19
  in ARDS, 248, 249f
  in sepsis, 591–593, 592f, 600
  neutralization of, in sepsis, 600
  transfusions contaminated with, 564t
Endotracheal aspirate stain, in ventilator-associated pneumonia, 179
Endotracheal intubation
  communication in, 201, 201f
  in spinal cord injury, 435
  of acutely unstable patient, 190
  of obese patients, 267–269, 268t
  pneumonia in, 81–83, 82b, 82t, 83f
  withdrawal of, at end-of-life, 220
Endovascular treatment, of intracranial aneurysm, 409, 409f
Energy balance, in respiratory muscle function, 275–277, 276f, 277f
Engineering controls, for infection control, 78
ENHANCE study, activated protein kinase C for inflammation, 11
Enoxaparin, for deep venous thrombosis, 260
Enteral nutrition, 202, 203f
  access for, 212
  advantages of, 212, 212f
  assessment for, 206, 206f
  difficult, 213, 213f, 214t
  for burns, 618
  for cardiac failure, 210, 211f
  for gut maintenance, 212
  for mechanical ventilation, 184, 184f
  for pancreatitis, 528
  in pregnancy, 635
  indications for, 212
  micronutrients in, 211
  postpyloric, 213, 213f
  solutions for, 213, 214t
  timing of, 207–208, 207f, 207t
Enterobacter pneumonia, 182t
Enterococcus faecalis infections, glycopeptides for, host defenses and, 68–69
Enteroscopy, in bleeding, 519
Environmental decontamination, from bioterrorism agents, 694–695
Eosinophils, in inflammation, 4t, 5
Epidural hematoma
  hypertensive crisis in, 351
  in brain injury, 395, 397f
Epilepsy, definition of, 415
Epinephrine
  for organ donors, 442
  in pregnancy, 635–636
  in stress response, 25
Epithelial cells, in inflammation, 3f, 5–6, 6b, 6f, 7f
Epithelial lining fluid, antibiotic levels in, 67
Epsilon-aminocaproic acid, for coagulopathy, 566
Eptifibatide, for myocardial infarction, 313
Equation of motion, for respiratory mechanics, 142
Equine antitoxin, for botulism, 690
Equipment, infection control and, 78
ERO₂ (oxygen extraction ratio), 46–48, 46f
ERV (expiratory reserve volume), in obesity, 264
Erythrocytes, transfusion of, 562
Erythropoietin-associated hypertensive crisis, 353
Escape, in stress response, 22–23
Escharotomy, for burns, 615, 616f
Escherichia coli pneumonia, 177, 177t, 182t
E-senc (inspiratory termination criteria), for pressure support ventilation, 112, 112f

Esmolol, for hypertensive crisis, 348t, 501
Esophageal pressure, measurement of, 141–142
Esophagus
  bleeding in. See Gastrointestinal bleeding, upper tract.
  injury of, 609
  spasm of, versus acute coronary syndromes, 308b
  temperature measurement in, 621
Ethanol use. See Alcohol use.
Ethical issues, in end-of-life care, 218–219, 218b
Ethylene glycol poisoning, 670–672, 671f, 671t
Eucapnia, in obesity, 264
Euglycemic ketoacidosis, 510, 511b
Euroscore, for cardiac surgery risk, 640
Euthanasia, 218
Exercise
  capacity for, in obesity, 265
  for myocardial infarction, 318
  heat stroke in, 622–623
  hyponatremia in, 466
Exhalation, in ARDS, 241–242, 241f
Expiratory reserve volume, in obesity, 264
Extended-spectrum beta-lactamases, bacteria producing, 84–85
Extracellular fluid
  antibiotic levels in, 66–67, 66t
  measurement of, in hypernatremia, 462–463, 463t
  osmolality of, 459–460
  volume of, in hyponatremia, 464–466
Extracorporeal Liver Assist Device, 540–541, 541t
Extracorporeal membrane oxygenation, for ARDS, 251
Extrinsic pathway, of coagulation cascade, 545–546, 546f
Eye care, 202
Eye protection, for infection control, 75t

F

Face masks, for noninvasive ventilation, in COPD, 230, 231f
Face shield, for infection control, 75t
Faces Scale, for pain assessment, 52
Factor(s), coagulation
  in hemostasis, 546–548, 546f, 547f
  transfusion of, 562–563
Factor VI Leiden mutation, 547–548
Factor VII
  in liver failure, 540
  replacement of, for coagulopathy, 566
Factor VIII, inhibitors of, 551
Famotidine, for gastrointestinal bleeding, 521
Fantoni tracheostomy technique, 133f
Fasciotomy, for compartment syndrome, 611
FAST examination, in abdominal injury, 610, 610f
Fasting, hypoglycemia in, 502–503
Fat embolism, 260
Fatty acids, polyunsaturated, in nutritional support, 210
Fatty liver of pregnancy, 533, 630–631, 630t
Fenoldopam, for hypertensive crisis, 347, 348t, 352
Fenoterol, for COPD, 228
Fentanyl, for pain, 53, 53t, 219
Fetomaternal hemorrhage, 633
Fetus
  injury of, 633
  oxygenation of, 627, 627f
  radiology risks to, 634, 634t, 636

FEV$_1$ (forced expiratory volume in one second), in obesity, 264–265
Fever
  after cardiac surgery, 647
  control of, in stress response, 29
  in systemic inflammatory response syndrome, 661–662, 662f
  transfusion-related, 564t
Fiber-optic systems, for ICP monitoring, 386t, 387
Fibrinogen, deficiency of, in liver failure, 534
Fibrinolysis, 543, 544f, 548–549, 548f
Fibroblasts, in inflammation, 3f, 7
Fick relationship, 44, 101, 388
Fisher grading scale, for subarachnoid hemorrhage, 406, 406f
Fistulas, in infective endocarditis, 360
Flail chest, 607
Fluconazole
  dosage of, during dialysis, 488t
  for postoperative infections, 661
Fludrocortisone, for subarachnoid hemorrhage, 412
Fluid responsiveness, measurement of, 105–107, 105f, 106f
Fluid therapy. *See also* Saline solutions.
  for burns, 614–617, 617b, 617t
  for diabetic ketoacidosis, 511–512, 512b, 512f, 513f
  for hepatorenal syndrome, 492–493, 493f, 493t
  for hyperosmolar nonketotic coma, 511–512, 512b, 512f, 513f
  for hyperthermia, 623
  for multiple trauma, 604–606, 606t
  for obstetric hemorrhage, 631
  for organ donors, 442–443
  for pheochromocytoma, 501
  for pneumonia, 577
  for preeclampsia, 629
  for sepsis, 598, 598f
  for spinal cord injury, 435
  for subarachnoid hemorrhage, 411
  for thyrotoxicosis, 498
  infusion-related acidosis in, 452
Fluid-filled catheter system, for ICP monitoring, 385–386, 386f, 386t
Flumazenil, as antidote, 668t, 672
Fluorocortisone, for sepsis, 599
Fluoroquinolones
  for ventilator-associated pneumonia, 182t, 661t
  host defenses and, 67–68, 68f
  tissue levels of, 66–67, 66t
Focal seizures, 420t
Folinic acid, as antidote, 668t, 670
Fomepizole, as antidote, 668t, 670
Fondaparinux, action of, 548
Forced expiratory volume in one second, in obesity, 264–265
Forced vital capacity, in obesity, 263–265, 265f
Formaldehyde formation, in methanol ingestion, 670
Formic acid formation, in methanol ingestion, 670
Forrest classification, of upper gastrointestinal tract bleeding lesions, 518, 519f
Fosphenytoin, for seizures, 426–427
FOXO transcription factors, for critical illness myopathy, 30
Fracture(s)
  fat embolism in, 260
  pelvic, 610–611
  rib, 607
  scapula, 607

Fracture(s)—cont'd
  skull, 399, 399f
  spinal, 432, 433f
  surgery for, postoperative care in, 660
Francisella tularensis infections (tularemia), 688t, 689, 689b
Frank-Starling law of the heart, 102, 104f, 284–286, 284f, 285f, 355
FRC (functional residual capacity)
  in obesity
    intraoperative, 266, 266f, 267
    postoperative, 270–272
    preoperative, 263–264
  in pregnancy, 625, 626f
Free fatty acids, in hyperglycemia, 507–508, 508f
Fresh frozen plasma, transfusion of, 562–563
Frova tracheostomy technique, 133f
Fulminant hepatic failure. *See* Liver failure.
Functional residual capacity
  in obesity
    intraoperative, 266, 266f, 267
    postoperative, 270–272
    preoperative, 263–264
  in partial ventilatory support, 152
  in pregnancy, 625, 626f
Fungal infections
  in liver failure, 536
  postoperative, 661
Futility, of treatment, 219
FVC (forced vital capacity), in obesity, 263–265, 265f

G

G proteins, in vascular tone control, 31, 32f
Gaeltec system, for ICP monitoring, 387
Gallstones, pancreatitis in, 525
Galveston formula, for burn resuscitation, 617t
Gamma-aminobutyric acid, in delirium, 55
Gamma-hydroxybutyrate (ecstasy)
  hyponatremia due to, 466
  poisoning from, 677
Ganciclovir, dosage of, during dialysis, 488t
Gaps, in acid-base disorders, 450–452, 450t, 451t
Gas embolism, from intra-aortic balloon pump, 357
Gas exchange
  evaluation of, in acutely unstable patient, 190
  in ARDS
    in diagnosis, 246
    pathophysiology and, 244–245, 245t
    positioning and, 242–243, 243f
  in mechanical ventilation, monitoring of, 146–148, 147f, 148t
  in obesity, 267
  in partial ventilatory support, 150, 151f, 152
  in pulmonary embolism, 256
Gastric lavage, for poisoning, 666, 666f
Gastric tonometry, in hypoxia, 48
Gastroduodenoscopy, in bleeding, 518, 519f, 520f
Gastrointestinal bleeding, 517–524
  complications of, 524b
  controversies in, 524b
  in sepsis, 595
  lower tract
    clinical features of, 518
    diagnosis of, 518–520
    epidemiology of, 517
    risk factors for, 517
    treatment of, 523–524, 523f
  pathogenesis of, 517
  pitfalls in, 524b
  postoperative, 662

Gastrointestinal bleeding—cont'd
  treatment of, 520–524
    in portal hypertension, 521–523, 522f, 523f
    lower tract, 523–524, 523f
    upper tract, 521–523, 522f, 523f
  upper tract
    clinical features of, 518, 518b, 518t
    diagnosis of, 518, 519f, 520f
    epidemiology of, 517
    prognosis for, 518, 518b
    rebleeding in, 522, 522f
    risk factors for, 517, 518t
    treatment of, 521–523, 522f, 523f
Gastrointestinal syndrome, bleeding in, in nutritional support, 214t
Gastrointestinal system
  decontamination of
    for antidepressant poisoning, 673
    for poisoning, 666, 666f
  maintenance of, enteral feeding for, 212, 212f
  physiology of, in pregnancy, 627
Gastroparesis, in nutritional support, 214t
Gatifloxacin, for ventilator-associated pneumonia, 183t
General anesthesia, for seizures, 427
Generalized convulsive status epilepticus, 418–419, 419t
Generalized seizures, 417, 420t, 423f, 426, 427t
Genetics, 13–19
  concepts of, 13, 14f
  for predisposition classification, 18
  future applications of, 19
  gene studies in, 14–17
    association, 14, 14f
    candidate genes for, 14–16, 15f, 15t, 16f
    genomic variations in, 15
    tumor necrosis factor as, 16–17, 17b, 17f
  genomic variations in, 13, 14f
  importance of, 13
  lessons learned in, 18
  Mendelian inheritance in, 13
  of anti-inflammatory cytokines, 17–18
  of asthma, 223–224
  of critical illness myopathy, 29–30, 29t
  of drug response, 18, 18t, 19t
  of pneumonia, 571, 572f, 572t
  of sepsis and septic shock, 571, 572f, 572t, 595–596, 596f, 596t
  promoter variants and, 17
Gentamicin
  for bioterrorist agents, 688t
  for ventilator-associated pneumonia, 182t, 183t
Gestational hypertension, 352–353
Gestational trophoblastic disease, 632
Glandular tularemia, 689
Glasgow Coma Scale
  in acutely unstable patient, 195, 195t
  in brain injury, 399, 399t
  in multiple trauma, 606, 606t
Glomerular filtration rate
  in kidney failure, 476–477
  in pregnancy, 627
Gloves, 75t
Glucagon
  as antidote, 668t
  for hypoglycemia, 502–503
  in stress response, 26
Glucocorticoids. *See* Corticosteroids.
Gluconeogenesis, in stress response, 26
Glucose
  as antidote, 668t
  for diabetic ketoacidosis, 512, 513
  for heart failure, 209–210
  for hyperosmolar nonketotic coma, 512, 513
  for hypoglycemia, 503

Glutamine
  for burns, 618
  for nutritional support, 212
  for stress response, 29
Glycemic control, in stress response, 29
Glycogenolysis, in stress response, 26
Glycolysis, anaerobic, 48
Glycopeptides, host defenses and, 68–69
Glycoprotein IIb/IIIA, in hemostasis, 544
Glycoprotein IIb/IIIA receptor antagonists
  for myocardial infarction, 313–314, 314f
  mechanism of action of, 544, 545f
Glycosuria, in diabetic ketoacidosis, 508–509,
    508f, 509f
Golden hours, in multiple trauma, 604
Gordon's syndrome, 469
Gowns, for infection control, 75t
Graft, for aortic dissection, 367
Graft versus host disease, transfusion-related,
    563
Gram stain, in ventilator-associated pneumonia,
    179
Gram-negative organisms, in ventilator-
    associated pneumonia, 177, 177t
Granulocyte colony-stimulating factor, for sepsis,
    601
Granulocyte transfusions, 563
Graves' disease, thyrotoxicosis in, 497–499
Grey-Turner's sign, in pancreatitis, 527
Griggs tracheostomy technique, 133f
Growth factors, in inflammation, 8, 9t
Growth hormone
  for critical illness myopathy, 30
  in stress response, 25–27, 26f, 28f
Growth hormone-releasing hormone, in stress
    response, 25–26, 26f
Guanethidine, for thyrotoxicosis, 498
Guanethine, for thyrotoxicosis, 498b
Guidewires, in tracheostomy, 131, 133f
Guillain-Barré syndrome
  hypertensive crisis in, 353
  respiratory failure in, 278–279
Gunshot wounds, multiple trauma in, 604
Guyton model for circulation, 286–288, 286f,
    288f

H

Haemophilus influenzae pneumonia, 177, 177t,
    182t
Haloperidol, for delirium, 59, 219
Hampton's hump, in pulmonary embolism,
    255
Hand hygiene, 75t, 76–78, 76b, 76f, 77f, 78b
  for bioterrorism agents, 694
  in vascular catheter care, 79
Head injury. See also Traumatic brain injury.
  hypertensive crisis in, 351
Headache
  in carbon monoxide poisoning, 680
  in hypertensive crisis, 344
  in pheochromocytoma, 500
  in subarachnoid hemorrhage, 406
Heart. See also subjects starting with
    Myocardial.
  arrhythmias of. See Arrhythmias.
  electrical injury of, 620
  function of. See Cardiac function.
  injury of, 359–360, 608
  lung interactions with. See Heart-lung
    interactions.
  rupture of
    left ventricular wall, 358
    traumatic, 359
  surgery on. See Cardiac surgery.
  valvular disease of. See Valvular heart disease.

Heart failure. See also Cardiovascular failure.
  after cardiac surgery, 648–652, 650f, 651f
  continuous positive airway pressure for, 374
  in COPD, 226
  in infective endocarditis, 360–362
  in multiorgan dysfunction syndrome, 591t
  in pregnancy, 635
  in prosthetic valve problems, 364
  nutritional support in, 209–210, 211f
  right, 291–293, 292f, 293f, 651–652, 651f
  versus cardiovascular failure, 283
Heart rate
  after cardiac surgery, 644
  in hepatorenal syndrome, 490
  in pregnancy, 625, 626t, 627
Heart-lung interactions, 369–382
  in cardiovascular dysfunction, 369–370, 370f
  in mechanical ventilation, 370–381
    airway pressure and, 370–374, 372f–374f
    intrathoracic pressure and, 377–381,
      377f–379f
    lung volume and, 374–377, 376f, 377f
    transpulmonary pressure and, 370–374,
      372f–374f
  mechanical considerations in, 376–377
Heart-lung machine, postoperative effects of,
    640
Heat loss, hypothermia in. See Hypothermia.
Heat stroke, 622–624, 623b
HELLP syndrome, 629–630, 630f
Helmet, for noninvasive ventilation, 128, 129f
Hemabate, for obstetric hemorrhage, 631
Hematemesis, in gastrointestinal bleeding, 518
Hematochezia, in gastrointestinal bleeding, 518
Hematologic system, physiology of, in pregnancy,
    627
Hematoma, epidural or subdural
  hypertensive crisis in, 351
  in brain injury, 395, 397f
Hematopoietic growth factors, for coagulopathy,
    567
Hematuria, in pelvic fractures, 610
Hemodialysis
  for ethylene glycol poisoning, 671t, 672
  for hepatorenal syndrome, 495
  for hyperkalemia, 471
  for lithium intoxication, 674
  for methanol poisoning, 671t
  for poisoning, 666–667, 667t
  intermittent, 482f, 483f, 486–487, 487f
  slow low-efficiency extended daily dialysis,
    481–482, 487, 487f
Hemodilution
  for cardiac surgery, 641
  for subarachnoid hemorrhage, 412
Hemodynamic(s)
  in ARDS, 247
  in liver failure, 539
  in pregnancy, 625, 626f, 626t, 627
  of heart-lung interactions. See Heart-lung
    interactions.
Hemodynamic monitoring, 101–108
  clinical trials of, 104, 104t
  complications of, 104, 104t
  controversies in, 108b
  equipment for, 104–105, 105b, 105f–107f
  in pregnancy, 636
  indications for, 101, 101b
  limitations of, 101
  minimally invasive, 105–107, 105b, 105f–107f
  outcome and, 102, 104, 104t
  oxygen delivery and, 102
  physiologic concepts of, 101–102, 103f
  postoperative, 658–659, 659t
  preload assessment, 102, 104f
  principles of, 101–104, 103f–104f, 104t

Hemodynamic monitoring—cont'd
  pulmonary artery catheter for, 105
  versus clinical examination, 102
Hemofiltration, continuous venovenous,
    481–482, 482f–486f, 484–486, 485b
Hemoglobin
  carbon monoxide binding to, 679, 680f–682f,
    681
  cerebral, near-infrared spectroscopy
    measurement of, 388t, 390–391
  in blood substitute products, 566, 566b
  in myocardial function, 294
  level of, in transfusion criteria, 562
Hemolysis
  in HELLP syndrome, 629–630
  in transfusion reactions, 563, 564t
Hemolytic anemia, autoimmune, transfusions
    for, 565
Hemoptysis
  in pneumonia, 574, 574t
  in pulmonary embolism, 254, 254t
Hemorrhage. See also Bleeding.
  after cardiac surgery, 646
  cerebral, hypertensive crisis in, 350–351
  estimation of, in multiple trauma, 604–605,
    606t
  fetomaternal, 633
  gastrointestinal. See Gastrointestinal
    bleeding.
  in pelvic fractures, 610–611
  liver, in HELLP syndrome, 629–630, 630f
  obstetric, 631
  Strich, 396
  subarachnoid. See Subarachnoid
    hemorrhage.
Hemorrhagic fevers, 688t, 691, 691b
Hemostasis
  coagulation cascade in, 545–548, 546f–548f
  disorders of. See Bleeding; Coagulopathy;
    Thrombosis.
  endothelium in, 549, 549f, 550f
  fibrinolytic system in, 548–549, 548f
  overview of, 543–544, 544f
  platelets in, 544, 545
  primary, 543
  secondary, 543
Hemostatic techniques, for gastrointestinal
    bleeding, 522–523, 523f
Hemothorax, 608
Henderson-Hasselbalch equation, 445
Heparan sulfate
  action of, 546
  in hemostasis regulation, 549, 549f, 550f
Heparin
  action of, 546
  for continuous renal replacement therapy, 485,
    485f
  for deep venous thrombosis, 260
  for myocardial infarction, 314–316
  for pulmonary embolism, 258–259, 634
  for venous thromboembolism prevention,
    662
  tissue factor pathway inhibitor interactions
    with, 548
Hepatassist bioartificial liver, 541, 541t
Hepatic encephalopathy. See Encephalopathy,
    hepatic.
Hepatitis A, liver failure in, 535
Hepatitis B
  liver failure in, 535
  transfusion-related, 563, 565t
Hepatitis C
  liver failure in, 535
  organ transplantation in, 441
  transfusion-related, 563, 565t
Hepatocytes, in artificial liver, 541, 541t

Index

Hepatorenal syndrome, 478–479, 539–540, 539b
  causes of, 489
  clinical features of, 491–492, 491b, 492f
  controversies in, 496b
  diagnosis of, 491–492, 491b, 492f, 539, 539b
  natural history of, 540
  pathogenesis of, 489–491, 491f
  prevention of, 495, 496b, 496f
  survival in, 492, 492f
  treatment of, 492–495
  type 1
    clinical features of, 491–492, 492f
    treatment of, 492–494, 493f, 493t, 494f
  type 2
    clinical features of, 491–492, 492f
    treatment of, 495, 495f
Heredity, laws of, 13
Heroin, poisoning from, 675
Hospice care
Host defenses, antibiotic action and, 67–69, 68f
Human immunodeficiency virus infection
  organ transplantation in, 441
  pneumonia in, 582, 586
  transfusion-related, 563, 565t
Human T-cell lymphocytic virus infections, transfusion-related, 563, 565t
Hunger, management of, in end-of-life care, 219
Hunt and Hess classification, of subarachnoid hemorrhage, 406, 406t
Hydatidiform mole, 632
Hydralazine
  for hypertensive crisis, 348t, 353
  for preeclampsia, 628
Hydrocephalus
  ICP monitoring in, 385, 385t
  in subarachnoid hemorrhage, 409–410, 410f
Hydrochloric acid, for metabolic alkalosis, 455
Hydrocortisone
  for adrenal crisis, 505
  for asthma, 233
  for inflammation, 10
  for sepsis, 599
  for subarachnoid hemorrhage, 412
  for thyrotoxicosis, 498b
Hydromorphone, for pain, 53, 53t
Hydroxocobalamin, as antidote, 668t
β-Hydroxybutyrate
  in diabetic ketoacidosis, 507–509
  in hyperosmolar nonketotic coma, 507–509
Hydroxyethyl starch, for subarachnoid hemorrhage, 411
Hyperammonemia, in liver failure, 534–537
Hyperbaric oxygen therapy, for carbon monoxide poisoning, 682
Hypercapnia
  acid-base disorders in, 452t
  definition of, 450t
  in asthma, 227, 233
  in COPD, 224, 226, 227
  in neuromuscular respiratory failure, 277–278, 280
  in obesity, 264, 265
Hypercoagulability, pulmonary embolism in, 253
Hyperglycemia
  critical illness polyneuropathy and myopathy in, 279
  in stress response, 29
  nutritional support and, 208–209, 210t
  of critical illness, 502
  pathogenesis of, 507–509, 508f, 509f
  severe, 502

Hyperinflation, 139–141, 139f–141f
  in asthma and COPD, 224–225, 233, 234
Hyperkalemia
  approach to, 469–470
  causes of, 468, 470b
  hyponatremia with, 465
  in Gordon's syndrome, 469
  in hyperthermia, 624
  in kidney failure, 481
  treatment of, 470–471
Hyperlactatemia, in liver failure, 534
Hypermetabolism
  in burns, 614, 618
  in sepsis, 595
  in stress response, 24, 24f, 26–27
Hypernatremia, 462–464
  assessment of, 462–463, 463t
  causes of, 462, 462b
  clinical approach to, 463
  definition of, 462
  in diabetic ketoacidosis, 509
  physiology of, 462, 462b
  treatment of, 463–464
Hyperosmolar nonketotic coma, 502
  clinical course of, 514
  clinical features of, 509–510, 510b
  complications of, 514–515, 514b
  controversies in, 515
  epidemiology of, 507
  pathogenesis of, 507–509
  pitfalls in, 514b
  prevention of, 514
  treatment of, 510–514, 511b, 512b, 512f, 513f
Hyperphosphatemia, in liver failure, 534
Hypertension
  intracranial. See Intracranial pressure, increased.
  portal. See Portal hypertension.
  pulmonary, in COPD, 227
  systemic. See also Hypertensive crisis.
    after cardiac surgery, 643, 643f, 644f
    aortic dissection in, 365
    in preeclampsia, 628–629, 629t
    in subarachnoid hemorrhage, 407, 412
Hypertensive crisis, 343–354
  aortic dissection in, 351
  catecholamine-associated, 352, 353f
  cerebral ischemia in, 350
  definition of, 343
  differential diagnosis of, 346, 346f
  encephalopathy in, 346, 350
  epidemiology of, 343
  erythropoietin-associated, 353
  evaluation in, 343–346, 346f
  gestational, 352–353
  in antiphospholipid antibody syndrome, 353
  in burns, 353
  in diabetes mellitus, 353
  in head trauma, 351
  in kidney transplantation, 353
  in myocardial infarction, 352
  in pheochromocytoma, 501
  in scleroderma, 353
  in spinal cord injury, 353
  intracerebral hemorrhage in, 350–351
  malignant hypertension as, 347, 349f, 350
  pathophysiology of, 343, 344f, 345f
  postoperative, 352
  pulmonary edema in, 351–352
  subarachnoid hemorrhage in, 350
  treatment of
    guidelines for, 346, 347f
    in pheochromocytoma, 501
    medications for, 346–347, 348t
  versus pseudohypertension, 344

Hyperthermia, 622–624
  diagnosis of, 623
  differential diagnosis of, 622, 623b
  in thyrotoxicosis, 497
  pathogenesis of, 623
  prevention of, 624
  risk factors for, 623, 623b
  treatment of, 623–624
Hyperthyroidism, life-threatening, 497–499, 497b, 499f
Hypertrophic cardiomyopathy, 358–359
Hyperventilation
  control of, in subarachnoid hemorrhage, 407
  for increased ICP, 400, 401
Hypervolemia, in subarachnoid hemorrhage, 411
Hypocapnia
  acid-base disorders in, 452t
  definition of, 450t
Hypoglycemia, 502–503
  in brain injury, 399
  in hypothyroidism, 500
  in liver failure, 534
Hypokalemia
  approach to, 471–473, 471b, 472f
  causes of, 471b, 472
  hyponatremia with, 465
  in anabolism, 468
  renal replacement therapy effects on, 483f
  treatment of, 472–473
Hypokalemic periodic paralysis, 472
Hypometabolic phase, of stress response, 24
Hyponatremia, 464–468
  after prostate surgery, 467
  approach to, 465–467, 466f, 467f
  assessment of, 464–465
  causes of, 464, 464b
  definition of, 464
  in ecstasy use, 466
  in exercise, 466
  in hepatorenal syndrome, 490
  in hypothyroidism, 500
  in liver failure, 534, 538
  in subarachnoid hemorrhage, 411–412, 412t
  laboratory tests in, 465
  physiology of, 464, 464b
  postoperative, 467
  renal replacement therapy and, 483f
  treatment of, 467–468
Hypotension
  after cardiac surgery, 642, 642t, 643t
  in burns, 617
  in decreased systemic vascular resistance, 284, 284b
  in hepatorenal syndrome, 490
  in liver failure, 539
  in pregnancy, 635
  in pulmonary embolism, 260
  in spinal cord injury, 435
  kidney failure in, 479, 480f
  treatment of, 298, 298f
Hypothalamic-pituitary-adrenal axis, in stress response, 24
Hypothermia
  brain death declaration and, 440
  classification of, 621, 622t
  diagnosis of, 621
  in blood transfusions, 563–564
  in cardiac surgery, 640–641
  in hypothyroidism, 499
  in liver failure, 538, 539
  in multiple trauma, 607, 607b
  in sepsis, 597
  prevention of, 622
  rewarming in, 607, 607b
  risk factors for, 621, 622b

Hypothermia—cont'd
  therapeutic, for brain injury, 401
  treatment of, 621–622
Hypothyroidism
  critical, 499–500, 499b
  hypothermia in, 622
Hypoventilation, control of, in subarachnoid
    hemorrhage, 407
Hypovolemia
  after cardiac surgery, 642
  in acutely unstable patient, 192–194, 193b,
    193f
  in burns, 614
  in diabetic ketoacidosis, 509, 511–512, 512b,
    512f
  in hyperosmolar nonketotic coma, 509,
    511–512, 512b, 512f
  in sepsis, 594–595, 594f
Hypovolemic shock
  in gastrointestinal bleeding, 518
  in multiple trauma, 605–606
Hypoxemia
  in acutely unstable patient, 190
  in ARDS, 244–245, 246t
  in neuromuscular respiratory failure, 277
  in obesity, 264, 265, 267
  in pneumonia, 572
  in pulmonary embolism, 256
  respiratory failure in, noninvasive ventilation
    for, 124–125
Hypoxemic hypoxia, 45, 45f
Hypoxia
  anaerobic metabolism in, 48
  anemic, 45
  assessment of, gastric tonometry in, 48
  cerebral vasodilation in, 392
  cytopathic, 595
  hypoxemic, 45, 45f
  in carbon monoxide poisoning, 680
  in COPD, 224, 227
  in diabetic ketoacidosis, 511, 511b
  in hyperosmolar nonketotic coma, 511, 511b
  in pregnancy, 625
  in sepsis, 594–595, 594f
  physiological, 44
  pulmonary vasoconstriction in, 375
  stagnant, 44–45, 44f, 45f

I

Ibuprofen, for pain, 53t
Ibutilide, for atrial fibrillation, 327
ICP. See Intracranial pressure.
Illness, severity of, measures of. See Severity of
    illness measures.
Imipenem
  dosage of, during dialysis, 488t
  for bioterrorist agents, 688t
  for ventilator-associated pneumonia, 180, 182t
  host defenses and, 67
Immobility, complications of, prevention of, 201
Immune cells. See also specific cell types.
  in inflammation, 2–5, 4t, 5f
Immunodeficiency
  isolation for, 75
  pneumonia in, 571, 572f, 572t, 581–587
Immunoglobulin(s)
  deficiency of, pneumonia in, 581, 582t, 586
  transfusion of, 563
Immunoglobulin E, in inflammation, 5
Immunomodulation, transfusion-related, 563
Indirect calorimetry
  in burns, 618
  in hemodynamic monitoring, 107
Indirect Fick method, in hemodynamic
    monitoring, 107

Indomethacin, for hepatic encephalopathy, 539
Infection(s)
  after hypothermia, 622
  catheter-related, 78–81, 78f, 80f, 80t, 81f,
    661
  control of. See Infection control.
  diabetic ketoacidosis in, 507, 510
  hepatorenal syndrome in, 492
  hyperosmolar nonketotic coma in, 507, 510
  hypothyroidism in, 499
  in pancreatitis, 526–528, 526f, 527t
  nosocomial. See Nosocomial infections.
  postoperative, 660–661, 660f, 661t
  transfusion-related, 563, 564t, 565t
  transmission routes for, 74–75
Infection control, 71–86. See also Antibiotics.
  antibiotic prophylaxis in. See Antibiotics,
    prophylactic.
  antibiotic resistance and. See Antibiotics,
    resistance to.
  benefits of, 73, 74f, 85, 85t
  catheter avoidance in, 78
  controversies in, 85, 85b
  educational programs for, 79–81, 80f, 80t, 81f
  equipment-related, 78
  hand hygiene for, 76–79, 76b, 76f, 77f, 78b
  implementation of, 74
  in bioterrorism attack, 693, 693b
  in burns, 618
  in central venous access lines, 78–79, 78f
  in mechanical ventilation, 81–83, 82b, 82t,
    83f, 183–185, 183b, 184f, 184t, 185f
  isolation precautions in, 75, 75t, 76b
  logistics for, 73, 74f
  nursing interventions for, 199–200
  nutrition for, 78
  of gram-negative rods, 84–85
  principles of, 74–78, 75t, 76b, 76f, 77f, 78b
  risks of, 85, 85t
  staffing issues in, 78
  surveillance in, 74
  transmission routes and, 74–75
  vaccination for, 78
Infective endocarditis
  native valve, 360–362, 360b, 361b, 361f
  prosthetic valve, 364
Inflammation, 1–12
  after cardiac surgery, 640
  clinical presentation of, 9
  coagulopathy interactions with, 555–557,
    556b, 556f, 557f
  diagnosis of, 9
  etiology of, 8–9, 9t
  in ARDS, 237–238, 238f
  in burns, 613–614, 614f
  in coronary artery disease, 306
  in mechanical ventilation, 164–166, 165f, 166f
  laboratory tests in, 9
  nutritional support in, 210
  pathophysiology of, 1–8, 2t, 3f, 4f, 661–662,
    662f
    endothelial cells in, 3f, 4f, 6–7
    epithelial cells in, 3f, 5–6, 6b, 6f, 7f
    fibroblasts in, 3f, 7
    immune cells in, 2–5, 4t, 5f
    inflammatory mediators in, 7–8, 7t, 9t
  radiography in, 9
  treatment of, 9–11, 10t, 11f
Inflammatory mediators. See also specific
    mediators.
  in inflammation, 7–8, 7t, 9t
  in mechanical ventilation, 165–166, 166f
Inflation, lung, in ARDS, 241, 241f
Influenza, vaccination for, 578, 578b
Informant Questionnaire on Cognitive Decline in
    the Elderly, 57

Informed consent, 219
Infusion-related acidosis, 452
Inhalation injuries, 619
Inhalational anthrax, 686–687, 687f, 688t
Inhalational tularemia, 689
Injury(ies)
  abdominal, 609–611, 610f, 633–634
  aortic, 608–609
  aortic valve, 359
  brain. See Traumatic brain injury.
  burn. See Burn(s).
  cardiac, 359–360, 608
  diaphragmatic, 609
  electrical, 619–620
  esophageal, 609
  fetal, 633
  in pregnancy, 633–634
  inhalation, 619
  irreversible, 22
  liver, 623
  lung. See Acute lung injury (ALI).
  multiple. See Multiple trauma.
  severe, nutritional support in, 211t
  spinal cord. See Spinal cord injury.
  thoracic, 605f, 606f, 607–609
  tracheal, 608
InnerSpace system, for ICP monitoring, 386t,
    387
Inotropic agents, for sepsis, 599
INR (international normalized ratio), 551
Inspiration
  detection of, in mechanical ventilation, 158
  in ARDS, 241, 241f
  in obesity, 265
  muscles involved in, dysfunction of, 275–277,
    276f, 277f
  right atrial pressure changes with, 290, 291f
Inspiratory duty cycle, 276
Inspiratory muscle dysfunction, 280
Inspiratory termination criteria, for pressure
    support ventilation, 112, 112f
Inspiratory time, in mechanical ventilation, lung
    injury and, 166–167
Insulin
  for diabetic ketoacidosis, 513–514, 513f
  for heart failure, 209–210
  for hyperkalemia, 470
  for hyperosmolar nonketotic coma, 513–514,
    513f
  for sepsis, 557–558
  in potassium movement, 468
  production of, after brain stem death, 442
  resistance to
    in sepsis, 595
    in severe hyperglycemia, 502
    in stress response, 27
  with nutritional support, 208–209, 210t
Insulin-like growth factor-1
  in critical illness myopathy, 30
  in inflammation, 9t
  in stress response, 25–26, 26f, 27
Insulinoma, hypoglycemia in, 502–503
Intensive Care Delirium Screening Checklist, 58
Interictal spikes, in EEG, 422, 423f
Interleukin(s)
  in inflammation, 8
  in sepsis, 593, 593t
Interleukin-1
  in inflammation, 17
  in pneumonia, 572
  in sepsis, 555–556, 556f
  inhibitors of, for sepsis, 600–601
Interleukin-6, in inflammation, 17
Interleukin-10, anti-inflammatory, 17
Intermittent hemodialysis, 482f, 483f, 486–487,
    487f

Intermittent mandatory pressure release
    ventilation, 150
Intermittent mandatory ventilation, 149, 156t
International Ascites Club, hepatorenal
    syndrome criteria of, 491b
International Classification of Spinal Cord Injury,
    432, 433f
International normalized ratio (INR), 551
Intestine, ischemia of, in nutritional support,
    214t
Intoxication. See Poisoning.
Intra-aortic balloon pump, 356–357, 356f, 357f,
    654–656, 655f
Intracellular fluid
    analysis of, in hypernatremia, 463–464
    potassium in, 468
    volume of, in hyponatremia, 464
Intracerebral hemorrhage, hypertensive crisis in,
    350–351
Intracranial compliance, 383–384
Intracranial pressure, 383–387
    control of, in subarachnoid hemorrhage, 407
    definition of, 383
    increased
        clinical features of, 384
        hypertensive crisis in, 351
        in brain injury, 399–401, 400f
        in liver failure, 537–539
        in subarachnoid hemorrhage, 409–410, 410f
        pathophysiology of, 383–384, 384f
        treatment of, 400–401, 400f
    monitoring of
        complications of, 387
        contraindications for, 384–385
        equipment for, 385–387, 386f, 386t
        in brain injury, 400–401, 400f
        in liver failure, 537–538
        indications for, 384–385, 385t
        sites for, 385
        techniques for, 385–387, 386f, 386t
    renal replacement therapy effects on, 483f
    uncontrollable, 384
Intraoperative risks, 658
Intrathoracic pressure, hemodynamic effects of,
    377–381, 377f, 378f
Intrinsic pathway, of coagulation cascade, 545
Iodine, for thyrotoxicosis, 498, 498b
Ion exchange resins, for hyperkalemia, 471–472
Iopanoic acid, for thyrotoxicosis, 498, 498b
Ipratropium bromide, for COPD, 228
Iron poisoning, 668t
Ischemia
    cerebral
        in hypertensive crisis, 350
        in injury, 398
    intestinal, in nutritional support, 214t
    myocardial. See Myocardial ischemia.
Ischemic penumbra, 350
Isolation precautions, 75, 75t, 76b, 693
Isoprenaline, for asthma, 233
Isopropanol poisoning, 669

J

Judgment, substituted, 218
Jugular bulb venous oxygen saturation, in
    cerebral blood flow measurement, 388t,
    389
Jugular veins, evaluation of, in hypovolemia,
    192–193, 193f

K

Kaliuresis, 470
Kayexalate, for hyperkalemia, 471–472

Ketoacidosis
    diabetic. See Diabetic ketoacidosis.
    euglycemic, 510, 511b
Ketonemia, in isopropanol poisoning, 669
Kety-Schmidt technique, in cerebral blood flow
    measurement, 388, 388t
Kidney
    dysfunction of
        dialysis for. See Dialysis.
        in cirrhosis, 489–490. See also Hepatorenal
            syndrome.
        postoperative, 659
        failure of. See Kidney failure.
    in acid-base balance compensation, 450
    ischemia of, in aortic dissection, 366
    perfusion of, in partial ventilatory support,
        153
    physiology of, in pregnancy, 627
    poisons excreted from, forcing methods for,
        666–667, 667t
    potassium excretion from, 468–469
    transplantation of, hypertensive crisis in,
        353
Kidney failure, 475–488
    assessment of, 476–477
    classification of, 477–479, 477f, 478b, 478t
    clinical features of, 479
    definition of, 475, 476f
    diagnosis of, 480–481
    epidemiology of, 475–476, 476f
    etiology of, 477–479, 477f, 478b, 478t
    in carbon monoxide poisoning, 680
    in ethylene glycol poisoning, 671–672, 671f
    in HELLP syndrome, 629
    in hepatorenal syndrome. See Hepatorenal
        syndrome.
    in hyperthermia, 623, 624
    in malignant hypertension, 347, 349f
    in multiorgan dysfunction syndrome, 591t
    in obstetric hemorrhage, 631
    in rhabdomyolysis, 479
    in sepsis, 595
    nutritional support in, 211t
    parenchymal, 477f, 478, 478b
    pathogenesis of, 479
    postrenal, 477f, 478
    prerenal, 477–478, 477f, 478t
    prevention of, 479–480, 480f
    radiocontrast-induced, 480
    treatment of, 481
        continuous, 484–486, 484f–486f, 485b
        continuous renal replacement therapy in,
            481–482, 482f–486f, 484–486, 485b
        drug prescription during, 487–488, 488t
        intermittent dialysis in, 482f, 483f,
            486–487, 487f
        methods for, 481–482, 481f, 482b,
            482f–484f
        transfusions in, 565
Killing rate, of antibiotics, 63, 64f
Kings College Hospital criteria, for liver failure,
    531, 532b
KIR2.2 channel, in vascular tone control, 35
Klebsiella pneumoniae pneumonia, 177, 177t,
    182t, 573
Krebs cycle, 41
Kussmaul breathing, in metabolic acidosis,
    510

L

Labetalol
    for aortic dissection, 367
    for hypertensive crisis, 348t
        gestational, 353
        in subarachnoid hemorrhage, 350

Lactic acid production
    in septic shock, 102
    in tissue hypoxia, 48
Lactic acidosis, 452–453, 454b
Langfitt curve, for intracranial pressure/volume,
    384, 384f
Laryngeal mask airway, for intubation, of obese
    patients, 268
Laryngoscopy, for intubation, of obese patients,
    268
Lavage
    gastric, for poisoning, 666, 666f
    peritoneal, for abdominal injury, 609
Left ventricular free wall rupture, 358
Legal issues
    in brain death, 439
    in end-of-life care, 218–219, 218b
Legionella pneumonia, 573, 573f, 575–576, 582,
    582f, 583f, 585t
Lenercept, for inflammation, 10
Lepirudin, for pulmonary embolism, 258
Leukemia, pneumonia in, 581
Leukocytosis, in pneumonia, 572
Leukopenia, in sepsis, 597
Levofloxacin, for ventilator-associated
    pneumonia, 182t, 183t
Liddle's syndrome, 469
Lidocaine
    for arrhythmias, 321b
    for hypertensive crisis, 501
Lifestyle modifications, for myocardial
    infarction, 318
Lightning injuries, 619–620
Limbic seizures, 418
Linezolid
    for pneumonia, 183t, 577, 661t
    tissue levels of, 66
Linton–Nachlas tube, for gastrointestinal
    bleeding, 523
Lipase, elevated, in pancreatitis, 527
Lipolysis
    in hyperglycemia, 507–508, 508f
    in stress response, 26
Lipopolysaccharide. See Endotoxin
    (lipopolysaccharide).
Lipopolysaccharide-binding protein, in sepsis,
    592, 592f
Liquid ventilation, in ARDS, 251
Lithium
    for thyrotoxicosis, 498
    poisoning from, 673–674
Lithium dilution, in cardiac output assessment,
    107
Liver
    artificial, 541, 541t
    cirrhosis of
        hepatorenal syndrome in. See Hepatorenal
            syndrome.
        portal hypertension in. See Portal
            hypertension.
    disease of, in pregnancy, differential diagnosis
        of, 630t
    dysfunction of, postoperative, 659
    failure of. See Liver failure.
    hemorrhage of, in HELLP syndrome,
        629–630, 630f
    injury of, in hyperthermia, 623
    shock, in sepsis, 595
    transplantation of, 493t, 494–495, 541, 542f,
        542t
Liver failure, 531–542
    biochemical changes in, 534–535
    definitions of, 531, 532t
    diagnosis of, 533–535, 533t, 534t, 535f
    encephalopathy in. See Encephalopathy,
        hepatic.

Liver failure—cont'd
  epidemiology of, 531
  etiology of, 531, 532f, 532t
  hematologic changes in, 534
  hepatorenal syndrome in. See Hepatorenal
    syndrome.
  ICP monitoring in, 385, 385t
  in acetaminophen poisoning, 674
  in Budd–Chiari syndrome, 533
  in multiorgan dysfunction syndrome, 591t
  in pregnancy, 533
  in sepsis, 595
  in Wilson's disease, 533, 535, 536f
  pathogenesis of, 531
  pathology of, 535–536, 535f, 536f
  prognosis for, 531–533, 532b, 533b
  scores for, 518, 518b
  transfusions for, 565
  transport to special centers in, 533, 533t
  treatment of, 536–542
    antibiotics in, 536
    controversies in, 541b
    liver support systems in, 540–541, 541t
    pitfalls in, 542b
    respiratory support in, 540
    transplantation in, 541, 542f, 542t
    with cardiovascular disorders, 539
    with coagulation disorders, 540
    with encephalopathy, 536–539, 537f
    with kidney failure, 539–540, 539b
    with sepsis, 536
Long QT syndrome, 333, 333b, 334b, 335
Lorazepam
  for agitation and anxiety, 55, 55t, 219
  for burns, 618
  for seizures, 426, 428t
Lower motor neuron disease, respiratory failure
  in, 278t
Lumbar puncture, in seizures, 422
Lund and Browder chart, for burn estimation,
  615, 615f
Lund approach, to brain injury treatment, 401
Lung. See also subjects starting with Pulmonary.
  auscultation of, in acutely unstable patient,
    190
  autonomic innervation of, 374
  "baby," in ARDS, 238, 239f, 240
  biopsy of, in pneumonia, 585, 586t
  contusion of, 608
  heart interactions with. See Heart-lung
    interactions.
  hyperinflation of
    in asthma, 224–225, 234
    in COPD, 224–225, 233
  inflammation of, in ARDS, 237–238, 238f
  inflation of
    hemodynamic effects of, 374–377, 376f,
      377f
    in ARDS, 241, 241f
  injury of. See also Acute lung injury (ALI).
    in mechanical ventilation. See Mechanical
      ventilation, lung injury in.
    inhalation, 619
  partitioning of, in ARDS, 247
  pressure-volume relationship of, in ARDS,
    247, 247f
  radial interstitial forces of, 376
  recruitment of, in ARDS, 241, 241f
  respirator. See Mechanical ventilation, lung
    injury in.
  volume of
    hemodynamics and, 374–377, 376f, 377f
    in ARDS, 238, 239f, 240, 247
    in COPD, 227
    in obesity, 264, 266, 266f, 271
    versus size of animal, 162–163, 162f

Lung compliance, in obesity, 264
Lung injury score, in ARDS, 245
Luteinizing hormone, in stress response, 27, 28
Lymphadenitis, in tularemia, 689
Lymphocyte(s), in inflammation, 3f, 4f

M
Macrophage(s)
  in inflammation, 2–3, 3f, 4t, 8
  in sepsis, 555, 556f
Magnesium
  for diabetic ketoacidosis, 513
  for hyperosmolar nonketotic coma, 513
Magnesium sulfate, for preeclampsia, 629
Magnetic resonance imaging
  in aortic dissection, 367
  in cerebral blood flow measurement, 391,
    391f
  in gastrointestinal bleeding, 520
  in pulmonary embolism, 257
  in spinal cord injury, 435, 435f
Malignant hypertension, 347, 349f, 350
Malnutrition
  nutritional support for. See Nutritional
    support.
  pneumonia in, 571
Mannitol
  for increased ICP, 400, 538–539
  for kidney protection, 480
Masks
  for infection control, 75t
  for noninvasive ventilation, 121, 128, 129f,
    230, 231f, 232f
Mast cell(s), in inflammation, 3f, 4t, 5
Matrix metalloproteinases, in inflammation, 8,
  165, 165f
Maximal transdiaphragmatic pressure, 276, 280
Maximal voluntary ventilation, in obesity,
  263–264
MD_2 protein, in sepsis, 592–593, 592f
Mean circulatory filling pressure, in
  cardiovascular failure, 286–289, 286f,
  288f, 289f, 298
Mean inspiratory flow, in obesity, 265
Mean inspiratory flow rate, 276
Mean tidal pressure, in respiratory muscle
  function, 275–276
Mechanical perfusion therapy, for myocardial
  infarction, 316–317, 316f, 317f
Mechanical ventilation
  airborne pathogens expired from, 694
  communication in, 201, 201f
  complications of, 169, 234–235, 235b,
    660–661, 661t
    lung injury as, 2f–6f, 161–167, 167b
    pneumonia as. See Mechanical ventilation,
      pneumonia in.
  delayed versus premature, 169, 170b
  diaphragmatic dysfunction in, 280
  dyssynchrony in, 109
  equipment for, infection control with, 184
  eye care in, 202
  for acute hypercapnic respiratory failure,
    121–122, 123f
  for acute hypoxemic respiratory failure,
    124–125
  for ARDS, 250–251
  for asthma, 127, 234
  for botulism, 690
  for brain injury, 400
  for bronchoscopy, 127
  for carbon monoxide poisoning, 681–682
  for COPD, 230, 230t, 231f, 232–233, 232f
  for flail chest, 607
  for hepatic encephalopathy, 540

Mechanical ventilation—cont'd
  for hypothyroidism, 500
  for inhalation injury, 619
  for liver failure, 540
  for pneumonia, 125–126, 586, 586f
  for pneumonia prevention, 184, 184t, 185f
  for pulmonary edema, 122–124
  for sepsis, 557–558, 598
  for tracheostomy procedure, 131
  for ventilator liberation, 126–127
  heart-lung interactions in. See Heart-lung
    interactions.
  iatrogenic cost of, 250
  in obesity, 269–270, 272, 272b
  in organ donors, 443
  in pregnancy, 636–637
  inflammatory response in, 6, 6f, 7f
  liberation from, noninvasive ventilation for,
    126–127
  lung injury in, 161–167
    alveolar overdistention in, 162–163, 162f
    atelectrauma in, 163–164, 164f
    barotrauma in, 162–163, 162f
    biotrauma in, 164–166, 165f, 166f
    first recognition of, 161
    forms of, 161, 162f
    inspiratory time and, 166–167
    monitoring for, 167, 167b
    oxygen concentration and, 166
    pathophysiology of, 162–167
    respiratory rate and, 166–167
    risk factors for, 162–167
    volutrauma in, 162–163, 162f
  modes of, 109–120
    adaptive support, 115–116, 115f
    airway pressure release, 118, 118f, 119f,
      150, 151f, 152–153, 156t, 157
    assist/control, 110, 111b, 111f, 142–146,
      145f–147f, 149, 171t
    automatic tube compensation, 116–117,
      116f, 149, 156–157, 156t
    bilevel pressure, 118, 119f
    biphasic positive airway pressure, 150,
      152–153, 154t, 157
    classic, 109, 110b
    continuous positive airway pressure. See
      Continuous positive airway pressure.
    control, 110, 110f, 111f
    intermittent mandatory, 149, 156t
    intermittent mandatory pressure release,
      150
    new, 109, 110b
    pressure, 109, 110b
    pressure support, 110–112, 112f, 113f,
      149–150, 152, 156t, 170, 171t
    pressure-regulated volume control, 114
    proportional assist, 117, 149, 155–158,
      156f, 156t, 157f
    synchronized intermittent mandatory,
      112–114, 113f–115f, 170, 171, 232
    T-piece, 170, 171, 171t
    volume, 109, 110b
    volume support, 114–115
    volume-assured pressure support, 117–118,
      117f
  monitoring of, 137–148
    during controlled ventilation, 137–142
    during partial support, 142–146
    dynamic intrinsic PEEP, 143–144, 145f
    equation of motion in, 142
    for lung injury, 167, 167b
    gas exchange, 146–148, 147f, 148t
    resistance, 138–139
    respiratory mechanics and, 137–138,
      138f
    static compliance, 141–142, 142f, 143f

Mechanical ventilation—cont'd
  monitoring of—cont'd
    static intrinsic positive end-expiratory
      pressure, 139–141, 139f–141f, 143–144,
      145f
    stress index, 142, 144f
    work of breathing, 144–145, 146f, 147f
  noninvasive, 82, 121–130
    contraindications for, 127, 127b
    equipment for, 128, 128f, 129f
    for acute hypercapnic respiratory failure,
      121–122, 123f
    for acute hypoxemic respiratory failure,
      124–125
    for asthma, 127, 234
    for bronchoscopy, 127
    for cardiogenic pulmonary edema, 122–124
    for COPD, 230, 230t, 231f, 232f
    for pneumonia, 125–126, 586, 586f
    for pneumonia prevention, 184, 184t, 185f
    for ventilator liberation, 126–127
    for weaning, 171, 172f
    in end-of-life care, 219
    in pregnancy, 636
    indications for, 127b
    techniques for, 128, 129f
    ventilator modes for, 128, 129f
  partial support with, 149–159, 156b
    cardiovascular effects of, 152
    classification of, 149–150
    contraindications for, 150
    controversies in, 158
    discontinuation of, 153–154, 153b–155b,
      157–158
    failure to wean from, 158
    indications for, 150–153, 151f
    inspiratory effort detection in, 158
    modes for, 154–157, 156b, 156f, 157f
    organ perfusion in, 153
    principles of, 149–150
    rationale for, 150, 151f, 152
    sedation for, 153
    spontaneous breathing in, 157
    tidal volumes for, 153
    ventilation pressures for, 153
    weaning from, 153–154, 154b, 155f, 156t
    work of breathing and, 152
  pneumonia in, 175–186, 660–661, 661t
    clinical course of, 181, 183
    clinical features of, 178–179, 179f, 180b
    complications of, 185, 185b
    controversies in, 185, 185b
    definition of, 175
    diagnosis of, 179–180, 180f, 181f, 583,
      583f
    differential diagnosis of, 178
    epidemiology of, 175–176
    morbidity and mortality in, 176
    pathogenesis of, 176–177, 176f, 177f, 177t
    pathogens causing, 177, 177t, 182t, 183t
    pitfalls in, 185, 185b
    prevention of, 81–83, 82b, 82t, 83f, 87–88,
      183–185, 183b, 184f, 184t, 185f
    risk factors for, 177–178, 178b, 178t, 185
    treatment of, 180–181, 182t, 183t
  premature versus delayed, 169, 170b
  "pseudocardiac" failure in, 297–298, 297f
  stressors in, 200b
  tracheostomy for, 131–135
  weaning from, 169–174
    at end-of-life, 220, 220t
    challenges of, 169, 170b
    controversies in, 173b
    failure of, 158, 369–370, 370f
    importance of, 169
    modes of, 170–171, 171t

Mechanical ventilation—cont'd
  weaning from—cont'd
    noninvasive, 171, 172f
    nursing interventions for, 202, 204t
    pharmacologic interventions for, 173, 173b
    predictors of, 169–170, 170b, 170t
    progression of, 169
    protocols for, 171–173, 172t, 173f, 174f
    sedation and, 173
    with partial support, 153–154, 154b, 155f,
      156t
Meckel's diverticulum, 524
Mediastinum, widened, in thoracic trauma, 607
Medical Algorithms Project, 96
MELD (Model for End-Stage Liver Disease)
    score, 518, 518b
Melena, in gastrointestinal bleeding, 518
Mendelian inheritance, 13
Mental status alterations, in hypothyroidism,
    499
Meropenem
    dosage of, during dialysis, 488t
    for ventilator-associated pneumonia, 182t
    host defenses and, 67
Metabolic acidosis
    clinical features of, 452–453, 453f, 453t,
      454b, 454f
    compensation in, 449t
    corrected anion gap, 452t
    definition of, 450t
    epidemiology of, 446t
    in acutely unstable patient, 195
    in anaerobic metabolism, 48
    in diabetic ketoacidosis, 508–509, 508f, 509f
    in ethylene glycol poisoning, 671–672
    in hyperosmolar nonketotic coma, 508–509,
      508f, 509f
    in kidney failure, 481
    in methanol poisoning, 670
    infusion-related, 452
    lactic, 452–453, 454b
    renal tubular, 452, 453t, 454f
    risk factors for, 452t
    treatment of, 453–454
Metabolic alkalosis, 454–455, 455f
    compensation in, 449t
    definition of, 450t
    epidemiology of, 446t
Metabolic compensation, in acid-base disorders,
    449t, 450
Metabolic rate, evaluation of, 206
Metabolism
    anaerobic, 48
    in stress response, 24, 24f, 26–27
    oxygen requirement for, 41–42, 42f
Metanephrine, in pheochromocytoma, 501
Methanol poisoning, 669–670, 670t, 671t
Methicillin, resistance to, Staphylococcus aureus,
    69, 73, 73f, 177, 177t, 182, 183t
Methimazole, for thyrotoxicosis, 498, 498b
Methyldopa, for hypertensive crisis,
    perioperative, 352
Methylene blue, as antidote, 668t
Methylergonovine, for obstetric hemorrhage,
    631
Methylprednisolone
    for asthma, 233
    for spinal cord injury, 436–437
Metronidazole
    dosage of, during dialysis, 488t
    prophylactic, 92
MIC (minimum inhibitory concentration),
    antibiotic, 62, 62f, 64, 67–69
Midazolam
    for agitation and anxiety, 55, 55t, 219
    for burns, 618

Midazolam—cont'd
    for seizures, 421f, 427, 428t
    in obesity, perioperative, 270
Midodrine, for hepatorenal syndrome, 493
Migraine, versus seizures, 421t
Mineralocorticoids, deficiency of, 503f–505f,
    504–505
Minerals, in nutritional support, 211
Minimum inhibitory concentration, antibiotic,
    62, 62f, 64, 67–69
Minocycline, catheters coated with, 79, 80f
Minute ventilation
    in pregnancy, 625, 626f
    in respiratory muscle function, 276
Minute volume, modulation of, in partial
    ventilatory support, 149–150
Missile blast effect, in pulmonary contusion,
    608
Mitochondrial respiration, 41–42, 42f, 43f
Mitogen-activated protein kinases, in sepsis,
    592f, 593
Mitral valve
    endocarditis of, 360, 360f
    regurgitation of, 295, 362–363, 362b, 363f
    stenosis of, 363–364, 364f
Model for End-Stage Liver Disease (MELD)
    score, 518, 518b
Modified Blessed Dementia Rating Scale, 57
MODS. See Multiorgan dysfunction syndrome
    (MODS).
Molar pregnancy, 632
Monobactam, for ventilator-associated
    pneumonia, 182t
Monocyte(s)
    in inflammation, 2–3
    in sepsis, 555, 556f
L-N-Monomethylarginine, for sepsis, 601
Monroe–Kellie theory, 383
Morphine
    for burns, 618
    for pain, 53, 53t, 219
    poisoning from, 675
Mortality
    in acute coronary syndromes
      epidemiology of, 301, 302f, 303f
      pathophysiology of, 304–306, 305f, 306f
    in anthrax, 686
    in aortic dissection, 351, 368
    in aortic trauma, 359–360
    in ARDS, 237, 237t, 252
    in asthma, 223
    in bioterrorist attack, 685–686, 686f
    in brain injury, 395, 401
    in burns, 613, 618–619
    in cardiac rupture, 359
    in COPD, 223, 224f
    in electrical injury, 620
    in hepatorenal syndrome, 495, 496b
    in ICU, 217
    in infective endocarditis, 362
    in malignant hypertension, 347
    in mechanical ventilation, 176
    in multiple trauma, 603, 603f
    in obese surgical patients, 271–272
    in pancreatitis, 525
    in plague, 687–688
    in pneumonia, 176, 569, 570f, 571f, 576–578,
      576f
    in preeclampsia, 628
    in pulmonary embolism, 260
    in sepsis, 590, 601, 601f
    in severe hyperglycemia, 502
    in smallpox, 690–691
    in status epilepticus, 428–429
    in surgery, prevention of, 663
    in thyrotoxicosis, 497

Mortality—cont'd
  in tularemia, 689
  in variceal bleeding, 517
Motion, equation of, for respiratory mechanics, 142
Motor Activity Assessment Scale, in agitation assessment, 53t, 54
Motor seizures, 418
Motor vehicle accidents, multiple trauma in, 604
Mouse bioassay test, in botulism, 690
Moxifloxacin, for ventilator-associated pneumonia, 183t
MRI. See Magnetic resonance imaging.
Multiorgan dysfunction syndrome (MODS), 2, 2f, 2t
  critical illness polyneuropathy and myopathy in, 279
  endocrine profile in, 27, 28f
  hypoxia in, 48–49
  in liver failure, 536
  in mechanical ventilation, 166, 166f
  in sepsis, 590
  nutritional support in, 211t
  treatment of, 10
Multiple Organ Dysfunction Score, 590, 591t
Multiple trauma, 603–611
  abdominal trauma in, 609–610, 610f
  blunt, 604
  epidemiology of, 603–604, 603f, 604f
  etiology of, 604
  in pregnancy, 633–634
  nutritional support in, 211t
  penetrating, 604
  peripheral compartment syndrome in, 611, 611b
  primary survey and treatment in, 604–607, 605f, 606f, 606t, 607b
  spinal cord injury in, 432–434
  thoracic trauma in, 607–609
Murmurs
  in aortic stenosis, 362
  in infective endocarditis, 360
Muscle(s). See also Myopathy.
  atrophy of, in starvation, 27
  degeneration of, in critical illness myopathy, 29–30, 29t
  disorders of, respiratory failure in, 278t
  proteolysis of, in stress response, 26–27
  wasting of, 206, 206f
Mutant protective concentration, of antibiotics, 64, 64f
Mutant selection window, of antibiotics, 64, 64f
MVV (maximal voluntary ventilation), in obesity, 263–264
Myasthenia gravis, respiratory failure in, 279, 281–282
Mycobacterium avium complex pneumonia, 582
Myeloperoxidase, in acute coronary syndromes, 304
Myocardial infarction
  anterior, 309b
  cardiogenic shock in, 355
  cardiovascular failure in, 297
  clinical course of, 317–318
  clinical features of, 306–308, 306b, 307f
  definition of, 306–307
  diagnosis of, 308–312, 308b, 308t, 309b, 309f–312f
  differential diagnosis of, 308b
  epidemiology of, 301, 302f, 303f
  hypertensive crisis in, 352
  inferior, 309b
  mitral regurgitation in, 362–363, 362b

Myocardial infarction—cont'd
  non–ST segment elevation (NSTEMI), 301, 302t
    clinical features of, 307–308, 307f
    diagnosis of, 308–312, 308b, 309f
    treatment of, 312–315, 313f–315f
  nutritional support in, 211t
  pathophysiology of, 304–306, 305f, 306f
  prevention of, 317–318
  risk factors for, 301, 304, 304b, 304f
  ST segment elevation (STEMI), 301, 302t
    clinical features of, 307–308, 307f
    diagnosis of, 308–312, 308t, 309b
    treatment of, 315–318, 316f–317f
  treatment of, 303f, 312–318, 313f–317f
  ventricular septal rupture in, 357–358
Myocardial ischemia
  bradycardia in, 339
  in obstetric hemorrhage, 631
  ventricular tachycardia in, 335, 335b
Myocardial stunning, in subarachnoid hemorrhage, 408
Myocarditis, 358
Myocardium
  contusion of, 359, 608
  dyskinetic segments in, 297
  energy supply-demand relationships in, 293–295, 293f, 294f
Myoclonic seizures, 418, 419
Myogenic control, of vascular tone, 38–39, 38f
Myoglobin, in myocardial infarction, 310, 310f
Myoneural junction, disorders of, respiratory failure in, 278t
Myopathy
  critical illness, 29–30, 29t, 279, 282
  necrotizing, in mechanical ventilation, 235
  quadriplegic, respiratory failure in, 279, 281–282
Myosin, in vascular smooth muscle mechanochemical cycle, 31, 32f
Myosin light chain kinase, in vascular tone control, 31–34, 32f, 33f
Myostatin, inhibitors of, for critical illness myopathy, 30
Myxedema coma, 499–500, 499b, 622

N

Naloxone, as antidote, 668t, 675
Nasal masks, for noninvasive ventilation, 128, 129f, 230, 231f, 232f
Nasotracheal intubation, blind, 268
National Laboratory Response Network, 692
Natriuretic peptides
  excess of, in hepatorenal syndrome, 489
  in vascular tone control, 37
Nausea and vomiting, in end-of-life care, 219
Near-infrared spectroscopy, in cerebral blood flow measurement, 388t, 390–391
Nebulizers, for asthma medication, 233
Necrosis
  muscle, in mechanical ventilation, 235
  warfarin-induced, 548, 548f
Necrotizing fasciitis, obstetric, 632
Neomycin, prophylactic, 91
Nested organization, of humans, 22
Neurologic disorders
  in aortic dissection, 366
  in botulism, 689–690
  in carbon monoxide poisoning, 680
  in electrical injury, 620
  in ethylene glycol poisoning, 671
  in hypoglycemia, 503
  in hypothyroidism, 499
  in lithium intoxication, 673–674
  in methanol poisoning, 670, 670t

Neurologic disorders—cont'd
  in multiorgan dysfunction syndrome, 591t
  in sepsis, 595
  respiratory failure in, 275–282
Neurologic examination
  in acutely unstable patient, 195–196
  in multiple trauma, 606, 606t
Neuromuscular blockade
  in pregnancy, 636
  prolonged, respiratory failure in, 280
Neurosurgery, postoperative care in, 658, 658b, 659
Neurotransmitters, in delirium, 55
Neutropenia, pneumonia in, 581, 582t
Neutrophil(s), in inflammation, 2, 3f–5f, 4t
New-onset angina, 308
Nicardipine, for hypertensive crisis, 348t
Nimodipine, for subarachnoid hemorrhage, 350, 407
Nitrates, for myocardial infarction, 315
Nitric oxide
  in hemostasis regulation, 549, 549f
  in pulmonary vasoconstriction, 375
  in sepsis, 594
  in vascular tone control, 37–38
  inhaled, for inflammation, 10
  neutralization of, for sepsis, 601
Nitrogen, metabolism of, in stress response, 24, 24f
Nitroglycerin
  for hypertensive crisis, 348t
    in pulmonary edema, 352
    perioperative, 352
  for organ donors, 443
Nitroprusside
  for aortic dissection, 367
  for hypertensive crisis, 346–347, 348t
    in aortic dissection, 351
    in cerebral ischemia, 350–351
    in pheochromocytoma, 501
    in pulmonary edema, 351–352
  for organ donors, 443
  for preeclampsia, 628
Noise, control of, 56
Nonconvulsive seizures, 420t, 427t
Noninvasive ventilation. See Mechanical ventilation, noninvasive.
Nonketotic hyperglycemia. See Hyperosmolar nonketotic coma.
Nonmaleficence, 218
Nonsteroidal anti-inflammatory drugs, for pain, 52–53
Nonvolatile weak acid (A_{TOT}), in acid-base balance, 445–448, 448f
Norepinephrine
  for hepatorenal syndrome, 493
  for sepsis, 599
  in pheochromocytoma, 501
  in pregnancy, 635–636
  in stress response, 25
Normotensive hydrocephalus, ICP monitoring in, 385, 385t
Nosocomial infections
  control of. See Infection control.
  epidemiology of, 71–73, 72f, 73f, 87
  from bioterrorist agents, 693, 693b
  mortality in, 71
  outbreaks of, 73, 73f, 91
  pathophysiology of, 71–72
  postoperative, 660–661, 660f, 661t
  risk factors for, 72–73, 87–88
  ventilator-associated pneumonia as. See Mechanical ventilation, pneumonia in.
  versus type of ICU, 71, 72f
Nuclear factor-κB, in sepsis, 592f, 593
Numeric Rating Scale, for pain assessment, 52

Nursing issues, 199–204
  bowel dysfunction, 202, 202b
  communication, 201, 201f
  ethos, 199
  eye care, 202
  immobility complications, 201
  infection control, 199–200
  mechanical ventilation weaning, 202, 204, 204f, 204t
  nutrition, 202, 203f
  oral hygiene, 201–202, 202f
  pain management, 201
  patient positioning, 202
  sensory imbalance, 200
  skills for, 199, 199t
  sleep management, 200
  stress management, 199, 200b
  teamwork, 199, 200f
  time allotments, 199, 200f
Nutritional support, 202, 203f, 205–215. See also Enteral nutrition; Parenteral nutrition.
  assessment for, 205–207, 206f, 207t, 209f
  diets for, 213, 214t
  energy targets of, 206–208, 207f
  goals of, 205
  history of, 205
  hyperglycemia and, 208–209, 210t
  in alcohol intoxication, 669
  in burns, 618
  in cardiac failure, 209–210, 211f
  in gut maintenance, 212
  in infection control, 78
  in inflammatory response, 210
  in kidney failure, 212, 481
  in mechanical ventilation, 184, 184f
  in pregnancy, 635
  in stress, 28, 29t
  micronutrients in, 211
  nursing interventions for, 202, 202b, 203f
  oral supplements in, 213
  problems with, 213, 213f, 214t
  routes for, 212–213, 212f
  timing of, 207–208, 207f–209f, 207t

O
Obesity
  anesthesia in, 270
  body mass index in, 263
  definition of, 263, 264f
  epidemiology of, 263
  intubation techniques in, 267–269, 268t
  mechanical ventilation in, 269–270
  morbid, 263, 264f
  mortality in, 271–272
  nutritional support in, 211t
  pancreatitis in, 525
  pneumonia in, 571
  postoperative care in, 660
  respiratory function in
    intraoperative, 266–270, 266f, 268t
    postoperative, 270–272, 271f, 272b, 272t
    preoperative, 263–266, 265f
Obesity hypoventilation syndrome, 263–266, 265f
Obidoxime, as antidote, 282, 668t
Oculoglandular tularemia, 689
Ohm's law, in gas flow resistance, 138–139
Omeprazole, for gastrointestinal bleeding, 521
Open pneumothorax, 608
Opening airway pressure
  in noncompartmental model versus patient, 138, 138f
  in work of breathing, 145, 145f, 146f

Opening airway pressure—cont'd
  measurement of, 142, 143f
    in ARDS, 142, 144f
    PEEP and, 143–144, 145f
    versus time, 137, 138f, 142, 144f
Opioids
  for burns, 618
  for pain, 53, 53t, 219
  poisoning from, 675
Oral hygiene, 201–202, 202f
Oral supplements, 213
Organ donor care, 441–443, 441b, 442t
Organ failure scores, 96
Organophosphate poisoning, respiratory failure in, 279, 281–282
Ornipressin, for hepatorenal syndrome, 492
Oropharyngeal tularemia, 689
Orthopedic surgery, postoperative care in, 660
Osler's maneuver, in hypertensive crisis, 344
Osmolal gap, in acid-base disorders, 450, 450t
Osmolality, of body fluids, 459–460, 460f
Osmotic diuresis, 461–462, 461t
Outcomes
  hemodynamic monitoring and, 102, 104
  prediction of. See Severity of illness measures.
Ovarian vein, thrombophlebitis of, 632
Oxandrolone, for critical illness myopathy, 30
Oximetry, pulse
  in acutely unstable patient, 190
  in mechanical ventilation, 147
Oxygen
  carriers for, as blood transfusion alternatives, 566, 566b
  deficiency of. See also Hypoxia.
    lactic acidosis in, 452–453, 454b
  extraction of, efficiency of, 46–48, 46f
  limited, cellular metabolism in, 48–49
  metabolic requirements for, 41–42, 42f
  partial pressure of
    cellular oxygen delivery and, 42, 43f
    in cerebral circulation regulation, 392
    in mechanical ventilation, 146–148, 147f, 148t
    in obesity, 264
    in pregnancy, 627, 627f
    in pulmonary embolism, 256
  shunting of, 47, 47f
  toxicity of, in mechanical ventilation, 166–167
  transport of, at tissue level, 46–47, 46f
Oxygen consumption
  at cellular level, 42–43, 43f
  determinants of, 101–102, 103f
  in ARDS, 48–49
  in multiorgan dysfunction syndrome, 48–49
  in obesity, 264
  in pregnancy, 625
  in tissue hypoxia, 44–45, 45f
  mitochondrial, 41, 42f, 43f
  of brain, 388
  of respiratory muscles, 369
Oxygen delivery
  assessment of. See Hemodynamic monitoring.
  at capillary level, 43–44, 43f
  at cellular level, 42–43, 43f
  determinants of, 101–102, 103f
  for fetus, 627, 627f
  in brain injury, 401
  versus consumption, 47, 47f
Oxygen demand
  myocardial, in left heart dysfunction, 293–295, 293f, 294f
  versus oxygen supply, 389
Oxygen extraction ratio, 46–48, 46f
Oxygen saturation, jugular bulb venous, in cerebral blood flow measurement, 388t, 389

Oxygen supply, versus oxygen demand, 389
Oxygen therapy
  as antidote, 668t
  for asthma, 233
  for carbon monoxide poisoning, 681–682, 683f
  for COPD, 228
  for dyspnea, 219
  for sepsis, 598
Oxygenation, in pregnancy, 627, 627f
Oxytocin, for obstetric hemorrhage, 631

P
Pacing
  after cardiac surgery, 643–644, 652–654, 652f, 652t, 653t, 654f
  for bradycardia, 339–341
Packed red blood cells, transfusion of, 562
Pain
  abdominal, in pancreatitis, 527
  assessment of, 51–52, 52b, 201
  behaviors in, 51, 52b
  causes of, 51
  definition of, 51
  in aortic dissection, 366
  in inflammation, 9
  management of, 52–53, 53t
    for burns, 617–618
    in end-of-life care, 219
    nursing interventions for, 201
Palliative care, 218–219, 218b
Palpitations, in pheochromocytoma, 500
Pancreatic duct, disruption of, pancreatitis in, 525–526, 526f
Pancreatitis, 525–530
  clinical course of, 529, 529b
  clinical features of, 527
  complications of, 529, 529b
  epidemiology of, 525
  in liver failure, 535
  in nutritional support, 214t
  necrosis in, 528–529, 529f, 568f
  pathogenesis of, 525–527, 526f, 527t
  risk factors for, 525, 526b
  spectrum of, 527
  treatment of, 527–529, 528f, 529f
Pantoprazole, for gastrointestinal bleeding, 521
Pao. See Opening airway pressure.
Papillary muscles, blood supply of, 363
Papworth regime, for hormone replacement, in organ donors, 442
Paracentesis, for hepatorenal syndrome, 495, 495f
Paracetamol. See Acetaminophen.
Paralysis
  in botulism, 689–690
  intraoperative, respiratory function in, in obesity, 266–270, 266f, 268t
Parenchymal renal failure, 477f, 478, 478b
Parenteral nutrition
  cautions with, 212–213, 212f
  complications of, 212–213, 212f
  for heart failure, 209–210
  glutamine in, 212
  in pregnancy, 635
  micronutrients in, 211
  timing of, 208, 208f, 208t
Parkinsonism, 420t
Parkland formula, for burn fluid resuscitation, 616, 617t
Paroxysmal supraventricular tachycardias, 328–329, 330f, 331f
Partial rebreathing technique, in hemodynamic monitoring, 107
Partial seizures, 417, 427t

Passy-Muir valve, 201, 201f
Patient Self-Determination Act, 219
Paw. See Airway pressure.
PCP (phencyclidine), 677
Peak expiratory flow rate
    in asthma, 227
    in COPD, 227
Pediatric patients
    brain death declaration in, 440
    burns in
        clinical course of, 618–619
        epidemiology of, 613
        fluid therapy for, 617t
        size and depth estimation in, 614–615, 615f
PEEP. See Positive end-expiratory pressure.
Pelvic fractures, 610–611
Penetrating trauma
    cardiac, 360
    multiple, 604
Penicillin(s), for bioterrorist agents, 688t
Penicillin G, as antidote, 668t
Pentobarbital, for seizures, 427, 428t
Pentoxifylline, for sepsis, 600
Peptic ulcer disease, bleeding in, 517
Percutaneous coronary intervention, for acute
        coronary syndromes, 315–317, 316f, 317f
Percutaneous tracheostomy
    complications of, 134f, 135
    contraindications for, 132
    history of, 131
    indications for, 132
    techniques for, 131–132, 132t, 133f
    timing of, 132–134
Perfluorocarbons, in blood substitutes, 566,
        566b
Perfusion, evaluation of, in acutely unstable
        patient, 194–195
Perfusion computed tomography, in cerebral
        blood flow measurement, 388t, 391
Perfusion weighted MRI, in cerebral blood flow
        measurement, 388t, 391, 391f
Pericardial pressure, lung interactions with, 371,
        374f
Pericardial tamponade, 364–366, 364b
Pericardiocentesis
    for cardiac penetrating wound, 360
    for cardiac tamponade, 365
Pericarditis, versus acute coronary syndromes,
        308b
Periodic epileptiform discharges, in EEG, 423,
        425f
Periodic lateralized epileptiform discharges, in
        EEG, 422–423, 424f
Peripheral compartment syndrome, in multiple
        trauma, 611, 611b
Peripheral neuropathy
    in critical illness, 279
    in sepsis, 595
    respiratory failure in, 278t
Peripheral vascular resistance, increase of,
        hypertensive crisis in, 343, 344f
Peritoneal dialysis, 487
Peritoneal lavage, in abdominal injury, 609
Personal protective equipment, for bioterrorism
        agents, 695
PET (positron emission tomography), in cerebral
        blood flow measurement, 388t, 389
pH
    arterial, normal, 450t
    carbon dioxide partial pressure relationship
        with, 445, 446f, 447–448, 448f, 452t
Pharmacogenetics, 18, 18t, 19t
Phencyclidine, 677
Phenobarbital
    for seizures, 421f, 427, 428t
    poisoning with, 672

Phenoxybenzamine, for hypertensive crisis, 352,
        501
Phentolamine, for hypertensive crisis, 348t, 501
Phenylephrine, for sepsis, 599
Phenytoin, for seizures, 408, 421f, 428t
Pheochromocytoma, 352, 500–501, 500b, 501b,
        501f
Phosphate
    for diabetic ketoacidosis, 513
    for hyperosmolar nonketotic coma, 513
    renal replacement therapy effects on, 484f
Phosphatidylinositol-3 kinase, in sepsis, 592f,
        593
Phospholipase A$_2$, inhibitors of, for sepsis, 601
Phospholipase C, in vascular tone control, 31,
        32f
Phrenic nerve, evaluation of, in respiratory
        failure, 280–281, 281f
pH-stat method, for arterial blood gas
        calculation, 450–451
Physician-assisted suicide, 218
Physiologic and Operative Severity Score for the
        Enumeration of Mortality and Morbidity
        (POSSUM), 96
Physiological hypoxia, 44
Physostigmine, as antidote, 668t
Phytomenadione, as antidote, 668t
Piperacillin, dosage of, during dialysis, 488t
Piperacillin/tazobactam, for ventilator-associated
        pneumonia, 182t
PIRO concept, in sepsis, 18, 596t
Pituitary gland, failure of, after brain stem death,
        442
Placenta previa, 631
Placental abruption, 631, 633
Plague, 687–689, 688t
Plaques, atherosclerotic, 304–305, 305f, 306f
Plasma, transfusion of, 562–563
Plasma mixing tests, in bleeding, 551
Plasmapheresis
    for Guillain-Barré syndrome, 281
    for liver failure, 540, 541t
Plasmin, action of, 548–549, 548f
Plasminogen activator, action of, 548–549, 548f
Plasminogen activator inhibitor, action of, 548f,
        549
Plateau airway pressure
    for asthma, 234
    for COPD, 232
Platelet(s)
    aggregation of, in coronary artery disease,
        305
    in hemostasis, 544, 545f
    transfusion of, 562
Platelet activating factor, inhibition of, for sepsis,
        601
Platelet count
    in bleeding, 550, 550t
    in multiorgan dysfunction syndrome, 591t
Plethysmography, in pulmonary embolism, 258
Pleural effusion
    in anthrax, 687
    in pulmonary embolism, 255
Pleural pain, versus acute coronary syndromes,
        308b
Pleural pressures, hemodynamics of, 371–373,
        372f, 373f
Pleural space, abnormal substances in. See also
        Pneumothorax.
    in multiple trauma, 607–608
Plugged telescoping catheter stain, in ventilator-
        associated pneumonia, 179
Pneumatic compression devices, for deep venous
        thrombosis, 260
Pneumocystis jiroveci pneumonia, 581–583,
        582f

Pneumomediastinum, in mechanical ventilation,
        163
Pneumonia
    community-acquired, 569–579
        clinical course of, 577–578
        clinical features of, 574, 574f, 574t
        diagnosis of, 574–575, 575b
        differential diagnosis of, 574, 574f, 574t
        epidemiology of, 569, 570f
        microbial spectrum of, 573, 573f, 575
        mortality in, 569, 570f, 571f, 576–578,
            576f
        pathogenesis of, 572–573, 573f
        phases of, 577–578
        Pneumonia Severity Index in, 569, 570t
        prevention of, 578, 578b
        recurrent, 571, 572f, 572t
        risk factors for, 569–571, 570b, 570f–572f,
            570t, 572t
        treatment of, 575–577, 576f, 577f
    in COPD, 226, 230
    in immunodeficiency, 581–587
        causes of, 581–582, 582f, 582t
        clinical course of, 585–586, 586f
        clinical features of, 582–583
        controversies in, 587, 587b
        diagnosis of, 583–585, 583f–585f, 585t
        epidemiology of, 581
        pathogenesis of, 581–582
        pitfalls in, 586–587, 586t
        treatment of, 585–586, 586f
    in mechanical ventilation. See Mechanical
        ventilation, pneumonia in.
    noninvasive ventilation for, 125–126
Pneumonic plague, 688–689
Pneumonic tularemia, 689
Pneumothorax
    after cardiac surgery, 646–647
    in diabetic ketoacidosis, 511
    in mechanical ventilation, 163
    in multiple trauma, 607–608
    open, 608
    tension, 608
    versus acute coronary syndromes, 308b
Poiseuille's law, in cardiovascular failure,
        283–290
Poisoning, 665–678
    acetaminophen, 674
    amphetamine, 677
    antiarrhythmic drugs, 674–675
    antidepressants, 672–673, 673f
    antidotes for, 667, 668t
    barbiturates, 672
    benzodiazepines, 672
    carbon monoxide, 679–683
    causes of, 665
    cocaine, 675–677, 676f
    controversies in, 678b
    drug
        of abuse, 675–677, 676f
        therapeutic, 672–675, 673f
    ecstasy, 677
    epidemiology of, 665
    ethanol, 667–669, 669f, 669t
    ethylene glycol, 670–672, 671f, 671t
    isopropanol, 669
    lithium, 673–674
    methanol, 669–670, 670t, 671t
    opioid, 675
    pathogenesis of, 665
    phencyclidine, 677
    pitfalls in, 678b
    risk factors for, 665
    salicylates, 674
    treatment of, 665–667, 666f, 667t, 668t
Poliomyelitis, respiratory failure in, 275

Polydipsia
in diabetic ketoacidosis, 509
in hyperosmolar nonketotic coma, 509
Polymeric diets, 213, 214t
Polymicrobial infections, pneumonia, 573
Polymyxin, prophylactic, 89, 89t, 90
Polyneuropathy, critical illness, respiratory failure
in, 279, 282
Polyuria, 459–462
assessment of, 460
clinical approach to, 460–462, 461f, 461t
definition of, 459
differential diagnosis of, 460, 461t
in diabetic ketoacidosis, 509
in hyperosmolar nonketotic coma, 509
physiology of, 459–460, 460f
Portal hypertension
bleeding in
clinical features of, 518, 518t
diagnosis of, 518
epidemiology of, 517
pathogenesis of, 518
treatment of, 521–523, 522f, 523f
definition of, 517
hepatorenal syndrome in. See Hepatorenal
syndrome.
Positioning, 202
in ARDS, 242–243, 243f
in pregnancy, 635
of obese persons, respiratory function and,
267
Positive end-expiratory pressure
atelectrauma in, 163–164, 164f, 165f
dynamic intrinsic, 143–144, 145f
equipment for, 128, 129f
for acute hypoxemic respiratory failure,
124
for ARDS, 250–251
chest wall compliance and, 243
gas exchange and, 244–246
lung opening in, 241–242, 241f, 242f
lung volume in, 238, 239f
tidal volume and, 242, 242f
ventilation–perfusion distribution and,
242
for asthma, 234
in anesthesia, 270
in heart-lung interactions, 371–374, 373f,
374f
in obesity, 265–266, 269–270, 272, 272b
static intrinsic, 139–141, 139f–141f, 143–144,
145f
systemic venous return and, 377–378, 379f
Positron emission tomography, in cerebral blood
flow measurement, 388f, 389
POSSUM (Physiologic and Operative Severity
Score for the Enumeration of Mortality
and Morbidity), 96
Postinjury Multiple Organ Failure Score, 96
Postoperative care, 657–663
after cardiac surgery. See Cardiac surgery,
postoperative care in.
after extensive procedures, 660
after neurosurgery, 658, 658b, 659
after organ transplantation, 660
after orthopedic surgery, 660
after vascular surgery, 659–660
circulatory dysfunction and, 658–659
complications of, 660–662, 660f, 661t, 662b,
662f
future of, 663
hypertensive crisis in, 352
hyponatremia in, 467
in obesity, 270–272, 271f, 272b, 272t
of high-risk patients, 657–659, 658b
outreach services in, 663

Postoperative care—cont'd
respiratory function in, 270–272, 271f, 272b,
272t, 659
risks in, 658
Postrenal kidney failure, 477f, 478
Posturing, 419, 420t
Potassium. See also Hyperkalemia; Hypokalemia.
distribution of
in diabetic ketoacidosis, 509, 509f
in hyperosmolar nonketotic coma, 509, 509f
for diabetic ketoacidosis, 513
for hyperosmolar nonketotic coma, 513
regulation of, 468–469
Potassium channels, in vascular tone control,
34–35, 36f
Potassium chloride, for hypokalemia, 472
Ppl (pleural pressures), hemodynamics of,
371–373, 372f, 373f
Pralidoxime, as antidote, 282, 668t
Prednisolone
for asthma, 233
for COPD, 229
for myasthenia gravis, 282
for sepsis, 599
Prednisone, for asthma, 233
Preeclampsia, 352–353, 628–629, 629t
Pregnancy, 625–637
acute fatty liver of, 533, 630–631, 630t
acute respiratory distress syndrome in,
634–635
amniotic fluid embolism in, 260, 627–628,
628f
asthma in, 635
carbon monoxide poisoning in, 682, 683f
cardiopulmonary resuscitation in, 636
critical care management in, 635–637, 635b
dilated cardiomyopathy in, 359
drug safety in, 635–636, 635b
fatty liver of, 533, 630–631, 630t
gestational trophoblastic disease in, 632, 633t
heart failure in, 635
HELLP syndrome in, 629–630, 630f
hemodynamic monitoring in, 636
hemorrhage in, 631
hypertensive crisis in, 352–353
mechanical ventilation in, 636–637
nutritional support in, 635
physiology of, 625–627, 626f, 626t, 627f
preeclampsia in, 352–353, 628–629, 629t
pulmonary thromboembolic disease in, 634,
634t
radiology in, 634, 634t, 636
sepsis in, 631–632, 632b
tocolytic pulmonary edema in, 632, 633t
trauma in, 633–634
Preload
assessment of, 102, 102f, 104f
factors affecting, 355
in right cardiovascular failure, 291–293, 293f
intrathoracic pressure effects on, 379–380
physiology of, 284–286, 284f
Preoperative period
respiratory function in, in obesity, 263–266,
265f
risk factors in, 657–658, 658b
Prerenal kidney failure, 477–478, 477f, 478t
Pressure support ventilation, 110–112, 112f,
113f, 149–150, 152, 156t
for COPD, 232
for weaning, 170
Pressure ventilation, 109, 109t, 110t
Pressure-regulated volume control ventilation,
114
Pressure-volume loop, in cardiac function,
284–286, 284f, 285f
Primary endogenous infections, 88, 88t

Procainamide, for arrhythmias, 321b
Prolactin, in stress response, 27, 28, 28f
Promoter genes, 15–16, 16f
Prone position
for ARDS, 242–243, 243f
in obesity, respiratory function and, 267
Propafenone, for arrhythmias, 321b
Prophylaxis, antibiotic. See Antibiotics,
prophylactic.
Propofol
for agitation and anxiety, 55, 55t
for burns, 618
for hepatic encephalopathy, 538
for seizures, 421f, 427, 428t
Proportional assist ventilation, 117, 149,
155–157, 156f, 156t, 157f
Propranolol
for aortic dissection, 351
for hypertensive crisis, 352
for thyrotoxicosis, 498, 498b
Propylthiouracil, for thyrotoxicosis, 498, 498b
Prospective Investigation of Pulmonary
Embolism Diagnosis (PIOPED), 256
Prostacyclin
in hemostasis regulation, 549, 549f
in vascular tone control, 34, 36f
Prostate surgery, hyponatremia after, 467
Prosthetic heart valves, complications of, 364
Protamine, for anticoagulant reversal, 641
Protective equipment, for bioterrorism agents,
695
Protein binding, of antibiotics, 64–66, 65f
Protein C
activated
for ARDS, 248
for disseminated intravascular coagulation,
553
for inflammation, 11, 11f
for pneumonia, 577
for sepsis, 557–558, 599–600
defects of, 547–548
in coagulation regulation, 547–548, 547f, 548f
Protein kinase A, in vascular tone control, 32,
33f
Protein kinase G, in vascular tone control, 32,
33f
Proteinuria, in preeclampsia, 628–629, 629t
Proteolysis, in stress response, 26–27
Proteus pneumonia, 182t
Prothrombin time
in bleeding, 550t, 551
in liver failure, 534
Prothrombinase complex, in hemostasis, 546
Proton pump inhibitors, for gastrointestinal
bleeding, 521
PROWESS study, activated protein kinase C for
inflammation, 11
"Pseudocardiac" failure, 297–298, 297f
Pseudohypertension, 344
Pseudohypoaldosteronism, hyperkalemia in, 469
Pseudomonas aeruginosa infections
beta-lactams for, host defenses and, 67
fluoroquinolones for, host defenses and, 68
pneumonia as, 177, 177t, 182t, 573, 581,
585t
Psychiatric disorders, versus seizures, 421t
Pugin clinical pulmonary infection score,
178–179, 180b
Pulmonary angiography, in pulmonary embolism,
258
Pulmonary artery catheter, 105, 617
Pulmonary artery occlusion pressure, 105, 370,
370f
Pulmonary artery pressure
in ARDS, 243–244, 244f
in pulmonary embolism, 254

Pulmonary aspiration
  in obesity, 267
  pneumonia due to, 572
Pulmonary circulation, vasoconstriction of, in
    hypoxia, 375
Pulmonary edema
  after brain stem death, 442
  airway resistance measurement in, 139
  cardiogenic, noninvasive ventilation for,
    122–124
  in ARDS, 238, 239f, 240, 240f, 244–245,
    251
  in carbon monoxide poisoning, 680
  in hypertensive crisis, 351–352
  in inhalation injury, 619
  in mechanical ventilation, 162, 162f
  in preeclampsia, 629
  in pregnancy, 632, 633t
  in subarachnoid hemorrhage, 407–408, 413
  neurogenic, 407–408
Pulmonary embolism, 253–261
  clinical course of, 260
  clinical features of, 254, 254t
  complications of, 260b
  controversies in, 260b
  diagnosis of, 254–258, 255f–257f
  epidemiology of, 253
  in pregnancy, 634, 634t
  massive, 258, 260
  mortality in, 260
  nonthrombotic, 260–261
  pathogenesis of, 253–254
  postoperative, 662
  prevention of, 260
  risk factors for, 253, 254t
  treatment of, 258–260, 259t
  versus acute coronary syndromes, 308b
Pulmonary function
  in acutely unstable patient, 189–191, 190b,
    196–197
  in asthma, 224–227, 226t
  in COPD, 224–225, 227
  in obesity
    intraoperative, 266–270, 266f, 268t
    postoperative, 270–272, 271f, 272b, 272t
    preoperative, 263–266, 265f
  in pregnancy, 625, 626f
Pulmonary hypertension, in COPD, 227
Pulmonary infiltrates, in mechanical ventilation,
    162, 162f
Pulmonary resistance, measurement of, 138–139
Pulmonary vascular resistance
  in ARDS, 243–244, 244f
  in pulmonary embolism, 253–254
  lung volume effects on, 374–376, 376f
Pulse, carotid, assessment of, 189, 189f
Pulse contour analysis, 107
Pulse oximetry
  in acutely unstable patient, 190
  in mechanical ventilation, 147
Pulse pressure, measurement of, 106, 106f
Pulseless electrical activity, in hypovolemia,
    194
Pulsus paradoxus, in cardiac tamponade, 365
Pump, intra-aortic balloon, 356–357, 356f, 357f,
    654–656, 655f
Push enteroscopy, in bleeding, 519
Pyridostigmine, for myasthenia gravis, 282
Pyridoxine, as antidote, 668t

Q

Quadriplegia, respiratory failure in, 279,
    281–282
Quality of care, severity of illness measures and,
    99–100

Quetelet's index, 263
Quinolones, tissue levels of, 66–67, 66t

R

Radioactive tracers, for cerebral blood flow
    measurement, 388–389, 388t
Radiocontrast agents, kidney failure due to, 480
Radiography
  in aortic dissection, 366
  in aortic stenosis, 362
  in asthma, 227–228, 229f
  in cardiac tamponade, 365
  in COPD, 227
  in inflammation, 9
  in pneumonia, 574–575, 583, 583f
  in pulmonary embolism, 255
  in spinal cord injury, 434
  in thoracic trauma, 607
  in ventilator-associated pneumonia, 178, 179f
Radiology, fetal exposure in, 634, 634t, 636
Radionuclide studies, in gastrointestinal bleeding,
    519–520
Ramsay Scale, for sedation assessment, 53, 53t
Ranitidine, for gastrointestinal bleeding, 521
Ranson's criteria, for pancreatitis, 527, 527t
Rapid antigen tests, in pneumonia, 575
Rapid occlusion method, for pulmonary
    resistance measurement, 139
Rapid shallow breathing index, for ventilator
    weaning, 170
Reactive nitrogen species, in inflammation, 6
Reactive oxygen species, in inflammation, 6
Recruitment, lung, in ARDS, 241, 241f
Rectum, bleeding in. See Gastrointestinal
    bleeding, lower tract.
Red blood cells, transfusion of, 562
Redness, in inflammation, 9
Regurgitation, in nutritional support, 214t
Rehau system, for ICP monitoring, 386t, 387
Relaxation, of vascular smooth muscle, 32–33,
    33f. See also Vasodilators.
  autoregulation of, 38–39, 38f
  circulating factors in, 35–38, 36t
  potential and, 34–35, 34f–36f
Renal failure. See Kidney failure.
Renal replacement therapy
  continuous, 481–482, 482f–486f, 484–486,
    485b
  drug prescription during, 487–488, 488t
  intermittent dialysis in, 482f, 483f, 486–487,
    487f
  methods for, 481–482, 481f, 482b, 482f–484f
  slow low-efficiency extended daily dialysis,
    481–482, 487, 487f
Renal tubular acidosis, 452, 453t, 454f
Renin-angiotensin system
  activation of, hypertensive crisis in, 343,
    344f
  dysfunction of, in hepatorenal syndrome,
    489–490
  in vascular tone control, 36
Repair, phases of, 24, 24f
Reporter genes, 15, 15f
Reserpine, for thyrotoxicosis, 498, 498b
Resistance
  antibiotic. See Antibiotics, resistance to.
  in mechanical ventilation, measurement of,
    138–139
Respiration
  blood flow changes with, 106, 106f
  mitochondrial, 41–42, 42f, 43f
  right atrial pressure changes with, 290, 291f
Respirator exchange ratio, in obesity, 264
Respirator lung. See Mechanical ventilation, lung
    injury in.

Respiratory acidosis, 456, 456t
  carbon dioxide partial pressure/pH
    relationship in, 448
  compensation in, 449t
  definition of, 450t
  epidemiology of, 446t
  in asthma, 227
Respiratory alkalosis, 456–457, 456b
  carbon dioxide partial pressure/pH
    relationship in, 448
  compensation in, 449t
  definition of, 450t
  epidemiology of, 446t
  in carbon monoxide poisoning, 680
  in pregnancy, 625
Respiratory drive, evaluation of, 280
Respiratory failure
  acute hypercapnic, noninvasive ventilation for,
    121–122, 123f
  acute hypoxemic, noninvasive ventilation for,
    124–125
  in hemothorax, 608
  in multiorgan dysfunction syndrome, 591t
  in open pneumothorax, 608
  in sepsis, 595
  neuromuscular, 275–282
    clinical course of, 282
    clinical features of, 277–280, 278t, 279f
    diagnosis of, 280–281, 281f
    epidemiology of, 275
    in acute quadriplegic myopathy, 279,
      281–282
    in botulism, 279, 281–282
    in critical illness polyneuropathy and
      myopathy, 279, 282
    in Guillain-Barré syndrome, 278–279
    in myasthenia gravis, 279, 281–282
    in organophosphate poisoning, 279,
      281–282
    in prolonged neuromuscular blockade, 280
    in ventilator-induced diaphragmatic
      dysfunction, 280
    pathophysiology of, 275–277, 276f, 277f
    prevention of, 282
    risk factors for, 275
    treatment of, 281–282
  postoperative, 659
Respiratory muscles
  dysfunction of, 275–277, 276f, 277f. See also
    Respiratory failure, neuromuscular.
  oxygen consumption of, 369
Respiratory rate
  in mechanical ventilation, lung injury and,
    166–167
  in obesity, 264–265
  in pneumonia, 574, 574f
Respiratory system. See also Lung; subjects
    starting with Airway.
  carbon monoxide poisoning effects on, 680
  in acid-base balance compensation, 449, 449t
  physiology of, in pregnancy, 625, 626f
  total pressure applied to, 142
Rest angina, 308
Resuscitation
  in acutely unstable patient, 189, 189f
  in brain injury, 399–400
  in burns, 614–617, 617b, 617t
  in diabetic ketoacidosis, 511–512, 511b, 512b,
    512f, 513f
  in electrical injury, 620
  in hyperosmolar nonketotic coma, 511–512,
    511b, 512b, 512f, 513f
  in multiple trauma, 604–606, 605f, 606f, 606t
  in pancreatitis, 527
  in poisoning, 666
  in pregnancy, 636

Resuscitation—cont'd
in sepsis, 598, 598f
in severe hyperglycemia, 502
in subarachnoid hemorrhage, 407
in sudden cardiac death, ventricular
arrhythmias after, 336
Retinopathy, in hypertensive crisis, 344–345,
347
Return function, in cardiovascular failure
cardiac function interactions with, 288, 288f
determinants of, 286–288, 286f, 288f
failure of, 288–289, 289f
Revascularization, for acute coronary syndromes,
315–317, 316f, 317f
Rewarming, in hypothermia, 607, 607b,
621–622
Rh immune globulin, in maternal injury, 633
Rhabdomyolysis
in carbon monoxide poisoning, 680
kidney failure in, 479
RhoA protein, in vascular tone control, 33, 33f
Rib fractures, 607
Ribavirin, for bioterrorist agents, 688t
Richmond Agitation–Sedation Scale, 54, 54t
Rifampin
catheters coated with, 79, 80f
for bioterrorist agents, 688t
for ventilator-associated pneumonia, 183t
RIFLE (Risk Injury Failure Loss End-Stage)
criteria, for kidney failure, 476f
Right atrial pressure
in cardiac function testing, 289f–291f, 290
in "pseudocardiac" failure, 297–298, 297f
in right heart failure, 291–293, 293f
intrathoracic pressure effects on, 377, 377f,
378f
physiology of, 285f, 287–288, 288f, 289f
Rigors, 420t
Riker Sedation–Agitation Scale, for sedation
assessment, 53–54, 53t
Rise time, for pressure support ventilation, 112,
113f
Risk Injury Failure Loss End-Stage (RIFLE)
criteria, for kidney failure, 476f
Rubor, in inflammation, 9
Rule of nines, for burn estimation, 614–615,
615f
Rules of thumb, for acid-base disorders, 449,
449t

S
SAH. See Subarachnoid hemorrhage.
Salbutamol
for asthma, 233
for COPD, 228
Salicylates, poisoning from, 674
Saline solutions
for adrenal crisis, 505
for burn resuscitation, 617t
for diabetic ketoacidosis, 511–512, 512b,
512f
for hyperglycemia, 502
for hyperosmolar nonketotic coma, 511–512,
512b, 512f
for hyponatremia, 467–468
for increased ICP, 400
for metabolic alkalosis, 455
infusion-related acidosis due to, 452
Scapula, fractures of, 607
SCIWORA (spinal cord injury without
radiological abnormality), 432
Scleroderma, hypertensive crisis in, 353
Sclerotherapy, for gastrointestinal bleeding,
521–522
Secondary endogenous infections, 88, 88t

Sedation
after cardiac surgery, 647
agents for, 54–55, 55t
assessment of, 53–54, 53t
for burns, 617–618
for hepatic encephalopathy, 538
for partial ventilatory support, 153
for subarachnoid hemorrhage, 407
in end-of-life care, 219
in obesity, 270
in pregnancy, 636
terminal, 218
ventilator weaning and, 173
Segregation analysis, in genetic studies, 14
Seizures, 415–430
algorithm for, 421f
classification of, 417–418
clinical course of, 428–429
clinical features of, 417–419, 419t
clonic, 418
complex, 418
complications of, 429b
controversies in, 429b
diagnosis of, 419, 422–423, 423f–426f, 427t
differential diagnosis of, 420t, 421t, 423,
427t
drug-induced, 415, 417t
electroencephalography in, 422, 423f–426f
epidemiology of, 415
focal, 420t
generalized, 417, 420t, 423f, 426, 427t
in hypothyroidism, 500
in subarachnoid hemorrhage, 406, 408
limbic, 418
motor, 418
myoclonic, 418, 419
nonconvulsive, 420t, 427
nonepileptic, 419, 427t
partial, 417, 427t
pathogenesis of, 415, 417, 418f
pitfalls in, 429b
prevention of, 429, 429f, 629
refractive. See Status epilepticus.
risk factors for, 415, 417t
sensory, 418
simple, 418
tonic, 418
treatment of, 421f, 426–428, 428t
triggers of, 415, 417t
versus ventricular tachycardia, 415, 416f
Seldinger technique, for percutaneous
tracheostomy, 131–135
Selective digestive decontamination
for pancreatitis, 528
for ventilator-associated pneumonia, 184
in mechanical ventilation, 82
Selenium supplementation, 211
Sengstaken–Blakemore tube, for gastrointestinal
bleeding, 522–523, 523f
Sensory imbalance, nursing interventions for,
200
Sensory seizures, 418
Sepsis and septic shock, 589–602
adrenal crisis in, 504
blood purification for, 487
cardiovascular failure in, 296
causes of, 589
clinical features of, 589, 590t, 594–595, 594f
comorbid conditions with, 596
continuum of, 589
controversies in, 602b
critical illness polyneuropathy and myopathy
in, 279
definitions of, 1–2, 2t, 589–590, 590f, 590t,
591t
diagnosis of, 597–598

Sepsis and septic shock—cont'd
differential diagnosis of, 589, 590t
disseminated intravascular coagulation and,
553
endothelial function and dysfunction in,
556–557, 556b, 557f
epidemiology of, 590, 591f
evaluation of, 196
genetic factors in, 571, 572f, 572t, 595–596,
596f, 596t
in liver failure, 536
in plague, 688
in pneumonia, 572, 575, 576f
in pregnancy, 631–632, 632b
kidney failure in, 477
mortality in, 589, 590, 601, 601f
multiorgan dysfunction syndrome in, 590,
591t
nutritional support in, 211t
obstetric, 631–632, 632b
pathogens causing, 597
pathophysiology of, 555, 556b, 556f, 557,
557f, 590–594, 592f, 593t
PIRO concept in, 18
pitfalls in, 602b
prognosis for, 601, 601f, 602t
staging of, 595–597, 596f, 596t
treatment of, 557–558, 558f, 598–601,
598f
Septic tularemia, 689
Septicemic plague, 688–689
Sequential Organ Failure Assessment score, 590,
591t
Serratia marcescens pneumonia, 182t
Severity of illness measures, 95–100
development of, 95–98, 97f
for individual patients, 98–99
for population, 99–100
future of, 100
ideal qualities of, 95, 96t
in clinical trials, 99
stepwise regression algorithm in, 96
validation of, 98, 98t
variables in, 96
Shakes, 420t
Shivering, 420t, 647
Shock
anaphylactic, tissue perfusion in, 194
brain death declaration in, 440
burn, 613–614, 614f
cardiogenic. See Cardiogenic shock.
hypovolemic
in gastrointestinal bleeding, 518
in multiple trauma, 605–606
in pregnancy, 633
septic. See Sepsis and septic shock.
treatment of, 298, 298f
Shock liver, in sepsis, 595
Signal transduction, in vascular tone control, 33,
33f
Silver sulfadiazine
catheters coated with, 79, 80f
for burns, 618
Simple seizures, 418
Single nucleotide polymorphisms (SNPs), 13,
14f
Single-photon emission computed tomography,
in cerebral blood flow measurement,
388t, 389
Sinus bradycardia, 337, 338f
Sinus rhythm, loss of, after cardiac surgery,
643–644
Sinusitis, postoperative, 661
Sir2 protein, in critical illness myopathy, 30
SIRS (systemic inflammatory response
syndrome), 1–2, 2f, 2t, 9

Skin
anthrax manifestations in, 687, 688f
burns of. See Burn(s).
carbon monoxide poisoning manifestations in, 680
substitutes for, in burn care, 617, 618f
tularemia manifestations in, 689
Skull, fractures of, 399, 399f
Sleep, promotion of, 200
Slow low-efficiency extended daily dialysis, 481–482, 487, 487f
Small intestine
bleeding in. See Gastrointestinal bleeding, lower tract.
perforation of, in nutritional support, 214t
Smallpox, 688t, 690–691, 691f
Smoke inhalation injury, 619
Smoking, COPD related to, 223, 224, 225f, 227
Smooth muscle, vascular. See Vascular smooth muscle; Vascular tone control.
SNPs (single nucleotide polymorphisms), 13, 14f
Sodium
deficit of. See Hyponatremia.
distribution of
in diabetic ketoacidosis, 509, 509f
in hyperosmolar nonketotic coma, 509, 509f
excess of (hypernatremia), 462–464, 462b, 463t, 509
retention of, in hepatorenal syndrome, 489–490
Sodium bicarbonate
as antidote, 668t
for hyperkalemia, 470
for metabolic acidosis, 453, 454t
Sodium nitroprusside. See Nitroprusside.
Sodium-potassium-ATPase, in potassium homeostasis, 468
Somatostatin
for gastrointestinal bleeding, 521
in stress response, 25–26, 26f
Somatotropic axis, in stress response, 25–27, 26f
Somatotropin. See Growth hormone.
Sotalol, for arrhythmias, 321b
Source control methods, for sepsis, 599
Spasticity, 420t
SPECT (single-photon emission computed tomography), in cerebral blood flow measurement, 388t, 389
Spectroscopy, near-infrared, in cerebral blood flow measurement, 388t, 390–391
Spiegelberg ICP monitoring system, 385–386, 386t
Spinal cord injury, 431–438
causes of, 431, 432t
clinical course of, 437
clinical examination in, 433–434, 433b
complications of, prevention of, 437
controversies in, 437b
epidemiology of, 431, 432t
hypertensive crisis in, 353
imaging in, 434–435, 434f–436f
injuries associated with, 432–433, 432t
level of, 432, 432t
physical signs of, 433–434, 433b
pitfalls in, 437b
severity of, 432, 432t, 433f
treatment of, 435–437, 437b
without radiological abnormality (SCIWORA), 432
Spiritual support, management of, 219–220
Splanchnic circulation, vasodilation of, in hepatorenal syndrome, 490
Sponge model, of ARDS, 240–242, 240f
Sputum culture, in pneumonia, 575

ST segment elevation, in myocardial infarction. See Myocardial infarction, ST segment elevation (STEMI).
Stagnant hypoxia, 44–45, 44f, 45f
Standard base excess, 448–449
Standard bicarbonate, 449
Standard precautions
in bioterrorism attack, 694
in normal situations, 75, 75t
Standardized mortality ratio, 98
Stanford classification, of aortic dissection, 366, 366f
Staphylococcus aureus infections
glycopeptides for, host defenses and, 68–69
methicillin-resistant, 69, 73, 73f, 177, 177t, 182t, 183t
pneumonia as, 177, 177t, 182t, 183t, 577, 581, 585t
Starling curve of ventricular function, 102, 104f, 355
Starvation, muscle atrophy in, 27
Static compliance, measurement of, 141–142, 142f
Static intrinsic positive end-expiratory pressure, 139–141, 139f–141f, 143–144, 145f
Statins, for myocardial infarction, 318
Status epilepticus
absence, 419
clinical course of, 428–429
clinical features of, 417
complex partial, 419
definition of, 418
electroencephalography in, 424f, 425f
epidemiology of, 415
generalized convulsive, 418–419, 419t
mortality in, 428–429
nonconvulsive, 419
prevention of, 429
risk factors for, 415, 417t
subtle, 419, 421f, 426–428, 428t
treatment of, 421f, 426–428, 428t
Stenotrophomonas maltophilia pneumonia, 182t
Stents, for aortic dissection, 367, 368f
Sternotomy, infection of, 641
Steroids. See Corticosteroids.
Stewart equations, for acid-base disorders, 445–450, 446f–448f, 447b
Stomach
bleeding in. See Gastrointestinal bleeding, upper tract.
stress ulcers of, 662
Streptococcal toxic shock syndrome, postpartum, 632
Streptococcus pneumoniae infections
pneumonia as, 177, 177t, 182t, 183t, 573, 577, 581
vaccination for, 578, 578b
Streptokinase
action of, 548–549, 548f
for pulmonary embolism, 259, 259t
Streptomycin, for bioterrorist agents, 688t
Stress and stress response, 21–30
additive, 22
biological, 21
chemical, 21
classification of, 21
critical illness myopathy in, 29–30, 29t
definition of, 21–22
distance scaling of, 22, 23f
dyadic relationship of, 21
endocrine profile in, 27, 28, 28f
escape in, 22–23
hypometabolic phase of, 24
in irreversible injury, 22
interventions for, 28–29

Stress and stress response—cont'd
normal physiology of, 24–28, 25f, 26f, 28f
nursing interventions for, 199, 200b
nutritional support in, 211t
physical, 21
repair phases in, 24, 24f
survival in, 23–24
temporal scaling of, 22, 23f
Stress index, in mechanical ventilation, 142, 144f
Stress ulcers, 662
Strich hemorrhage, 396
Stridor, in acutely unstable patient, 189
Stroke
cerebrovascular
in hypertensive crisis, 350
in subarachnoid hemorrhage. See Subarachnoid hemorrhage.
seizures in, 415
thrombosis in, 543
heat, 622–624, 623b
Stroke volume, determinants of, 284, 284f
Strong anion gaps, in acid-base disorders, 450, 450t, 451t
Strong ion concept, acid-base disorders, 445–449, 446f–448f, 447b
Study to Understand Prognoses and Preferences for Outcomes and Risks of Treatments (SUPPORT) model, 96, 99, 217–218, 218b
Subarachnoid hemorrhage, 405–414
classification of, 406, 406f, 406t
clinical course of, 413–414
clinical features of, 406, 406t
epidemiology of, 405
ICP monitoring in, 385, 385t
in hypertensive crisis, 350
nonaneurysmal, 405
outcome of, 405–406
pathogenesis of, 406
perimesencephalic, 405
prevention of, 414
risk factors for, 405–406
treatment of, 407–413
aneurysm clipping or coiling in, 409, 409f
cardiovascular management in, 407–408, 408f
hydrocephalus, 409–410, 410f
initial, 407
pulmonary management in, 407, 408f
rebleeding prevention in, 408–409, 409f
seizures, 408
"triple H" therapy, 410–413, 411f, 412b, 412t, 413f, 414f
vasospasm, 407, 410–413, 411f, 412b, 412t, 413f, 414f
Subdural hematoma
hypertensive crisis in, 351
in brain injury, 395, 397f
Substituted judgment, 218–219
Subtle status epilepticus, 419, 421f, 426–428, 428t
Sudden cardiac death
epidemiology of, 301, 302f, 303f
in asthma, 234
in electrical injury, 620
in hypothermia, 622
in pregnancy, 636
pathophysiology of, 304–306, 305f, 306f
resuscitation from, ventricular arrhythmias after, 336
Suicide
physician-assisted, 218
poisoning in, 665
Supine hypotensive syndrome, in pregnancy, 635

SUPPORT (Study to Understand Prognoses and Preferences for Outcomes and Risks of Treatments) model, 96, 99, 217–218, 218b
Supraventricular arrhythmias. *See* Arrhythmias, supraventricular.
Surfactant
    abnormal, in mechanical ventilation, 163
    for ARDS, 251
Surgery. *See also specific procedures.*
    cardiac. *See* Cardiac surgery.
    postoperative care in. *See* Postoperative care.
    preoperative period in. *See* Preoperative period.
Surrogates, for treatment decision making, 218–219
Surveillance, for nosocomial infections, 74
Survival, in stress response, 23–24
Sweating, in heat stroke, 623
Swelling, in inflammation, 9
Sympathetic nervous system
    in cerebral circulation autoregulation, 392–393
    in stress response, 25
Sympathomimetic agents, hypertension due to, 352
Synchronized intermittent mandatory ventilation, 112–114, 113f–115f
    for COPD, 232
    for weaning, 170, 171
Syncope, in pulmonary embolism, 254, 254t
Systemic inflammatory response syndrome, 1–2, 2f, 2t
    causes of, 590
    clinical features of, 590t
    clinical presentation of, 9
    critical illness polyneuropathy and myopathy in, 279
    definition of, 589
    differential diagnosis of, 589, 590t
    in burns, 613–614, 614f
    in liver failure, 536, 537
    in pancreatitis, 526
    mortality in, 595
    pathophysiology of, 590
    postoperative, 661–662, 662f
Systemic vascular resistance
    in cardiovascular failure, 284, 284b, 298, 298f
    maintenance of, in organ donors, 443

T

T lymphocytes
    defects of, pneumonia in, 581–582, 582t
    in inflammation, 5
Tachy-brady syndrome, 337
Tachycardia
    after cardiac surgery, 644
    in hypovolemia, 192–193
    in pulmonary embolism, 254
Tachypnea
    in ARDS, 245
    in COPD, 227
    in pulmonary embolism, 254, 254t
Tamponade, cardiac, 364–365, 364b
    after cardiac surgery, 644, 646
    in aortic dissection, 366
TBI. *See* Traumatic brain injury.
Teamwork
    in burn care, 613
    nursing care in, 199, 200f
Technetium-99 scan, in gastrointestinal bleeding, 519–520
Teicoplanin, host defenses and, 68–69
Temperature, body
    abnormal. *See* Hyperthermia; Hypothermia.
    control of, 29, 621, 621f

Tenase, in hemostasis, 546
Tension pneumothorax, 608
Tension time index, in respiratory muscle function, 276
Teratogenicity, of radiation, 636
Terbutaline
    for asthma, 233
    for COPD, 228
Terlipressin
    for gastrointestinal bleeding, 521, 522
    for hepatorenal syndrome, 492–493, 493f
Terminal illness. *See* End-of-life care.
Terminal sedation, 218
Terrorism. *See* Bioterrorism agents.
Testosterone, in stress response, 27
THAM, for metabolic acidosis, 453–454
Theophylline, for asthma, 233–234
Thermal injuries. *See* Burn(s).
Thermodilution techniques, in hemodynamic monitoring, 107
Thermoregulation, 621, 621f
    abnormal. *See* Hyperthermia; Hypothermia.
Thiopentone, for hepatic encephalopathy, 539
Thirst
    in end-of-life care, 219
    in hypernatremia, 462, 463
Thoracentesis, for pneumonia, 577
Thoracic trauma, 605f, 606f, 607–609
Thoracotomy, for hemothorax, 608
Thrombin, in hemostasis, 544
Thrombin clotting time, in bleeding, 550t, 551
Thrombocytopenia, 551
    in HELLP syndrome, 629–630
    in liver failure, 534
    platelet transfusion in, 562
Thromboembolism, postoperative, 662, 662b
Thrombolytic therapy
    for myocardial infarction, 316, 357–358
    for pulmonary embolism, 259, 259t, 634
Thrombomodulin
    action of, 547, 547f
    in hemostasis regulation, 549, 549f, 550f
Thrombophilia
    familial, 547
    laboratory assessment of, 551–552
Thrombophlebitis, ovarian vein, 632
Thrombosis
    coronary, pathophysiology of, 304–305, 305f, 306f
    in disseminated intravascular coagulation, 565
    in protein C defects, 547
    laboratory assessment of, 551–552
    of prosthetic heart valves, 364
    pathogenesis of, 543–544, 544f
    prevention of, in pregnancy, 635
    risk factors for, 551, 552b
    treatment of, 552
Thrombotic microangiopathy, in HELLP syndrome, 629–630
Thymectomy, for myasthenia gravis, 282
Thyroid hormone
    deficiency of, myxedema coma in, 499–500, 499b
    replacement of, in hypothyroidism, 500
Thyroid storm, 497–499, 497b, 499f
Thyroiditis, thyrotoxicosis in, 497–499
Thyroid-stimulating hormone, in stress response, 27, 28f
Thyrotoxicosis, 497–499, 497b, 499f
Ticarcillin
    dosage of, during dialysis, 488t
    for obstetric sepsis, 632
Ticlopidine, mechanism of action of, 544, 545f
Tidal volume
    in ARDS, 242, 242f

Tidal volume—cont'd
    in mechanical ventilation
        in obesity, 270
        lung injury due to, 162–163, 162f
        partial support, 149–150
    in obesity, 265
Tiotropium, for COPD, 228
TIP. *See* Transpulmonary pressure.
Tirofiban, for myocardial infarction, 313
Tissue factor
    in hemostasis, 545–546
    in sepsis, 555–556, 556f
Tissue factor pathway inhibitor, 548, 549, 549f
Tissue hypoxia. *See* Hypoxia.
Tissue plasminogen activator, for pulmonary embolism, 259, 259t
TLC (total lung capacity), in obesity, 263–264
Tobramycin
    for ventilator-associated pneumonia, 182t
    prophylactic, 89, 89t, 90, 91
Tocolytic therapy, pulmonary edema due to, 632, 633t
Todd's paralysis, 422
Toll-like receptors
    in inflammation, 5
    in sepsis, 592–593, 592f
Tongue, airway obstruction from, 190
Tonic seizures, 418
Tonicity balance, in hypernatremia, 463
Tonometry, gastric, in hypoxia, 48
Torsade des pointes, 333
Total lung capacity, in obesity, 263–264
Toxic exposures. *See* Poisoning.
Toxins, anthrax, 687
T-piece ventilation, for weaning, 170
Trace elements, in nutritional support, 211
Tracers, in cerebral blood flow measurement, 388–389, 388t
Trachea, rupture of, 608
Tracheal pressure, measurement of, 139
Tracheostomy
    for COPD, 233
    in spinal cord injury, 435
    percutaneous. *See* Percutaneous tracheostomy.
Train-of-four stimulation test, evaluation of, 281
Tranexamic acid
    for coagulopathy, 566
    for subarachnoid hemorrhage, 408–409
Transdiaphragmatic pressure, maximal, 276, 280
Transducers, in catheter tip system, for ICP monitoring, 386t, 387
Transesophageal Doppler monitoring, 107, 107f
Transesophageal echocardiography, in thoracic trauma, 607
Transforming growth factor-β, in inflammation, 9t
Transfusions, 561–567
    allogenic versus autologous, 561
    alternatives to, 565–567, 566b
    autologous, 561
    blood components for, 561–563
    blood substitutes in, 566, 566b
    donor-directed, 561
    for autoimmune hemolytic anemia, 565
    for disseminated intravascular coagulation, 565
    for liver failure, 565
    for uremia, 565
    granulocyte, 563
    history of, 561
    immunoglobulin, 563
    in organ donors, 443
    massive, 563
    plasma, 562–563
    platelet, 562
    reactions to, 563–564, 564t
    red blood cell, 562
    risks of, 563–564, 564t

Transient ischemic attack, versus seizures, 421t
Transjugular intrahepatic portocaval shunt
  for hepatorenal syndrome, 493–494, 494f
  for variceal bleeding, 522–523, 523f
Transmission disequilibrium test, 14
Transplantation
  donors for, management of, 441–443, 441b,
    442t
  kidney, hypertensive crisis in, 353
  liver, 493t, 494–495, 541, 542f, 542t
  pneumonia in, 582, 582f
  postoperative care in, 660
Transpulmonary pressure
  cardiovascular effects of, 370–376, 372f–374f,
    376f
  hemodynamic effects of, 377–381, 377f, 378f
  in ARDS, 250
  in obesity, 269
Transthoracic bioimpedance, in hemodynamic
    monitoring, 107
Transthoracic echocardiography
  in aortic dissection, 367, 367f
  in infective endocarditis, 360, 361f
  in pulmonary embolism, 257, 257f
Transvenous pacing, for bradycardia, 339–340
Trauma. See also Injury(ies).
  multiple. See Multiple trauma.
  seizures in, 415
Traumatic brain injury, 395–403
  clinical course of, 401–402
  clinical features of, 399, 399t, 400f
  complications of, 402–403
  controversies in, 403
  epidemiology of, 395
  evaluation of, 606, 606t
  hypertensive crisis in, 351
  ICP monitoring in, 384–385, 385t
  mortality in, 395, 401
  nutritional support in, 211t
  pathogenesis of, 395–399, 396f–398f
  prevention of, 402
  primary, 395, 396f
  risk factors for, 395
  secondary, 395, 396f, 398
  treatment of, 399–401, 402f
Triage, in brain injury, 399–400
Triiodothyronine, in stress response, 27
Trimethaphan, for hypertensive crisis, 349t,
  351
Trimethoprim-sulfamethoxazole, for ventilator-
    associated pneumonia, 182t
Triphasic waves, in EEG, 423, 425f
"Triple H" therapy, for subarachnoid
    hemorrhage, 410–413
  algorithm for, 410, 413f
  cardiac output maintenance in, 412–413
  electrolyte correction in, 411–412, 412t
  failure of, 413, 414f
  goals of, 410
  hemodilution in, 412
  hypertension induction in, 412
  hypervolemia correction in, 411
Tris buffer, for metabolic acidosis, 453–454
Tromethamine buffer (THAM)
  for metabolic acidosis, 453–454
  for obstetric hemorrhage, 631
Trophoblastic disease, gestational, 632
Troponins
  in myocardial infarction, 307, 307b, 307f,
    310, 310f–312f
  in pulmonary embolism, 256
  in subarachnoid hemorrhage, 407–408
TSH (thyroid-stimulating hormone), in stress
    response, 27, 28f
Tube(s), chest, for pneumothorax, 608
Tube feeding. See Enteral nutrition.

Tuberculosis
  in immunodeficiency, 581
  pneumonia in, 585
Tularemia, 688t, 689, 689b
Tumor, in inflammation, 9
Tumor necrosis factor-α
  gene of, variations in, 16–17, 17b, 17f
  in inflammation, 8
  in pneumonia, 572
  in sepsis, 555–556, 556f
  inhibitors of, for inflammation, 10–11
  neutralization of, in sepsis, 600
Twitch Pdi test, in respiratory failure, 280–281,
    281f
Tyramine-containing foods, hypertension due to,
    352, 353f

U
Ulcer(s)
  peptic, bleeding in, 517
  stress, 662
Ulceroglandular tularemia, 689
Ultrasonography
  in abdominal injury, 610, 610f, 633
  in liver failure, 535
  in pulmonary embolism, 258
Unconsciousness. See Consciousness alterations.
Uniform Determination of Death Act, 439
Unstable patient. See Acutely unstable patient.
Upper motor neuron disease, respiratory failure
    in, 278t
Upper respiratory infections, pneumonia
    preceding, 569, 571
Uremia, transfusions for, 565
Urinary output
  in acutely unstable patient, 194
  in hypernatremia, 463
  in organ donors, 443
Urinary tract
  infections of, postoperative, 661
  obstruction of, kidney failure in, 478
Urine
  concentration of, 460
  electrolytes in, in hyponatremia, 465
  flow rate of, 460
  osmolality of, 460–462
Urokinase
  action of, 548–549, 548f
  for pulmonary embolism, 259, 259t
Urticaria, transfusion-related, 564t
Uterine blood flow, 627, 627f

V
Vaccination
  for bioterrorism agents, 694
  for infection control, 78
  for pneumonia, 578, 578b
  for smallpox (vaccinia), 691
Vaccinia vaccination, 691
Vagal tone, bradycardia and, 339, 340f
Valproic acid, for seizures, 427, 428t
Valvotomy, balloon
  for aortic stenosis, 362
  for mitral stenosis, 364
Valvular heart disease
  aortic regurgitation, 295–296, 362
  aortic stenosis, 296, 362
  cardiovascular failure in, 295–296
  infective endocarditis, 360–362, 360b, 361b,
    361f, 364
  mitral regurgitation, 295, 362–363, 362b,
    363f
  mitral stenosis, 363–364, 364f

Valvular heart disease—cont'd
  prosthetic, 364
  traumatic, 359
Vancomycin
  dosage of, during dialysis, 488t
  for bioterrorist agents, 688t
  for ventilator-associated pneumonia, 180,
    183t, 661t
  host defenses and, 68–69
  prophylactic, 90, 91
Vanillyl-mandelic acid, in pheochromocytoma,
    501
Variable numbers of tandem repeats, 13, 14f
Variceal band ligation, for gastrointestinal
    bleeding, 522
Variceal bleeding. See Portal hypertension,
    bleeding in.
Variola virus infections (smallpox), 688t,
    690–691, 691f
Vascular endothelial growth factor (VEGF), in
    inflammation, 9t
Vascular smooth muscle
  constriction mechanisms of, 31–32, 32f
  mechanochemical cycle of, 31, 32f
  membrane potential of, 34–35, 34f–36f
  receptors on, for vasodilators and
    vasoconstrictors, 35–36, 36t
  relaxation mechanisms of, 32–33, 33f
Vascular tone control, 31–39
  autoregulation in, 38–39, 38f
  calcium sensitization in, 31–35, 32f–36f
  cellular mechanisms of, 31–35, 32f–36f
  circulating factors in, 35–38, 36t
Vasoactive intestinal peptide, in vascular tone
    control, 34, 36f
Vasoconstriction and vasoconstrictors
  for hepatorenal syndrome, 492–493, 493f,
    493t
  in ARDS, 243–244, 244f
  in hepatorenal syndrome, 490
  pulmonary, in hypoxia, 375
Vasodilation, in sepsis, 594–595, 594f
Vasodilators
  failure of, 348t
  for hypertensive crisis, 352
Vasoplegia, after cardiac surgery, 643
Vasopressin
  for sepsis, 599
  in hypernatremia, 462
  in hyponatremia, 464, 464b, 465
  in urine concentration, 460–461, 461f
  in vascular tone control, 36–37
Vasospasm, in subarachnoid hemorrhage, 407,
    410–413, 411f, 412b, 412t, 413f, 414f
VC (vital capacity)
  in COPD, 227
  in Guillain-Barré syndrome, 278–279
  in neuromuscular respiratory failure, 280
Vegetations, in infective endocarditis, 360–361,
    361f
Vegetative state, 440
VEGF (vascular endothelial growth factor), in
    inflammation, 9t
Vena cava, filter placement in, for pulmonary
    embolism, 259
Venography, in pulmonary embolism, 258
Venous resistance, in cardiovascular failure, 287,
    289, 289f
Venous return, intrathoracic pressure effects on,
    377–378, 377f, 378f
Venous stasis, pulmonary embolism in, 253
Venous thromboembolism, postoperative, 662,
    662b
Ventilation
  liquid, in ARDS, 251
  mechanical. See Mechanical ventilation.

Ventilation/perfusion
  mismatch of
    in COPD, 224
    in inhalation injury, 619
    in obesity, 264
    in pulmonary embolism, 253, 256, 256f
  redistribution of, in ARDS, 242
Ventilator-associated lung injury. *See* Mechanical ventilation, lung injury in.
Ventilator-associated pneumonia. *See* Mechanical ventilation, pneumonia in.
Ventilator-induced diaphragmatic dysfunction, 280
Ventricle(s) (brain), dysfunction of, in subarachnoid hemorrhage, 407–408
Ventricle(s) (heart)
  interdependence of, 376, 376f, 377f
  left
    hypertrophy of, in hypertensive crisis, 345
    wall rupture in, 358
  right, filling of, intrathoracic pressure effects on, 378–379, 379f
Ventricular arrhythmias. *See* Arrhythmias, ventricular.
Ventricular fibrillation, 333–335, 333b, 334f
Ventricular flutter, 330b
Ventricular septum, rupture of 357–358
Ventricular tachycardia
  monomorphic, 331–333, 332b, 332f, 333f
  polymorphic, 333–335, 333b, 334f
Verapamil
  for aortic dissection, 367
  for cardiomyopathy, 359
Vertebrae, fractures of, 432, 433f
Videolaryngoscopy, for intubation of obese patients, 268
Viral hemorrhagic fevers, 688t, 691, 691b
Virchow's triad, in pulmonary embolism, 253
Visual Analogue Scale, for pain assessment, 52
Visual disorders, in methanol poisoning, 670, 670t

Vital capacity
  in COPD, 227
  in Guillain-Barré syndrome, 278–279
  in neuromuscular respiratory failure, 280
Vitamin(s), in nutritional support, 211
Vitamin B_6, as antidote, 668t
Vitamin K
  as antidote, 668t
  for coagulopathy, 567
  in liver failure, 540
VO_2. *See* Oxygen consumption.
Volume mode, for mechanical ventilation, 109, 109t, 110t
Volume status, evaluation of, in acutely unstable patient, 192–194, 193b, 193f
Volume support ventilation, 114–115
Volume ventilation, versus pressure ventilation, 109, 109t, 110t
Volume-assured pressure support ventilation, 117–118, 117f
Volutrauma
  in diabetic ketoacidosis, 511
  in mechanical ventilation, 162–163, 162f, 163f
Vomiting. *See* Nausea and vomiting.
von Willebrand factor, in hemostasis, 544

W

Wall tension, in left heart dysfunction, 293
Wallace's rule of nines, for burn estimation, 614–615, 615f
Warfarin
  for pulmonary embolism, 258
  necrosis due to, 548, 548f
Wasting syndrome, in stress response, 27, 29–30, 29t
Water
  disorders of. *See also* Hypernatremia; Hyponatremia.
    polyuria as, 459–462, 460f, 461f, 461t
  physiology of, 459–460, 460f

Water diuresis, 460–461, 461t
Weak ions, in acid-base disorders, 446–447, 447b, 447f
Weaning, from mechanical ventilation. *See* Mechanical ventilation, weaning from.
Weight
  excessive. *See* Obesity.
  in obesity definition, 263
  measurement of, in nutritional assessment, 205–206, 206f
Wheezing, in COPD, 227
Wilson's disease, liver failure in, 533, 535, 536f
Withholding and withdrawal of treatment, 218, 218b, 220, 220b
Wolff-Parkinson-White syndrome, 329
Work of breathing
  in obesity, 265
  in partial ventilatory support, 152
  measurement of, 144–145, 146f, 147f
World Federation of Neurological Surgeons Grading Scale, for subarachnoid hemorrhage, 406, 406t

X

Xenon-enhanced computed tomography, in cerebral blood flow measurement, 388–389
Ximelagatran, for pulmonary embolism, 258

Y

Yersinia pestis infections (plague), 687–689, 688t

Z

Zinc supplementation, 211